The American Psychiatric Association Publishing

TEXTBOOK OF
GERIATRIC PSYCHIATRY

SIXTH EDITION

The American Psychiatric Association Publishing

TEXTBOOK OF

GERIATRIC PSYCHIATRY

SIXTH EDITION

EDITED BY

David C. Steffens, M.D., M.H.S.
Kristina F. Zdanys, M.D.

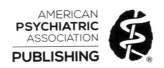

AMERICAN
PSYCHIATRIC
ASSOCIATION
PUBLISHING

If you wish to buy 50 or more copies of the same title, please go to www.appi.org/specialdiscounts for more information.

Copyright © 2023 American Psychiatric Association Publishing

ALL RIGHTS RESERVED

Sixth Edition

Manufactured in the United States of America on acid-free paper
26   25   24   23   22   5   4   3   2   1

American Psychiatric Association Publishing
800 Maine Avenue SW, Suite 900
Washington, DC 20024-2812
www.appi.org

Library of Congress Cataloging-in-Publication Data
Names: Steffens, David C., 1962- editor. | Zdanys, Kristina, editor. | American Psychiatric Association Publishing.
Title: The American Psychiatric Association Publishing textbook of geriatric psychiatry / edited by David C. Steffens, Kristina F. Zdanys.
Other titles: Textbook of geriatric psychiatry
Description: Sixth edition. | Washington, DC : American Psychiatric Association Publishing, [2023] | Includes bibliographical references and index.
Identifiers: LCCN 2021061105 (print) | LCCN 2021061106 (ebook) | ISBN 9781615373406 (hardcover) | ISBN 9781615374373 (ebook)
Subjects: MESH: Mental Disorders | Aged | Aging—physiology | Geriatric Psychiatry—methods
Classification: LCC RC451.4.A5 (print) | LCC RC451.4.A5 (ebook) | NLM WT 150 | DDC 618.97/689—dc23/eng/20220118
LC record available at https://lccn.loc.gov/2021061105
LC ebook record available at https://lccn.loc.gov/2021061106

British Library Cataloguing in Publication Data
A CIP record is available from the British Library.

Contents

Contributors

David H. Adamowicz, M.D., Ph.D.
Resident, Department of Psychiatry, University of California San Diego, San Diego, California

Marc Agronin, M.D.
Senior Vice President for Behavioral Health, Miami Jewish Health; Chief Medical Officer, MIND Institute at Miami Jewish Health; Affiliate Associate Professor of Psychiatry and Neurology, University of Miami Miller School of Medicine, Miami, Florida

Patricia Andrews, M.D.
Assistant Professor of Psychiatry and Behavioral Sciences, Vanderbilt University Medical Center, Nashville, Tennessee

Lisa Barry, Ph.D., M.P.H.
Associate Professor of Psychiatry, University of Connecticut School of Medicine, Farmington, Connecticut

John L. Beyer, M.D.
Professor of Psychiatry, Duke University Medical Center, Durham, North Carolina

Dan G. Blazer, M.D., Ph.D.
J.P. Gibbons Professor of Psychiatry Emeritus, Department of Psychiatry and Behavioral Sciences, Duke University Medical Center, Durham, North Carolina

Kecia-Ann Blissett, D.O.
Assistant Professor, Department of Psychiatry, Mount Sinai Beth Israel, New York, New York

Amy Byers, Ph.D.
Professor of Psychiatry and Behavioral Sciences, Department of Medicine and Division of Geriatrics, University of California, San Francisco, California

Benjamin P. Chapman, Ph.D., M.P.H.
Associate Professor, Department of Psychiatry, University of Rochester Medical Center, Rochester, New York

Michelle L. Conroy, M.D.
Assistant Professor of Psychiatry, Yale University School of Medicine, New Haven; VA Connecticut Healthcare System, West Haven, Connecticut

Joan M. Cook, Ph.D.
Professor of Psychiatry, Yale University School of Medicine, New Haven, Connecticut

Breno S. Diniz, M.D., Ph.D.
Department of Psychiatry and UConn Center on Aging, School of Medicine, University of Connecticut Health Center, Farmington, Connecticut

Laura B. Dunn, M.D.
Professor, Department of Psychiatry and Behavioral Sciences, Stanford University, Stanford, California

Richard H. Fortinsky, Ph.D.
Professor and Health Net Inc. Chair in Geriatrics and Gerontology, UConn Center on Aging, Departments of Medicine and Public Health Sciences, University of Connecticut School of Medicine, Farmington, Connecticut

Mary Ganguli, M.D., M.P.H.
Professor of Psychiatry, Epidemiology, and Neurology, University of Pittsburgh, Pittsburgh, Pennsylvania

Sarah A. Graham, Ph.D.
Clinical Research Manager, Lark Health, Mountain View, California

Lisa P. Gwyther, M.S.W., L.C.S.W.
Associate Professor Emeritus, Department of Psychiatry and Behavioral Sciences and Center for Aging, Duke School of Medicine, Durham, North Carolina

Elizabeth Hathaway, M.D.
Geriatric Psychiatry Fellow, Department of Psychiatry, Indiana University School of Medicine, Indianapolis, Indiana

Mustafa M. Husain, M.B.B.S.
Professor of Psychiatry, Neurology, and Internal Medicine, UT Southwestern Medical Center, Dallas, Texas; Adjunct Professor, Department of Psychiatry and Behavioral Sciences, Duke University School of Medicine, Durham, North Carolina

Sharon K. Inouye, M.D., M.P.H.
Professor of Medicine, Department of Medicine, Beth Israel Deaconess Medical Center, Harvard Medical School; Director and Milton and Shirley F. Levy Family Chair, Aging Brain Center, Institute for Aging Research, Hebrew SeniorLife, Boston, Massachusetts

Mini Elizabeth Jacob, M.D., Ph.D.
Psychiatry Resident, University of Washington, Seattle, Washington

Jaclyn Olsen Jaeger, D.O., C.M.D.
Assistant Professor of Medicine, University of Connecticut Center on Aging, Farmington, Connecticut

Dilip V. Jeste, M.D.
Senior Associate Dean for Health Aging and Senior Care; Estelle and Edgar Levi Chair in Aging; Director, Sam and Rose Stein Institute for Research on Aging; Distinguished Professor of Psychiatry and Neurosciences; Co-Director, UCSD-IBM Center on Artificial Intelligence for Healthy Living; Department of Psychiatry, University of California, San Diego, San Diego, California

Elisa Kallioniemi, Ph.D.
Postdoctoral Researcher, Department of Psychiatry, University of Texas Southwestern Medical Center, Dallas, Texas

Heejung J. Kim, B.A.
Research Assistant, Department of Geriatric Psychiatry, McLean Hospital, Belmont, Massachusetts

Daniel S. Kim, M.D.
Clinical Assistant Professor, Department of Psychiatry and Behavioral Sciences, Stanford University, Stanford, California

Dimitris N. Kiosses, Ph.D.
Professor of Psychology in Psychiatry, Emotion, Cognition, and Psychotherapy Lab, Weill-Cornell Institute of Geriatric Psychiatry, Weill Cornell Medicine, White Plains, New York

George A. Kuchel, M.D.C.M.
Professor of Medicine, University of Connecticut Center on Aging, Farmington, Connecticut

Chadrick E. Lane, M.D.
Assistant Professor of Psychiatry, Peter O'Donnell Jr. Brain Institute, UT Southwestern Medical Center, Dallas, Texas

Melinda Lantz, M.D.
Vice Chair, Department of Psychiatry, Mount Sinai Beth Israel, New York, New York

Ellen E. Lee, M.D.
Assistant Professor of Psychiatry, and Chief, Division of Geriatric Psychiatry, University of California, San Diego; Staff Psychiatrist, VA San Diego Healthcare System, San Diego, California

Constantine G. Lyketsos, M.D., M.H.S.
The Elizabeth Plank Althouse Professor and Chair of Psychiatry for Johns Hopkins Bayview, Department of Psychiatry and Behavioral Sciences, Johns Hopkins University School of Medicine, Baltimore, Maryland

Tanya Mailhot, R.N., Ph.D.
Assistant Professor, Faculty of Nursing, Université de Montréal; Researcher, Montreal Heart Institute Research Center, Montreal, Quebec, Canada

Kevin J. Manning, Ph.D.
Department of Psychiatry, University of Connecticut Health Center, Farmington, Connecticut

Phelan E. Maruca-Sullivan, M.D.
Assistant Professor of Psychiatry, Yale University School of Medicine, New Haven; VA Connecticut Healthcare System, West Haven, Connecticut

Shahrzad Mavandadi, Ph.D.
VISN4 Mental Illness Research, Education, and Clinical Center; Department of Psychiatry, Perelman School of Medicine, University of Pennsylvania, Philadelphia, Pennsylvania

Benoit H. Mulsant, M.D., M.S.
Centre for Addiction and Mental Health, Department of Psychiatry, Temerty Faculty
of Medicine, University of Toronto, Toronto, Ontario, Canada

David W. Oslin, M.D.
VISN4 Mental Illness Research, Education, and Clinical Center; Department of Psychiatry, Perelman School of Medicine, University of Pennsylvania, Philadelphia, Pennsylvania

David T. Plante, M.D., Ph.D.
Associate Professor, Department of Psychiatry, University of Wisconsin, Madison,
Wisconsin

Bruce G. Pollock, M.D., Ph.D.
Centre for Addiction and Mental Health, Department of Psychiatry, Temerty Faculty
of Medicine, University of Toronto, Toronto, Ontario, Canada

Wendy Qiu, M.D., Ph.D.
Psychiatrist, Department of Psychiatry, Boston Medical Center, Boston, Massachusetts

Aniqa T. Rahman, B.A.
Research Assistant, Department of Geriatric Psychiatry, McLean Hospital, Belmont,
Massachusetts

Meredith E. Rumble, Ph.D.
Associate Professor, Department of Psychiatry, University of Wisconsin, Madison,
Wisconsin

Jane S. Saczynski, Ph.D.
Department of Pharmacy and Health System Sciences, Northeastern University, Boston, Massachusetts

Stephanie A. Schuette, M.A.
Department of Psychology and Neuroscience, Duke University, Durham, North Carolina

Adam Simning, M.D., Ph.D.
Assistant Professor, Department of Psychiatry, University of Rochester Medical Center, Rochester, New York

Miranda D. Skurla, B.S.
Research Assistant, Department of Geriatric Psychiatry, McLean Hospital, Belmont,
Massachusetts

Moria J. Smoski, Ph.D.
Associate Professor, Department of Psychiatry and Behavioral Sciences, Duke University Medical Center, Durham, North Carolina

Beth Springate, Ph.D.
Department of Psychiatry, University of Connecticut Health Center, Farmington,
Connecticut

David C. Steffens, M.D., M.H.S.
Professor and Chair of Psychiatry, University of Connecticut School of Medicine, Farmington, Connecticut

Joel Streim, M.D.
Professor of Psychiatry, Perelman School of Medicine, University of Pennsylvania, Philadelphia, Pennsylvania

Rajesh R. Tampi, M.D., M.S.
Professor Adjunct, Department of Psychiatry, Yale School of Medicine, New Haven, Connecticut; Chairman, Department of Psychiatry and Behavioral Sciences, Cleveland Clinic Akron General, Akron; Professor, Department of Medicine, Cleveland Clinic Lerner College of Medicine of Case Western Reserve University, Cleveland, Ohio

Warren D. Taylor, M.D., M.H.Sc.
James G. Blakemore Professor of Psychiatry, Department of Psychiatry and Behavioral Sciences, Vanderbilt University Medical Center; Physician-Scientist, The Geriatric Research, Education, and Clinical Center, Veterans Affairs Tennessee Valley Health System, Nashville Tennessee

Larry W. Thompson, Ph.D.
Professor Emeritus, Department of Medicine; Professor, Active Duty, Department of Psychiatry and Behavioral Sciences; Stanford University School of Medicine, Stanford, California

Ipsit V. Vahia, M.D.
McLean Hospital, Belmont; Harvard Medical School, Boston, Massachusetts

Sophia Wang, M.D.
Assistant Professor of Clinical Psychiatry, Department of Psychiatry, Indiana University School of Medicine; Indiana Alzheimer's Disease Research Center, Indianapolis, Indiana

Richard D. Weiner, M.D., Ph.D.
Professor Emeritus of Psychiatry and Behavioral Sciences, Duke University School of Medicine, Durham, North Carolina

Elizabeth A. Wise, M.D.
Assistant Professor, Department of Psychiatry and Behavioral Sciences, Johns Hopkins University School of Medicine, Baltimore, Maryland

Jonathan R. Young, M.D.
Staff Psychiatrist, Durham VA Health Care System; Consulting Associate, Department of Psychiatry and Behavioral Sciences, Duke University School of Medicine, Durham, North Carolina

Juan Joseph Young, M.D.
Postdoctoral Fellow, Department of Psychiatry, Yale School of Medicine, New Haven, Connecticut

Kristina F. Zdanys, M.D.
Associate Professor of Psychiatry and Chief, Division of Geriatric Psychiatry and Behavioral Health, University of Connecticut School of Medicine; Director, Geriatric Psychiatry Fellowship Program, UConn Health, Farmington, Connecticut

Disclosures

The following contributors to this book have indicated financial interest in or other affiliation with a commercial supporter, manufacturer of commercial products, provider of commercial services, nongovernmental organization, and/or government agency, as listed.

Mustafa M. Husain, M.B.B.S.

Research support: National Institutes of Health, National Alliance for Research on Schizophrenia and Depression, Stanley Medical Foundation, Cyberonics, Neuronetics, St. Jude Medical/Abbott, Brainsway, NeoSync, Alkermes, Assurex, Avanir Pharmaceuticals; *Equipment support:* MagStim, MagVenture.

Constantine G. Lyketsos, M.D., M.H.S.

Grants: National Institute of Mental Health, National Institute on Aging, Associated Jewish Federation of Baltimore, Weinberg Foundation, Forest, Glaxo-Smith-Kline, Eisai, Pfizer, Astra-Zeneca, Lilly, Ortho-McNeil, Bristol-Myers, Novartis, National Football League, Elan, Functional Neuromodulation, Bright Focus Foundation; *Consultant/Advisor:* Astra-Zeneca, Glaxo-Smith Kline, Eisai, Novartis, Forest, Supernus, Adlyfe, Takeda, Wyeth, Lundbeck, Merz, Lilly, Pfizer, Genentech, Elan, NFL Players Association, NFL Benefits Office, Avanir, Zinfandel, BMS, Abvie, Janssen, Orion, Otsuka, Servier, Astellas; *Honorarium or travel support:* Pfizer, Forest, Glaxo-Smith Kline, Health Monitor.

David T. Plante, M.D., Ph.D.

Grants: National Institute of Mental Health, National Institute on Aging, Brain and Behavior Research Foundation, University of Illinois at Chicago Occupational and Environmental Health and Safety Education and Research Center/National Institute for Occupational Safety and Health, Madison Education Partnership; *Consultant:* Teva Australia, Jazz Pharmaceuticals.

Meredith E. Rumble, Ph.D.

Grants: National Institute of Mental Health, Merck.

David C. Steffens, M.D., M.H.S.

Consultant: Janssen Research and Development, LLC.

Sophia Wang, M.D.

Royalties: American Psychiatric Association Publishing.

Jonathan R. Young, M.D.

Grants: VA Clinical Science Research and Development Career Development Award (CDA-1) IK1 CX002187.

Preface

With this sixth edition of *The American Psychiatric Publishing Textbook of Geriatric Psychiatry*, Dr. David Steffens welcomes Dr. Kristina Zdanys as a coeditor. Dr. Zdanys is an experienced clinician and educator with broad knowledge in geriatric psychiatry. This edition of the textbook builds on prior editions led by Drs. Ewald Busse and Dan G. Blazer and most recently coedited by Dr. Mugdha Thakur. In the present edition, Drs. Steffens and Zdanys have sought to maintain the multidisciplinary and developmental perspectives that have characterized the *Textbook* while keeping pace with the latest scientific advances and clinical developments in the field.

This edition captures recent advances in the assessment, treatment, and biological understanding of late-life neuropsychiatric disorders. Readers will find new information and updates or alterations to previous material. The first edition of this textbook, entitled *Geriatric Psychiatry*, was published in 1989; the second edition was published in 1996, with the title *The American Psychiatric Press Textbook of Geriatric Psychiatry*. The third, fourth, and fifth editions were published in 2004, 2009, and 2015, respectively, as *The American Psychiatric Publishing Textbook of Geriatric Psychiatry*, and the sixth edition retains this title. The fifth edition of the textbook provided an update for DSM-5 (American Psychiatric Association 2013), highlighting areas particularly salient for older adults. The present edition includes new material exploring the use of technology and legal and ethical issues in the psychiatric care of older adults. We sought to equip both the scholar and clinician with the current state of scientific understanding, as well as the practical skills and knowledge base required for dealing with mental disorders in late life.

As in previous editions, the chapters are organized in a sequential and logical fashion, which we have found enhances the accessibility and utility of the material presented. We feature both new and established contributors, both clinical and basic science scholars, who have a clear ability to make complex information understandable to the reader. We have maintained an eclectic orientation regarding theory and practice in geriatric psychiatry. Although most contributors are psychiatrists, we called on colleagues from relevant biomedical and behavioral disciplines because of their expertise and ability to incorporate such knowledge into a comprehensive approach to patient care.

Also of note, nearly all of the chapters in this edition were written during the first surge of the coronavirus disease 2019 (COVID-19) pandemic in the United States. We are indebted to those authors who completed their work under the most trying of circumstances. Contributors to this edition provided insights learned about telepsychiatry and care in nursing homes during the early days of the pandemic. We anticipate that future editions of the *Textbook* will include more information about COVID-19, as well as the epidemiology and care of mental disorders related to epidemics and pandemics.

We targeted this text to psychiatrists and other mental health professionals who have an interest in and a commitment to older adults. This book is of particular value to candidates seeking certification in geriatrics from the American Board of Psychiatry and Neurology, the American Board of Internal Medicine, and the American Board of Family Practice. All these bodies' examinations place considerable emphasis on geriatric psychiatry and the behavioral aspects of aging.

David C. Steffens, M.D., M.H.S.
Kristina F. Zdanys, M.D.
Farmington, Connecticut

References

American Psychiatric Association: Diagnostic and Statistical Manual of Mental Disorders, 5th Edition. Arlington, VA, American Psychiatric Association, 2013

CHAPTER 1

Epidemiology of Psychiatric Disorders in Later Life

Lisa Barry, Ph.D., M.P.H.

Amy Byers, Ph.D.

Mini Elizabeth Jacob, M.D., Ph.D.

Mary Ganguli, M.D., M.P.H.

Demography of Aging

The primary responsibility of clinical geriatric psychiatrists is to take care of their individual patients; why, then, should they concern themselves with the demography of aging in the population at large? Because the size, structure, distribution, and trends in the aging population are highly relevant to current and future clinical practice. Globally, including in the United States, the population is aging rapidly. The U.S. Census Bureau (2020) estimated that in 2020, about 56 million older adults were living in the United States and formed 17% of the total U.S. population. In 2030, as the current decade draws to a close, another 18 million older adults will be added to this segment, raising the proportion to 21% (Mather et al. 2015). This accelerated growth rate of older adults is driven by the aging of the Baby Boomers, born during the post–World War II "baby boom" between 1946 and 1964. The oldest Baby Boomers turned 65 years old in 2011, whereas the youngest will turn 65 in 2030. This demographic trend is not unique to the United States and other high-income countries. With substantial increases in life expectancy and declining fertility across the world, individuals older than 65 are now the fastest-growing segment in all world regions. They numbered 500 million (8%) in 2006 and will number 1 billion (13%, or one in every eight persons) in 2030 (National Institute on Aging et al. 2007). In fact, the most rapid increases in the older adult population are occurring in low- and middle-income countries, where there will be 140% growth between 2006 and 2030, compared with 51% in high-income countries.

The older adult population is also undergoing dynamic changes in terms of sex and race structure. In the United States, women still live longer than men and account for approximately 56% of the population age 65 years and older and 66% of those age 85 years and older (Federal Interagency Forum on Aging-Related Statistics 2016). However, the 7-year sex gap in life expectancy among those age 65 and older in 1990 narrowed to <5 years in 2013; the difference in life expectancy is <3 years among those who survive to age 85. One reason might be that smoking-related deaths decreased among men and increased among women (Mather 2015). The U.S. population is also becoming increasingly diverse in terms of race and ethnicity, with diversity concentrated in the youngest age groups. In 2014, 78% of the older adult population was non-Hispanic white, whereas only 50% of children younger than 18 were non-Hispanic white (Mather et al. 2015). However, between 2030 and 2060, the percentage of older adults who are non-Hispanic white will decrease from 72% to 55%, and the percentage of those who are Hispanic will double from 11% to 22%. During this same period, the percentage of Blacks and Asians in the older adult population is expected to rise from 10% to 12% and 5% to 9%, respectively (Mather et al. 2015).

Global aging represents a success story, a triumph of public health medical advancement and economic development over disease and poverty. However, it also brings major challenges. Although mortality due to malnutrition and infectious diseases has diminished, larger proportions of the population are living with one or more chronic diseases and cognitive and functional disabilities. Thus, the number of older adults living with psychiatric disorders, with or without other comorbid medical conditions, is rising, thereby also increasing the demand for mental health services. This is why appropriate policymaking and planning for mental health service delivery in the future will require a fundamental understanding of the demography and epidemiology of psychiatric disorders in the older population.

Epidemiology

Epidemiology is the study of the "distribution and determinants" of disease in the population and their application to prevent and control disease. The classic "seven uses" of epidemiology include community diagnosis, completing the clinical picture of disease, computing individual risk, charting historical trends, evaluating health services, delineating new syndromes, and identifying the causal and risk factors (Morris 1955). This chapter primarily discusses 1) community diagnosis—that is, how psychiatric disorders are distributed in the general population and selected clinical settings, and 2) causal and risk factors, briefly reviewing the factors in the population that appear to increase and decrease the risk of these disorders and thus determine their distribution. Examples of the other uses of epidemiology are provided for illustration. This chapter specifically focuses on the epidemiology of neurocognitive disorders, depression, and anxiety disorders in late life. Epidemiology of other psychiatric disorders is covered separately in their respective chapters in this textbook.

Increasingly, the epidemiology of brain disorders is seen as "population neuroscience" (Falk et al. 2013; Ganguli et al. 2018; Paus 2010), merging the perspectives and contributions of the population sciences with those of clinical and basic neuroscience. This approach, by incorporating the study of brain disease mechanisms into epidemiology, enhances our ability to contribute to precision medicine and population health.

Completing the Clinical Picture of Disease

Geriatric psychiatrists and other specialists must recognize that the patients who present to them for care of a particular disorder are only a subgroup of people in the community with that disorder. Other subgroups with the same disorder may be seen solely by their primary care providers or may not be receiving diagnoses or care at all, and these various subgroups may not all have the same clinical presentation. An excellent illustration is the example of Alzheimer's disease (AD). In 1906, Professor Alois Alzheimer published a single case report about a 51-year-old woman who was admitted to the mental hospital in Frankfurt with delusions, general disorganization, and cognitive deterioration (Cipriani et al. 2011). When she died 5 years later, he performed the autopsy and published a report about what he described as a new disease of the cerebral cortex. The condition named after him was then regarded as a rare disease of middle-aged people. This perception did not change until 1964, when Professor Sir Martin Roth and his colleagues published the results of an epidemiological study of older adults in Newcastle-Upon-Tyne in England (Roth et al. 1966). This population study showed that AD was a common disease of older people and not just a rare disease of middle-aged people. By completing the clinical picture of AD, this epidemiological study influenced both the clinical diagnosis and the known prevalence of the disease, leading to our current understanding of the massive public health burden it imposes. This example illustrates the importance of studying mental disorders outside of the specialty psychiatric setting. More people with depression and anxiety disorders are seen in the primary care sector than in the mental health sector (Shapiro et al. 1984) and may present differently in different care settings.

Community diagnosis refers to the detection and diagnosis of psychiatric disorders in the community at large to allow us to estimate how common a given disorder is within a given population (prevalence) and how rapidly new cases of the disorder develop in that population (incidence). More precisely, *prevalence* is the proportion of cases of a psychiatric disorder within a clearly defined population at a given time or over a given period, regardless of how long the subjects have lived with that disorder. The true prevalence of a disorder may vary across different populations (e.g., different countries, different parts of the country, different age or sex groups) at different periods in history. Prevalence estimates will differ further depending on the assessment methods and diagnostic criteria used, which vary across places and times. The precision of a prevalence estimate, indicated by the confidence interval around that estimate, is most often a function of how large a sample was studied. Prevalence is usually determined by cross-sectional surveys, although for rare disorders that typically do not go undiagnosed, prevalence may be estimated based on individuals receiving treatment for the disorder in clinical settings (treatment prevalence). *Incidence*, on the other hand, is the rate at which new cases of the disorder develop in a given population; it is calculated as the proportion of new cases during a given period, usually 1 year, among a defined population of persons at risk (i.e., people who did not already have the disorder). Incidence is estimated by longitudinal studies of cohorts of people who were determined to be free of the disorder when they entered the study. Such studies are labor-intensive, expensive, and particularly challenging in populations that are mobile and transient. Incidence of rare conditions has also been estimated by the occurrence of new patients seeking care for the disorder for the first time (treatment incidence).

The relationship between incidence and prevalence is simple but important. The formula is Incidence×Duration=Prevalence. The incidence of a disorder in a given population depends on characteristics, such as the age structure of that population, and on the presence of risk and protective factors for that disorder. Once a new (incident) case has developed, the key issue becomes how long that person lives with the disorder (duration). If the condition is short-lived, for example, 1 year or less, the prevalence will be the same as the incidence.

Throughout this chapter, we illustrate these points using tables of prevalence and incidence estimates from selected studies of various disorders.

Risk and Protective Factors

In epidemiological parlance, *risk factors* are factors associated with higher subsequent incidence of the disease/disorder/condition of interest, whereas *protective factors* are associated with lower subsequent incidence. Risk represents the probability of disease onset taking place at all or, more often, of onset occurring earlier rather than later. Risk factors defined in this way are not necessarily causal or directly within the causal pathway of the disease; they may be mediators or moderators of other relationships. Depending on how close in time they are observed in relation to disease onset, they might also be preclinical or subclinical markers of disease rather than true independent risk factors. Nonetheless, they allow us to identify and target subgroups with elevated probabilities of having or developing the disease or condition of interest.

Neurocognitive Disorders

In DSM-5 (American Psychiatric Association 2013), new terminology was introduced. The *neurocognitive disorders* are acquired conditions in which the primary deficits are in cognitive functioning, recognizing that cognition is also impaired as a secondary feature in many other categories of mental disorders. DSM-5 recognized three subgroups of neurocognitive disorders: delirium, major neurocognitive disorder, and mild neurocognitive disorder. Further details are available in Chapter 7, "Delirium," and Chapter 8, "Dementia and Mild Neurocognitive Disorders."

Delirium

Delirium is typically an acute mental condition characterized by changes in attention and awareness that develop over a short period of time and fluctuate in severity over the course of the day. There are often additional cognitive disturbances, such as in memory, executive function, visuospatial function, or language. The syndrome must be shown as being the result of another medical condition, drug intoxication or withdrawal, another toxin, or multiple causes (American Psychiatric Association 2013).

Prevalence and Incidence

Being an acute, fluctuating, and transient condition, delirium is difficult to detect reliably in community- or population-based studies. Clinical epidemiology studies indicate that delirium is common among older adults admitted to medical and surgical hospital wards, emergency departments, intensive care units, and postoperative wards. The range of prevalence of delirium in these settings varies hugely depending on the setting; details are beyond the scope of this chapter but are discussed in Chapter 7 and have been amply reviewed elsewhere (Cheung et al. 2018; Vasilevskis et al. 2012).

Risk Factors

The risk factors for delirium are generally classified into *predisposing* and *precipitating* factors. Predisposing factors include older age, less education, underlying dementia and its severity, cerebrovascular and cardiovascular disease, other medical comorbidity, visual impairment, malnutrition, smoking, or alcohol and substance use, including opioid and benzodiazepine use. Precipitating factors include infections, the type and duration of surgery, and the type of anesthesia used. Chapter 7 also elaborates on these factors.

Major Neurocognitive Disorder (Dementia)

In DSM-5, the term *major neurocognitive disorder* subsumes what is generally called *dementia* in older adults, with severe acquired loss of function in at least two cognitive domains (and, rarely, severe loss in a single domain) that is sufficient to interfere with independent everyday functioning and is not attributable to another mental disorder (American Psychiatric Association 2013). Typically, the clinician first diagnoses the syndrome of major neurocognitive disorder/dementia and then diagnoses the etiological subtype, such as AD, cerebrovascular disease, traumatic brain injury, or another neurodegenerative dementing disorder, such as frontotemporal lobar degeneration, dementia with Lewy bodies, or Huntington's disease. In the research setting, these distinctions are usually made in clinical studies for which imaging and fluid biomarker data are available, and neuropathological data often are obtained from autopsy. In most population studies, prevalence and incidence have been estimated for overall dementia or for AD or vascular dementia (VaD); the other etiological subtypes are insufficiently common in the community at large or require diagnostic testing beyond the capacity of most population studies.

Prevalence and Incidence

Prevalence estimates for dementia have varied based on the age structure of the population studied, the specific diagnostic criteria used, the region where the study was done, and the time when the study was done, because diagnostic criteria have evolved over the years. Some studies have used the DSM criteria of that period, some have used *International Classification of Disease* criteria, and still others have used Clinical Dementia Rating (Morris 1993) criteria. Where response (participation) from the community is low, there are concerns not only about lowered precision of the estimates but also about systematically biased estimates (e.g., if people with dementia were less likely to participate than those without dementia) (Hall et al. 2009). Incidence estimates have varied for the same reasons, but relatively few incidence studies have been done. Table 1–1 lists some studies that have reported both prevalence and incidence estimates.

The studies shown in Table 1–1 demonstrate that incidence and prevalence increase with age and are higher in high-income countries, where life expectancy is longer and people survive longer with dementia (i.e., disease duration is longer) than in low and

TABLE 1–1.   Prevalence and incidence of all-cause dementia: selected studies

Study, location	Sampling method	Diagnosis (diagnostic criteria)	Sample size (age range, years; mean age, years)	Prevalence (year)*	Incidence (time period)
Alzheimer's Disease International (Ferri et al. 2005), global data	Systematic review data	Dementia (Delphi consensus)	Global population (≥60)	24.3 million (2005); 42.3 million (2020, as projected in 2005); 81.1 million (2040, projected)	4.6 million per year
Global Burden of Disease Study (GBD 2016 Disease and Injury Incidence and Prevalence Collaborators 2017), global data	Vital registration systems, scientific literature, health service data	Dementia	Global population (all ages)	20.2 million (1990); 43.8 million (2016)	
Indianapolis Ibadan Dementia Project (Gao et al. 2016; Hall et al. 2009; Ogunniyi et al. 2000), Indianapolis, Indiana, and Ibadan, Nigeria	Older African Americans randomly sampled from a defined urban U.S. population; two cohorts (1992 and 2001)	Dementia (DSM-III-R, ICD 10)	1,500 (≥65; 77)	1992 cohort: 6.8% (1992)	
			1,892 (≥70; 77)	1992 cohort: 7.5% (2001)	
			1,440 (≥70; 78)		3.6% per year (1992–2009)
			1,835 (≥70; 77)		1.4% per year (2001–2009)
	Older adults randomly sampled from a defined urban Nigerian population; two cohorts (1992 and 2001)	Dementia (DSM-III-R, ICD-10)	2,494 (≥65; 72)	2.3% (1992, age adjusted)	
			1,174 (≥70; 78)		1.7% per year (1992–2009)
			1,895 (≥70; 76)		1.4% per year (2001–2009)

TABLE 1-1. Prevalence and incidence of all-cause dementia: selected studies *(continued)*

Study, location	Sampling method	Diagnosis (diagnostic criteria)	Sample size (age range, years; mean age, years)	Prevalence (year)*	Incidence (time period)
Health and Retirement Study (Langa et al. 2017), all census tracts, United States	U.S. nationwide random sample of older adults in both community and institutions	Dementia, assumed based on score from telephone interview for cognitive status	10,546 (≥65; 75) 10,511 (≥65; 75)	11.6% (2000) 8.6% (2012; age and sex adjusted)	
Aging, Demographics, and Memory Study (Plassman et al. 2007), all census tracts, United States	Subsample from Health and Retirement Study	Dementia (DSM-III-R, DSM-IV, clinical consensus)	856 (≥70)	13.9% (2002)	
Framingham Heart Study (Bachman et al. 1992; Satizabal et al. 2016), Framingham, Massachusetts	Longitudinal cohorts of people in a specific geographical region, original cohort	Dementia (moderate-severe)	2,180 (61–93)	Men 3%, women 4.8% (1982)	
	Original cohort and offspring cohort	Dementia (DSM-IV)	2,457 (60–89; 69) 2,135 (60–96; 72) 2,333 (60–101; 72) 2,090 (60–101; 72)		5-year rates, age and sex adjusted 3.6% (1977–1983) 2.8% (1986–1991) 2.2% (1992–1998) 2.0% (2004–2008)
Rotterdam Study (Schrijvers et al. 2012), Rotterdam, Netherlands	Longitudinal cohorts of people in a specific geographical region	Dementia (DSM-III-R)	5,727 (60–90) 1,769 (60–90)		6.6 per 1,000 person-years (1990–1995) 4.9 per 1,000 person-years (2000–2005)

TABLE 1–1. Prevalence and incidence of all-cause dementia: selected studies *(continued)*

Study, location	Sampling method	Diagnosis (diagnostic criteria)	Sample size (age range, *years*; mean age, *years*)	Prevalence (year)*	Incidence (time period)
Hisayama Study (Sekita et al. 2010), Hisayama, Japan	All older adults in a specific geographical region	Dementia (DSM-III in 1985, DSM-III-R in 1992, 1998, 2005)	887 (≥65; 74) / 1,189 (≥65; 74) / 1,437 (≥65; 75) / 1,566 (≥65; 76)	6% (1985, age and sex adjusted) / 4.4% (1992) / 5.3% (1998) / 8.3% (2005)	
Indo-U.S. Study (Chandra et al. 1998, 2001), Ballabgarh, India	Older adults from a defined rural geographical area; prevalence survey and 2-year follow-up for incidence	Dementia (DSM-IV, Clinical Dementia Rating ≥1)	2,698 (≥65)	1.14% (1996)	3.2 per 1,000 person-years (1996–1998)
Canadian Study of Health and Aging Working Group (1994, 2000), Canada (all 10 provinces)	Age-stratified random sample of older Canadian adults, including community and institutional populations	Dementia (DSM-III-R)	10,263 (≥65) / 9,131 (≥65; 74)	8% (1991–1992)	Men: 19.1 per 1,000 person-years (1991–1996); women: 21.8 per 1,000 person-years (1991–1996)

*Factors adjusted for.

middle-income countries. Furthermore, when diagnosis is restricted to moderate and severe dementia (Bachman et al. 1992), prevalence will be lower than when diagnosis also includes mild cases. Predictably, these estimates will be lower if they are based on individuals ages 55–60 years or older versus those age 65 or older because prevalence increases markedly with age. A systematic review and meta-analysis of the global prevalence of dementia showed that age-standardized prevalence for those aged ≥60 years varied in a narrow band, 5%–7% in most world regions, with a higher prevalence in Latin America (8.5%) and a distinctively lower prevalence in the four sub-Saharan African regions (2%–4%) (Prince et al. 2013).

As noted, some studies have reported prevalence and incidence estimates for etiological subtypes of dementia, principally AD and VaD. The challenge in comparing these studies, particularly when they were performed during different decades, is that definitions and diagnostic criteria for both AD and VaD have evolved over time. These changes became increasingly pronounced as neuroimaging techniques improved in resolution and became more accessible and now as research diagnoses lean increasingly on biomarkers (e.g., levels and ratios of brain and cerebrospinal fluid amyloid-β and tau proteins for AD diagnosis) (Jack et al. 2018). In an earlier period, the presence of any vascular pathology was regarded as representing VaD, excluding the possibility of a primary neurodegenerative dementia, such as AD. We now understand that neurodegenerative and cerebrovascular diseases are more frequently comorbid than not. Based on autopsy studies comparing brains of individuals diagnosed with AD from a clinical research sample with those from a community research sample, it has become clear that mixed neuropathology is the most common picture in the community at large, in contrast to the predominance of typical Alzheimer-type pathology in clinical research centers (Schneider et al. 2009). Furthermore, we now know that in the ninth and tenth decades of life, the predominant pathology in individuals with dementia is neither AD nor VaD but, rather, limbic-predominant age-related transactive response DNA-binding protein (TDP)-43 encephalopathy and hippocampal sclerosis (Nelson et al. 2019). The neuropathology underlying dementia is relevant to clinicians because, at least in theory, treatment should be specific to the disease entity; it is also relevant to epidemiologists' ability to identify independent risk factors for dementia because these factors likely vary depending on the specific pathological processes causing dementia.

Time Trends in Incidence of Dementia

Demonstrating the third of the classic seven uses of epidemiology, the charting of historical trends, an intriguing finding from several North American and European sites, all high-income countries, is that the incidence of dementia seems to be declining over successive birth cohorts (Matthews et al. 2016; Satizabal et al. 2016; Schrijvers et al. 2012; Sullivan et al. 2019). While increasing education, better cardiovascular disease management, and decreasing smoking rates have been invoked as potential reasons, the data available thus far do not fully explain the trend. One study showed that the incidence declined in African Americans but not in Africans (Gao et al. 2016).

Mild Neurocognitive Disorder (Mild Cognitive Impairment)

According to DSM-5, mild neurocognitive disorder (more commonly referred to as mild cognitive impairment, or MCI) is a condition of mild acquired impairment in at least one domain of cognition that is not severe enough to interfere with independence in everyday functioning and is not attributable to another mental disorder (American Psychiatric Association 2013). It is intermediate, but not necessarily transitional, between normal aging and dementia. In specialty research and clinical settings, MCI is often a precursor to dementia; in population-based studies, however, most individuals with MCI remain mildly impaired, whereas one minority progresses to dementia and another minority reverts to normal aging (Mitchell and Shiri-Feshki 2009).

Prevalence and Incidence

Prevalence of MCI varies greatly across population studies depending on the specific diagnostic criteria used for MCI and how they were operationalized. Table 1–2 illustrates some of these studies. In 1999, a group at the Mayo Clinic published criteria for diagnosis of amnestic MCI that included memory complaint, normal activities of daily living (ADLs), normal general cognitive function, abnormal memory for age by objective testing, and no dementia (Petersen et al. 1999). In 2004, an international working group on MCI expanded the working definition to encompass impairments in all cognitive domains. MCI was defined as having neither dementia nor normal cognition, with normal functional abilities, cognitive decline as indicated by self- or informant report, and objective evidence of cognitive impairment in one or more domains (Winblad et al. 2004). Studies focused on isolated amnestic MCI, with only memory deficits, tend to have the lowest prevalence in population studies. Another concept, known as *cognitive impairment, no dementia* (CIND), is defined a little differently (Graham et al. 1997), and thus its prevalence also varies. CIND is based on the exclusion of dementia and the presence of various categories of functional or cognitive impairment identified by clinical examination and neuropsychological tests. This is a heterogeneous classification that does not exclude delirium, depression, and other psychiatric disorders. Relatively few longitudinal studies have been able to follow large population-based cohorts of cognitively healthy older adults until they developed MCI/CIND and thus to generate incidence estimates.

Risk Factors

Multiple studies have reported risk and protective factors; they vary as to whether the measured outcome is incident dementia, incident MCI, progression from MCI/CIND to dementia, cognitive decline over time, or changes in brain structure as viewed by neuroimaging. They also vary in whether the risk factors are measured in early life, midlife, or later life. Results vary accordingly; key points are highlighted here.

Risk factors for dementia. Age is the strongest risk factor for dementia; the exponential increase in risk associated with age (Jorm and Jolley 1998) continues beyond age 90 (Corrada et al. 2010). Evidence regarding sex as a risk factor, on the other hand, continues to be debated, despite the fact that two-thirds of diagnosed cases are women (Alzheimer's Association 2013). The extent to which sex differences are caused by higher longevity among women and by women being more likely to seek diagnosis and care, relative to men, is not fully understood. Black and Latinx populations have higher prevalence and incidence of dementia than European Americans, whereas Native Americans have lower rates and Asian Americans have rates similar to those of European Americans (National Research Council [U.S.] Panel on Race 2004). Methodological variation, including inadequate adjustment for socioeconomic status and ed-

TABLE 1–2. Prevalence and incidence of mild cognitive impairment (mild neurocognitive disorder): selected studies

Study, location	Sampling	Diagnostic criteria	Sample size (mean age/age range, years)	Prevalence (year)	Incidence
Monongahela-Youghiogheny Healthy Aging Team (Ganguli et al. 2010, 2013), Pennsylvania	Age-stratified random sample of older adults from a defined U.S. small-town population	CDR 0.5 1999 amnestic MCI 2004 expanded MCI Objective cognitive criteria only MCI (objective cognitive criteria only) CDR 0.5	1,982 (78)	26.8% (2010) 2.2% 17.1% 33.7%	95 per 1,000 person-years 55 per 1,000 person-years
Pittsburgh Cardiovascular Health Study–Cognition Study (Lopez et al. 2012), Pennsylvania	Subsample of a U.S. population-based cohort; mean follow-up 10 years	1999 amnestic MCI	285 (79)		111 per 1,000 person-years (1998–2008, age adjusted)
Cognitive Function and Ageing Studies (CFAS; Richardson et al. 2019), United Kingdom	Random sample of older adults from six U.K. geographical regions	2004 expanded MCI	CFAS 1: 7,635 (≥65) CFAS 2: 7,796 (≥65)	17.6% (1991) 15.2% (2011)	
Aging, Demographics, and Memory Study (Plassman et al. 2008, 2011), United States	Stratified (by cognitive scores) random sample of nationally representative Health and Retirement Study subjects; mean follow-up of 5 years	CIND	856 (≥70) 456 (≥72)	22.2% (2001)	60.4 per 1,000 person-years (2001–2009)

CDR=Clinical Dementia Rating; CIND=cognitive impairment, no dementia; MCI=mild cognitive impairment.

ucational attainment, different levels of acculturation, and linguistic issues in testing, may contribute to a significant portion of the observed differences.

Mendelian forms of dementia, such as Huntington's disease and early-onset AD (EOAD) are autosomal dominant, with high penetrance and usually a typical family history. For EOAD, the three currently known causative genetic mutations are the amyloid precursor protein (APP) gene on chromosome 21, the presenilin 1 (PSEN1) gene on chromosome 14, and the presenilin 2 (PSEN2) gene on chromosome 1. Together, these three genes account for about 70%–80% of EOAD, PSEN1 being the most frequent (Campion et al. 1999; Raux et al. 2005). The vast number of individuals with late-onset AD, however, do not have these genetic mutations but may have one or more genetic variations (polymorphisms) that increase risk. The ε4 allele of apolipoprotein E (APOE*4) on chromosome 19 is the most important of these; compared with the common APOE ε3/ε3 genotype, homozygous APOE ε4/ε4 carriers have eight times higher risk for AD (Corder et al. 1993). However, most heterozygous carriers remain disease free, and more than half of patients with AD do not have the APOE ε4 allele, which is why APOE genotyping is not recommended for routine clinical use in the diagnosis of AD (American College of Medical Genetics/American Society of Human Genetics Working Group on ApoE and Alzheimer Disease 1995). Candidate gene association studies and genome-wide association studies have identified additional genes with small effects, but relatively few of these findings have been replicated.

Potentially modifiable risk factors identified in longitudinal studies include early life factors (e.g., fewer years of schooling), midlife factors (e.g., hearing loss, hypertension, diabetes, obesity), and late-life factors (e.g., smoking, depression, social isolation, physical inactivity, diabetes). One-third of dementia is, in theory, considered potentially preventable by, for example, increasing childhood education and physical exercise, maintaining social engagement, or reducing smoking. Management of hearing loss, depression, diabetes, and obesity may delay or prevent dementia in one-third of the population. Hypertension (McGrath et al. 2017), hypercholesterolemia (Kivipelto et al. 2001), and obesity in midlife (Fitzpatrick et al. 2009) appear to increase risk of dementia in late life; paradoxically, when measured in late life, lower blood pressure (Qiu et al. 2009), cholesterol (Mielke et al. 2005), and BMI (Fitzpatrick et al. 2009) seem to be associated with subsequent late-life dementia. The latter associations may reflect independent risk—for example, lower blood pressure may be associated with heart failure and hypoxia, which accelerate cognitive decline—however, they may also be epiphenomena of the disease processes that cause dementia. This example also illustrates the nuances of prevention and treatment implications of risk factors, such as how tightly blood pressure should be controlled in older adults.

Cardiovascular and cerebrovascular disease, further downstream on the causal pathway from modifiable lifestyle and behavioral factors, are obvious risk factors for VaD, but these also increase risk for AD in older members of both sexes (Hofman et al. 1997). Among women, the role of hormone replacement therapy following menopause has been debated. Observational studies consistently showed that estrogen-containing hormone replacement therapy was associated with lower risk for dementia (LeBlanc et al. 2001); however, a randomized clinical trial demonstrated that conjugated equine estrogens plus medroxyprogesterone acetate increased dementia risk in older females (Shumaker et al. 2003). The divergent results between the observational studies and the clinical trial were likely related to the timing of estrogen therapy; hormone replacement initiated later in life is associated with increased risk, whereas initiation at an age closer to menopause appears to confer protection (Shao et al. 2012).

Among those older than 85 years, very few risk factors are discernible, although the risk of dementia continues to increase with aging. The role of many traditional risk factors in this age group is unclear, possibly because underlying neuropathology appears to be mixed and heterogeneous (Gardner et al. 2013).

Risk factors for mild cognitive impairment.   To the extent that MCI is sometimes a prodrome of dementia, risk factors for MCI would be the same as those for dementia. A systematic review found that higher age, hypertension, and lower education were consistent risk factors (Luck et al. 2010). Studies have shown risk for MCI increases with age (Ward et al. 2012) and may be higher among men (Roberts et al. 2012). Higher educational achievement has been found to be protective (Tervo et al. 2004). Vascular risk factors, including hypertension, *APOE*4* genotype, diabetes, obesity, overt vascular disease (stroke, heart failure) with end-organ damage, and clustering of factors, as in metabolic syndrome and stroke risk profile, have been found to increase risk significantly (Ganguli et al. 2013; Llewellyn et al. 2008; Tervo et al. 2004).

Risk factors for progression to dementia.   In clinical research studies, the annualized progression rate from MCI to dementia is about 10%. However, population-based studies consistently show that, annually, most individuals in the community with MCI remain mildly impaired, a minority revert to normal cognition, and another minority progress to dementia (Ganguli et al. 2011).

Consistently, both clinical research and population studies have shown that those who progress from MCI to dementia are older and have specific memory deficits and worse overall cognitive function, the *APOE*4* genotype, and cerebrovascular disease (Ganguli et al. 2015). Patients with MCI in the clinical setting are more likely to progress than are those identified in the population at large (Snitz et al. 2018). In neuroimaging studies, global and medial temporal atrophy and rate of atrophy, reflecting the underlying neurodegenerative process, predict progression to dementia (Geroldi et al. 2006; Korf et al. 2004; Sluimer et al. 2009) but are not independent risk factors. Risk factors for progression among the oldest-old are elusive, indicating the potential for unexplored risk and protective factors in this age group (Ganguli et al. 2015).

Brain/Cognitive reserve and resilience.   The concepts of brain reserve, cognitive reserve, and resilience are they frequently are found in the literature and are often the basis for risk factor models and prevention studies (Stern et al. 2020). *Brain reserve* and *cognitive reserve* refer to the individual's premorbid brain structure and brain function capacity (analogous to hardware and software) (Montine et al. 2019). They might offer protection against disease development and be associated either with no disease or with delayed onset of disease or disease manifestations. *Resilience* is the ability of the brain to maintain its cognitive functioning despite the presence of disease or injury. Thus, factors that promote reserve and resilience may be considered protective factors, whereas those that reduce reserve and resilience may be considered risk factors.

Behavioral/Psychological symptoms.   Psychiatrists and patients' families have long been aware that MCI and dementia have prominent behavioral and psychological symptoms, also referred to as neuropsychiatric symptoms. These symptoms are often more distressing to patients and families than the cognitive symptoms and are frequently the reason that clinical services are sought. However, for many decades, mainstream AD research has regarded these symptoms as peripheral and nonspecific to the disease process. They have been more systematically recognized in research on frontotemporal lobar degeneration and dementia with Lewy bodies, which are common in clinical settings but relatively rare at the population level. Since 2000, however, epidemiological work has shown that apathy is possibly an early sign of cognitive decline (Rattinger et al. 2019), that neuropsychiatric symptoms are associated with CIND (Peters et al. 2012), and that severity of neuropsychiatric symptoms is associated with severity of dementia (Rozum et al. 2019). More recently, the concept of *mild behavioral impairment* has emerged, suggesting a syndrome of behavioral symptoms that represents a prodrome of dementia, with or without concomitant MCI. Although the specifications and criteria are still evolving, mild behavioral impairment was shown to have a 10% prevalence in a cognitively normal U.K. volunteer sample with a mean age of 62 years (Creese et al. 2019) and an overall 34% prevalence in an Australian population sample with a mean age of 75 years and a range of cognitive levels (Mortby et al. 2018).

Screening for Cognitive Impairment and Dementia

In public health terminology, *screening* refers to testing everyone regardless of symptoms, setting, or risk factors. The U.S. Preventive Services Task Force has repeatedly concluded that insufficient evidence exists either for or against routine cognitive screening of older adults (Owens et al. 2020). Cognitive screening in clinical and research settings is typically undertaken with a brief global or general mental status test such as the Mini-Mental State Examination (Folstein et al. 1975), the Montreal Cognitive Assessment (Nasreddine et al. 2005), or the Mini-Cog (Borson et al. 2005). On these tests, a higher score reflects better cognitive functioning. There is no absolute threshold for a normal or abnormal test score; the ideal cut point depends upon the population being studied or the individual's demographic and other characteristics. Furthermore, a low score does not necessarily indicate a diagnosis of MCI or dementia; it only suggests that a detailed clinical examination is warranted. Finally, although a screening test's sensitivity and specificity should be established before it is used, its predictive value will depend on how prevalent dementia or cognitive impairment are in the population being screened.

Late-Life Depression

Epidemiology of Late-Life Depression

Late-life depression (LLD) encompasses a wide spectrum marked by severity of symptoms. The 12-month prevalence of major depressive disorder (MDD) among community-based samples of adults age 65 and older is approximately 1%–5% and increases with age. A meta-analysis of community-living persons age 75 and older reported prevalence estimates between 4.6% and 9.3%, with a pooled prevalence of 7.2% (Luppa et al. 2012). Whereas some studies indicate that approximately half of older persons with MDD experience their first onset of depression in late life (i.e., late-onset depression) (Brodaty et al. 2001; Bruce et al. 2002), it is difficult to provide accurate

TABLE 1–3. **Prevalence of major depression among older adults in selected treatment settings**

Study	Sample	N	Age, years	Diagnostic criteria	Prevalence
Lyness et al. 1999	Primary care sample in New York	224	60+	DSM-III-R	6.5%
Teresi et al. 2001	Nursing home sample in New York	319	46+	DSM-III-R	14.4%
Bruce et al. 2002	Elderly home health care patients in New York	539	65+	PHQ–9	13.5%
Harralson et al. 2002	Four nursing homes in Philadelphia	208	60+	ICD-9	–
Anderson et al. 2003	Minimum dataset, nursing home residents	145	60+	DSM-IV	28%
Jongenelis et al. 2004	Nursing home residents in The Netherlands	333	55+	DSM-IV	8.1%
Hasin et al. 2005	NESARC	43,093	65+	DSM-IV	2.7%
Kessler et al. 2005	NCS-R	9,282	60+	DSM-IV	10.6%
McCusker et al. 2005	Two acute care hospitals in Montreal, Canada	380	65+	DSM-IV	14.2%–44.5%
Smalbrugge et al. 2005	Various nursing homes in The Netherlands	333	55+	DSM-IV	17.1%
George et al. 2007	Various residential facilities in Melbourne, Australia	300	65+	DSM-IV	18%
Trollor et al. 2007	Australian National Mental Health and Well-Being Survey	1,792	65+	DSM-IV ICD-10	1.2%
Gum et al. 2009	NCS-R	9,282	65+	DSM-IV	2.3%
Boorsma et al. 2012	Various nursing homes in The Netherlands	864	85+	DSM-IV	13.6%
Davison et al. 2012	Various nursing homes in Melbourne, Australia	100	64+	DSM-IV	–

NCS-R=National Comorbidity Survey–Replication; NESARC=National Epidemiological Survey on Alcohol and Related Conditions; PHQ-9=Patient Health Questionnaire–9.

estimates because most studies of depression in later life do not distinguish early from late onset. However, general consensus indicates that those with early-onset depression are more likely to have a genetic predisposition to depression or a personality disorder (Brodaty et al. 2001). Prevalence estimates of MDD also differ according to the source of the data. For example, the point prevalence of MDD is considerably higher in nursing home samples. Among nursing home residents without dementia, point prevalence ranges from approximately 12% in cross-sectional studies to 44% in prospective studies (Fornaro et al. 2020). Table 1–3 shows some examples of studies that have reported prevalence estimates of MDD in specialized samples.

Subsyndromal depression is the presence of depressive symptoms that do not meet DSM criteria for MDD. Also referred to as *minor depression* or *subthreshold depression*, subsyndromal depression is more common than MDD. Prevalence estimates among community-living persons age 65 and older range from 8% to 30%, with 25%–49% of these individuals experiencing persistent symptoms (Barry et al. 2012; Blazer 2003; Forlani et al. 2014; Mackenzie et al. 2014; Meeks et al. 2011; Smits et al. 2008). Both subsyndromal depression and MDD are similarly associated with adverse outcomes in older adults, including increased health care costs (Katon et al. 2003; Schousboe et al. 2019), exacerbation of coexisting medical illness (Carnethon et al. 2007), onset of disability in ADLs (Barry et al. 2009, 2011; Murphy et al. 2016; Penninx et al. 1999b), and higher mortality risk (Penninx et al. 1999a; Unützer et al. 2002). Complications and consequences of LLD are elaborated upon in Chapter 9, "Depressive Disorders."

Sociodemographic Risk Factors

Sex

Across the adult life span, the burden of depression (which includes MDD and subsyndromal depression) is disproportionately higher in females. The most recent estimates indicate that among those age 65 years and older in the United States, the prevalence of depression is 10% among males and 15% among females (Federal Interagency Forum on Aging-Related Statistics 2016). In addition to experiencing a higher prevalence of depression, females are also more likely to have more severe depressive symptoms (Shanmugasegaram et al. 2012). The preponderance of depression in older females does not appear to be an artifact of greater symptom reporting; rather, females' greater likelihood of having been exposed to risk factors for depression, including lower income and having one or more chronic illnesses (Sonnenberg et al. 2000), and their higher likelihood of experiencing depression onset and persistence of depressive symptoms (Barry et al. 2008) explain this sex difference. However, whereas females have higher rates of depression in older age, males are at considerably higher risk of dying by suicide. Suicide rates among males are highest for those age 75 years or older, at 39.9 per 100,000 people. In contrast, suicide rates in females were highest for those ages 45–64 years; those age 75 years or older had a lower risk compared with all other age groups except early adolescence (Hedegaard et al. 2020).

Race

The population of adults 65 years of age or older in the United States is becoming increasingly diverse. Whereas members of one or more minority groups comprised ~22% of older adults in 2014, projections indicate that by 2060 the composition of the older population will be 55% non-Hispanic white, 22% Hispanic, 12% Black, and 9% Asian (Federal Interagency Forum on Aging-Related Statistics 2016). Despite growing numbers of minorities living to older ages, whether race is a risk factor for mood disorders in later life is uncertain. Most studies focusing on race differences in mood disorders in later life have evaluated Black/white differences in depression. However, how studies define depression contributes to the uncertainty about the role of Black/white race in LLD. Whereas the 12-month prevalence of MDD has been reported to be higher among older whites than older Blacks (Byers et al. 2010), some studies report that Blacks are more likely to experience clinically significant depressive symptoms, even after controlling for factors such as socioeconomic status (Barry et al. 2014; Jang et al. 2005; Murphy et al. 2016; Vyas et al. 2020). Longitudinal studies evaluating race differences in trajectories of depression symptoms indicate that, compared with older whites, older Blacks are more likely to experience an increase in depressive symptoms (Skarupski et al. 2005) and an increase in depression onset (Barry et al. 2014) over time. In accordance with the "race paradox," which posits that throughout their lives Blacks experience more risk factors for psychiatric disorders, including more poverty, poorer health, and discrimination, some studies report that older Blacks are less likely than whites to experience depressive symptoms or that there is no association between race and depression (Cohen et al. 2005; Gallo et al. 1998; Taylor and Chatters 2020). Moreover, findings from the Health and Retirement Study and its companion study, the Asset and Health Dynamics Among the Oldest Old, indicate that the rate of change in depressive symptoms over time is lower for older Black and Latinx individuals than for older white individuals (Xu et al. 2010). Among those with depressive symptoms, the lower rate of increase over time for minorities as compared with whites, particularly among Latinx, may be explained by minority persons' effective use in old age of coping strategies learned throughout life for dealing with racial discrimination (Ferraro and Farmer 1996).

Biological and Clinical Risk Factors for Depression

A large body of literature has evaluated the relationship between physical functioning and depression in older persons, with physical functioning assessed subjectively via self-reported disability in ADLs (e.g., bathing, walking, dressing) and objectively through assessments of mobility and gait. Across all studies, there is general consensus that these conditions are inextricably linked. However, some research points to a stronger influence of disability on subsequent depression than of depression on disability (Chen et al. 2012; Ormel et al. 2002). The relationship between compromised physical function and depression may be explained by stress theory (Avison and Turner 1988; Pearlin et al. 1981), which says that new disability or the ongoing psychological and physical stress of chronic disability alters homeostasis, thereby leading to depression. In turn, depression may alter neural, hormonal, or immunological function, subsequently resulting in disability.

Whereas cross-sectional studies have been critical to establishing the relationship between physical function and depression in older persons (Bruce 2001; Harris et al. 2006; Ormel et al. 2002), findings from large prospective cohort studies have contributed significantly to our understanding of this relationship (Table 1–4).

Psychosocial Risk Factors for Depression

Social Support

Cassel (1976) and Cobb (1976) were the first investigators to suggest that it was critical to evaluate the relationship between social support and depression in older persons. Nearly two decades after the publication of their studies, research regarding the impact of social support on the mental health of older persons began to emerge. Early findings from the New Haven Established Populations for Epidemiologic Study of the Elderly reported that perceptions of having emotional support (e.g., love and caring from another) and instrumental support (e.g., help and assistance with tasks such as getting to appointments) were independently associated with fewer depressive symptoms in older persons (Berkman and Kawachi 2000; Oxman et al. 1992; Thoits 1995).

TABLE 1–4.   Selected prospective studies that evaluated the relationship between depression and subsequent disability in older persons

Study	Sample	N	Age, years	Functional assessment	Depression assessment	Measure of association
Barry et al. 2013	Community-dwelling adults from the Precipitating Events Project with no ADL disability at baseline	754	70+	Self-reported ADL disability every month up to 108 months	11-item CES-D every 18 months up to 108 months	Any vs. no disability, OR 1.65 (95% CI 1.34–2.02)
Demakakos et al. 2013	Community-dwelling adults from the English Longitudinal Study of Ageing	4,581	60+	8-foot gait speed measured at baseline and every 4 years	8-item CES-D at baseline and yearly for 4 years	Slowed gait speed, OR 0.42 (95% CI 0.30–0.59)
Sanders et al. 2016	Community-dwelling adults in The Netherlands	271	55+	3-meter gait speed measured at baseline	20-item CES-D every 5 months and 3 years	Slowed gait speed, OR 0.56 (95% CI 0.41–077)
Li and Dong 2017	Community-dwelling adults from the Population Study of Chinese Elderly	3,157	60+	Self-reported ADL disability, SPPB	PHQ-9	ADLs, OR 1.29 (95% CI 1.14–1.45) IADLs, OR 1.17 (95% CI 1.13–1.22) Index of Basic Physical Activities scale, OR 1.22 (95% CI 1.19–1.26) Index of Mobility scale, OR 1.52 (95% CI 1.39–1.66) SPPB, OR 1.16 (95% CI 1.12–1.19)
Veronese et al. 2017	Participants from the Progetto Veneto Anziani study with no depression at baseline	970	65+	SPPB, leg extension and flexion, handgrip strength, 6-minute walk	30-item GDS	Low SPPB scores; OR 1.79 (95% CI 1.18–2.71)
Briggs et al. 2018	Community-dwelling adults from the Irish Longitudinal Study on Ageing	2,638	60+	The Timed Up and Go test	20-item CES-D at baseline and 2-year follow-up	Gait abnormality; IRR 2.00 (95% CI 1.18–3.40)

ADL=activity of daily living; CES-D=Center for Epidemiological Studies–Depression; GDS=Geriatric Depression Scale; IADL=instrumental activity of daily living; IRR=incidence rate ratio; PHQ-9=Patient Health Questionnaire–9; SPPB=Short Physical Performance Battery.

Numerous studies now have evaluated the association between social support and depression in older persons, with social support encompassing related concepts such as social network, social integration/connectedness, and social participation (Schwarzbach et al. 2014). However, the research largely points toward qualitative aspects of social support (e.g., perceived emotional support, quality of relationships) having a greater impact on depression in late life than quantitative aspects (e.g., size of one's social network). Of note, perceiving social support as excessive or unhelpful, often in regard to instrumental support, has been found to be associated with increased depressive symptoms in older persons (Nagumey et al. 2004).

Bereavement

Bereavement is a normal response to death accompanied by acute grief symptoms that typically attenuate over time. Yet bereavement can precipitate a mental health disorder, with a meta-analysis of prospective studies of those age 50 and older reporting that bereaved people have more than a threefold risk of experiencing depression (Cole and Dendukuri 2003). However, although this risk is high, bereavement still confers a lower risk of depression in older persons than in younger and middle-aged adults. Regarding spousal death, which is common in older age, the risk difference between younger and older persons is largely attributed to the greater expectedness of a spouse's death in late life as compared with early or midlife (Blazer and Hybels 2005). In addition, for more than two decades investigators have debated whether severe and chronic forms of grief can be distinguished clinically from bereavement-related depression (Prigerson et al. 1995). This question led to considerable deliberation regarding whether complicated grief or prolonged grief disorder should be included in DSM-5 (Lichtenthal et al. 2004; Prigerson et al. 2009; Shear et al. 2011). Because of a lack of consensus, the "bereavement exclusion" was removed from the clinical criteria for depression and adjustment disorders (Wakefield and First 2012). However, the removal of this exclusion raised concerns that grief will become "medicalized" and that grieving individuals may be inappropriately prescribed antidepressant medications. Consequently, DSM-5 included "persistent complex bereavement disorder" in a chapter on conditions needing further study. Following a DSM Steering Committee workshop on prolonged grief disorder and period of public commentary in April and May 2020, the Steering Committee released the proposed criteria. The American Psychiatric Association approved inclusion of prolonged grief disorder in DSM-5-TR (American Psychiatric Association 2022) on November 20, 2020 (Prigerson et al. 2021).

Late-Life Anxiety Disorder

Epidemiology

The anxiety disorders include panic disorder, agoraphobia without panic, specific phobia, social phobia, generalized anxiety disorder (GAD), and PTSD. Nationally representative 12-month prevalence estimates from the National Comorbidity Survey–Replication (NCS-R) determined that nearly 12% of older adults age 55 years and older had any anxiety disorder, compared with 5% having any mood disorder (Byers et al. 2010). When U.S. respondents were stratified into young-old (55–64 years), mid-old (65–74), old-old (75–84), and oldest-old (≥85), the prevalences for any anxiety disorder were 16.6%, 8.9%, 6.0%, and 8.1%, respectively (Byers et al. 2010). For any mood disorder, the 12-month prevalences were 7.6%, 3.6%, 1.8%, and 2.4%, respectively. Among the NCS-R adults age 55 and older, the most prevalent anxiety disorder was specific phobia (6.5%), followed by social phobia (3.5%), PTSD (2.1%), GAD (2.0%), panic disorder (1.3%), and agoraphobia (0.8%). Similarly, anxiety disorders were the most prevalent disorders in participants age 65 years and older in the Epidemiologic Catchment Area Survey (5.5%), with phobic disorder the most prevalent disorder (4.8%) (Hybels and Blazer 2003). Chapter 12, "Anxiety, Obsessive-Compulsive, and Trauma-Related Disorders," elaborates further on the epidemiology of late-life anxiety disorders.

Risk Factors

Despite the high prevalence of anxiety disorders in late life, risk factors associated with late-life anxiety are not well conceptualized. Yet what is known suggests that risk factors for anxiety and depression are similar. This is not surprising given the strong overlap between anxiety and depression seen throughout adult life and in late life. Shared genetic risk has been found between GAD and depression (Kendler et al. 2007), and research from the NCS-R has shown that anxiety disorders throughout the life span are associated with female gender, higher number of comorbid chronic medical conditions, being unmarried or divorced, and having less than a high school education (Gum et al. 2009). Furthermore, research suggests that cognitive impairment and dementia may be major risk factors for anxiety in late life (Seignourel et al. 2008); however, the overlap of symptoms between anxiety and dementia complicates assessment of this association. Older adults with VaD have also been found to have a higher prevalence of anxiety than older adults with Alzheimer's-type dementia (Seignourel et al. 2008), which suggests that anxiety in dementia may be related to the vascular risk for depression in late life.

Late-Life Coexisting Mood and Anxiety Disorders

Epidemiology

Late-life mood and anxiety disorders have similar risk factors and overlapping symptom profiles and frequently co-occur. These disorders are also often difficult to disentangle from other conditions that affect older adults, making diagnosis and treatment challenging. However, given that persons with mental illness are living longer and that the incidence of late-onset mood and anxiety disorders is expected to increase with the rapid aging of the population, the prevalence of older adults with these disorders is expected to increase.

Most U.S. studies of coexisting mood and anxiety disorders have been clinically based and have found a high prevalence of comorbid anxiety in patients with depression (Lenze 2003; Lenze et al. 2000, 2001). Twenty-three percent of older subjects (age ≥60 years) with depressive disorders had a current anxiety disorder diagnosis (Lenze et al. 2000). The most common current coexisting anxiety disorders were panic (9.3%), specific phobia (8.8%), and social phobia (6.6%). Interestingly, 27.5% of older subjects with depression had symptoms that met criteria for GAD. The prevalence of GAD symptoms went up to 45% for those in the inpatient psychiatric subgroup. In contrast, nationally representative estimates from population-based research in NCS-R respondents documented that the 12-month prevalence of any coexisting mood or anxiety disorder was 3% among adults age 55 years and older (Byers et al. 2010).

Risk Factors

Risk factors for coexisting mood and anxiety disorders in late life appear to be largely associated with severity of somatic symptoms related to the primary mood or anxiety disorder, a decline in function, or a particularly high accumulation of individual risk factors for mood or anxiety. In older adults with depressive disorders, poorer social functioning and a higher level of somatic symptoms (e.g., sweating, nausea, and palpitations) were associated with a greater likelihood of a comorbid anxiety disorder, excluding symptoms of GAD (Lenze et al. 2000). Greater severity of depressive symptoms was associated with greater likelihood of GAD symptoms.

Conclusion

In the coming years, the number of adults living past the age of 65 will increase significantly, forming an ethnically and racially more diverse group that will make up a larger percentage of the overall population relative to decades past. The corresponding increasing need for delivery of effective geriatric mental health services can only be addressed with an understanding of current and future epidemiological trends, with an emphasis on identifying relevant modifiable risk factors that, if addressed, may reduce the incidence, prevalence, and severity of cognitive, mood, anxiety, and other psychiatric disorders facing older adults in the future.

Key Points

- Epidemiology is the study of the "distribution and determinants" of disease in the population and their application for preventing and controlling disease.

- Understanding risk and protective factors allows the identification of subgroups with an elevated probability of having or developing a disease or condition of interest.

- Estimates of incidence and prevalence of neurocognitive disorders vary depending on factors such as age of population studied, geography, socioeconomic variables, and level of care.

- A small subset of patients with mild cognitive impairment progress to dementia annually; most remain mildly impaired.

- Modifiable risk factors for dementia are present in early, mid-, and late life.

- The 12-month prevalence of major depressive disorder among community-based samples of adults age 65 and older is approximately 1%–5% and increases with age; rates of subsyndromal depression are higher.

- Risk factors for late-life depression include impaired physical functioning, lack of social support, and bereavement.

- Anxiety disorders are more common among older adults than mood disorders, although these frequently co-occur.

References

Alzheimer's Association: 2013 Alzheimer's disease facts and figures. Alzheimers Dement 9(2):208–245, 2013 23507120

American College of Medical Genetics/American Society of Human Genetics Working Group on ApoE and Alzheimer Disease: Statement on use of apolipoprotein E testing for Alzheimer disease. JAMA 274(20):1627–1629, 1995 7474250

American Psychiatric Association: Diagnostic and Statistical Manual of Mental Disorders, 5th Edition. Arlington, VA, American Psychiatric Association, 2013

American Psychiatric Association: Diagnostic and Statistical Manual of Mental Disorders, 5th Edition, Text Revision. Arlington, VA, American Psychiatric Association, 2022

Anderson RL, Buckwalter KC, Buchanan RJ, et al: Validity and reliability of the Minimum Data Set Depression Rating Scale (MDSDRS) for older adults in nursing homes. Age Ageing 34(4):435–438, 2003 12851189

Avison WR, Turner RJ: Stressful life events and depressive symptoms: disaggregating the effects of acute stressors and chronic strains. J Health Soc Behav 29(3):253–264, 1988 3241066

Bachman DL, Wolf PA, Linn R, et al: Prevalence of dementia and probable senile dementia of the Alzheimer type in the Framingham Study. Neurology 42(1):115–119, 1992 1734291

Barry LC, Allore HG, Guo Z, et al: Higher burden of depression among older women: the effect of onset, persistence, and mortality over time. Arch Gen Psychiatry 65(2):172–178, 2008 18250255

Barry LC, Allore HG, Bruce ML, Gill TM: Longitudinal association between depressive symptoms and disability burden among older persons. J Gerontol A Biol Sci Med Sci 64(12):1325–1332, 2009 19776217

Barry LC, Murphy TE, Gill TM: Depressive symptoms and functional transitions over time in older persons. Am J Geriatr Psychiatry 19(9):783–791, 2011 21873834

Barry LC, Abou JJ, Simen AA, Gill TM: Under-treatment of depression in older persons. J Affect Disord 136(3):789–796, 2012 22030136

Barry LC, Soulos PR, Murphy TE, et al: Association between indicators of disability burden and subsequent depression among older persons. J Gerontol A Biol Sci Med Sci 68(3):286–292, 2013 22967459

Barry LC, Thorpe RJ Jr, Penninx BW, et al: Race-related differences in depression onset and recovery in older persons over time: the Health, Aging, and Body Composition study. Am J Geriatr Psychiatry 22(7):682–691, 2014 24125816

Berkman LF, Kawachi I: Social Epidemiology. New York, Oxford University Press, 2000

Blazer DG: Depression in late life: review and commentary. J Gerontol A Biol Sci Med Sci 58(3):249–265, 2003 12634292

Blazer DG II, Hybels CF: Origins of depression in later life. Psychol Med 35(9):1241–1252, 2005 16168147

Boorsma M, Karlijn J, Dussel M, et al: The incidence of depression and its risk factors in Dutch nursing homes and residential care homes. Am J Geriatr Psychiatry 20(11):932–942, 2012

Borson S, Scanlan JM, Watanabe J, et al: Simplifying detection of cognitive impairment: comparison of the Mini-Cog and Mini-Mental State Examination in a multiethnic sample. J Am Geriatr Soc 53(5):871–874, 2005 15877567

Briggs R, Carey D, Kenny RA, Kennelley SP: What is the longitudinal relationship between gait abnormalities and depression in a cohort of community-dwelling older people? Data from the Irish Longitudinal Study on Ageing (TILDA). Am J Geriatr Psychiatry 26(1):75–86, 2018

Brodaty H, Luscombe G, Parker G, et al: Early and late onset depression in old age: different aetiologies, same phenomenology. J Affect Disord 66(2–3):225–236, 2001 11578676

Bruce ML: Depression and disability in late life: directions for future research. Am J Geriatr Psychiatry 9(2):102–112, 2001 11316615

Bruce ML, McAvay GJ, Raue PJ, et al: Major depression in elderly home health care patients. Am J Psychiatry 159(8):1367–1374, 2002 12153830

Byers AL, Yaffe K, Covinsky KE, et al: High occurrence of mood and anxiety disorders among older adults: the National Comorbidity Survey Replication. Arch Gen Psychiatry 67(5):489–496, 2010 20439830

Campion D, Dumanchin C, Hannequin D, et al: Early onset autosomal dominant Alzheimer disease: prevalence, genetic heterogeneity, and mutation spectrum. Am J Hum Genet 65(3):664–670, 1999 10441572

Canadian Study of Health and Aging Working Group: Canadian Study of Health and Aging: study methods and prevalence of dementia. CMAJ 150(6):899–913, 1994 8131123

Canadian Study of Health and Aging Working Group: The incidence of dementia in Canada. Neurology 55(1):66–73, 2000 10891908

Carnethon MR, Biggs ML, Barzilay JI, et al: Longitudinal association between depressive symptoms and incident type 2 diabetes mellitus in older adults: the Cardiovascular Health Study. Arch Intern Med 167(8):802–807, 2007 17452543

Cassel J: The contribution of the social environment to host resistance: the Fourth Wade Hampton Frost Lecture. Am J Epidemiol 104(2):107–123, 1976 782233

Chandra V, Ganguli M, Pandav R, et al: Prevalence of Alzheimer's disease and other dementias in rural India: the Indo-US study. Neurology 51(4):1000–1008, 1998 9781520

Chandra V, Pandav R, Dodge HH, et al: Incidence of Alzheimer's disease in a rural community in India: the Indo-US study. Neurology 57(6):985–989, 2001 11571321

Chen M, Tse LA, Au RK, et al: Mesothelioma and lung cancer mortality: a historical cohort study among asbestosis workers in Hong Kong. Lung Cancer 76(2):165–170, 2012 22129857

Cheung ENM, Benjamin S, Heckman G, et al: Clinical characteristics associated with the onset of delirium among long-term nursing home residents. BMC Geriatr 18(1):39, 2018 29394886

Cipriani G, Dolciotti C, Picchi L, Bonuccelli U: Alzheimer and his disease: a brief history. Neurol Sci 32(2):275–279, 2011 21153601

Cobb S: Presidential Address 1976: social support as a moderator of life stress. Psychosom Med 38(5):300–314, 1976 981490

Cohen CI, Magai C, Yaffee R, Walcott-Brown L: Racial differences in syndromal and subsyndromal depression in an older urban population. Psychiatr Serv 56(12):1556–1563, 2005 16339618

Cole MG, Dendukuri N: Risk factors for depression among elderly community subjects: a systematic review and meta-analysis. Am J Psychiatry 160(6):1147–1156, 2003 12777274

Corder EH, Saunders AM, Strittmatter WJ, et al: Gene dose of apolipoprotein E type 4 allele and the risk of Alzheimer's disease in late onset families. Science 261(5123):921–923, 1993 8346443

Corrada MM, Brookmeyer R, Paganini-Hill A, et al: Dementia incidence continues to increase with age in the oldest old: the 90+ Study. Ann Neurol 67(1):114–121, 2010 20186856

Creese B, Brooker H, Ismail Z, et al: Mild behavioral impairment as a marker of cognitive decline in cognitively normal older adults. Am J Geriatr Psychiatry 27(8):823–834, 2019 30902566

Davison T, Snowdon J, Castle N, et al: An evaluation of a national program to implement the Cornell Scale for Depression in Dementia into routine practice in aged care facilities. Int Psychogeriatr 24(4):631–641, 2012

Demakakos P, Cooper R, Hamer M, et al: The bidirectional association between depressive symptoms and gait speed: evidence from the English Longitudinal Study of Ageing (ELSA). PLoS ONE 8(7):1–9, 2013

Falk EB, Hyde LW, Mitchell C, et al: What is a representative brain? Neuroscience meets population science. Proc Natl Acad Sci USA 110(44):17615–17622, 2013 24151336

Federal Interagency Forum on Aging-Related Statistics: Older Americans 2016: Key Indicators of Well-Being. Washington, DC, U.S. Government Printing Office, 2016

Ferraro KF, Farmer MM: Double jeopardy, aging as leveler, or persistent health inequality? A longitudinal analysis of white and black Americans. J Gerontol B Psychol Sci Soc Sci 51(6):S319–S328, 1996 8931631

Ferri CP, Prince M, Brayne C, et al: Global prevalence of dementia: a Delphi consensus study. Lancet 366(9503):2112–2117, 2005 16360788

Fitzpatrick AL, Kuller LH, Lopez OL, et al: Midlife and late-life obesity and the risk of dementia: Cardiovascular Health Study. Arch Neurol 66(3):336–342, 2009 19273752

Folstein MF, Folstein SE, McHugh PR: "Mini-mental state": a practical method for grading the cognitive state of patients for the clinician. J Psychiatr Res 12(3):189–198, 1975 1202204

Forlani C, Morri M, Ferrari B, et al: Prevalence and gender differences in late-life depression: a population-based study. Am J Geriatr Psychiatry 22(4):370–380, 2014 23567427

Fornaro M, Solmi M, Stubbs B, et al: Prevalence and correlates of major depressive disorder, bipolar disorder and schizophrenia among nursing home residents without dementia: systematic review and meta-analysis. Br J Psychiatry 216(1):6–15, 2020 30864533

Gallo JJ, Cooper-Patrick L, Lesikar S: Depressive symptoms of whites and African Americans aged 60 years and older. J Gerontol B Psychol Sci Soc Sci 53(5):277–286, 1998 9750564

Ganguli M, Chang CC, Snitz BE, et al: Prevalence of mild cognitive impairment by multiple classifications: the Monongahela-Youghiogheny Healthy Aging Team (MYHAT) project. Am J Geriatr Psychiatry 18(8):674–683, 2010 20220597

Ganguli M, Snitz BE, Saxton JA, et al: Outcomes of mild cognitive impairment by definition: a population study. Arch Neurol 68(6):761–767, 2011 21670400

Ganguli M, Fu B, Snitz BE, et al: Mild cognitive impairment: incidence and vascular risk factors in a population-based cohort. Neurology 80(23):2112–2120, 2013 23658380

Ganguli M, Lee CW, Snitz BE, et al: Rates and risk factors for progression to incident dementia vary by age in a population cohort. Neurology 84(1):72–80, 2015 25471390

Ganguli M, Albanese E, Seshadri S, et al: Population neuroscience: dementia epidemiology serving precision medicine and population health. Alzheimer Dis Assoc Disord 32(1):1–9, 2018 29319603

Gao S, Ogunniyi A, Hall KS, et al: Dementia incidence declined in African-Americans but not in Yoruba. Alzheimers Dement 12(3):244–251, 2016 26218444

Gardner RC, Valcour V, Yaffe K: Dementia in the oldest old: a multi-factorial and growing public health issue. Alzheimers Res Ther 5(4):27, 2013 23809176

GBD 2016 Disease and Injury Incidence and Prevalence Collaborators: Global, regional, and national incidence, prevalence, and years lived with disability for 328 diseases and injuries for 195 countries, 1990–2016: a systematic analysis for the Global Burden of Disease Study 2016. Lancet 390(10100):1211–1259, 2017 28919117

George K, Davison TE, McCabe M, et al: Treatment of depression in low-level residential care facilities for the elderly. Int Psychogeriatr 19(6):1153–1160, 2007

Geroldi C, Rossi R, Calvagna C, et al: Medial temporal atrophy but not memory deficit predicts progression to dementia in patients with mild cognitive impairment. J Neurol Neurosurg Psychiatry 77(11):1219–1222, 2006 16891386

Graham JE, Rockwood K, Beattie BL, et al: Prevalence and severity of cognitive impairment with and without dementia in an elderly population. Lancet 349(9068):1793–1796, 1997 9269213

Gum AM, King-Kallimanis B, Kohn R: Prevalence of mood, anxiety, and substance-abuse disorders for older Americans in the National Comorbidity Survey–Replication. Am J Geriatr Psychiatry 17(9):769–781, 2009 19700949

Hall KS, Gao S, Baiyewu O, et al: Prevalence rates for dementia and Alzheimer's disease in African Americans: 1992 versus 2001. Alzheimers Dement 5(3):227–233, 2009 19426950

Harralson TL, White TM, Regenberg AC, et al: Similarities and differences in depression among black and white nursing home residents. Am J Geriatr Psychiatry 10(2):175–184, 2002

Harris T, Cook DG, Victor C, et al: Onset and persistence of depression in older people: results from a 2-year community follow-up study. Age Ageing 35(1):25–32, 2006 16303774

Hasin DS, Goodwin RD, Stinson FS, et al: Epidemiology of major depressive disorder: results from the National Epidemiologic Survey on Alcoholism and Related Conditions. Arch Gen Psychiatry 62(10):1097–1106, 2005 16203955

Hedegaard H, Curtin SC, Warner M: Increase in Suicide Mortality in the United States, 1999–2018. NCHS Data Brief, No 362. Hyattsville, MD, National Center for Health Statistics, 2020

Hofman A, Ott A, Breteler MM, et al: Atherosclerosis, apolipoprotein E, and prevalence of dementia and Alzheimer's disease in the Rotterdam Study. Lancet 349(9046):151–154, 1997 9111537

Hybels CF, Blazer DG: Epidemiology of late-life mental disorders. Clin Geriatr Med 19(4):663–696, 2003 15024807

Jack CR Jr, Bennett DA, Blennow K, et al: NIA-AA research framework: toward a biological definition of Alzheimer's disease. Alzheimers Dement 14(4):535–562, 2018 29653606

Jang Y, Borenstein AR, Chiriboga DA, Mortimer JA: Depressive symptoms among African American and white older adults. J Gerontol B Psychol Sci Soc Sci 60(6):P313–P319, 2005

Jongenelis K, Pot AM, Eisses AMH, et al: Prevalence and risk indicators of depression in elderly nursing home patients: the AGED study. J Affect Disord 83(2–3):135–142, 2004 15555706

Jorm AF, Jolley D: The incidence of dementia: a meta-analysis. Neurology 51(3):728–733, 1998 9748017

Katon WJ, Lin E, Russo J, Unutzer J: Increased medical costs of a population-based sample of depressed elderly patients. Arch Gen Psychiatry 60(9):897–903, 2003 12963671

Kendler KS, Gardner CO, Gatz M, Pedersen NL: The sources of co-morbidity between major depression and generalized anxiety disorder in a Swedish national twin sample. Psychol Med 37(3):453–462, 2007 17121688

Kessler RC, Berglund P, Demler O, et al: Lifetime prevalence and age-of-onset distributions of DSM-IV disorders in the National Comorbidity Survey Replication. Arch Gen Psychiatry 62(6):593–602, 2005 15939837

Kivipelto M, Helkala EL, Laakso MP, et al: Midlife vascular risk factors and Alzheimer's disease in later life: longitudinal, population based study. BMJ 322(7300):1447–1451, 2001 11408299

Korf ES, Wahlund LO, Visser PJ, Scheltens P: Medial temporal lobe atrophy on MRI predicts dementia in patients with mild cognitive impairment. Neurology 63(1):94–100, 2004 15249617

Langa KM, Larson EB, Crimmins EM, et al: A comparison of the prevalence of dementia in the United States in 2000 and 2012. JAMA Intern Med 177(1):51–58, 2017 27893041

LeBlanc ES, Janowsky J, Chan BK, Nelson HD: Hormone replacement therapy and cognition: systematic review and meta-analysis. JAMA 285(11):1489–1499, 2001 11255426

Lenze EJ: Comorbidity of depression and anxiety in the elderly. Curr Psychiatry Rep 5(1):62–67, 2003 12686004

Lenze EJ, Mulsant BH, Shear MK, et al: Comorbid anxiety disorders in depressed elderly patients. Am J Psychiatry 157(5):722–728, 2000 10784464

Lenze EJ, Mulsant BH, Shear MK, et al: Comorbidity of depression and anxiety disorders in later life. Depress Anxiety 14(2):86–93, 2001 11668661

Li M, Dong X: Association between both self-reported and directly observed physical function and depressive symptoms in a US Chinese population: findings from the PINE Study. SOJ Psychol 3(1):1–8, 2017

Lichtenthal WG, Cruess DG, Prigerson HG: A case for establishing complicated grief as a distinct mental disorder in DSM-V. Clin Psychol Rev 24(6):637–662, 2004 15385092

Llewellyn DJ, Lang IA, Xie J, et al: Framingham Stroke Risk Profile and poor cognitive function: a population-based study. BMC Neurol 8:12, 2008 18430227

Lopez OL, Becker JT, Chang YF, et al: Incidence of mild cognitive impairment in the Pittsburgh Cardiovascular Health Study–Cognition Study. Neurology 79(15):1599–1606, 2012 23019262

Luck T, Luppa M, Briel S, Riedel-Heller SG: Incidence of mild cognitive impairment: a systematic review. Dement Geriatr Cogn Disord 29(2):164–175, 2010 20150735

Luppa M, Sikorski C, Luck T, et al: Age- and gender-specific prevalence of depression in latest-life: systematic review and meta-analysis. J Affect Disord 136(3):212–221, 2012 21194754

Lyness JM, King DA, Cox C, et al: The importance of subsyndromal depression in older primary care patients: prevalence and associated functional disability. J Am Geriatr Soc 47(6):647–652, 1999 10366161

Mackenzie CS, El-Gabalawy R, Chou KL, Sareen J: Prevalence and predictors of persistent versus remitting mood, anxiety, and substance disorders in a national sample of older adults. Am J Geriatr Psychiatry 22(9):854–865, 2014 23800537

Mather M: Narrowing old-age gender gap in U.S. linked to smoking trends. PRB Resource Library (online). July 13, 2015. Available at: https://www.prb.org/resources/narrowing-old-age-gender-gap-in-u-s-linked-to-smoking-trends. Accessed November 2021.

Mather M, Jacobsen LA, Pollard KM: Aging in the United States. Population Bulletin 70, No 2. Washington, DC, Population Reference Bureau, 2015

Matthews FE, Stephan BC, Robinson L, et al: A two decade dementia incidence comparison from the Cognitive Function and Ageing Studies I and II. Nat Commun 7:11398, 2016 27092707

McCusker J, Cole M, Dufouil C, et al: The prevalence and correlates of major and minor depression in older medical inpatients. J Am Geriatr Soc 53(8):1344–1353, 2005 16078960

McGrath ER, Beiser AS, DeCarli C, et al: Blood pressure from mid- to late life and risk of incident dementia. Neurology 89(24):2447–2454, 2017 29117954

Meeks TW, Vahia IV, Lavretsky H, et al: A tune in "a minor" can "b major": a review of epidemiology, illness course, and public health implications of subthreshold depression in older adults. J Affect Disord 129(1–3):126–142, 2011 20926139

Mielke MM, Zandi PP, Sjögren M, et al: High total cholesterol levels in late life associated with a reduced risk of dementia. Neurology 64(10):1689–1695, 2005 15911792

Mitchell AJ, Shiri-Feshki M: Rate of progression of mild cognitive impairment to dementia: meta-analysis of 41 robust inception cohort studies. Acta Psychiatr Scand 119(4):252–265, 2009 19236314

Montine TJ, Cholerton BA, Corrada MM, et al: Concepts for brain aging: resistance, resilience, reserve, and compensation. Alzheimers Res Ther 11(1):22, 2019 30857563

Morris JC: The Clinical Dementia Rating (CDR): current version and scoring rules. Neurology 43(11):2412–2414, 1993 8232972

Morris JN: Uses of epidemiology. BMJ 2(4936):395–401, 1955 13240122

Mortby ME, Ismail Z, Anstey KJ: Prevalence estimates of mild behavioral impairment in a population-based sample of pre-dementia states and cognitively healthy older adults. Int Psychogeriatr 30(2):221–232, 2018 28931446

Murphy RA, Hagaman AK, Reinders I, et al: Depressive trajectories and risk of disability and mortality in older adults: longitudinal findings from the Health, Aging, and Body Composition Study. J Gerontol A Biol Sci Med Sci 71(2):228–235, 2016 26273025

Nagumey AJ, Reich JW, Newsom J: Gender moderates the effects of independence and dependence desires during the social support process. Psychol Aging 19(1):215–218, 2004 15065946

Nasreddine ZS, Phillips NA, Bedirian V, et al: The Montreal Cognitive Assessment, MoCA: a brief screening tool for mild cognitive impairment. J Am Geriatr Soc 53(4):695–699, 2005 15817019

National Institute on Aging, National Institutes of Health, U.S. Department of Health and Human Services, U.S. Department of State: Why Population Aging Matters: A Global Perspective (Publ No 07-6134). Bethesda, MD, National Institutes of Health, 2007

National Research Council (US) Panel on Race: Ethnic differences in dementia and Alzheimer's disease, in Critical Perspectives on Racial and Ethnic Differences in Health in Late Life. Edited by Anderson N, Bulatao R, Cohen B. Washington, DC, National Academies Press, 2004, pp 95–142

Nelson PT, Dickson DW, Trojanowski JQ, et al: Limbic-predominant age-related TDP-43 encephalopathy (LATE): consensus working group report. Brain 142(6):1503–1527, 2019 31039256

Ogunniyi A, Baiyewu O, Gureje O, et al: Epidemiology of dementia in Nigeria: results from the Indianapolis-Ibadan Study. Eur J Neurol 7(5):485–490, 2000 11054131

Ormel J, Rijsdijk FV, Sullivan M, et al: Temporal and reciprocal relationship between IADL/ADL disability and depressive symptoms in late life. J Gerontol B Psychol Sci Soc Sci 57(4):P338–P347, 2002 12084784

Owens DK, Davidson KW, Krist AH, et al: Screening for cognitive impairment in older adults: US Preventive Services Task Force Recommendation Statement. JAMA 323(8):757–763, 2020 32096858

Oxman TE, Berkman LF, Kasl S, et al: Social support and depressive symptoms in the elderly. Am J Epidemiol 135(4):356–368, 1992 1550090

Paus T: Population neuroscience: why and how. Hum Brain Mapp 31(6):891–903, 2010 20496380

Pearlin LI, Lieberman MA, Menaghan EG, Mullan JT: The stress process. J Health Soc Behav 22(4):337–356, 1981 7320473

Penninx BW, Geerlings SW, Deeg DJ, et al: Minor and major depression and the risk of death in older persons. Arch Gen Psychiatry 56(10):889–895, 1999a 10530630

Penninx BW, Leveille S, Ferrucci L, et al: Exploring the effect of depression on physical disability: longitudinal evidence from the established populations for epidemiologic studies of the elderly. Am J Public Health 89(9):1346–1352, 1999b 10474551

Peters ME, Rosenberg PB, Steinberg M, et al: Prevalence of neuropsychiatric symptoms in CIND and its subtypes: the Cache County Study. Am J Geriatr Psychiatry 20(5):416–424, 2012 22522960

Petersen RC, Smith GE, Waring SC, et al: Mild cognitive impairment: clinical characterization and outcome. Arch Neurol 56(3):303–308, 1999 10190820

Plassman BL, Langa KM, Fisher GG, et al: Prevalence of dementia in the United States: the Aging, Demographics, and Memory Study. Neuroepidemiology 29(1–2):125–132, 2007 17975326

Plassman BL, Langa KM, Fisher GG, et al: Prevalence of cognitive impairment without dementia in the United States. Ann Intern Med 148(6):427–434, 2008 18347351

Plassman BL, Langa KM, McCammon RJ, et al: Incidence of dementia and cognitive impairment, not dementia in the United States. Ann Neurol 70(3):418–426, 2011 21425187

Prigerson HG, Frank E, Kasl SV, et al: Complicated grief and bereavement-related depression as distinct disorders: preliminary empirical validation in elderly bereaved spouses. Am J Psychiatry 152(1):22–30, 1995 7802116

Prigerson HG, Horowitz MJ, Jacobs SC, et al: Prolonged grief disorder: psychometric validation of criteria proposed for DSM-V and ICD-11. PLoS Med 6(8):e1000121, 2009 19652695

Prigerson HG, Boelen PA, Xu J, et al: Validation of the new DSM-5-TR criteria for prolonged grief disorder and the PG-13-Revised (PG-13-R) scale. World Psychiatry 20(1):96–106, 2021 33432758

Prince M, Bryce R, Albanese E, et al: The global prevalence of dementia: a systematic review and metaanalysis. Alzheimers Dement 9(1):63–75, 2013 23305823

Qiu C, Winblad B, Fratiglioni L: Low diastolic pressure and risk of dementia in very old people: a longitudinal study. Dement Geriatr Cogn Disord 28(3):213–219, 2009 19752556

Rattinger GB, Sanders CL, Vernon E, et al: Neuropsychiatric symptoms in patients with dementia and the longitudinal costs of informal care in the Cache County population. Alzheimers Dement 5:81–88, 2019 30911601

Raux G, Guyant-Maréchal L, Martin C, et al: Molecular diagnosis of autosomal dominant early onset Alzheimer's disease: an update. J Med Genet 42(10):793–795, 2005 16033913

Richardson C, Stephan BCM, Robinson L, et al: Two-decade change in prevalence of cognitive impairment in the UK. Eur J Epidemiol 34(11):1085–1092, 2019 31489532

Roberts RO, Geda YE, Knopman DS, et al: The incidence of MCI differs by subtype and is higher in men: the Mayo Clinic Study of Aging. Neurology 78(5):342–351, 2012 22282647

Roth M, Tomlinson BE, Blessed G: Correlation between scores for dementia and counts of "senile plaques" in cerebral grey matter of elderly subjects. Nature 209(5018):109–110, 1966 5927229

Rozum WJ, Cooley B, Vernon E, et al: Neuropsychiatric symptoms in severe dementia: associations with specific cognitive domains the Cache County Dementia Progression Study. Int J Geriatr Psychiatry 34(7):1087–1094, 2019 30945374

Sanders JB, Bremmer MA, Comijs HC, et al: Gait speed and the natural course of depressive symptoms in late life: an independent association with chronicity? J Am Med Dir Assoc 17(4):331–335, 2016

Satizabal CL, Beiser AS, Chouraki V, et al: Incidence of dementia over three decades in the Framingham Heart Study. N Engl J Med 374(6):523–532, 2016 26863354

Schneider JA, Arvanitakis Z, Leurgans SE, Bennett DA: The neuropathology of probable Alzheimer disease and mild cognitive impairment. Ann Neurol 66(2):200–208, 2009 19743450

Schousboe JT, Vo TN, Kats AM, et al: Depressive symptoms and total healthcare costs: roles of functional limitations and multimorbidity. J Am Geriatr Soc 67(8):1596–1603, 2019 30903701

Schrijvers EM, Verhaaren BF, Koudstaal PJ, et al: Is dementia incidence declining? Trends in dementia incidence since 1990 in the Rotterdam Study. Neurology 78(19):1456–1463, 2012 22551732

Schwarzbach M, Luppa M, Forstmeier S, et al: Social relations and depression in late life: a systematic review. Int J Geriatr Psychiatry 29(1):1–21, 2014 23720299

Seignourel PJ, Kunik ME, Snow L, et al: Anxiety in dementia: a critical review. Clin Psychol Rev 28(7):1071–1082, 2008 18555569

Sekita A, Ninomiya T, Tanizaki Y, et al: Trends in prevalence of Alzheimer's disease and vascular dementia in a Japanese community: the Hisayama Study. Acta Psychiatr Scand 122(4):319–325, 2010 20626720

Shanmugasegaram S, Russell KL, Kovacs AH, et al: Gender and sex differences in prevalence of major depression in coronary artery disease patients: a meta-analysis. Maturitas 73(4):305–311, 2012 23026020

Shao H, Breitner JC, Whitmer RA, et al: Hormone therapy and Alzheimer disease dementia: new findings from the Cache County Study. Neurology 79(18):1846–1852, 2012 23100399

Shapiro S, Skinner EA, Kessler LG, et al: Utilization of health and mental health services: three Epidemiologic Catchment Area sites. Arch Gen Psychiatry 41(10):971–978, 1984 6477055

Shear MK, Simon N, Wall M, et al: Complicated grief and related bereavement issues for DSM-5. Depress Anxiety 28(2):103–117, 2011 21284063

Shumaker SA, Legault C, Rapp SR, et al: Estrogen plus progestin and the incidence of dementia and mild cognitive impairment in postmenopausal women: the Women's Health Initiative Memory Study: a randomized controlled trial. JAMA 289(20):2651–2662, 2003 12771112

Skarupski KA, Mendes de Leon CF, Bienias JL, et al: Black-white differences in depressive symptoms among older adults over time. J Gerontol B Psychol Sci Soc Sci 60(3):P136–P142, 2005

Sluimer JD, van der Flier WM, Karas GB, et al: Accelerating regional atrophy rates in the progression from normal aging to Alzheimer's disease. Eur Radiol 19(12):2826–2833, 2009 19618189

Smalbrugge M, Pot AM, Jongenelis K, et al: Prevalence and correlates of anxiety among nursing home patients. J Affect Disord 88(2):145–153, 2005 16122811

Smits F, Smits N, Schoevers R, et al: An epidemiological approach to depression prevention in old age. Am J Geriatr Psychiatry 16(6):444–453, 2008 18515688

Snitz BE, Wang T, Cloonan YK, et al: Risk of progression from subjective cognitive decline to mild cognitive impairment: the role of study setting. Alzheimers Dement 14(6):734–742, 2018 29352855

Sonnenberg CM, Beekman AT, Deeg DJ, van Tilburg W: Sex differences in late-life depression. Acta Psychiatr Scand 101(4):286–292, 2000 10782548

Stern Y, Arenaza-Urquijo EM, Bartrés-Faz D, et al: Whitepaper: defining and investigating cognitive reserve, brain reserve, and brain maintenance. Alzheimers Dement 16(9):1305–1311, 2020 30222945

Sullivan KJ, Dodge HH, Hughes TF, et al: Declining incident dementia rates across four population-based birth cohorts. J Gerontol A Biol Sci Med Sci 74(9):1439–1445, 2019 30312371

Taylor RJ, Chatters LM: Psychiatric disorders among older Black Americans: within- and between-group differences. Innov Aging 4(3):igaa007, 2020

Teresi J, Abrams R, Holmes D, et al: Prevalence of depression and depression recognition in nursing homes. Soc Psychiatry Psychiatr Epidemiol 36(12):613–620, 2001 11838834

Tervo S, Kivipelto M, Hänninen T, et al: Incidence and risk factors for mild cognitive impairment: a population-based three-year follow-up study of cognitively healthy elderly subjects. Dement Geriatr Cogn Disord 17(3):196–203, 2004 14739544

Thoits PA: Stress, coping, and social support processes: where are we? What next? J Health Soc Behav (spec no):53–79, 1995 7560850

Trollor JN, Anderson TM, Sachdev PS, et al: Prevalence of mental disorders in the elderly: the Australian National Mental Health and Well-Being Survey. Am J Geriatr Psychiatry 15(6):455–466, 2007 17545446

Unützer J, Patrick DL, Marmon T, et al: Depressive symptoms and mortality in a prospective study of 2,558 older adults. Am J Geriatr Psychiatry 10(5):521–530, 2002 12213686

U.S. Census Bureau: 2017 National Population Projections Tables: Main Series. Washington, DC, U.S. Census Bureau, Updated February 2020. Available at: https://www.census.gov/data/tables/2017/demo/popproj/2017-summary-tables.html. Accessed April 12, 2020.

Vasilevskis EE, Han JH, Hughes CG, Ely EW: Epidemiology and risk factors for delirium across hospital settings. Best Pract Res Clin Anaesthesiol 26(3):277–287, 2012 23040281

Veronese N, Stubbs B, Trevisan C, et al: Poor physical performance predicts future onset of depression in elderly people: Progetto Veneto Anziani Longitudinal Study. Phys Ther 97(6):659–668, 2017

Vyas CM, Donneyong M, Mischoulon D, et al: Association of race and ethnicity with late-life depression severity, symptom burden, and care. JAMA Netw Open 3(3):e201606, 2020 32215634

Wakefield JC, First MB: Validity of the bereavement exclusion to major depression: does the empirical evidence support the proposal to eliminate the exclusion in DSM-5? World Psychiatry 11(1):3–10, 2012 22294996

Ward A, Arrighi HM, Michels S, Cedarbaum JM: Mild cognitive impairment: disparity of incidence and prevalence estimates. Alzheimers Dement 8(1):14–21, 2012 22265588

Winblad B, Palmer K, Kivipelto M, et al: Mild cognitive impairment—beyond controversies, towards a consensus: report of the International Working Group on Mild Cognitive Impairment. J Intern Med 256(3):240–246, 2004 15324367

Xu X, Liang J, Bennett JM, et al: Ethnic differences in the dynamics of depressive symptoms in middle-aged and older Americans. J Aging Health 22(5):631–652, 2010 20495153

CHAPTER 2

Physiological and Clinical Considerations of Geriatric Patient Care

Jaclyn Olsen Jaeger, D.O., C.M.D.

George A. Kuchel, M.D.C.M.

The scope and potential impact of aging demographics in the United States and across the globe have been increasingly well documented (Crimmins 2015). Since 2012, each day more than 10,000 persons living in the United States turn 65 years of age. By 2030, one-fifth of the U.S. population will be 65 or older (Crimmins 2015; U.N. Department of Economic and Social Affairs 2019). Despite common public misperceptions, the aging population is highly heterogeneous. Many older adults maintain their independence and lead productive, healthy lives well into their 80s, 90s, and beyond, whereas others develop multimorbidity, frailty, and functional changes (Crimmins 2015). Many older adults require varying amounts of assistance in the setting of physical and cognitive impairments, ranging from intermittent or daily home care to institutional support. According to the Centers for Disease Control and Prevention (CDC), in 2016 more than 1.3 million persons in the United States lived in institutions and another 8 million received long-term care services (Harris-Kojetin et al. 2019).

We would like to thank Robert M. Kaiser, M.D., M.H.Sc., for his work in developing the prior version of this book chapter.

All of these issues are critical to the care of older adults that is provided by psychiatrists because in this population, behavioral and cognitive issues typically develop on a background of and in close association with other important clinical issues (Brinkley et al. 2018) that, in many cases, may not represent the areas of typical psychiatric expertise. These conditions include most chronic conditions, such as diabetes, osteoporosis, cancer, and heart disease, for which aging represents a dominant risk factor (Burch et al. 2014). Moreover, these also include geriatric syndromes—common multifactorial conditions with complex multisystem clinical presentations, such as falls, delirium, polypharmacy, physical frailty, voiding disorders, and incontinence (Inouye et al. 2007).

The multifactorial complexity and interindividual heterogeneity seen in the geriatric population contribute to the need for increased communication and collaboration between geriatric psychiatrists and geriatricians who are trained in internal or family medicine. Optimal care of older patients with multiple morbidities requires an emphasis on patient preferences and function, considerations that frequently cross traditional organ-, disease-, and discipline-based boundaries. Multidisciplinary clinics and team-based care represent attractive alternatives to silo-based clinical practice because care of such patients often becomes fragmented and suboptimal when each issue is dealt with in isolation from other considerations (Bierman and Tinetti 2016; Inouye et al. 2007; Tisminetzky et al. 2017). Emergence of the field of geroscience has demonstrated the transformational potential of interventions that seek to delay the onset and progression of multiple chronic conditions by targeting biological aging (Burch et al. 2014; Justice et al. 2018); for example, the Targeting Aging Through Metformin trial is seeking to delay the onset of an aggregate of three chronic disease categories (cardiovascular disease, cancer, dementia), with a secondary focus on measures of physical and cognitive performance (Justice et al. 2018; Kulkarni et al. 2020). Moreover, growing numbers of psychiatrists have begun to highlight accelerated biological aging as a target for future geroscience-guided therapies, seeking to further expand the human health span by innovatively addressing common mental health conditions of old age (Bersani et al. 2019; Diniz et al. 2017; Mendes-Silva et al. 2019; Rutherford et al. 2017). As a result, opportunities for multidisciplinary clinical, educational, and research collaborations between geriatric psychiatrists and geriatricians are undergoing unprecedented growth.

With these considerations in mind, this chapter provides a brief overview of the various physiological changes that occur with typical aging to whatever extent they are separate from the pathological development of disease, emphasizing aspects that may be particularly useful from the perspective of a practicing psychiatrist. To that end, we discuss the following topics:

- Physiological changes in major organ systems
- Geriatric syndromes
- Pharmacodynamic and pharmacokinetic changes and needed prescribing considerations in older adults
- Core principles of a geriatric assessment within the setting of typical physiological changes

Physiological Changes in Major Organ Systems

Although aging in humans is both a universal and inevitable phenomenon, the rate at which individuals age in terms of underlying biological and physiological processes is highly heterogeneous, with distinct aging trajectories observed between those who experience healthy and productive aging and those with evidence of multiple chronic diseases, frailty, and disability (Hadley et al. 2017; Keck Futures Initiative 2008; Kuchel 2017; Navaratnarajah and Jackson 2013). Although the precise nature of physiological changes with aging varies across different tissues and organ systems, several common shared features tend to be conserved. These are listed in Table 2–1 and include the observation that aging-related declines are less likely to be seen under basal resting conditions as opposed to when the individual is being challenged. Also, older adults tend to experience other global aging changes that span multiple organ systems, such as changes in homeostenosis and resilience, among others.

Stress can manifest itself as a physical, psychological, or emotional challenge. Psychiatrists and others working in the behavioral sciences are familiar with the concept of *resilience*, which the American Psychological Association (2015) defined as "the process of adapting well in the face of adversity, trauma, tragedy, threats, or significant sources of stress." Resilience is a dynamic, mutable process that can be developed and enhanced. However, in more recent years, attention has been also brought to *physical resilience*, which has been defined as the capacity to maintain normal homeostasis, with delayed or partial return to baseline, when confronted with physiological stressors (Hadley et al. 2017). A common finding in persons who have aged successfully is high resilience. *High resilience* is the ability to rebound from challenging experiences. The concept of *homeostenosis* refers to decreased physiological reserve in the setting of a stress response, with resultant increased physiological vulnerability and greater consequences. This phenomenon, along with resilience and frailty, is a common motif observed across different organ systems (see Table 2–1).

Sensory Systems: Vision, Hearing, Taste and Oral Cavity, Smell

Many important physiological changes occur with aging in the sensory systems. Anatomical changes occur in many of the major structures of the eye, including the lids, lens, pupil, and retina. Periorbital tissues atrophy, and eyelids become more relaxed. Lower lid flaccidity can lead to ectropion or entropion. Lacrimal gland function, tear production, and goblet cell function all decrease (Van Haeringen 1997). The lens becomes thicker and more opaque, commonly causing cataract formation and need for extraction and lens replacement. Half of all Americans will have cataracts by age 75 (Lee et al. 2003). Cataract surgery is the most commonly performed elective surgery in older adults, with ~1.7 million procedures performed in 2012 (Schein et al. 2012). The overall rates of routine cataract surgery in 2014 increased 24% from a decade earlier, when the age-adjusted rate was 618 per 10,000 beneficiaries (French et al. 2017). In addition to changes in the lens, the pupil becomes increasingly miotic due to dilator

TABLE 2–1.   Common features of physiological aging

Concept	Illustration
Stressors bring out some aging-related declines not evident under resting or basal conditions	Aging by itself does not influence serum sodium levels but decreases the ability to prevent hypo- or hypernatremia when confronted with osmotic or volume stressors
Homeostenosis	Declines with aging in ability to maintain normal homeostasis
Diminished physiological resilience	Decreased capacity to maintain normal homeostasis with delayed or partial return to baseline when confronted with physiological stressors
Diminished physiological reserve	Increased homeostatic vulnerability as a result of critical loss in numbers of neurons or decline in glomerular filtration rate
Loss of complexity	Declines in bone or neuronal architecture; narrowing of hearing frequency responses or loss of long-range correlations in blood pressure readings
Enhanced heterogeneity	Greater inter- and intraindividual variability over time in sympathetic activity or blood pressure readings
Higher basal activity	Basal sympathetic activity elevated in older adults
Excessive responses to some stressors	Sympathetic responses to common challenges are excessively large and prolonged
Diminished end-organ responsiveness	Ability of peripheral catecholamines to increase heart rate via β-adrenergic receptors or to mediate arterial vasoconstriction via α-adrenergic receptors is decreased
Loss of negative feedback	Ability of corticosteroids to downregulate activity of the hypothalamic-pituitary-adrenal system via negative feedback is diminished
Allostatic load	Increased biological burden in terms of estimates of cumulative exposure exacted by attempts to adapt to life's demands predicts future mortality, as well as declines in cognitive and physical function
Frailty as a phenotype	Increased vulnerability to adverse events and stressors conceptualized as a syndrome with elements of weakness, slow walking speed, low physical activity, exhaustion, and unintentional weight loss
Frailty as a cumulative deficit index	Proxy measure of aging and vulnerability to poor outcomes calculated from index of accumulation of stochastic (random) deficits involving diseases, signs, symptoms, laboratory abnormalities, cognitive impairments, and disabilities in activities of daily living

Source.   Adapted from Kuchel GA: "Aging and Homeostatic Regulation," in *Hazzard's Geriatric Medicine and Gerontology,* 7th Edition. Edited by Halter JB, Ouslander JG, Studenski S, et al. New York, McGraw-Hill, 2017, pp 681–690. Used with permission.

muscle fiber atrophy and increased iris blood vessel rigidity. These pupillary and lenticular changes contribute to difficulty with visual performance and light adaptation. Changes that can occur in the retina include drusen deposition in the retinal pigmented epithelium, which results in central vision loss, clinically known as macular degeneration. Age-related macular degeneration affects females more often and is the most common cause of blindness in older adults in the United States. By age 80, more than 10% of persons will have late age–related macular degeneration (Lee et al. 2003).

Anatomical and physiological changes in the ear may lead to both high- and low-frequency hearing loss. Changes in the middle ear include ossicle degeneration and tympanic membrane thickening, although neither change has a significant impact on hearing capability. In the inner ear, changes in multiple structures can cause difficulties with hearing and word discrimination. Changes in the organ of Corti are associated with high-frequency sensorineural hearing loss, and changes in the stria vascularis can cause hearing loss across all frequencies. Stiffening of the basilar membrane and atrophy of the spiral ligament can cause difficulties with speech discrimination (Huang and Tang 2010). Hearing loss is very prevalent in older adults and has been independently associated with incident dementia, falls, and social isolation (Lin et al. 2011). Yet multiple studies have shown that many older adults who would benefit from hearing amplification do not use hearing aids (Chien and Lin 2012; McCormack and Fortnum 2013). Furthermore, up to 40% of people fitted with a hearing aid either fail to use it or may not gain optimal benefit from it (Barker et al. 2014). Barriers to hearing aid use include lack of appreciation of hearing loss consequences, physical discomfort, high cost (if not reimbursed by insurance), and fear of social stigmatization (Pacala and Yueh 2012).

In the oral cavity, the number of tongue papillae decreases, and the visual appearance of taste buds is altered. Quantity of taste buds has no impact on gustatory acuity, although taste sensitivity decreases. Many older adults report that food tastes bland and seek to correct this by adding more sugar and salt to their diet. Production of saliva decreases and gums recede, making teeth more susceptible to decay, dental caries, and tooth loss. Up to 50% of older adults endorse dry mouth, which can affect chewing and swallowing; it is important to differentiate whether complaints of dry mouth are due to age-related change, medication side effects, or a disease process, such as Sjögren's syndrome (Nagler and Hershkovich 2005).

Loss of taste in older adults is intimately linked to decreased olfaction (Hall et al. 2005). The etiology is of this loss unclear, but the quantity of sensing neurons, sensation area, and ability to replenish olfactory receptor neurons are decreased. Detection thresholds are increased more than 50%, and familiar smell recognition decreases (Boyce and Shone 2006).

Cardiovascular System

Many structural and physiological changes occur in the heart and blood vessels with usual aging. Both the myocardium and vessels stiffen with decreased compliance, which results in increased afterload and impaired early diastolic filling. Although the number of myocytes decreases, myocyte volume increases. Regardless of cardiovascular risk factors, left ventricular (LV) wall thickness progressively increases with age due to hypertrophy rather than hyperplasia, based on histomorphometric analysis. The LV ejection fraction ([LV end-diastolic volume–LV end-systolic volume]/LV end-diastolic volume) is relatively preserved with aging, although ejection fraction during exhaustive upright exercise (maximum LV ejection fraction) decreases (Fleg and Kennedy 1992). The number of sinoatrial node pacemaker cells decreases. The prevalence of premature atrial and isolated ventricular ectopic beats is not associated with increased cardiac risk and is part of the typical aging process (Busby et al. 1989; Fleg and Kennedy 1992). The responsiveness of β-adrenergic receptors declines, limiting the maximum achievable heart rate, although resting heart rate is unaffected by aging. Exercise training does not modify the age-associated decline in maximum heart rate (Ozemek et al. 2016). Because of intrinsically lower heart rates, the heart compensates with exercise-induced dilation of the left ventricle. Although stroke volume is unchanged with the aging process, maximum cardiac output (stroke volume × heart rate) decreases, along with overall cardiac reserve.

The vasculature throughout the body stiffens due to arterial wall changes. Arterial intima endothelial cells become more heterogeneous in size, shape, and axial orientation, which causes intraluminal blood flow to become less laminar. In the media, smooth muscle layers thicken, elastin has a greater degree of fragmentation, and calcification increases. Aorta diameter, length, and stiffness increase, which increases the load on the heart. Vasculature changes likely contribute to compensatory myocyte loss and heart hypertrophy (Wei 1992).

Pulmonary System

The three components of the pulmonary system—the thoracic cage, diaphragm, and lungs—all undergo changes that impact function. Degenerative joint diseases and costal cartilage calcification contribute to thoracic cage stiffening. Osteoporosis may result in vertebral fracture, which can contribute to kyphosis and increased anteroposterior diameter that can affect chest wall mechanics. Chest wall compliance decreases by about one-third from age 30 to age 75. Abdominal muscles have a greater contribution to respiration due to less input from intercostal contraction. The diaphragm flattens and becomes less efficient, contributing to increased work of breathing with exercise. Lung elastic tissue and recoil decrease, alveolar duct and respiratory bronchioles enlarge, and the collagen fiber network is altered. Less tissue is available for gas exchange. Partial pressure of oxygen and diffusion capacity decrease in a nonlinear fashion. Ventilation-perfusion mismatch increases with age as airways in dependent portions of the lung are closed during all or part of the respiratory cycle. Carbon dioxide excretion is not compromised with age. Coughing is less vigorous in the setting of muscle weakness. Mucociliary clearance is reduced and slowed in large and small airways (Ho et al. 2001; Svartengren et al. 2005). Peak aerobic performance decreases but is not constant, especially in males.

Gastrointestinal System

Functional and anatomical changes occur throughout the gastrointestinal system. The number of myenteric ganglion cells that coordinate peristalsis decreases, which can affect swallowing coordination and predispose some older adults to higher aspiration risk. Esophageal changes include decreased contraction during peristalsis and decreased lower esophageal sphincter tone, the latter leading to increased gastric acid exposure. Food movement is not impaired (Hall et al. 2005). Gastric changes include delayed gastric emptying, decreased prostaglandin production, lower bicarbonate and nonparietal fluid excretion, and impaired microcirculation (Guslandi et al. 1999). The small bowel's ability to absorb vitamins and nutrients such as calcium, iron, folic acid, and vitamin B_{12} is impaired (Saltzman and Russell 1998). The large bowel's motor function is not significantly affected by aging. Liver mass decreases up to 40%, and blood flow decreases up to 50% (McLean and Le Couteur 2004). The liver synthesizes fewer vitamin K–dependent clotting factors, and lower doses of coumadin are needed for anticoagulation in older adults. Typical liver function tests (alkaline phosphatase, transaminases) are not significantly affected by aging. Minimal anatomical changes occur in the gallbladder, although bile composition changes, which predisposes older adults to cholesterol gallstone production (Valdivieso et al. 1978). The exocrine pancreas becomes more fibrotic, fatty, and atrophic, which has no real impact on function.

Renal System

Aging has multiple effects on the renal system. Renal mass decreases up to 30%, and the remaining composition becomes fattier and more fibrotic, most especially in the renal cortex. Functional glomeruli decrease by almost 50%, primarily due to atrophy and absorption of nephrons rather than diffuse sclerosis (Denic et al. 2017; Nyengaard and Bendtsen 1992). Glomerular filtration rate (GFR) changes are heterogeneous; one-third of older adults have no decline, one-third have a slight decline, and one-third have a significant decline. Creatinine production decreases, but tubular creatinine secretion increases, with a net result of serum creatinine remaining stable despite decreased GFR (Giannelli et al. 2007). Creatinine clearance decreases 7.5 to 10 mL/minute/decade, although decline is variable in healthy older adults (Lindeman 1990). In the absence of stressors, fluid and electrolyte homeostasis are well maintained. In the setting of physiological challenge, water excretion and maximal urine dilution are impaired. The renin-angiotensin system response is less robust in the setting of decreased renin activity and production. Erythropoietin synthesis is preserved, but vitamin D hydroxylation decreases. The aged kidney is more prone to nephrotoxic effects due to medications, chemotherapy, or intravenous contrast (Pucelikova et al. 2008; Toprak 2007).

Endocrine System

Three different hormonal systems show decreasing circulating hormone concentrations during normal aging, including estrogen and testosterone, which are involved in menopause and andropause, respectively. Dehydroepiandrosterone (DHEA) and its sulfate form (DHEA-S) reflect adrenopause, whereas declines in the growth hormone/insulin-like growth factor 1 (IGF-1) axis have been referred as the *somatopause* (Lamberts et al. 1997).

Estrogen

Menopause is accompanied by a dramatic and rapid decline in serum 17β-estradiol (E2) levels, with cycling E2 levels replaced by very low and constant levels of both this estrogen and also the lower-potency estrone (E1) (Lamberts et al. 1997). Moreover, the primary source of estrogen production shifts from ovaries to adipose tissues, where adrenally produced androgens are converted to estrone. The Women's Health Initiative trial demonstrated the risks of estrogen hormone replacement in older females and a lack of benefit for primary or chronic disease prevention (Manson et al. 2003; Shifren et al. 2019). Since then, estrogen replacement is only recommended on an individual basis, such as for older females with severe menopausal vasomotor symptoms with hot flashes and night sweats who have no absolute contraindications and are ideally <10 years from menopause (Shifren et al. 2019). Also, very low doses of intravaginal estrogens can be used for dyspareunia and other selected menopausal genitourinary symptoms of menopause with minimal systemic absorption and risk (Shifren et al. 2019).

Testosterone

With aging, males experience a gradual decline in both serum total and free testosterone (T) levels (Lamberts et al. 1997). This is accompanied by a decrease in testicular Leydig cell numbers and their secretory capacity, together with declines in normal episodic and stimulated gonadotropin secretion (Lamberts et al. 1997). Given its broad biological effects, there has been great interest in the use of testosterone for various chronic conditions of aging. However, testosterone replacement should not be initiated in asymptomatic older males. In contrast, in symptomatic males age 65 years and older, raising testosterone concentrations for 1 year from moderately low to the midnormal range for males age 19–40 has been shown to provide a moderate benefit with respect to sexual function and some benefit with respect to mood and depressive symptoms, but without any apparent benefit with respect to vitality or walking distance (Snyder et al. 2016). In older males with low testosterone levels without well-established medical conditions known to cause hypogonadism, testosterone therapy has been shown to provide small improvement in sexual functioning and quality of life but little or no benefit for other common symptoms of aging, such as declines in cognitive performance (Resnick et al. 2017). Long-term efficacy and safety remain unknown (Diem et al. 2020).

Dehydroepiandrosterone

The adrenal steroid DHEA is a prohormone for the synthesis of biologically active androgens and estrogens, with DHEA and DHEA-S levels declining approximately 70% between the ages of 20 and 60 years (Orentreich et al. 1984). Because DHEA-S circulates as an inactive prohormone that is converted to biologically active sex steroids in a tissue-specific manner, it has been proposed as a potentially safer alternative for preserving muscle and bone mass in females as compared with the use of estrogen (Jankowski et al. 2019).

Growth Hormone and Insulin-Like Growth Factor 1

Mean pulse amplitude, duration, and fraction of growth hormone secreted—but not pulse frequency—decline with age, along with circulating levels of IGF-1 (Lamberts et al. 1997). Treatment of clinical symptomatic deficiency of growth hormone should be considered at all ages (Melmed 2019). At the same time, the off-label use of growth hormone for antiaging purposes is neither justified nor supported by the evidence (Melmed 2019). While such treatments may result in modest effects in body composition, they have no clear and consistent impact on function and other relevant outcomes and have adverse side effects to consider, such as diabetes and cancer (Melmed 2019).

Thyroid

The distribution curve for thyroid-stimulating hormone (TSH) levels shifts to higher values with age, and many older individuals with subclinical hypo- or hyperthyroidism revert to normal values over time without any intervention (Tabatabaie and Surks 2013). Even when elevated TSH levels do persist, there is no conclusive evidence that subclinical hypothyroidism has any adverse cognitive, metabolic, or cardiovascular outcomes in older adults (Tabatabaie and Surks 2013), and thyroid therapy does not appear to be of benefit in this particular population (Mooijaart et al. 2019), leading to the recommendation that TSH reference values for older adults should be changed (Cappola 2019).

Glucose Metabolism and Diabetes Mellitus

Nearly half of adults 65 years and older have impaired glucose tolerance or diabetes mellitus, and more than half of all people with diabetes are 60 years and older (Lamberts et al. 1997; Morley 2008). Of note, 25%–41% of those with diabetes remain undiagnosed (Lamberts et al. 1997; Morley 2008). The physiological factors underlying this predisposition include peripheral insulin resistance related to aging, poor diet, physical inactivity, increased abdominal fat mass and decreased lean body mass, and decreased (relative) insulin secretion by pancreatic β cells, which all contribute to the decreased ability to uptake and metabolize glucose (Lamberts et al. 1997; Longo et al. 2019). Diabetes in older adults, especially when combined with obesity, greatly enhances the risk of various chronic diseases and geriatric syndromes contributing to frailty and declines in physical and cognitive performance (Longo et al. 2019; Stout et al. 2017). Diet, exercise, oral hypoglycemic drugs, and insulin represent key elements of diabetes care in older adults. There is also a growing recognition that older adults, especially those who are frail, benefit from less intense diabetes control (Brown et al. 2003), given the lack of evidence linking intense control to improved outcomes in this population, combined with the decreased capacity to physiologically recognize and respond to hypoglycemia in old age.

Musculoskeletal System

Bones and muscle undergo changes that affect function. Although these changes are heterogeneous, muscle mass decreases relative to weight in both sexes, and this loss increases with age. *Age-related sarcopenia*, or the age-related loss of muscle mass and strength, is defined as a decrease in appendicular muscle mass two standard deviations from the average in young healthy adults (Baumgartner et al. 1999). Type II fast-twitch fibers are fewer, and slow muscle fibers predominate. Muscle loss is greater in the lower than in the upper extremities and is most striking in the intrinsic muscles of the hands and feet. The composition of muscle changes, with increased fat and connective tissue deposition, is termed *myosteatosis*. There are fewer and smaller myofibrils. The number of motor units decreases, but their size increases. Age-related muscle loss contributes to insulin resistance and changes in the volumes of distribution for water-soluble drugs. Strength also decreases with age, more so in the lower extremities than the upper extremities. Grip strength decreases with age by up to 60% by age 80. Activity can be a strong mitigating factor because sarcopenia and decreased strength can lead to physical debility and functional impairment (Ryall et al. 2008).

In terms of bone changes, cortical and trabecular bone loss occurs at ~0.5% per year within the setting of a proinflammatory environment (Chan and Duque 2002). These changes are enhanced with coexisting vitamin D deficiency and, for females, menopausal changes. Osteoblast activity and quantity decrease, with osteoblast precursors having a decreased likelihood of forming bone and a higher tendency to form fat (Ganguly et al. 2017; Stolzing et al. 2008). Osteoclast activity increases with menopause and, to a more variable extent, with aging. Aging increases fracture risk, and, if fracture occurs, healing is less robust due to impaired repair mechanisms.

Hematological System

The function of the hematological system is mostly maintained throughout the lifetime. Bone marrow mass decreases, and fat content increases nonuniformly (French et al. 2002; Kirkland et al. 2002). Older adults maintain the ability to manufacture normal numbers of major cell lines. In the setting of stressors such as hypoxia or blood loss, the aged bone marrow has a less robust and timely response, consistent with homeostenosis (Boggs and Patrene 1985). Platelet count remains unchanged with typical aging, but responsiveness to clot-forming triggers heightens. Multiple clotting factors, including fibrinogen, factor V, factor VII, factor VIII, and factor IX, among others, increase with age in the setting of age-related inflammation (Franchini 2006). Fibrin degradation fragment (D-dimer) levels also increase with typical aging, without associated thrombosis; levels may be even higher in hospitalized older adults and thus should be interpreted with caution.

Immune System

The aging of the immune system, called *immunosenescence*, is one of the most important physiological changes that occur with aging. Total hematopoietic tissue in the bone marrow declines. Telomere attrition occurs with loss of telomeric DNA and a resultant increase in cell apoptosis. Both the innate and adaptive immune systems are affected by these changes. Some innate immune system mechanisms are decreased, but some are more active in older adults, with an increased tendency toward chronic inflammatory states. Macrophages and the phagocytic ability of neutrophils decrease, but neutrophil numbers are preserved. Natural killer cell numbers tend to increase with age (Panda et al. 2009).

In adaptive immunity, the thymus undergoes consistent decline with age, and naive T cells decline in number, repertoire, and function. This change makes older adults more susceptible to new infections (Naylor et al. 2005). The number and diversity of B cells also decrease with age, although immunoglobulin levels remain stable or increase. The amount of specific antibody production after exposure to antigen declines with age (Frasca et al. 2008; Lazuardi et al. 2005); however, memory responses are mostly preserved.

Integumentary System

Aging skin becomes increasingly atrophic and fragile, with compromised elasticity, resilience, and restorative capabilities. The epidermis thins and has decreased turnover. The dermoepidermal intersection becomes flatter. The dermis also thins, with decreased vascularity. Subdermal fat decreases, which contributes to wrinkling and sagging (McCullough and Kelly 2006). Decreased dermal fat also leads to difficulty with thermoregulation. Skin xerosis is more common due to decreased nutrient transfer and lipid content (Montagna and Carlisle 1990). Sensory perception, including touch and low-frequency vibratory sense, decreases due to decreases in Messiner's and Pacinian corpuscles, respectively (Gescheider et al. 1994; Matsuoka et al. 1983; Perry 2006).

Neurological System

Structural changes involving the aging CNS include brain volume loss, which is most profoundly seen in the frontal and temporal lobes (Driscoll et al. 2009). Synaptic connections and new neurons continue to be formed throughout the life span, although age-related neuronal loss, especially in more vulnerable brain regions, outpaces neuronal production (van der Zee 2015). There is associated neuronal loss in the cerebellum and cerebral cortex but only modest or no losses in the hypothalamus, pons, and medulla with typical aging (Lee et al. 2009; Moreno-Torres et al. 2005; Walhovd et al. 2011). Neuronal loss is attributed to apoptosis rather than inflammation, ischemia, or etiologies not yet described (Sastry and Rao 2000). The formation of neurofibrillary tangles and age-related plaques has also been noted in certain areas of the brain, but to a lesser extent than in persons with Alzheimer's disease (AD). Levels of neurotransmitters such as acetylcholine, dopamine, and serotonin decrease, as do their synthesis, receptors, and, in some cases, signaling.

Age-related peripheral nervous system changes include decreases in the number of myelinated fibers, vibration perception, pain and temperature sensation, and proprioception. Reflexes overall remain present or mildly decreased, with the exception of the Achilles reflex, which can be absent or have a more marked decrease (Odenheimer et al. 1994).

Geriatric Syndromes

Geriatric syndromes, including conditions such as frailty, polypharmacy, falls, urinary incontinence, and delirium, represent a conglomeration of conditions that occur more commonly in older adults. In contrast to most typical diseases, geriatric syndromes pose some special clinical considerations and challenges for the clinician (Inouye et al. 2007). First, for each geriatric syndrome, multiple underlying and precipitating risk factors and multiple organ systems typically contribute. Second, diagnostic strategies for identifying a single unifying underlying cause can be ineffective, burdensome, dangerous, and costly. Third, clinical manifestations may not respect traditional boundaries between organ systems and professional disciplines, whereby the chief complaint may not represent the specific pathological condition underlying the change in health status, with a disconnect between the site of the underlying physiological insult (e.g., infection in the urinary tract) and the resulting clinical symptoms (e.g., delirium with behavioral and cognitive manifestations). Finally, in spite of being highly multifactorial, geriatric syndromes often share both common risk factors (e.g., declines in mobility raising risk of falls, incontinence, and functional dependence) (Tinetti et al. 1995) and common ultimate universal outcomes in terms of declining function and independence (Tinetti et al. 2011).

Frailty

Frailty has been conceptualized as both a phenotype (Clegg et al. 2013) reflective of a defined state or syndrome and as a more random process related to the accumulation of random deficits (Clegg et al. 2013). Despite the similarity in the terms used, these two approaches need to be viewed as offering complementary as opposed to competing insights into aging and evidence-based care of older adults (Kuchel 2018). Both approaches to frailty predict adverse events in older individuals, such as multimorbidity, disability, hospitalization, complications following procedures, and death. Nevertheless, with phenotypic frailty it is possible to identify individuals with this phenotype with or without the presence of disability and varied morbidities (Clegg et al. 2013). Moreover, all these conditions contribute to declines in resilience in terms of the capacity to maintain normal homeostasis and function in the face of varied stressors (Kuchel 2018).

Although there is no consensus on which tool to use, many different tools exist to evaluate frailty, including the frailty index, clinical frailty scale, and FRAIL (Fatigue, Resistance, Ambulation, Illness, and Loss of weight) scale. *Phenotypic frailty* is defined as having three or more (and prefrail with two or more) of the following characteristics: unintentional weight loss (10 lb in the past year), self-reported exhaustion, weakness (grip strength), slow walking speed, and low physical activity (Buigues et al. 2015; Fried et al. 2001). Evaluating frailty has become and should continue to be a standardized part of geriatric patient assessment in all care settings, including preoperative, hospital, community, and institutionalized settings.

Frailty and mental health disorders often overlap, especially depression (Buigues et al. 2015) and dementia (Wallace et al. 2019). While neither of these is considered a normal part of aging, depression and dementia frequently coexist with physical frailty. Either can contribute to worse health outcomes, and although suggested causation has only recently been described, it is imperative to treat both frailty and depression when identified (Buigues et al. 2015). The best strategies for treating frailty are still largely unknown, although interventions are largely supportive, individual, and multifactorial based on the patient's medical conditions, care preferences, and life expectancy. The one intervention with the strongest benefit is exercise, particularly strength and resistance training.

Polypharmacy

Medication use, both prescription and nonprescription, is common in older adults. Although no specific number of medications defines polypharmacy, a primary goal is to identify medications that have suboptimal effect, no indication, or a high risk of adverse events. Polypharmacy is associated with increased risk of falls, delirium, cognitive impairment, morbidity, mortality, adverse drug reactions, and worse medication adherence. Etiologies of polypharmacy include multimorbidity, higher health care utilization, and multiple prescribers.

Within a national sample of community-dwelling individuals ages 57–85 years, 81% were taking one or more prescription medications, with those ages 75–85 years accounting for 89.7%. In addition to prescription medications, 68% of older adults use nonprescription medications, dietary supplements, or both, and more than 50% use five or more medications and supplements (Qato et al. 2008). Most ambulatory community dwellers have also been found to be taking suboptimal medications or ones without appropriate indications. Thus, medication management in the older adult is a complex balancing act, with polypharmacy being a common occurrence and concern. Polypharmacy should be assessed and addressed at every patient visit to assess opportunities for dosage reduction and deprescribing.

Falls

Falls are a common and feared occurrence in older adults. According to the CDC, on average, one in four older adults reports falling annually. The fall rate is even higher in long-term care settings, with an average of 2.6 falls per resident per year. Falls can have many deleterious effects, including hip fracture, head trauma, loss of function or independence, and even death. Falls account for the largest percentage of deaths from unintentional injuries, which are the seventh leading cause of death in older adults (Burns and Kakara 2018). Fall-related care involves significant cost to the health care system, resulting in $31 billion in Medicare costs annually. Clinicians should assess fall risk and implement fall prevention measures for high-risk older adults.

The etiology of falls is usually multifactorial and typically divided into intrinsic and extrinsic factors. *Intrinsic factors* are patient-specific etiologies, such as sensory impairment (especially vision and hearing), vestibular dysfunction with balance impairment, cognitive impairment with poor safety awareness, neurological or systemic diseases, polypharmacy, high-risk medications, muscle weakness, poor proprioception, vitamin D deficiency, and more. *Extrinsic factors* are environmental hazards and situational concerns that can impact a patient's fall risk, such as the home milieu. Evaluation of a fall requires careful consideration of both intrinsic and extrinsic factors, starting with a comprehensive history. The circumstances surrounding the fall should always be assessed. Medications should be reviewed and reconciled, with special attention paid to high-risk or new medications. A complete review of systems should be discussed because a fall may be a manifestation of a serious underlying condition, such as ischemia, infection, or other systemic illness. Physical examination should also be detailed and include vision, cardiac, joint, and neurological assessment, including balance, sensation, gait, and cerebellar testing.

Fall prevention should also address both intrinsic and extrinsic factors. Routine vision, hearing, and cognitive examinations (or at least screening) should be encouraged at least annually for community-dwelling older adults. Medications should be thoughtfully reviewed and reconciled at each visit to confirm indications and implement dosage reduction or deprescribing as clinically appropriate. Chronic medical conditions should be treated as optimally as possible depending on the patient's age, cognitive status, and frailty status and available evidence-based guidelines. Physical exercise, such as tai chi, has been shown to improve balance and decrease fall risk. Environmental hazards should be eliminated, and the living environment should be tidy and free of clutter. In some individuals, vitamin D supplementation may be effective in primary and secondary fall prevention (Annweiler et al. 2010).

Voiding Disorders and Incontinence

Lower urinary tract aging is associated with an increased prevalence of overactive bladder, which is diagnosed based on symptoms involving a sudden uncontrollable urge to void and detrusor overactivity, which represents a urodynamic diagnosis (Wagg et al. 2015). Detrusor underactivity resulting in either prolonged or inefficient voiding is also seen in some older adults, with the combination of both conditions representing the most common urodynamic finding in incontinent nursing home residents (Resnick et al. 1989). Decreased bladder sensation is also very common (Pfisterer et al. 2006). Nevertheless, urinary incontinence in older adults needs to be viewed as a geriatric syndrome because many risk factors outside of the genitourinary tract collectively determine whether an individual is able to remain continent in the face of a stressor represented by bladder filling in the context of everyday life (Markland et al. 2011; Wagg et al. 2015).

Antispasmodic medications are widely used to manage symptoms of overactive bladder, yet their efficacy is variable, and their use is often accompanied by significant side effects in older adults because of their potent anticholinergic properties (Markland et al. 2011; Wagg et al. 2015). With these considerations in mind, efforts to identify and mitigate the role of risk factors, such as polyuria, nocturia, offending medications, uncontrolled endocrine conditions (e.g., diabetes mellitus and insipidus), and decreased mobility, assume great importance. As a result, it is not surprising that interventions including prompted voiding, mobility training, and perineal biofeedback have been shown to offer benefits that often exceed those of antispasmodics and with fewer adverse effects, particularly in nursing home residents and cognitively impaired individuals (Goode et al. 2010; Ouslander et al. 2005).

Delirium and Dementia

Delirium

Delirium and dementia are two distinct disease processes for which age is the major risk factor, yet they are not parts of typical aging. Delirium has many synonyms, including acute confusional state, toxic metabolic encephalopathy, acute brain syndrome, and acute cerebral insufficiency, although *delirium* should be used as the standard terminology when the phenomenon is identified. Delirium is generally defined by inattention and acute cognitive dysfunction. The DSM-5 (American Psychiatric Association 2013) definition is based on disturbance in attention; acute fluctuating change from baseline; additional disturbance in cognition; change not better explained by another preexisting, evolving, or established neurocognitive disorder or coma; and no evidence that a medical condition, substance intoxication or withdrawal, or medication side effect is present.

Delirium risk factors can be divided into two categories: nonmodifiable and modifiable. Nonmodifiable factors include baseline dementia or cognitive impairment, older age (>65 years), male sex, chronic renal or hepatic impairment, multimorbidity, and history of delirium, stroke, neurological disease, fall, or gait disorder. Modifiable risk factors are numerous and include sensory impairment, immobilization, medications (polypharmacy, high-risk, intoxication, or withdrawal), acute neurological insult, metabolic derangement, surgery, pain, constipation, urinary retention, emotional distress, sustained sleep deprivation, new environment, and intercurrent illness.

Multiple tools exist to identify delirium, but the Confusion Assessment Method, or CAM, is most commonly used. The CAM is a four-item instrument that requires inattention, acute onset with fluctuating course, and either disorganized thinking or change in consciousness to meet delirium criteria. Tests of attention can include digit span or recitation of the days of the week backward. Delirium prevention is key; an estimated 30%–40% of delirium cases are thought to be preventable. Medications, including benzodiazepines and anticholinergics, and other known precipitants of delirium should be avoided. The Hospital Elder Life Program has been shown to decrease delirium and days of delirium in hospitalized older adults. This program has a specialized focus on providing sensory aids; addressing nutrition, fluid, and sleep management; promoting mobility within physical limitations; and maintaining orientation to surroundings.

Routine pharmacotherapy has no role in delirium prophylaxis. Haloperidol has been demonstrated to decrease delirium incidence in a small group of postoperative patients, but the reduction was not statistically confirmed in a larger study, although the severity and duration of delirium and length of hospital stay were decreased in some patients. These results should be interpreted cautiously in the setting of methodological limitations and small sample sizes; further research is warranted. Nonpharmacological treatment strategies are the cornerstone of delirium management for all patients and include frequent reorientation, sensory aids, environmental interventions such as a quiet care environment (especially at night), and avoidance of physical restraints. In terms of acute drug treatment, few high-quality randomized controlled trials have been performed, and current clinical practice is thus based on retrospective analyses or case series. Antipsychotics are typically reserved for patients with delirium-associated behaviors that inhibit needed medical care or who are a danger to staff or themselves. Thus, use of these medications should be a last resort due to possible further clouding of mental status and QT prolongation, among other unwanted effects (Fong et al. 2009).

Dementia

Dementia, also called *major neurocognitive disorder*, is a common condition that is not a part of the typical aging process. Expected cognitive changes in older adults include decline in information processing speed and mild memory changes that are nonprogressive and do not typically impact daily functioning. Neither the U.S. Preventive Services Task Force nor the American Academy of Neurology (AAN) recommend for or against routine dementia screening due to insufficient evidence; however, any patient or family concerns about cognitive changes require thorough evaluation. Only 16% of older adults receive regular cognitive assessments during routine examinations (Alzheimer's Association 2019).

Dementia diagnosis, as defined by DSM-5, includes

- Evidence from history and clinical assessment of a significant cognitive impairment in at least one cognitive domain
- Impairment must be acquired and represent a decline from previous level of functioning
- Cognitive deficit must interfere with independence in everyday activities
- Deficit does not occur exclusively during the course of delirium
- Disturbances are not better accounted for by another mental disorder

There are many dementia syndromes, including AD, vascular dementia, Lewy body dementia, Parkinson's disease dementia, progressive supranuclear palsy, multiple system atrophy, corticobasal degeneration, normal pressure hydrocephalus, and Creutzfeldt-Jakob disease. AD and vascular dementia account for the most cases of dementia. According to the Alzheimer's Association (2019), every 65 seconds a person in the United States develops AD. This equates to nearly 6 million persons in 2019 in the United States living with AD or another dementia, at an annual health care expenditure of $290 billion. By 2050, this number is projected to skyrocket to nearly 14 million persons, with annual costs reaching $1.1 trillion. Most persons with dementia are community dwelling; unpaid caregivers or family in this setting provide 18.5 billion hours of care valued at nearly $234 billion.

Evaluation of dementia should include a comprehensive history and physical examination, ideally with a person who knows the patient well. Patients with cognitive changes often do not recognize or report impairment. A depression screen should be performed. Laboratory work, including vitamin B_{12} level and thyroid function evaluation, should be ordered if not recently obtained, based on AAN recommendations, although data are limited as to whether treating any abnormality improves cognitive function. Screening for neurosyphilis should not be a routine part of cognitive impairment evaluation unless high-risk sexual practices or travel to regions where exposure may be more common is elicited in the history. No clear data support or refute the use of "routine" laboratory tests, although ideally these should be reserved for specific patient populations in which abnormalities are suspected, such as red blood cell folate levels in persons with alcoholism. In general, yield is low and cost effectiveness is questionable when ordering routine laboratory work. Neuroimaging is controversial as part of a dementia evaluation. Many guidelines do not recommend routine neuroimaging unless there is a focal neurological finding or concern of neurological insult, such as stroke, subdural hematoma, or normal pressure hydrocephalus. However, the AAN recommends structural neuroimaging with either noncontrast CT or MRI as part of routine initial evaluation. Serial imaging is not recommended or clinically useful unless a new focal finding, seizure, or abrupt or unexpected clinical change is identified. Neuropsychological testing is also an available option to aid in dementia diagnosis when bedside testing is equivocal, although most patients do not require a full neuropsychological examination as part of a dementia evaluation.

Treatment of dementia is multimodal. An appropriate care environment that can provide the needed supportive care is essential. Adequate nutrition support, cognitive and physical exercise, risk factor control, and alcohol moderation are key. Pharmacotherapy with a cholinesterase inhibitor such as donepezil, galantamine, or rivastigmine, in addition to the NMDA receptor antagonist memantine, has modest effectiveness in patients with mild to moderate AD.

Considerations in Geriatric Prescribing

It is important to define and differentiate pharmacokinetic and pharmacodynamic changes that occur in typical aging. *Pharmacokinetics* is the way the body affects a drug, whereas *pharmacodynamics* is the way a drug affects the body. There are four major components of pharmacokinetics: absorption, distribution, metabolism, and excretion. Absorption is not usually affected by typical aging, although it can be altered by drug interactions or disease. Distribution is significantly affected. Water content decreases and fat content increases, which increases the concentration of water-soluble drugs and prolongs the action of fat-soluble drugs, respectively. Serum proteins such as albumin decrease, resulting in increased concentration of active drug. Metabolism slows phase I reactions such as oxidation, reduction, and dealkylation. Phase II reactions, such as conjugation, acetylation, and methylation, are unchanged. Decreased creatinine clearance and hepatic blood flow lead to decreased renal and hepatic clearance, respectively, resulting in decreased excretion. These age-related changes require judicious use and monitoring of many medication classes (Lotrich and Pollock 2005).

Pharmacodynamic changes are profound in older adults and require special consideration with regard to selection, dosing, and frequency. Examples of these medications are found on the Beers List (Blanco-Reina et al. 2014). Older adults often develop deleterious adverse side effects, such as delirium, constipation, urinary retention, and drug toxicity, more frequently or with greater severity.

Geriatric Assessment

Geriatric assessment represents a multidimensional evaluation of older adults that emphasizes functional status and involves physical, cognitive, psychological, and social domains (Carlson et al. 2015; Inouye et al. 2007). This emphasis on a whole-person assessment, functional performance, and quality of life allows clinicians to move beyond the traditional single-organ/single-disease paradigm for appropriately evaluating and managing geriatric syndromes. Although geriatric assessment should represent the cornerstone of comprehensive care of older adults by all providers, consultations for comprehensive geriatric assessment are typically provided by geriatricians who are often functioning within multidisciplinary clinics. Assessment is most indicated when concerns have been raised regarding recent functional declines, when dealing with competing risk factors and decisions in the context of multimorbidities, and in anticipation of decisions and optimal clinical stewardship during elective surgery, dialysis, and chemotherapy regimens, among others.

In addition to the usual clinical elements involving history and physical examination, comprehensive geriatric assessment includes a strong emphasis on assessment of function using validated instruments. Psychiatrists are generally very knowledgeable about tools used to evaluate affect, behavior, and cognition, with likely less experience in the use of instruments or approaches for evaluating mobility performance, balance, flexibility, or frailty. Nonetheless, a simple observation of a person's ability to walk and turn can provide extremely useful screening information regarding fall risk, mobility disability, undiagnosed pathology, and frailty. Moreover, asking patients to rise five times from a chair with their arms crossed offers important insights into core muscle strength.

Key Points

- Although aging in humans is both a universal and inevitable phenomenon, the rate at which individuals age in terms of underlying biological and physiological processes is highly heterogeneous.

- Older adults tend to experience other global aging changes that span multiple organ systems, such as changes in homeostenosis and resilience.

- Geriatric syndromes represent a conglomeration of conditions that occur more commonly in older adults and pose special considerations and challenges for the clinician.

- Geriatric assessment represents a multidimensional evaluation of older adults that emphasizes a whole-person assessment, functional performance, and quality of life.

References

Alzheimer's Association: New Alzheimer's Association report shows significant disconnect between seniors, physicians when it comes to cognitive assessment (press release). Chicago, IL, Alzheimer's Association, March 4, 2019. Available at: https://www.alz.org/news/2019/new-alzheimer-s-association-report-shows-signifi. Accessed October 19, 2021.

American Psychiatric Association: Diagnostic and Statistical Manual of Mental Disorders, 5th Edition. Arlington, VA, American Psychiatric Association, 2013

American Psychological Association: The Road to Resilience (online). Washington, DC, American Psychological Association, 2015. Available from: http://www.apa.org/helpcenter/road-resilience.aspx. Accessed August 1, 2020.

Annweiler C, Montero-Odasso M, Schott AM, et al: Fall prevention and vitamin D in the elderly: an overview of the key role of the non-bone effects. J Neuroeng Rehabil 7:50, 2010 20937091

Barker F, Mackenzie E, Elliott L, et al: Interventions to improve hearing aid use in adult auditory rehabilitation. Cochrane Database Syst Rev (7):CD010342, 2014 25019297

Baumgartner RN, Waters DL, Gallagher D, et al: Predictors of skeletal muscle mass in elderly men and women. Mech Ageing Dev 107(2):123–136, 1999 10220041

Bersani FS, Mellon SH, Reus VI, Wolkowitz OM: Accelerated aging in serious mental disorders. Curr Opin Psychiatry 32(5):381–387, 2019 31145144

Bierman AS, Tinetti ME: Precision medicine to precision care: managing multimorbidity. Lancet 388(10061):2721–2723, 2016 27924764

Blanco-Reina E, Ariza-Zafra G, Ocaña-Riola R, León-Ortiz M: 2012 American Geriatrics Society Beers criteria: enhanced applicability for detecting potentially inappropriate medications in European older adults? A comparison with the Screening Tool of Older Person's Potentially Inappropriate Prescriptions. J Am Geriatr Soc 62(7):1217–1223, 2014 24917083

Boggs DR, Patrene KD: Hematopoiesis and aging III: anemia and a blunted erythropoietic response to hemorrhage in aged mice. Am J Hematol 19(4):327–338, 1985 4025313

Boyce JM, Shone GR: Effects of ageing on smell and taste. Postgrad Med J 82(966):239–241, 2006 16597809

Brinkley TE, Berger M, Callahan KE, et al: Workshop on synergies between Alzheimer's research and clinical gerontology and geriatrics: current status and future directions. J Gerontol A Biol Sci Med Sci 73(9):1229–1237, 2018 29982466

Brown AF, Mangione CM, Saliba D, et al: Guidelines for improving the care of the older person with diabetes mellitus. J Am Geriatr Soc 51(5 suppl):S265–S280, 2003 12694461

Buigues C, Padilla-Sánchez C, Garrido JF, et al: The relationship between depression and frailty syndrome: a systematic review. Aging Ment Health 19(9):762–772, 2015 25319638

Burch JB, Augustine AD, Frieden LA, et al: Advances in geroscience: impact on healthspan and chronic disease. J Gerontol A Biol Sci Med Sci 69(suppl 1):S1–S3, 2014 24833579

Burns E, Kakara R: Deaths from falls among persons aged ≥65 years—United States, 2007–2016. MMWR Morb Mortal Wkly Rep 67(18):509–514, 2018 29746456

Busby MJ, Shefrin EA, Fleg JL: Prevalence and long-term significance of exercise-induced frequent or repetitive ventricular ectopic beats in apparently healthy volunteers. J Am Coll Cardiol 14(7):1659–1665, 1989 2479667

Cappola AR: The thyrotropin reference range should be changed in older patients. JAMA 322(20):1961–1962, 2019 31664455

Carlson C, Merel SE, Yukawa M: Geriatric syndromes and geriatric assessment for the generalist. Med Clin North Am 99(2):263–279, 2015 25700583

Chan GK, Duque G: Age-related bone loss: old bone, new facts. Gerontology 48(2):62–71, 2002 11867927

Chien W, Lin FR: Prevalence of hearing aid use among older adults in the United States. Arch Intern Med 172(3):292–293, 2012 22332170

Clegg A, Young J, Iliffe S, et al: Frailty in elderly people. Lancet 381(9868):752–762, 2013 23395245

Crimmins EM: Lifespan and healthspan: past, present, and promise. Gerontologist 55(6):901–911, 2015 26561272

Denic A, Lieske JC, Chakkera HA, et al: The substantial loss of nephrons in healthy human kidneys with aging. J Am Soc Nephrol 28(1):313–320, 2017 27401688

Diem SJ, Greer NL, MacDonald R, et al: Efficacy and safety of testosterone treatment in men: an evidence report for a clinical practice guideline by the American College of Physicians. Ann Intern Med 172(2):105–118, 2020 31905375

Diniz BS, Reynolds CF III, Sibille E, et al: Enhanced molecular aging in late-life depression: the senescent-associated secretory phenotype. Am J Geriatr Psychiatry 25(1):64–72, 2017 27856124

Driscoll I, Davatzikos C, An Y, et al: Longitudinal pattern of regional brain volume change differentiates normal aging from MCI. Neurology 72(22):1906–1913, 2009 19487648

Fleg JL, Kennedy HL: Long-term prognostic significance of ambulatory electrocardiographic findings in apparently healthy subjects greater than or equal to 60 years of age. Am J Cardiol 70(7):748–751, 1992 1381549

Fong TG, Tulebaev SR, Inouye SK: Delirium in elderly adults: diagnosis, prevention and treatment. Nat Rev Neurol 5(4):210–220, 2009 19347026

Franchini M: Hemostasis and aging. Crit Rev Oncol Hematol 60(2):144–151, 2006 16860994

Frasca D, Landin AM, Lechner SC, et al: Aging down-regulates the transcription factor E2A, activation-induced cytidine deaminase, and Ig class switch in human B cells. J Immunol 180(8):5283–5290, 2008 18390709

French DD, Margo CE, Behrens JJ, Greenberg PB: Rates of routine cataract surgery among Medicare beneficiaries. JAMA Ophthalmol 135(2):163–165, 2017 28056119

French RA, Broussard SR, Meier WA, et al: Age-associated loss of bone marrow hematopoietic cells is reversed by GH and accompanies thymic reconstitution. Endocrinology 143(2):690–699, 2002 11796526

Fried LP, Tangen CM, Walston J, et al: Frailty in older adults: evidence for a phenotype. J Gerontol A Biol Sci Med Sci 56(3):M146–M157, 2001 11253156

Ganguly P, El-Jawhari JJ, Giannoudis PV, et al: Age-related changes in bone marrow mesenchymal stromal cells: a potential impact on osteoporosis and osteoarthritis development. Cell Transplant 26(9):1520–1529, 2017 29113463

Gescheider GA, Bolanowski SJ, Hall KL, et al: The effects of aging on information-processing channels in the sense of touch: I. Absolute sensitivity. Somatosens Mot Res 11(4):345–357, 1994 7778411

Giannelli SV, Patel KV, Windham BG, et al: Magnitude of underascertainment of impaired kidney function in older adults with normal serum creatinine. J Am Geriatr Soc 55(6):816–823, 2007 17537080

Goode PS, Burgio KL, Richter HE, Markland AD: Incontinence in older women. JAMA 303(21):2172–2181, 2010 20516418

Guslandi M, Pellegrini A, Sorghi M: Gastric mucosal defences in the elderly. Gerontology 45(4):206–208, 1999 10394077

Hadley EC, Kuchel GA, Newman AB, et al: Report: NIA workshop on measures of physiologic resiliencies in human aging. J Gerontol A Biol Sci Med Sci 72(7):980–990, 2017 28475732

Hall KE, Proctor DD, Fisher L, Rose S: American gastroenterological association future trends committee report: effects of aging of the population on gastroenterology practice, education, and research. Gastroenterology 129(4):1305–1338, 2005 16230084

Harris-Kojetin L, Sengupta M, Lendon JP, et al: Long-Term Care Providers and Services Users in the United States, 2015–2016 (Series 3, No 43). Washington, DC, National Center for Health Statistics, 2019

Ho JC, Chan KN, Hu WH, et al: The effect of aging on nasal mucociliary clearance, beat frequency, and ultrastructure of respiratory cilia. Am J Respir Crit Care Med 163(4):983–988, 2001 11282777

Huang Q, Tang J: Age-related hearing loss or presbycusis. Eur Arch Otorhinolaryngol 267(8):1179–1191, 2010 20464410

Inouye SK, Studenski S, Tinetti ME, Kuchel GA: Geriatric syndromes: clinical, research, and policy implications of a core geriatric concept. J Am Geriatr Soc 55(5):780–791, 2007 17493201

Jankowski CM, Wolfe P, Schmiege SJ, et al: Sex-specific effects of dehydroepiandrosterone (DHEA) on bone mineral density and body composition: A pooled analysis of four clinical trials. Clin Endocrinol (Oxf) 90(2):293–300, 2019 30421439

Justice JN, Niedernhofer L, Robbins PD, et al: Development of clinical trials to extend healthy lifespan. Cardiovasc Endocrinol Metab 7(4):80–83, 2018 30906924

Keck Futures Initiative: The Future of Human Healthspan: Demography, Evolution, Medicine and Bioengineering. Washington, DC, National Academies Press, 2008

Kirkland JL, Tchkonia T, Pirtskhalava T, et al: Adipogenesis and aging: does aging make fat go MAD? Exp Gerontol 37(6):757–767, 2002 12175476

Kuchel GA: Aging and homeostatic regulation, in Hazzard's Geriatric Medicine and Gerontology, 7th Edition. Edited by Halter JB, Ouslander JG, Studenski S, et al. New York, McGraw-Hill, 2017, pp 681–690

Kuchel GA: Frailty and resilience as outcome measures in clinical trials and geriatric care: are we getting any closer? J Am Geriatr Soc 66(8):1451–1454, 2018 30094816

Kulkarni AS, Gubbi S, Barzilai N: Benefits of metformin in attenuating the hallmarks of aging. Cell Metab 32(1):15–30, 2020 32333835

Lamberts SW, van den Beld AW, van der Lely AJ: The endocrinology of aging. Science 278(5337):419–424, 1997 9334293

Lazuardi L, Jenewein B, Wolf AM, et al: Age-related loss of naïve T cells and dysregulation of T-cell/B-cell interactions in human lymph nodes. Immunology 114(1):37–43, 2005 15606793

Lee NJ, Park IS, Koh I, et al: No volume difference of medulla oblongata between young and old Korean people. Brain Res 1276:77–82, 2009 19393230

Lee PP, Feldman ZW, Ostermann J, et al: Longitudinal prevalence of major eye diseases. Arch Ophthalmol 121(9):1303–1310, 2003 12963614

Lin FR, Thorpe R, Gordon-Salant S, Ferrucci L: Hearing loss prevalence and risk factors among older adults in the United States. J Gerontol A Biol Sci Med Sci 66(5):582–590, 2011 21357188

Lindeman RD: Overview: renal physiology and pathophysiology of aging. Am J Kidney Dis 16(4):275–282, 1990 2220770

Longo M, Bellastella G, Maiorino MI, et al: Diabetes and aging: from treatment goals to pharmacologic therapy. Front Endocrinol (Lausanne) 10:45, 2019 30833929

Lotrich FE, Pollock BG: Aging and clinical pharmacology: implications for antidepressants. J Clin Pharmacol 45(10):1106–1122, 2005 16172176

Manson JE, Hsia J, Johnson KC, et al: Estrogen plus progestin and the risk of coronary heart disease. N Engl J Med 349(6):523–534, 2003 12904517

Markland AD, Vaughan CP, Johnson TM, et al: Incontinence. Med Clin North Am 95(3):539–554, 2011

Matsuoka S, Suzuki H, Morioka S, et al: Quantitative and qualitative studies of Meissner's corpuscles in human skin, with special reference to alterations caused by aging. J Dermatol 10(3):205–216, 1983 6358309

McCormack A, Fortnum H: Why do people fitted with hearing aids not wear them? Int J Audiol 52(5):360–368, 2013 23473329

McCullough JL, Kelly KM: Prevention and treatment of skin aging. Ann N Y Acad Sci 1067:323–331, 2006 16804006

McLean AJ, Le Couteur DG: Aging biology and geriatric clinical pharmacology. Pharmacol Rev 56(2):163–184, 2004 15169926

Melmed S: Pathogenesis and diagnosis of growth hormone deficiency in adults. N Engl J Med 380(26):2551–2562, 2019 31242363

Mendes-Silva AP, Mwangi B, Aizenstein H, et al: Molecular senescence is associated with white matter microstructural damage in late-life depression. Am J Geriatr Psychiatry 27(12):1414–1418, 2019 31320246

Montagna W, Carlisle K: Structural changes in ageing skin. Br J Dermatol 122(suppl 35):61–70, 1990 2186788

Mooijaart SP, Du Puy RS, Stott DJ, et al: Association between levothyroxine treatment and thyroid-related symptoms among adults aged 80 years and older with subclinical hypothyroidism. JAMA 322(20):1977–1986, 2019 31664429

Moreno-Torres A, Pujol J, Soriano-Mas C, et al: Age-related metabolic changes in the upper brainstem tegmentum by MR spectroscopy. Neurobiol Aging 26(7):1051–1059, 2005 15748785

Morley JE: Diabetes and aging: epidemiologic overview. Clin Geriatr Med 24(3):395–405, 2008 18672179

Nagler RM, Hershkovich O: Age-related changes in unstimulated salivary function and composition and its relations to medications and oral sensorial complaints. Aging Clin Exp Res 17(5):358–366, 2005 16392409

Navaratnarajah A, Jackson SHD: The physiology of ageing. Medicine 41(1):5–8, 2013

Naylor K, Li G, Vallejo AN, et al: The influence of age on T cell generation and TCR diversity. J Immunol 174(11):7446–7452, 2005 15905594

Nyengaard JR, Bendtsen TF: Glomerular number and size in relation to age, kidney weight, and body surface in normal man. Anat Rec 232(2):194–201, 1992 1546799

Odenheimer G, Funkenstein HH, Beckett L, et al: Comparison of neurologic changes in "successfully aging" persons vs the total aging population. Arch Neurol 51(6):573–580, 1994 8198468

Orentreich N, Brind JL, Rizer RL, Vogelman JH: Age changes and sex differences in serum dehydroepiandrosterone sulfate concentrations throughout adulthood. J Clin Endocrinol Metab 59(3):551–555, 1984 6235241

Ouslander JG, Griffiths PC, McConnell E, et al: Functional incidental training: a randomized, controlled, crossover trial in Veterans Affairs nursing homes. J Am Geriatr Soc 53(7):1091–1100, 2005 16108924

Ozemek C, Whaley MH, Finch WH, Kaminsky LA: High cardiorespiratory fitness levels slow the decline in peak heart rate with age. Med Sci Sports Exerc 48(1):73–81, 2016 26258854

Pacala JT, Yueh B: Hearing deficits in the older patient: "I didn't notice anything." JAMA 307(11):1185–1194, 2012 22436959

Panda A, Arjona A, Sapey E, et al: Human innate immunosenescence: causes and consequences for immunity in old age. Trends Immunol 30(7):325–333, 2009 19541535

Perry SD: Evaluation of age-related plantar-surface insensitivity and onset age of advanced insensitivity in older adults using vibratory and touch sensation tests. Neurosci Lett 392(1–2):62–67, 2006 16183200

Pfisterer MH, Griffiths DJ, Schaefer W, Resnick NM: The effect of age on lower urinary tract function: a study in women. J Am Geriatr Soc 54(3):405–412, 2006 16551306

Pucelikova T, Dangas G, Mehran R: Contrast-induced nephropathy. Catheter Cardiovasc Interv 71(1):62–72, 2008 17975790

Qato DM, Alexander GC, Conti RM, et al: Use of prescription and over-the-counter medications and dietary supplements among older adults in the United States. JAMA 300(24):2867–2878, 2008 19109115

Resnick NM, Yalla SV, Laurino E: The pathophysiology of urinary incontinence among institutionalized elderly persons. N Engl J Med 320(1):1–7, 1989 2909873

Resnick SM, Matsumoto AM, Stephens-Shields AJ, et al: Testosterone treatment and cognitive function in older men with low testosterone and age-associated memory impairment. JAMA 317(7):717–727, 2017 28241356

Rutherford BR, Taylor WD, Brown PJ, et al: Biological aging and the future of geriatric psychiatry. J Gerontol A Biol Sci Med Sci 72(3):343–352, 2017 27994004

Ryall JG, Schertzer JD, Lynch GS: Cellular and molecular mechanisms underlying age-related skeletal muscle wasting and weakness. Biogerontology 9(4):213–228, 2008 18299960

Saltzman JR, Russell RM: The aging gut: nutritional issues. Gastroenterol Clin North Am 27(2):309–324, 1998 9650019

Sastry PS, Rao KS: Apoptosis and the nervous system. J Neurochem 74(1):1–20, 2000 10617101

Schein OD, Cassard SD, Tielsch JM, Gower EW: Cataract surgery among Medicare beneficiaries. Ophthalmic Epidemiol 19(5):257–264, 2012 22978526

Shifren JL, Crandall CJ, Manson JE: Menopausal hormone therapy. JAMA 321(24):2458–2459, 2019 31145419

Snyder PJ, Bhasin S, Cunningham GR, et al: Effects of testosterone treatment in older men. N Engl J Med 374(7):611–624, 2016 26886521

Stolzing A, Jones E, McGonagle D, Scutt A: Age-related changes in human bone marrow-derived mesenchymal stem cells: consequences for cell therapies. Mech Ageing Dev 129(3):163–173, 2008 18241911

Stout MB, Justice JN, Nicklas BJ, Kirkland JL: Physiological aging: links among adipose tissue dysfunction, diabetes, and frailty. Physiology 32(1):9–19, 2017 27927801

Svartengren M, Falk R, Philipson K: Long-term clearance from small airways decreases with age. Eur Respir J 26(4):609–615, 2005 16204590

Tabatabaie V, Surks MI: The aging thyroid. Curr Opin Endocrinol Diabetes Obes 20(5):455–459, 2013 23974775

Tinetti ME, Inouye SK, Gill TM, Doucette JT: Shared risk factors for falls, incontinence, and functional dependence: unifying the approach to geriatric syndromes. JAMA 273(17):1348–1353, 1995 7715059

Tinetti ME, McAvay GJ, Chang SS, et al: Contribution of multiple chronic conditions to universal health outcomes. J Am Geriatr Soc 59(9):1686–1691, 2011 21883118

Tisminetzky M, Bayliss EA, Magaziner JS, et al: Research priorities to advance the health and health care of older adults with multiple chronic conditions. J Am Geriatr Soc 65(7):1549–1553, 2017 28555750

Toprak O: Risk markers for contrast-induced nephropathy. Am J Med Sci 334(4):283–290, 2007 18030185

U.N. Department of Economic and Social Affairs: World Population Ageing 2019: Highlights (ST/ESA/SER.A/430). New York, United Nations, 2019

Valdivieso V, Palma R, Wünkhaus R, et al: Effect of aging on biliary lipid composition and bile acid metabolism in normal Chilean women. Gastroenterology 74(5 Pt 1):871–874, 1978 640341

van der Zee EA: Synapses, spines and kinases in mammalian learning and memory, and the impact of aging. Neurosci Biobehav Rev 50:77–85, 2015 24998408

Van Haeringen NJ: Aging and the lacrimal system. Br J Ophthalmol 81(10):824–826, 1997 9486019

Wagg A, Gibson W, Ostaszkiewicz J, et al: Urinary incontinence in frail elderly persons: report from the 5th International Consultation on Incontinence. Neurourol Urodyn 34(5):398–406, 2015 24700771

Walhovd KB, Westlye LT, Amlien I, et al: Consistent neuroanatomical age-related volume differences across multiple samples. Neurobiol Aging 32(5):916–932, 2011 19570593

Wallace LMK, Theou O, Godin J, et al: Investigation of frailty as a moderator of the relationship between neuropathology and dementia in Alzheimer's disease: a cross-sectional analysis of data from the Rush Memory and Aging Project. Lancet Neurol 18(2):177–184, 2019 30663607

Wei JY: Age and the cardiovascular system. N Engl J Med 327(24):1735–1739, 1992 1304738

CHAPTER 3

Genomics in Geriatric Psychiatry

Breno S. Diniz, M.D., Ph.D.
Wendy Qiu, M.D., Ph.D.

For decades, psychiatric clinical diagnoses, including those in geriatric psychiatry, have relied on the description of clinical syndromes. The flow of events leading from variation in a gene sequence to the development of various cognitive, behavioral, and emotional symptoms that encompass psychiatric disorders of later life is not straightforward. However, the understanding of these processes is well under way and will significantly influence the practice of geriatric psychiatry in the 21st century. In 2015, the Precision Medicine Initiative (Terry 2015) established a new direction for medical research and practice, including geriatric psychiatry. The completion of the Human Genome Project in the mid-2000s marked a milestone in genomics. Since then, the field has rapidly moved forward, with the first genomic mapping of a living human followed by the more recent availability of direct-to-consumer genome sequencing. Personalized genome sequencing (Ceyhan-Birsoy et al. 2019; D'Angelo et al. 2016) is a reality that will have a profound impact on the field. Family, twin, and adoption studies have demonstrated robust genetic influences in schizophrenia, bipolar disorders, and Alzheimer's disease (AD), and conventional and newer approaches have advanced the understanding of the specific genetic components of these disorders. In this chapter, we have attempted to 1) summarize key advances in genomic science, 2) introduce the growing field of genomic medicine (especially as it relates to genetic testing), and 3) review the current state of understanding of the genetics of mental disorders of aging and later life.

Advances in Genomic Science: Background and Context

The field of genomic science has come a long way since Gregor Mendel's first work with pea plants in the mid-19th century. Given this rapid evolution, it is important to understand and appreciate the general framework of genomic science, especially as the groundwork is laid for new genetically informed diagnoses and interventions that likely will arrive in the coming years. With this in mind, we have briefly summarized recent advances in the field and have provided a table of important terminology and definitions (Table 3–1) to assist readers in understanding this somewhat technical yet important topic.

One of the fundamental insights arising from human genome sequencing was the discovery that the number of protein-coding genes (around 20,000) was severalfold less than expected, encompassing <2% of human DNA. With the subsequent discovery that genes are surprisingly conserved across mammalian species, investigators have begun to look within and across species for other sources of variation within the genome. Novel information has shed light on the remainder of the genome's functional role, the so-called silent or noncoding DNA (ncDNA), which is never translated into protein. This process has also led to the realization that structural variation—including deletions and replications of segments of chromosomes—makes up the largest proportion (as measured in base pairs) of variation within humans and between humans and other primates (Levy et al. 2007; Samonte and Eichler 2002). Epigenetic modifications of the genome, such as DNA methylation and histone modifications, have also been reported to play a role in psychiatric and neurodegenerative diseases (Wen et al. 2016).

It has become apparent that a large degree of complexity in the human genome results from the regulation of gene transcription (the conversion of DNA to RNA) and gene splicing (which alters the isoform of the resulting translated protein). This regulation was known to occur via sites within nontranscribed DNA sequences (e.g., promoter sequences) and within transcribed yet noncoding portions of the messenger RNA sequence (e.g., splice sites at the boundaries of introns and exons). Such evidence has recently been supplemented by a novel understanding of the extent to which ncDNA sequences are transcribed into noncoding RNA (ncRNA) (Carninci et al. 2005) and the breadth of cellular mechanisms under the control of ncRNA. It is now known, for example, that ncRNAs serve critical roles as transcriptional and posttranscriptional regulators, facilitating normal development and physiology and, when dysfunctional, contributing to disease (Pu et al. 2019). These recent discoveries emphasize the need to move beyond the confines of protein-coding genes and highlight that continued investigation of ncRNA functions will be necessary for a comprehensive understanding of genetic diseases.

Single-Nucleotide Polymorphisms

Single-nucleotide polymorphisms (SNPs; i.e., the change of a single DNA base in the gene sequence in one or two chromosomes) are common in the human genome. If an SNP is located in a coding gene, it can alter the amino acid sequence of proteins and

TABLE 3–1.	Glossary of important terms for genomic science
Allele	One of a number of different forms of the same gene. Alleles may or may not result in different observable phenotypic traits.
Base pair	The building blocks of the DNA double helix, each containing two complementary nucleotides.
Complex disease	A disease that arises from complex interactions between multiple genes and/or environmental factors.
CRISPR	A gene editing technology that allows the manipulation and editing of DNA sequences, with high precision, in living cells or organisms.
DNA epigenetic modifications	Includes DNA methylation and histone modifications. Epigenetic modifications can regulate gene transcription without changing the DNA sequence.
Dominance	Key concept in Mendelian inheritance referring to the relationship between alleles of a single gene. In a dominant gene, one allele (dominant) masks the phenotypic expression of a second allele (recessive) at the same location.
Gene expression	General process by which information from a nucleotide sequence is synthesized into a functional gene product (e.g., a protein). Includes processes of transcription, splicing, translation, and posttranslational modification.
Gene splicing	Regulated process during gene expression that results in a single gene coding for multiple proteins. During splicing, particular portions of a gene are included in (or excluded from) the final messenger RNA produced from the nucleotide sequence. Because proteins translated from alternatively spliced RNAs contain different amino acid sequences, splicing allows the synthesis of many more proteins than would be expected from the human genome's approximately 20,000 protein-coding genes.
Gene transcription	First step of gene expression, during which a segment of DNA is copied into RNA by the enzyme RNA polymerase. During transcription, a DNA sequence is read by RNA polymerase, which produces a complementary, antiparallel RNA strand called a primary transcript.
Gene translation	Part of the process of gene expression during which the primary transcript is decoded to produce a specific amino acid chain that will later fold into an active protein.
Genome-wide association study	An examination of many common genetic variants in different individuals to determine if any variant is associated with the disease of interest.
Genotype	Genetic makeup of an organism.
Haplotype	Combination of alleles that are often inherited together due to their close physical proximity on a chromosome.
Mendelian disease	Disease that displays a predictable, single-gene pattern of inheritance (e.g., autosomal dominant, autosomal recessive).
Mutation	Change in the nucleotide sequence of a genome. Results from unrepaired damage to nucleotides, errors in replication, or insertion or deletion of segments by mobile genetic units. Considered to be rare events and may or may not result in discernible changes in phenotype.
Noncoding RNA (ncRNA)	RNA sequences that do not function as messenger, transfer, or ribosomal RNAs. Includes long ncRNA and microRNAs. Serves many functions (e.g., regulation of gene expression).

TABLE 3–1.	Glossary of important terms for genomic science *(continued)*
Nonsynonymous substitution (mutation)	Substitution of one base pair for another in an exon of a gene coding for protein, such that the produced amino acid sequence is modified. In a synonymous substitution, on the other hand, base pair substitution does not result in a change in the amino acid sequence.
Penetrance	Proportion of individuals carrying a particular genotype that also expresses an associated phenotype. In medical genetics, the proportion of individuals with the mutation who exhibit clinical symptoms.
Phenotype	Observable composite of an organism's genetic characteristics and traits.
Polygenic risk score	Summarizes the estimated effect of many genetic variants on an individual's phenotype, reflecting the estimated genetic predisposition for a given trait in an individual.
Polymorphism	Simultaneous occurrence in the same population of two or more forms of a gene in proportions not maintained by spontaneous mutation or immigration. Actively and steadily maintained by natural selection and considered more common than mutations.
Single-nucleotide polymorphism	Sequence variation occurring when a single nucleotide in the genome differs between members of a species or paired chromosomes.
Structural variation	Variation in the structure of an organism's chromosome, usually involving changes such as deletions, duplications (copy number variants), insertions, and translocations.
Single-cell sequencing	Sequence information from individual cells provides a higher resolution of cellular differences and a better understanding of the function of an individual cell in the context of its microenvironment.
Telomere	Repetitive nucleotide sequences (TTAGGG) at the end of chromosomes. Erosion after each cell division is a marker of cellular senescence.
Trinucleotide repeat (or microsatellite expansion)	Special type of mutation in which repeats of three nucleotides increase in copy numbers. If the repeats cross a threshold, they can cause defects in proteins, change in the gene expression, or lead to chromosomal instability.

lead to changes in protein function. Many early case-control studies aimed to identify genetic polymorphisms associated with psychiatric disorders, including in geriatric psychiatry. For example, researchers found a significant association of SNPs in genes related to serotonin function (serotonin transporter gene [5-HTTLPR]); inflammatory activation (tumor necrosis factor alpha [TNFA] and C-reactive protein [CRP]); neurotrophic support (brain-derived neurotrophic factor [BDNF]); and late-life depression (Ancelin et al. 2015; Cerri et al. 2010; Taylor et al. 2007). Recent genome-wide association studies (GWASs) did not replicate most of the genes previously associated with major depressive disorder (MDD) (Wray et al. 2018), raising questions about their relevance to the pathophysiology of depression. Nonetheless, the investigation of individual SNPs can still be relevant for psychiatric disorders of late life, for example, to identify individuals who may respond better to specific drugs (see discussion of genetic testing later in the chapter).

There is now growing recognition of the contribution of SNPs in ncDNA sequences to disease risk and expression. A study mapped more than 9 million SNPs to gene sequences and ncDNA sequences of functional significance, including transcription factor binding sites, exon splicing enhancers or silencers, transcribed ncRNA, regulatory potential sequences, and ncRNA binding sites (Miller et al. 2005). The authors found that SNPs in coding DNA that altered protein structure had significantly decreased allele frequencies and increased population specificity (providing evidence of a functional effect, subject to natural selection). Furthermore, they observed the same pattern among SNPs in ncDNA that mapped to transcription factor binding sites, ncRNA binding elements, regulatory-potential sequences, and splice sites, with substitutions in ncRNA binding or splice sites being more likely to show evidence of selection than coding SNPs. Subsequent discoveries have led ncRNA to be implicated in several diseases that affect the brain, such as schizophrenia, bipolar disorder, and MDD (Schizophrenia Psychiatric Genome-Wide Association Study Consortium 2011).

Copy Number Variations

Efforts to screen the human genome have shown that large segments of DNA may also be deleted or duplicated (Lupski 2007), resulting in changes in the number of genes within these regions and disrupting gene structure at deletion or duplication breakpoints. Diseases caused by genomic rearrangements that result in an altered number of gene copies (copy number variants [CNVs]) are often referred to as genomic disorders. To date, CNVs have been identified in more than 900,000 regions that overlap with approximately 5%–20% of protein-encoding genes and genes associated with human disease (Database of Genomic Variants 2020; Redon et al. 2006). CNVs are associated with several psychiatric disorders and neurodegenerative conditions, including schizophrenia, autism spectrum disorder (ASD), OCD, and Parkinson's disease (PD).

Genome-Wide Association Studies

The efforts of the International HapMap Consortium (2007) to identify contiguous blocks within the genome that are relatively invariant across individuals and populations have been critical to recent successes in identifying genetic variants associated with complex diseases. The relative constancy of each haplotype block allows all genetic sequences contained within it to be represented by a single tag SNP, such that the entire genome can be thoroughly interrogated for association with disease (genomewide association) by about 10^6 tag SNPs, a number substantially smaller than the ~3 billion nucleotides within the genome. Advances in DNA sequencing technologies (e.g., next-generation sequencing technologies) have allowed sequencing of the whole genome at unprecedented speed, and lower costs have allowed the inclusion of thousands of participants in GWASs, significantly increasing the power to detect genetic variants with small effects. Psychiatric disorders have benefited from these technological advances, and several worldwide research consortiums have been established to investigate the genetic underpinnings of psychiatric and neurodegenerative disorders (e.g., Psychiatric Genomics Consortium, U.K. Biobank, Alzheimer's Disease Neuroimaging Initiative).

De Novo Mutations

Although genetic risk is thought to be passed down through families, it is also true that new mutations (i.e., de novo mutations, or DNMs) or structural rearrangements may occur in a parental gamete (sperm or egg) and thus first manifest in an affected offspring. Rates of DNMs are increased, for example, by increasing paternal age, whereas increasing maternal age is a risk factor for de novo structural alterations such as trisomy 21, which results in Down syndrome. DNMs can lead to changes in gene function (e.g., loss of function), leading to different medical conditions in offspring that were not present in their progenitors.

Recent studies have implicated DNMs in the etiology of psychiatric disorders, mostly those with neurodevelopmental features (e.g., ASD, schizophrenia) (Wang et al. 2019). Nonetheless, the proportion of cases related to DNMs is probably small, and it is not clear to what extent they contribute to the pathophysiological processes related to these neurodevelopmental disorders.

Genetics of Mental Disorders of Aging and Later Life

Alzheimer's Disease

AD, or neurocognitive disorder due to AD, is the predominant cause of dementia in the United States, with more than 5 million people affected. Its etiology remains unclear, although significant strides have been made using gene mapping efforts. Success has been most notable for Mendelian familial early-onset AD (EOAD), which comprises a minority (<5%) of all AD cases (Goldman et al. 2011). However, recent success in identifying genetic variants in AD has led to a deeper understanding of the biology of the disorder and has potential therapeutic implications for both EOAD and late-onset AD (LOAD).

Early-Onset Alzheimer's Disease

Rare nonsynonymous mutations at three genetic loci associated with EOAD have been identified. The first was the amyloid precursor protein (*APP*), located on chromosome 21 (Goate et al. 1991). Since then, more than 30 different mutations in *APP* have been identified, each of which may contribute to the development of EOAD. Individuals with one of these mutations generally experience the onset of disease between the ages of 40 and 60 years, although later age at onset can occur (Theuns et al. 2006). Families with duplications of *APP*—leaving the mutation carrier with three copies of the gene on their two chromosomes—have also been reported (Rovelet-Lecrux et al. 2006; Sleegers et al. 2006). Carriers of *APP* duplications experience EOAD associated with cerebral amyloid angiopathy and intracerebral hemorrhage. Although the identification of mutations in *APP* has been important in advancing our understanding of AD's genetic causes, all *APP* mutations and duplications reported to date account for the disease in fewer than 100 families worldwide (VIB Center for Molecular Neurology 2021).

A second AD locus was found on chromosome 14 (St George-Hyslop et al. 1992) and is now called presenilin 1 (*PSEN1*) (Sherrington et al. 1995). More than 180 mutations in the *PSEN1* locus have been reported in hundreds of families worldwide (VIB Center for Molecular Neurology 2021). The onset of symptoms for those with *PSEN1* mutations is often before age 50, but later ages have also been reported. As with *APP* mutations, *PSEN1* mutations appear to act as autosomal dominant traits with nearly complete penetrance (Cruts et al. 1998). However, there is at least one report of possible nonpenetrance of a *PSEN1* mutation in a healthy 68-year-old member of a pedigree with multiple affected members (Rossor et al. 1996).

A third EOAD gene has been localized to chromosome 1, known as presenilin 2 (*PSEN2*) (Levy-Lahad et al. 1995). Mutations in *PSEN2* appear to be rare, with only a few families of varying ethnicity identified. Although *PSEN2* mutations are autosomal dominant, they may not be fully penetrant, with demonstrated penetrance rates of about 95% (Goldman et al. 2011). *PSEN2* mutations generally lead to the onset of AD symptoms before age 65. The proportion of EOAD cases attributable to mutations in *APP*, *PSEN1*, and *PSEN2* remains unclear. Some reports have suggested that *PSEN1* mutations account for most familial EOAD cases (Campion et al. 1999), whereas others have reported that a more realistic estimate is 20% or fewer of such cases, with *PSEN2* and *APP* accounting for 1% and 5%, respectively (Cruts et al. 1998). Because not all families with autosomal dominant EOAD have identifiable mutations in *PSEN1*, *PSEN2*, or *APP*, it is likely that additional genes influence the pathophysiology of EOAD (Goldman et al. 2011).

Although an appreciation for the role of amyloid-β (Aβ) protein in AD preceded the identification of AD genes, the identification of causative mutations in EOAD has confirmed the primacy of this mechanism. Aβ is generated by the processing of APP protein, the product of *APP*. In some families, AD results from simple duplication of *APP*. Also, AD pathology develops in individuals with Down syndrome unless the trisomy of chromosome 21 occurs distal to *APP*'s location (Prasher et al. 1998). As evidenced by the results of animal and in vitro studies, the expressions of the identified mutations in *APP*, *PSEN1*, and *PSEN2* that lead to EOAD all result in overproduction of the toxic 42 amino acid species of Aβ (i.e., the $A\beta_{42}$) (Hardy 2006). The discovery of genes associated with EOAD and their role in Aβ protein metabolism has contributed to the development and investigation of anti-amyloid therapeutic strategies for both EOAD and LOAD (Huang et al. 2020).

Late-Onset Alzheimer's Disease

In contrast to EOAD variants, LOAD is a complex disorder that results from the effects of multiple genes, likely interacting with pertinent environmental risk factors. As a result, LOAD can present as either a familial disorder or a sporadic disorder. Many genes appear to be associated with LOAD. Interestingly, pathway analysis implicates immunity, lipid metabolism, tau binding proteins, and *APP* metabolism, showing that genetic variants affecting *APP* and Aβ processing are associated not only with EOAD but also with LOAD (Kunkle et al. 2019; Wang et al. 2019). The most well-known risk allele, apolipoprotein E (*APOE*), is clearly associated with LOAD, with increased risk of AD found in individuals carrying *APOE*E4* in both familial and sporadic cases (Saunders et al. 1993). Although *APOE*E4* is most associated with an increased risk for LOAD, it has also been associated with EOAD (see Goldman et al. 2011). As the number of ε4 alleles increases from 0 to 2, the risk for AD increases and the mean age at onset of AD is earlier (Corder et al. 1993). These findings were confirmed in a meta-analysis of more than 14,000 subjects recruited from clinical, community, and brain bank sources (Farrer et al. 1997). Although the effect of *APOE*E4* on the increased risk for LOAD was evident in both sexes and in all age and ethnic groups, the magnitude of the risk varied by age and ethnicity. The risk appeared to be attenuated in older individuals and in Black and Latinx (relative to whites) individuals, whereas the risk conferred by *APOE*E4* was increased in persons of Japanese ethnicity.

The strength of the relationship between *APOE*E4* and risk for LOAD cannot be overstated. Approximately 50%–70% of people with AD carry at least one ε4 allele, and *APOE*E4* accounts for up to 50% of the genetic contribution to LOAD. Typical estimates suggest a two- to threefold increased risk for ε4 heterozygotes (with estimates for homozygotes varying from a two- to tenfold increased risk). Many studies have suggested that the ε4 allele influences the age at which AD occurs rather than the overall lifetime risk. Studies have also suggested that the ε2 allele may play a protective role against the development of AD. Nevertheless, carrying one or two *APOE*E4* alleles does not translate into the development of AD. It has been estimated that of *APOE*E4* homozygotes who are disease-free at age 65, at most 50% will develop AD within their lifetime (Henderson et al. 1995).

At least half of the genetic contribution to LOAD is due to genes other than *APOE*. Many linkage analyses of families with multiple individuals affected by LOAD have been conducted, and many regions in the genome have been implicated as possibly harboring LOAD-relevant genes. Recent large GWASs have identified, in addition to *APOE*, other potential genetic loci for LOAD. Recent studies have shown that genes related to Aβ metabolism, tau, immunity, and lipid processing are also associated with LOAD (Kunkle et al. 2019). Another recent analysis that included 71,880 cases and 383,378 control subjects from the Psychiatric Genomics Consortium, the Alzheimer's Disease Sequencing Project, the International Genomics of Alzheimer's Project, and the U.K. Biobank extended previous GWAS findings and further identified 29 risk loci, implicating 215 potential causative genes. Gene set analyses indicated that immune response, lipid-related processes, and the degradation of *APP* were the most represented biological pathways for the associated risk genes (Jansen et al. 2019).

The availability of large databases, including genomic information, also allowed the development of polygenic risk scores (PRSs) to estimate the individual genetic predisposition to AD. An AD-PRS could identify mild cognitive impairment (MCI) in adults who were only in their 50s (Logue et al. 2019). A recent analysis focused on developing AD-PRS using the summary statistics from the International Genomics of Alzheimer's Project study to evaluate the risk of progression from MCI to clinical AD (Chaudhury et al. 2019). This study showed that individuals with MCI who progressed to AD had a significantly higher AD-PRS compared with nonconverters. The AD-PRS predicted the conversion from MCI to AD with 61% accuracy. The AD-PRS also predicted the AD risk in cognitively unimpaired older adults over 17 years of follow-up (Stocker et al. 2020) and faster cognitive decline (Kauppi et al. 2020). Despite the success of large GWASs in identifying novel loci and genes that can be related to AD and in identifying those at higher risk for cognitive decline, these studies also shed light on the high heterogeneity of AD genetics and the significant overlap of estimated AD predisposition, based on PRS, between patients with AD and cognitively unimpaired subjects. These are important topics for investigation in future studies to improve our understanding of the biological mechanisms of AD and to aid in the development of prediction models to identify individuals at the highest risk for developing this disorder.

Neuropsychiatric Symptoms in Alzheimer's Disease

Nearly all individuals with AD will develop neuropsychiatric symptoms at some point in their illness, with depression, aggression, and psychosis being the most common (Devanand et al. 1997). Such symptoms invariably cause distress for the person who experiences them and for family and caregivers. Psychotic symptoms occur in ~50% of individuals with AD, and pharmacotherapies for AD with psychosis have limited efficacy and may increase short-term mortality (Murray et al. 2014). Also, psychosis in AD indicates a more severe phenotype, with more rapid cognitive decline beginning even before the onset of psychotic symptoms (Murray et al. 2014).

Several investigators have been interested in whether psychosis and other behavioral disturbances in LOAD may result from the interaction of genetic variation with the neurodegenerative process. For example, Tunstall et al. (2000) reported significant genotypic influence on mood disorder manifestations in AD but found the evidence for familial aggregation of AD-related psychosis to be equivocal. In contrast, Sweet et al. (2002) found a significant association between the presence of psychotic symptoms in probands and siblings in a cohort of 371 patients with AD and 461 siblings also diagnosed with AD who were recruited and characterized as part of the National Institute of Mental Health AD Genetics Initiative. Such work has resulted in an estimated heritability of psychosis in AD of 61% (Bacanu et al. 2005). The familial aggregation of psychosis in AD has been confirmed in independent samples (Sweet et al. 2010). Furthermore, this study also found that psychosis in AD was significantly—albeit modestly—correlated with the severity of other behavioral symptoms, which raises the possibility of some overlapping genetic determinants. Synaptic proteins, especially postsynaptic ones, have been shown to be linked with resilience to psychosis in AD (Krivinko et al. 2018).

Motivated by the observation of the heritability of psychosis in AD, Hollingworth et al. (2012) undertook an analysis of three GWASs to identify loci that increase susceptibility to psychosis in AD. The strongest evidence for an association was observed in an intergenic region on chromosome 4. Additional SNPs upstream of *SLC2A9* and within *VSNL1* showed strong evidence for an association when compared with control subjects without psychosis. More recent works have found strong associations between three SNPs within the antisense transcript *RP11-541P9.3* and risk of psychosis in AD (Ballard et al. 2020; DeMichele-Sweet et al. 2018). This antisense transcript is a likely regulator of cyclin G1 expression and may act to inhibit tau phosphorylation by cyclin-dependent kinases. Another study that investigated the association of a schizophrenia PRS and risk of psychosis in AD showed that a higher PRS increased the risk of psychosis in AD cases by 18% (Creese et al. 2019). These results suggested a shared genetic liability between schizophrenia and psychosis in AD.

Other Neurodegenerative Illnesses of Later Life

Substantial progress has been made in identifying genetic variation that contributes to the risk of other common neurodegenerative diseases of later life. In AD, much of this progress has resulted from the identification of variants that contribute to the risk of highly heritable, familial forms of this illness.

Frontotemporal Dementia

Frontotemporal dementia (FTD)—or, in DSM-5 (American Psychiatric Association 2013), neurocognitive disorder due to frontotemporal lobar degeneration—comprises a clinically and pathologically heterogeneous group of non-AD dementias whose underlying pathology includes progressive degeneration of the prefrontal and anterior temporal lobes (Neary et al. 2005). There are three main clinical syndromes of FTD, characterized by leading features at presentation (Sivasathiaseelan et al. 2019). About half of FTD cases present with behavioral changes, referred to as *behavioral variant FTD*. The remainder present with language decline (primary progressive aphasia) characterized by either impaired speech production (progressive nonfluent aphasia) or impaired word comprehension and semantic memory (semantic dementia).

Nearly all FTD cases result from one of two major types of neurodegenerative lesions: 1) tau-positive inclusions and 2) ubiquitin-positive inclusions, shown to contain transactive response DNA-binding protein 43 (TDP-43) (Neumann et al. 2006). The neuropathological findings of FTD overlap with those of several other neurodegenerative disorders; for example, tau-positive inclusions are also seen in progressive supranuclear palsy and corticobasal degeneration, and TDP-43-positive inclusions are often seen with motor neuron disease.

FTD has been the subject of extensive genetic investigation. Positive family history is present in up to 50% of cases (Chow et al. 1999). Mutations in one of several genes can result in FTD, which typically demonstrates an autosomal dominant pattern of transmission. Major causes of FTD include mutations in the following genes: *MAPT*, *PGRN* or *GRN*, and *C9orf72* (Wang et al. 2013). A minority of cases are caused by mutations in *TDP-43*, *VCP*, *CHMP2B*, *TBK1*, and *FUS* (Sivasathiaseelan et al. 2019). In addition, the involvement of the *APOE* locus has been reported (Wang et al. 2013). A significant discovery identified mutation in *C9orf72* (DeJesus-Hernandez et al. 2011) as perhaps the most common genetic risk factor in both familial FTD (25% of cases) and sporadic FTD (5%) (Sivasathiaseelan et al. 2019). This new mutation is an expansion of a noncoding GGGGCC hexanucleotide repeat located on chromosome 9p (Dobson-Stone et al. 2012). A recent study showed that increased *CYLD* activity reduced autophagy function, suggesting that *CYLD* may be a causative gene in the pathogenesis of FTD (Dobson-Stone et al. 2020).

Parkinson's Disease

PD is a progressive neurodegenerative disorder that affects 1%–2% of the population age 65 years and older. The global prevalence is expected to double from 6.2 million cases in 2015 to 12.9 million cases by 2040 (Blauwendraat et al. 2020). PD is characterized by motor symptoms that include akinesia, rest tremor, rigidity, and disturbance of postural reflexes. Genetic risk is often divided into two categories: rare DNA variants with high effect sizes, which are typically associated with monogenic or familial PD, and more common, smaller effect variants that are usually identified in apparently sporadic PD (Blauwendraat et al. 2020). Many cases of PD are thought to arise sporadically; as a result, the risk for first-degree family members of individuals with PD is increased only two- to threefold, and only in families with an early age at onset (Gasser 2005). Mutations in multiple genes have been identified that appear to cause PD via a Mendelian mode of inheritance. As with AD, however, these mutations account for a small number of affected families and are primarily associated with earlier lifetime onset (Gasser 2005).

To date, GWASs have identified 90 independent risk-associated variants (Blauwendraat et al. 2020). Autosomal dominant PD has been robustly associated with mutations in *SNCA*, *LRRK2*, *EIF4G1*, and *VPS35*. Recessive PD has been associated with mutations in *PARK2*, *PINK1*, *DJ1/PARK*, and *VPS13C* (Puschmann 2013). Changes in a long list of additional genes have been suggested, including the genes for hereditary ataxias, FTD, dopa-responsive dystonia, and other conditions. Point mutations and multiplications in *SNCA*, the gene encoding the protein α-synuclein, cause cognitive or psychiatric symptoms and parkinsonism, with widespread α-synuclein pathology in the central and peripheral nervous systems (Puschmann 2013). *LRRK2* mutations may lead to a clinical phenotype closely resembling idiopathic PD, with a variety of neuropathology. Mutations in *PARK2*, *PINK1*, and *DJ1/PARK7*, on the other hand, may cause early-onset parkinsonism with limited risk for cognitive decline. Carriers of mutations in the other genes may develop parkinsonism with or without additional symptoms but rarely develop a disease resembling PD. Although some mutations occur with higher frequency in specific populations, all are very rare. Therefore, the genetic etiology of most cases of sporadic or hereditary PD remains unknown on a more global scale.

In a two-stage meta-analysis, the International Parkinson's Disease Genomics Consortium and Wellcome Trust Case Control Consortium 2 (2011) identified several new potential genetic loci for PD. The researchers identified five additional PD risk loci—*PARK16*/1q32, *FGF20*/8p22, *STX1B*/16p11, *STBD1*/4q21, and *GPNMB*/7p15—the first two of which had been suggested by previous association studies. Using data from postmortem brain samples assayed for gene expression and methylation, the investigators were able to identify methylation and expression changes associated with PD risk variants within *PARK16*/1q32, *GPNMB*/7p15, and *STX1B*/16p11, suggesting potential molecular mechanisms and candidate genes at these locations.

Psychiatric Disorders of Adulthood: Schizophrenia, Bipolar Disorders, and Major Depressive Disorder

The major idiopathic psychiatric disorders of adulthood—schizophrenia, the bipolar disorders, and MDD—are complex disorders with complex genetic contributions to their etiologies. MDD shows evidence of a moderate genetic contribution, with estimates of its heritability at around 37% (Bienvenu et al. 2011). In contrast, schizophrenia and bipolar disorders demonstrate substantially greater heritability, estimated at 81% and 85%, respectively (Bienvenu et al. 2011; Rajarajan et al. 2020). However, these three diagnostic categories are not genetically distinct. Family studies have shown a substantial overlap in risk for schizophrenia and bipolar disorders and bipolar disorders and MDD, although the overlap between schizophrenia and MDD is more modest. These findings are consistent with the notion that common genetic variants have a nonspecific effect increasing the risk for psychiatric disorders. Such findings have led to further attempts to pool diagnoses to enhance the power to detect shared variants (Cross-Disorder Group of the Psychiatric Genomics Consortium 2013). Similarly, studies have revealed evidence of a shared liability to rare structural variation (CNV) among schizophrenia, bipolar disorders, ASD, and intellectual disability (Malhotra and Sebat 2012).

Because the search for specific underlying genetic contributions to these disorders is an area of substantial ongoing research effort (and, as such, is rapidly evolving), we have not attempted to generate a comprehensive summary of all recent findings. Instead, we have focused on findings that are well established or will guide future studies. It should be noted that studies summarized here are not specific to late-life (or late-onset) disease but instead focus on schizophrenia, bipolar disorders, and MDD across the lifespan.

Rare Mutations

Efforts to identify rare variants with high penetrance leading to Mendelian diseases have proved successful for neurodegenerative disorders but have not yielded definitive results for schizophrenia, bipolar disorders, or MDD. In recent years, efforts have shifted to detecting rare de novo variants, with most studies to date having focused on schizophrenia. This shift has been motivated in part by the recognition that many individuals with schizophrenia do not have family histories of the disorder and the fact that schizophrenia has persisted in the population despite conferring lower reproductive success. These observations may be explained by an excess of DNMs (Xu et al. 2012). Efforts in this area have met with some preliminary success, suggesting there may be enrichment of DNMs that disrupt genes involved in brain development or synaptic function (Kenny et al. 2014; Rees et al. 2020). However, these studies have been limited because most identified mutations are both individually rare and not fully penetrant, meaning they occur to some extent in unaffected individuals. The result is that substantially larger numbers of subjects need to be genotyped for many of these rare variants before clear evidence of causality for any of these genes can be established. However, even in large cohorts, interindividual variability reduces statistical power. Thus, the need for genetically informed patient selection in human induced pluripotent stem cell (iPSC) model-based studies is increasingly recognized by the field (Rajarajan et al. 2020). For instance, recent studies combining CRISPR-engineering of iPSC model-based studies with single-cell RNA sequencing show promising results for evaluating large numbers of genomic perturbations (Rajarajan et al. 2020).

Structural Variants

Several studies have established that individuals with schizophrenia have a greater frequency of genetic structural variation than those without schizophrenia; data for bipolar disorders are less striking and consistent with a greater frequency of structural variation (Malhotra and Sebat 2012). Such loci have included confirmation of a previously known association of increased risk for schizophrenia in individuals with a large deletion at chromosome 22q11.2, which is associated with the developmental disorder velocardiofacial syndrome (i.e., DiGeorge syndrome). Twenty-five percent of patients with DiGeorge syndrome develop schizophrenia. Other loci with replicated structural variations associated with increased risk of schizophrenia, and in some cases with bipolar disorders and recurrent depression, include deletions at chromosomes 1q21.1, 3q29, and 15q13.3. However, the implications of these and other similar findings for a more specific biological understanding of schizophrenia and bipolar disorders are not entirely clear because these deletions are also associated with increased risk for intellectual disability, developmental disorders, and ASD. Besides, these loci contain many genes within the deleted regions, and therefore determining the actual genetic changes that lead to neuropsychiatric impairment remains a challenge.

Concerning the latter issue, several structural variants seem to implicate a single gene or a limited set of genes. Among the most intensively studied of these has been a reciprocal translocation between chromosomes 1 and 11 that disrupts *DISC1* and ncRNAs *DISC2* and *DISC1FP1* (Thomson et al. 2013). This translocation has been found in a single large Scottish family in which carriers of the translocation have increased rates of schizophrenia, recurrent MDD, and bipolar disorders (Blackwood et al. 2001). However, the translocation is not fully penetrant because carriers are unaffected. This finding has spurred extensive examination of the genetics of *DISC1* in other individuals and families. These studies, which have encompassed the assessment of structural variation, rare mutations, and common variants, have provided supportive but not unequivocal evidence for an association of *DISC1* with schizophrenia, depressive disorders, and ASD (Thomson et al. 2013). A recent meta-analysis confirmed that *DISC1* polymorphisms increase schizophrenia risk, especially in the Chinese population (Wang et al. 2018). Nevertheless, as one of the best single-gene candidates for mental illness causation, *DISC1* has been the subject of increasingly extensive investigation of its functionality and its implications for therapeutic interventions (Weng et al. 2018).

Deletions and duplications affecting the gene neurexin 1 (*NRXN1*) have likewise been described in schizophrenia but are also known to occur in ASD, intellectual disability, and seizure disorder (Hu et al. 2019). Similarly, a duplication affecting the vasoactive intestinal peptide receptor 2 gene (*VIPR2*)—which, despite its name, is expressed and functions in the brain, not the intestine—has been associated with schizophrenia and ASD but has not been associated with bipolar disorders (Vacic et al. 2011). The fact that these duplications increase the amount of *VIPR2* expressed raises the question of whether antagonists could be developed as potential targeted therapeutics for schizophrenia.

Common Variants

Until recently, most studies of common variants focused on candidate genes identified by their known function or position within chromosomal regions showing linkage to disease in gene mapping studies. However, the extent to which these earlier reports may represent true associations remains unclear due to many biases inherent in such approaches. The field has since moved toward the use of GWASs, which, by controlling for multiple hypothesis testing, increases the confidence that significant associations are true positives. However, GWASs also require large samples to detect significant associations. Therefore, recent international efforts to combine all moderate-sized GWASs in psychiatric illness into a large analysis via the Psychiatric Genomics Consortium are under way and have generated a series of analyses with increasing sample size. The most recent meta-analysis of common variation in schizophrenia involved 41,000 subjects and 65,000 control subjects (Pardiñas et al. 2018). Investigators found 145 significantly associated genomic risk loci, implicating multiple genes and ncRNAs as possibly associated with increased risk for schizophrenia, adding 50 new loci to an earlier study (Ripke et al. 2013). First and foremost has been the significant association of schizophrenia and bipolar disorders with genes involved in calcium signaling, including *CACNA1C* and *CACNB2*. Brain-relevant functional gene sets significantly associated with schizophrenia included targets of fragile X mental retardation protein and long-term potentiation. These findings have clear potential therapeutic implications (e.g., for agents active at these receptors), although much work remains necessary to elucidate the biological mechanisms underlying these associations. A second important and consistent finding was the identification of associations with variants in the dopamine receptor *DRD2* and in genes affecting glutamate signaling (e.g., *GRM3*, *GRIN2A*, *SRR*, *GRIA1*), supporting prior hypothesized dopaminergic and glutamatergic mechanisms in disease.

Genetic studies have also found schizophrenia to be associated with the ncRNA miR-137, a microRNA that acts to reduce expression of multiple gene targets and is associated with increased risk for schizophrenia (Ripke et al. 2013). In addition, many genes associated with schizophrenia are themselves potentially regulated by miR-137. This publication also found many potential associations of another class of RNA—long ncRNA—with risk for schizophrenia. The functions of long ncRNA are still being uncovered but are expected to have a role in the regulation of gene transcription, further highlighting the extent to which genetic variation in schizophrenia may act through complex regulation of gene expression rather than through alterations in specific protein sequences (Cookson et al. 2009). Finally, as in previous studies, recent studies have found the major histocompatibility complex to be associated with schizophrenia, although the complicated genetics of the histocompatibility complex make the implications of this association somewhat unclear at this time. New integrative studies on postmortem brains used deep machine learning techniques coupled with mapping of active enhancers in gene regulatory networks and were able to predict the presence or absence of disease based on a subject's brain transcriptome and chromatin profiles (Rajarajan et al. 2020).

The efforts of the Psychiatric Genomics Consortium have also led to the aforementioned discovery of shared common genetic variation among individuals with schizophrenia, bipolar disorders, MDD, and other disorders, and efforts to identify genetic variation that may contribute to risk across disorders have since been under way. The largest of these to date examined 33,332 individual subjects diagnosed with bipolar disorders, MDD, schizophrenia, ASD, or ADHD, as well as 27,888 healthy control subjects of European ancestry (Cross-Disorder Group of the Psychiatric Genomics Consortium 2013). Significant associations with SNPs in *ITIH3*, *AS3MT*, and *CACNB2* were found, with similar associations to risk for all five disorders. Also, a significant association with an SNP in *CACNA1C* was driven by the schizophrenia and bipolar groups. A recent GWAS of endophenotypes from the Consortium on the Genetics of Schizophrenia Study (Greenwood et al. 2019) demonstrated the utility of endophenotypes for resolving the genetic architecture of schizophrenia and characterizing the underlying biological dysfunctions. Understanding the molecular basis of these endophenotypes may help identify novel treatment targets and pave the way for precision-based medicine in schizophrenia and related psychotic disorders.

Recent large GWASs have identified novel genetic loci related to MDD. A study analyzing sequencing data from 44 independent cohorts found many genetic loci associated with MDD. New genes identified included *OLFM4*, *NEGR1*, *RBFOX1*, *LRFN5*, *CACNA2D1*, *DRD2*, *GRM5*, and *PCLO* (Wray et al. 2018). These genes are related to body mass and metabolism regulation, hypothalamus-pituitary-adrenal axis, gene expression regulation, and neurotransmission. A more recent meta-analysis, including data on 807,553 individuals (246,363 cases and 561,190 controls) and independent replication in 1,306,354 individuals (414,055 cases and 892,299 controls) confirmed the association of 87 genetic loci with MDD (Howard et al. 2019). Fewer GWASs address the genetics of late-life depression; a recent GWAS identified novel genes potentially associated with cognitive impairment and decline in late-life depression (i.e., *SLC27A1* and *GRXCR1*) (Steffens et al. 2020).

Despite the robustness of recent findings concerning the genetic underpinnings of MDD, the genetic polymorphisms explain <15% of the variance in MDD diagnosis. Together with the low heritability, these findings indicate that environmental factors and the gene × environment interaction play major roles in the pathophysiology of MDD across the lifespan. For example, a study that attracted a great deal of attention in studies of MDD reported that the short alleles of a 44-base-pair insertion/deletion polymorphism in serotonin transporter *SLC6A4* moderated environmental effects on depression, increasing the risk for depression induced by stressful life events or childhood maltreatment (Caspi et al. 2003). The possibility that genetic variation in *SLC6A4* might influence stress reactivity has been supported by several smaller studies using different approaches (Levinson 2006). However, two subsequent large-scale studies were unable to replicate these findings (Gillespie et al. 2005; Surtees et al. 2006). More recent meta-analyses have continued to provide conflicting results, adding uncertainty to the relationship between genetic variation in *SLC6A4*, stressful life events, and MDD (Park et al. 2019).

The consideration of specified environmental factors may have relevance for the study of the genetics of late-life depression. Whereas some environmental stressors that are common in late life (e.g., bereavement) may share mechanisms with early-life stressors, other important environmental contributors to late-life depression, such as cerebrovascular disease, are likely to interact with a different set of genetic variants. Some efforts have been made to detect common variants that may interact with cerebrovascular disease to alter the risk for late-life depression (reviewed in Chapter 9, "Depressive Disorders"). At present, these studies have been limited by sample size and evaluation of a few candidate genes. Thus, they must be interpreted with caution because these designs are prone to generate both false-positive and false-negative results when common variants are considered.

Genomic Medicine and Genetic Testing: A Guide for the Clinician

Despite advances in the knowledge of the genetic basis of psychiatric disorders, we still face a large "translational gap" in clinical settings. Other fields of medicine, such as oncology, have incorporated genetic testing as part of their day-to-day clinical operations. Genetic testing helps improve diagnosis and prognosis and helps determine the best treatment strategy for different tumors (Hudson 2013). Routine genetic testing is still in its infancy in psychiatry and confined mostly to research settings. Nonetheless, the increasing availability of direct-to-consumer genetic tests poses an additional challenge to clinicians in how to use such information when available. Before genetic testing is ordered, the patient, family, and health care team must discuss several issues (Goldman 2012):

- Will the test contribute to the diagnosis or treatment of the disorder?
- Does the patient have the capacity to consent?
- Who else in the family should be present (or consulted) for a discussion of possible genetic etiology and testing?
- What will be the effect of testing on other family members, and do they want to know?

Other relevant issues to consider when requesting genetic testing include costs, often with limited coverage and reimbursement by health insurance plans, and how this information can be used by insurance companies or in legal disputes. For example, the 2008 Genetic Information Nondiscrimination Act protects against genetic discrimination by health insurance companies and employers, but it does not protect against genetic discrimination related to long-term care or life insurance (Goldman 2012). Deciding whether genetic testing is appropriate for a particular clinical scenario involves a balance of benefit and risk. Furthermore, testing requires informed consent and must be guided by an experienced genetic counselor. The impact of genetic results often differs for each member of the family, and the counselor should explain the importance of identifying who should be privy to the results and educate the patient about how a negative result relates to diagnosis.

Testing for Genes Associated With Early-Onset Alzheimer's Disease

Mutations in *APP*, *PSEN1*, and *PSEN2* have been identified in ~50% of familial cases of EOAD. Although EOAD is rare, the identification of mutations in any of these genes is part of its current diagnostic criteria (McKhann et al. 2011), even in those who are still asymptomatic or who present with MCI. Genetic testing can be recommended in those individuals who have a clear family history of EOAD (e.g., at least three generations) and are currently experiencing cognitive impairment. In this scenario, the presence of mutations in *APP*, *PSEN1*, or *PSEN2* can help diagnose EOAD.

Genetic testing for asymptomatic probands of autosomal mutation carriers is more controversial and should be considered on a case-by-case basis. In this scenario, genetic testing should be accompanied by pretest genetic counseling, with a clear explanation of the meaning of AD-related autosomal genetic mutations. Important considerations when disclosing positive genetic test results include the lack of clear genotype-phenotype correlations between genetic mutations and the age at onset of dementia, because it can vary by more than 20 years within the same family. Also, there is the possibility that mutations may have variable expression across individuals (Goldman et al. 2011). Another critical aspect is the lack of disease-modifying therapies currently approved for the treatment of AD. However, recent advances in the anti-amyloid immunotherapies raise hopes that this soon will no longer be a limitation (Tolar et al. 2020).

Testing for *APOE*E4* in Late-Onset Alzheimer's Disease

In general, the addition of *APOE*E4* testing to a clinical dementia assessment lowers the sensitivity and enhances the specificity of an AD diagnosis (Ertekin-Taner 2007), ultimately reducing the false-positive rate. However, in individuals with normal cognition or MCI, *APOE*E4* testing appears to be an insufficient predictor (on its own) of subsequent AD and may offer little benefit over cognitive testing in predicting a subsequent dementia diagnosis (Cervilla et al. 2004). For this reason and others, *APOE* genotyping is not routinely offered in the clinical setting. Because the ε4 allele is neither necessary nor sufficient to cause AD, numerous consensus statements have recommended against using *APOE* genotyping for predicting AD risk. The primary reasons for this recommendation are the low sensitivity of testing, the limited availability of treatment options, and the difficult nature of effectively conveying probabilistic risk (Goldman et al. 2011).

Testing for Genes Associated With Frontotemporal Dementia

The definitive diagnosis of FTD can be made only at autopsy, but genetics may increase diagnostic and prognostic accuracy (Farlow and Foroud 2013). *MAPT*, *GRN*, and *C9orf72* are easily sequenced for mutations that lead to FTD and account for most familial cases. Families concerned about the possibility of FTD developing in future generations frequently ask their physician to order genetic testing. As always, a referral to a genetic counselor should precede the collection of samples for testing.

The first step in determining the order for genetic testing for FTD is to take a detailed family history. As with AD, testing for autosomal dominant genes is less likely to yield a mutational finding without a known or suspected family history of FTD. However, *PGRN* and *C9orf72* mutations have been found in sporadic cases (Goldman 2012). Genetic testing for FTD is also greatly facilitated by having a pathological diagnosis in an affected family member because autopsy results can guide genetic testing by eliminating the need to test certain genes. If the parents are deceased, ages at death should be documented (Sivasathiaseelan et al. 2019).

FTD genotyping may soon play a role in treatment selection. Several preliminary reports have proposed the use of antisense oligonucleotides (short synthetic single DNA strands designed to bind their complementary sequence) to reduce levels of RNA containing the pathological hexanucleotide repeat on chromosome 9p (Lagier-Tourenne et al. 2013). Antisense oligonucleotide therapies may treat gain-of-function disorders by silencing the causative gene, either by acting on both alleles for nonessential genes or by selectively acting on the mutant allele in the case of essential genes (Fernandes et al. 2013). For certain loss-of-function diseases, antisense oligonucleotides might also be used for splice modulation, which in certain cases can restore gene function or otherwise compensate for its loss. In contrast, tau PET imaging has yet to show promise in genetic FTD. Three key fluid biomarkers have been identified that are likely to be helpful in clinical trials: cerebrospinal fluid or blood neurofilament light chain levels, cerebrospinal fluid or blood progranulin levels (in *GRN* carriers), and cerebrospinal fluid poly(GP) dipeptide repeat protein levels (in *C9orf72* carriers) (Greaves and Rohrer 2019). The heterogeneity of FTD makes biomarker development a more challenging proposition in this group of diseases than in, for example, AD. New methods, such as molecular ligand neuroimaging that can capture protein tau in vivo, and wet biomarkers from cerebrospinal fluid and blood assays, such as tau and its metabolites (neurofilament light chain, *TREM2*, and progranulin), offer promise for future research and treatment opportunities.

Testing for Genes Associated With Parkinson's Disease

Genetic testing is currently available for several PD-related genes, including *SNCA*, *LRRK2* (*PARK8*), *PARK2*, *PARK7*, and *PINK1*. Because a universal therapy for PD is unlikely to be found, clinical trials are under way for *GBA*-related PD (NCT02906020) and *LRRK2*-related PD (NCT3710707) (Blauwendraat et al. 2020). Routine testing is not recommended due to the lack of disease-modifying therapies and still-evolving research on the role and utility of testing in clinical decision-making. Approaches such as deep brain stimulation and treatment with levodopa-carbidopa enteral suspension can help patients with medication-resistant tremors, worsening symptoms when the medication wears off, and dyskinesias (Armstrong and Okun 2020). If an individual or family is interested in pursuing testing, this should be guided by a genetic counselor with experience working with patients who have a family history of PD.

Pharmacogenomics

Pharmacogenomics is the study of how genetic factors relate to interindividual variability of drug response (Kitzmiller et al. 2011). In recent years, the field of pharmacogenomics has rapidly evolved, with a positive impact on clinical outcomes for patients taking psychiatric medications (Lauschke and Ingelman-Sundberg 2020). In psychiatry, the main goals of pharmacogenomics are to evaluate if a medication will be effective in a given person (i.e., to guide individualized medication choice); to determine ideal dosages for a particular drug (i.e., to guide individualized dose-finding of a medication); and to evaluate the potential risk of severe side effects from medication (i.e., to guide treatment safety). There is a growing selection of commercially available pharmacogenomic tests to guide psychopharmacological treatment, and health insurance companies have started to cover these. Pharmacogenomic tests primarily have focused on genes related to drug metabolism (i.e., cytochrome P450 [*CYP*]), the transport through the blood-brain barrier (e.g., *ABCB1*), or the drug action in target cells (e.g., serotonin receptor in neurons [*HT2RA*]) or used to evaluate the risk of severe, life-threatening side effects (e.g., *HLA-B*1502* variant and risk of life-threatening side effects with carbamazepine).

Most psychotropic drugs commonly used in geriatric psychiatry are metabolized in the liver by the CYP450 enzymes. Other drug metabolism pathways are the uridine glucuronyl transferases (UGT) enzymes in the liver (e.g., lamotrigine) and the renal excretion of unmetabolized drugs (e.g., pregabalin and oxcarbazepine). Gene variants in the CYP450 and UGT enzyme complexes can significantly alter the rate of drug metabolism and bioavailability and, consequently, affect treatment response. Table 3–2 shows a list of the main CYP450 and UGT enzymes and their substrates (focusing on psychotropic medications).

An important question for clinicians is whether the routine use of pharmacogenomic tests would improve clinical outcomes in their daily practice. Recent clinical trials have addressed this question. These studies were designed to have one group of participants in which the clinician could use the pharmacogenomic information to guide treatment decisions (e.g., which drug to start treatment or to switch to in case of side effects, i.e., guided treatment decision) and another group that was managed as usual

TABLE 3–2. **Most commonly prescribed psychotropic medications and their respective metabolizing CYP enzymes**

Enzyme	Antidepressants	Benzodiazepines	Antipsychotics	Mood stabilizers/ Anticonvulsants
CYP1A2	Duloxetine Fluvoxamine Mirtazapine Tricyclics		Asenapine Clozapine Haloperidol Olanzapine	Carbamazepine Phenytoin
CYP2B6	Bupropion			
CYP2C9	Amitriptyline Fluoxetine Sertraline	All		Phenytoin Valproic acid
CYP2C19	Amitriptyline Citalopram Clomipramine Escitalopram Fluoxetine Imipramine Sertraline	Diazepam		Phenytoin
CYP2D6	Amitriptyline Atomoxetine Citalopram Clomipramine Desipramine Duloxetine Escitalopram Fluoxetine Imipramine Mirtazapine Paroxetine Venlafaxine		Aripiprazole Chlorpromazine Haloperidol Olanzapine Risperidone Sertindole Thioridazine Zuclopenthixol	
CYP3A4	Amitriptyline Buspirone Citalopram Mirtazapine Nefazodone Paroxetine Sertraline	All	Aripiprazole Asenapine Lurasidone Quetiapine Risperidone	Carbamazepine

(treatment as usual group, i.e., unguided treatment decision). In general, participants in the guided treatment decision group had better outcomes (i.e., higher response and remission rates; better tolerability and fewer side effects) compared with those in the treatment as usual group (Bradley et al. 2018; Greden et al. 2019; Pérez et al. 2017). The results from the individual clinical trials were confirmed in recent meta-analyses, although the authors pointed to elevated heterogeneity among the trials that can significantly impact the results (Bousman et al. 2019; Tanner et al. 2019). A post hoc analysis of one of the largest clinical trials to date showed that the benefit of guided treatment decisions extended to those with previous treatment failures (Lauschke and Ingelman-Sundberg 2020). Despite the higher rates of response and remission in the guided treatment decision groups, it is worth mentioning that the absolute rates of response and remission are still low. For example, in the Bradley et al. (2018) study, the remission rates in the guided treatment group ranged from 25% to 35% after 8 and 12 weeks of treatment, respectively. Response rates were higher, ranging from 49% to 64% after 8 and 12 weeks of treatment, respectively.

Current evidence on the benefits of making pharmacogenomic-guided treatment decisions is restricted to young and middle-aged adults, and there are no clinical trial data from older adults (Marshe et al. 2020). Also, it is not clear how other age-related changes that can affect drug pharmacokinetics, such as reduced volume distribution, increase in fat distribution, or changes in CYP enzymatic efficiency, may interact with pharmacogenomic characteristics and influence the treatment outcomes. Therefore, pharmacogenomic testing to guide treatment choices is recommended only in select cases, especially in patients who do not have a satisfactory response to treatment or those with severe side effects from medications at low dosages.

Conclusion

Medical genetics has entered the postgenomics era. The pace at which genetic variants are being discovered continues to accelerate, and such discoveries are beginning to inform the development of novel and much-needed interventions. With faster and increasingly inexpensive genomic approaches becoming available, untangling the genetic underpinnings of some of the more complex disorders in geriatric psychiatry will ideally soon follow. Although the impact of these developments on practicing geriatric psychiatrists has so far been limited, it will soon be felt. The potential for genomics to contribute to individualized clinical care has long been recognized, and many optimistic scenarios for its use have been proposed. In fact, several academic medical centers and integrated health systems have already begun implementing genomic medicine in clinical practice.

Although advancements in medical genomics continue, identifying the genes that lead to the development of complex disorders remains a challenging process. The flow of events leading from variation in the sequence of a gene to the development of multiple cognitive, emotional, and behavioral criteria that define the complex neuropsychiatric disorders of later life is not linear or straightforward. Genes encode proteins, which act within extensive biochemical networks in which changes may be amplified or compensated for by the effects of other proteins or environmental factors. The net result is that the magnitude of an increase in disease risk for a complex disorder due to any single genetic variation will be relatively small, suggesting that the ability to predict clinical outcomes for individual patients will be quite limited, even if one knows that a patient carries a genetic variation associated with the disease of interest.

Given current limitations in the availability of disease-modifying therapies for several neurodegenerative illnesses and the complex ethical considerations involved in genomic medicine, clinicians must carefully consider the appropriateness of ordering genetic tests for their patients. Because both positive and negative findings may have significant implications for patients and their families, thorough genetic counseling is advised before and after genetic testing is performed. Methods for screening and diagnosing neurodegenerative illnesses will continue to improve as additional genes are identified and correlated with increasingly specific phenotypes, and such discoveries will hopefully inform the development of preventive and disease-modifying therapies. Geriatric psychiatrists will need to be familiar with these developments to effectively counsel their patients and continue to provide state-of-the-art care.

Key Points

- The discovery of rare disease-causing mutations has been instrumental in further understanding the neurobiology of several neuropsychiatric disorders of later life, including Alzheimer's disease, frontotemporal dementia, and Parkinson's disease. Furthermore, the pace of discovery in these areas continues to accelerate.

- Many neuropsychiatric disorders of later life—including the most common presentations of the dementias—are genetically complex diseases resulting from the interaction of multiple genes and environmental factors. Such complexity limits the definitive identification of contributory genes and reduces the ability to use genetic information to predict clinical outcomes. Nevertheless, important strides in this area are continuing to be made.

- Genetic testing may be useful for detection of some of the aforementioned disorders, including early-onset Alzheimer's disease and frontotemporal dementia, and to help guide treatment in older adults (pharmacogenomic testing).

Suggested Reading

GeneCards (www.genecards.org): Searchable, integrated database providing comprehensive information on all known and predicted human genes.

References

American Psychiatric Association: Diagnostic and Statistical Manual of Mental Disorders, 5th Edition. Arlington, VA, American Psychiatric Association, 2013

Ancelin ML, Farre A, Carriere I, et al: C-reactive protein gene variants: independent association with late-life depression and circulating protein levels. Transl Psychiatry 5:e499, 2015

Armstrong MJ, Okun MS: Diagnosis and treatment of Parkinson disease: a review. JAMA 323(6):548–560, 2020 32044947

Bacanu SA, Devlin B, Chowdari KV, et al: Heritability of psychosis in Alzheimer disease. Am J Geriatr Psychiatry 13(7):624–627, 2005 16009739

Ballard C, Kales HC, Lyketsos C, et al: Psychosis in Alzheimer's disease. Curr Neurol Neurosci Rep 20(12):57, 2020 33048274

Bienvenu OJ, Davydow DS, Kendler KS: Psychiatric "diseases" versus behavioral disorders and degree of genetic influence. Psychol Med 41(1):33–40, 2011 20459884

Blackwood DH, Fordyce A, Walker MT, et al: Schizophrenia and affective disorders: cosegregation with a translocation at chromosome 1q42 that directly disrupts brain-expressed genes: clinical and P300 findings in a family. Am J Hum Genet 69(2):428–433, 2001 11443544

Blauwendraat C, Nalls MA, Singleton AB: The genetic architecture of Parkinson's disease. Lancet Neurol 19(2):170–178, 2020 31521533

Bousman CA, Arandjelovic K, Mancuso SG, et al: Pharmacogenetic tests and depressive symptom remission: a meta-analysis of randomized controlled trials. Pharmacogenomics 20(1):37–47, 2019 30520364

Bradley P, Shiekh M, Mehra V, et al: Improved efficacy with targeted pharmacogenetic-guided treatment of patients with depression and anxiety: a randomized clinical trial demonstrating clinical utility. J Psychiatr Res 96:100–107, 2018 28992526

Campion D, Dumanchin C, Hannequin D, et al: Early onset autosomal dominant Alzheimer disease: prevalence, genetic heterogeneity, and mutation spectrum. Am J Hum Genet 65(3):664–670, 1999 10441572

Carninci P, Kasukawa T, Katayama S, et al: The transcriptional landscape of the mammalian genome. Science 309(5740):1559–1563, 2005 16141072

Caspi A, Sugden K, Moffitt TE, et al: Influence of life stress on depression: moderation by a polymorphism in the 5-HTT gene. Science 301(5631):386–389, 2003 12869766

Cerri AP, Arosio B, Viazzoli C, et al: The –308 (G/A) single nucleotide polymorphism in the TNF-α gene and the risk of major depression in the elderly. Int J Geriatr Psychiatry 25(3):219–223, 2010 19618378

Cervilla J, Prince M, Joels S, et al: Premorbid cognitive testing predicts the onset of dementia and Alzheimer's disease better than and independently of APOE genotype. J Neurol Neurosurg Psychiatry 75(8):1100–1106, 2004 15258208

Ceyhan-Birsoy O, Murry JB, Machini K, et al: Interpretation of genomic sequencing results in healthy and ill newborns: results from the BabySeq Project. Am J Hum Genet 104(1):76–93, 2019 30609409

Chaudhury S, Brookes KJ, Patel T, et al: Alzheimer's disease polygenic risk score as a predictor of conversion from mild-cognitive impairment. Transl Psychiatry 9(1):154, 2019 31127079

Chow TW, Miller BL, Hayashi VN, Geschwind DH: Inheritance of frontotemporal dementia. Arch Neurol 56(7):817–822, 1999 10404983

Cookson W, Liang L, Abecasis G, et al: Mapping complex disease traits with global gene expression. Nat Rev Genet 10(3):184–194, 2009 19223927

Corder EH, Saunders AM, Strittmatter WJ, et al: Gene dose of apolipoprotein E type 4 allele and the risk of Alzheimer's disease in late onset families. Science 261(5123):921–923, 1993 8346443

Creese B, Vassos E, Bergh S, et al: Examining the association between genetic liability for schizophrenia and psychotic symptoms in Alzheimer's disease. Transl Psychiatry 9(1):273, 2019 31641104

Cross-Disorder Group of the Psychiatric Genomics Consortium: Identification of risk loci with shared effects on five major psychiatric disorders: a genome-wide analysis. Lancet 381(9875):1371–1379, 2013 23453885

Cruts M, van Duijn CM, Backhovens H, et al: Estimation of the genetic contribution of presenilin-1 and -2 mutations in a population-based study of presenile Alzheimer disease. Hum Mol Genet 7(1):43–51, 1998 9384602

D'Angelo D, Lebon S, Chen Q, et al: Defining the effect of the 16p11.2 duplication on cognition, behavior, and medical comorbidities. JAMA Psychiatry 73(1):20–30, 2016 26629640

Database of Genomic Variants, 2020. Available at http://dgv.tcag.ca/dgv/app/home. Accessed March 7, 2021.

DeJesus-Hernandez M, Mackenzie IR, Boeve BF, et al: Expanded GGGGCC hexanucleotide repeat in noncoding region of C9ORF72 causes chromosome 9p-linked FTD and ALS. Neuron 72(2):245–256, 2011 21944778

DeMichele-Sweet MAA, Weamer EA, Klei L, et al: Genetic risk for schizophrenia and psychosis in Alzheimer disease. Mol Psychiatry 23(4):963–972, 2018 28461698

Devanand DP, Jacobs DM, Tang MX, et al: The course of psychopathologic features in mild to moderate Alzheimer disease. Arch Gen Psychiatry 54(3):257–263, 1997 9075466

Dobson-Stone C, Hallupp M, Bartley L, et al: C9ORF72 repeat expansion in clinical and neuro-pathologic frontotemporal dementia cohorts. Neurology 79(10):995–1001, 2012 22875086

Dobson-Stone C, Hallupp M, Shahheydari H, et al: CYLD is a causative gene for frontotemporal dementia—amyotrophic lateral sclerosis. Brain 143(3):783–799, 2020 32185393

Ertekin-Taner N: Genetics of Alzheimer's disease: a centennial review. Neurol Clin 25(3):611–667, 2007 17659183

Farlow JL, Foroud T: The genetics of dementia. Semin Neurol 33(4):417–422, 2013 24234360

Farrer LA, Cupples LA, Haines JL, et al: Effects of age, sex, and ethnicity on the association between apolipoprotein E genotype and Alzheimer disease: a meta-analysis. JAMA 278(16):1349–1356, 1997 9343467

Fernandes SA, Douglas AG, Varela MA, et al: Oligonucleotide-based therapy for FTD/ALS caused by the C9orf72 repeat expansion: a perspective. J Nucleic Acids 2013:208245, 2013 24349764

Gasser T: Genetics of Parkinson's disease. Curr Opin Neurol 18(4):363–369, 2005 16003110

Gillespie NA, Whitfield JB, Williams B, et al: The relationship between stressful life events, the serotonin transporter (5-HTTLPR) genotype and major depression. Psychol Med 35(1):101–111, 2005 15842033

Goate A, Chartier-Harlin MC, Mullan M, et al: Segregation of a missense mutation in the amyloid precursor protein gene with familial Alzheimer's disease. Nature 349(6311):704–706, 1991 1671712

Goldman JS: New approaches to genetic counseling and testing for Alzheimer's disease and frontotemporal degeneration. Curr Neurol Neurosci Rep 12(5):502–510, 2012 22773362

Goldman JS, Hahn SE, Catania JW, et al: Genetic counseling and testing for Alzheimer disease: joint practice guidelines of the American College of Medical Genetics and the National Society of Genetic Counselors. Genet Med 13(6):597–605, 2011 21577118

Greaves CV, Rohrer JD: An update on genetic frontotemporal dementia. J Neurol 266(8):2075–2086, 2019 31119452

Greden JF, Parikh SV, Rothschild AJ, et al: Impact of pharmacogenomics on clinical outcomes in major depressive disorder in the GUIDED trial: a large, patient- and rater-blinded, randomized, controlled study. J Psychiatr Res 111:59–67, 2019 30677646

Greenwood TA, Lazzeroni LC, Maihofer AX, et al: Genome-wide association of endophenotypes for schizophrenia from the Consortium on the Genetics of Schizophrenia (COGS) Study. JAMA Psychiatry 76(12):1274–1284, 2019 31596458

Hardy J: A hundred years of Alzheimer's disease research. Neuron 52(1):3–13, 2006 17015223

Henderson AS, Easteal S, Jorm AF, et al: Apolipoprotein E allele epsilon 4, dementia, and cognitive decline in a population sample. Lancet 346(8987):1387–1390, 1995 7475820

Hollingworth P, Sweet R, Sims R, et al: Genome-wide association study of Alzheimer's disease with psychotic symptoms. Mol Psychiatry 17(12):1316–1327, 2012 22005930

Howard DM, Adams MJ, Clarke TK, et al: Genome-wide meta-analysis of depression identifies 102 independent variants and highlights the importance of the prefrontal brain regions. Nat Neurosci 22(3):343–352, 2019 30718901

Hu Z, Xiao X, Zhang Z, Li M: Genetic insights and neurobiological implications from NRXN1 in neuropsychiatric disorders. Mol Psychiatry 24(10):1400–1414, 2019 31138894

Huang LK, Chao SP, Hu CJ: Clinical trials of new drugs for Alzheimer disease. J Biomed Sci 27(1):18, 2020 31906949

Hudson TJ: Genome variation and personalized cancer medicine. J Intern Med 274(5):440–450, 2013 23751076

International HapMap Consortium: A second generation human haplotype map of over 3.1 million SNPs. Nature 449:851–862, 2007

International Parkinson's Disease Genomics Consortium, Wellcome Trust Case Control Consortium 2: a two-stage meta-analysis identifies several new loci for Parkinson's disease. PLoS Genet 7(6):e1002142, 2011

Jansen IE, Savage JE, Watanabe K, et al: Genome-wide meta-analysis identifies new loci and functional pathways influencing Alzheimer's disease risk. Nat Genet 51(3):404–413, 2019 30617256

Kauppi K, Rönnlund M, Nordin Adolfsson A, et al: Effects of polygenic risk for Alzheimer's disease on rate of cognitive decline in normal aging. Transl Psychiatry 10(1):250, 2020 32709845

Kenny EM, Cormican P, Furlong S, et al: Excess of rare novel loss-of-function variants in synaptic genes in schizophrenia and autism spectrum disorders. Mol Psychiatry 19(8):872–879, 2014 24126926

Kitzmiller JP, Groen DK, Phelps MA, Sadee W: Pharmacogenomic testing: relevance in medical practice: why drugs work in some patients but not in others. Cleve Clin J Med 78(4):243–257, 2011 21460130

Krivinko JM, Erickson SL, Ding Y, et al: Synaptic proteome compensation and resilience to psychosis in Alzheimer's disease. Am J Psychiatry 175(10):999–1009, 2018 30021459

Kunkle BW, Grenier-Boley B, Sims R, et al: Genetic meta-analysis of diagnosed Alzheimer's disease identifies new risk loci and implicates Aβ, tau, immunity and lipid processing. Nat Genet 51(3):414–430, 2019 30820047

Lagier-Tourenne C, Baughn M, Rigo F, et al: Targeted degradation of sense and antisense C9orf72 RNA foci as therapy for ALS and frontotemporal degeneration. Proc Natl Acad Sci USA 110(47):E4530–E4539, 2013 24170860

Lauschke VM, Ingelman-Sundberg M: Emerging strategies to bridge the gap between pharmacogenomic research and its clinical implementation. NPJ Genom Med 5:9, 2020

Levinson DF: The genetics of depression: a review. Biol Psychiatry 60(2):84–92, 2006 16300747

Levy S, Sutton G, Ng PC, et al: The diploid genome sequence of an individual human. PLoS Biol 5(10):e254, 2007 17803354

Levy-Lahad E, Wijsman EM, Nemens E, et al: A familial Alzheimer's disease locus on chromosome 1. Science 269(5226):970–973, 1995 7638621

Logue MW, Panizzon MS, Elman JA, et al: Use of an Alzheimer's disease polygenic risk score to identify mild cognitive impairment in adults in their 50s. Mol Psychiatry 24(3):421–430, 2019 29487403

Lupski JR: Structural variation in the human genome. N Engl J Med 356(11):1169–1171, 2007 17360997

Malhotra D, Sebat J: CNVs: harbingers of a rare variant revolution in psychiatric genetics. Cell 148(6):1223–1241, 2012 22424231

Marshe VS, Islam F, Maciukiewicz M, et al: Pharmacogenetic implications for antidepressant pharmacotherapy in late-life depression: a systematic review of the literature for response, pharmacokinetics and adverse drug reactions. Am J Geriatr Psychiatry 28(6):609–629, 2020 32122803

McKhann GM, Knopman DS, Chertkow H, et al: The diagnosis of dementia due to Alzheimer's disease: recommendations from the National Institute on Aging–Alzheimer's Association workgroups on diagnostic guidelines for Alzheimer's disease. Alzheimers Dement 7(3):263–269, 2011 21514250

Miller RD, Phillips MS, Jo I, et al: High-density single-nucleotide polymorphism maps of the human genome. Genomics 86(2):117–126, 2005 15961272

Murray PS, Kumar S, Demichele-Sweet MA, Sweet RA: Psychosis in Alzheimer's disease. Biol Psychiatry 75(7):542–552, 2014 24103379

Neary D, Snowden J, Mann D: Frontotemporal dementia. Lancet Neurol 4(11):771–780, 2005 16239184

Neumann M, Sampathu DM, Kwong LK, et al: Ubiquitinated TDP-43 in frontotemporal lobar degeneration and amyotrophic lateral sclerosis. Science 314(5796):130–133, 2006 17023659

Pardiñas AF, Holmans P, Pocklington AJ, et al: Common schizophrenia alleles are enriched in mutation-intolerant genes and in regions under strong background selection. Nat Genet 50(3):381–389, 2018 29483656

Park C, Rosenblat JD, Brietzke E, et al: Stress, epigenetics and depression: a systematic review. Neurosci Biobehav Rev 102:139–152, 2019 31005627

Pérez V, Salavert A, Espadaler J, et al: Efficacy of prospective pharmacogenetic testing in the treatment of major depressive disorder: results of a randomized, double-blind clinical trial. BMC Psychiatry 17(1):250, 2017 28705252

Prasher VP, Farrer MJ, Kessling AM, et al: Molecular mapping of Alzheimer-type dementia in Down's syndrome. Ann Neurol 43(3):380–383, 1998 9506555

Pu M, Chen J, Tao Z, et al: Regulatory network of miRNA on its target: coordination between transcriptional and post-transcriptional regulation of gene expression. Cell Mol Life Sci 76(3):441–451, 2019 30374521

Puschmann A: Monogenic Parkinson's disease and parkinsonism: clinical phenotypes and frequencies of known mutations. Parkinsonism Relat Disord 19(4):407–415, 2013 23462481

Rajarajan P, Flaherty E, Akbarian S, Brennand KJ: CRISPR-based functional evaluation of schizophrenia risk variants. Schizophr Res 217:26–36, 2020 31277978

Redon R, Ishikawa S, Fitch KR, et al: Global variation in copy number in the human genome. Nature 444(7118):444–454, 2006 17122850

Rees E, Han J, Morgan J, et al: De novo mutations identified by exome sequencing implicate rare missense variants in SLC6A1 in schizophrenia. Nat Neurosci 23(2):179–184, 2020 31932766

Ripke S, O'Dushlaine C, Chambert K, et al: Genome-wide association analysis identifies 13 new risk loci for schizophrenia. Nat Genet 45(10):1150–1159, 2013 23974872

Rossor MN, Fox NC, Beck J, et al: Incomplete penetrance of familial Alzheimer's disease in a pedigree with a novel presenilin-1 gene mutation. Lancet 347(9014):1560, 1996 8684135

Rovelet-Lecrux A, Hannequin D, Raux G, et al: APP locus duplication causes autosomal dominant early onset Alzheimer disease with cerebral amyloid angiopathy. Nat Genet 38(1):24–26, 2006 16369530

Samonte RV, Eichler EE: Segmental duplications and the evolution of the primate genome. Nat Rev Genet 3(1):65–72, 2002 11823792

Saunders AM, Strittmatter WJ, Schmechel D, et al: Association of apolipoprotein E allele ε4 with late-onset familial and sporadic Alzheimer's disease. Neurology 43(8):1467–1472, 1993 8350998

Schizophrenia Psychiatric Genome-Wide Association Study Consortium: Genome-wide association study identifies five new schizophrenia loci. Nat Genet 43(10):969–976, 2011 21926974

Sherrington R, Rogaev EI, Liang Y, et al: Cloning of a gene bearing missense mutations in early onset familial Alzheimer's disease. Nature 375(6534):754–760, 1995 7596406

Sivasathiaseelan H, Marshall CR, Agustus JL, et al: Frontotemporal dementia: a clinical review. Semin Neurol 39(2):251–263, 2019 30925617

Sleegers K, Brouwers N, Gijselinck I, et al: APP duplication is sufficient to cause early onset Alzheimer's dementia with cerebral amyloid angiopathy. Brain 129(Pt 11):2977–2983, 2006 16921174

St George-Hyslop P, Haines J, Rogaev E, et al: Genetic evidence for a novel familial Alzheimer's disease locus on chromosome 14. Nat Genet 2(4):330–334, 1992 1303289

Steffens DC, Garrett ME, Soldano KL, et al: Genome-wide screen to identify genetic loci associated with cognitive decline in late-life depression. Int Psychogeriatr 1–9, 2020 32641180

Stocker H, Perna L, Weigl K, et al: Prediction of clinical diagnosis of Alzheimer's disease, vascular, mixed, and all-cause dementia by a polygenic risk score and APOE status in a community-based cohort prospectively followed over 17 years. Mol Psychiatry 2020 32404947 Epub ahead of print

Surtees PG, Wainwright NW, Willis-Owen SA, et al: Social adversity, the serotonin transporter (5-HTTLPR) polymorphism and major depressive disorder. Biol Psychiatry 59(3):224–229, 2006 16154545

Sweet RA, Bennett DA, Graff-Radford NR, Mayeux R: Assessment and familial aggregation of psychosis in Alzheimer's disease from the National Institute on Aging Late Onset Alzheimer's Disease Family Study. Brain 133(Pt 4):1155–1162, 2010 20147454

Sweet RA, Nimgaonkar VL, Devlin B, et al: Increased familial risk of the psychotic phenotype of Alzheimer disease. Neurology 58(6):907–911, 2002 11914406

Tanner JA, Davies PE, Voudouris NC, et al: Adequate evidence to support improved outcomes in depression by primary care physicians compared to psychiatrists when using combinatorial pharmacogenomics. J Psychiatr Res 117:151–152, 2019 30522850

Taylor WD, Züchner S, McQuoid DR, et al: Allelic differences in the brain-derived neurotrophic factor Val66Met polymorphism in late-life depression. Am J Geriatr Psychiatry 15(10):850–857, 2007 17911362

Terry SF: Obama's Precision Medicine Initiative. Genet Test Mol Biomarkers 19(3):113–114, 2015 25751403

Theuns J, Marjaux E, Vandenbulcke M, et al: Alzheimer dementia caused by a novel mutation located in the APP C-terminal intracytosolic fragment. Hum Mutat 27(9):888–896, 2006 16917905

Thomson PA, Malavasi EL, Grünewald E, et al: DISC1 genetics, biology and psychiatric illness. Front Biol (Beijing) 8(1):1–31, 2013 23550053

Tolar M, Abushakra S, Hey JA, et al: Aducanumab, gantenerumab, BAN2401, and ALZ-801: the first wave of amyloid-targeting drugs for Alzheimer's disease with potential for near term approval. Alzheimers Res Ther 12(1):95, 2020 32787971

Tunstall N, Owen MJ, Williams J, et al: Familial influence on variation in age of onset and behavioural phenotype in Alzheimer's disease. Br J Psychiatry 176:156–159, 2000 10755053

Vacic V, McCarthy S, Malhotra D, et al: Duplications of the neuropeptide receptor gene VIPR2 confer significant risk for schizophrenia. Nature 471(7339):499–503, 2011 21346763

VIB Center for Molecular Neurology: Alzheimer Disease and Frontotemporal Dementia Mutation Database (website). Gent, Belgium, VIB Center for Molecular Neurology, 2021. Available at: https://uantwerpen.vib.be/ADMutations. Accessed March 7, 2021.

Wang HY, Liu Y, Yan JW, et al: Gene polymorphisms of DISC1 is associated with schizophrenia: evidence from a meta-analysis. Prog Neuropsychopharmacol Biol Psychiatry 81:64–73, 2018 29031911

Wang W, Corominas R, Lin GN: De novo mutations from whole exome sequencing in neurodevelopmental and psychiatric disorders: from discovery to application. Front Genet 10:258, 2019 31001316

Wang X, Shen Y, Chen W: Progress in frontotemporal dementia research. Am J Alzheimers Dis Other Demen 28(1):15–23, 2013 23221030

Wen KX, Miliç J, El-Khodor B, et al: The role of DNA methylation and histone modifications in neurodegenerative diseases: a systematic review. PLoS One 11(12):e0167201, 2016 27973581

Weng YT, Chien T, Kuan II, Chern Y: The TRAX, DISC1, and GSK3 complex in mental disorders and therapeutic interventions. J Biomed Sci 25(1):71, 2018 30285728

Wray NR, Ripke S, Mattheisen M, et al: Genome-wide association analyses identify 44 risk variants and refine the genetic architecture of major depression. Nat Genet 50(5):668–681, 2018 29700475

Xu B, Ionita-Laza I, Roos JL, et al: De novo gene mutations highlight patterns of genetic and neural complexity in schizophrenia. Nat Genet 44(12):1365–1369, 2012 23042115

CHAPTER 4

The Psychiatric Interview of Older Adults

Dan G. Blazer, M.D., Ph.D.

Despite the proliferation of standardized questions and laboratory procedures, the diagnostic interview is the foundation of the diagnostic workup of the older adult experiencing a psychiatric disorder. Each year, time pressures push clinicians to rely more on standardized techniques that, in turn, limit their ability to employ the art of the interview. Standardized procedures such as interview schedules and diagnostic tests can always complement the interview and in some cases "make" the diagnosis for us (e.g., neurocognitive disorder with Lewy bodies). Even so, an in-person interview by a clinician saves valuable time over the course of an older adult's illness. In this chapter, I review the core of the psychiatric interview, including history taking, family assessment, and the mental status examination; describe selected rating scales; and outline techniques for communicating effectively with older adults.

History

The elements of a diagnostic workup for elderly patients are presented in Table 4–1. To obtain historical information, the clinician should first interview the patient, if that is feasible, and then ask the patient's permission to interview family members. Members from at least two generations, if available, can expand the perspective on the older adult's impairment. If the patient has difficulty providing an accurate or understandable history, the clinician should concentrate especially on eliciting the symptoms or problems that the patient perceives as being most disabling, then fill the historical gap with data from the family.

TABLE 4–1.	Psychiatric interview of the elderly patient

History
  Present illness
  Past history
  Family history
  Social functioning
  Context
  Medication history
  Medical history
Family assessment
Mental status examination or subjective cognitive assessment

Present Illness

DSM-5 (American Psychiatric Association 2013) provides a useful catalog of symptoms and behaviors of psychiatric interest that are relevant to the diagnosis of the present illness. *Symptoms* are bits of data—the most visible part of the clinical picture and generally the part clinicians most easily agree upon. They should be defined in such a way that if multiple clinicians independently obtained equivalent information, they would have minimal disagreement about the presence or absence of those symptoms. The decision about whether the symptoms form a syndrome or derive from a particular etiology must be determined independently of data collection.

Even so, the clinical interaction may be confounded by bias when a clinician communicates with an older adult about psychiatric symptoms. As many insightful clinicians, such as Eisenberg (1977), have noted, physicians diagnose and treat *diseases*—that is, abnormalities in the structure and function of body organs and systems. Patients have *illnesses*—experiences of disvalued changes in states of being and in social function. Disease and illness do not maintain a one-to-one relationship. Factors that determine who becomes a patient and who does not can be understood only by expanding horizons beyond symptoms. During the process of becoming a patient, the older adult, usually with the advice of others, forms a self-diagnosis of the problem and judges the degree of illness perceived. For some, illness is perceived when a specific level of discomfort is experienced. For others, it reflects a general perception of physical or social alienation and despair. Illness also means different things to different people. The historical background, values, social class, and culture of the older adult contribute to the formation of constructs regarding the nature of the problem, cause, and possibility for recovery.

For these reasons, clinicians must take care to avoid accepting patients' explanations for a given problem or set of problems. Statements such as "I guess I'm just getting old, and there's nothing really to worry about" or "Most people slow down when they get to be my age" can lull clinicians into complacency about what may be a treatable psychiatric disorder. On the other hand, the advent of new and disturbing symptoms in an older adult patient between office visits can exhaust a clinician's patience, thereby derailing pursuit of the problem. For example, an older adult with illness anxiety disorder whose awakenings during the night are increasing may insist that this symptom be treated with a sedative and plead with the clinician not to allow continual suffering. In the clinician's view, however, the symptom is a normal accompaniment of older age and therefore should be accepted.

To prevent attitudinal biases when eliciting reports from older individuals (which may result in missing the symptoms and signs of a treatable psychiatric disorder), clinicians should include in the initial interview a review of the more important psychiatric symptoms in a relatively structured format. Common symptoms to be reviewed include excessive weakness or lethargy; depressed mood or "the blues"; memory problems; difficulty concentrating; feelings of helplessness, hopelessness, and uselessness; isolation; suspicion of others; anxiety and agitation; sleep problems; and appetite problems and weight loss. Less common yet critical symptoms that should be reviewed include the presence or absence of suicidal thoughts, profound anhedonia, impulsive behavior ("I can't control myself"), confusion, delusions, and hallucinations. The review of symptoms is most valuable when it is considered within the context of symptom presentation: When did these symptoms begin? How long have they lasted? Has their severity changed over time? Are there physical or environmental events that precipitate them? What steps, if any, have been taken to try to correct the symptoms? Have any of these interventions proved successful? Do the symptoms vary during the day (diurnal variation)? Do they vary during the week or with the seasons? Do they form clusters—that is, are they associated with one another? Which symptoms appear to be ego-syntonic, and which appear ego-dystonic? As symptoms are reviewed, a specific time frame facilitates focus on the present illness. Having a 1-month or 6-month window enables the patient to review symptoms and events temporally—an approach not usually taken by distressed older persons, who tend to concentrate on immediate suffering.

Critical to the assessment of the present illness is an assessment of function and change in function. The two parameters that are most important (and are not included in usual assessments of physical and psychiatric illness) are social functioning and activities of daily living. Many scales have been developed to assess activities of daily living; however, in the interview, the clinician can simply ask about the patient's ability to get around (e.g., walk inside and outside the house), to perform certain physical activities independently (e.g., bathe, dress, shave, brush teeth, select clothes), and to do instrumental activities (e.g., cook, maintain a bank account, shop, drive). It is also important to assess how often the patient engages in these activities; for example, being able to walk outside does not always translate to exercising outside.

Past History

Next, the clinician must review the past history of symptoms and episodes. Has the patient had similar episodes in the past? How long did those episodes last? When did they occur? How many times in the patient's lifetime have such episodes occurred? Unfortunately, the older adult may not equate present distress with past episodes that are symptomatically similar, so the perspective of the family is especially valuable in the attempt to link current and past episodes. Other psychiatric and medical problems should be reviewed as well, especially medical illnesses that have led to hospitalization and the use of medication. Not infrequently, an older adult has experienced a major illness or trauma in childhood or as a younger adult but views this information as irrelevant to the present episode and therefore dismisses it. Eliciting these data is essential. Older adults may ignore or even forget past psychiatric difficulties, especially if these difficulties were disguised. For example, mood swings in early or mid-life may have occurred during periods of excessive and productive activity, episodes of excessive alcohol intake, or periods of vague, undiagnosed physical problems. An older person sometimes becomes angry or irritated when the clinician continues to probe. Reassurance regarding the importance of obtaining this information will generally suffice, except when dealing with a patient who cannot tolerate the discomfort and distress even for brief periods. Older persons who have chronic and moderately severe anxiety or a histrionic personality style, as well as distressed cognitive disorder, tolerate their symptoms poorly.

Family History

The distribution of psychiatric symptoms and illnesses in the family should be determined next. The older person with symptoms consistent with major neurocognitive impairment may have a family history of a disorder such as major neurocognitive disorder due to Alzheimer's disease. The genogram can be valuable for charting the distribution of mental illness and other relevant behaviors throughout the family tree. This genogram should include parents, blood-related aunts and uncles, brothers and sisters, spouse(s), children, grandchildren, and great-grandchildren (recognizing that data from many family members will not be complete). A history should be obtained about institutionalization, significant memory problems in family members, hospitalization for a nervous breakdown or depressive disorder, suicide, alcohol abuse and dependence, electroconvulsive therapy, long-term residence in a mental health facility (and possibly a diagnosis of schizophrenia), and use of mental health services by family members (Blazer 1984).

Of relevance to the pharmacological treatment of certain disorders—especially depression—in older adults is the tendency of family members to respond therapeutically to the same pharmacological agent. If the patient has a depressive disorder, and biological relatives have been treated effectively for depression, the clinician should determine what pharmacological agent was used to treat a relative's depression. For example, a positive response to sertraline in a family member could make sertraline the initial drug of choice for treating this patient, assuming that side effects are not an issue (Ayd 1975).

Accurate genetic information can be better obtained when family members from more than one generation are interviewed. Many psychiatric disorders are characterized by a variety of symptoms, so asking only the patient or one family member for the family's history of depression is insufficient. Research on the genetic expression of psychiatric disorders in families requires the psychiatric investigator to interview directly as many family members as possible to determine accurately the distribution of disorders throughout the family. Such a detailed family assessment is not feasible for clinicians, yet a telephone call to a relative—with permission from the patient—may become a standard of clinical assessment as the genetics of psychiatric disorders are clarified.

Social Functioning

Questions should be asked about the social interaction of the older adult, such as the frequency of visits made outside the home, telephone calls received or made, and visits from family and friends, as well as the quality of these interactions. Social isolation and loneliness are frequent and serious problems for many older adults. Forty-three percent of adults in the United States who are 60 years of age and older report feeling lonely, and one-quarter of those who live in community settings are lonely (National Academies of Sciences, Engineering, and Medicine 2020). Social isolation can be assessed using the Berkman-Syme Social Network Index (Berkman and Syme 1979), and loneliness can be assessed using the UCLA Loneliness Scale (Russell 1996). Both social isolation and loneliness (which are not identical constructs) lead to significant risk of several psychiatric disorders and of premature mortality.

Context

Psychiatric disorders occur in a biomedical and psychosocial context. Although the clinician will try to determine what medical problems the patient has experienced, it is possible to overlook a variation in the relative contribution of these medical disorders to psychopathology or to overlook the psychosocial contribution to the onset and continuance of the problem. Has the spouse of the older adult undergone a change? Are the middle-aged children managing high stress, such as simultaneously caring for an emotionally disturbed child and the loss of employment? Are the grandchildren placing emotional stress on the elderly patient, perhaps by requesting money? Has the economic status of the older adult deteriorated? Has the availability of medical care changed? Although many psychiatric disorders are biologically driven, they do not occur in a psychosocial vacuum. Environmental precipitants remain important in the web of causation that leads to the onset of emotional distress and are critical to the assessment of the older adult.

Medication History

A careful review of the older patient's current and past medications by the clinician, a nurse, or a physician's assistant is essential. The patient should be asked to bring to the appointment all pill bottles, a list of medications taken, and the dosage schedule. A comparison between the written schedule and the pill containers will frequently expose some discrepancy. Both prescription and over-the-counter drugs, such as laxatives and vitamins, should be recorded. The clinician can then identify medications that potentially lead to drug–drug interactions and ask about these during subsequent patient visits. Most elderly persons take a variety of medicines simultaneously, and the potential for drug–drug interaction is high. For example, concomitant use of escitalopram and aspirin can lead to an increased risk of bleeding. Some medications prescribed for older persons—such as the β-blocker metoprolol and calcium channel blockers—can exacerbate or produce depressive symptoms.

Older persons are less likely than younger persons to have a substance use disorder, but a careful history of alcohol and drug intake (especially nonprescription use of prescription medications) is essential to the diagnostic workup. Although older persons do not usually volunteer information about their substance intake, they are generally forthcoming when asked about their drinking habits.

Medical History

Given the high likelihood of comorbid medical problems associated with psychiatric disorders in late life, a comprehensive medical history is essential. Most older persons see a primary care physician regularly (although decreasing payments from Medicare render this assumption less accurate each year). The geriatric psychiatrist should obtain medical records if possible (much easier today with the use of the electronic health record). Major illnesses should be recorded. A brief contact with the patient's primary care physician can be extremely useful.

Family Assessment

Clinicians working with older adults must be equipped to evaluate the family—both its functionality and its potential as a resource for the patient. Geriatric psychiatry, almost by definition, is family psychiatry. The family assessment is best done, if possible, in conjunction with a family member who is providing care and support for the older adult (Blazer 1984). Social workers can be of great help in gathering family history. The purpose of a comprehensive diagnostic family workup is to determine the nature of the family structure regarding interaction, the presence or absence of a crisis in the family, and the type and amount of support available to the older adult. A primary goal of the clinician, as advocate for the older adult with psychiatric disturbance, is to facilitate family support for the patient during a time of disability. At least four parameters of support are important for clinicians to evaluate as the treatment plan evolves: 1) the availability of family members to the older person over time; 2) the tangible services provided by the family to the older person; 3) the perception of family support by the older patient (and therefore the patient's willingness to cooperate and accept support); and 4) tolerance by the family of specific behaviors that derive from the psychiatric disorder.

What specific "tangible services" can be provided to older adults by family members? Even the most devoted spouse can be limited in delivering certain services. For example, he or she may not drive and therefore cannot provide transportation or is not physically strong enough to provide certain types of nursing care. Generic services of special importance to at-home support of the older adult with psychiatric impairment include transportation; nursing services (e.g., administering medications at home); physical therapy; checks on or continuous supervision of the patient; homemaker and household services; meal preparation; administrative, legal, and protective services; financial assistance; living quarters; and coordination of the delivery of services. These services are considered generic because they can be defined by their activities, regardless of who provides each service. Assessing the range and extent of service delivery by the family to the older person with functional impairment provides a convenient barometer of the economic, social, and emotional burdens placed on the family.

Intangible supports include the perception of a dependable network, participation or interaction in the network, a sense of belonging to the network, intimacy with network members, and a sense of usefulness to the family (Blazer and Kaplan 1983). The sense of usefulness may be of less importance to some older adults who believe they have contributed to the family for many years and therefore deserve reciprocal services in their waning years. Unfortunately, family members, frequently stressed across generations, may not recognize this reciprocal responsibility. Family tolerance of specific behaviors may not correlate with overall support; every person has a level of tolerance for behaviors that are especially difficult to manage. Sanford (1975) found that the following behaviors were tolerated by families of older persons with impairments (in decreasing percentages): incontinence of urine (81%), personality conflicts (54%), falls (52%), physically aggressive behavior (44%), inability to walk unaided (33%), daytime wandering (33%), and sleep disturbance (16%). These relative frequencies may appear counterintuitive, because incontinence is generally considered particularly aversive to family members; however, although the outcome can be corrected easily enough, a few nights of no sleep can easily push family members beyond their capabilities for serving a parent, sibling, or spouse.

Mental Status Examination

Although physicians and other clinicians are sometimes hesitant to perform a structured mental status examination, it is central to the diagnostic workup. Many aspects of this examination can be assessed during the history-taking interview.

Appearance may be affected by the older patient's psychiatric symptoms (e.g., a patient with depression may neglect grooming), cognitive status (e.g., a patient with dementia may be unable to match clothing or dress him- or herself appropriately), and environment (e.g., a nursing home patient may not be groomed as well as a patient living at home with a spouse). Affect and mood can usually be assessed by observing the patient during the interview. *Affect* is the emotional tone that accompanies the patient's cognitive output (Linn 1980). This may fluctuate during the interview, but the older person is more likely to demonstrate a constriction of affect. *Mood*, the state that underlies overt affect and is sustained over time, is usually apparent by the end of the interview. For example, the affect of an older adult with depression may not reach the degree of dysphoria seen in younger persons (as evidenced by crying spells or protestations of uncontrollable despair), yet the depressed mood is usually sustained and discernible from beginning to end.

Psychomotor activity may be agitated or retarded and is especially important to determine in the evaluation of mood disorders, neurocognitive disorders, and delirium. Psychiatrically impaired older adults, except some with advanced neurocognitive disorder, are more likely to exhibit hyperactivity or agitation. Those who are depressed will appear uneasy, move their hands frequently, and have difficulty remaining seated during the interview. Pacing is often observed when the older adult is admitted to a hospital ward. Occasionally, the older adult with psychomotor retardation may be experiencing a disturbance in consciousness and may even reach an almost stuporous state, as in delirium. He or she may not be easily aroused, but when aroused, may respond with grimacing or withdrawal.

Perception is the awareness of objects in relation to each other and follows stimulation of the peripheral sense organs (Linn 1980). Disturbances of perception include hallucinations—that is, false sensory perceptions that are not associated with real or external stimuli. For example, an older person experiencing paranoia may perceive nighttime invasions of his or her home by individuals who disarrange belongings and abuse the patient sexually. Hallucinations often take the form of false auditory perceptions, false perceptions of movement or body sensation (e.g., palpitations), and false perceptions of smell, taste, or touch. Older patients with severe depression may have frank auditory hallucinations that condemn or encourage self-destructive behavior.

Disturbances in thought content are the most prominent disturbances of cognition noted in older patients with psychosis. Patients with severe depression often develop beliefs that are inconsistent with objective information obtained from family members about their abilities and social resources. Meyers and Greenberg (1986) found delusional depression to be more prevalent among older patients with depression than among middle-aged adults. Of 161 patients with endogenous depression, 72 (45%) were found to be delusional. Delusions included beliefs such as "I've lost my mind," "My body is disintegrating," "I have an incurable illness," and "I have caused some great harm." Even after elderly persons recover from depression, they may still experience periodic recurrences of delusional thoughts, which can be disturbing to otherwise rational older adults. Older patients appear to be less likely to feel delusional remorse, guilt, or persecution. Even if delusions are not obvious, preoccupation with a particular thought or idea is common among elderly persons with depression. Such preoccupation is closely associated with obsessional thinking or the irresistible intrusion of thoughts into the conscious mind. Although older adults rarely act on these thoughts compulsively, guilt-provoking or self-accusing thoughts may occasionally become so difficult to bear that the person considers, attempts, or dies by suicide.

Disturbances of thought progression accompany disturbances of content. Evaluation of the content and process of cognition may uncover disturbances such as problems with the structure or speed of associations and the content of thought. Thinking is a goal-directed flow of ideas, symbols, and associations initiated in response to environmental stimuli, a perceived problem, or a task that requires progression to a logical or reality-based conclusion (Linn 1980). The older adult who is compulsive or has schizophrenia may pathologically repeat the same word or idea in response to various probes, as may the patient who has major neurocognitive disorder. Some older adults with a neurocognitive disorder exhibit circumstantiality—that is, the introduction of many apparently irrelevant details to cover a lack of clarity and memory problems. Interviews with patients who have this problem can be frustrating because they proceed very slowly. On other occasions, elderly patients may appear incoherent, with no logical connection to their thoughts, or may produce irrelevant answers. The intrusion of thoughts from previous conversations into a current conversation is a prime example of the disturbance in association found in patients with major neurocognitive disorder.

Suicidal thoughts are critical to assess in the elderly patient with psychiatric impairment. Although thoughts of death are common in late life, spontaneous revelations of suicidal thoughts are rare. A stepwise probe is the best means of assessing the presence of suicidal ideation (Blazer 1982). The clinician should ask if the patient has ever thought that life was not worth living. If so, has the patient considered acting on that thought? If so, how would the patient attempt to inflict such harm? If definite plans are revealed, the clinician should probe to determine whether the implements for a suicide attempt are available. For example, if a patient has considered shooting himself, the clinician should ask, "Do you have a gun available and loaded at home?" Suicidal ideation in an older adult is always of concern, but intervention is necessary when suicide has been considered seriously and the implements are available.

Memory and cognitive status are most accurately assessed through neuropsychological testing. However, the psychiatric interview of the older adult should include a reasonable assessment. Although they may not complain of memory dysfunction, older adults are more likely than younger patients to have problems with memory, concentration, and intellect. Brief, informal means of testing cognitive functioning should be included in the diagnostic workup. The clinician proceeding through an evaluation of memory and intellect must also remember that poor performance may reflect psychic distress or a lack of education as opposed to intellectual disability or neurocognitive disorder. Testing can also be performed on more than one occasion to rule out the potential confounding of agitation and anxiety. More formal brief testing, such as with the Mini-Mental State Examination (MMSE; Folstein et al. 1975), provides a baseline from which performance can be documented over time.

Memory testing is based on three essential processes: 1) registration (the ability to record an experience in the CNS), 2) retention (the persistence and permanence of a registered experience), and 3) recall (the ability to summon consciously the registered experience and report it) (Linn 1980). *Registration*, apart from recall, is difficult to evaluate directly. Occasionally, events or information that the older adult denies remembering will appear spontaneously during other parts of the interview. Registration usually is not impaired except in patients with a major neurocognitive disorder. *Retention*, on the other hand, can be blocked by both psychic distress and brain dysfunction. Lack of retention is especially relevant to the unimportant data often requested in a mental status examination. For example, asking the older adult to remember three objects for 5 minutes frequently reveals a deficit if the patient has little motivation to attempt the task.

Disturbances of *recall* can be tested directly in several ways. The most common are tests of orientation to time, place, person, and situation. Most persons continually orient themselves through radio, television, and reading material and through conversations with others. Some elderly persons may be isolated due to sensory impairment or lack of social contact; poor orientation in these patients may represent deficits in the physical and social environment rather than brain dysfunction. Immediate recall can be tested by asking the older person to repeat a word, phrase, or series of numbers or be tested in conjunction with cognitive skills by requesting that a word be spelled backward or that elements of a story be recalled.

During the mental status examination, *intelligence* can be assessed only superficially. Tests of simple arithmetic calculation and fund of knowledge, supplemented by portions of well-known psychiatric tests, are helpful. The classic test for calculation is to ask a patient to subtract 7 from 100 and to repeat this operation on the succession of remainders. Usually, five calculations are sufficient to determine the older adult's ability to complete this task. If the older adult fails the task, a less exacting test is to ask the patient to subtract 3 from 20 and to repeat this operation until 0 is reached. These examinations must not be rushed because older persons may not perform as well when they perceive time pressure. A capacity for *abstract thinking* is often tested by asking the patient to interpret a well-known proverb, such as "A rolling stone gathers no moss." A more accurate test, however, is to ask the patient to classify objects in a common category, for example, asking the patient to state the similarity between an apple and a pear. Whereas naming objects from a category, such as fruits, is retained despite moderate and sometimes marked declines in cognition, the opposite process of classifying two different objects in a common category is not retained as well.

The older adult being examined may meet usual standards during the assessment of cognitive functioning. However, evaluating "cognitive aging" is critical during the examination. *Cognitive aging* is the lifelong progression of change in cognitive capacity. It is not a disease or a quantifiable level of function, and the process is gradual and ongoing. For example, episodic memory and executive function exhibit, on average, a gradual decline over many years that accelerates in later life. Yet this process is highly variable within and between individuals. Some individuals may do well on a typical cognitive status questionnaire, such as the MMSE, yet have difficulty with tasks such as paying monthly bills. Driving skills may decrease to the point that the older adult cannot drive safely due to slowed reaction time. Once again, a discussion with the family regarding their concerns about the independent functioning of their older member is critical to identify these deficits. One area receiving increased attention is the role of fraud and abuse, because older persons are especially at risk of receiving soliciting calls and email attempts to obtain vital information.

Rating Scales and Standardized Interviews

Rating scales and standardized interviews have progressively been incorporated into the diagnostic assessment of elderly psychiatric patients. Such rating procedures have increased in popularity as the need has increased for systematic, reproducible assessments for third-party carriers and for a standard means of assessing change in clinical status. The scores or even the scales themselves can be incorporated into the electronic health record. A thorough review of all instruments used is beyond the scope of this chapter; therefore, selected instruments are presented and evaluated, chosen either because they have special relevance to geriatric patients or because they are widely utilized.

Screens for Neurocognitive Disorders

A number of standardized assessment methods for delirium have emerged. Perhaps the best and the most easily used is the Confusion Assessment Method (CAM; Inouye et al. 1990). The CAM assesses nine characteristics of delirium, such as acute onset (evidence of such onset), fluctuating course (behavior change during the day), inattention (trouble in focusing), disorganized thinking (presence of rambling or irrelevant conversations and illogical flow of ideas), and altered level of consciousness (rated from alert to comatose). Diagnosis of delirium according to DSM-5 criteria can be derived from the CAM.

Two interviewer-administered cognitive screens for neurocognitive disorder have been popular in both clinical and community studies. The Montreal Cognitive Assessment (MoCA; Nasreddine et al. 2005), a one-page, 30-point assessment, is used to assess several cognitive domains relevant to neurocognitive disorders. The short-term memory recall task includes two learning trials of five nouns and delayed recall after approximately 5 minutes. Visuospatial abilities are assessed using the Clock Drawing Test and a three-dimensional cube copy. Multiple aspects of executive functions are assessed using an alternation task (e.g., moving from numbers to letters in a systematic process), a phonemic fluency task, and a two-item verbal abstraction task. Attention, concentration, and working memory are evaluated using a sustained attention task, a serial subtraction task, and digits forward and backward. Language is assessed using a three-item confrontation naming task with low-familiarity animals (e.g., lion, camel, rhinoceros), repetition of two syntactically complex sentences, and the aforementioned fluency task. Finally, orientation to time and place is evaluated. The MMSE is a 30-item screening instrument that assesses orientation, registration, attention and calculation, recall, and language. It requires 5–10 minutes to administer. Making 7–12 errors suggests mild to moderate cognitive impairment, and 13 or more errors indicates severe impairment. The MMSE is perhaps the most frequently used standardized screening instrument in clinical practice.

Depression Rating Scales

A number of self-rating depression scales have been used to screen for depression in patients at all stages of the life cycle, and most of these scales have been studied in older populations. The instrument currently most widely used in community studies is the Center for Epidemiological Studies–Depression Scale (CES-D; Radloff 1977), which consists of 20 behaviors and feelings. Patients indicate how frequently each was experienced over the past week (from no days to most days). In a factor-analytic study of the CES-D in a community population, four factors were identified: somatic symptoms, positive affect, negative affect, and interpersonal relationships (Ross and Mirowsky 1984). The disaggregation of these factors and exploration of their interaction are significant steps forward in understanding the results derived from symptom scales such as the CES-D in older populations. For example, the somatic items (e.g., loss of interest, poor appetite) are more likely to be associated with a course of depressive episodes similar to that described for major depression with melancholia, and the positive-affect items are more likely to be associated with life satisfaction scores.

The Geriatric Depression Scale (GDS) was developed because the CES-D presents problems for older persons who have difficulty selecting one of four forced-response items (Yesavage et al. 1982–1983). The GDS is a 30-item scale that permits patients to rate items as either present or absent; it includes questions about symptoms such as cognitive complaints, self-image, and losses. Items selected are thought to have relevance to late-life depression. The GDS has not been used extensively in community populations and is not as well standardized as the CES-D, but many clinicians prefer its Yes/No format to the CES-D's frequency ratings.

A scale that has received considerable attention clinically, having been standardized in clinical but not community populations, is the Montgomery-Åsberg Depression Rating Scale (MADRS; Montgomery and Åsberg 1979). This scale concentrates on 10 symptoms of depression; the clinician rates each symptom on a scale of 0–6 (for a range of total scores between 0 and 60). The symptoms include apparent sadness, reported sadness, inattention, reduced sleep, reduced appetite, concentration difficulties, lassitude, inability to feel, pessimistic thoughts, and suicidal thoughts.

The Patient Health Questionnaire–9 (PHQ-9; Kroenke et al. 2001) is a brief clinical screen for depression widely used in primary care but probably not applicable to psychiatric practice given that the clinician's assessment of depressive symptoms almost always would be in greater depth than that obtained by this instrument.

General Assessment Scales

Some general assessment scales of psychiatric status (occasionally combined with functioning in other areas) have been found to be useful in both community and clinical populations. DSM-5 has adopted the World Health Organization Disability Assessment Schedule (WHODAS) 2.0 to assess disability in adults age 18 years and older (World Health Organization 2010; the scale is also available in DSM-5 Section III, "Emerging Measures and Models"). This 36-item self-assessment is divided into six areas of functioning: understanding and communicating, getting around, self-care, getting along with people, life activities (i.e., household, work, or school activities), and participation in society.

Any discussion of clinical rating scales is not complete without a discussion of the Abnormal Involuntary Movement Scale (AIMS; National Institute of Mental Health 1975). The incidence of tardive dyskinesia has increased among older adults, coupled with the need for better documentation of this outcome due to prolonged use of antipsychotic agents. Regular ratings of patients with the AIMS by clinicians have therefore become essential to the practice of inpatient and outpatient geriatric psychiatry. The AIMS consists of seven movement disorders; the presence and severity of each is rated from *none* to *severe*. Three items require a global judgment: severity of abnormal movements, incapacitation due to abnormal movements, and patient awareness of abnormal movements. Current problems with teeth or dentures are also assessed. Procedures are described to increase the reliability of this rating scale.

Structured Diagnostic Interviews

Several structured interview schedules are available for both clinical and community diagnosis. These interview schedules have allowed increased reliability of the identification of symptoms and psychiatric diagnoses; however, if one adheres closely to the structured interview, the richness inherent in the unstructured interview tends to be lost. Comments made by the patient during the evaluation that could be used to trace relevant associations must be ignored in order to push through the interview schedule. Most of these interviews require more time than the traditional unstructured first session with the patient.

The most frequently used structured interview instrument in the United States is the Structured Clinical Interview for DSM-5 (SCID; First et al. 2016). This instrument is tailored to DSM-5. Although specific questions are suggested for probing most areas of interest, the interviewer using the SCID has the flexibility to ask additional questions and can use any available data to assign a diagnosis. The interviewer must have clinical training but does not have to be a psychiatrist. Many of the symptoms may not be relevant to older adults (especially the extensive probes for psychotic symptoms), and the interview frequently takes 2.5–3 hours to administer. Nevertheless, the experience gained by the clinician in using this instrument can contribute to a more effective clinical practice.

Effective Communication With the Older Adult

Clinicians who work with older adults should be cognizant of factors relating to both patients and themselves that may produce barriers to effective communication (Blazer 1978). Many older persons experience a relatively high level of anxiety yet do not complain of this symptom. Stress deriving from a new situation, such as visiting a clinician's office or being interviewed in a hospital, may intensify such anxiety and subsequently impair effective communication. Perceptual problems, such as hearing and visual impairment, may exacerbate disorientation and complicate the communication of problems to the clinician. Elderly persons are more likely to withhold information than to hazard answers that may be incorrect—in other words, older persons tend to be more cautious. Elderly persons frequently take longer to respond to inquiries and resist the clinician who attempts to rush through the history-taking interview.

The elderly patient may perceive the physician unrealistically based on previous life experiences (i.e., transference may occur). Although older patients sometimes accept the role of child, viewing the physician as parent, they are initially more likely to view the clinician as the idealized child providing reciprocal care to the previously capable but now impaired parent. Splitting between the physician (idealized) and the child of the patient (devalued) may subsequently occur. Also, clinicians may perceive older adult patients incorrectly because of fears of aging and death or because of previous negative experiences with their own parents. For clinicians to work effectively with older adults, these personal feelings should be discussed during training and afterward.

Once physician and patient attitudes have been recognized and acknowledged, certain techniques have generally proved to be valuable in communicating with elderly patients. These techniques should not be implemented indiscriminately, however, because the variation in the population of older adults is significant. First, the older person should be approached with respect. The clinician should knock before entering the patient's room and should greet the patient by surname (e.g., Mr. Jones, Mrs. Smith) rather than by a given name, unless the clinician also wishes to be addressed by a given name. After taking a position near the patient—near enough to reach out and touch him or her—the clinician should speak clearly and slowly and use simple sentences in case the person's hearing is impaired. Because of hearing problems, older patients may understand conversation better over the telephone than in person. By placing the receiver against the mastoid bone, the patient with otosclerosis can take advantage of preserved bone conduction.

The interview should be paced so that the patient has enough time to respond to questions. Most older individuals are not uncomfortable with silence because it gives them a welcome opportunity to formulate their answers to questions and to elaborate certain points they may wish to emphasize. Nonverbal communication is frequently a key to effective communication with elderly individuals because they may be reticent about revealing affect verbally. The patient's facial expressions, gestures, postures, and long silences may provide clues to the clinician about issues that are unspoken. One key to successful communication with an older adult is a willingness to continue working as a professional with that person. Older adults—possibly unlike some of their children and grandchildren—place a great deal of stress on loyalty and continuity. Most elderly patients do not require large amounts of time from clinicians, and those who are more demanding can usually be controlled through the structure of the interview.

Conclusion

The psychiatric interview is critical to the evaluation and eventual treatment of psychiatric disorders in older adults. Over the past few years, many measures have become available to clinicians to assist in this diagnostic effort. Nevertheless, sitting down with the patient and family, engaging them in a semistructured interview, and simply "getting to know them" remain the key components of the evaluation. In our busy clinical world, time has become increasingly scarce, and therefore, skimping on diagnostic interview is quite tempting. In the long run, however, a thorough psychiatric interview at patient intake will save the entire team much time, ensure a better therapeutic relationship, and improve therapeutic outcomes.

Key Points

- The diagnostic interview is the cornerstone of assessment and treatment assignment for the older adult with psychiatric impairment.

- A thorough medication history, although it takes time to obtain, saves valuable time and avoids complications in the treatment of psychiatric disorders in older adults.

- Functional status (i.e., the ability to perform usual activities of daily living) is often as important as diagnosis in tracking the progress of treatment of psychiatric disorders in older adults.

- Geriatric psychiatry is family psychiatry.

- What is gained in reliability by using a structured diagnostic interview is offset by the loss of valuable information about the subjective feelings of the older adult and the context of symptom emergence.

- Speak clearly and slowly but not in a patronizing way to the older adult, who might have a hearing impairment.

Suggested Readings

Blazer DG: Techniques for communicating with your elderly patient. Geriatrics 33:79–80, 83–84, 1978 710895

Inouye SK: Clarifying confusion: the Confusion Assessment Method: a new method for detection of delirium. Ann Intern Med 113:941–950, 1990 2240918

Nasreddine ZS, Phillips NA, Bédirian V, et al: The Montreal Cognitive Assessment (MoCA): a brief screening tool for mild cognitive impairment. J Am Geriatr Soc 53:695–699, 2005 15817019

Othmer E, Othmer SC, Othmer JP: Psychiatric interview, history and mental status examination, in Kaplan and Sadock's Comprehensive Textbook of Psychiatry, Vol 1. Edited by Sadock BJ, Sadock VA. Philadelphia, PA, Lippincott Williams and Wilkins, 2005, pp 794–826

References

American Psychiatric Association: Diagnostic and Statistical Manual of Mental Disorders, 4th Edition. Washington, DC, American Psychiatric Association, 1994

American Psychiatric Association: Diagnostic and Statistical Manual of Mental Disorders, 4th Edition, Text Revision. Washington, DC, American Psychiatric Association, 2000

American Psychiatric Association: Diagnostic and Statistical Manual of Mental Disorders, 5th Edition. Arlington, VA, American Psychiatric Association, 2013

Ayd FJ: Treatment-resistant patients: a moral, legal and therapeutic challenge, in Rational Psychopharmacotherapy and the Right to Treatment. Edited by Ayd FJ. Baltimore, MD, Ayd Medical Communications, 1975, pp 3–15

Berkman LF, Syme SL: Social networks, host resistance, and mortality: a nine-year follow-up study of Alameda County residents. Am J Epidemiol 109(2):186–204, 1979 425958

Blazer DG: Techniques for communicating with your elderly patient. Geriatrics 33:79–80, 83–84, 1978 710895

Blazer DG: Depression in Late Life. St Louis, MO, CV Mosby, 1982

Blazer DG: Evaluating the family of the elderly patient, in A Family Approach to Health Care in the Elderly. Edited by Blazer D, Siegler IC. Menlo Park, CA, Addison-Wesley, 1984, pp 13–32

Blazer DG, Kaplan BH: The assessment of social support in an elderly community population. American Journal of Social Psychiatry 3:29–36, 1983

Eisenberg L: Disease and illness: distinctions between professional and popular ideas of sickness. Cult Med Psychiatry 1(1):9–23, 1977 756356

First MB, Williams JBW, Karg RS, Spitzer RL: Structured Clinical Interview for DSM-5 Disorders, Clinician Version. Arlington, VA, American Psychiatric Association, 2016

Folstein MF, Folstein SE, McHugh PR: "Mini-mental state": a practical method for grading the cognitive state of patients for the clinician. J Psychiatr Res 12(3):189–198, 1975 1202204

Inouye SK, van Dyck CH, Alessi CA, et al: Clarifying confusion: the Confusion Assessment Method: a new method for detection of delirium. Ann Intern Med 113(12):941–948, 1990 2240918

Kroenke K, Spitzer RL, Williams JB: The PHQ-9: validity of a brief depression severity measure. J Gen Intern Med 16(9):606–613, 2001 11556941

Linn L: Clinical manifestations of psychiatric disorders, in Comprehensive Textbook of Psychiatry, 3rd Edition, Vol 1. Edited by Kaplan HI, Freedman AM, Sadock BJ. Baltimore, MD, Williams and Wilkins, 1980, pp 990–1034

Meyers BS, Greenberg R: Late-life delusional depression. J Affect Disord 11(2):133–137, 1986 2948986

Montgomery SA, Åsberg M: A new depression scale designed to be sensitive to change. Br J Psychiatry 134:382–389, 1979 444788

Nasreddine ZS, Phillips NA, Bédirian V, et al: The Montreal Cognitive Assessment, MoCA: a brief screening tool for mild cognitive impairment. J Am Geriatr Soc 53(4):695–699, 2005 15817019

National Academies of Sciences, Engineering, and Medicine: Social Isolation and Loneliness in Older Adults: Opportunities for the Health Care System. Washington, DC, National Academies Press, 2020

National Institute of Mental Health: Development of a Dyskinetic Movement Scale (Publ No 4). Rockville, MD, National Institute of Mental Health, Psychopharmacology Research Branch, 1975

Radloff LS: The CES-D Scale: a self-report depression scale for research in the general population. Appl Psychol Meas 1:385–401, 1977

Ross CE, Mirowsky J: Components of depressed mood in married men and women: the Center for Epidemiologic Studies' Depression Scale. Am J Epidemiol 119(6):997–1004, 1984 6731436

Russell DW: UCLA Loneliness Scale (Version 3): reliability, validity, and factor structure. J Pers Assess 66(1):20–40, 1996 8576833

Sanford JRA: Tolerance of debility in elderly dependents by supporters at home: its significance for hospital practice. BMJ 3(5981):471–473, 1975 1156826

World Health Organization: Measuring Health and Disability: Manual for WHO Disability Assessment Schedule (WHODAS 2.0). Edited by Üstün TB, Kostanjsek N, Chatterji S, Rehm J. Geneva, Switzerland, World Health Organization, 2010. Available at: http://whqlibdoc.who.int/publications/2010/9789241547598_eng.pdf. Accessed October 2014.

Yesavage JA, Brink TL, Rose TL, et al: Development and validation of a geriatric depression screening scale: a preliminary report. J Psychiatr Res 17(1):37–49, 1982–1983 7183759

Use of the Laboratory in the Diagnostic Workup of Older Adults

Elizabeth Hathaway, M.D.

Sophia Wang, M.D.

Laboratory testing is an essential component of the psychiatric evaluation of elderly individuals, who often present with comorbid medical illnesses. The laboratory does not replace the clinician; no test is pathognomonic for a primary psychiatric illness. However, laboratory testing does aid in the evaluation of comorbidities that complicate or contribute to a psychiatric diagnosis. The number and quality of diagnostic tools available have grown significantly. Progress in research and technology, particularly in imaging technology and genetic testing, has advanced rapidly over the past decade. Regardless of the tools available, however, we must balance what we *can* do with what we *should* do, as guided by our clinical judgment, relative risk to the patient, and cost expenditure. When all risks are considered, the decision to proceed with a test should be based on the clinical presentation and on how the test results may change a treatment plan.

The following discussion of specific diagnostic tests is not an exhaustive review. We focus on tests currently being used or being considered for clinical use. We hope this chapter will assist the clinician in selecting laboratory tests that are appropriate for the individual patient.

Serological Tests

Basic clinical chemistry and hematological screens are routine for all hospital admissions and many outpatient evaluations. These screens are critical for identifying any previously undiagnosed or poorly controlled medical illnesses that may contribute to mental status changes, such as in dementia or delirium. These tests should also be monitored when patients are taking medications that may result in potentially dangerous abnormalities. For most tests, the only risks are those associated with blood draws, which may result in transient pain, bruising, and occasional bleeding or fainting. These risks can be significantly reduced, however, when the draws are performed by skilled phlebotomists.

Hematological Tests

A complete blood count (CBC) is a standard part of any evaluation. It screens for multiple problems, including infections and anemia, and provides a platelet count, which is important to monitor in patients taking psychiatric medications associated with thrombocytopenia, such as divalproex sodium or carbamazepine. This concern is particularly important in elderly patients because the risk of drug-induced thrombocytopenia may increase with age. Lithium, in contrast, may result in mild leukocytosis. Because of the risk of agranulocytosis, CBC testing is required weekly or biweekly for patients taking clozapine and may be needed more frequently if the patient develops signs of infection. Mirtazapine can also lead to agranulocytosis in rare cases, and although routine CBC monitoring is not indicated, it should be pursued if a patient develops sore throat, fever, stomatitis, or other signs of infection.

Chemistry Tests

Most general chemistry panels have a variety of values that may be helpful in medical evaluations. Blood glucose values may reveal hypoglycemia, which may produce anxiety and weakness; more commonly, these tests show hyperglycemia, which may be associated with diabetes and may result in lethargy or, in severe cases, delirium, diabetic coma, or ketoacidosis. This testing is critical for the diagnosis of diabetes, which can be diagnosed with a hemoglobin A1C level ≥6.5%, a fasting plasma glucose level >126 mg/dL, a random plasma glucose level ≥200 mg/dL in a patient with symptoms of diabetes, or an oral glucose tolerance test showing a plasma glucose level ≥200 mg/dL 2 hours after a 75-g glucose load (American Diabetes Association 2020). Kidney function tests are also important. Blood urea nitrogen and creatinine will be elevated in kidney failure and in hypovolemic states such as dehydration. Kidney tests also must be performed before initiating lithium therapy because of that drug's potential for nephrotoxicity. General chemistry panels also measure serum sodium, potassium, and other electrolytes.

Hyponatremia—defined as a serum sodium concentration <135 mEq/L—has been reported with selective serotonin reuptake inhibitors (SSRIs), particularly in elderly patients. The signs and symptoms of hyponatremia result from neurological dysfunction secondary to cerebral edema. Acute hyponatremia can start with nausea and malaise when the plasma sodium concentration falls below 125–130 mEq/L and progress rapidly to coma and respiratory arrest if the plasma sodium concentration falls below 115–120 mEq/L. In chronic hyponatremia, the brain cells adapt to the edema, and symptoms are much less severe. Patients may be asymptomatic despite a plasma sodium concentration that is persistently as low as 115–120 mEq/L. When symptoms occur in individuals with such low sodium concentrations, they are relatively nonspe-

TABLE 5–1. **Guidelines for screening and monitoring of patients taking second-generation antipsychotics[a]**

Assessment	Frequency
Personal and family history[b]	At baseline and annually
Weight	At baseline, every 4 weeks for 12 weeks, then quarterly
Waist circumference[c]	At baseline and annually
Blood pressure	At baseline, at 12 weeks, and annually
Fasting plasma glucose	At baseline, at 12 weeks, and annually
Fasting lipid profile	At baseline, at 12 weeks, and every 5 years

[a]More frequent assessments may need to be done based on clinical status.
[b]Personal and family history includes obesity, diabetes, dyslipidemia, hypertension, and cardiovascular disease.
[c]Waist circumference is measured at umbilicus.
Source. American Diabetes Association et al. 2004.

cific (e.g., fatigue, nausea, dizziness, gait disturbances, forgetfulness, confusion, lethargy, muscle cramps). The clinician should be vigilant to this risk in older adults who begin taking SSRIs. Of all the electrolyte abnormalities, potassium disorders may be the most crucial to identify. These rarely cause psychiatric symptoms but may result in severe cardiac arrhythmias. Although not always included in routine chemistry screens, calcium and magnesium levels are also important to consider, because abnormal levels may result in paranoid ideation or frank psychosis. Any or all of these results may be abnormal in patients undergoing hemodialysis.

Because second-generation antipsychotics can lead to weight gain and diabetes, a set of guidelines has been proposed to screen and monitor patients who are taking these drugs (Table 5–1) (American Diabetes Association et al. 2004). These guidelines should be routinely incorporated into clinical practice by all psychiatrists caring for older adults. Additionally, when patients develop abdominal pain while being treated with atypical antipsychotics or valproic acid, their amylase and lipase levels should be checked to rule out pancreatitis. Liver function tests should be monitored periodically in patients taking valproic acid. There have been case reports of both venlafaxine and duloxetine causing elevated hepatic enzymes and even hepatic failure. Liver function tests should be obtained in patients taking these drugs who develop symptoms of liver disease.

Serological Tests for Syphilis

Although syphilis rates in the United States were at historical lows in 2000 and 2001, the rate of primary and secondary syphilis cases has steadily increased since then, mainly due to higher rates among gay, bisexual, and other men who have sex with men (Centers for Disease Control and Prevention 2019b). Men from this demographic group who are infected with HIV and are of lower socioeconomic status are at especially high risk of syphilis infection. According to the American Academy of Neurology's guidelines for diagnosis of dementia, unless the patient has some specific risk factor (e.g., another sexually transmitted disease) or evidence of prior syphilitic infection, or the patient resides in one of the few areas in the United States with high numbers of syphilis cases, screening for the disorder in patients with dementia is not justified (Knopman et al. 2001). If a clinician suspects syphilis infection, the Venereal Disease Research Laboratory and rapid plasmin reagin tests are screening tools for infection with *Treponema pallidum*, the cause of syphilis. These tests are unfortunately nonspecific; false-positive results may occur in acute infections and chronic illnesses such as systemic lupus erythematosus. More specific tests, the fluorescent treponemal antibody and the microhemagglutination assay for *T. pallidum*, may distinguish false-positive from true-positive results and may aid in diagnosing late syphilis when blood and even cerebrospinal fluid (CSF) reagin tests are negative.

HIV Testing

According to the Centers for Disease Control and Prevention (2019a), HIV infection is a significant issue in the geriatric population. Individuals age 50 years and older account for almost 50% of known HIV infections, and 17% of new HIV diagnoses are made in this age group. The diagnosis of AIDS in elderly individuals is complicated; like syphilis, AIDS has been described as a "great imitator" because its clinical presentation may mimic that of other diseases (Sabin 1987). AIDS may mimic not only medical illnesses but also neuropsychiatric disorders, because AIDS may result in dementia.

There is no evidence that HIV treatment for elderly patients with AIDS should differ from that for younger patients. The geriatric psychiatrist must therefore assist the internist by screening for risk factors, such as a history of sexually transmitted diseases, intravenous drug use, risky sexual behavior, or a history of blood transfusions, particularly prior to the early 1990s. We recommend HIV testing for individuals who have these risk factors or who present with atypical neuropsychiatric symptoms. The guidelines for the upper age limit of universal screening for individuals vary from age 65 (Branson et al. 2006; Owens et al. 2019) to 75 (Qaseem et al. 2009). For patients in whom testing is warranted, the psychiatrist will also play an important role in counseling them about the reasons behind testing and providing further counseling as the test results are reported.

Thyroid Function Tests

To understand the significance of thyroid test results, one must first understand the hormones themselves. Secretion of the thyroid hormones thyroxine (T_4) and triiodothyronine (T_3) is regulated by pituitary gland secretion of thyroid-stimulating hormone (TSH). TSH secretion, in turn, is controlled via negative feedback by thyroid hormones. Both T_4 and T_3 are reversibly bound to the plasma protein thyroxine-binding globulin, and only the small unbound fraction exerts its physiological effects.

A serum TSH test is the most frequently used screening test for thyroid disease; it is an excellent screen because of its high negative predictive value (Klee and Hay 1997). However, many medications may result in increased TSH levels (amiodarone, estrogens) or decreased TSH levels (glucocorticoids, phenytoin), and altered TSH levels may also be seen in patients with acute nonthyroidal illness or systemic stress. A physical examination and measurement of T_4, T_3, and TSH may be required for a definitive diagnosis of thyroid disease (Table 5–2). TSH testing should be performed in all older patients presenting with neuropsychiatric symptoms because hypothyroidism may

TABLE 5–2.	Patterns of thyroid function tests		
TSH	**Free T$_4$**	**T$_3$**	**Suggested diagnosis**
Normal	Normal	Normal	Euthyroid
High	Low	Low or normal	Primary hypothyroidism
High	Normal	Normal	Subclinical hypothyroidism
Low	High or normal	High	Hyperthyroidism

T$_3$=triiodothyronine; T$_4$=thyroxine; TSH=thyroid-stimulating hormone.

cause symptoms of depression, fatigue, and impaired cognition, and hyperthyroidism can cause symptoms of anxiety or even psychosis. Older women have a high prevalence of hypothyroidism. Patients who are taking lithium should have their TSH level checked every 6 months.

Vitamin B$_{12}$, Folate, and Homocysteine

Measurement of serum vitamin B$_{12}$ and folate levels is an integral part of the laboratory evaluation. The prevalence of B$_{12}$ deficiency increases with age; the deficiency is present in up to 15% of the elderly population. Although macrocytic anemia is a well-known sign of B$_{12}$ deficiency, it is a later presentation in most cases, with neuropsychiatric symptoms presenting much earlier. Vitamin B$_{12}$ and folate deficiencies may result in neuropsychiatric disturbances, including depression, psychosis, or cognitive deficits. In patients with dementia, B$_{12}$ deficiencies often result in delirium or disorientation. Low levels of these vitamins may also result in visuospatial and word fluency deficits (Robins Wahlin et al. 2001) and even greater behavioral disturbances in patients with Alzheimer's disease (AD) (Meins et al. 2000). In a longitudinal study of 965 older individuals, a lower incidence of AD was noted among subjects in the highest quartile of total folate intake, after adjustments for age, sex, education, ethnicity, and other comorbidities. No significant association was found between vitamin B$_6$ or vitamin B$_{12}$ intake and risk of AD (Luchsinger et al. 2007).

Vitamin B$_{12}$ and folate levels may not tell the entire story, however; there is also considerable interest in homocysteine. Serum homocysteine levels may serve as a functional indicator of B$_{12}$ and folate status because both vitamins are needed to convert homocysteine to methionine in one-carbon metabolism in brain tissue. Hyperhomocysteinemia is prevalent in elderly persons, and high serum levels of homocysteine can be attributed to an inadequate supply of B$_{12}$ and folate, even in the presence of low to normal serum levels (Selhub et al. 2000). High levels of homocysteine have been associated with an increased risk of occlusive vascular disease, thrombosis, and stroke (Boushey et al. 1995). Hyperhomocysteinemia is further associated with cognitive dysfunction (Hooshmand et al. 2010; Leblhuber et al. 2000; Selhub et al. 2000). A recent consensus statement reflects the current thinking that hyperhomocysteinemia is a modifiable risk factor for cognitive decline and dementia (Smith et al. 2018), with some evidence supporting benefit from vitamin B supplementation (Durga et al. 2007; Smith and Refsum 2016), although this is disputed (Ford and Almeida 2012). Recent work has also explored whether a higher methionine-to-homocysteine ratio may reduce risk of brain atrophy and dementia (Hooshmand et al. 2019).

Toxicology

When an acute change occurs in an individual's mental status, investigation of the cause must include the possible ingestion of a substance. This consideration is particularly important in individuals with a history of substance abuse or with a history of depression, for whom there is the risk of medication overdose. When mental status changes in an individual who is taking medications such as lithium, phenytoin, tricyclic antidepressants (TCAs), or any medication that requires blood level monitoring, those levels should be checked. Toxic levels of many pharmacological agents may cause psychiatric or life-threatening medical conditions. Levels for common over-the-counter medications, such as acetaminophen and salicylates, can also be tested. A serum alcohol level should also be drawn. Depending on the individual's history, even a negative result may be critical if withdrawal is a possibility. Finally, urine can be tested for prescription medications, such as benzodiazepines, barbiturates, and opioids, as well as illicit substances, such as cocaine and marijuana. Advanced age does not preclude addiction. Clinicians should also be attentive to the possibility of false-positives or false-negatives. For example, sertraline may trigger a positive screen for benzodiazepines, and a positive result for amphetamines may stem from trazodone or bupropion use (Smith and Bluth 2016), whereas testing may *not* detect synthetic substances (Castellanos and Thornton 2012).

Urinalysis

A urinalysis is an inexpensive, noninvasive test that provides a significant amount of information. It determines the urine's specific gravity, which may indicate dehydration, and tests for glucose and ketones, which are important in the evaluation of patients with diabetes. In the elderly population, the most important use of urinalysis may be as a screening tool for urinary tract infections (UTIs). A UTI is suggested when a microscopic examination shows high levels of white blood cells, bacteria, positive leukocyte esterase and nitrite, and possibly red blood cells; high numbers of epithelial cells make the results difficult to interpret because their presence suggests contamination. A urine culture is a definitive means of diagnosing a UTI and will identify the infecting organism and its susceptibility to antimicrobial treatments. Approximately 20% of patients admitted to geropsychiatry units may have UTIs, and many cases of UTI result in a delirium that improves with appropriate antibiotic treatment (Levkoff et al. 1991; Manepalli et al. 1990).

Cerebrospinal Fluid Analysis
and Plasma Assays for Dementia

Although one of the most common diagnostic uses of CSF analysis is the workup of suspected CNS infections (e.g., meningitis), CSF analysis is now playing an increasingly important role of the assessment of patients with dementia. In patients with AD and mild cognitive impairment (MCI) due to AD, CSF levels of amyloid-β (Aβ) peptide

1–42 are reduced, whereas levels of phosphorylated tau (p-tau) and total tau (t-tau) are increased (Blennow et al. 2010; Hansson et al. 2006). Increased p-tau is more specific for AD than Aβ but is less sensitive (Hansson et al. 2006; Maddalena et al. 2003). Tau elevations may be less pronounced in Black populations (Morris et al. 2019), however, and can also be found in other conditions, such as frontotemporal lobar degeneration (FTLD) and Parkinson-plus syndromes. Other promising assays for AD include CSF measurement of Aβ oligomers and amyloid precursor proteins. The combination of these CSF biomarkers may improve accuracy in the diagnosis of AD.

Although CSF biomarkers are not part of the routine dementia workup, they may be collected when dementia specialists are clarifying the etiology of an atypical presentation of suspected MCI or dementia. National Institute on Aging–Alzheimer's Association guidelines for diagnosing AD have also focused on the use of plasma and CSF biomarkers and neuroimaging for the early detection of preclinical AD and MCI due to AD (Jack et al. 2011a). Research studies, most notably the Alzheimer's Disease Neuroimaging Initiative (ADNI) 3, are under way to better characterize the utility of these biomarkers in the context of neuropsychological testing and neuroimaging. Research on blood-based assays to predict risk of conversion to MCI and AD and to confirm AD pathology as the etiology for cognitive impairment is rapidly evolving.

Assays have been developed for early-onset and rapidly progressive dementias. Potentially promising biomarkers for FTLD include transactive response DNA-binding protein of 43 kDa molecular weight (TDP-43), neurofilament light chain, progranulin, tau, Aβ, and poly(GP) dipeptide repeat protein (Feneberg et al. 2018; Greaves and Rohrer 2019; Zetterberg et al. 2019), but a clinical biomarker has been elusive for this heterogeneous group of disorders. Lower plasma levels of progranulin are predictive of progranulin-encoding *GRN* mutations in patients with FTLD and asymptomatic family members (Finch et al. 2009). TDP-43 proteinopathy has also been associated with both FTLD and amyotrophic lateral sclerosis, which suggests these are two processes on a disease continuum (Neumann et al. 2006). Elevated levels of TDP-43 in the CSF and plasma are seen in FTLD, amyotrophic lateral sclerosis, and AD; plasma levels of phosphorylated TDP-43 may be more specific for FTLD (Foulds et al. 2009).

Hsich et al. (1996) described an immunoassay for detecting the 14-3-3 protein in CSF that had a specificity of 99% and a sensitivity of 96% for the diagnosis of Creutzfeldt-Jakob disease (CJD) among patients with dementia. CSF 14-3-3 protein assay has been found to be superior to electroencephalography or MRI in identifying cases of CJD (Poser et al. 1999). However, other acute neurological conditions such as stroke, viral encephalitis, and paraneoplastic neurological disorders can provide false-positive results. Nevertheless, the American Academy of Neurology recommends testing for CSF 14-3-3 protein to confirm or reject the diagnosis of CJD in clinically appropriate circumstances (Knopman et al. 2001).

Electrocardiogram

An electrocardiogram (ECG) provides a graphic representation of the heart's electrical activity, obtained via surface electrodes placed in specific locations on the patient's chest and limbs. This placement makes possible a graph of electrical activity from a variety of spatial perspectives. In psychiatry, the most important roles of the ECG in-

TABLE 5–3.	Common electrocardiographic abnormalities associated with psychotropic medications
Medication	Electrocardiographic change
Antipsychotics (typical or atypical agents)	Increased QTc interval
	Potential for torsades de pointes
β-Blockers	Bradycardia
Lithium	Sick sinus syndrome
	Sinoatrial block
Tricyclic antidepressants	Increased PR, QRS, or QT intervals
	Atrioventricular block

clude screening for cardiovascular disease that may preclude the use of specific medications and monitoring for drug-induced electrocardiographic changes, either from standard doses or from overdose. Electrocardiographic changes associated with specific psychotropic medications are summarized in Table 5–3.

TCAs are known to be cardiotoxic in overdose; even at therapeutic dosages, their use is considered unsafe in individuals with cardiovascular disease, particularly ischemic disease. Although the most common cardiovascular complication of TCAs is orthostatic hypotension, TCAs have the same pharmacological properties as type IA antiarrhythmics such as quinidine and procainamide. TCAs slow conduction at the bundle of His; patients with preexisting bundle branch block who take TCAs are at increased risk for atrioventricular block. Even therapeutic levels are associated with prolonged PR intervals and QRS complexes; these results may be more pronounced in elderly individuals because the incidence and severity of adverse drug reactions increase with age. If TCAs are used, baseline and frequent follow-up ECGs should be obtained.

Lithium may also result in electrocardiographic changes, and ECGs are recommended before starting lithium in those who are older than 40 (Bowden et al. 2002) or who have cardiovascular disease risk factors (National Institute for Health and Care Excellence 2014). Lithium appears to most affect the sinus node, and even at therapeutic levels it may result in sick sinus syndrome or sinoatrial block, either of which may occur early or later in treatment. At higher levels, there have been reports of sinus arrest and asystole.

Antipsychotics also result in electrocardiographic changes; ~25% of individuals receiving antipsychotics exhibit electrocardiographic abnormalities (Thomas 1994). Although many of these changes have historically been considered benign, there is increased concern that prolongation of the QT interval (when corrected for heart rate, the QTc interval) may contribute to potentially fatal ventricular arrhythmias, particularly torsades de pointes. QTc values are typically around 400 ms in duration; values lower than this are considered normal. Because the greater the duration, the greater the risk of torsades de pointes, clinicians should be attentive to abnormal QTc prolongation, suggested as the ninety-ninth percentile or ~470 ms for males and 480 ms for females, with 500 ms viewed as "highly abnormal" in both sexes (Drew et al. 2010) and frequently used as a cutoff. Other medications also affect the QTc interval and produce an additive effect when combined with an antipsychotic. This phenomenon may be seen with almost any antipsychotic agent but is most likely to be associated with thioridazine and haloperidol among typical antipsychotics and with ziprasidone among atypical antipsychotics. Unfortunately, there are currently concerns about QTc prolongation for all atypical antipsychotic agents.

Routine ECGs for all patients receiving antipsychotics are not currently recommended, but it is wise to be prudent. A detailed history of cardiac illness, family history, or syncope should be obtained for all patients. ECGs should be considered more carefully when patients have other risk factors, such as heart failure, bradycardia, electrolyte imbalance (particularly with low levels of potassium and magnesium), female sex, old age, hepatic or renal impairment, and slow metabolizer status. ECG and/or electrolyte testing should be performed in patients with risk factors.

In 2011, the FDA posted a black box warning recommending against dosages of citalopram >40 mg/day (20 mg/day in patients age ≥60 years) because of the risk of QTc prolongation and torsades de pointes. Further studies have had mixed findings; one study questioned whether there was truly a concern with citalopram (Zivin et al. 2013), whereas another found modest prolongation for not only citalopram but also escitalopram and amitriptyline (Castro et al. 2013). Further studies are needed to address the effects of citalopram and other antidepressants on QTc and risk of torsades de pointes. Until more data are available, physicians should continue to discuss the black box warning with patients prior to initiating citalopram (and possibly escitalopram), and citalopram should be discontinued if the QTc persistently exceeds 500 ms.

There are various methodologies for correctly calculating a patient's QTc interval. For each person, the QT decreases as the heart rate increases. The formula for correction is QT/RR^c, in which RR=the RR interval and c=the correction factor. According to the FDA, the most accurate proposed method is to calculate this correction factor for the patient based on 50–100 pretreatment ECGs, and this is the recommended approach for Phase I ECG trials (U.S. Food and Drug Administration 2005). Other methodologies for calculation include population-based approaches, such as the Bazett, Fridericia, linear regression, and nonlinear regression techniques. The Bazett QT correction formula is most frequently used in clinical practice and in the medical literature, but clinicians should be aware that this type of correction tends to be inaccurate at the extreme ranges (both elevated and low). With few exceptions, an ECG should always be obtained in cases of potential medication overdose, even when the medication used is not associated with arrhythmia. ECGs are important because some medications may affect heart rhythm in overdose when they would not do so at the usual dosage. Also, suicidal patients often do not report all the medications that they have used to overdose; suicide attempts may be impulsive, and patients who have an altered mental status may not be able to provide a complete report.

Imaging Studies

Plain film radiographs remain an integral piece of the diagnostic imaging performed in geriatric psychiatry. Such techniques are most often used to detect lung pathology that may contribute to mental status changes or to detect bone fractures. Plain film radiographs are critical for individuals who have both severe dementia and either a recent history of falls or newly developed limb immobility.

More recently developed imaging techniques have greatly enhanced diagnostic abilities. These techniques are costly, so they should not be used without a good rationale that includes why they are needed and how the specific findings may affect a patient's treatment plan. Two commonly used structural imaging techniques, CT and MRI, are also discussed in other chapters of this book, so our focus is on the scientific basis behind these tools and information to support their clinical use, particularly in brain imaging, and to facilitate providing informed consent. PET is an active area of research, with improvements in tracers for detection of amyloid or tau facilitating recent use criteria, clinical trial data, and evolving clinical utility, as we discuss later. Other imaging techniques such as single-photon emission computed tomography and functional MRI are used mostly in research and have limited clinical use and therefore are not discussed here.

Computed Tomography

Computed tomography is a general term for several radiographic techniques that result in the computer-assisted generation of a series of images showing slices of an organ or body region, such as the brain or abdomen. The CT scanner uses a small X-ray device that rotates around the body region of interest in a fixed plane; these signals are sent to a computer that produces the corresponding cross-sectional slice for that plane. The computer can create sections in axial, coronal, and sagittal alignments. More recent advances in software and display systems have led to many useful clinical applications, including virtual CT colonoscopy or angiography.

When used to examine brain structure, CT can allow for the ready identification of many structures, although it does have limitations. By measuring differences in density, it can distinguish among CSF, blood, bone, gray matter, and white matter. CT is particularly useful for demonstrating bone abnormalities (e.g., skull fractures), areas of hemorrhage (e.g., subdural hematoma), and the mass effect from various lesions. It can also display atrophy or ventricular enlargement. However, CT is not very useful for visualizing posterior fossa or brain stem structures because of surrounding bone.

A typical concern of patients is radiation exposure. CT scans require the use of a limited amount of radiation; any given CT procedure results in a radiation exposure, but that exposure is well below governmental recommendations for individuals who work around radiation. However, these recommendations do not consider multiple CT scans (thus multiple radiation exposures) or CT studies that overlap scanned regions, a technique that increases the radiation dose. CT imaging should be used when appropriate, but other assessment techniques that may result in lower radiation exposure should also be considered.

Magnetic Resonance Imaging

Whereas CT scanners rely on radiation, in MRI, the scanner creates a magnetic field that is 3,000–25,000 times the strength of the Earth's natural magnetic field. The underlying principle behind MRI is that the nuclei of identifiable endogenous isotopes (e.g., hydrogen or phosphorus) behave like tiny spinning magnets. Strong magnetic fields alter this behavior, and an MRI scanner can identify the resultant change. When patients are put into the strong, static magnetic field generated by the MRI scanner, their nuclei align parallel to the field. Because the nuclei are also spinning, they wobble

TABLE 5–4.	Neuroimaging in geriatric psychiatry
Suspected condition	**Indicated neuroimaging study**
Sudden loss of consciousness	Noncontrast CT scan
Pituitary tumor (hyperprolactinemia)	MRI
Old vs. new lacunar infarct	Diffusion-weighted imaging
Hippocampal atrophy	Coronal thin slice MRI
Wernicke's encephalopathy	MRI to rule out midbrain hemorrhage

randomly around the field; different molecules can be identified because their nuclei wobble at different frequencies. A second, oscillating magnetic field is then applied at a right angle to the first. This field affects only the nuclei that are in resonance with it—that is, the nuclei that wobble at the field's frequency. This second field forces those resonant nuclei to wobble in unison. When this field is deactivated, the nuclei return to their original positions, and the synchronized movement creates a voltage that can be measured and displayed. Measurements taken at various times during the procedure produce the different magnetic resonance images.

MRI has advantages and disadvantages compared with CT. MRI produces higher-resolution images and can obtain good detail in regions (e.g., the posterior fossa) that are poorly visualized on CT. It is versatile, with applications in structural, functional, and molecular imaging (Risacher and Saykin 2019). Additionally, no radiation is involved in MRI. Unfortunately, the procedure is more burdensome than CT because the patient must remain motionless for a longer period in a smaller, enclosed space. This may be difficult for individuals who are claustrophobic. Additionally, the magnetic device must be housed in an area devoid of iron, and staff and patients must not carry or wear certain metals or have them embedded in their bodies. Moreover, MRI tends to be more costly than CT imaging in most institutions.

In the psychiatric workup of a geriatric patient (Table 5–4), MRI should be considered when the clinician suspects small lesions in regions that are difficult to visualize—for example, to obtain evidence of midbrain hemorrhage in an individual with suspected Wernicke's encephalopathy or to confirm a suspected pituitary tumor in a patient with hyperprolactinemia, which may be seen in association with risperidone and other high-potency antipsychotic agents. Hyperprolactinemia carries the risks of osteopenia, sexual dysfunction, amenorrhea, breast enlargement, and possibly cardiac disease and breast cancer. Switching from high-potency to low-potency antipsychotic drugs such as quetiapine or aripiprazole has been shown not only to normalize prolactin but also, in some instances, to reverse menstrual dysfunction or other symptoms (Shim et al. 2007). MRI can also easily identify vascular pathology, including lacunar infarcts, and it is better than CT for defining exact anatomical localization.

A limitation of CT and MRI is that neither can differentiate between acute and chronic lesions. Diffusion-weighted imaging (DWI) overcomes this difficulty. DWI is based on the capacity of fast MRI to detect a signal related to the movement of water molecules between two closely spaced radiofrequency pulses (diffusion). This technique can detect abnormalities due to ischemia within 3–30 minutes of onset, whereas conventional MRI and CT images would still appear normal. Therefore, DWI is helpful in defining the clinically appropriate infarct when multiple subcortical infarcts of various ages are present.

The American Academy of Neurology recommends routine use of structural neuroimaging (noncontrast head CT or MRI) in the initial evaluation of all patients with dementia (Knopman et al. 2001). Recent studies also suggest novel uses for MRI in dementia. Schuff et al. (2009) showed that in the ADNI cohort, patients with MCI and AD showed progressive hippocampal loss over 6 months and then accelerated loss over 1 year. However, standardization of volumetric measurement techniques is necessary for the structure to be established as a formal diagnostic biomarker (Jack et al. 2011b). NeuroQuant, an FDA-approved software program, automatically quantifies volumes of brain structures; it may be useful for measuring progressive hippocampal loss in patients and has been investigated as a means to distinguish AD from non-dementia and non-AD dementia through volumetry of the hippocampus, cerebellum, and other structures (Persson et al. 2017). MRI measurements of cortical thickness, ventricular volume, and mean diffusivity may also help distinguish normal pressure hydrocephalus from other neurodegenerative disorders (Ivkovic et al. 2013; Moore et al. 2012). DWI also shows promise for dementia diagnosis because its techniques can provide information about white matter tracts, including their myelination and mean diffusivity, which are altered in neurodegeneration (Kehoe et al. 2014; Mori and Zhang 2006).

Positron Emission Tomography Imaging

As detailed by Risacher and Saykin (2019), PET imaging uses a compound with a radioactive isotope to investigate the distribution of metabolic activity or a selected protein of interest. The radioactive tracer is administered prior to the scan and distributes across the region of interest in proportion to its metabolic utilization or protein binding. The varying tracer concentrations emit varying levels of energy via radioactive decay. Detection of this radiation with a PET scan enables computer reconstruction of the tracer distribution with high sensitivity. PET imaging may be coupled with additional imaging studies, such as CT or MRI, and has an expanding range of applications as new tracers are developed for various targets with research or clinical utility. The main risk of PET imaging is exposure from the radioactive imaging agents, which are mostly ^{18}fluorodeoxyglucose (FDG)-based and have a half-life of ~110 minutes.

The role of PET imaging in the clinical workup of dementia continues to evolve. A nuanced discussion of recent developments, particularly those relating to amyloid PET and tau PET imaging, first requires situating the modalities within the relevant diagnostic framework for AD. In 2011, recommendations from the National Institute on Aging and the Alzheimer's Association put forth a diagnostic framework for the clinically defined conditions of MCI (Albert et al. 2011) and dementia (McKhann et al. 2011). Associated work groups also proposed the notion of preclinical AD, expanding the concept of AD from only the clinical disease stages to a long-term pathophysiological process with amyloid accumulation, synaptic dysfunction, tau-mediated neuronal injury, and structural changes to the brain all preceding detectable impacts to cognition and eventual dementia (Sperling et al. 2011). This was a research-driven rather than clinical concept but carries significant potential for real-world impact because the rapidly evolving research on disease-modifying therapy offers hope for targeting pathology prior to significant cognitive and functional decline.

The amyloid cascade hypothesis underlying the concept of preclinical AD implies that the pathophysiological processes leading to Alzheimer's dementia begin decades before dementia onset. This has been supported by findings of the ADNI throughout its progression from ADNI-1 to ADNI-3 and shifts the time frame for potential early detection and intervention in AD to well before the emergence of clinical symptoms. To better investigate preclinical AD, in 2018 a biologically based research framework called the AT(N) system was developed (Jack et al. 2018), suitable to accommodate future investigation of various biomarkers of amyloid deposition (A), pathologic tau (T), and neurodegeneration (N). Further discussion of PET imaging can thus be conceptualized as incorporating all AT(N) biomarkers; before exploring evolving PET techniques using agents that specifically bind amyloid or tau, we first focus on the techniques of FDG-PET, a test for neurodegeneration with established clinical utility.

FDG-PET Imaging

FDG-PET imaging can be useful in distinguishing AD from frontotemporal dementia (FTD) when the clinical diagnosis is unclear. On FDG-PET imaging, AD causes hypometabolism predominantly in the posterior temporoparietal association and posterior cingulate cortices, whereas FTD causes hypometabolism in the frontal lobes and anterior temporal and anterior cingulate cortices. In one study, visual interpretation of FDG-PET metabolic and statistical maps was superior to clinical assessment, with a diagnostic accuracy of 89.6% (Foster et al. 2007). Medicare has approved payment for FDG-PET imaging in patients who meet the criteria for both AD and FTD and who need clarification of their diagnosis.

Amyloid PET Imaging

Florbetapir, flumetamol, and florbetaben (a chemical cousin of florbetapir) are fluorine-based radioactive PET imaging agents that bind to brain Aβ plaque. They are approved by the FDA for detecting the presence of Aβ neuritic plaques in people with progressive cognitive decline. There are no major differences among these agents. Because amyloid PET scans expose patients to radioactivity (equivalent to 100 or more X-ray examinations), it is not recommended that patients have multiple scans during their lifetime.

Patients must be carefully counseled before and after undergoing an amyloid PET scan because the results may generate confusion. The scans are interpreted visually as positive, negative, or indeterminate by an experienced reader. A negative scan only indicates the state at the time of the scan and does not preclude the possibility that a scan would be positive a year or so later. Aβ plaques are currently required for a confirmatory diagnosis of Alzheimer's dementia; a negative scan indicating a low probability of Aβ plaques may point to other causes for the person's dementia. The negative predictive value of amyloid scans for future progression is high. The positive predictive value of amyloid scans is close to 50%; therefore, positive scans themselves do not necessarily mean that the patient has AD (Zannas et al. 2012). Positive scans can be seen in numerous conditions such as dementia with Lewy bodies, late-stage Parkinson's dementia, prion disorders, and even in cognitively normal elderly individuals, particularly those who carry an allele producing the ε4 type of apolipoprotein E. Patients must also be counseled on other limitations of the findings; although the findings may help inform advance planning, a positive scan does not indicate anticipated rate of progression. Given these considerations and the potential psychological impact of amyloid PET results, particularly during the preclinical period, disclosure protocols merit careful thought and research (de Wilde et al. 2018a).

Appropriate use criteria have been published to help guide clinicians considering amyloid PET. Current criteria limit the use of amyloid PET to those who have been determined by a dementia expert to have persistent or progressive unexplained MCI, possible AD with an atypical or mixed presentation, or early-onset progressive dementia (Johnson et al. 2013). It is not appropriate to use the technology for screening asymptomatic individuals, even those with a significant family history of AD, or for evaluation of subjective cognitive complaints.

Use of amyloid PET scans is further limited by reimbursement in light of questions surrounding its clinical value, given the evolving status of disease-modifying treatments. Currently, Medicare and insurance companies do not reimburse for these scans except in special circumstances. Initial results from the Imaging Dementia–Evidence for Amyloid Scanning (IDEAS) study demonstrated that amyloid PET, when used in accordance with the appropriate criteria, impacted management in almost two-thirds of cases and changed the diagnosis in more than one-third (Rabinovici et al. 2019). The optimal clinical practice standards and models for reimbursement based on analyses of costs and clinical benefits will depend on further research into clinical utilization and outcomes, particularly for minority populations, and the availability of disease-modifying treatments. Aside from these factors, the population included in the appropriate use criteria may evolve; the Alzheimer's Biomarkers in Daily Practice project has suggested that even in an unselected memory clinic sample, suspected etiology and treatment each changed in about one-quarter of patients following an amyloid PET scan (de Wilde et al. 2018b).

Tau PET Imaging

Tau PET imaging is also actively being researched; in 2020, the FDA approved the tau PET tracer flortaucipir. Tau PET imaging has been incorporated into data collection for ADNI-3 given the proposed role of tau in the neurodegenerative cascade of the AT(N) framework. Tau burden has been found to correlate more closely than amyloid burden with structural degeneration (Cho et al. 2016) and clinical severity (Bejanin et al. 2017; Bierer et al. 1995) of AD, suggesting promise as a biomarker. Tau PET signal is also more closely linked than that of amyloid PET with the spatial pattern of neurodegeneration and specific clinical deficits in AD (Ossenkoppele et al. 2016). One recent longitudinal study found that mean baseline global signal intensity on tau PET was predictive of future atrophy rates, whereas that of amyloid PET was more weakly and nonsignificantly correlated, and spatial correlation with atrophy was significantly higher for tau PET than amyloid PET binding (La Joie et al. 2020). Future studies will need to study the clinical utility of both tau PET and amyloid PET imaging.

Electroencephalography

Electroencephalography is a technique in which scalp electrodes allow the measurement of cortical electrical activity. A skilled reader can interpret the electroencephalographic waveforms to identify the presence of epileptic activity, the slowing of electrical activity, or a patient's sleep stage. Electroencephalography is most useful in a psychiatric evaluation of individuals with known or suspected seizure disorders. Although a history of brain injury or trauma with mental status changes or psychosis may be an important indication for an electroencephalographic evaluation, imaging studies are generally preferred for diagnostic clarification in these situations.

In elderly patients, electroencephalographic changes occur in both delirium and dementia, but these changes are not specific to a given diagnosis. In delirium, except that caused by alcohol or sedative-hypnotic withdrawal, electroencephalograms (EEGs) typically display slowing of the posterior dominant rhythm and increased generalized slow-wave activity. Electroencephalography has limited clinical use in this area because the diagnosis of delirium is typically made clinically, increased slow-wave activity is seen in other disorders, and the EEG provides minimal information about the causes of delirium. However, electroencephalography is useful for distinguishing between depression and "quiet" delirium because no electroencephalographic changes are seen in depression, whereas generalized slowing is seen in delirium.

There are also electroencephalographic changes in dementia. AD results in multiple changes in electroencephalographic parameters. Although Kowalski et al. (2001) reported that the degree of change (slowing of normal background activity) is correlated with cognitive impairment, there are also reports that worsening of electroencephalographic results does not always parallel clinical deterioration. Various treatments, including cholinesterase inhibitors, may mitigate electroencephalographic changes in patients with mild dementia (Kogan et al. 2001). However, significant negative correlations have been found between frontal theta activity and hippocampal volumes (Grunwald et al. 2001). Although electroencephalography currently has limited clinical utility, it has recently been explored as a possible noninvasive correlate of CSF biomarkers for AD (Smailovic et al. 2018) and as a way to distinguish types of dementia (Garn et al. 2017).

Electroencephalographic testing may be useful, however, when CJD is a consideration in the differential diagnosis. CJD is a rare, rapidly progressive prion disease characterized by dementia and neurological signs that may include gait disturbances and myoclonus. Electroencephalography may play an important role in diagnosing this disease: periodic sharp-wave complexes are strongly associated with CJD, with a sensitivity of 67% and a specificity of 86% (Steinhoff et al. 1996). Although electroencephalography is an important diagnostic tool when considering CJD, it is important to remember that periodic sharp-wave complexes may also occur in AD and dementia with Lewy bodies.

Genetic Testing

Genetics in geriatric psychiatry is covered in more detail in Chapter 3, "Genomics in Geriatric Psychiatry." In this section, intended to serve as an introduction to genetic testing, we briefly discuss a well-researched test for apolipoprotein E (*APOE*) alleles, pharmacogenomics, and ethical and psychological concerns related to genetic testing.

APOE Testing

Extensive research has attempted to identify genetic markers for AD. Mutations on chromosomes 1, 14, and 21 have been linked to rare forms of early-onset familial AD. One of the most studied genes for AD is *APOE*. This gene encodes for an astrocyte-secreted plasma protein that is involved in cholesterol transport. *APOE* may also play a role in the regeneration of injured nerve tissue. There are three possible alleles (ε2, ε3, ε4) of the *APOE* gene that may be combined in either a heterozygous (ε2/ε3, ε2/ε4, ε3/ε4) or homozygous (ε2/ε2, ε3/ε3, ε4/ε4) fashion.

Multiple epidemiological studies have documented that the presence of the ε4 allele is a risk factor for AD. The ε4 allele may impact racial groups differently, with Blacks showing a weaker link between the ε4 allele and AD (Farrer et al. 1997; Morris et al. 2019). In the past, clinical guidelines have not recommended *APOE* genotyping in asymptomatic individuals. However, as the research evolves, a clinical role for *APOE* testing may emerge. *APOE* status may eventually help stratify risk for certain clearly-defined clinical situations; for example, *APOE* status has been found to impact the risk of amyloid-related imaging abnormalities during antibody treatments targeting Aβ (VandeVrede et al. 2020). In terms of potential risks, survey data suggest a hypothetical risk of suicidal ideation if cognitively normal participants were informed of high-risk status for AD (Caselli et al. 2014, 2015), although studies of *APOE* genotype disclosure have largely been reassuring (Ashida et al. 2010; Christensen et al. 2011; Green et al. 2009).

Pharmacogenomics

Pharmacogenetic testing is progressing into mainstream psychiatric practice, and psychiatrists are increasingly expected to know and discuss genetic principles with patients (Nurnberger et al. 2018). Most pharmacogenetic tests are designed to detect certain alleles correlated with psychotropic metabolism or serious psychotropic-related adverse events. For example, assessment of the cytochrome P450 gene *CYP2D6* allele is purportedly helpful for clinicians who are trying to determine an appropriate starting dosage for numerous psychotropic drugs (including several SSRIs, TCAs, and antipsychotics) that are metabolized by *CYP2D6*. Ultrarapid metabolizers (~1% of the population) may require higher dosages to reach therapeutic levels, whereas poor metabolizers (~7%–10% of whites and 1% of Asians) may require lower dosages to reach similar levels, and the FDA has recommended limiting the daily dosage of citalopram in this population (U.S. Food and Drug Administration 2017). Testing has expanded from *CYP2D6* to various proprietary panels incorporating multiple genes, but the evidence base for clinically actionable findings from pharmacogenetic testing is variable. Currently, based on the available studies, the FDA recommends performing the HLA-B*1502 allele test for carbamazepine-induced Stevens-Johnson syndrome only for individuals of Asian descent. The FDA also recommends limiting vortioxetine dosage for *CYP2C19* slow metabolizers (Takeda Pharmaceuticals America 2016). Several studies have examined various alleles to try to detect those individuals at higher risk for serious adverse events while taking antipsychotics, such as metabolic syndrome (Malhotra et al. 2012).

Psychiatrists should ask themselves a few questions before ordering the results of a pharmacogenetics test for clinical purposes. First, is the patient from the specific population in which the test has been shown to be valid? For example, the HLA-B*1502 allele test was recommended in Asian but not white populations. Second, what is the evidence for predictive power of the test in the clinical (vs. the laboratory) setting? Demonstration of biologically accurate results and quality control is an essential part of any laboratory test but does not necessarily equate to clinical validity. Third, what is the likelihood that the pharmacogenomic test will sufficiently explain the observed phenotype? Although an allele may be associated with a high risk of an adverse outcome, it may not explain the majority of cases seen.

Additionally, as discussed in the next section, ethical and psychological concerns must be considered. Does the patient fully appreciate the implications of undergoing such tests in the clinical setting? For example, a patient may agree to the release of test results to a health insurance company or another third party, believing at the time that the test is designed for a particular purpose (e.g., detection of risk of weight gain from antipsychotics). However, future studies may show that this allele is associated with development of an unrelated disease process such as cancer, and this discovery may have consequences that the patient did not anticipate if proper counseling was not received. Clinicians and researchers should be prepared to discuss such considerations with patients considering genetic testing, and collaboration with a genetic counselor may be appropriate.

Ethical and Psychological Concerns in Genetic Testing

The results of genetic testing may have significant psychological, social, and personal repercussions. These possible effects are likely to be of less concern for someone already diagnosed with dementia than for family members who are faced with the risk of inheriting the disease. The offspring of a patient with AD are at increased risk for the disease based on family history alone. If a parent with AD is found to be homozygous for the *APOE* ε4 allele, the children, who will have at least one copy of the allele, have at least two to three times the average risk of developing AD. Unfortunately, this knowledge does not allow offspring to anticipate with certainty whether and when they will develop AD. Also, no treatment is available for *APOE* ε4 allele carriers to prevent the disease.

A positive family history of late-onset AD has been associated with a distinctive phenotype in MCI—namely, lower levels of $A\beta_{42}$ and higher levels of t-tau in the CSF—suggesting that other genetic factors are present besides *APOE* (Lampert et al. 2013). Previously, family members were discouraged from being tested due to stigmatization because of or worry about their increased risk of AD. However, given that several AD trials are now being geared toward asymptomatic individuals at higher risk for dementia (usually with a family history) and the AT(N) framework raises the prospect of earlier detection and intervention, such ethical questions will remain relevant, and interested individuals may wish to discuss the issue with their physicians and genetic counselors.

Beyond personal and psychological concerns, there are also financial concerns. Genetic testing should be confidential. The inappropriate release of such information could result in job loss or lack of insurability. Although the Genetic Information Nondiscrimination Act of 2008 prohibited health insurers from engaging in genetic discrimination, some health insurance organizations and providers of long-term-care insurance, life insurance, or disability insurance are exempt from this prohibition (National Human Genome Research Institute 2020). Medical and life insurance in particular might be exceedingly difficult to obtain if insurance agencies gain access to this information. In the end, however, genetic testing is yet another tool at the disposal of patients and clinicians. It is a tool with much untapped potential. It also carries significant risks that are different from those associated with other laboratory tests described in this chapter. As with other procedures, clinicians must ensure that patients or their families clearly understand not only the benefits but also the risks before they proceed with testing.

Omics Technologies

Since the inception of the Human Genome Project, high-throughput omics technologies have shown immense promise for revolutionizing medicine in the decades to come. There is, however, an absence of widespread use and acceptance of these tests in the clinical setting for various reasons, including the need for replication, the need to demonstrate validity in the general population, and costs. Nevertheless, given the high likelihood that psychiatrists will see patients who ask to have these tests performed or who bring in results of these tests from elsewhere, clinicians should have a basic conceptual understanding of the general purpose and challenges that may arise in the interpretation of these omics technologies. Given the rapid development of this field, an exhaustive review is not possible. Nevertheless, many of the same questions regarding the clinical interpretation of pharmacogenetic tests (see earlier section "Pharmacogenomics") can also be applied to the other omics technologies.

The purpose of the omics technologies is to examine the changes that can occur at different levels within an organism due to both physiological and pathophysiological processes. Table 5–5 briefly describes various omics technologies (Valdes et al. 2013). The overall concept is that these technologies sample the process of how the organism is functioning from the beginning product (the genome) to the end product (its metabolites), as well as in between (epigenomics, transcriptomics, and proteomics). This offers the potential for improved pathophysiological understanding of diseases beyond the current symptom-based or syndromal definitions (Bragazzi 2013; Fernandes et al. 2017), along the lines of the National Institute of Mental Health Research Domain Criteria. Findings could be used to determine at which stage(s) critical differences or modifications associated with certain types of outcomes (particularly in diseases or adverse medication effects) may arise. Biomarkers may play an increasing role as technology enables progression toward personalized medicine (Sethi and Brietzke 2015). As with genetic testing, however, ethical considerations are critical for this emerging technology because increased knowledge may bring unanticipated or undesired consequences.

Conclusion

Laboratory testing can provide invaluable information in both the diagnosis and treatment of geriatric psychiatry patients. Clinicians should carefully interpret laboratory values in the context of patients' histories and other available data. The roles of neuroimaging, CSF biomarkers, and various omics in clinical care are the focus of future research and will revolutionize the care of the geriatric psychiatric patient. Future directions for laboratory values include detection of populations that may be at risk for certain psychiatric disorders (e.g., dementia) and prediction of which individuals may or may not respond to certain treatments for psychiatric disorders.

TABLE 5–5.   **Omics technologies**

Omics technology	Example
Genomics	Examination of somatic differences in the nucleus and mitochondria genomes
Epigenomics	Examination of epigenetic changes (including DNA methylation and histone modification) that affect whether parts of the DNA sequences can be transcribed
Transcriptomics (expression profiling)	Examination of RNA transcripts, namely the expression of genomic material, including microRNAs, which can negatively regulate or degrade transcripts
Proteomics	Examination of proteins, including posttranslational modifications such as phosphorylation, ubiquination, and glycosylation that can affect the proteins' functioning
Metabolomics	Examination of metabolic content of a cell or organism (including changes in proteins, nucleic acid, carbohydrates, and lipids)

Source.   Valdes et al. 2013.

Key Points

- Laboratory testing is an essential component of the psychiatric evaluation of elderly individuals, who often present with comorbid medical illnesses.

- Laboratory tests are also useful in monitoring medication side effects, such as for monitoring patients taking atypical antipsychotics.

- Neuroimaging is useful in the evaluation of various neuropsychiatric illnesses, including dementia.

- Genetic testing has great potential in geriatric psychiatry but currently has limited clinical utility. Important ethical issues should be considered when using genetic testing.

Suggested Reading

Knopman DS, DeKosky ST, Cummings JL, et al: Practice parameter: diagnosis of dementia (an evidence-based review): report of the Quality Standards Subcommittee of the American Academy of Neurology. Neurology 56:1143–1153, 2001 11342678

References

Albert MS, DeKosky ST, Dickson D, et al: The diagnosis of mild cognitive impairment due to Alzheimer's disease: recommendations from the National Institute on Aging-Alzheimer's Association workgroups on diagnostic guidelines for Alzheimer's disease. Alzheimers Dement 7(3):270–279, 2011 21514249

American Diabetes Association: 2. Classification and diagnosis of diabetes: Standards of Medical Care in Diabetes–2020. Diabetes Care 43(suppl 1):S14–S31, 2020 31862745

American Diabetes Association, American Psychiatric Association, American Association of Clinical Endocrinologists, North American Association for the Study of Obesity: Consensus development conference on antipsychotic drugs and obesity and diabetes. Diabetes Care 27(2):596–601, 2004 14747245

Ashida S, Koehly LM, Roberts JS, et al: The role of disease perceptions and results sharing in psychological adaptation after genetic susceptibility testing: the REVEAL Study. Eur J Hum Genet 18(12):1296–1301, 2010 20664629

Bejanin A, Schonhaut DR, La Joie R, et al: Tau pathology and neurodegeneration contribute to cognitive impairment in Alzheimer's disease. Brain 140(12):3286–3300, 2017 29053874

Bierer LM, Hof PR, Purohit DP, et al: Neocortical neurofibrillary tangles correlate with dementia severity in Alzheimer's disease. Arch Neurol 52(1):81–88, 1995 7826280

Blennow K, Hampel H, Weiner M, Zetterberg H: Cerebrospinal fluid and plasma biomarkers in Alzheimer disease. Nat Rev Neurol 6(3):131–144, 2010 20157306

Boushey CJ, Beresford SA, Omenn GS, Motulsky AG: A quantitative assessment of plasma homocysteine as a risk factor for vascular disease: probable benefits of increasing folic acid intakes. JAMA 274(13):1049–1057, 1995 7563456

Bowden CL, Gitlin MJ, Keck PE, et al: Practice guideline for the treatment of patients with bipolar disorder (revision). Am J Psychiatry 159(4 suppl):1–50, 2002 11958165

Bragazzi NL: Rethinking psychiatry with OMICS science in the age of personalized P5 medicine: ready for psychiatome? Philos Ethics Humanit Med 8:4, 2013 23849623

Branson BM, Handsfield HH, Lampe MA, et al: Revised recommendations for HIV testing of adults, adolescents, and pregnant women in health-care settings. MMWR Recomm Rep 55(RR-14):1–17, quiz CE1–CE4, 2006 16988643

Caselli RJ, Langbaum J, Marchant GE, et al: Public perceptions of presymptomatic testing for Alzheimer disease. Mayo Clin Proc 89(10):1389–1396, 2014 25171823

Caselli RJ, Marchant GE, Hunt KS, et al: Predictive testing for Alzheimer's disease: suicidal ideation in healthy participants. Alzheimer Dis Assoc Disord 29(3):252–254, 2015 25984909

Castellanos D, Thornton G: Synthetic cannabinoid use: recognition and management. J Psychiatr Pract 18(2):86–93, 2012 22418399

Castro VM, Clements CC, Murphy SN, et al: QT interval and antidepressant use: a cross sectional study of electronic health records. BMJ 346:f288, 2013 23360890

Centers for Disease Control and Prevention: HIV and older Americans, in HIV (online). Atlanta, GA, Centers for Disease Control and Prevention, 2019a. Available at https://www.cdc.gov/hiv/group/age/olderamericans/index.html. Accessed April 29, 2020.

Centers for Disease Control and Prevention: Syphilis, in Sexually Transmitted Disease Surveillance 2018 (online). Atlanta, GA, Centers for Disease Control and Prevention, 2019b. Available at: https://www.cdc.gov/std/stats18/syphilis.htm. Accessed April 29, 2020.

Cho H, Choi JY, Hwang MS, et al: Tau PET in Alzheimer disease and mild cognitive impairment. Neurology 87(4):375–383, 2016 27358341

Christensen KD, Roberts JS, Uhlmann WR, Green RC: Changes to perceptions of the pros and cons of genetic susceptibility testing after APOE genotyping for Alzheimer disease risk. Genet Med 13(5):409–414, 2011 21270636

de Wilde A, van Buchem MM, Otten RHJ, et al: Disclosure of amyloid positron emission tomography results to individuals without dementia: a systematic review. Alzheimers Res Ther 10(1):72, 2018a 30055660

de Wilde A, van der Flier WM, Pelkmans W, et al: Association of amyloid positron emission tomography with changes in diagnosis and patient treatment in an unselected memory clinic cohort: the ABIDE project. JAMA Neurol 75(9):1062–1070, 2018b 29889941

Drew BJ, Ackerman MJ, Funk M, et al: Prevention of torsade de pointes in hospital settings: a scientific statement from the American Heart Association and the American College of Cardiology Foundation. Circulation 121(8):1047–1060, 2010 20142454

Durga J, van Boxtel MP, Schouten EG, et al: Effect of 3-year folic acid supplementation on cognitive function in older adults in the FACIT trial: a randomised, double blind, controlled trial. Lancet 369(9557):208–216, 2007 17240287

Farrer LA, Cupples LA, Haines JL, et al: Effects of age, sex, and ethnicity on the association between apolipoprotein E genotype and Alzheimer disease: a meta-analysis. JAMA 278(16):1349–1356, 1997 9343467

Feneberg E, Gray E, Ansorge O, et al: Towards a TDP-43-based biomarker for ALS and FTLD. Mol Neurobiol 55(10):7789–7801, 2018 29460270

Fernandes BS, Williams LM, Steiner J, et al: The new field of 'precision psychiatry'. BMC Med 15(1):80, 2017 28403846

Finch N, Baker M, Crook R, et al: Plasma progranulin levels predict progranulin mutation status in frontotemporal dementia patients and asymptomatic family members. Brain 132(Pt 3):583–591, 2009 19158106

Ford AH, Almeida OP: Effect of homocysteine lowering treatment on cognitive function: a systematic review and meta-analysis of randomized controlled trials. J Alzheimers Dis 29(1):133–149, 2012 22232016

Foster NL, Heidebrink JL, Clark CM, et al: FDG-PET improves accuracy in distinguishing frontotemporal dementia and Alzheimer's disease. Brain 130(Pt 10):2616–2635, 2007 17704526

Foulds PG, Davidson Y, Mishra M, et al: Plasma phosphorylated-TDP-43 protein levels correlate with brain pathology in frontotemporal lobar degeneration. Acta Neuropathol 118(5):647–658, 2009 19823856

Garn H, Coronel C, Waser M, et al: Differential diagnosis between patients with probable Alzheimer's disease, Parkinson's disease dementia, or dementia with Lewy bodies and frontotemporal dementia, behavioral variant, using quantitative electroencephalographic features. J Neural Transm 124(5):569–581, 2017 28243755

Greaves CV, Rohrer JD: An update on genetic frontotemporal dementia. J Neurol 266(8):2075–2086, 2019 31119452

Green RC, Roberts JS, Cupples LA, et al: Disclosure of APOE genotype for risk of Alzheimer's disease. N Engl J Med 361(3):245–254, 2009 19605829

Grunwald M, Busse F, Hensel A, et al: Correlation between cortical theta activity and hippocampal volumes in health, mild cognitive impairment, and mild dementia. J Clin Neurophysiol 18(2):178–184, 2001 11435810

Hansson O, Zetterberg H, Buchhave P, et al: Association between CSF biomarkers and incipient Alzheimer's disease in patients with mild cognitive impairment: a follow-up study. Lancet Neurol 5(3):228–234, 2006 16488378

Hooshmand B, Solomon A, Kåreholt I, et al: Homocysteine and holotranscobalamin and the risk of Alzheimer disease: a longitudinal study. Neurology 75(16):1408–1414, 2010 20956786

Hooshmand B, Refsum H, Smith AD, et al: Association of methionine to homocysteine status with brain magnetic resonance imaging measures and risk of dementia. JAMA Psychiatry 76(11):1198–1205, 2019 31339527

Hsich G, Kenney K, Gibbs CJ, et al: The 14-3-3 brain protein in cerebrospinal fluid as a marker for transmissible spongiform encephalopathies. N Engl J Med 335(13):924–930, 1996 8782499

Ivkovic M, Liu B, Ahmed F, et al: Differential diagnosis of normal pressure hydrocephalus by MRI mean diffusivity histogram analysis. AJNR Am J Neuroradiol 34(6):1168–1174, 2013 23257611

Jack CR Jr, Albert MS, Knopman DS, et al: Introduction to the recommendations from the National Institute on Aging–Alzheimer's Association workgroups on diagnostic guidelines for Alzheimer's disease. Alzheimers Dement 7(3):257–262, 2011a 21514247

Jack CR Jr, Barkhof F, Bernstein MA, et al: Steps to standardization and validation of hippocampal volumetry as a biomarker in clinical trials and diagnostic criterion for Alzheimer's disease. Alzheimers Dement 7(4):474–485, 2011b 21784356

Jack CR Jr, Bennett DA, Blennow K, et al: NIA-AA research framework: toward a biological definition of Alzheimer's disease. Alzheimers Dement 14(4):535–562, 2018 29653606

Johnson KA, Minoshima S, Bohnen NI, et al: Appropriate use criteria for amyloid PET: a report of the Amyloid Imaging Task Force, the Society of Nuclear Medicine and Molecular Imaging, and the Alzheimer's Association. J Nucl Med 54(3):476–490, 2013 23359661

Kehoe EG, McNulty JP, Mullins PG, Bokde ALW: Advances in MRI biomarkers for the diagnosis of Alzheimer's disease. Biomarkers Med 8(9):1151–1169, 2014 25402585

Klee GG, Hay ID: Biochemical testing of thyroid function. Endocrinol Metab Clin North Am 26(4):763–775, 1997 9429859

Knopman DS, DeKosky ST, Cummings JL, et al: Practice parameter: diagnosis of dementia (an evidence-based review): report of the Quality Standards Subcommittee of the American Academy of Neurology. Neurology 56(9):1143–1153, 2001 11342678

Kogan EA, Korczyn AD, Virchovsky RG, et al: EEG changes during long-term treatment with donepezil in Alzheimer's disease patients. J Neural Transm 108(10):1167–1173, 2001 11725819

Kowalski JW, Gawel M, Pfeffer A, Barcikowska M: The diagnostic value of EEG in Alzheimer disease: correlation with the severity of mental impairment. J Clin Neurophysiol 18(6):570–575, 2001 11779971

La Joie R, Visani AV, Baker SL, et al: Prospective longitudinal atrophy in Alzheimer's disease correlates with the intensity and topography of baseline tau-PET. Sci Transl Med 12(524):eaau5732, 2020 31894103

Lampert EJ, Roy Choudhury K, Hostage CA, et al: Prevalence of Alzheimer's pathologic endophenotypes in asymptomatic and mildly impaired first-degree relatives. PLoS One 8(4):e60747, 2013 23613741

Leblhuber F, Walli J, Artner-Dworzak E, et al: Hyperhomocysteinemia in dementia. J Neural Transm 107(12):1469–1474, 2000 11458999

Levkoff S, Cleary P, Liptzin B, Evans DA: Epidemiology of delirium: an overview of research issues and findings. Int Psychogeriatr 3(2):149–167, 1991 1811770

Luchsinger JA, Tang MX, Miller J, et al: Relation of higher folate intake to lower risk of Alzheimer disease in the elderly. Arch Neurol 64(1):86–92, 2007 17210813

Maddalena A, Papassotiropoulos A, Müller-Tillmanns B, et al: Biochemical diagnosis of Alzheimer disease by measuring the cerebrospinal fluid ratio of phosphorylated tau protein to β-amyloid peptide42. Arch Neurol 60(9):1202–1206, 2003 12975284

Malhotra AK, Zhang JP, Lencz T: Pharmacogenetics in psychiatry: translating research into clinical practice. Mol Psychiatry 17(8):760–769, 2012 22083729

Manepalli J, Grossberg GT, Mueller C: Prevalence of delirium and urinary tract infection in a psychogeriatric unit. J Geriatr Psychiatry Neurol 3(4):198–202, 1990 2073307

McKhann GM, Knopman DS, Chertkow H, et al: The diagnosis of dementia due to Alzheimer's disease: recommendations from the National Institute on Aging-Alzheimer's Association workgroups on diagnostic guidelines for Alzheimer's disease. Alzheimers Dement 7(3):263–269, 2011 21514250

Meins W, Müller-Thomsen T, Meier-Baumgartner H-P: Subnormal serum vitamin B12 and behavioural and psychological symptoms in Alzheimer's disease. Int J Geriatr Psychiatry 15(5):415–418, 2000 10822240

Moore DW, Kovanlikaya I, Heier LA, et al: A pilot study of quantitative MRI measurements of ventricular volume and cortical atrophy for the differential diagnosis of normal pressure hydrocephalus. Neurol Res Int 2012:718150, 2012 21860791

Mori S, Zhang J: Principles of diffusion tensor imaging and its applications to basic neuroscience research. Neuron 51(5):527–539, 2006 16950152

Morris JC, Schindler SE, McCue LM, et al: Assessment of racial disparities in biomarkers for Alzheimer disease. JAMA Neurol 76(3):264–273, 2019 30615028

National Human Genome Research Institute: Genetic Discrimination (online). Bethesda, MD, National Human Genome Research Institute, 2020. Available at: http://www.genome.gov/10002077#al-3. Accessed April 29, 2020.

National Institute for Health and Care Excellence: Bipolar Disorder: Assessment and Management. Clinical Guideline CG185. London, National Institute for Health and Care Excellence, September 24, 2014. Available at https://www.nice.org.uk/guidance/cg185. Accessed April 29, 2020.

Neumann M, Sampathu DM, Kwong LK, et al: Ubiquitinated TDP-43 in frontotemporal lobar degeneration and amyotrophic lateral sclerosis. Science 314(5796):130–133, 2006 17023659

Nurnberger JI Jr, Austin J, Berrettini WH, et al: What should a psychiatrist know about genetics? Review and recommendations from the Residency Education Committee of the International Society of Psychiatric Genetics. J Clin Psychiatry 80(1):17nr12046, 2018 30549495

Ossenkoppele R, Schonhaut DR, Schöll M, et al: Tau PET patterns mirror clinical and neuroanatomical variability in Alzheimer's disease. Brain 139(Pt 5):1551–1567, 2016 26962052

Owens DK, Davidson KW, Krist AH, et al: Screening for HIV infection: US Preventive Services Task Force recommendation statement. JAMA 321(23):2326–2336, 2019 31184701

Persson K, Selbæk G, Braekhus A, et al: Fully automated structural MRI of the brain in clinical dementia workup. Acta Radiol 58(6):740–747, 2017 27687251

Poser S, Mollenhauer B, Kraubeta A, et al: How to improve the clinical diagnosis of Creutzfeldt-Jakob disease. Brain 122(Pt 12):2345–2351, 1999 10581227

Qaseem A, Snow V, Shekelle P, et al: Screening for HIV in health care settings: a guidance statement from the American College of Physicians and HIV Medicine Association. Ann Intern Med 150(2):125–131, 2009 19047022

Rabinovici GD, Gatsonis C, Apgar C, et al: Association of amyloid positron emission tomography with subsequent change in clinical management among medicare beneficiaries with mild cognitive impairment or dementia. JAMA 321(13):1286–1294, 2019 30938796

Risacher SL, Saykin AJ: Neuroimaging in aging and neurologic diseases, in Geriatric Neurology. Edited by Dekosky ST, Asthana S (Handbook of Clinical Neurology, Vol 167; Aminoff MJ, Boller F, and Swaab DF, series eds). Amsterdam, Elsevier, 2019, pp 191–227

Robins Wahlin TB, Wahlin A, Winblad B, Bäckman L: The influence of serum vitamin B12 and folate status on cognitive functioning in very old age. Biol Psychol 56(3):247–265, 2001 11399353

Sabin TD: AIDS: the new "great imitator." J Am Geriatr Soc 35(5):467–468, 1987 3571794

Schuff N, Woerner N, Boreta L, et al: MRI of hippocampal volume loss in early Alzheimer's disease in relation to ApoE genotype and biomarkers. Brain 132(pt 4):1067–1077, 2009 19251758

Selhub J, Bagley LC, Miller J, Rosenberg IH: B vitamins, homocysteine, and neurocognitive function in the elderly. Am J Clin Nutr 71(2):614S–620S, 2000 10681269

Sethi S, Brietzke E: Omics-based biomarkers: application of metabolomics in neuropsychiatric disorders. Int J Neuropsychopharmacol 19(3):pyv096, 2015 26453695

Shim JC, Shin JG, Kelly DL, et al: Adjunctive treatment with a dopamine partial agonist, aripiprazole, for antipsychotic-induced hyperprolactinemia: a placebo-controlled trial. Am J Psychiatry 164(9):1404–1410, 2007 17728426

Smailovic U, Koenig T, Kåreholt I, et al: Quantitative EEG power and synchronization correlate with Alzheimer's disease CSF biomarkers. Neurobiol Aging 63:88–95, 2018 29245058

Smith AD, Refsum H: Homocysteine, B vitamins, and cognitive impairment. Annu Rev Nutr 36:211–239, 2016 27431367

Smith AD, Refsum H, Bottiglieri T, et al: Homocysteine and dementia: an international consensus statement. J Alzheimers Dis 62(2):561–570, 2018 29480200

Smith MP, Bluth MH: Common interferences in drug testing. Clin Lab Med 36(4):663–671, 2016 27842784

Sperling RA, Aisen PS, Beckett LA, et al: Toward defining the preclinical stages of Alzheimer's disease: recommendations from the National Institute on Aging-Alzheimer's Association workgroups on diagnostic guidelines for Alzheimer's disease. Alzheimers Dement 7(3):280–292, 2011 21514248

Steinhoff BJ, Räcker S, Herrendorf G, et al: Accuracy and reliability of periodic sharp wave complexes in Creutzfeldt-Jakob disease. Arch Neurol 53(2):162–166, 1996 8639066

Takeda Pharmaceuticals America: Trintellix: Highlights of Prescribing Information. Deerfield, IL, Takeda Pharmaceuticals, May 2016. Available at: https://www.accessdata.fda.gov/drugsatfda_docs/label/2016/204447s007lbl.pdf. Accessed April 16, 2020.

Thomas SHL: Drugs, QT interval abnormalities and ventricular arrhythmias. Adverse Drug React Toxicol Rev 13(2):77–102, 1994 7918900

U.S. Food and Drug Administration: Guidance for Industry: E14 Clinical Evaluation of QT/QTc Interval Prolongation and Proarrhythmic Potential for Non-Antiarrhythmic Drugs. Rockville, MD, U.S. Food and Drug Administration, October 2005. Available at: https://www.fda.gov/media/71372/download. Accessed April 29, 2020.

U.S. Food and Drug Administration: Revised recommendations for Celexa (citalopram hydro-
     bromide) related to a potential risk of abnormal heart rhythms with high doses. FDA Drug
     Safety Communication, December 2017. Available at: https://www.fda.gov/drugs/drug-
     safety-and-availability/fda-drug-safety-communication-revised-recommendations-celexa-
     citalopram-hydrobromide-related. Accessed April 16, 2020.
Valdes AM, Glass D, Spector TD: Omics technologies and the study of human ageing. Nat Rev
     Genet 14(9):601–607, 2013 23938363
VandeVrede L, Gibbs DM, Koestler M, et al: Symptomatic amyloid-related imaging abnormal-
     ities in an APOE ε4/ε4 patient treated with aducanumab. Alzheimers Dement (Amst)
     12(1):e12101, 2020 33072846
Zannas AS, Wong TZ, Doraiswamy PM: How much is a picture worth? Putting amyloid imag-
     ing to the test. Dement Geriatr Cogn Disord Extra 2(1):649–651, 2012 23341830
Zetterberg H, van Swieten JC, Boxer AL, Rohrer JD: Review: Fluid biomarkers for frontotem-
     poral dementias. Neuropathol Appl Neurobiol 45(1):81–87, 2019 30422329
Zivin K, Pfeiffer PN, Bohnert AS, et al: Evaluation of the FDA warning against prescribing cit-
     alopram at doses exceeding 40 mg. Am J Psychiatry 170(6):642–650, 2013 23640689

CHAPTER 6

Neuropsychological Assessment of Late-Life Cognitive Disorders

Kevin J. Manning, Ph.D.
Beth Springate, Ph.D.

Neuropsychiatric illnesses—especially in later life—are commonly associated with perceived or objective changes in cognitive functioning. Neuropsychological assessment offers a sensitive, reliable, and noninvasive approach to documenting cognitive changes (Welsh-Bohmer et al. 2003). Neuropsychological evaluations are utilized in several contexts (e.g., academic, forensic, rehabilitation). Our goals in this chapter are 1) to describe in detail the instances in which neuropsychological assessment can be most useful in geriatric settings, 2) to discuss the neuropsychological examination process and common instruments applied in this context, and 3) to summarize the neurobehavioral presentations of common disorders in geriatric practices, specifically the profiles of normal aging, common neurodegenerative disorders of later life, and late-life depression.

Neuropsychological Assessment in Geriatric Settings

Patients in geriatric clinics are commonly referred for neuropsychological evaluation for three reasons. The first and by far most frequent reason for referral is to assist in the diagnosis of a cognitive disorder. Specifically, the examination is used to verify the presence or absence of a cognitive syndrome (e.g., mild cognitive impairment [MCI] or dementia) and to determine the likely differential diagnostic possibilities based on the behavioral profile (e.g., Alzheimer's disease [AD] vs. vascular cognitive impairment). Follow-up examinations may be recommended to enhance diagnostic clarification of neurodegenerative diseases when the establishment of progression is helpful in making a diagnosis. For example, the certainty of a probable AD diagnosis is increased with evidence of progressive cognitive decline on subsequent evaluations (McKhann et al. 2011). The second reason for referral to testing is to guide clinical care decisions, including the determination of functional capacities and competency (see Koltai and Welsh-Bohmer 2000). Issues typically confronted in a geriatric evaluation include the patient's ability to live independently, and increasing empirical evidence supports the use of neuropsychological tests as proxies for assessing instrumental activities of daily living such as medication management, automobile driving, and financial capacity (Manning et al. 2012; Ott et al. 2013; Papandonatos et al. 2015; Sherod et al. 2009). Finally, the neuropsychological evaluation can be used to guide appropriate therapeutic interventions, such as rehabilitation efforts or psychiatric management. Identified cognitive strengths and weaknesses can be used for designing appropriate rehabilitation approaches (see Attix and Welsh-Bohmer 2006) or to alert providers to the likelihood of poor antidepressant treatment response (Morimoto et al. 2011, 2012).

The actual neuropsychological evaluation process varies in form and length of administration across clinical practices. This depends in part on the populations typically served and in part on the training emphasis of the neuropsychologist administering the examination. Our practice at the University of Connecticut School of Medicine begins with a diagnostic interview to identify the major referral issues and presenting symptoms. During the interview, a patient's orientation to situation, language, behavioral organization, memory, mood, and affect are observed in a naturalistic context. With patient consent, family members are also interviewed to determine changes in the patient's functional ability and to clarify historical and medical information. In the formal testing session, 10 central domains of cognition and behavior are generally assessed: orientation, intelligence, language expression and comprehension, episodic learning and memory, attention and concentration, higher executive functions, spatial abilities, sensorimotor integration, personality and behavior, and mood and anxiety. Neuropsychological tests commonly used to assess these various functional domains are listed in Table 6–1.

The neuropsychological evaluation results in a profile of performance that is interpreted relative to the established behavioral profiles of known neurobehavioral syndromes. Comprehensive neuropsychological evaluations go beyond routine screening of cognitive functioning and benefit from well-established normative data. Although normative data stratified by various races, age groups, and education levels are increasingly available for screening tests, it is still commonplace to interpret cognitive screening tests as an absolute score. Case in point: a score of <26 on the Montreal Cognitive Assessment may be useful in distinguishing MCI from healthy aging in a well-educated white sample, but such a score may not be appropriate when used with other racial groups or patients with lower education backgrounds (Milani et al. 2018; Rossetti et al. 2019). Screening tests also may not capture the subtle cognitive deficits associated with the very earliest stages of a neurodegenerative disorder or neuropsychiatric illness associated with modest cognitive changes (e.g., geriatric depression). As an example from the domain of memory, the length of the word list asked to be recalled and the number of repetition trials impact the sensitivity of the measure in detecting MCI; 16-item word list learning and recall tests appear to be more sensitive to

TABLE 6–1.   **Common neuropsychological tests used in geriatric assessment**

Domain	Tests commonly used	References
Orientation/Global mental status	Mini-Mental State Examination	Folstein et al. 1975
	Montreal Cognitive Assessment	Nasreddine et al. 2005
Intellect	Wechsler Adult Intelligence Scale, 4th Edition, Wechsler Test of Adult Reading	Wechsler 2009a
Language	Boston Naming Test	Kaplan et al. 1978
	Category/Semantic fluency (e.g., animal fluency)	Strauss et al. 2006
	Lexical fluency (e.g., F-A-S or C-F-L; Controlled Oral Word Association Test)	Benton and Hamsher 1983
	Multilingual Naming Test	Gollan et al. 2012
Memory	Brief Visuospatial Memory Test–Revised	Benedict 1997
	Buschke Selective Reminding Test	Strauss et al. 2006
	California Verbal Learning Test, 2nd Edition	Delis et al. 2000
	Hopkins Verbal Learning Test–Revised	Brandt and Benedict 2001
	Rey Auditory Verbal Learning Test	Ivnik et al. 1992
	Wechsler Memory Scale, 4th Edition	Wechsler 2009b
Attention/Concentration	Subtests from the Wechsler Memory Scale–IV and Wechsler Adult Intelligence Scale–IV	Lezak et al. 2012
Executive function	Color Trail Making Test	D'Elia et al. 1996
	Stroop Color and Word Test	Golden and Freshwater 2002
	Symbol Digit Modalities Test	Smith 1968
	Trail Making Test	Reitan 1958
	Wisconsin Card Sorting Test	Berg 1948
Visuoperception	Benton Facial Recognition Test	Benton et al. 1983
	Judgment of Line Orientation Test	Benton et al. 1981
Sensorimotor abilities	Grooved pegboard	Strauss et al. 2006
	Finger oscillation	Heaton et al. 1991
Personality and behavior	Frontal Systems Behavior Rating Scale	Grace et al. 1999
	Minnesota Multiphasic Personality Inventory–2	Hathaway and McKinley 1951
Mood and anxiety	Beck Anxiety Inventory	Beck and Steer 1993
	Beck Depression Inventory–II	Beck et al. 1996
	Geriatric Depression Scale	Yesavage et al. 1982–1983
Everyday functioning	Dementia Severity Rating Scale	Clark and Ewbank 1996
	Everyday Cognition Test	Farias et al. 2008
	Functional Activities Questionnaire	Pfeffer et al. 1982

MCI than 10-item word lists or other composite measures of memory (Duff et al. 2010; Rabin et al. 2009).

Neuropsychological examination is not simply a process of actuarial comparisons to normative tables. Like other forms of clinical diagnosis, this examination rests on an inferential process. The neuropsychological diagnosis is an iterative process incorporating multiple sources of information to arrive at diagnostic impressions (see Potter and Attix 2006). When assessing a geriatric patient, the psychologist must first determine the patient's likely premorbid ability to determine if any observed changes are newly acquired or reflect long-standing weaknesses. Once this has been established, the presence of cognitive impairment is determined in reference to appropriate normative values. Any potential confounding influences on test performance are considered, including the patient's motivation, effort, and other behaviors that might interfere with optimal function (e.g., anxiety). Interpretation of likely medical and psychological contributions to the cognitive profile requires a good appreciation of brain-behavior organization. The neuropsychologist must consider whether the results obtained make sense from a functional anatomical perspective and then analyze the profile to determine its conformity to known neurobehavioral syndromes, such as normal aging, MCI, AD, and depression. Other attendant data are considered, such as medical history, ancillary studies (including imaging data), and informant report of functional change. In the following sections, we summarize the neuropsychology of normal aging and the differentiation of various common forms of late-life neurocognitive disorder (NCD). We begin by reviewing the concept of effort as it applies to interpreting neuropsychological evaluations. We end by considering in some detail the neuropsychology of geriatric mood disorders and the contribution of depressive disorders to the NCD presentation.

Symptom Validity Testing

Symptom validity testing is a major component of the neuropsychological evaluation. It attempts to address the critical question of whether the patient's neuropsychological performance is at or below the patient's true capacity (Bianchini et al. 2001). The answer to this question directly influences the interpretation of the entire evaluation. Symptom validity testing is a predominant part of medicolegal neuropsychological evaluations but is also relevant to clinical evaluation of older adults, including patients from memory disorder clinics—of whom a small but significant percentage may exhibit a performance that is not considered valid in the context of presenting complaints, symptom history, and cognitive profile (Rienstra et al. 2013).

Neuropsychologists traditionally frame equivocal or substandard symptom validity findings in terms of "effort." Thus, the terms *insufficient effort, inadequate effort*, or *poor effort* are often used to describe patients performing below expectations on symptom validity or "effort" tests. These effort tests require very little effort or ability and are typically performed with few or no errors by a wide range of patients with bona fide neurological, psychiatric, or developmental problems (Bigler 2012). Performance below an established threshold on such measures suggests that not enough effort was expended in the direction of capable performance. Clinical investigation is needed to understand the cause of the suboptimal effort, and this may not be ascertained from a single neuropsychological evaluation. Certainly, factitious disorder, malingering, and symptom exaggeration are potential considerations. Careful administration and interpretation of effort tests are required when working with older adults, perhaps more so than with other populations; clinicians should be mindful that patients with mild cognitive problems can appear to exhibit "poor effort" on symptom validity testing due to their NCD. Several studies have reported that patients with mild dementia often perform below effort testing thresholds that, if interpreted at face value, would suggest the patient demonstrated inadequate effort (Dean et al. 2009; Teichner and Wagner 2004).

Neuropsychology of Normal Aging

Most cognitive abilities naturally decline with age, including abilities broadly lumped into the domains of memory, reasoning, and speed of information processing (Salthouse 2010). By contrast, learned information such as vocabulary continues to improve into the sixth decade of life before slightly declining and then plateauing (Salthouse 2010). Some cognitive theorists have posited that decreases in a specific cognitive domain may account for the more general cognitive changes accompanying age. Empirical studies support slowed central processing as a leading cause of cognitive change with aging (Finkel et al. 2007). Another explanation posits that the profile of cognitive change in normal aging is due to a loss in fluid abilities—that is, skills that require novel problem solving and flexible thought (Botwinick 1977; Horn 1982). By contrast, well-rehearsed verbal abilities—so-called crystalized skills—are less susceptible to age-associated change. Refinements of this hypothesis have conceptualized normal aging as a selective vulnerability in frontal dysexecutive processes (Daigneault and Braun 1993). This notion is consistent with the behavioral difficulties observed, suggesting subtle impairments in integrative and retrieval functions, and is also supported by neuroimaging (Coffey et al. 1992; Gur et al. 1987; Langley and Madden 2000; Tisserand 2003). Indeed, cognitive changes in normal aging are likely in part brought about by neuronal cell loss in prefrontal regions and the hippocampus, as well as the accumulation of small vessel ischemia.

Despite declines in several cognitive abilities, the cognitive profile of normal aging is distinct from that seen in dementia. For example, although learning and recall abilities decline in both normal aging and AD, the principal memory problem in normal aging is difficulty efficiently accessing stored information, as opposed to the difficulty consolidating or conserving new information into long-term memory stores seen in patients with AD. Thus, recognition memory testing usually helps facilitate the retrieval process in normal aging but not in AD. Elsewhere, normal aging can be distinguished from other cognitive disorders by the magnitude of cognitive impairments. For example, whereas both normal aging and vascular cognitive impairment are characterized by slowed processing speed and changes in executive functioning, the severity of cognitive slowing and executive dysfunction is much greater in vascular cognitive impairment.

Differentiating Common Forms of Neurocognitive Disorder in Late Life

To some extent, the cognitive profiles of various NCD subtypes are overlapping, but many of them have unique features that can be of diagnostic utility. When attempting to differentiate common forms of NCD, we find it useful to begin our case conceptualization with two key questions in mind: 1) What are the most prominent symptoms? and 2) What is the severity of the presented difficulties? In other words, does the patient or family report symptoms suggestive of normal aging, mild impairment, or more severe impairment? The cognitive profiles of NCD subtypes are described in Table 6–2. Prominent symptoms for each NCD are discussed in the sections that follow.

Regarding symptom severity, considerable time should be spent gathering information about a patient's everyday functioning. Despite incredible advances in the in vivo identification of disease pathology, dementia remains a clinical diagnosis for which impaired everyday functioning is a critical and necessary component. Thus, diagnostic interviewing should seek to understand whether a patient can successfully complete basic and instrumental activities of daily living necessary for independent living. Where mild impairment is in question, we find a detailed understanding of the patient's ability to manage finances, use transportation, and take medications as prescribed to be particularly important. Several good brief questionnaires can be administered to an informant to help quantify the nature of the patient's cognitive and functional performance (see Table 6–1). Normative data are available for several measures, and the Dementia Severity Rating Scale can be converted to a Clinical Dementia Rating Sum of Box Score, a common metric in determining dementia severity (Moelter et al. 2015).

Alzheimer's Disease

AD is the leading cause of dementia in older adults, accounting for 50%–75% of all dementia cases identified in community-based cohorts and population-based series (Breitner 2006; Ebly et al. 1994; Gascón-Bayarri et al. 2007). AD is primarily a disorder of memory, although there are exceptions, as in cases of posterior cortical atrophy and certain types of primary progressive aphasia in which the initial cognitive symptoms associated with AD are visuospatial and language difficulties (de Souza et al. 2011; Santos-Santos et al. 2018). By and large, however, the initial presenting symptom is memory impairment, with family members of patients often providing examples of forgetfulness (e.g., patient is increasingly repetitive or appears to forget conversations after a brief period). This difficulty arises from the selective involvement of the medial temporal lobe early in the illness (Braak and Braak 1991; Hyman et al. 1984) giving rise to impaired consolidation of newly learned information into more permanent memory stores located across interconnected neocortical structures. From a neuropsychological perspective, the patient with AD has considerable difficulty learning new information and an inability to recall that information following a delay, and provided cues do not "jog" the patient's recall. This degree of memory difficulty may not be obvious on cognitive screening tests but often becomes readily apparent when assessed with a word list memory test.

AD is an insidious illness whereby neuropathology might accumulate for upward of 20 years or longer before clinical symptoms appear (Bateman et al. 2012). The diagnosis of MCI was developed to label older adults at risk of developing AD and described patients with memory impairment who did not exhibit functional difficulties indicative of gross dementia (Petersen et al. 1999). As a clinical syndrome, MCI is independent of etiology. However, with advances in biomarkers, research criteria suggest it is possible to definitively attribute MCI to AD's pathological change (based on the presence of amyloid in

TABLE 6–2.   Clinical neurocognitive syndromes and associated neuropsychological profiles

Neurocognitive syndrome and characteristics	Neuropsychological profile	Examples of tests fit for purpose*
Normal aging Annoying but not disabling problems Frequent problems with name retrieval Minor difficulties in recalling detailed events Subjective memory complaints	Deficiencies in memory retrieval Decreased general speed of processing Impaired fluid abilities (novel problem solving) Lowered performance on executive tasks and visuospatial skills/visuomotor speed	Lexical fluency, immediate recall of word lists Timed tests from WAIS-IV Symbol substitution tasks WAIS-IV Digit Span Backward, Trail Making Test WAIS-IV Performance IQ tests
Mild cognitive impairment—amnesic form CDR score of 0.5 (mild, questionable dementia) (Hughes et al. 1982) Noticeable change in memory as noted by informants Problem not disabling Subjective memory complaints	Functional disorder limited to mild interference from the memory difficulty Memory performance 1.0 or 1.5 SD below age-matched peers Otherwise-intact neurocognitive function or only minimal losses (<1.5 SD)	Buschke Selective Reminding Test CVLT-II Hopkins Verbal Learning Test–Revised Rey Auditory Verbal Learning Test Wechsler Memory Scale, 4th Edition
Alzheimer's disease Insidious onset Progressive impairment Prominent memory impairment Possible disorders: aphasia, apraxia, agnosia	Diminished executive skills Impaired memory consolidation with rapid forgetting Impaired semantic fluency and naming Impaired visuospatial analysis and praxis	Episodic memory tests (e.g., CVLT-II, Brief Visuospatial Memory Test–Revised) Tests of novel problem solving and abstraction (WAIS-IV) Constructional praxis (copying figures), Trail Making Test, WAIS-IV Digit Span
Frontotemporal neurocognitive disorder Disinhibition or apathy Impaired judgment/insight Normal mental status initially	Less obvious memory impairments Pronounced executive impairments	Frontal Assessment Battery Short Category Test Stroop Color Word Test

TABLE 6–2. Clinical neurocognitive syndromes and associated neuropsychological profiles *(continued)*

Neurocognitive syndrome and characteristics	Neuropsychological profile	Examples of tests fit for purpose*
Frontotemporal neurocognitive disorder *(continued)*		
Prominent personality/behavioral change	Cognitive inflexibility Impaired sequencing Perseverative, imitative utilization behaviors Poor use of feedback Prone to interference	Wisconsin Card Sorting Test
Lewy body neurocognitive disorder		
Fluctuations in alertness/acute confusional state Falls resulting from orthostatic hypotension Memory impairment Neuroleptic sensitivity Parkinsonian signs Visual hallucinations	Memory impairment of AD, but with some partial saving Pronounced apraxia, visuospatial difficulties Rapidly increasing quantifiable deficits in many cases	Tests of visuospatial organization, e.g., constructional praxis tests (clock drawing, copy of the Rey-Osterrieth figure [Osterrieth 1944]), WAIS-IV Performance subtests
Vascular neurocognitive disorder		
Abrupt onset Focality on examination In multi-infarct neurocognitive disorder, stepwise progression Variation of symptoms with subtype	Asymmetric motor speed/dexterity Benefit from structural support/cueing Executive inefficiencies Language/memory retrieval difficulties common	Particular attention to discrepancies on memory test (CVLT-II) between intact recognition and cued recall but impaired free recall Trail Making Test, WAIS-IV Digit Span Backward
Parkinson's disease neurocognitive disorder		
Bradykinesia Bradyphrenia	Constructional deficits Executive deficiencies (slowed sequencing, impaired lexical fluency)	Benton Visual Retention Test or similar copy test; Judgment of Line Orientation Test

TABLE 6–2.   Clinical neurocognitive syndromes and associated neuropsychological profiles (continued)

Neurocognitive syndrome and characteristics	Neuropsychological profile	Examples of tests fit for purpose*
Parkinson's disease neurocognitive disorder (*continued*)		
Extrapyramidal motor disturbance	Impaired fine motor speed (asymmetry common)	Trail Making Test, WAIS-IV Digit Span Backward, and animal and other verbal fluency tests
Gait dysfunction and frequent falls	Retrieval memory deficit; Slowed performance	Wisconsin Card Sorting Test
Huntington's disease		
Bradyphrenia	Benefit from retrieval supports (recognition okay)	CVLT-II
Choreiform movements	Executive compromises	Motor testing: finger oscillation, grooved pegboard
Early age at onset (midlife)	Memory difficulty in retrieval	Trail Making Test, WAIS-IV Digit Span Backward, Wisconsin Card Sorting Test, and animal and other verbal fluency tests
Neurocognitive disorder	Poor verbal fluency/preserved naming; Slowed performance	
Progressive supranuclear palsy		
Axial rigidity	Memory weakness characterized as inefficiencies in storage and retrieval	Benton Visual Retention Test or similar copy test; Judgment of Line Orientation Test
Extrapyramidal syndrome but no tremor	Mild dysexecutive symptoms: impaired sequencing, fluency, flexibility	Trail Making Test, WAIS-IV Digit Span Backward, Wisconsin Card Sorting Test, and animal and other verbal fluency tests
Frequent falls	Motor slowing	
Ophthalmic abnormalities (limited downgaze)		
Pseudobulbar palsy		
Normal-pressure hydrocephalus		
Gait disturbance	Benefit from retrieval supports	Naming and verbal fluency
Incontinence	Memory retrieval problems	Special attention to CVLT-II (recall vs. recognition)
Memory impairment	Slowed information processing	

TABLE 6–2.   Clinical neurocognitive syndromes and associated neuropsychological profiles *(continued)*

Neurocognitive syndrome and characteristics	Neuropsychological profile	Examples of tests fit for purpose*
Creutzfeldt-Jakob disease		
Neurocognitive disorder with pyramidal and extrapyramidal signs	Rapidly evolving neurocognitive disorder	Constructional tasks
Transient spikes on electroencephalogram	Subtypes with a profile akin to AD or a pronounced complex visuospatial disorder (Balint's syndrome)	Judgment of Line Orientation Test
Typically, rapid onset and course		WAIS-IV processing speed and perceptual organization tasks
Neurocognitive disorder associated with geriatric depression		
Affective disorder	Behavioral tendencies to abandon tasks, poor motivation	Effort across all tests
Cognitive complaints linked temporally to the depressive disorder	Impaired attention, concentration, sequencing, cognitive flexibility, and executive control	Naming and verbal fluency
Memory complaints	Impaired performance on effortful processing tasks	Special attention to CVLT-II (recall vs. recognition)
Psychomotor slowing	Memory improvement with cueing/recognition	
	Retrieval memory difficulty	

AD=Alzheimer's disease; CDR=Clinical Dementia Rating; CVLT-II=California Verbal Learning Test, 2nd Edition; WAIS-IV=Wechsler Adult Intelligence Scale, 4th Edition.
*Author citations are included in this table only for tests not listed in Table 6–1.

the absence of tau) or prodromal AD (based on the presence of amyloid and tau) (Jack et al. 2018). With the increasing availability of biomarkers, greater precision in linking MCI with an etiology such as AD may soon be clinically commonplace, but for most practitioners this is not the case. There is also a considerable literature on "reversible" MCI (Grande et al. 2016), although empirical evidence suggests MCI definitions based on consistent impairment in memory or another domain (e.g., where the patient clearly exhibits impairment across two or more memory measures) result in a reliable definition of MCI that very rarely reverts to normal (Jak et al. 2009).

As AD progresses, other areas of cognition become progressively more involved, reflecting the spread of neuropathological involvement to the lateral temporal areas, parietal cortex, and frontal neocortical areas (Small et al. 2000; Storandt et al. 2006; Welsh et al. 1992). The prototypical changes appear in expressive language, visuospatial function, higher executive control, and semantic knowledge (Weintraub et al. 2012). At later stages of the illness, anomia with impaired semantic fluency (e.g., generation of animal names) is generally seen on examination. Word search and circumlocution tendencies are common in conversational speech, whereas speech comprehension is better preserved, as are all other fundamental elements of communication (Weintraub et al. 2012). Visuospatial problems become more prominent in later stages of illness, resulting in dressing apraxia, difficulty recognizing objects or people, and problems performing familiar motor acts (Cronin-Golomb and Amick 2001). Subtle problems in spatial processing and visual motion detection can occur early and may be detectable only on formal examination (Mapstone et al. 2003). Visuospatial problems can be illuminated by tests of spatial judgment and visual organization (Rizzo et al. 2000). In everyday settings, visuospatial problems may manifest as intermittent topographical disorientation, leading to difficulties in finding familiar routes while driving (Rizzo et al. 1997). Figure 6–1 compares the memory loss characterizing AD and MCI with that characterizing normal aging.

Cerebrovascular Disease

Cerebrovascular disease is an independent contributor to cognitive decline and frequently co-occurs with AD and other dementias (Schneider et al. 2007). Traditionally, neuropsychological investigations into the cognitive sequelae of cerebrovascular disease have focused on vascular dementia subsequent to "overt" cerebrovascular disease—that is, clinically relevant infarcts. Reference was often made to the stepwise cognitive decline of vascular dementia accompanying additional infarcts as a prime aspect differentiating it from AD. Although this remains true, it is also increasingly clear that "covert" cerebrovascular disease—small vessel ischemia, lacunar infarcts, microbleeds—contribute to cognitive decline in older adults and may otherwise be clinically silent (Black 2011). The term *vascular cognitive impairment* describes patients with cognitive impairment related to cerebrovascular disease that is not severe enough to warrant a diagnosis of dementia.

Vascular cognitive impairment or dementia in the absence of a clinical history of stroke or available neuroimaging can be challenging to differentiate from AD. Small vessel cerebrovascular disease may insidiously increase over time and detrimentally impact a wide range of cognitive abilities, including memory (Kennedy and Raz 2009). However, the more common cognitive profile associated with small vessel disease reflects the disruption in the dorsolateral prefrontal and subcortical circuitry (Kramer

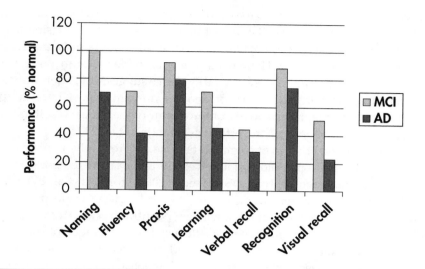

FIGURE 6–1. Profiles of neuropsychological test performance by patients with mild cognitive impairment (MCI) and patients with moderate Alzheimer's disease (AD).

Bars indicate the performance of patients with MCI (*n*=153) and moderately impaired patients with AD (*n*=277) on subtests of the Consortium to Establish a Registry for Alzheimer's Disease (CERAD; Tariot 1996) neuropsychological battery compared with the performance of nonimpaired elderly control subjects (*n*=158) of similar age, sex, and education. The overall neuropsychological test performance of the sample with AD is well below that of both patients with MCI and subjects experiencing normal aging. Patients with MCI performed at normal levels on naming and praxis. Learning and verbal fluency were mildly affected in this group, falling at 71% of normal. Memory was particularly affected in both AD and MCI. Verbal recall on the CERAD Word List Memory Task was 45% of normal in the sample with MCI and only 28% for the sample with AD. Visual memory was 51% of normal in MCI and 23% in AD.
Source. Data from the Cache County Study of Memory sample (K.A. Welsh-Bohmer, unpublished).

et al. 2002). Memory is involved, but deficits are often patchy in nature. Patients may show impaired recollection of some recent events but a surprising memory of some other occurrence transpiring in the same time frame. With formal neuropsychological testing, the pattern on memory testing is usually one of inefficient acquisition of new information leading to a flattened learning curve over repeating trials (Looi and Sachdev 1999; Padovani et al. 1995). Recall performance can be quite low, similar to that seen in AD and MCI, but rapid forgetting is not a typical feature (Hayden et al. 2005; Matsuda et al. 1998). The information acquired, albeit limited, is generally retained, so that savings scores between a final learning trial and a later delayed recall trial generally are high. Finally, recall improves dramatically with a recognition format, suggesting a primary difficulty in retrieval rather than in the storage or consolidation of new information (Hayden et al. 2005). Beyond memory, dysexecutive functions are typically involved (Prins et al. 2005), leading to slowed sequencing, cognitive inflexibility, and decreased verbal fluency (Mathias and Burke 2009). Asymmetries in sensory motor function or deficits in coordination also are frequently demonstrated.

Frontotemporal Lobar Degeneration

Frontotemporal lobar degeneration (FTLD) represents one of the major non-AD neurodegenerative disorders. Methodological limitations have led to varying estimates of its incidence and prevalence, with a recent review noting a point prevalence of 0.01–

4.6 per 1,000 persons and an incidence of 0.0–0.3 per 1,000 person-years (Hogan et al. 2016). With average age at onset in the mid- to late 50s (Johnson et al. 2005), FTLD is one of the more common causes of early-onset dementia. Patients often present with changes in behavior and language, which contrasts with AD's typical amnestic presentation. FTLD is typically divided into three subtypes: behavioral variant (bvFTLD) and the primary progressive aphasias (PPAs)—semantic variant PPA (svPPA) and nonfluent variant PPA (nfvPPA). bvFTLD is the most common variant, with patients typically presenting with early changes in socioemotional behavior, including disinhibition, apathy, obsessions and compulsions, hyperorality, and lack of empathy (Rascovsky et al. 2011). Although executive dysfunction is often present (e.g., inflexibility, decreased abstract reasoning and problem solving), a significant number of patients with bvFTLD perform normally on brief mental status examinations or formal neuropsychological testing in early stages of the disease (Gregory et al. 1999). Insight into their behavioral changes is often limited. Misdiagnosis with primary psychiatric disorders early in the disease course is not uncommon (Landqvist Waldö et al. 2015).

svPPA and nfvPPA represent the language manifestations of FTLD, meaning language is the primary impairment within the first 2 years of the disease process. Logopenic PPA is a third PPA variant but is primarily associated with AD pathology and thus is not discussed here. Patients with svPPA display a slow loss of semantic knowledge over time, with the core clinical features being anomia and single-word comprehension deficits, with spared speech production, syntax, and grammar. In contrast, patients with nfvPPA initially present with effortful speech and changes in grammar but intact comprehension (Gorno-Tempini et al. 2011; Mesulam 2003)

The underlying neuropathology of FTLD involves frontal or anterior temporal lobe abnormalities, which is expected because these regions support language and behavioral functioning. The aggregation of three major proteins is key in FTLD's pathology: phosphorylated tau, transactive response DNA-binding protein 43 (TDP-43), and fused in sarcoma (FUS). Evidence suggests that 30%–50% of FTLD cases are familial in origin (Goldman et al. 2005), and multiple genetic mutations have been linked to FTLD, with the most common being mutations in *MAPT*, *GRN*, and *C9orf72* (Sieben et al. 2012).

Parkinson's Disease and Lewy Body Disease

Cognitive changes are commonplace in Parkinson's disease (PD) and gradually progress. Subtle decline in cognitive functioning and instrumental activities of daily living occurs several years before patients receive an official diagnosis of PD (Darweesh et al. 2017; Fereshtehnejad et al. 2019). For most patients, cognitive abilities continue to deteriorate throughout the course of the illness until cognitive and functional impairments are severe enough to warrant a diagnosis of dementia. It is estimated that 75% of patients with PD who live 10 years past their initial diagnosis will develop PD dementia (PDD) (Aarsland and Kurz 2010). Related to PDD is dementia with Lewy bodies (DLB), with both dementia syndromes overlapping in many clinical features and neuropathology (Friedman 2018). The temporal sequence of movement and cognitive symptoms has traditionally been used to differentiate these disorders. DLB is diagnosed when cognitive impairment precedes parkinsonism or begins within 1 year of its onset, whereas in PDD the cognitive impairment begins in the setting of well-established PD (McKeith et al. 2017). The cognitive profiles of these two disorders are similar, and on autopsy, both clinical syndromes reveal a mix of cortical and subcortical Lewy bodies, α-synuclein pathology, and significant plaques and tangles (Jellinger and Korczyn 2018).

On neuropsychological evaluation, the cognitive impairments of PDD and DLB are similar, but the profiles can often be differentiated from those typically observed in AD (Tröster 2008; Welsh-Bohmer and Warren 2006). Both PDD and DLB are characterized by a pattern of memory retrieval problems and mild dysexecutive disturbances, which early in the course are less dramatic and globally impairing than the cognitive deficits of AD (Hamilton et al. 2004). Visuospatial disturbances are often observed early in the course of the Lewy body dementias (Ballard et al. 1999; Hansen et al. 1990; Salmon et al. 1996), but expressive language such as naming tends to be better preserved than in AD (Ballard et al. 1999; Heyman et al. 1999). Despite these differences on neuropsychological testing, making a solid differential diagnosis based solely on the cognitive profile will be difficult (Monza et al. 1998; Soliveri et al. 2000; Testa et al. 2001), particularly in the very early stages. The integration of the clinical examination findings (which include history and review of systems, motor examination, cognitive findings, behavioral ratings, psychiatric interview, and supportive laboratory studies such as neuroimaging) is necessary to clarify these disorders from each other and to make an accurate diagnosis early in the process (Litvan et al. 2012).

In this context, particular attention to the history of symptoms (e.g., fluctuations in ability throughout the day) and to the presence or absence of defined behavioral impairments is crucial to diagnosis (Geser et al. 2005; Pillon et al. 1991). The presence of visual hallucinations not associated with treatment can help distinguish DLB from PDD (Aarsland et al. 2001). Although visual hallucinations can occur in AD, they are uncommon in the earliest stages; hence, their presence in a neurocognitive process signals another etiological cause, such as DLB. Finally, rapid eye movement sleep behavior disorder—now a core symptom of DLB (McKeith et al. 2017)—is recognized as a prodromal stage of synucleinopathies (DLB and PD) (Galbiati et al. 2019) but is seemingly much less likely to occur in AD (Galbiati et al. 2018).

Geriatric Depression and Neurocognitive Disorders

Two of the most common uses of neuropsychological assessment for elderly patients are evaluating memory disorders and determining the role of depression. Depression is common in elderly persons and associated with various medical conditions and increased mortality. Major depressive disorder (MDD) in elderly persons has a point prevalence of about 4% and a lifetime prevalence of about 16% (Steffens et al. 2000). Symptoms subthreshold to MDD are even more common, with some epidemiologically based studies suggesting that nearly one-third (28%) of adults age 65 and older exhibit prominent affective syndromes (Lyketsos et al. 2001). Depression severity may have a modest impact on the extent of cognitive dysfunction, but even mild levels of depressive symptoms are associated with cognitive weaknesses in older adults (Dotson et al. 2008).

Geriatric depression in the absence of other neuropsychiatric disorders can result in disabling cognitive functioning (Kiosses et al. 2001) and exacerbate the cognitive impairment observed in other neurocognitive disorders (Mackin et al. 2012). In years past, the term *pseudodementia* was used to describe older adults with depression and significant cognitive impairment—like that seen in dementia—who experienced an apparent improvement in cognition following depression remission. Over time, the use of *pseudodementia* as a descriptive label has become antiquated for several reasons. First—and of major relevance to this chapter—the neuropsychological profile of older adults with MDD largely involves mild weaknesses (i.e., low average performance) in processing speed and executive functioning, whereas other cognitive abilities are generally not significantly different from older adults without depression. Diffuse cognitive difficulties in patients with geriatric depression likely reflect bona fide dementia or its prodrome, psychosis, or issues related to effort. Indeed, early longitudinal studies of older adults with pseudodementia found that they were more likely to develop "irreversible" dementia after a relatively brief follow-up period of 2 years (Alexopoulos et al. 1993). Finally, many older adults with depression have cognitive weaknesses that do not always improve following treatment of depression, even if the depression has remitted (Bhalla et al. 2006; Koenig et al. 2015).

The neuropsychological profile of geriatric depression tends to be one of executive dysfunction. Cross-sectionally, mild weaknesses (i.e., low average performances) in processing speed and attention, response inhibition, working memory, planning and organization, and cognitive flexibility may be observed (Lockwood et al. 2002). Longitudinally, a recent study by Riddle et al. (2017) also found that patients with late-life MDD experienced a more rapid cognitive decline in various attention and memory measures over 5 years when compared with cognitively normal older adults without depression. Although the extent of cognitive change over time in this study was modest, these and other findings bolster the argument that late-life MDD increases the statistical likelihood of cognitive decline and eventual dementia. In fact, meta-analytic evidence suggests that older adults with MDD are about twice as likely to develop dementia (both AD and vascular dementia) as older adults without depression (Diniz et al. 2013).

Executive dysfunction may contribute to weaknesses in verbal learning and constructional praxis (Elderkin-Thompson et al. 2004, 2006; Mesholam-Gately et al. 2012). For example, older adults with MDD may exhibit weaknesses in word list learning and demonstrate a memory profile characterized by a flattened learning curve and impaired free recall of previously learned information after brief delays. Successful performance on word list learning tasks often involves working memory and organizational skills, two weaknesses commonly observed in geriatric depression. Thus, although older adults with geriatric depression may show weaknesses in learning and recall on word list tasks, a similar degree of difficulty may not be observed on memory tests in which information is presented in context (e.g., short stories). Furthermore, recognition memory testing is also often preserved in geriatric depression.

Conclusion

The neuropsychological evaluation provides a useful and cost-effective management approach for the diagnosis and management of the growing geriatric population with memory complaints. Neuropsychological evaluations are not needed for most major NCDs in which symptoms are obvious and the diagnosis is secure. They can be enormously useful, however, in more complex, less straightforward diagnostic situations, such as early AD detection or geriatric depression. By its objective nature, the neuropsychological examination has strong applications in medical management, providing information about patient capacities and deficits that is important for choosing intervention approaches and for guiding future decision-making with respect to competency and safety.

Key Points

- The neuropsychological presentation of Alzheimer's disease (AD) is characterized by a pronounced deficit in the consolidation of new information from short-term, immediate memory to more permanent storage. Thus, the deficit early in the disorder is a problem of rapidly forgetting newly learned information.

- The profile of normal cognitive aging is characterized by modest declines on executive function tests, in large measure because of inefficiencies in multi-task processing and declines in perceptual motor speed.

- Frontotemporal lobar degeneration is characterized by profound functional and behavioral changes. The neurocognitive deficits associated with the disorder, particularly in the early stages, may be difficult to discern with mental status instruments. Neuropsychological testing targeting executive functions can tease out the impairments in behavioral regulation, disinhibition, perseveration, judgment, and abstraction.

- The neuropsychological deficits associated with neurocognitive disorder due to Parkinson's disease are clinically similar to those of a closely aligned condition, neurocognitive disorder with Lewy bodies. However, the neuropsychological profiles of these conditions can be distinguished from that of neurocognitive disorder due to AD. Visuospatial deficits are common early in neurocognitive disorder due to Parkinson's disease and neurocognitive disorder with Lewy bodies, and the memory deficits are less severe than those of AD.

- Geriatric depression can cause significant impairments in the efficiency of cognitive processing, leading to selective problems in sustained attention, concentration, and memory. It is a risk factor for cognitive decline to dementia. When co-occurring with progressive neurological disorders, such as AD or vascular neurocognitive disorder, depression can lead to excess disability and an overall reduction in the quality of life that might otherwise be achieved.

References

Aarsland D, Kurz MW: The epidemiology of dementia associated with Parkinson's disease. Brain Pathol 20(3):633–639, 2010 20522088

Aarsland D, Cummings JL, Larsen JP: Neuropsychiatric differences between Parkinson's disease with dementia and Alzheimer's disease. Int J Geriatr Psychiatry 16(2):184–191, 2001 11241724

Alexopoulos GS, Meyers BS, Young RC, et al: The course of geriatric depression with "reversible dementia": a controlled study. Am J Psychiatry 150(11):1693–1699, 1993 8105707

Attix DK, Welsh-Bohmer KA: Geriatric Neuropsychology: Assessment and Intervention. Edited by Attix DK, Welsh-Bohmer KA. New York, Guilford, 2006

Ballard CG, Ayre G, O'Brien J, et al: Simple standardised neuropsychological assessments aid in the differential diagnosis of dementia with Lewy bodies from Alzheimer's disease and vascular dementia. Dement Geriatr Cogn Disord 10(2):104–108, 1999 10026383

Bateman RJ, Xiong C, Benzinger TL, et al: Clinical and biomarker changes in dominantly inherited Alzheimer's disease. N Engl J Med 367(9):795–804, 2012 22784036

Beck AT, Steer RA: Beck Anxiety Inventory. San Antonio, TX, Psychological Corporation, 1993

Beck AT, Steer RA, Brown GK: Beck Depression Inventory, II. San Antonio, TX, Psychological Corporation, 1996

Benedict RHB: Brief Visuospatial Memory Test–Revised. Lutz, FL, Psychological Assessment Resources, 1997

Benton AL, Hamsher K: Multilingual Aphasia Examination. Iowa City, IA, AJA Associates, 1983

Benton AL, Eslinger PJ, Damasio AR: Normative observations on neuropsychological test performances in old age. J Clin Neuropsychol 3(1):33–42, 1981 7276195

Benton AL, Hamsher K, Varney NR, et al: Contributions to Neuropsychological Assessment. New York, Oxford University Press, 1983

Berg EA: A simple objective technique for measuring flexibility in thinking. J Gen Psychol 39:15–22, 1948 18889466

Bhalla RK, Butters MA, Mulsant BH, et al: Persistence of neuropsychologic deficits in the remitted state of late-life depression. Am J Geriatr Psychiatry 14(5):419–427, 2006 16670246

Bianchini KJ, Mathias CW, Greve KW: Symptom validity testing: a critical review. Clin Neuropsychol 15(1):19–45, 2001 11778576

Bigler ED: Symptom validity testing, effort, and neuropsychological assessment. J Int Neuropsychol Soc 18(4):632–640, 2012 23057080

Black SE: Vascular cognitive impairment: epidemiology, subtypes, diagnosis and management. J R Coll Physicians Edinb 41(1):49–56, 2011 21365068

Botwinick J: Intellectual abilities, in The Handbook of the Psychology of Aging. Edited by Birren JE, Schaie KW. New York, Van Nostrand Reinhold, 1977, pp 508–605

Braak H, Braak E: Neuropathological stageing of Alzheimer-related changes. Acta Neuropathol 82(4):239–259, 1991 1759558

Brandt J, Benedict RHB: Hopkins Verbal Learning Test–Revised. Lutz, FL, Psychological Assessment Resources, 2001

Breitner JCS: Dementia: epidemiological considerations, nomenclature, and a tacit consensus definition. J Geriatr Psychiatry Neurol 19(3):129–136, 2006 16880354

Clark CM, Ewbank DC: Performance of the dementia severity rating scale: a caregiver questionnaire for rating severity in Alzheimer disease. Alzheimer Dis Assoc Disord 10(1):31–39, 1996 8919494

Coffey CE, Wilkinson WE, Parashos IA, et al: Quantitative cerebral anatomy of the aging human brain: a cross-sectional study using magnetic resonance imaging. Neurology 42(3 pt 1):527–536, 1992 1549213

Cronin-Golomb A, Amick M: Spatial abilities in aging, Alzheimer's disease, and Parkinson's disease, in Handbook of Neuropsychology, Vol 6: Aging and Dementia, 2nd Edition. Edited by Boller F, Cappa S. Amsterdam, Elsevier, 2001, pp 119–143

Daigneault S, Braun CM: Working memory and the Self-Ordered Pointing Task: further evidence of early prefrontal decline in normal aging. J Clin Exp Neuropsychol 15(6):881–895, 1993 8120125

Darweesh SK, Verlinden VJ, Stricker BH, et al: Trajectories of prediagnostic functioning in Parkinson's disease. Brain 140(2):429–441, 2017 28082300

Dean AC, Victor TL, Boone KB, et al: Dementia and effort test performance. Clin Neuropsychol 23(1):133–152, 2009 18609332

D'Elia LF, Satz P, Uchiyama CL, et al: Color Trails Test. Lutz, FL, Psychological Assessment Resources, 1996

Delis DC, Kramer JH, Kaplan E, et al: California Verbal Learning Test, Adult Version, 2nd Edition. San Antonio, TX, Psychological Corporation, 2000 de Souza LC, Corlier F, Habert MO, et al: Similar amyloid-β burden in posterior cortical atrophy and Alzheimer's disease. Brain 134(Pt 7):2036–2043, 2011 21705422

Diniz BS, Butters MA, Albert SM, et al: Late-life depression and risk of vascular dementia and Alzheimer's disease: systematic review and meta-analysis of community-based cohort studies. Br J Psychiatry 202(5):329–335, 2013 23637108

Dotson VM, Resnick SM, Zonderman AB: Differential association of concurrent, baseline, and average depressive symptoms with cognitive decline in older adults. Am J Geriatr Psychiatry 16(4):318–330, 2008 18378557

Duff K, Hobson VL, Beglinger LJ, O'Bryant SE: Diagnostic accuracy of the RBANS in mild cognitive impairment: limitations on assessing milder impairments. Arch Clin Neuropsychol 25(5):429–441, 2010 20570820

Ebly EM, Parhad IM, Hogan DB, Fung TS: Prevalence and types of dementia in the very old: results from the Canadian Study of Health and Aging. Neurology 44(9):1593–1600, 1994 7936280

Elderkin-Thompson V, Kumar A, Mintz J, et al: Executive dysfunction and visuospatial ability among depressed elders in a community setting. Arch Clin Neuropsychol 19(5):597–611, 2004 15271406

Elderkin-Thompson V, Mintz J, Haroon E, et al: Executive dysfunction and memory in older patients with major and minor depression. Arch Clin Neuropsychol 21(7):669–676, 2006 16908116

Farias ST, Mungas D, Reed BR, et al: The measurement of everyday cognition (ECog): scale development and psychometric properties. Neuropsychology 22(4):531–544, 2008 18590364

Fereshtehnejad SM, Yao C, Pelletier A, et al: Evolution of prodromal Parkinson's disease and dementia with Lewy bodies: a prospective study. Brain 142(7):2051–2067, 2019 31111143

Finkel D, Reynolds CA, McArdle JJ, Pedersen NL: Age changes in processing speed as a leading indicator of cognitive aging. Psychol Aging 22(3):558–568, 2007 17874954

Folstein MF, Folstein SE, McHugh PR: "Mini-mental state": a practical method for grading the cognitive state of patients for the clinician. J Psychiatr Res 12(3):189–198, 1975 1202204

Friedman JH: Dementia with Lewy bodies and Parkinson disease dementia: it is the same disease! Parkinsonism Relat Disord 46(suppl 1):S6–S9, 2018 28756177

Galbiati A, Carli G, Hensley M, Ferini-Strambi L: REM sleep behavior disorder and Alzheimer's disease: definitely no relationship? J Alzheimers Dis 63(1):1–11, 2018 29578489

Galbiati A, Verga L, Giora E, et al: The risk of neurodegeneration in REM sleep behavior disorder: a systematic review and meta-analysis of longitudinal studies. Sleep Med Rev 43:37–46, 2019 30503716

Gascón-Bayarri J, Reñé R, Del Barrio JL, et al: Prevalence of dementia subtypes in El Prat de Llobregat, Catalonia, Spain: the PRATICON study. Neuroepidemiology 28(4):224–234, 2007 17878737

Geser F, Wenning GK, Poewe W, McKeith I: How to diagnose dementia with Lewy bodies: state of the art. Mov Disord 20(suppl 12):S11–S20, 2005 16092075

Golden CJ, Freshwater SM: Stroop Color and Word Test: Revised Examiners Manual. Woodale, IL, Stoeling, 2002

Goldman JS, Farmer JM, Wood EM, et al: Comparison of family histories in FTLD subtypes and related tauopathies. Neurology 65(11):1817–1819, 2005 16344531

Gollan TH, Weissberger GH, Runnqvist E, et al: Self-ratings of spoken language dominance: a Multilingual Naming Test (MINT) and preliminary norms for young and aging Spanish-English bilinguals. Biling (Camb Engl) 15(3):594–615, 2012 25364296

Gorno-Tempini ML, Hillis AE, Weintraub S, et al: Classification of primary progressive aphasia and its variants. Neurology 76(11):1006–1014, 2011 21325651

Grace J, Stout JC, Malloy PF: Assessing frontal lobe behavioral syndromes with the frontal lobe personality scale. Assessment 6(3):269–284, 1999 10445964

Grande G, Cucumo V, Cova I, et al: Reversible mild cognitive impairment: the role of comorbidities at baseline evaluation. J Alzheimers Dis 51(1):57–67, 2016 26836169

Gregory CA, Serra-Mestres J, Hodges JR: Early diagnosis of the frontal variant of frontotemporal dementia: how sensitive are standard neuroimaging and neuropsychologic tests? Neuropsychiatry Neuropsychol Behav Neurol 12(2):128–135, 1999 10223261

Gur RC, Gur RE, Obrist WD, et al: Age and regional cerebral blood flow at rest and during cognitive activity. Arch Gen Psychiatry 44(7):617–621, 1987 3606327

Hamilton JM, Salmon DP, Galasko D, et al: A comparison of episodic memory deficits in neuropathologically confirmed dementia with Lewy bodies and Alzheimer's disease. J Int Neuropsychol Soc 10(5):689–697, 2004 15327716

Hansen L, Salmon D, Galasko D, et al: The Lewy body variant of Alzheimer's disease: a clinical and pathologic entity. Neurology 40(1):1–8, 1990 2153271

Hathaway SR, McKinley JC: Minnesota Multiphasic Personality Inventory: Manual (Revised). San Antonio, TX, Psychological Corporation, 1951

Hayden KM, Warren LH, Pieper CF, et al: Identification of VaD and AD prodromes: the Cache County Study. Alzheimers Dement 1(1):19–29, 2005 19595812

Heaton RK, Grant I, Matthews CG: Comprehensive Norms for an Expanded Halstead-Reitan Battery: Demographic Corrections, Research Findings, and Clinical Applications. Odessa, FL, Psychological Assessment Resources, 1991

Heyman A, Fillenbaum GG, Gearing M, et al: Comparison of Lewy body variant of Alzheimer's disease with pure Alzheimer's disease: Consortium to Establish a Registry for Alzheimer's Disease, Part XIX. Neurology 52(9):1839–1844, 1999 10371532

Hogan DB, Jetté N, Fiest KM, et al: The prevalence and incidence of frontotemporal dementia: a systematic review. Can J Neurol Sci 43(suppl 1):S96–S109, 2016 27307130

Horn J: The theory of fluid and crystallized intelligence in relation to concepts of cognitive psychology and aging in adulthood, in Aging and Cognitive Processes. Edited by Craik F, Trehub S. New York, Plenum, 1982, pp 237–278

Hughes CP, Berg L, Danziger WL, et al: A new clinical scale for the staging of dementia. Br J Psychiatry 140:566–572, 1982 7104545

Hyman BT, Van Hoesen GW, Damasio AR, Barnes CL: Alzheimer's disease: cell-specific pathology isolates the hippocampal formation. Science 225(4667):1168–1170, 1984 6474172

Ivnik RJ, Malec JF, Smith GE, et al: Mayo's older Americans normative studies: updated AVLT norms for ages 56–97. Clin Neuropsychol 6:83–104, 1992

Jack CR Jr, Bennett DA, Blennow K, et al: NIA-AA research framework: toward a biological definition of Alzheimer's disease. Alzheimers Dement 14(4):535–562, 2018 29653606

Jak AJ, Bondi MW, Delano-Wood L, et al: Quantification of five neuropsychological approaches to defining mild cognitive impairment. Am J Geriatr Psychiatry 17(5):368–375, 2009 19390294

Jellinger KA, Korczyn AD: Are dementia with Lewy bodies and Parkinson's disease dementia the same disease? BMC Med 16(1):34, 2018 29510692

Johnson JK, Diehl J, Mendez MF, et al: Frontotemporal lobar degeneration: demographic characteristics of 353 patients. Arch Neurol 62(6):925–930, 2005 15956163

Kaplan EF, Goodglass H, Weintraub S: The Boston Naming Test, 2nd Edition. Philadelphia, PA, Lea and Febiger, 1978

Kennedy KM, Raz N: Aging white matter and cognition: differential effects of regional variations in diffusion properties on memory, executive functions, and speed. Neuropsychologia 47(3):916–927, 2009 19166865

Kiosses DN, Klimstra S, Murphy C, Alexopoulos GS: Executive dysfunction and disability in elderly patients with major depression. Am J Geriatr Psychiatry 9(3):269–274, 2001 11481135

Koenig AM, DeLozier IJ, Zmuda MD, et al: Neuropsychological functioning in the acute and remitted States of late-life depression. J Alzheimers Dis 45(1):175–185, 2015 25471193

Koltai DC, Welsh-Bohmer KA: Geriatric neuropsychological assessment, in Clinician's Guide to Neuropsychological Assessment, 2nd Edition. Edited by Vanderploeg RD. Mahwah, NJ, Erlbaum Associates, 2000, pp 383–415

Kramer JH, Reed BR, Mungas D, et al: Executive dysfunction in subcortical ischaemic vascular disease. J Neurol Neurosurg Psychiatry 72(2):217–220, 2002 11796772

Landqvist Waldö M, Gustafson L, Passant U, Englund E: Psychotic symptoms in frontotemporal dementia: a diagnostic dilemma? Int Psychogeriatr 27(4):531–539, 2015 25486967

Langley LK, Madden DJ: Functional neuroimaging of memory: implications for cognitive aging. Microsc Res Tech 51(1):75–84, 2000 11002355

Lezak MD, Howieson DB, Biegler ED, et al: Neuropsychological Assessment, 5th Edition. New York, Oxford University Press, 2012

Litvan I, Goldman JG, Tröster AI, et al: Diagnostic criteria for mild cognitive impairment in Parkinson's disease: Movement Disorder Society Task Force guidelines. Mov Disord 27(3):349–356, 2012 22275317

Lockwood KA, Alexopoulos GS, van Gorp WG: Executive dysfunction in geriatric depression. Am J Psychiatry 159(7):1119–1126, 2002 12091189

Looi JC, Sachdev PS: Differentiation of vascular dementia from AD on neuropsychological tests. Neurology 53(4):670–678, 1999 10489025

Lyketsos CG, Sheppard JM, Steinberg M, et al: Neuropsychiatric disturbance in Alzheimer's disease clusters into three groups: the Cache County study. Int J Geriatr Psychiatry 16(11):1043–1053, 2001 11746650

Mackin RS, Insel P, Aisen PS, et al: Longitudinal stability of subsyndromal symptoms of depression in individuals with mild cognitive impairment: relationship to conversion to dementia after 3 years. Int J Geriatr Psychiatry 27(4):355–363, 2012 21744390

Manning KJ, Clarke C, Lorry A, et al: Medication management and neuropsychological performance in Parkinson's disease. Clin Neuropsychol 26(1):45–58, 2012 22150514

Mapstone M, Steffenella TM, Duffy CJ: A visuospatial variant of mild cognitive impairment: getting lost between aging and AD. Neurology 60(5):802–808, 2003 12629237

Mathias JL, Burke J: Cognitive functioning in Alzheimer's and vascular dementia: a meta-analysis. Neuropsychology 23(4):411–423, 2009 19586206

Matsuda O, Saito M, Sugishita M: Cognitive deficits of mild dementia: a comparison between dementia of the Alzheimer's type and vascular dementia. Psychiatry Clin Neurosci 52(1):87–91, 1998 9682939

McKeith IG, Boeve BF, Dickson DW, et al: Diagnosis and management of dementia with Lewy bodies: fourth consensus report of the DLB Consortium. Neurology 89(1):88–100, 2017 28592453

McKhann GM, Knopman DS, Chertkow H, et al: The diagnosis of dementia due to Alzheimer's disease: recommendations from the National Institute on Aging-Alzheimer's Association workgroups on diagnostic guidelines for Alzheimer's disease. Alzheimers Dement 7(3):263–269, 2011 21514250

Mesholam-Gately RI, Giuliano AJ, Zillmer EA, et al: Verbal learning and memory in older adults with minor and major depression. Arch Clin Neuropsychol 27(2):196–207, 2012 22189596

Mesulam MM: Primary progressive aphasia: a language-based dementia. N Engl J Med 349(16):1535–1542, 2003 14561797

Milani SA, Marsiske M, Cottler LB, et al: Optimal cutoffs for the Montreal Cognitive Assessment vary by race and ethnicity. Alzheimers Dement 10:773–781, 2018 30505927

Moelter ST, Glenn MA, Xie SX, et al: The Dementia Severity Rating Scale predicts clinical dementia rating sum of boxes scores. Alzheimer Dis Assoc Disord 29(2):158–160, 2015 24770371

Monza D, Soliveri P, Radice D, et al: Cognitive dysfunction and impaired organization of complex motility in degenerative parkinsonian syndromes. Arch Neurol 55(3):372–378, 1998 9520011

Morimoto SS, Gunning FM, Murphy CF, et al: Executive function and short-term remission of geriatric depression: the role of semantic strategy. Am J Geriatr Psychiatry 19(2):115–122, 2011 20808124

Morimoto SS, Gunning FM, Kanellopoulos D, et al: Semantic organizational strategy predicts verbal memory and remission rate of geriatric depression. Int J Geriatr Psychiatry 27(5):506–512, 2012 21618287

Nasreddine ZS, Phillips NA, Bédirian V, et al: The Montreal Cognitive Assessment, MoCA: a brief screening tool for mild cognitive impairment. J Am Geriatr Soc 53(4):695–699, 2005 15817019

Osterrieth PA: Le test de copie d'une figure complexe. Arch Psychol 30:206–356, 1944

Ott BR, Davis JD, Papandonatos GD, et al: Assessment of Driving-Related Skills prediction of unsafe driving in older adults in the office setting. J Am Geriatr Soc 61(7):1164–1169, 2013 23730836

Padovani A, Di Piero V, Bragoni M, et al: Patterns of neuropsychological impairment in mild dementia: a comparison between Alzheimer's disease and multi-infarct dementia. Acta Neurol Scand 92(6):433–442, 1995 8750107

Papandonatos GD, Ott BR, Davis JD, et al: Clinical utility of the Trail-Making Test as a predictor of driving performance in older adults. J Am Geriatr Soc 63(11):2358–2364, 2015 26503623

Petersen RC, Smith GE, Waring SC, et al: Mild cognitive impairment: clinical characterization and outcome. Arch Neurol 56(3):303–308, 1999 10190820

Pfeffer RI, Kurosaki TT, Harrah CH Jr, et al: Measurement of functional activities in older adults in the community. J Gerontol 37(3):323–329, 1982 7069156

Pillon B, Dubois B, Agid Y: Severity and specificity of cognitive impairment in Alzheimer's, Huntington's, and Parkinson's diseases and progressive supranuclear palsy. Ann NY Acad Sci 640:224–227, 1991 1837977

Potter GG, Attix DK: An integrated model for geriatric neuropsychological assessment, in Geriatric Neuropsychology: Assessment and Intervention. Edited by Attix DK, Welsh-Bohmer KA. New York, Guilford, 2006, pp 5–26

Prins ND, van Dijk EJ, den Heijer T, et al: Cerebral small-vessel disease and decline in information processing speed, executive function and memory. Brain 128(Pt 9):2034–2041, 2005 15947059

Rabin LA, Paré N, Saykin AJ, et al: Differential memory test sensitivity for diagnosing amnestic mild cognitive impairment and predicting conversion to Alzheimer's disease. Neuropsychol Dev Cogn B Aging Neuropsychol Cogn 16(3):357–376, 2009 19353345

Rascovsky K, Hodges JR, Knopman D, et al: Sensitivity of revised diagnostic criteria for the behavioural variant of frontotemporal dementia. Brain 134(Pt 9):2456–2477, 2011 21810890

Reitan RM: Validity of the Trail Making Test as an indicator of organic brain damage. Percept Mot Skills 8:271–276, 1958

Riddle M, Potter GG, McQuoid DR, et al: Longitudinal cognitive outcomes of clinical phenotypes of late-life depression. Am J Geriatr Psychiatry 25(10):1123–1134, 2017 28479153

Rienstra A, Groot PF, Spaan PE, et al: Symptom validity testing in memory clinics: hippocampal-memory associations and relevance for diagnosing mild cognitive impairment. J Clin Exp Neuropsychol 35(1):59–70, 2013 23228141

Rizzo M, Reinach S, McGehee D, Dawson J: Simulated car crashes and crash predictors in drivers with Alzheimer disease. Arch Neurol 54(5):545–551, 1997 9152111

Rizzo M, Anderson SW, Dawson J, Nawrot M: Vision and cognition in Alzheimer's disease. Neuropsychologia 38(8):1157–1169, 2000 10838150

Rossetti HC, Smith EE, Hynan LS, et al: Detection of mild cognitive impairment among community-dwelling African Americans using the Montreal Cognitive Assessment. Arch Clin Neuropsychol 34(6):809–813, 2019 30517598

Salmon DP, Galasko D, Hansen LA, et al: Neuropsychological deficits associated with diffuse Lewy body disease. Brain Cogn 31(2):148–165, 1996 8811990

Salthouse TA: Selective review of cognitive aging. J Int Neuropsychol Soc 16(5):754–760, 2010 20673381

Santos-Santos MA, Rabinovici GD, Iaccarino L, et al: Rates of amyloid imaging positivity in patients with primary progressive aphasia. JAMA Neurol 75(3):342–352, 2018 29309493

Schneider JA, Arvanitakis Z, Bang W, Bennett DA: Mixed brain pathologies account for most dementia cases in community-dwelling older persons. Neurology 69(24):2197–2204, 2007 17568013

Sherod MG, Griffith HR, Copeland J, et al: Neurocognitive predictors of financial capacity across the dementia spectrum: normal aging, mild cognitive impairment, and Alzheimer's disease. J Int Neuropsychol Soc 15(2):258–267, 2009 19203439

Sieben A, Van Langenhove T, Engelborghs S, et al: The genetics and neuropathology of frontotemporal lobar degeneration. Acta Neuropathol 124(3):353–372, 2012 22890575

Small BJ, Fratiglioni L, Viitanen M, et al: The course of cognitive impairment in preclinical Alzheimer disease: three- and 6-year follow-up of a population-based sample. Arch Neurol 57(6):839–844, 2000 10867781

Smith A: The Symbol Digit Modalities Test: a neuropsychologic test for economic screening of learning and other cerebral disorders. Learning Disorders 3:83–91, 1968

Soliveri P, Monza D, Paridi D, et al: Neuropsychological follow up in patients with Parkinson's disease, striatonigral degeneration-type multisystem atrophy, and progressive supranuclear palsy. J Neurol Neurosurg Psychiatry 69(3):313–318, 2000 10945805

Steffens DC, Skoog I, Norton MC, et al: Prevalence of depression and its treatment in an elderly population: the Cache County study. Arch Gen Psychiatry 57(6):601–607, 2000 10839339

Storandt M, Grant EA, Miller JP, Morris JC: Longitudinal course and neuropathologic outcomes in original vs revised MCI and in pre-MCI. Neurology 67(3):467–473, 2006 16894109

Strauss E, Sherman EM, Spreen O: A Compendium of Neuropsychological Tests: Administration, Norms, and Commentary, 3rd Edition. New York, Oxford University Press, 2006

Tariot PN: CERAD Behavior Rating Scale for Dementia. Int Psychogeriatr 8(suppl 3):317–320, discussion 351–354, 1996 9154581

Teichner G, Wagner MT: The Test of Memory Malingering (TOMM): normative data from cognitively intact, cognitively impaired, and elderly patients with dementia. Arch Clin Neuropsychol 19(3):455–464, 2004 15033228

Testa D, Monza D, Ferrarini M, et al: Comparison of natural histories of progressive supranuclear palsy and multiple system atrophy. Neurol Sci 22(3):247–251, 2001 11731878

Tisserand DJ: Structural and Functional Changes Underlying Cognitive Aging. Maastricht, The Netherlands, Maastricht University, 2003

Tröster AI: Neuropsychological characteristics of dementia with Lewy bodies and Parkinson's disease with dementia: differentiation, early detection, and implications for "mild cognitive impairment" and biomarkers. Neuropsychol Rev 18(1):103–119, 2008 18322801

Wechsler D: Wechsler Intelligence Scale, 4th Edition. San Antonio, TX, Psychological Corporation, 2009a

Wechsler D: Wechsler Memory Scale, 4th Edition. San Antonio, TX, Psychological Corporation, 2009b

Weintraub S, Wicklund AH, Salmon DP: The neuropsychological profile of Alzheimer disease. Cold Spring Harb Perspect Med 2(4):a006171, 2012 22474609

Welsh KA, Butters N, Hughes JP, et al: Detection and staging of dementia in Alzheimer's disease: use of the neuropsychological measures developed for the Consortium to Establish a Registry for Alzheimer's Disease. Arch Neurol 49(5):448–452, 1992 1580805

Welsh-Bohmer KA, Warren LH: Neurodegenerative dementias, in Geriatric Neuropsychology: Assessment and Intervention. Edited by Attix DK, Welsh-Bohmer KA. New York, Guilford, 2006, pp 56–88

Welsh-Bohmer KA, Koltai DC, Mason DJ: The clinical utility of neuropsychological evaluation of patients with known or suspected dementia, in Clinical Neuropsychology and Cost Outcome Research. Edited by Prigatano G, Pliskin N. Philadelphia, PA, Psychology Press-Taylor and Francis Group, 2003, pp 177–200

Yesavage JA, Brink TL, Rose TL, et al: Development and validation of a geriatric depression screening scale: a preliminary report. J Psychiatr Res 17(1):37–49, 1982–1983 7183759

CHAPTER 7

Delirium

Tanya Mailhot, R.N., Ph.D.
Sharon K. Inouye, M.D., M.P.H.
Jane S. Saczynski, Ph.D.

Delirium, defined as an acute and sudden change in attention and overall cognitive function, is a serious medical problem for older individuals—and one that is often fatal (Inouye et al. 2013; Marcantonio 2017; Oh et al. 2017). Delirium is the most frequent complication affecting hospitalized patients age 65 and older and, despite its high prevalence and incidence, often remains unrecognized. Patients with delirium have a worse prognosis than those without delirium, and they are at an increased risk of developing long-term cognitive and functional decline, which leads to additional post-hospitalization treatment costs, including institutionalization, rehabilitation services, and home health care (Gou et al. 2021; Inouye et al. 2013; Pandharipande et al. 2013; Rengel et al. 2019; Saczynski et al. 2012; Salluh et al. 2015; Shi et al. 2019). In addition to the increased risk of mortality, patients in the intensive care unit (ICU) who present with delirium have longer durations of mechanical ventilation and lengths of stay, thereby further complicating their recovery (Falsini et al. 2018; Salluh et al. 2015). Because it is preventable, delirium is increasingly the target for interventions to prevent its associated burden of downstream complications and costs, and it is now included on the patient safety agenda (Wachter 2012) and as an indicator of health care quality for older patients (Agency for Healthcare Research and Quality 2021; Siddiqi et al. 2016). Delirium and its complications are costly, with total annual health care costs estimated at more than $164 billion (Leslie et al. 2008). In critical care patients, the development of delirium is associated with a 20% increase in health care costs (Vasilevskis et al. 2018).

Epidemiology

Delirium is often the only sign of an acute and serious medical condition affecting a patient, and it most often occurs in frail older persons with an underlying disease process. More than 300 studies have been published with sample sizes of more than 100 subjects and in which screeners for delirium were trained and using validated methods of identifying delirium. These methodologically strong studies highlight that, across patient populations, delirium affects between 7% and 80% of patients, making it a highly common neuropsychiatric syndrome. The highest rates of delirium were observed in ICUs, with an observed prevalence between 7% and 80% and incidence between 16% and 82%, the upper range being attributed to patients who are ventilated (Chan et al. 2017; Mesa et al. 2017; Ng et al. 2020; Tsuruta et al. 2014; Wøien et al. 2013). More than half of surgical patients may present with prevalent (observed range between 8% and 58%) or incident (observed range between 8% and 58%) delirium (Cahill et al. 2017; Freter et al. 2016; Hewitt et al. 2019; Hov et al. 2016; Smulter et al. 2013). Studies among general medicine patients have reported a range of prevalence between 11% and 48% and an incidence range between 11% and 26%, whereas geriatric unit patients experience prevalent delirium at rates between 14% and 26% and incident delirium at rates between 16% and 29% (Bellelli et al. 2018; Blandfort et al. 2020; Boettger et al. 2018; Diwell et al. 2018; Hshieh et al. 2020; Pinkhasov et al. 2017; Thomas et al. 2012).

Although these prevalent and incident delirium rates are high, they likely represent underestimates of true incidence rates because many studies of delirium exclude patients with cognitive impairment or dementia at baseline. Delirium is extremely common among patients who have dementia at baseline, with a prevalence rate between 8% and 28% and an incidence rate between 25% and 56% (Avelino-Silva et al. 2017; Fick et al. 2013; Fong et al. 2012; Hasegawa et al. 2013; Morandi et al. 2014; Sepúlveda et al. 2015; Steensma et al. 2019; Steis et al. 2012). The prevalence of delirium in the community setting is relatively low (1%–2%), but its onset usually brings patients to emergency care. Among patients presenting to the emergency department, delirium is present in 7%–27% of all seniors and develops in between 8% and 12% during their stay, resulting in up to 39% of emergency department patients experiencing this serious condition (Émond et al. 2018; Giroux et al. 2018; Goldberg et al. 2012; Hasemann et al. 2018; Holt et al. 2013; Hsieh et al. 2015; Mailhot et al. 2020; Mariz et al. 2013; Singler et al. 2014; Sri-on et al. 2016). Finally, more than one-third of nursing home residents present with delirium on admission, and up to 48% develop it during their nursing home stay (Cole et al. 2016; Morichi et al. 2018).

Delirium is consistently associated with higher mortality rates across all surgical and nonsurgical populations, including cardiac and noncardiac surgery populations as well as general medical, geriatric, ICU, stroke, dementia, nursing home, and emergency department populations (Falsini et al. 2018; Fick et al. 2013; Fong et al. 2012; Honda et al. 2018; Hshieh et al. 2020; Moon and Park 2018; Morandi et al. 2014; Moskowitz et al. 2017; Noriega et al. 2015; Turco et al. 2013; van den Boogaard et al. 2012b). Delirium in the ICU is associated with up to a fourfold increased risk of in-hospital death and up to a sixfold increased risk of dying within up to 6 months following hospitalization (Falsini et al. 2018; Pauley et al. 2015; Sanson et al. 2018; van den Boogaard et al. 2012c). Longer lengths of stay have also been reported in general medical and surgical patients, as well as patients in the ICU and emergency department (Fick et al. 2013; Hshieh et al. 2020; Mariz et al. 2013; Mitasova et al. 2012; Pauley et al. 2015; van den Boogaard et al. 2012a, 2012b).

Delirium is also related to important cognitive and functional sequelae. Postoperative cognitive impairment is common among surgical patients who develop delirium, with impairments lasting up to 1 year postoperatively, and physical function is impaired for ≥30 days after discharge among surgical and nonsurgical patients who develop delirium (Brown et al. 2018; Hshieh et al. 2020; Noriega et al. 2015; Qu et al. 2018). Therefore, not only do patients experiencing delirium see their risk of dying severely increased, but their autonomy is also threatened, with up to a fivefold increased risk of institutionalization in surgical and nonsurgical patients who develop delirium compared with those who do not (Fong et al. 2012; Freter et al. 2016; Hshieh et al. 2020; Mariz et al. 2013; Miu and Yeung 2013; Morandi et al. 2014; Turco et al. 2013). For patients with dementia, the risk of institutionalization increases by up to ninefold in patients with delirium compared with those without delirium (Fong et al. 2012; Morandi et al. 2014; van Roessel et al. 2019).

Diagnosis, Assessment, and Workup

The diagnostic criteria for delirium that appear in DSM-5 (American Psychiatric Association 2013) and the ICD-10 (World Health Organization 1993) are generally accepted as the current diagnostic standard. Expert consensus was used to develop the DSM-5 criteria, which include an impairment in attention (i.e., inability to sustain attention) and awareness that represents a change from baseline and develops within hours or days and fluctuates during the day. At least another impairment in cognition should accompany the impaired attention and awareness (i.e., disorientation). These impairments are not the result of a neurocognitive disorder or related to a coma. In contrast to DSM-5, the ICD-10 diagnostic criteria suggest that impaired consciousness and attention should be paired with impaired cognition, which can take the form of altered perceptions resulting in illusions and hallucinations, incoherence, and deficit in recent memory. The ICD-10 criteria also indicate that psychomotor disruptions should accompany the impaired mental state. Finally, a disrupted sleep pattern and altered emotional state are also included in the diagnostic criteria.

More than 42 delirium instruments have been used in published studies (Gélinas et al. 2018; Helfand et al. 2021; Jones et al. 2019). The Confusion Assessment Method (CAM; Inouye et al. 1990) is the most widely used instrument for the identification of delirium and provides a simple diagnostic algorithm (Table 7–1) (Green et al. 2019). The CAM algorithm has been validated in high-quality studies of more than 1,000 patients and has a sensitivity of 94%, specificity of 89%, and high interrater reliability. The CAM has been translated into at least 15 languages, has been used in more than 4,000 published studies, and has been adapted for use in ICUs (Ely et al. 2001), emergency departments (Han et al. 2009), and nursing homes and is now included as part of the Minimum Data Set (Centers for Medicare and Medicaid Services 2010). Several behavioral checklists for symptoms of delirium, such as the Delirium Observation Screening Scale (Schuurmans et al. 2003), the Nursing Delirium Screening Checklist

TABLE 7–1.   Confusion Assessment Method (CAM) diagnostic algorithm*

Feature 1: Acute onset and fluctuating course	Usually obtained from a reliable reporter, such as a family member, caregiver, or nurse, and shown by a positive response to this question: Is there evidence of an acute change in mental status from the patient's baseline?
Feature 2: Inattention	Shown by a positive response to this question: Did the patient have difficulty focusing attention, for example, being easily distractible, or have difficulty keeping track of what was being said?
Feature 3: Disorganized thinking	Shown by a positive response to this question: Was the patient's thinking disorganized or incoherent, such as rambling or irrelevant conversation, unclear or illogical flow of ideas, or unpredictable switching from subject to subject?
Feature 4: Altered level of consciousness	Shown by any answer other than "alert" to this question: Overall, how would you rate this patient's level of consciousness—alert (normal), vigilant (hyperalert), lethargic (drowsy, easily aroused), stupor (difficult to arouse), or coma (unarousable)?

*CAM ratings should be completed following brief cognitive assessment of the patient, for example, with the Mini-Mental State Examination (Folstein et al. 1975). The diagnosis of delirium by the CAM requires the presence of both features 1 and 2 plus either 3 or 4.

(Gaudreau et al. 2005), and the Neecham Confusion Scale (Neelon et al. 1996), are utilized, particularly in nursing-based studies. Delirium severity is most widely measured using the Delirium Rating Scale (Trzepacz et al. 1988, 2001) and the Memorial Delirium Assessment Scale (Breitbart et al. 1997). The CAM also has a severity rating, CAM-Severity, which has strong psychometric properties and has been validated against clinical outcomes (Inouye et al. 2014). A chart method for retrospective identification of delirium has been validated (Inouye et al. 2005), but its sensitivity is limited compared with interview-based methods. A combined method that includes both chart review and direct patient interview captures the broadest number of patients with delirium (Saczynski et al. 2014).

The development of brief screening tools with high sensitivity and specificity has also changed the landscape of delirium detection. There is increasing interest in these brief delirium assessments because they can be easily incorporated into clinical care and are scalable due to the minimal training required to administer, score, and interpret the test results. As presented in Table 7–2, seven of these brief tools have been validated in several patient populations. Brief delirium screening tools are valuable to clinicians because they can be completed in <5 minutes and require very little training to administer and score. These tools have moderate to high sensitivity (78%–95%) and moderate to high specificity (64%–97%) in a wide range of patient populations, including medical, surgical, emergency department, stroke, dementia, palliative care, geriatric units, and nursing homes. They are typically used as a first step in delirium detection and are followed up by a more comprehensive assessment. Information on these tools and classic delirium screening tools can easily be found in the Network for Investigation of Delirium: Unifying Scientists measurement tool information cards (https://deliriumnetwork.org/measurement/adult-delirium-info-cards).

Two of these brief tools were created based on the CAM. The 3-Minute Diagnostic Confusion Assessment Method (3D-CAM; Marcantonio et al. 2014) and the Brief Con-

TABLE 7–2. Brief delirium screening tools

Tool	Description	Populations validated in
3-Minute Diagnostic Confusion Assessment Method (3D-CAM; Marcantonio et al. 2014)	Twenty items (10 interview questions, 10 observational items) and two supplementary questions. Assesses four features of delirium.* Each item is scored as positive or negative. Score is considered positive for delirium if three of four features are present (features 1 *and* 2 and *either* 3 or 4).	Surgery, medicine, inpatient, rehabilitation facility
4AT Rapid Clinical Test for Delirium (4AT; Bellelli et al. 2014)	Four items. Assesses four features of delirium.* Attention is assessed by reciting months of the year backward, acute change, or fluctuating course. Items are rated on a scale of either 0–4 or 0–2. Total is calculated by adding the score of each item. Total score >4 indicates possible delirium.	Medicine, postanesthesia care unit, emergency department, dementia, stroke
Recognizing Acute Delirium As Routine (RADAR; Voyer et al. 2015)	Three items (all observational, no formal assessment). Assesses three features of delirium: consciousness, attention/hyperactivity, and psychomotor retardation. Each item is rated as present or absent. Delirium is likely when at least one of the three items is present.	Dementia/Nursing home, emergency department
Delirium Triage Screen (DTS; Han et al. 2013)	Two items. Assesses two features of delirium*: altered level of consciousness and attention. Altered level of consciousness is rated as present or absent. Delirium is likely if feature 1 is present and should be confirmed using another validated delirium detection tool. If feature 1 is not present, attention should be assessed using the "LUNCH" backward spelling test. Attention is rated as present or absent; 0–1 error rated as negative and >1 error as positive. If positive, delirium is likely and should be confirmed using another validated tool.	Emergency department

TABLE 7–2.　Brief delirium screening tools (continued)

Tool	Description	Populations validated in
Simple Question for Easy Evaluation of Consciousness (SQEEC; Lin et al. 2015)	Two items (questions). Assesses two features of delirium*: disturbance of awareness and consciousness. Awareness is assessed by the answer to question 1: "Name a place you would like to visit that you have never been before." Consciousness is assessed by the answer to question 2: "How would you make the journey?" If patient is unable to answer question 1 and/or answer to question 2 is not logical, score is considered positive.	General medicine
Ultra-Brief 2-Item Screener (UB-2; Fick et al. 2015)	Two items. Question 1: "Please tell me the day of the week." Question 2: "Please tell me the months of the year backward; say December as your first month." Each question is scored as correct or incorrect. For question 2, answer is incorrect if patient misses ≥1 month or is unable to name the months after either one reminder of instructions or two prompts. If one or both items is incorrect, delirium is likely, and the patient should be assessed formally using a diagnostic interview.	Delirium superimposed on dementia

*See Table 7–1.
Source. Data from original papers and the Network for Investigation of Delirium: Unifying Scientists measurement tool information cards (https://deliriumnetwork.org/measurement/adult-delirium-info-cards).

fusion Assessment Method (bCAM; Han et al. 2013) include 20 and 7 items, respectively. Both assess the four features of delirium described in Table 7–1. Each item is scored as positive or negative and, as in the CAM algorithm, a score is positive for delirium if three of four features are present (*both* features 1 and 2, and *either* 3 or 4). The 3D-CAM includes 10 interview questions and 10 observational items and has been validated in surgical, medicine, inpatient, and rehabilitation populations, whereas the bCAM has been validated in emergency department and palliative care populations.

Another brief tool that has been validated in several patient populations, including general medicine, postanesthesia care unit, emergency department, dementia, and stroke, is the 4AT Rapid Clinical Test for Delirium (4AT; Bellelli et al. 2014). The 4AT includes four items that target alertness, orientation (assessed with the Abbreviated Mental Test–4), attention (assessed by having the patient recite the months of the year backward), and acute change or fluctuating course. Two other brief tools have been validated among patients with dementia: the Recognizing Acute Delirium As Routine (RADAR; Voyer et al. 2015) and the Ultra-Brief 2-Item Screener (UB2; Fick et al. 2015). These tools include only three and two items, respectively. The RADAR targets hypoactive delirium by assessing consciousness, attention/hyperactivity, and psychomotor retardation, whereas the UB2 asks two questions focusing on the day of the week and the months of the year backward. Finally, the Delirium Triage Screen (Han et al. 2013) and the Simple Question for Easy Evaluation of Consciousness (SQEEC; Lin et al. 2015) each include two items and have been validated in emergency department and general medicine populations, respectively. The Delirium Triage Screen assesses altered level of consciousness (feature 1) and attention using the "LUNCH" backward spelling test (feature 2). The SQEEC assesses disturbance of awareness (feature 1) or consciousness (feature 2). Feature 1 is assessed using question 1: "Name a place you would like to visit that you have never been before." Feature 2 is assessed using question 2: "How would you make the journey?"

Delirium goes unrecognized by clinicians in up to 85% of older patients who develop this condition in the emergency department and in nursing homes and in up to 68% of other patient populations (Boucher et al. 2019; Inouye et al. 2001; Numan et al. 2017; Sepúlveda et al. 2019); therefore, careful clinical assessment for this condition is imperative. Identification of these factors relies on insightful clinical judgment combined with a thorough medical evaluation. Clinicians should also assess any recent changes or updates in medication regimen, new infections, or recent development of medical illnesses that may contribute to delirium. Sudden and acute onset, alteration in attention, and fluctuating course are the central features of delirium. Therefore, it is important to establish a patient's level of baseline cognitive functioning and the course of cognitive change when evaluating for the presence of delirium. A detailed and in-depth background interview with a proxy informant, such as a family member, caregiver, or medical professional who knows the patient, proves invaluable when documenting change in the patient's mental status. To distinguish delirium from dementia, which can be very challenging, it is important to differentiate between 1) cognitive changes that increase and decrease in severity over a period of days, which is indicative of delirium, and 2) changes that are more chronic and progressive over a period of months to years, which is indicative of dementia.

In addition to using the family to help determine whether there has been a change in the patient's mental status, there are also delirium assessments designed for use by family members. These instruments are designed to support clinician detection of delirium. The Family Confusion Assessment Method (FAM-CAM) is an 11-item tool developed and validated to identify delirium from reports of informal caregivers (Martins et al. 2014; Steis et al. 2012). The FAM-CAM has a sensitivity between 57% and 86% and a specificity between 83% and 98% among elderly patients with preexisting cognitive impairment (Steis et al. 2012), hospitalized older patients (Martins et al. 2014), orthopedic surgery patients (Bull et al. 2017), and emergency department patients with and without dementia (Mailhot et al. 2020). The FAM-CAM is based on the CAM and is considered positive for delirium using the CAM diagnostic algorithm: presence of acute onset or fluctuating course *and* inattention and *either* disorganized thinking or altered level of consciousness. The FAM-CAM does not require training for informal caregivers and can be completed independently.

Four other informant-based tools have also been validated in medical-surgical, oncology, dementia, and geriatric unit populations (Rosgen et al. 2018). The Single Question in Delirium (Sands et al. 2010) and Single Screening Question–Delirium (Hendry et al. 2015a, 2015b) are one-item tools that yield a positive or negative result for delirium. The Informant Assessment of Geriatric Delirium (Rhodius-Meester et al. 2013) and the Sour Seven (Shulman et al. 2016) each have between 7 and 10 items associated with symptoms of delirium that can be observed by family members. These tools performed well against the CAM, with sensitivities ranging from 67% to 90% and specificities ranging from 56% to 90%. Families should be considered an untapped resource and an ally in the detection of delirium, and these tools can help families communicate delirium symptoms to the relevant health care professionals.

Clinicians also typically perform a thorough cognitive evaluation. For delirium, this evaluation should encompass the following domains: global cognitive changes, impairment in attention, disorganized thought process, and altered level of consciousness. Global cognitive changes associated with delirium can be assessed through simple cognitive testing and close clinical observation during test administration for the patient's completion of tasks. Brief cognitive screening should be conducted with formal cognitive screening tests, such as the Short Portable Mental Status Questionnaire (Pfeiffer 1975), the Mini-Cog (Borson et al. 2000), or the Montreal Cognitive Assessment (Nasreddine et al. 2005). If time is extremely limited, then an assessment of orientation, along with an attention task such as naming days of the week (allow no errors) or months of the year backward (allow one error), serial 7s (allow one error on five subtractions), or reciting digit spans backward (normal=three or more digits backward), can provide a basic screening. In fact, "months of the year backward" has been shown to have good sensitivity and specificity, respectively, of 83% and 69%, for detecting possible delirium in general medicine inpatients age 75 years and older (Fick et al. 2015). Moreover, when the "months of the year backward" test was combined with the "naming the day of the week" test, the sensitivity increased from 83% to 93% (Fick et al. 2015).

The waxing and waning periods of delirium should not be underestimated because periods of lucidity and reversal of symptoms can often be deceiving. Impairment in attention, a hallmark feature of delirium, is clinically manifested by the patient's difficulty focusing on the task at hand, maintaining or following a conversation, or shifting attention, often leading to perseveration on a previous topic or task. Disorganized thought is present when the patient's speech is incoherent or jumbled and when the patient lacks a clear or logical presentation of ideas; this problem can be similar to the "word salad" phenomenon seen in schizophrenia and other formal thought disorders. Alteration in consciousness is highly variable and can range from an agitated or aggressive state to one of lethargy or stupor. Other clinical features commonly associated with delirium that are not included in the current diagnostic criteria are psychomotor agitation, paranoid delusions, sleep-wake cycle disruption, and emotional lability.

Clinically, delirium typically presents in one of three major forms: hypoactive, hyperactive, or mixed. The hypoactive form, which is more common in older patients, is characterized by lethargy and reduced psychomotor functioning. The hypoactive form of delirium is associated with overall poorer prognosis and often goes unrecognized by clinicians and caregivers (Inouye et al. 2001; Krewulak et al. 2018). The reduced level of patient activity associated with hypoactive delirium is often attributed to low mood or fatigue, which may contribute to its misdiagnosis or underrecognition. The hyperactive form of delirium is characterized by agitation and increased vigilance and often by concomitant hallucinations. The hyperactive form rarely goes unnoticed by caregivers or clinicians. Clinicians should be aware of a mixed form of delirium in which patients fluctuate between the hypo- and hyperactive forms. The mixed form creates a challenge in distinguishing symptoms of delirium from symptoms of other psychotic or mood disorders.

Figure 7–1 summarizes the suggested workup for delirium. Several fundamental points in the evaluation of delirium are worthy of special emphasis. Often, delirium may be the initial and only sign of a serious and life-threatening underlying illness, such as sepsis, pneumonia, or myocardial infarction. Further complicating the evaluation of older patients is the occult or atypical presentation of disease in older persons; for instance, an octogenarian with myocardial infarction presents more often with delirium than with classic symptoms of chest pain or shortness of breath. Thus, a patient presenting with delirium should be screened for acute physiological disturbance such as hypoxemia, low blood glucose, and high arterial carbon dioxide. Another important principle is that the diagnostic evaluation (e.g., laboratory testing, neuroimaging) must be targeted based on the history and physical examination; an untargeted battery of testing is likely to be low-yield (Hirano et al. 2006). For example, in patients with an identified medical etiology of delirium or with preexisting dementia, more than 98% will have a normal brain scan (Hufschmidt and Shabarin 2008).

The clinician's most important and difficult task is to differentiate delirium from dementia. Dementia and cognitive impairment are strong risk factors for delirium, increasing the risk two- to sixfold (Fick et al. 2013; Heim et al. 2015; Kim et al. 2016; Pasinska et al. 2018; Rudolph et al. 2016; Wassenaar et al. 2015). Patients with dementia who develop a superimposed delirium experience a more rapid progression of cognitive dysfunction and worse long-term prognosis (Avelino-Silva et al. 2017; Fick and Foreman 2000; Fick et al. 2013; Fong et al. 2012; Jackson et al. 2004; Morandi et al. 2014). The key diagnostic feature that aids in distinguishing these two conditions is that delirium has an acute and rapid onset, whereas dementia is much more gradual in progression. Alterations in attention and in level of consciousness also point to a diagnosis of delirium. However, establishing the occurrence of these changes can be difficult in the face of missing baseline cognitive data or if preexisting cognitive deficits are reported by an informant. If the differentiation cannot be made with certainty,

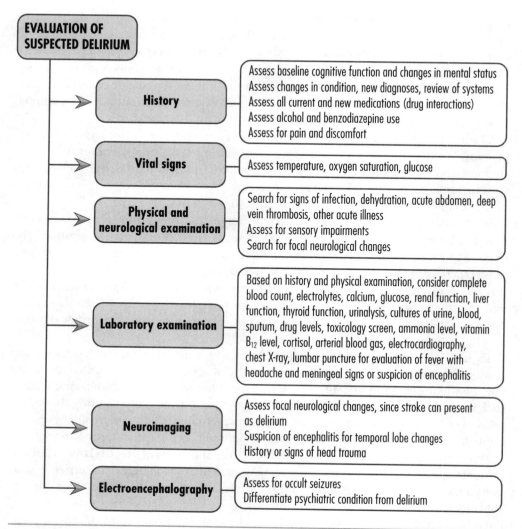

EVALUATION OF SUSPECTED DELIRIUM

History
- Assess baseline cognitive function and changes in mental status
- Assess changes in condition, new diagnoses, review of systems
- Assess all current and new medications (drug interactions)
- Assess alcohol and benzodiazepine use
- Assess for pain and discomfort

Vital signs
- Assess temperature, oxygen saturation, glucose

Physical and neurological examination
- Search for signs of infection, dehydration, acute abdomen, deep vein thrombosis, other acute illness
- Assess for sensory impairments
- Search for focal neurological changes

Laboratory examination
- Based on history and physical examination, consider complete blood count, electrolytes, calcium, glucose, renal function, liver function, thyroid function, urinalysis, cultures of urine, blood, sputum, drug levels, toxicology screen, ammonia level, vitamin B_{12} level, cortisol, arterial blood gas, electrocardiography, chest X-ray, lumbar puncture for evaluation of fever with headache and meningeal signs or suspicion of encephalitis

Neuroimaging
- Assess focal neurological changes, since stroke can present as delirium
- Suspicion of encephalitis for temporal lobe changes
- History or signs of head trauma

Electroencephalography
- Assess for occult seizures
- Differentiate psychiatric condition from delirium

FIGURE 7–1. Evaluation of suspected delirium.

then, given the life-threatening nature of delirium, the patient should be treated as delirious until proven otherwise.

Other important diagnoses that must be differentiated from delirium include psychiatric conditions such as depression and mania and nonorganic psychotic disorders such as schizophrenia. In general, these conditions do not develop suddenly in the context of a medical illness. Although hallucinations and perceptual disturbances can occur in the context of delirium, alterations in attention and global cognitive impairment are the key features that help to differentiate delirium from psychiatric conditions. Differentiating among diagnoses is critical because delirium carries a more serious prognosis without proper evaluation and management. For example, treatment for certain conditions such as depression or affective disorders may involve the use of drugs with anticholinergic activity, which in turn could exacerbate an unrecognized case of delirium. Establishing the diagnosis can be difficult when the symptoms are subtle, a background history is unavailable, or the patient is uncooperative. Given the seriousness of delirium and the fact that certain medical treatments may worsen symptoms, clinicians should assume that delirium is present until further diagnostic information is available.

The electroencephalogram (EEG) has limited sensitivity and specificity in the diagnosis of delirium. However, delirium does result in a characteristic pattern of diffuse slowing, with increased theta and delta activity and poor organization of background rhythm that correlates with severity (Kimchi et al. 2019; Nielsen et al. 2020; van der Kooi et al. 2015). An EEG can be particularly useful for differentiating organic etiologies from functional or psychiatric disorders in patients who are difficult to assess, for evaluating deteriorating mental status in patients with dementia, and for identifying occult seizures (e.g., nonconvulsive status epilepticus or atypical complex partial seizures) (Palanca et al. 2017).

No specific laboratory tests currently exist that will aid in the definitive identification of delirium. The laboratory evaluation for delirium is intended to identify contributing factors that need to be addressed, and the approach should be guided by astute clinical judgment and tailored to the individual situation. Laboratory tests that should be considered in the delirium evaluation include complete blood count, electrolytes, kidney and liver function, oxygen saturation, and glucose levels. Evaluation of occult infection can be obtained through blood cultures, urinalysis, and urine culture. Other laboratory tests, such as thyroid function, arterial blood gas, vitamin B_{12} level, cortisol level, drug levels, toxicology screen, and ammonia levels, may be helpful in identifying factors that contribute to delirium. An electrocardiogram or chest radiograph may prove useful in patients with cardiac or respiratory diseases.

In general, the routine use of neuroimaging in delirium is not recommended because the overall diagnostic yield is low and the findings from neuroimaging change the management of patients in <10% of cases (Scottish Intercollegiate Guidelines Network 2019). Neuroimaging in patients with delirium has the potential to worsen the episode because an agitated patient may need to be sedated for testing. Brain imaging using CT, PET, single-photon emission computed tomography, or MRI is low-yield in unselected patients and is recommended in cases of head trauma or injury, evaluation of new focal neurological symptoms, evaluation for suspected encephalitis, development of fever of unknown origin, epileptic activity, or nonconvulsive status epilepticus as a potential cause for delirium (Scottish Intercollegiate Guidelines Network 2019). Cerebrospinal fluid examination, accomplished through lumbar puncture, may be useful in cases in which the suspicion of meningitis, encephalitis, or subarachnoid hemorrhage is high (Engelborghs et al. 2017; Scottish Intercollegiate Guidelines Network 2019). Although data are sparse, neuroimaging and functional neuroimaging may be informative when delirium is persistent or where no etiology can be identified (Haggstrom et al. 2017; Lai and Wong Tin Niam 2012).

Pathophysiology of Delirium

Although important work is ongoing to further clarify the mechanisms involved in the development of delirium, the fundamental pathophysiology of delirium remains unclear (Vlisides and Avidan 2019). With each episode of delirium having a unique set of contributors representing different causal mechanisms, it is unlikely that a single cause or pathophysiological mechanism for delirium will be identified. There is increasing evidence that the multiple hypotheses proposed to explain delirium are most likely complementary, thereby resulting in several sets of biological factors that interact to cause the disruption of large-scale neuronal networks in the brain (Flaherty et al. 2017; Fong et al. 2015; Oldham et al. 2018; Vlisides and Avidan 2019). To date, a number of pathways are thought to result in delirium via neurotransmitter dysregulation or network dysconnectivity. These include neuronal aging, neuroinflammation, oxidative stress, neuroendocrine regulation and circadian dysregulation, neuronal injury, and the implication of genetic factors.

The neuroinflammation hypothesis suggests that the peripheral system and CNS work closely when responding to infectious and inflammatory abnormalities. Data support the idea that macrophages and brain endothelial cells release inflammatory mediators (e.g., interleukin [IL]-1β, tumor necrosis factor–α, interferon [IFN]-α/β, prostaglandin E2) as a response to systemic inflammation (Maclullich et al. 2013; Vasunilashorn et al. 2015, 2019). Several prospective and retrospective studies in general medicine, surgery, oncology, stroke, and ICU populations have highlighted different inflammatory biomarkers involved in the development of delirium, thereby supporting the neuroinflammation theory (Alexander et al. 2014; Dillon et al. 2017; Duceppe et al. 2019; Erikson et al. 2019; Guo et al. 2016; Kalantar et al. 2018; Lee et al. 2019; Levy et al. 2017; Liu et al. 2013, 2018; McNeil et al. 2019; Vasunilashorn et al. 2015, 2019). A recent meta-analysis of 54 observational studies among surgery populations concluded that significant increases in C-reactive protein and IL-6 are associated with the development of delirium (Liu et al. 2018).

The inflammatory mediators highlighted in the neuroinflammation hypothesis are thought to affect neuronal function temporarily in the case of delirium and irreversibly in the case of long-term cognitive decline. Whereas some mediators can result in abnormal functioning of neurons, others are thought to result in neuronal injury (Fong et al. 2019). The study of biomarkers of neuronal injury is a growing field of research that not only informs on new risk factors for delirium but also provides information on the interrelationship among delirium, Alzheimer's disease, and related dementias (Fong et al. 2015, 2017, 2019). In recent years, several biomarkers of neuronal injury have been researched in Alzheimer's disease and delirium, including neuron-specific enolase and plasma S100B (Fong et al. 2019). Currently, existing data yield conflicting results and highlight the need for further research in this area.

Another important area of ongoing investigation relates to the involvement of genetic factors in the development of delirium. Apolipoprotein E (*APOE*) is a biomarker that has been related to Alzheimer's disease and is currently being investigated in delirium. To date, two meta-analyses assessing the role of *APOE* in the risk of developing delirium have concluded, with conflicting results. The first meta-analysis (van Munster et al. 2009) included four studies, pooling data from 1,099 patients, and supported a relationship between *APOE* and longer duration of delirium but not between *APOE* and the incidence of delirium. The second meta-analysis (Adamis et al. 2016) included eight studies, pooling data from 1,762 participants, and concluded that the *APOE*E4* allele had a small and nonsignificant effect on the presence of delirium. Since then, in a recent study among 282 knee surgery patients age 65 years or older, the *APOE*E4* allele was not associated with postoperative delirium (Cunningham et al. 2019). However, a novel way to explore the role of the *APOE*E4* allele in delirium has resulted in findings indicating that *APOE* may play a role in delirium by acting as a modulator in the relationship between C-reactive protein and delirium (Vasunilashorn et al. 2020). These recent findings highlight the importance of continued exploration of the role of genetics in the development of delirium.

Finally, chronic stress induced by severe illness, trauma, or surgery involves sympathetic and immune system activation that may lead to delirium; this activation may include increased activity of the hypothalamic-pituitary-adrenal axis with hypercortisolism, release of cerebral cytokines that alter neurotransmitter systems, alterations in the thyroid axis, and modification of blood-brain barrier permeability (Hov et al. 2016; Hughes et al. 2012). Neuroimaging studies using either CT or MRI have demonstrated structural abnormalities in the brains of patients with delirium, especially in the splenium of the corpus callosum, thalamus, and right temporal lobe (Bogousslavsky et al. 1988; Doherty et al. 2005; Naughton et al. 1997; Ogasawara et al. 2005; Takanashi et al. 2006). Advanced neuroimaging techniques identify overall and regional perfusion abnormalities in the brains of people with delirium (Nitchingham et al. 2018). Functional imaging has highlighted cerebral hemodynamics and connectivity abnormalities related to delirium while also distinguishing structural damage resulting from an episode of delirium due to preexisting changes (Choi et al. 2012; Haggstrom et al. 2017).

Risk Factors for Delirium

Although a single factor may lead to delirium, more commonly delirium is multifactorial in older persons (Inouye and Charpentier 1996). To facilitate immediate and effective diagnosis and treatment of delirium, all multifactorial contributors must be identified. The development of delirium involves a complex interrelationship between a vulnerable patient with multiple predisposing factors and exposure to noxious insults or precipitating factors (Figure 7–2). For example, a single dose of a sedative given to a patient who is cognitively impaired or severely ill may lead to delirium. However, a patient without severe illness or cognitive impairment has greater resistance to developing delirium unless the patient is repeatedly exposed to multiple insults, such as surgery, anesthesia, and psychoactive medications (Marcantonio 2017). Addressing only a single noxious insult or factor may not aid in improving delirium. Rather, multicomponent approaches will be most effective for both prevention and treatment (Marcantonio 2017; Siddiqi et al. 2016).

Several predisposing and precipitating factors have been identified in prospectively validated prediction models (Table 7–3). The leading risk factors consistently identified at admission in both general medical and noncardiac surgery populations were dementia or cognitive impairment, history of delirium, functional impairment, vision impairment, history of alcohol abuse, and advanced age (>70 years) (Caplan et al. 2010; Heim et al. 2015; Hirano et al. 2006; Hufschmidt and Shabarin 2008; Jadad et al. 1996; Jacobson and Jerrier 2000; Jenssen 2005; Lai and Wong Tin Niam 2012; Kumar et al. 2017; Marcantonio 2011; McDowell et al. 1998; Park and Tang 2007; Wong et al. 2010). Comorbidity burden or the presence of specific comorbidities (e.g., stroke, depression) was associated with an increased risk in all patient populations. In the ICU study, younger patients were included, and baseline factors (e.g., dementia, functional

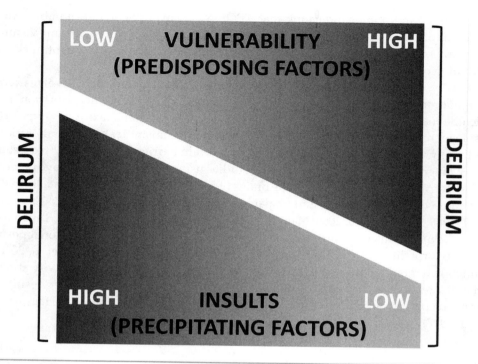

FIGURE 7–2.   Multifactorial model of delirium in older persons.
The onset of delirium involves a complex interaction between the patient's baseline vulnerability (predisposing factors) present on admission and precipitating factors or noxious insults occurring during hospitalization. See text for details.

impairment) were not significant independent predictors. Precipitating factors varied more across patient populations. In medical patients, polypharmacy, psychoactive medication use, and physical restraints were the leading precipitating factors, conferring up to a 4.5-fold increased risk. Abnormal laboratory values were precipitating risk factors in medical and surgical populations, conferring up to fivefold increased risk.

Medications and Delirium

Medication use contributes to delirium. Medications identified by the 2019 American Geriatrics Society Beers Criteria as causing or exacerbating delirium are listed in Table 7–4. The medications most frequently associated with delirium are those with psychoactive effects, such as sedative-hypnotics, anxiolytics, narcotics, and histamine (H_2) blockers. Drugs with anticholinergic effects, including antipsychotics, antihistamines, antidepressants, antiparkinsonian agents, and anticonvulsants, are also commonly associated with delirium.

Previous studies, including validated risk prediction models, have shown that the use of psychoactive medication results in a fourfold greater risk of delirium, whereas the use of two or more psychoactive medications is associated with a fivefold greater risk (Burry et al. 2016, 2017, 2018, 2019). Sedative-hypnotic drugs are associated with a 3- to 12-fold increased risk of delirium, narcotics with a 3-fold risk, and anticholiner-

TABLE 7–3.   **Risk factors for delirium from validated predictive models**

Predisposing factors	Precipitating factors
Dementia	Medications
Cognitive impairment	Multiple medications added
History of delirium	Psychoactive medication use
Functional impairment	Sedative-hypnotics
Vision impairment	Use of physical restraints
Hearing impairment	Use of bladder catheter
Comorbidity/severity of illness	Physiological
Depression	Elevated serum urea
History of transient ischemia/stroke	Elevated blood urea nitrogen/creatinine ratio
Alcohol abuse	Abnormal serum albumin
Older age	Abnormal sodium, glucose, or potassium
History of hypertension	Metabolic acidosis
Carotid artery disease	Infection
	Any iatrogenic event
	Surgery
	Aortic aneurysm
	Noncardiac thoracic
	Neurosurgery
	Trauma admission
	Urgent admission
	Coma
	Intensive care unit stay >10 days
	Pain
	Noninvasive ventilation

gic drugs with a 5- to 12-fold risk (Chaiwat et al. 2019; Chen et al. 2017; Fan et al. 2019). In observational studies among older adults in critical care, palliative care, surgery, and general medicine, the anticholinergic burden as measured by the Anticholinergic Risk Scale, the Anticholinergic Cognitive Burden Scale, or the Anticholinergic Drug Burden Score has been associated with the occurrence of delirium (Egberts et al. 2017; Kolanowski et al. 2015; Mueller et al. 2020; Pasina et al. 2019; Zimmerman et al. 2014). Finally, systematic reviews of prospective studies identified opioids, benzodiazepines, dihydropyridines, and antihistamines as increasing the risk of delirium (Clegg and Young 2011; Zaal et al. 2015).

Polypharmacy leads to a proportionately greater increased risk for developing delirium. This is related to the direct toxicity of the medications themselves, as well as the increased risk of drug–drug and drug–disease interactions. Some homeopathic or herbal therapies, particularly those used for mood disorders (e.g., St. John's wort, kava kava), may increase the risk of delirium, especially when used in combination with prescribed psychoactive medications. Given the role of medications in contributing to the development of delirium, it is essential to conduct a complete review of all prescription and over-the-counter medications a patient is taking. Most older patients take sev-

TABLE 7–4.   **Drugs to avoid in delirium: Beers Criteria**

All tricyclic antidepressants

Anticholinergics

Antidepressants	Antiparkinson agents	Antispasmodics
Antihistamines	Antipsychotics	Muscle relaxants
Antimuscarinics		

Antipsychotics, first- (conventional) and second-generation (atypical)

Benzodiazepines, short- and intermediate-acting

Alprazolam	Lorazepam	Temazepam
Estazolam	Oxazepam	Triazolam

Benzodiazepines, long-acting

Chlordiazepoxide	Clorazepate	Flurazepam
Clonazepam	Diazepam	

Nonbenzodiazepine, benzodiazepine receptor agonist hypnotics (i.e., Z drugs)

Eszopiclone	Zaleplon	Zolpidem

Corticosteroids

Histamine receptor (H$_2$) antagonist

Meperidine

Sedative-hypnotics

Thioridazine

Source.   American Geriatrics Society: "2019 Updated AGS Beers Criteria for Potentially Inappropriate Medication Use in Older Adults." *Journal of the American Geriatrics Society* 67(4):674–694, 2019.

eral prescribed medications during hospitalization, increasing the risk for interactions. Medications with known psychoactive effects should be discontinued or minimized whenever possible. At the very least, steps should be taken to reduce dosage or to substitute medications with less toxic potential. In aging adults, medications may cause adverse effects even when given at recommended dosages and when serum drug levels are within the "therapeutic range." Determining whether the patient has a history of chronic sedative use or alcohol dependence is critical in assessing for withdrawal risk.

Prevention and Management of Delirium

Pharmacological Prevention and Management

Although clinical trials have used various pharmacological approaches, at present no convincing, reproducible evidence has shown any of these treatments to be effective for either the prevention or treatment of delirium (Burry et al. 2018; Finucane et al. 2020; Li et al. 2020; Yu et al. 2018). Many published pharmacological trials report no difference in delirium rates (Herling et al. 2018). In most trials that do show a reduced rate of delirium following targeted pharmacological treatment, there is either no corresponding impact on clinical outcomes, such as ICU or hospital length of stay, hospital complications, or mortality, or the clinical outcomes were not measured. For instance, a double-blind, randomized controlled trial of haloperidol versus ziprasidone versus placebo in 1,183 medical or surgical ICU patients showed no significant differences in the number of patient days alive without delirium or coma (median number of days without delirium: haloperidol, 7.9 days [95% CI 4.4–9.6]; ziprasidone, 8.7 days [5.9–10]; placebo, 8.5 days [5.6–9.9]) (Girard et al. 2018).

Recent systematic reviews have concluded that among hospitalized non-ICU patients, antipsychotics did not improve outcomes of delirium incidence, duration, or severity and had no effect on cognitive functioning, hospital length of stay, or mortality (Burry et al. 2018; Nikooie et al. 2019; Oh et al. 2020). Similarly, several trials have reported that treatment resulted in potentially worse outcomes: olanzapine reduced incidence of delirium compared with placebo in 400 patients receiving hip replacement but resulted in a greater duration and severity of delirium (Larsen et al. 2010); rivastigmine resulted in greater delirium duration and mortality in 104 ICU patients (van Eijk et al. 2010).

The use of dexmedetomidine, an α_2-receptor agonist, to lower the delirium burden is an area of research that still demands work. Although some systematic reviews and meta-analyses have supported that dexmedetomidine sedation was associated with a decreased incidence and duration of delirium, shorter mechanical ventilation, and shorter ICU length of stay (Burry et al. 2019; Chen et al. 2015; Pieri et al. 2020; Zhang et al. 2013), others have concluded that it does not decrease the risk of delirium (Chen et al. 2015). A recent Cochrane review among critically ill patients could only find three dexmedetomidine trials that met their inclusion criteria, and only one could be used to assess the impact of dexmedetomidine on delirium duration (Burry et al. 2019). This double-blind, placebo-controlled, parallel-group randomized clinical trial included 71 intubated patients who presented with severe agitation or delirium and found that dexmedetomidine, compared with placebo, may shorten delirium duration (Reade et al. 2016). Published trials in this area of research have utilized different approaches to assess delirium and have evaluated diverse patient populations; thus, generalizing findings is difficult. To date, the American Geriatrics Society and the Society of Critical Care Medicine were either unable to publish recommendations or have yet to evaluate this option (American Geriatrics Society Expert Panel on Postoperative Delirium in Older Adults 2015; Devlin et al. 2018).

Other work among postoperative patients has highlighted a potential modifiable precipitating factor in the development of delirium: anesthesia guided by intraoperative processed electroencephalography, such as the Bispectral Index. Two recent systematic reviews support that monitoring the depth of anesthesia using processed electroencephalography in cardiac and noncardiac surgery patients reduces the risk of postoperative delirium (MacKenzie et al. 2018; Punjasawadwong et al. 2018). MacKenzie et al. (2018) included five studies conducted with both cardiac and noncardiac surgical patients, pooling data from 2,654 patients. They found a reduction of 38% in the odds for developing postoperative delirium when anesthesia was optimized using processed electroencephalography. In their Cochrane review, Punjasawadwong et al. (2018) included four studies among noncardiac and nonneurological surgery patients, pooling data from 2,929 patients. They concluded that Bispectral Index–guided anesthesia reduced the risk of postoperative delirium. Both reviews highlighted the moderate quality of the evidence supporting their conclusions.

In contrast to these meta-analyses, two recent studies found conflicting results. A randomized clinical trial in 1,232 adults age 60 years and older undergoing major surgery did not find evidence that anesthesia guided by processed EEG reduced the risk of postoperative delirium (Wildes et al. 2019). Similarly, another randomized clinical trial among 200 adults age 65 and older who were undergoing hip surgery found that the risk of delirium was reduced by processed EEG anesthesia only for the subgroup of patients with low comorbidity and not for the subgroup with heavier comorbidity (Sieber et al. 2018). Moreover, within that same trial, investigators studied mortality or functional level 1 year post surgery and found that heavier sedation did not impact these outcomes (Sieber et al. 2019). Ongoing work may shed some light on this potentially modifiable risk factor for postoperative delirium (Punjasawadwong et al. 2018).

Given the preponderance of currently available evidence on the pharmacological prevention and management of delirium, pharmacological approaches are not recommended at this time in any patient population, and nonpharmacological interventions remain the important first step (Barr et al. 2013; Devlin et al. 2018).

Nonpharmacological Prevention and Management

Primary prevention—that is, preventing delirium before it develops—is the most effective strategy to alleviate symptoms associated with delirium. The Hospital Elder Life Program (HELP; www.hospitalelderlifeprogram.org) uses a multidisciplinary team approach to aid in preventing delirium and is the most widely disseminated approach to delirium prevention in hundreds of hospitals worldwide (Hshieh et al. 2018; Inouye et al. 2006). HELP is a hospital-wide program designed to implement delirium prevention strategies and to promote an overall increase in quality of medical care. HELP interventions include reorientation, therapeutic activities, reduction of psychoactive medications, early mobilization, sleep promotion, maintenance of hydration and nutrition, and provision of vision and hearing adaptations. The program is implemented by a skilled interdisciplinary team assisted by either nursing staff or trained volunteers.

In general, nonpharmacological approaches, as used in the HELP protocols, should be implemented as the first-line treatment of delirium (Figure 7–3). Nonpharmacological treatment approaches include reorientation (e.g., using orientation boards, clocks, calendars), behavioral interventions, encouraging the presence of family members, and transferring a disruptive patient to a private room or closer to the nurse's station for increased supervision. Consistent and compassionate staff are essential in facilitating contact and communication with the patient through frequent verbal reorienting strategies, clear instructions, frequent eye contact, and the inclusion of patients as much as possible in all decisions regarding their daily and medical care. Sensory deficits should be assessed and then corrected by ensuring that all assistive devices, such as eyeglasses and hearing aids, are readily available, functioning, and being used properly by the patient. The use of physical restraints should be minimized due to their role in prolonging delirium, worsening agitation, and increasing complications such as strangulation (Inouye et al. 2007; Pan et al. 2018). Strategies that increase the patient's mobility, self-care, and independence should be promoted. Family involvement in HELP interventions (rather than volunteers) has been demonstrated to be effective in delirium prevention (Wang et al. 2020).

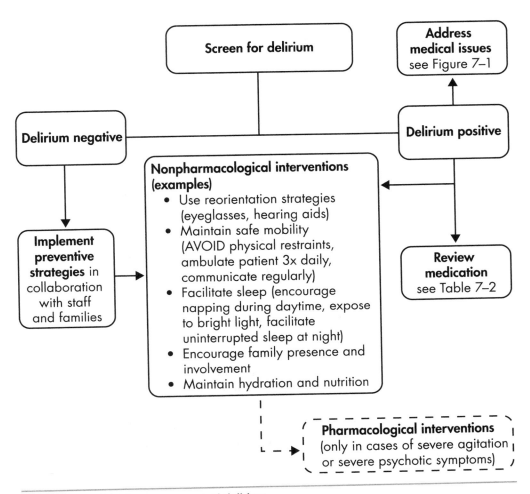

FIGURE 7–3. Initial management of delirium.

Multifactorial targeted interventions have also been successful in preventing and treating delirium (Siddiqi et al. 2016). For instance, a trial of a proactive geriatric consultation resulted in a 40% reduction in the risk of delirium in patients following hip fractures (Marcantonio et al. 2001). The targeted multifactorial strategy focused on 10 domains: adequate brain oxygen delivery, fluid and electrolyte balance, pain management, reduction in psychoactive medications, bowel and bladder function, nutrition, early mobilization, prevention of postoperative complications, appropriate environmental stimuli, and treatment of delirium. Among ICU patients, implementation of a multicomponent clinical approach named the ABCDEF (A2F) bundle was associated with a lower likelihood of developing delirium (Balas et al. 2014; Pun et al. 2019). The A2F bundle consists of the following six components:

- A=Assess, prevent, manage pain
- B=Both spontaneous awakening and spontaneous breathing trials
- C=Choice of analgesic and sedation
- D=Delirium assessment, prevention, and management

- E=Early mobility and exercise
- F=Family engagement and empowerment

Controlled trials of educational strategies targeted toward training staff in assessing, preventing, identifying, and treating delirium have demonstrated positive results in increasing recognition and reducing episodes and duration of delirium (Marcantonio et al. 2010; Milisen et al. 2001; Tabet et al. 2005). Controlled trials of multifactorial interventions, which usually consist of a combination of staff education and treatments tailored to meet the specific needs of patients, have demonstrated reductions in rate of delirium and duration of delirium episode (Deschodt et al. 2012; Lundström et al. 2005; Naughton et al. 2005; Pitkälä et al. 2006). Approaches include interventions delivered by family members and mobility or rehabilitation interventions, both of which were shown to be effective for prevention of delirium (Caplan et al. 2006; Martinez et al. 2012; Schweickert et al. 2009). Family caregiver involvement in delirium management has shown to improve family and patient outcomes, such as reducing anxiety in family members and lengths of stay in patients (Mailhot et al. 2017; McKenzie and Joy 2020).

Conclusion

Delirium is a common, serious, and potentially preventable source of morbidity and mortality for hospitalized older persons. Delirium affects as many as half of all hospitalized older adults and, importantly, is preventable in up to 50% of cases. Delirium often initiates a cascade of events in older persons, leading to a downward spiral of functional and cognitive decline, loss of independence, institutionalization, and, ultimately, death and is thus a critical risk factor for identifying patients at high risk for poor outcomes.

Key Points

- Delirium is a common problem for older hospitalized persons.

- Delirium is the most frequent complication affecting surgical and nonsurgical older patient populations and often goes unrecognized.

- Patients with delirium have a worse prognosis than those without delirium and an increased risk of developing long-term cognitive and functional decline.

- It is important to establish a patient's level of baseline cognitive functioning and course of cognitive change when evaluating for delirium.

- The Confusion Assessment Method provides a simple diagnostic algorithm and has become widely used for identification of delirium.

- Family members can play an important role in identification of symptoms of delirium, and validated instruments exist to facilitate systematic reporting by family members and caregivers.

- Although delirium can be caused by a single factor, it is usually multifactorial.

- Existing cognitive impairment and dementia are the leading risk factors for the development of delirium.

- Although the fundamental pathophysiology of delirium remains unclear, neuroinflammation, neuronal injury, and genetic factors are being explored as potential mechanisms.

- Nonpharmacological approaches should be implemented as the first line of treatment for delirium.

- Certain medications can induce or exacerbate an episode of delirium.

- Pharmacological management of delirium should be used only in patients with severe agitation.

Suggested Readings

American Geriatrics Society 2019 Beers Criteria Update Expert Panel: American Geriatrics Society 2019 updated Beers criteria for potentially inappropriate medication use in older adults. J Am Geriatr Soc 67:674–694, 2019

Fong TG, Jones RN, Marcantonio ER, et al: Adverse outcomes after hospitalization and delirium in persons with Alzheimer disease. Ann Intern Med 156:848–856, 2012

Inouye SK, Westendorp RGJ, Saczynski J: Delirium in elderly people. Lancet 383:911–922, 2014

Marcantonio ER: Delirium in hospitalized older adults. N Engl J Med 377:1456–1466, 2017

Oh ES, Fong TG, Hshieh TT, Inouye SK: Delirium in older persons: advances in diagnosis and treatment (systematic review). JAMA 318:1161–1174, 2017

References

Adamis D, Meagher D, Williams J, et al: A systematic review and meta-analysis of the association between the apolipoprotein E genotype and delirium. Psychiatr Genet 26(2):53–59, 2016 26901792

Agency for Healthcare Research and Quality: National Quality Measures: Delirium: Proportion of Patients Meeting Diagnostic Criteria on the Confusion Assessment Method (CAM), n.d. Available at: http://qualityindicators.ahrq.gov/Downloads/Modules/PSI/v2020/TechSpecs/PSI_08_In_Hospital_Fall_with_Hip_Fracture_Rate.pdf. Accessed November 16, 2021.

Alexander SA, Ren D, Gunn SR, et al: Interleukin 6 and apolipoprotein E as predictors of acute brain dysfunction and survival in critical care patients. Am J Crit Care 23(1):49–57, 2014 24382617

American Geriatrics Society Expert Panel on Postoperative Delirium in Older Adults: American Geriatrics Society abstracted clinical practice guideline for postoperative delirium in older adults. J Am Geriatr Soc 63(1):142–150, 2015 25495432

American Psychiatric Association: Diagnostic and Statistical Manual of Mental Disorders, 5th Edition. Arlington, VA, American Psychiatric Association, 2013

Avelino-Silva TJ, Campora F, Curiati JA, Jacob-Filho W: Association between delirium superimposed on dementia and mortality in hospitalized older adults: a prospective cohort study. PLoS Med 14(3):e1002264, 2017 28350792

Balas MC, Vasilevskis EE, Olsen KM, et al: Effectiveness and safety of the awakening and breathing coordination, delirium monitoring/management, and early exercise/mobility bundle. Crit Care Med 42(5):1024–1036, 2014 24394627

Barr J, Fraser GL, Puntillo K, et al: Clinical practice guidelines for the management of pain, agitation, and delirium in adult patients in the intensive care unit: executive summary. Am J Health Syst Pharm 70(1):53–58, 2013 23261901

Bellelli G, Morandi A, Davis DH, et al: Validation of the 4AT, a new instrument for rapid delirium screening: a study in 234 hospitalised older people. Age Ageing 43(4):496–502, 2014 24590568

Bellelli G, Zambon A, Volpato S, et al: The association between delirium and sarcopenia in older adult patients admitted to acute geriatrics units: results from the GLISTEN multicenter observational study. Clin Nutr 37(5):1498–1504, 2018 28918171

Blandfort S, Gregersen M, Rahbek K, et al: Single-bed rooms in a geriatric ward prevent delirium in older patients. Aging Clin Exp Res 32(1):141–147, 2020 30900213

Boettger S, Garcia Nuñez D, Meyer R, et al: Screening for delirium with the Intensive Care Delirium Screening Checklist (ICDSC): a re-evaluation of the threshold for delirium. Swiss Med Wkly 148:w14597, 2018 29537480

Bogousslavsky J, Ferrazzini M, Regli F, et al: Manic delirium and frontal-like syndrome with paramedian infarction of the right thalamus. J Neurol Neurosurg Psychiatry 51(1):116–119, 1988 3258356

Borson S, Scanlan J, Brush M, et al: The Mini-Cog: a cognitive 'vital signs' measure for dementia screening in multi-lingual elderly. Int J Geriatr Psychiatry 15(11):1021–1027, 2000 11113982

Boucher V, Lamontagne ME, Nadeau A, et al: Unrecognized incident delirium in older emergency department patients. J Emerg Med 57(4):535–542, 2019 31353267

Breitbart W, Rosenfeld B, Roth A, et al: The Memorial Delirium Assessment Scale. J Pain Symptom Manage 13(3):128–137, 1997 9114631

Brown CH IV, Probert J, Healy R, et al: Cognitive decline after delirium in patients undergoing cardiac surgery. Anesthesiology 129(3):406–416, 2018 29771710

Bull MJ, Boaz L, Maadooliat M, et al: Preparing family caregivers to recognize delirium symptoms in older adults after elective hip or knee arthroplasty. J Am Geriatr Soc 65(1):e13–e17, 2017 27861701

Burry LD, Hutton B, Guenette M, et al: Comparison of pharmacological and non-pharmacological interventions to prevent delirium in critically ill patients: a protocol for a systematic review incorporating network meta-analyses. Syst Rev 5(1):153, 2016 27609018

Burry LD, Williamson DR, Mehta S, et al: Delirium and exposure to psychoactive medications in critically ill adults: A multi-centre observational study. J Crit Care 42:268–274, 2017 28806561

Burry L, Mehta S, Perreault MM, et al: Antipsychotics for treatment of delirium in hospitalised non-ICU patients. Cochrane Database Syst Rev (6):CD005594, 2018 29920656

Burry L, Hutton B, Williamson DR, et al: Pharmacological interventions for the treatment of delirium in critically ill adults. Cochrane Database Syst Rev (9):CD011749, 2019 31479532

Cahill A, Pearcy C, Agrawal V, et al: Delirium in the ICU: what about the floor? J Trauma Nurs 24(4):242–244, 2017 28692620

Caplan GA, Coconis J, Board N, et al: Does home treatment affect delirium? A randomised controlled trial of rehabilitation of elderly and care at home or usual treatment (the REACH-OUT trial). Age Ageing 35(1):53–60, 2006 16239239

Caplan GA, Kvelde T, Lai C, et al: Cerebrospinal fluid in long-lasting delirium compared with Alzheimer's dementia. J Gerontol A Biol Sci Med Sci 65(10):1130–1136, 2010

Centers for Medicare and Medicaid Services: Minimum Data Set, Version 3.0. Washington, DC, Centers for Medicare and Medicaid Services, 2010

Chaiwat O, Chanidnuan M, Pancharoen W, et al: Postoperative delirium in critically ill surgical patients: incidence, risk factors, and predictive scores. BMC Anesthesiol 19(1):39, 2019 30894129

Chan KY, Cheng LS, Mak IW, et al: Delirium is a strong predictor of mortality in patients receiving non-invasive positive pressure ventilation. Lung 195(1):115–125, 2017 27787611

Chen K, Lu Z, Xin YC, et al: Alpha-2 agonists for long-term sedation during mechanical ventilation in critically ill patients. Cochrane Database Syst Rev (1):CD010269, 2015 25879090

Chen Y, Du H, Wei BH, et al: Development and validation of risk-stratification delirium prediction model for critically ill patients: a prospective, observational, single-center study. Medicine 96(29):e7543, 2017 28723773

Choi SH, Lee H, Chung TS, et al: Neural network functional connectivity during and after an episode of delirium. Am J Psychiatry 169(5):498–507, 2012 22549209

Clegg A, Young JB: Which medications to avoid in people at risk of delirium: a systematic review. Age Ageing 40(1):23–29, 2011 21068014

Cole MG, Bailey R, Bonnycastle M, et al: Frequency of full, partial and no recovery from subsyndromal deliriumin older hospital inpatients. Int J Geriatr Psychiatry 31(5):544–550, 2016 26526733

Cunningham EL, McGuinness B, McAuley DF, et al: CSF beta-amyloid 1–42 concentration predicts delirium following elective arthroplasty surgery in an observational cohort study. Ann Surg 269(6):1200–1205, 2019 31082921

Deschodt M, Braes T, Flamaing J, et al: Preventing delirium in older adults with recent hip fracture through multidisciplinary geriatric consultation. J Am Geriatr Soc 60(4):733–739, 2012 22429099

Devlin JW, Skrobik Y, Gélinas C, et al: Clinical practice guidelines for the prevention and management of pain, agitation/sedation, delirium, immobility, and sleep disruption in adult patients in the ICU. Crit Care Med 46(9):e825–e873, 2018 30113379

Dillon ST, Vasunilashorn SM, Ngo L, et al: Higher C-reactive protein levels predict postoperative delirium in older patients undergoing major elective surgery: a longitudinal nested case-control study. Biol Psychiatry 81(2):145–153, 2017 27160518

Diwell RA, Davis DH, Vickerstaff V, Sampson EL: Key components of the delirium syndrome and mortality: greater impact of acute change and disorganised thinking in a prospective cohort study. BMC Geriatr 18(1):24, 2018 29370764

Doherty MJ, Jayadev S, Watson NF, et al: Clinical implications of splenium magnetic resonance imaging signal changes. Arch Neurol 62(3):433–437, 2005 15767508

Duceppe MA, Williamson DR, Elliott A, et al: Modifiable risk factors for delirium in critically ill trauma patients: a multicenter prospective study. J Intensive Care Med 34(4):330–336, 2019 28335673

Egberts A, van der Craats ST, van Wijk MD, et al: Anticholinergic drug exposure is associated with delirium and postdischarge institutionalization in acutely ill hospitalized older patients. Pharmacol Res Perspect 5(3):e00310, 2017 28603629

Ely EW, Margolin R, Francis J, et al: Evaluation of delirium in critically ill patients: validation of the Confusion Assessment Method for the Intensive Care Unit (CAM-ICU). Crit Care Med 29(7):1370–1379, 2001 11445689

Émond M, Boucher V, Carmichael PH, et al: Incidence of delirium in the Canadian emergency department and its consequences on hospital length of stay: a prospective observational multicentre cohort study. BMJ Open 8(3):e018190, 2018 29523559

Engelborghs S, Niemantsverdriet E, Struyfs H, et al: Consensus guidelines for lumbar puncture in patients with neurological diseases. Alzheimers Dement 8:111–126, 2017 28603768

Erikson K, Ala-Kokko TI, Koskenkari J, et al: Elevated serum S-100? in patients with septic shock is associated with delirium. Acta Anaesthesiol Scand 63(1):69–73, 2019 30079511

Falsini G, Grotti S, Porto I, et al: Long-term prognostic value of delirium in elderly patients with acute cardiac diseases admitted to two cardiac intensive care units: a prospective study (DELIRIUM CORDIS). Eur Heart J Acute Cardiovasc Care 7(7):661–670, 2018 29064263

Fan H, Ji M, Huang J, et al: Development and validation of a dynamic delirium prediction rule in patients admitted to the intensive care units (DYNAMIC-ICU): a prospective cohort study. Int J Nurs Stud 93:64–73, 2019 30861455

Fick D, Foreman M: Consequences of not recognizing delirium superimposed on dementia in hospitalized elderly individuals. J Gerontol Nurs 26(1):30–40, 2000 10776167

Fick DM, Steis MR, Waller JL, Inouye SK: Delirium superimposed on dementia is associated with prolonged length of stay and poor outcomes in hospitalized older adults. J Hosp Med 8(9):500–505, 2013 23955965

Fick DM, Inouye SK, Guess J, et al: Preliminary development of an ultrabrief two-item bedside test for delirium. J Hosp Med 10(10):645–650, 2015 26369992

Finucane AM, Jones L, Leurent B, et al: Drug therapy for delirium in terminally ill adults. Cochrane Database Syst Rev (1):CD004770, 2020 31960954

Flaherty JH, Yue J, Rudolph JL: Dissecting delirium: phenotypes, consequences, screening, diagnosis, prevention, treatment, and program implementation. Clin Geriatr Med 33(3):393–413, 2017 28689571

Folstein MF, Folstein SE, McHugh PR: "Mini-mental state": a practical method for grading the cognitive state of patients for the clinician. J Psychiatr Res 12(3):189–198, 1975 1202204

Fong TG, Jones RN, Marcantonio ER, et al: Adverse outcomes after hospitalization and delirium in persons with Alzheimer disease. Ann Intern Med 156(12):848–856, 2012

Fong TG, Davis D, Growdon ME, et al: The interface between delirium and dementia in elderly adults. Lancet Neurol 14(8):823–832, 2015 26139023

Fong TG, Inouye SK, Jones RN: Delirium, dementia, and decline. JAMA Psychiatry 74(3):212–213, 2017 28114516

Fong TG, Vasunilashorn SM, Libermann T, et al: Delirium and Alzheimer disease: a proposed model for shared pathophysiology. Int J Geriatr Psychiatry 34(6):781–789, 2019

Freter S, Dunbar M, Koller K, et al: Prevalence and characteristics of pre-operative delirium in hip fracture patients. Gerontology 62(4):396–400, 2016 26667308

Gaudreau JD, Gagnon P, Harel F, et al: Fast, systematic, and continuous delirium assessment in hospitalized patients: the nursing delirium screening scale. J Pain Symptom Manage 29(4):368–375, 2005 15857740

Gélinas C, Bérubé M, Chevrier A, et al: Delirium assessment tools for use in critically ill adults: a psychometric analysis and systematic review. Crit Care Nurse 38(1):38–49, 2018 29437077

Girard TD, Exline MC, Carson SS, et al: Haloperidol and ziprasidone for treatment of delirium in critical illness. N Engl J Med 379(26):2506–2516, 2018 30346242

Giroux M, Sirois MJ, Boucher V, et al: Frailty assessment to help predict patients at risk of delirium when consulting the emergency department. J Emerg Med 55(2):157–164, 2018 29764723

Goldberg SE, Whittamore KH, Harwood RH, et al: The prevalence of mental health problems among older adults admitted as an emergency to a general hospital. Age Ageing 41(1):80–86, 2012 21890483

Gou RY, Hshieh TT, Marcantonio ER, et al: One-year Medicare costs associated with delirium in older patients undergoing major elective surgery. JAMA Surg 156(5):430–442, 2021

Green JR, Smith J, Teale E, et al: Use of the confusion assessment method in multicentre delirium trials: training and standardisation. BMC Geriatr 19(1):107, 2019 30991945

Guo Y, Sun L, Li L, et al: Impact of multicomponent, nonpharmacologic interventions on perioperative cortisol and melatonin levels and postoperative delirium in elderly oral cancer patients. Arch Gerontol Geriatr 62:112–117, 2016 26547518

Haggstrom L, Welschinger R, Caplan GA: Functional neuroimaging offers insights into delirium pathophysiology: a systematic review. Australas J Ageing 36(3):186–192, 2017 28519903

Han JH, Zimmerman EE, Cutler N, et al: Delirium in older emergency department patients: recognition, risk factors, and psychomotor subtypes. Acad Emerg Med 16(3):193–200, 2009 19154565

Han JH, Wilson A, Vasilevskis EE, et al: Diagnosing delirium in older emergency department patients: validity and reliability of the delirium triage screen and the Brief Confusion Assessment Method. Ann Emerg Med 62(5):457–465, 2013 23916018

Hardy JE, Brennan N: Computerized tomography of the brain for elderly patients presenting to the emergency department with acute confusion. Emerg Med Australas 20(5):420–424, 2008

Hasegawa N, Hashimoto M, Yuuki S, et al: Prevalence of delirium among outpatients with dementia. Int Psychogeriatr 25(11):1877–1883, 2013 23870331

Hasemann W, Grossmann FF, Stadler R, et al: Screening and detection of delirium in older ED patients: performance of the modified Confusion Assessment Method for the Emergency Department (mCAM-ED): a two-step tool. Intern Emerg Med 13(6):915–922, 2018 29290048

Heim N, van Fenema EM, Weverling-Rijnsburger AW, et al: Optimal screening for increased risk for adverse outcomes in hospitalised older adults. Age Ageing 44(2):239–244, 2015 25432981

Helfand BKI, D'Aquila ML, Tabloski P, et al: Detecting delirium: a systematic review of identification instruments for non-ICU settings. J Am Geriatr Soc 69:547–555, 2021

Hendry K, Hill E, Quinn TJ, et al: Single screening questions for cognitive impairment in older people: a systematic review. Age Ageing 44(2):322–326, 2015a 25385272

Hendry K, Quinn TJ, Evans JJ, Stott DJ: Informant single screening questions for delirium and dementia in acute care: a cross-sectional test accuracy pilot study. BMC Geriatr 15:17, 2015b 25885022

Herling SF, Greve IE, Vasilevskis EE, et al: Interventions for preventing intensive care unit delirium in adults. Cochrane Database Syst Rev (11):CD009783, 2018 30484283

Hewitt J, Owen S, Carter BR, et al: The prevalence of delirium in an older acute surgical population and its effect on outcome. Geriatrics 4(4):E57, 2019 31623269

Hirano LA, Bogardus ST Jr, Saluja S, et al: Clinical yield of computed tomography brain scans in older general medical patients. J Am Geriatr Soc 54(4):587–592, 2006 16686867

Holt R, Young J, Heseltine D: Effectiveness of a multi-component intervention to reduce delirium incidence in elderly care wards. Age Ageing 42(6):721–727, 2013 23978407

Honda S, Furukawa K, Nishiwaki N, et al: Risk factors for postoperative delirium after gastrectomy in gastric cancer patients. World J Surg 42(11):3669–3675, 2018 29850948

Hov KR, Berg JP, Frihagen F, et al: Blood-cerebrospinal fluid barrier integrity in delirium determined by Q-albumin. Dement Geriatr Cogn Disord 41(3–4):192–198, 2016 27058253

Hshieh TT, Yang T, Gartaganis SL, et al: Hospital Elder Life Program: systematic review and meta-analysis of effectiveness. Am J Geriatr Psychiatry 26(10):1015–1033, 2018 30076080

Hshieh TT, Fong TG, Schmitt EM, et al: Does Alzheimer's disease and related dementias modify delirium severity and hospital outcomes? J Am Geriatr Soc 68(8):1722–1730, 2020 32255521

Hsieh SJ, Madahar P, Hope AA, et al: Clinical deterioration in older adults with delirium during early hospitalisation: a prospective cohort study. BMJ Open 5(9):e007496, 2015 26353866

Hufschmidt A, Shabarin V: Diagnostic yield of cerebral imaging in patients with acute confusion. Acta Neurol Scand 118(4):245–250, 2008 18336626

Hughes CG, Patel MB, Pandharipande PP: Pathophysiology of acute brain dysfunction: what's the cause of all this confusion? Curr Opin Crit Care 18(5):518–526, 2012 22941208

Inouye SK, Charpentier PA: Precipitating factors for delirium in hospitalized elderly persons: predictive model and interrelationship with baseline vulnerability. JAMA 275(11):852–857, 1996 8596223

Inouye SK, van Dyck CH, Alessi CA, et al: Clarifying confusion: the Confusion Assessment Method: a new method for detection of delirium. Ann Intern Med 113(12):941–948, 1990 2240918

Inouye SK, Foreman MD, Mion LC, et al: Nurses' recognition of delirium and its symptoms: comparison of nurse and researcher ratings. Arch Intern Med 161(20):2467–2473, 2001 11700159

Inouye SK, Leo-Summers L, Zhang Y, et al: A chart-based method for identification of delirium: validation compared with interviewer ratings using the confusion assessment method. J Am Geriatr Soc 53(2):312–318, 2005 15673358

Inouye SK, Baker DI, Fugal P, Bradley EH: Dissemination of the Hospital Elder Life Program: implementation, adaptation, and successes. J Am Geriatr Soc 54(10):1492–1499, 2006 17038065

Inouye SK, Zhang Y, Jones RN, et al: Risk factors for delirium at discharge: development and validation of a predictive model. Arch Intern Med 167(13):1406–1413, 2007 17620535

Inouye SK, Westendorp RG, Saczynski JS: Delirium in elderly people. Lancet 383(9920):911–922, 2013 23992774

Inouye SK, Kosar CM, Tommet D, et al: The CAM-S: development and validation of a new scoring system for delirium severity in 2 cohorts. Ann Intern Med 160(8):526–533, 2014 24733193

Jackson JC, Gordon SM, Hart RP, et al: The association between delirium and cognitive decline: a review of the empirical literature. Neuropsychol Rev 14(2):87–98, 2004 15264710

Jacobson S, Jerrier H: EEG in delirium. Semin Clin Neuropsychiatry 5(2):86–92, 2000

Jadad AR, Moore RA, Carroll D, et al: Assessing the quality of reports of randomized clinical trials: is blinding necessary? Controlled Clinical Trials 17(1):1–12, 1996

Jenssen S: Electroencephalogram in the dementia workup. Am J Alzheimers Dis Other Demen 20(3):159–166, 2005

Jones RN, Cizginer S, Pavlech L, et al: Assessment of instruments for measurement of delirium severity: a systematic review. JAMA Intern Med 179(2):231–239, 2019 30556827

Kalantar K, LaHue SC, DeRisi JL, et al: Whole-genome mRNA gene expression differs between patients with and without delirium. J Geriatr Psychiatry Neurol 31(4):203–210, 2018 29991314

Kim MY, Park UJ, Kim HT, Cho WH: DELirium Prediction Based on Hospital Information (Delphi) in general surgery patients. Medicine 95(12):e3072, 2016 27015177

Kimchi EY, Neelagiri A, Whitt W, et al: Clinical EEG slowing correlates with delirium severity and predicts poor clinical outcomes. Neurology 93(13):e1260–e1271, 2019 31467255

Kolanowski A, Mogle J, Fick DM, et al: Anticholinergic exposure during rehabilitation: cognitive and physical function outcomes in patients with delirium superimposed on dementia. Am J Geriatr Psychiatry 23(12):1250–1258, 2015 26419732

Krewulak KD, Stelfox HT, Leigh JP, et al: Incidence and prevalence of delirium subtypes in an adult ICU: a systematic review and meta-analysis. Crit Care Med 46(12):2029–2035, 2018 30234569

Kumar AK, Jayant A, Arya VK, et al: Delirium after cardiac surgery: a pilot study from a single tertiary referral center. Ann Card Anaesth 20(1):76–82, 2017 28074801

Lai MM, Wong Tin Niam DM: Intracranial cause of delirium: computed tomography yield and predictive factors. Intern Med J 42(4):422–427, 2012 21118407

Larsen KA, Kelly SE, Stern TA, et al: Administration of olanzapine to prevent postoperative delirium in elderly joint-replacement patients: a randomized, controlled trial. Psychosomatics 51(5):409–418, 2010 20833940

Lee C, Lee J, Cho H, et al: The association of perioperative serum lactate levels with postoperative delirium in elderly trauma patients. BioMed Res Int 2019:3963780, 2019 31828102

Leslie DL, Marcantonio ER, Zhang Y, et al: One-year health care costs associated with delirium in the elderly population. Arch Intern Med 168(1):27–32, 2008 18195192

Levy I, Attias S, Ben-Arye E, et al: Complementary medicine for treatment of agitation and delirium in older persons: a systematic review and narrative synthesis. Int J Geriatr Psychiatry 32(5):492–508, 2017 28239906

Li Y, Ma J, Jin Y, et al: Benzodiazepines for treatment of patients with delirium excluding those who are cared for in an intensive care unit. Cochrane Database Syst Rev (2):CD012670, 2020 32108325

Lin HS, Eeles E, Pandy S, et al: Screening in delirium: a pilot study of two screening tools, the Simple Query for Easy Evaluation of Consciousness and Simple Question in Delirium. Australas J Ageing 34(4):259–264, 2015 26059554

Liu P, Li YW, Wang XS, et al: High serum interleukin-6 level is associated with increased risk of delirium in elderly patients after noncardiac surgery: a prospective cohort study. Chin Med J 126(19):3621–3627, 2013 24112153

Liu X, Yu Y, Zhu S: Inflammatory markers in postoperative delirium (POD) and cognitive dysfunction (POCD): a meta-analysis of observational studies. PLoS One 13(4):e0195659, 2018 29641605

Lundström M, Edlund A, Karlsson S, et al: A multifactorial intervention program reduces the duration of delirium, length of hospitalization, and mortality in delirious patients. J Am Geriatr Soc 53(4):622–628, 2005 15817008

MacKenzie KK, Britt-Spells AM, Sands LP, Leung JM: Processed electroencephalogram monitoring and postoperative delirium: a systematic review and meta-analysis. Anesthesiology 129(3):417–427, 2018 29912008

Maclullich AM, Anand A, Davis DH, et al: New horizons in the pathogenesis, assessment and management of delirium. Age Ageing 42(6):667–674, 2013 24067500

Mailhot T, Cossette S, Côté J, et al: A post cardiac surgery intervention to manage delirium involving families: a randomized pilot study. Nurs Crit Care 22(4):221–228, 2017 28371230

Mailhot T, Darling C, Ela J, et al: Family identification of delirium in the emergency department in patients with and without dementia: validity of the Family Confusion Assessment Method (FAM-CAM). J Am Geriatr Soc 68(5):983–990, 2020 32274799

Marcantonio ER: In the clinic: delirium. Ann Intern Med 154(11):ITC6-1–ITC6-16, 2011

Marcantonio ER: Delirium in hospitalized older adults. N Engl J Med 377(15):1456–1466, 2017 29020579

Marcantonio ER, Flacker JM, Wright RJ, Resnick NM: Reducing delirium after hip fracture: a randomized trial. J Am Geriatr Soc 49(5):516–522, 2001 11380742

Marcantonio ER, Bergmann MA, Kiely DK, et al: Randomized trial of a delirium abatement program for postacute skilled nursing facilities. J Am Geriatr Soc 58(6):1019–1026, 2010 20487083

Marcantonio ER, Ngo LH, O'Connor M, et al: 3D-CAM: derivation and validation of a 3-minute diagnostic interview for CAM-defined delirium: a cross-sectional diagnostic test study. Ann Intern Med 161(8):554–561, 2014 25329203

Mariz J, Santos NC, Afonso H, et al: Risk and clinical-outcome indicators of delirium in an emergency department intermediate care unit (EDIMCU): an observational prospective study. BMC Emerg Med 13:2, 2013 23360089

Martinez FT, Tobar C, Beddings CI, et al: Preventing delirium in an acute hospital using a non-pharmacological intervention. Age Ageing 41(5):629–634, 2012 22589080

Martins S, Conceição F, Paiva JA, et al: Delirium recognition by family: European Portuguese validation study of the Family Confusion Assessment Method. J Am Geriatr Soc 62(9):1748–1752, 2014 25039562

McDowell JA, Mion LC, Lydon TJ, Inouye SK: A nonpharmacologic sleep protocol for hospitalized older patients. J Am Geriatr Soc 46(6):700–705, 1998

McKenzie J, Joy A: Family intervention improves outcomes for patients with delirium: systematic review and meta-analysis. Australas J Ageing 39(1):21–30, 2020 31250961

McNeil JB, Hughes CG, Girard T, et al: Plasma biomarkers of inflammation, coagulation, and brain injury as predictors of delirium duration in older hospitalized patients. PLoS One 14(12):e0226412, 2019 31856187

Mesa P, Previgliano IJ, Altez S, et al: Delirium in a Latin American intensive care unit: a prospective cohort study of mechanically ventilated patients. Rev Bras Ter Intensiva 29(3):337–345, 2017 29044304

Milisen K, Foreman MD, Abraham IL, et al: A nurse-led interdisciplinary intervention program for delirium in elderly hip-fracture patients. J Am Geriatr Soc 49(5):523–532, 2001 11380743

Mitasova A, Kostalova M, Bednarik J, et al: Poststroke delirium incidence and outcomes: validation of the Confusion Assessment Method for the Intensive Care Unit (CAM-ICU). Crit Care Med 40(2):484–490, 2012 22001583

Miu DK, Yeung JC: Incidence of post-stroke delirium and 1-year outcome. Geriatr Gerontol Int 13(1):123–129, 2013 22672215

Moon KJ, Park H: Outcomes of patients with delirium in long-term care facilities: a prospective cohort study. J Gerontol Nurs 44(9):41–50, 2018 30148531

Morandi A, Davis D, Fick DM, et al: Delirium superimposed on dementia strongly predicts worse outcomes in older rehabilitation inpatients. J Am Med Dir Assoc 15(5):349–354, 2014 24566447

Morichi V, Fedecostante M, Morandi A, et al: A point prevalence study of delirium in Italian nursing homes. Dement Geriatr Cogn Disord 46(1–2):27–41, 2018 30092581

Moskowitz EE, Overbey DM, Jones TS, et al: Post-operative delirium is associated with increased 5-year mortality. Am J Surg 214(6):1036–1038, 2017 28947274

Mueller A, Spies CD, Eckardt R, et al: Anticholinergic burden of long-term medication is an independent risk factor for the development of postoperative delirium: a clinical trial. J Clin Anesth 61:109632, 2020 31668693

Nasreddine ZS, Phillips NA, Bédirian V, et al: The Montreal Cognitive Assessment, MoCA: a brief screening tool for mild cognitive impairment. J Am Geriatr Soc 53(4):695–699, 2005 15817019

Naughton BJ, Moran M, Ghaly Y, Michalakes C: Computed tomography scanning and delirium in elder patients. Acad Emerg Med 4(12):1107–1110, 1997 9408423

Naughton BJ, Saltzman S, Ramadan F, et al: A multifactorial intervention to reduce prevalence of delirium and shorten hospital length of stay. J Am Geriatr Soc 53(1):18–23, 2005 15667371

Neelon VJ, Champagne MT, Carlson JR, Funk SG: The NEECHAM Confusion Scale: construction, validation, and clinical testing. Nurs Res 45(6):324–330, 1996 8941300

Ng SY, Phua J, Wong YL, et al: Singapore SPICE: sedation practices in intensive care evaluation in Singapore—a prospective cohort study of the public healthcare system. Singapore Med J 61(1):19–23, 2020 31197381

Nielsen RM, Urdanibia-Centelles O, Vedel-Larsen E, et al: Continuous EEG monitoring in a consecutive patient cohort with sepsis and delirium. Neurocrit Care 32(1):121–130, 2020 30891696

Nikooie R, Neufeld KJ, Oh ES, et al: Antipsychotics for treating delirium in hospitalized adults: a systematic review. Ann Intern Med 171(7):485–495, 2019 31476770

Nitchingham A, Kumar V, Shenkin S, et al: A systematic review of neuroimaging in delirium: predictors, correlates and consequences. Int J Geriatr Psychiatry 33(11):1458–1478, 2018 28574155

Noriega FJ, Vidán MT, Sánchez E, et al: Incidence and impact of delirium on clinical and functional outcomes in older patients hospitalized for acute cardiac diseases. Am Heart J 170(5):938–944, 2015 26542502

Numan T, van den Boogaard M, Kamper AM, et al: Recognition of delirium in postoperative elderly patients: a multicenter study. J Am Geriatr Soc 65(9):1932–1938, 2017 28497575

Ogasawara K, Komoribayashi N, Kobayashi M, et al: Neural damage caused by cerebral hyperperfusion after arterial bypass surgery in a patient with moyamoya disease: case report. Neurosurgery 56(6):E1380, discussion E1380, 2005 15918959

Oh ES, Fong TG, Hshieh TT, Inouye SK: Delirium in older persons: advances in diagnosis and treatment. JAMA 318(12):1161–1174, 2017 28973626

Oh ES, Needham DM, Wilson LM, et al: Antipsychotics for preventing delirium in hospitalized adults. Ann Intern Med 172(5):366, 2020 32120390

Oldham MA, Flaherty JH, Maldonado JR: Refining delirium: a transtheoretical model of delirium disorder with preliminary neurophysiologic subtypes. Am J Geriatr Psychiatry 26(9):913–924, 2018 30017237

Palanca BJA, Wildes TS, Ju YS, et al: Electroencephalography and delirium in the postoperative period. Br J Anaesth 119(2):294–307, 2017 28854540

Pan Y, Jiang Z, Yuan C, et al: Influence of physical restraint on delirium of adult patients in ICU: a nested case-control study. J Clin Nurs 27(9–10):1950–1957, 2018 29495083

Pandharipande PP, Girard TD, Jackson JC, et al: Long-term cognitive impairment after critical illness. N Engl J Med 369(14):1306–1316, 2013 24088092

Park M, Tang JH: Changing the practice of physical restraint use in acute care. J Gerontol Nurs 33(2):9–16, 2007

Pasina L, Colzani L, Cortesi L, et al: Relation between delirium and anticholinergic drug burden in a cohort of hospitalized older patients: an observational study. Drugs Aging 36(1):85–91, 2019 30484239

Pasinska P, Kowalska K, Klimiec E, et al: Frequency and predictors of post-stroke delirium in PROspective Observational POLIsh Study (PROPOLIS). J Neurol 265(4):863–870, 2018 29423616

Pauley E, Lishmanov A, Schumann S, et al: Delirium is a robust predictor of morbidity and mortality among critically ill patients treated in the cardiac intensive care unit. Am Heart J 170(1):79–86, 2015

Pfeiffer E: A short portable mental status questionnaire for the assessment of organic brain deficit in elderly patients. J Am Geriatr Soc 23(10):433–441, 1975 1159263

Pieri M, De Simone A, Rose S, et al: Trials focusing on prevention and treatment of delirium after cardiac surgery: a systematic review of randomized evidence. J Cardiothorac Vasc Anesth 34(6):1641–1654, 2020 31668634

Pinkhasov A, James SA, Fazzari M, et al: Role of ramelteon in reduction of as-needed antipsychotics in elderly patients with delirium in a general hospital setting. Clin Drug Investig 37(12):1137–1141, 2017 28933013

Pitkälä KH, Laurila JV, Strandberg TE, Tilvis RS: Multicomponent geriatric intervention for elderly inpatients with delirium: a randomized, controlled trial. J Gerontol A Biol Sci Med Sci 61(2):176–181, 2006 16510862

Pun BT, Balas MC, Barnes-Daly MA, et al: Caring for critically ill patients with the ABCDEF Bundle: results of the ICU Liberation Collaborative in over 15,000 adults. Crit Care Med 47(1):3–14, 2019 30339549

Punjasawadwong Y, Chau-In W, Laopaiboon M, et al: Processed electroencephalogram and evoked potential techniques for amelioration of postoperative delirium and cognitive dysfunction following non-cardiac and non-neurosurgical procedures in adults. Cochrane Database Syst Rev (5):CD011283, 2018 29761891

Qu J, Chen Y, Luo G, et al: Delirium in the acute phase of ischemic stroke: incidence, risk factors, and effects on functional outcome. J Stroke Cerebrovasc Dis 27(10):2641–2647, 2018 30172676

Reade MC, Eastwood GM, Bellomo R, et al: Effect of dexmedetomidine added to standard care on ventilator-free time in patients with agitated delirium: a randomized clinical trial. JAMA 315(14):1460–1468, 2016 26975647

Rengel KF, Hayhurst CJ, Pandharipande PP, Hughes CG: Long-term cognitive and functional impairments after critical illness. Anesth Analg 128(4):772–780, 2019 30883422

Rhodius-Meester HFM, van Campen JPCM, Fung W, et al: [Development and validation of the Informant Assessment of Geriatric Delirium Scale (I-AGeD): recognition of delirium in geriatric patients]. Tijdschr Gerontol Geriatr 44(5):206–214, 2013 23943558

Rosgen B, Krewulak K, Demiantschuk D, et al: Validation of caregiver-centered delirium detection tools: a systematic review. J Am Geriatr Soc 66(6):1218–1225, 2018 29671281

Rudolph JL, Doherty K, Kelly B, et al: Validation of a delirium risk assessment using electronic medical record information. J Am Med Dir Assoc 17(3):244–248, 2016 26705000

Saczynski JS, Marcantonio ER, Quach L, et al: Cognitive trajectories after postoperative delirium. N Engl J Med 367(1):30–39, 2012 22762316

Saczynski JS, Kosar CM, Xu G, et al: A tale of two methods: chart and interview methods for identifying delirium. J Am Geriatr Soc 62(3):518–524, 2014 24512042

Salluh JI, Wang H, Schneider EB, et al: Outcome of delirium in critically ill patients: systematic review and meta-analysis. BMJ 350:h2538, 2015 26041151

Sands MB, Dantoc BP, Hartshorn A, et al: Single Question in Delirium (SQiD): testing its efficacy against psychiatrist interview, the Confusion Assessment Method and the Memorial Delirium Assessment Scale. Palliat Med 24(6):561–565, 2010 20837733

Sanson G, Khlopenyuk Y, Milocco S, et al: Delirium after cardiac surgery: incidence, phenotypes, predisposing and precipitating risk factors, and effects. Heart Lung 47(4):408–417, 2018 29751986

Schuurmans MJ, Shortridge-Baggett LM, Duursma SA: The Delirium Observation Screening Scale: a screening instrument for delirium. Res Theory Nurs Pract 17(1):31–50, 2003 12751884

Schweickert WD, Pohlman MC, Pohlman AS, et al: Early physical and occupational therapy in mechanically ventilated, critically ill patients: a randomised controlled trial. Lancet 373(9678):1874–1882, 2009 19446324

Scottish Intercollegiate Guidelines Network: Risk Reduction and Management of Delirium (Publ No 157). Edinburgh, SIGN, 2019

Sepúlveda E, Franco JG, Trzepacz PT, et al: Performance of the Delirium Rating Scale-Revised-98 against different delirium diagnostic criteria in a population with a high prevalence of dementia. Psychosomatics 56(5):530–541, 2015 26278338

Sepúlveda E, Franco JG, Leunda A, et al: Delirium clinical correlates and underdiagnosis in a skilled nursing home. Eur J Psychiatry 33(4):152–158, 2019

Shi Z, Mei X, Li C, et al: Postoperative delirium is associated with long-term decline in activities of daily living. Anesthesiology 131(3):492–500, 2019 31335550

Shulman RW, Kalra S, Jiang JZ: Validation of the Sour Seven Questionnaire for screening delirium in hospitalized seniors by informal caregivers and untrained nurses. BMC Geriatr 16:44, 2016 26879927

Siddiqi N, Harrison JK, Clegg A, et al: Interventions for preventing delirium in hospitalised non-ICU patients. Cochrane Database Syst Rev (3):CD005563, 2016 26967259

Sieber F, Neufeld KJ, Gottschalk A, et al: Effect of depth of sedation in older patients undergoing hip fracture repair on postoperative delirium: the STRIDE randomized clinical trial. JAMA Surg 153(11):987–995, 2018 30090923

Sieber F, Neufeld KJ, Gottschalk A, et al: Depth of sedation as an interventional target to reduce postoperative delirium: mortality and functional outcomes of the Strategy to Reduce the Incidence of Postoperative Delirium in Elderly Patients randomised clinical trial. Br J Anaesth 122(4):480–489, 2019 30857604

Singler K, Thiem U, Christ M, et al: Aspects and assessment of delirium in old age: first data from a German interdisciplinary emergency department. Z Gerontol Geriatr 47(8):680–685, 2014 24733451

Smulter N, Lingehall HC, Gustafson Y, et al: Delirium after cardiac surgery: incidence and risk factors. Interact Cardiovasc Thorac Surg 17(5):790–796, 2013 23887126

Sri-on J, Tirrell GP, Vanichkulbodee A, et al: The prevalence, risk factors and short-term outcomes of delirium in Thai elderly emergency department patients. Emerg Med J 33(1):17–22, 2016 25805897

Steensma E, Zhou W, Ngo L, et al: Ultra-brief screeners for detecting delirium superimposed on dementia. J Am Med Dir Assoc 20(11):1391–1396, 2019 31279670

Steis MR, Evans L, Hirschman KB, et al: Screening for delirium using family caregivers: convergent validity of the Family Confusion Assessment Method and interviewer-rated Confusion Assessment Method. J Am Geriatr Soc 60(11):2121–2126, 2012 23039310

Tabet N, Hudson S, Sweeney V, et al: An educational intervention can prevent delirium on acute medical wards. Age Ageing 34(2):152–156, 2005 15713859

Takanashi J, Barkovich AJ, Shiihara T, et al: Widening spectrum of a reversible splenial lesion with transiently reduced diffusion. AJNR Am J Neuroradiol 27(4):836–838, 2006 16611774

Thomas C, Kreisel SH, Oster P, et al: Diagnosing delirium in older hospitalized adults with dementia: adapting the Confusion Assessment Method to International Classification of Diseases, Tenth Revision, diagnostic criteria. J Am Geriatr Soc 60(8):1471–1477, 2012 22881707

Trzepacz PT, Baker RW, Greenhouse J: A symptom rating scale for delirium. Psychiatry Res 23(1):89–97, 1988 3363018

Trzepacz PT, Mittal D, Torres R, et al: Validation of the Delirium Rating Scale-Revised-98: comparison with the Delirium Rating Scale and the Cognitive Test for Delirium. J Neuropsychiatry Clin Neurosci 13(2):229–242, 2001 11449030

Tsuruta R, Oda Y, Shintani A, et al: Delirium and coma evaluated in mechanically ventilated patients in the intensive care unit in Japan: a multi-institutional prospective observational study. J Crit Care 29(3):472.e1–472.e5, 2014 24602999

Turco R, Bellelli G, Morandi A, et al: The effect of poststroke delirium on short-term outcomes of elderly patients undergoing rehabilitation. J Geriatr Psychiatry Neurol 26(2):63–68, 2013 23504308

van den Boogaard M, Pickkers P, Slooter AJ, et al: Development and validation of PRE-DELIRIC (PREdiction of DELIRium in ICu patients) delirium prediction model for intensive care patients: observational multicentre study. BMJ 344:e420, 2012a 22323509

van den Boogaard M, Schoonhoven L, Evers AW, et al: Delirium in critically ill patients: impact on long-term health-related quality of life and cognitive functioning. Crit Care Med 40(1):112–118, 2012b 21926597

van den Boogaard M, Schoonhoven L, van der Hoeven JG, et al: Incidence and short-term consequences of delirium in critically ill patients: a prospective observational cohort study. Int J Nurs Stud 49(7):775–783, 2012c 22197051

van der Kooi AW, Zaal IJ, Klijn FA, et al: Delirium detection using EEG: what and how to measure. Chest 147(1):94–101, 2015 25166725

van Eijk MM, Roes KC, Honing ML, et al: Effect of rivastigmine as an adjunct to usual care with haloperidol on duration of delirium and mortality in critically ill patients: a multicentre, double-blind, placebo-controlled randomised trial. Lancet 376(9755):1829–1837, 2010 21056464

van Munster BC, Korevaar JC, Zwinderman AH, et al: The association between delirium and the apolipoprotein E epsilon 4 allele: new study results and a meta-analysis. Am J Geriatr Psychiatry 17(10):856–862, 2009 19910874

van Roessel S, Keijsers CJPW, Romijn MDM: Dementia as a predictor of morbidity and mortality in patients with delirium. Maturitas 125:63–69, 2019 31133220

Vasilevskis EE, Chandrasekhar R, Holtze CH, et al: The cost of ICU delirium and coma in the intensive care unit patient. Med Care 56(10):890–897, 2018 30179988

Vasunilashorn SM, Ngo L, Inouye SK, et al: Cytokines and postoperative delirium in older patients undergoing major elective surgery. J Gerontol A Biol Sci Med Sci 70(10):1289–1295, 2015 26215633

Vasunilashorn SM, Ngo LH, Chan NY, et al: Development of a dynamic multi-protein signature of postoperative delirium. J Gerontol A Biol Sci Med Sci 74(2):261–268, 2019 29529166

Vasunilashorn SM, Ngo LH, Inouye SK, et al: Apolipoprotein E genotype and the association between C-reactive protein and postoperative delirium: importance of gene-protein interactions. Alzheimers Dement 16(3):572–580, 2020 31761478

Vlisides P, Avidan M: Recent advances in preventing and managing postoperative delirium. F1000Res 8:F1000, 2019 31105934

Voyer P, Champoux N, Desrosiers J, et al: Recognizing acute delirium as part of your routine [RADAR]: a validation study. BMC Nurs 14:19, 2015 25844067

Wachter RM: Understanding Patient Safety, 2nd Edition. New York, McGraw-Hill Medical, 2012

Wang Y-Y, Yue J-R, Xie D-M, et al: Effect of the tailored, family involved Hospital Elder Life Program on postoperative delirium and function in older adults: a randomized clinical trial. JAMA Intern Med 180(1):17–25, 2020 31633738

Wassenaar A, van den Boogaard M, van Achterberg T, et al: Multinational development and validation of an early prediction model for delirium in ICU patients. Intensive Care Med 41(6):1048–1056, 2015 25894620

Wildes TS, Mickle AM, Ben Abdallah A, et al: Effect of electroencephalography-guided anesthetic administration on postoperative delirium among older adults undergoing major surgery: the ENGAGES randomized clinical trial. JAMA 321(5):473–483, 2019 30721296

Wøien H, Balsliemke S, Stubhaug A: The incidence of delirium in Norwegian intensive care units: deep sedation makes assessment difficult. Acta Anaesthesiol Scand 57(3):294–302, 2013 23075027

Wong CL, Holroyd-Leduc J, Simel DL, Straus SE: Does this patient have delirium? Value of bedside instruments. JAMA 304(7):779–786, 2010

World Health Organization: The ICD-10 Classification of Mental and Behavioural Disorders: Diagnostic Criteria for Research. Geneva, World Health Organization, 1993

Yu A, Wu S, Zhang Z, et al: Cholinesterase inhibitors for the treatment of delirium in non-ICU settings. Cochrane Database Syst Rev (6):CD012494, 2018 29952000

Zaal IJ, Devlin JW, Hazelbag M, et al: Benzodiazepine-associated delirium in critically ill adults. Intensive Care Med 41(12):2130–2137, 2015 26404392

Zhang H, Lu Y, Liu M, et al: Strategies for prevention of postoperative delirium: a systematic review and meta-analysis of randomized trials. Crit Care 17(2):R47, 2013 23506796

Zimmerman KM, Salow M, Skarf LM, et al: Increasing anticholinergic burden and delirium in palliative care inpatients. Palliat Med 28(4):335–341, 2014 24534725

CHAPTER 8

Dementia and Mild Neurocognitive Disorders

Elizabeth A. Wise, M.D.

Constantine G. Lyketsos, M.D., M.H.S.

Dementia is a clinical syndrome that can be caused by a range of diseases or injuries to the brain. Although it can affect young people, it is most common among older persons because dementia prevalence increases with age. Alzheimer's Disease International estimates that approximately 35.6 million people were living with dementia worldwide in 2010 (Prince et al. 2013). Considering its high prevalence and worldwide distribution, dementia should be considered a pandemic. By 2050, the number of people age 60 years and older worldwide will have increased by 1.25 billion and will account for 22% of the world's population. Accordingly, the number of people living with dementia worldwide is expected to approximately double every 20 years to 65.7 million in 2030 and 115.4 million in 2050 (Prince et al. 2013) (Figure 8–1). The Alzheimer's Association (2019) estimates that 5.8 million Americans are living with Alzheimer's disease (AD), the single most common cause of dementia. About 10% of people age 65 years and older and about 32% of the oldest-old (those age ≥85 years) have AD, and it is the sixth leading cause of death in the United States (Heron 2018). Given the chronicity of dementia, with estimates of its duration ranging from 3 to 4 years in community settings (Graham et al. 1997) to 10 to 12 years in clinical settings (Rabins et al. 2016), it poses a unique public health problem with serious effects on those who have it, their families, and society at large. For example, the Alzheimer's Association (2019) estimated that in the United States, annual direct and indirect expenses of caring for people with AD and other dementias will soar from an estimated $290 billion in 2019 to a projected $1.1 trillion annually by 2050.

In this chapter, we discuss definitions, clinical presentation, evaluation, and differential diagnosis of dementia and related cognitive disorders, describe specific dementia syndromes according to their etiology, and discuss treatment approaches, including treatments that may be on the horizon. For an in-depth discussion of the clinical management of dementia, we recommend *Practical Dementia Care* by Rabins et al. (2016).

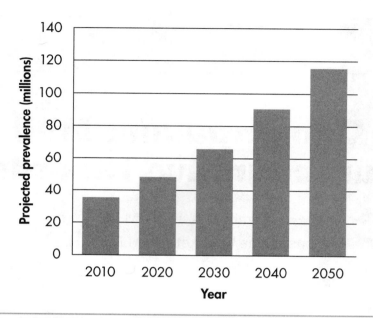

FIGURE 8–1. Projected prevalence of dementia worldwide.
Source. Data from Prince et al. 2013.

Definitions

Clinical syndromes such as dementia and cognitive impairment, no dementia (CIND) are differentiated from clinical subsyndromes such as mild cognitive impairment (MCI). *Alzheimer's disease* refers to a process of characteristic pathological changes in the brain that presumably causes (or influences) the observed dementia syndrome. Although these definitions are important to the clinical world, uncertainty remains about linking cognitive decline to brain pathology. Many studies demonstrate relationships between specific anatomical distributions of neuropathological markers and specific domains of cognitive function (e.g., the presence of medial temporal neurofibrillary tangles affects primarily episodic memory) (Dowling et al. 2011). Other studies show that even older adults without cognitive impairment can accumulate significant neuropathological changes of AD, cerebral infarctions, and Lewy bodies (Bennett et al. 2012; Negash et al. 2011). In fact, in a study undertaken to examine the relationship of AD pathology, cerebral infarcts, and Lewy body pathology to cognition in individuals without cognitive impairment, nearly all of the patients had AD pathology (>75% exhibiting amyloid) and a significant percentage had macroscopic infarctions (22%), microscopic infarctions (24%), and Lewy body pathology (13%) (Bennett et al. 2012). Furthermore, up to one-third of individuals without dementia can have AD lesions that meet the criteria for intermediate or even high likelihood of AD (Negash et al. 2011). In community settings, up to 88% of individuals with dementia or cognitive impairment who come to autopsy have mixed rather than unitary brain pathologies, including a combination of AD lesions (neocortical neurofibrillary tangles and neuritic plaques), microvascular infarcts (microinfarcts and lacunar infarcts), neocortical Lewy bodies, hippocampal

TABLE 8–1.   **Four key elements of the dementia syndrome**

1. Dementia affects cognition.
2. Cognition is affected globally.
3. Decline from prior baseline significantly affects functioning.
4. Delirium is absent.

sclerosis, and generalized brain atrophy (White 2009). Although microvascular infarcts predominate as the sole or dominant lesion in 33.8% of patients with dementia or cognitive impairment, AD lesions predominate in 18.6%, and codominant lesions (most often AD and microvascular) predominate in 14.2% (White 2009).

Clinical Presentation, Evaluation, and Differential Diagnosis

Clinical Presentation of the Dementia Syndrome

Dementia, being a syndrome, is defined entirely on clinical grounds. Table 8–1 lists the four critical elements of the dementia syndrome. First, it affects *cognition*, which is defined as the mental processes used to obtain knowledge or to become aware of and interact with the environment. These processes include perception, imagination, judgment, memory, and language, as well as the processes people use to think, organize, and learn. Second, cognition is affected globally, meaning that for the dementia syndrome to be present, several areas of cognition (e.g., complex attention, learning, procedural or explicit memory, language, social awareness) must be affected. Third, to differentiate dementia from intellectual disability, the cognitive symptoms must represent a cognitive decline for the individual. The decline must be substantial enough to be of concern to the individual, a knowledgeable informant, or the clinician; be quantitatively demonstrable by standardized neuropsychological testing or clinical assessment; and affect the person's daily functioning, operationalized as basic activities of daily living (ADLs) or instrumental activities of daily living (IADLs). Fourth, because delirium can cause the full range of cognitive symptoms associated with dementia, the cognitive syndrome must be present in the absence of delirium.

DSM-5 (American Psychiatric Association 2013) has largely moved away from the term *dementia* in favor of *major neurocognitive disorder* (NCD). However, it acknowledges that the two terms are substantially congruent. The diagnostic criteria for major NCD, which parallel the key elements of the dementia syndrome, are listed in Box 8–1. Clinicians have recently started to deemphasize the concept of the four A's of cognitive impairment (i.e., amnesia, aphasia, apraxia, and agnosia) in favor of the following cognitive domains: complex attention, executive function, learning and memory, language, perceptual-motor, and social cognition. Patients must demonstrate significant decline in cognitive function in one or more of these cognitive domains for a diagnosis of major or mild NCD. The exception is major NCD due to AD, in which a decline in at least two domains is required. DSM-5 primarily subtypes major NCDs based on the known or presumed etiology or pathological entity (e.g., AD, frontotemporal lobar degeneration, Lewy body disease) underlying the cognitive decline. The degree of functional impairment determines the severity of the dementia (mild, moderate, or severe).

Although the dementia syndrome is defined by cognitive disturbances, patients with dementia have a wider range of impairments that are of relevance to themselves, their daily lives, and their caregivers. These include functional, neuropsychiatric (behavioral), and neurological impairments.

Box 8–1.   DSM-5 Diagnostic Criteria for Major Neurocognitive Disorder

A. Evidence of significant cognitive decline from a previous level of performance in one or more cognitive domains (complex attention, executive function, learning and memory, language, perceptual-motor, or social cognition) based on:
1. Concern of the individual, a knowledgeable informant, or the clinician that there has been a significant decline in cognitive function; and
2. A substantial impairment in cognitive performance, preferably documented by standardized neuropsychological testing or, in its absence, another quantified clinical assessment.

B. The cognitive deficits interfere with independence in everyday activities (i.e., at a minimum, requiring assistance with complex instrumental activities of daily living such as paying bills or managing medications).
C. The cognitive deficits do not occur exclusively in the context of a delirium.
D. The cognitive deficits are not better explained by another mental disorder (e.g., major depressive disorder, schizophrenia).

Specify whether due to:
Alzheimer's disease
Frontotemporal lobar degeneration
Lewy body disease
Vascular disease
Traumatic brain injury
Substance/medication use
HIV infection
Prion disease
Parkinson's disease
Huntington's disease
Another medical condition
Multiple etiologies
Unspecified

Note.   Criteria set above contains only the diagnostic criteria and specifiers; refer to DSM-5 for the full criteria set, including specifier descriptions and coding and reporting procedures.
Source.   Reprinted from *Diagnostic and Statistical Manual of Mental Disorders*, 5th Edition. Arlington, VA, American Psychiatric Association, 2013, pp. 602–603. Used with permission. Copyright © 2013 American Psychiatric Association.

Functional Impairments

Patients with dementia have problems in their social and interpersonal functioning and in their ability to live independently. Patients with milder dementia have difficulties with IADLs, such as preparing a meal, balancing a checkbook, shopping, and driving. Patients with more severe dementia develop impairments in their basic ADLs, such as eating, toileting, dressing, and transferring. Changes in functional abilities are associated with cognitive decline (Royall et al. 2007) and have prognostic significance because declining functional abilities impact caregiver burden and are associated with institutionalization (Massoud 2007).

Neuropsychiatric Impairments

Dementia has also been associated with neuropsychiatric symptoms (NPS), which affect ≤97% of individuals with dementia. These are generally grouped into four types: 1) affective and motivational symptoms, such as depression, apathy, anxiety, and irritability; 2) psychotic symptoms, such as delusions or perceptual disturbances; 3) disturbances of basic drives, including feeding, sleep, and sexuality; and 4) unexpected, socially inappropriate, or disinhibited behaviors. The latter behaviors, such as spontaneous verbal or physical aggression, uncharacteristic vocalizations, intrusiveness, and wandering, typically arise in more severe dementia; they represent behavioral manifestations of loss of executive control, sometimes referred to as *executive dysfunction syndrome* (Lyketsos et al. 2004). Over the course of a progressive dementia, essentially all patients develop one or more of the NPS (Okura et al. 2010; Steinberg et al. 2008). These symptoms are associated with a decline in function and cognition among patients that may ultimately lead to increased mortality (Levy et al. 2012). Furthermore, the severity of NPS is a strong predictor of caregiver burden (Bergvall et al. 2011), with increased rates of depression, anxiety, stress, loss of sleep, medical illness, and mortality among caregivers (Levy et al. 2012). Caregiver burden, in turn, results in greater use of institutionalization for patients with dementia (Levy et al. 2012).

Neurological Impairments

Patients with dementia develop a range of neurological impairments. Depending on the cause of dementia and specifically on the parts of the brain affected over time, a range of neurological symptoms may occur. The most common of these are gait disorders, especially unstable, ataxic, or labored gait. Other symptoms include incontinence, focal findings, seizures, and, less commonly, cranial nerve findings.

Clinical Presentation of Milder Cognitive Syndromes

Epidemiological studies have found that large numbers of older people experience mild decline in one or more cognitive domains, such as memory, attention, and thinking, that does not compromise their everyday activities and functioning (i.e., independence is preserved) and thus does not satisfy the criteria for dementia. Nevertheless, the cognitive impairment is greater than expected for the person's age and education, such that tasks require more time or effort to complete than previously. Impairments may be demonstrable on cognitive assessments and are often troubling to the person or to family members. The population-based Mayo Clinic Study of Aging reported the prevalence of mild impairments to be 16% in elderly individuals who were ages 70–89 years and were free of dementia (Petersen et al. 2009). Several terms have evolved for these impairments: age-associated memory impairment, age-associated cognitive decline, CIND, and MCI. Impairments can be further divided into *amnestic* or *nonamnestic* subtypes, depending on whether significant memory impairments are present.

Population-based studies have found a range of MCI prevalence estimates, depending on the criteria utilized for classification (Ganguli et al. 2010; Lopez et al. 2003; see Chapter 1, "Epidemiology of Psychiatric Disorders in Later Life" for further incidence and prevalence data).

The core clinical features of MCI, as identified by the National Institute on Aging–Alzheimer's Association (NIA-AA), are listed in Table 8–2 (Albert et al. 2011). Paralleling the change of preference for the term *major neurocognitive disorder* over *dementia*, DSM-5 has largely moved away from the term *mild cognitive impairment* in favor of *mild neurocognitive disorder*, while acknowledging the congruency of the terms. The DSM-5 diagnostic criteria for mild NCD are listed in Box 8–2. NPS are more common in patients with MCI than in individuals with normal cognition. These symptoms include depression (most common), irritability, anxiety, agitation, apathy, and delusions. In one population-based study in Cache County, Utah, the presence of at least one NPS (even of mild severity) was a risk factor for progression from CIND to all-cause dementia (Peters et al. 2013). Few individual NPS were predictive of progression; however, nighttime behaviors were a risk factor for all-cause dementia and for AD, and hallucinations were a risk factor for vascular dementia (VaD). Several prior studies have also linked specific NPS, such as major depression and anxiety, to progression of CIND/MCI to dementia. For instance, in one study, increasing levels of anxiety doubled the risk of progression (Palmer et al. 2007). Given the risk of cognitive decline in individuals with NPS, researchers have proposed a diagnostic construct of mild behavioral impairment to capture the syndrome of late-life onset of NPS that are early manifestations of neurodegenerative disease in people without dementia who may or may not have MCI (Ismail et al. 2016).

Long-term follow-up studies suggest that although one-third of individuals with MCI improve to the point that their cognitive impairments are no longer detectable in the subsequent few years, most go on to develop dementia (Rosenberg et al. 2006). Approximately 46% of individuals with MCI developed dementia within 3 years, compared with only 3% of individuals of the same age who did not have MCI at the beginning of the study (Tschanz et al. 2006). These findings are consistent with the idea that most patients who develop progressive dementia do so in stages and typically go through a prodromal period of milder cognitive impairment. Pathological studies have confirmed that after long-term follow-up, large numbers of patients who met criteria for MCI have AD pathology. Risk factors for progression of MCI to dementia include greater cognitive and functional impairment, advancing age, male sex, marital status (never married), years of education (inverse relationship), being a carrier of the allele producing the ε4 type of apolipoprotein E (*APOE*E4*), cerebrospinal fluid (CSF) markers or PET scan patterns compatible with AD, positive amyloid imaging, and the presence of anxiety and other NPS (Palmer et al. 2007; Peters et al. 2013; Petersen et al. 2009; Tschanz et al. 2006; Yu et al. 2019). Although statins carry a black-box FDA warning that they could cause cognitive change, most data do not support this effect, and a recent multicenter cohort study found no association between statin use and progression from MCI to AD. Rather, the data demonstrated an association between statin use and a significantly slower rate of decline on a composite memory score among participants with early MCI (Kemp et al. 2020).

TABLE 8–2. **National Institute on Aging–Alzheimer's Association's proposed clinical and cognitive criteria for mild cognitive impairment**

Cognitive concern reflecting a historical or observed decline in cognition over time as reported by a patient, informant, or clinician

Objective evidence of impairment in one or more cognitive domains (typically including memory)

Preservation of independence in functional abilities

No dementia

Source. Adapted from Albert et al. 2011.

Box 8–2. DSM-5 Diagnostic Criteria for Mild Neurocognitive Disorder

A. Evidence of modest cognitive decline from a previous level of performance in one or more cognitive domains (complex attention, executive function, learning and memory, language, perceptual-motor, or social cognition) based on:
1. Concern of the individual, a knowledgeable informant, or the clinician that there has been a mild decline in cognitive function; and
2. A modest impairment in cognitive performance, preferably documented by standardized neuropsychological testing or, in its absence, another quantified clinical assessment.
B. The cognitive deficits do not interfere with capacity for independence in everyday activities (i.e., complex instrumental activities of daily living such as paying bills or managing medications are preserved, but greater effort, compensatory strategies, or accommodation may be required).
C. The cognitive deficits do not occur exclusively in the context of a delirium.
D. The cognitive deficits are not better explained by another mental disorder (e.g., major depressive disorder, schizophrenia).

Specify whether due to:
Alzheimer's disease
Frontotemporal lobar degeneration
Lewy body disease
Vascular disease
Traumatic brain injury
Substance/medication use
HIV infection
Prion disease
Parkinson's disease
Huntington's disease
Another medical condition
Multiple etiologies
Unspecified

Coding note: For mild neurocognitive disorder due to any of the medical etiologies listed above, code **331.83 (G31.84).** Do *not* use additional codes for the presumed etiological medical conditions. For substance/medication-induced mild neurocognitive disorder, code based on type of substance; see "Substance/Medication-Induced Major or Mild Neurocognitive Disorder." For unspecified mild neurocognitive disorder, code **799.59 (R41.9).**

Specify:
Without behavioral disturbance: If the cognitive disturbance is not accompanied by any clinically significant behavioral disturbance.

With behavioral disturbance *(specify disturbance)*: If the cognitive disturbance is accompanied by a clinically significant behavioral disturbance (e.g., psychotic symptoms, mood disturbance, agitation, apathy, or other behavioral symptoms).

Source. Reprinted from *Diagnostic and Statistical Manual of Mental Disorders*, 5th Edition. Arlington, VA, American Psychiatric Association, 2013, pp. 605–606. Used with permission. Copyright © 2013 American Psychiatric Association.

The prodromal period most often, but not exclusively, starts with cognitive symptoms characteristic of the specific cause of dementia. For example, amnestic MCI (Petersen et al. 2009) appears to be a precursor to AD. In fact, the NIA-AA (Albert et al. 2011) has proposed terminology for classifying patients with MCI due to AD with varying degrees of certainty based on the presence or absence of AD biomarkers. As with major NCDs, DSM-5 primarily subtypes mild NCDs based on the known or presumed etiology underlying the cognitive decline. The term *vascular cognitive impairment* (Bowler and Hachinski 1995; Hachinski 1994, 2007) was coined to refer to nondementia disturbances associated with cerebrovascular disease, likely the prodrome of VaD. Whereas MCI, the prodrome of AD, appears to have primarily cortical features, vascular cognitive impairment, the prodrome of VaD, typically affects executive functions (Hayden et al. 2006).

Conducting an Evaluation

Although a detailed discussion of how to evaluate patients with suspected dementia is beyond the scope of this chapter, we highlight critical aspects of the evaluation, with a focus on taking a history, conducting a cognitive assessment, and using diagnostic tests. A thorough discussion of the evaluation of patients with suspected dementia, including reasons for doing an evaluation, the setting for the evaluation, and ways to communicate the diagnosis to patients and caregivers, is provided in *Practical Dementia Care* (Rabins et al. 2016).

History Taking

Because dementia is diagnosed clinically, a thorough medical history is essential. A patient with suspected dementia may have difficulty providing history due to language problems, memory disturbance, or anosognosia (lack of insight). Therefore, it is critical during history taking to involve a reliable informant who knows the patient well, such as family members. Because informants themselves can be influenced by their own mental states, such as depression or denial of the situation, it is often useful to speak with more than one informant to confirm or challenge discrepancies between the history and the patient evaluation.

Clinicians should date and elucidate the type of onset of cognitive symptoms (e.g., insidious onset, abrupt onset following traumatic brain injury [TBI]) and establish the progression of symptoms over time (e.g., gradual, stepwise, or nonprogressive decline). Comparing the severity of the patient's current impairment with its duration often influences the differential diagnosis. For instance, a slowly progressive dementia over years with insidious onset may point to Alzheimer's dementia, whereas a rapidly progressive dementia over months may point to dementia due to prion disease. Clinicians must resolve discrepancies in reports of severity and duration because they portend different prognoses and recommendations. It is often more feasible to determine when the patient was last well rather than when symptoms first started. Informants often minimize early symptoms by attributing them to "normal aging." The history should also systematically evaluate for the presence or absence of the broader dementia syndrome presentation, as discussed earlier (see "Clinical Presentation of the Dementia Syndrome"), assessing for cortical and subcortical cognitive symptoms; functional losses in social, interpersonal, and daily functioning; the full range of NPS; and neurological deficits.

Cognitive Assessment

Conducting a cognitive assessment is the central aspect of the evaluation. Many specialists tend to use the Mini-Mental State Examination (MMSE; Folstein et al. 1975) as their primary tool because it is brief, easy to use, and well-known. The MMSE, however, is inefficient in evaluating patients with milder cognitive symptoms or mild dementia, especially those with subcortical features. This is because the MMSE has ceiling effects, especially for premorbidly well-educated and intelligent individuals, and limitations in evaluating executive control function. Furthermore, it is unable to discriminate subtle degrees of impairment in severe dementia. We recommend specialists in geriatric psychiatry and other clinicians who work with patients broaden their use of bedside standardized assessments and consider the Montreal Cognitive Assessment (MoCA; Nasreddine et al. 2005) as an alternative first-line test. Advantages of the MoCA include that it has several available translations and has been validated in various languages; it assesses abstract thinking, delayed recall, and verbal fluency better than the MMSE; and it has well-known population norms. The Modified Mini-Mental State (Teng and Chui 1987) is another bedside cognitive test that can provide a more comprehensive assessment of cognition and has been validated with several language translations. In addition, for closer assessments of executive functioning, geriatric psychiatrists should consider incorporating the following three measures in every dementia evaluation: the Clock Drawing Test (van der Burg et al. 2004), the Frontal Assessment Battery (Dubois et al. 2000), and the Mental Alternation Test (Jones et al. 1993).

Neuropsychological testing is often useful for differentiating dementia from milder cognitive syndromes or normal aging or for clarifying the etiology of the cognitive disorder. However, neuropsychological testing is not needed in every case, assuming the clinician conducts a standardized assessment using tools such as those discussed here. If neuropsychological testing is needed, clinicians should have in mind specific questions that they wish to address, such as how to clarify the differential diagnosis or how to set the stage for monitoring prognosis or response to treatment.

Differential Diagnosis and Diagnostic Testing

A key aspect of the dementia evaluation is forming a complete differential diagnosis of the syndrome. Figure 8–2 provides a useful flowchart for this purpose. The first decision is whether any of the observed cognitive changes are disproportionate to normal aging. This can be determined by reviewing the patient's history or by assessing the patient's performance against well-known norms for age and education. If the cognitive changes are beyond an age-appropriate level, the next question is whether the patient meets criteria for major NCD, such as those listed in DSM-5. If the patient does not meet these criteria, then either CIND (which might be further subtyped as MCI or

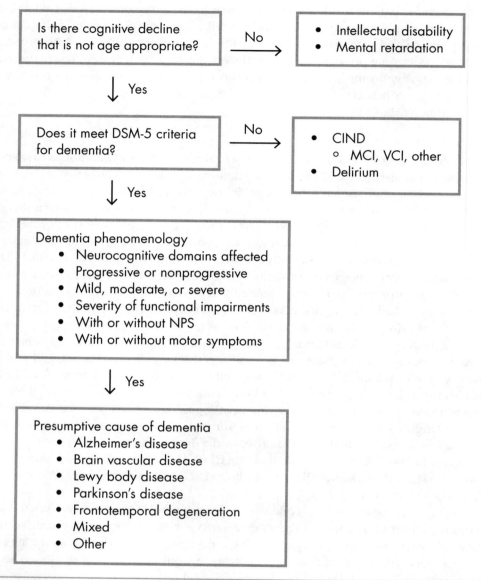

FIGURE 8–2. Flowchart in the diagnosis of dementia.

CIND=cognitive impairment, no dementia; MCI=mild cognitive impairment; NPS=neuropsychiatric symptoms; VCI=vascular cognitive impairment.

vascular cognitive impairment) or delirium is present. If dementia is present, the geriatric psychiatrist will determine whether it is cortical or subcortical, consider whether it is progressive or nonprogressive, rate its severity, and assess the degree of functional impairment, the presence or absence of NPS and their specific phenomenology, and the presence or absence of motor and other neurological symptoms. Finally, the clinician establishes the presumptive cause of the dementia.

The severity of the dementia, typically labeled mild, moderate, or severe, is guided by the score on the MMSE (or equivalent, such as the MoCA) or degree of functional impairment. An MMSE score of 20–24 or difficulties with IADLs suggest mild dementia; an MMSE score of 13–20 or difficulties with basic ADLs suggest moderate dementia; and an MMSE score ≤12 or complete functional dependence indicates severe dementia. NPS can be assessed by history, mental status examination, and standardized tools such as the Neuropsychiatric Inventory–Clinician rating scale (de Medeiros et al. 2010). Occupational therapists are skilled at assessing functional impairment and often use scales such as the Assessment of Motor and Processing Skills (Fisher 2003). A complete neurological evaluation is central to assessing neurological conditions that may cause or be the sequelae of a cognitive disorder.

Further workup using laboratory studies and brain imaging is needed in most cases of dementia. A basic dementia screening typically involves laboratory studies and brain imaging. The American Academy of Neurology (Knopman et al. 2001) and the National Institute for Health and Care Excellence (2011) recommend obtaining a metabolic panel, liver function test, complete blood count, thyroid function study, and vitamin B_{12} level. In at-risk populations or if the clinical picture indicates, clinicians may consider additional tests, such as heavy metal screening, HIV, syphilis serology, toxicology, electrocardiogram, and chest radiograph, to determine possible underlying pathology.

Urinalysis is useful when the clinician suspects delirium as part of the differential diagnosis. CSF analysis is not routinely part of a dementia workup unless the clinician suspects Creutzfeldt-Jakob disease (CJD) or other forms of rapidly progressive dementias. Likewise, electroencephalography is not part of a routine dementia workup unless frontotemporal lobar degeneration (FTLD), CJD, or delirium is suspected. Brain biopsies are indicated only in rare cases in which dementia is thought to be secondary to a potentially reversible condition that cannot be diagnosed in any other way (Manix et al. 2015).

The type of brain imaging to use remains controversial. Most clinicians suggest that CT scanning of the head is adequate to exclude other cerebral pathologies, whereas others think it is important to perform an MRI, especially when cortical or subcortical vascular disease may be involved. In the near future, the quantification of specific MRI components, such as hippocampal or medial parietal cortical atrophy, will provide information that is important to the differential diagnosis, prognosis, and treatment options. Currently, however, no standardization method for hippocampal volume measures has been widely accepted because normative data are lacking. Functional brain imaging using functional MRI, PET, or single-photon emission computed tomography (SPECT) has come into broader use and is reimbursed by Medicare under specific circumstances. These types of imaging reveal distinct regions of low metabolism and hypoperfusion and are most useful in the differential diagnosis of dementia caused by AD, cerebrovascular disease, Lewy body disease, or FTLD, if the rest of the clinical picture is inconclusive. SPECT of alterations of the dopamine transporter system can help distinguish dementia with Lewy bodies from AD.

Various amyloid PET tracers, such as ^{18}F-AV-45 (also known as florbetapir) and Pittsburgh compound B (PiB), which measure amyloid lesion burden in the brain by binding to amyloid-β (Aβ), can aid in the diagnosis and prognosis of AD and differentiate AD from other causes of dementia. In 2012, the FDA approved florbetapir for this purpose. The long half-life of ^{18}F allows florbetapir to accumulate considerably more in the brains of patients with AD (Wong et al. 2010). In 2013, the FDA also approved ^{18}F-flutemetamol, an ^{18}F-labeled derivative of the parent molecule PiB. Some studies have demonstrated the utility of amyloid PET in diagnostic clarification and in the management of patients with atypical neuropsychological testing, structural imaging, or biomarker profiles (Barthel and Sabri 2017; Boccardi et al. 2016; Ceccaldi et al. 2018; Leuzy et al. 2019). Researchers initiated the Imaging Dementia–Evidence for Amyloid Scanning (IDEAS) study in 2015 to evaluate the utility and clinical impact of amyloid PET in diagnosis, diagnostic confidence, and management changes for patients who meet appropriate use criteria. The results of the IDEAS study will inform whether Medicare reimburses amyloid PET (Kim et al. 2018). A recent large, multisite, practice-based study found that dementia care specialists did change their management within 90 days after PET in a majority of patients with MCI and dementia, specifically involving the use of AD drugs (Rabinovici et al. 2019).

Furthermore, with the introduction of tracers that bind to neurofibrillary tangles composed of hyperphosphorylated tau protein, PET-derived measurement of brain tau is another potentially useful clinical biomarker for diagnosis and assessment of disease progression in AD (Chien et al. 2013; Cho et al. 2016; Gordon et al. 2019). Using the tracer ^{18}F-AV-1451 (flortaucipir), investigators have found an association among elevated tau binding with clinical impairment in AD, severity of regional atrophy, and glucose hypometabolism (Cho et al. 2016; Gordon et al. 2019; Johnson et al. 2016; Ossenkoppele et al. 2016).

Investigators have proposed AT(N) staging as a way for researchers to describe and communicate AD biomarker profiles. In this framework, "A" refers to the value of an Aβ biomarker, either amyloid PET or CSF Aβ$_{42}$; "T" refers to tau pathology biomarker value, either CSF phosphorylated tau or tau PET; and "N" is a quantitative or topographical biomarker of neurodegeneration or neuronal injury (Jack et al. 2016). See Chapter 5, "Use of the Laboratory in the Diagnostic Workup of Older Adults," for further detail of the system. At this time, AT(N) staging is not clinically useful because it has not been validated and practitioners do not have universal access to widely agreed-upon, standard, age-appropriate measures to underpin biomarker cut points.

The same is true for genetic testing. Although *APOE* genotyping is not used in clinical settings universally, it might soon have greater utility for tailoring treatment options. Some studies suggest that certain medications may be more effective in specific *APOE* subgroups (Petersen et al. 2005). Testing for specific genetic mutations associated with AD also has its place in the rare instances of a clear familial autosomal dominant case of Alzheimer's dementia, and knowledge of the specific genetic mutation involved might be useful to the patient or the patient's progeny following appropriate counseling.

More than 100 different disease processes have been associated with dementia (Rabins et al. 2016). Most cases of dementia can be adequately assessed through the patient's history and the diagnostic testing approach discussed previously in this section. In the past, dementias were often categorized as either *treatable* or *nontreatable*. This differentiation is no longer useful for two reasons. First, the reversibility of a "treatable dementia" depends on the severity of brain damage that has occurred. For example, dementia resulting from moderate to severe vitamin B$_{12}$ deficiency, hypothyroidism, or normal-pressure hydrocephalus does not reverse when treated. Second, the implication that AD, VaD, and other dementias are not treatable is incorrect. Although these cases tend to be progressive despite available treatments, applying treatments

TABLE 8–3.   **The most common causes of dementia**

Causes	Hallmark features
Alzheimer's disease (AD)	Brain disease characterized by plaques, tangles, and neuronal loss. Insidious onset with slow progressive cognitive and functional decline. Neuropsychiatric symptoms nearly universal.
Cerebrovascular disease	Known as vascular dementia or multi-infarct dementia. Controversial nosological entity due to lack of agreed-upon neuropathological definition. Heterogeneous group of dementias. Stepwise progression with variable rates of decline. Symptoms overlap with those of AD. Focal neurological signs. Apathy and depression common.
Lewy body disorders	Examples include Parkinson's disease dementia and dementia with Lewy bodies. α-Synuclein aggregates in neurons. Progressive cognitive decline, fluctuating cognition, visual hallucinations, parkinsonian features, rapid eye movement sleep disorder, and severe neuroleptic sensitivity are common.
Frontotemporal lobar degeneration	Previously referred to as Pick's disease. Clinically and pathologically heterogeneous. Most commonly presents as behavioral variant frontotemporal dementia and primary progressive aphasia. Focal degeneration of frontal and temporal lobes. Hyperphosphorylated tau protein or transactive response DNA binding protein (TDP)-43 inclusions. Knife-edge atrophy on MRI. Progressive change in personality, behavior, and language; motor impairment syndromes co-occur. Typically a more rapid rate of decline than with AD.

makes a big difference to patients, caregivers, and families because treatments may attenuate progression, reduce symptoms, and improve quality of life.

Specific Dementias

The more common causes of dementia are listed in Table 8–3. AD is generally considered to be the most prevalent cause of dementia. Other common causes include cerebrovascular disease, Lewy body disease, and FTLD. Less common causes include normal-pressure hydrocephalus, prion diseases (e.g., CJD), TBI (more common in the young, however), AIDS, Huntington's disease, primary progressive aphasia, corticobasal degeneration, and dementia of depression (previously referred to as pseudodementia). In this section, we highlight the most common, as well as some of the less common, causes of dementia. An extended discussion of these causes is beyond the scope of this chapter.

Dementia Due to Alzheimer's Disease

Alzheimer's dementia is the most common form of dementia. Depending on the population series, 50%–70% of people with dementia are diagnosed clinically as having dementia due to AD (Ranginwala et al. 2008). Experts can typically make a reliable clinical diagnosis of AD; however, although most patients meet pathological criteria for AD, a significant number have other pathological findings, such as cerebrovascular infarcts, Lewy bodies, and lacunes.

The prevalence of Alzheimer's dementia is closely tied to age, which is the primary risk factor. Other reported risk factors include head injury or TBI, reduced cognitive reserve capacity of the brain, limited educational or occupational attainment, cerebrovascular disease, hyperlipidemia, hypertension, atherosclerosis, coronary heart disease, atrial fibrillation, smoking, obesity, and diabetes. A possible risk factor is homocysteinemia. Some but not all epidemiological studies have suggested that dietary intake of folate and vitamin B_{12}, antioxidants (especially vitamins C and D), moderate alcohol (especially red wine), nonsteroidal anti-inflammatory drugs (NSAIDs), and estrogen during the perimenopausal period are associated with reduced risk of AD.

Genetics

A major risk factor for AD is genetics, with 70%–80% of the disease being heritable, as supported by twin studies (Blennow et al. 2006). AD is a heterogeneous genetic disorder with familial and sporadic forms. The familial forms follow classical autosomal dominant inheritance and typically have their onset before age 65 years. The familial forms are linked with several mutations in genes associated with amyloid precursor protein (APP) on chromosome 21; presenilin 1 (PSEN1), on chromosome 14; or presenilin 2 (PSEN2), on chromosome 1. Mutations in PSEN1 account for 18%–55% of early-onset familial AD cases, whereas mutations in PSEN2 and APP are less common (Nowrangi et al. 2011). Taken together, these genes account for one-half to two-thirds of familial cases, suggesting that many autosomal dominant genes are unknown. Researchers are currently studying the mechanisms by which these genetic loci interact.

Many genes, most unidentified, likely increase risk but do not determine the absolute occurrence of sporadic, late-onset AD (LOAD). The most well-known gene, APOE, is a genetic risk factor for LOAD. APOE*E4 is associated with >50% of cases of AD (Nowrangi et al. 2011). Individuals who are heterozygous carriers of APOE*E4 have three times the risk of developing AD, whereas individuals who are homozygous APOE*E4 carriers have 15 times the risk compared with non–APOE*E4 carriers. APOE*E4 probably operates mainly by modifying the age at onset through uncertain molecular mechanisms (Breitner et al. 1999). Another major gene associated with LOAD is the sortilin-related receptor SORL1. This gene, which is probably involved in amyloid clearance, has also been identified as a risk factor (Rogaeva et al. 2007). The SORL1 protein may alter intracellular trafficking of APP, causing aggregated Aβ to accumulate and ultimately causing cell death (Nowrangi et al. 2011).

Since 2009, genome-wide association studies (GWASs) have revolutionized the ability to identify biological pathways potentially involved in AD (Medway and Morgan 2014). GWASs compare the entire genome of patients with a disease with the genome of those without the disease to determine whether specific alleles occur in greater frequency in those with the disease and are thus more likely to be associated with that disease. Determining a causal allele strengthens the ability to identify candidate genes that increase the risk of specific disease phenotypes and to attribute risk to each gene. GWASs have led to the discovery of new LOAD alleles, each common (minor allele frequency >5%) and transmitting modest genetic effects (Medway and Morgan 2014). In the largest GWAS meta-analysis of LOAD to date, the International Genomics of Alzheimer's Project recently reported 11 new Alzheimer's susceptibility loci (CASS4, CELF1, FERMT2, HLA-DRB5/HLA-DRB1, INPP5D, MEF2C, NME8, PTK2B, SLC24A4/RIN3, SORL1, and ZCWPW1) (Lambert et al. 2013). The study also confirmed eight

(*CR1, BIN1, CD2AP, EPHA1, CLU, MS4A6A, PICALM, ABCA7*) of the nine previously reported genome-wide associations in addition to *APOE*. Drawing on more than 74,000 samples, this meta-analysis was sufficiently powered to reveal new risk alleles previously concealed due to low frequency or weak genetic effects.

Although some genes cannot be attributed to pathways that are biologically relevant to LOAD, many susceptibility loci can be linked to pathways involving cholesterol metabolism, synaptic vesicle recycling/endocytosis, and immune system function (see Figure 8–3 in the previous edition of this textbook; Steffens et al. 2015). These pathways may modify amyloid aggregation or clearance. Alternatively, some of these genes may act through non-amyloid mechanisms. Although GWASs are useful for detecting common variants with weak to modest effects, these studies have limitations in detecting rare variants that may confer large genetic effects. Alternative technology (e.g., next-generation sequencing) may be used in tandem with GWASs to detect these uncommon variants in small cohorts (Medway and Morgan 2014). Genetic research findings highlight the diversity in AD molecular pathways, and continued investigation can contribute to a precision medicine approach with successful interventions based on molecular or genetic subtypes (Cuyvers and Sleegers 2016). Dourlen et al. (2019) published a comprehensive review of the genetic landscape of AD, highlighting the impact of GWAS-defined genes on AD pathophysiology beyond the amyloid cascade hypothesis. In particular, a focal adhesion pathway involved in synapse dynamics could be core to AD pathophysiology and a target of future therapies.

The current hypothesis is that Alzheimer's dementia is a heterogeneous condition representing a range of etiologies involving different interactions between different sets of genetic and environmental risk factors (Blennow et al. 2006). At one end of the spectrum are individuals with familial disease, for whom genes such as *APOE* influence the age at onset and who will develop the disease if they live long enough. At the other end of the spectrum are individuals with a weak predisposition, perhaps carriers of few or no risk genes, in whom the occurrence of environmental risk factors is critical to the onset of Alzheimer's pathology and later dementia. As an example of gene×environment interactions, individuals with TBI may be at increased risk of progressive dementia if they also carry one or more *APOE*E4* alleles (Isoniemi et al. 2006).

Progression

The natural history of Alzheimer's dementia has been well described from tertiary clinical centers. Time from diagnosis to death in these settings is on the order of 10–12 years, with considerable variability around this median estimate. Population studies from Canada and the United States suggest that a significant proportion of patients with dementia do not make it to clinical centers and that if all patients in this group are included, the median time from onset of symptoms to death in patients with dementia is on the order of 3–5 years (Wolfson et al. 2001). A significant number of patients exhibit slow progression after dementia onset. In the Cache County Memory Study (CCMS), 25%–30% of individuals with AD exhibited limited to no progression from milder stages of dementia, even 3–5 years after onset (Tschanz et al. 2011). Likewise, only ~25% of individuals with AD ever progressed to severe dementia, with most dying prior to that point (Rabins et al. 2013).

Cognitive and functional decline in Alzheimer's dementia also vary significantly. For instance, although the annual rate of cognitive decline on the MMSE reported in most studies is 3 points, the mean rate of decline in the CCMS was 1.5 points (Tschanz et al. 2013). Furthermore, 30%–56% of individuals in this study exhibited a slow rate of decline in one or more domains (cognitive, functional, and behavioral), declining no more than 1 point per year on the measure of each domain (Tschanz et al. 2011).

In the CCMS, many factors appeared to influence the cognitive, functional, and behavioral progression of Alzheimer's dementia. Women and individuals in both the youngest and oldest age-at-onset cohorts exhibited faster declines (Rabins et al. 2013; Tschanz et al. 2013). Factors such as a more severe form of AD in younger persons or greater comorbidity in the oldest cohort may influence the rate of progression. Neither being a carrier of APOE*E4 nor having fewer years of education affected the rate of progression in any of the three domains (Rabins et al. 2013). Other studies reported mixed results for both risk factors (Tschanz et al. 2013). Individuals with unstable or poorly controlled general health performed cognitively and behaviorally worse over the course of dementia (Tschanz et al. 2013). Specifically, hypertension, atrial fibrillation, angina, and myocardial infarctions were all associated with faster cognitive and functional decline, particularly in older adults. Several medical treatments—statins, antihypertensive medications, and history of coronary artery bypass graft—were associated with slower rates of cognitive and functional decline in AD. In general, cholinesterase inhibitors and memantine, taken by ~22% of the cohort, were associated with higher baseline cognitive scores but did not affect the rate of decline (Tschanz et al. 2011). However, among female APOE*E4 carriers, a longer duration of treatment with a cholinesterase inhibitor was associated with a slower cognitive and functional decline (Tschanz et al. 2013).

Caregiver and care environment factors influenced the clinical course of subjects with AD in the CCMS (Tschanz et al. 2013). Participant engagement in more cognitively stimulating activities was associated with slower cognitive decline early in the course of AD. Likewise, a closer caregiver and care recipient relationship was associated with slower cognitive and functional decline. AD participants who were being cared for by an adult child with a neurotic personality trait exhibited faster cognitive decline. Conversely, AD participants being cared for by an adult child with high extroversion scores exhibited slower rates of decline, and AD participants whose caregivers reported regular use of problem-solving coping strategies had a slower rate of cognitive and functional decline.

Despite the variability in their rate of decline, patients who progress show a typical pattern, with loss of memory occurring early, followed by the development of agnosia, apraxia, and aphasia. Patients also follow a predictable progression in functional impairments and, in later stages, universally develop problems with mobility and continence. In terminal stages, patients with AD may live a long time, sometimes years, in near-vegetative states if they are in good general health and receive good care.

NPS are nearly universal, affecting as many as 97% of individuals (Steinberg et al. 2008). They also tend to be persistent, and ~80% of those with NPS at baseline will show at least one symptom over an 18-month interval (Tschanz et al. 2013). Over time, the prevalence of NPS increases; the most common symptoms are depression, apathy, agitation, and restlessness (at least one of these symptoms is manifested in ~75% of individuals), followed by sundowning and verbal outbursts (manifested in ~50%) (Scarmeas et al. 2007; Steinberg et al. 2008; Tschanz et al. 2011). Several cohort studies suggest that affective, psychotic, and sleep symptoms relapse and remit throughout the course of Alzheimer's dementia and are very troubling for patients and caregivers (Rabins et al. 2016; Steinberg et al. 2008). Apathy, in contrast, appears to be a steadily accumulating symptom; many, but not all, patients gradually develop persistent and pervasive apathy (Steinberg et al. 2008). Overall, the presence of NPS tends to increase over time (Scarmeas et al. 2007).

During the past several decades, studies have explored the possibility of neuropsychiatric subsyndromes in Alzheimer's dementia (Canevelli et al. 2013). For example, increasing evidence suggests that AD with psychosis may be a distinct phenotype with a genetic basis (Geda et al. 2013). By examining the internal structure of the Neuropsychiatric Inventory, researchers have classified NPS into specific clusters. The practical implications of identifying clusters or subsyndromes include more adequately comprehending the neurobiological correlates and psychosocial determinants of NPS and tailoring interventions to specific phenotypes and subsyndromes (Canevelli et al. 2013). Neurobiological data support the notion of specific clusters of NPS by recognizing three major neurobiological models relevant to NPS in AD: the frontal-subcortical circuits, corticocortical networks, and monoaminergic system (Geda et al. 2013). Specific NPS have been associated with lesions involving crucial structures or tracks in a network that mediat a particular behavior (Geda et al. 2013). For instance, disinhibition or apathy can result from lesions involving the frontal-subcortical circuits, even if the lesions are far from the frontal cortex (Geda et al. 2013). Reflecting the evidence that NPS tend to cluster into distinct groups, the Neuropsychiatric Syndromes of AD Professional Interest Area (NPS-PIA) of the International Society to Advance Alzheimer's Research and Treatment organized NPS around five syndromic areas: depression, apathy, sleep, agitation, and psychosis (Geda et al. 2013). The NPS-PIA has prepared specific reviews and recommendations for each syndrome, while recognizing that these syndromes will overlap (Geda et al. 2013).

Depression. Depression affects up to 50% of persons with dementia over the course of the illness (Schwarz et al. 2012). It is the most common symptom early in the course of dementia, affecting 29% of individuals (Tschanz et al. 2013). Potentially devastating and debilitating, depression tends to be underrecognized and highly correlated with increased health care utilization, increased risk of suicide, decreased quality of life for the affected person and caregiver, and greater severity and acceleration of cognitive impairment (Sepehry et al. 2012). Among individuals with AD, the risk for depression increases with older age, female sex, and less education (Treiber et al. 2008).

Apathy. Apathy affects a large proportion of persons with dementia. In the CCMS, apathy was among the most frequently reported NPS, with 20% of individuals exhibiting apathy at baseline and 51% at 5-year follow-up (Steinberg et al. 2008). It was consistently the most severe symptom at each evaluated time point. Apathy affects up to 70% of individuals with mild to moderate AD and up to 90% of those with late-stage AD (Berman et al. 2012). It tends to appear early in dementia, increase with illness severity, and persist throughout the illness. Risk factors include greater severity of cognitive and functional impairment, older age, and stroke (Treiber et al. 2008). Strokes may damage areas such as the prefrontal cortex or related neural pathways involved in the planning and execution of goal-directed behaviors (Treiber et al. 2008). Apathy is significantly associated with subsequent development of depression, consisting of inactivity, loss of confidence, learned helplessness, and poor response to rehabilitation due to lack of motivation (Berman et al. 2012). Understandably, apathy is associated with poorer quality of life for patients and caregivers (Berman et al. 2012).

Sleep disorders.   Up to half of all individuals with AD experience sleep disorders (Camargos et al. 2014; Roth 2012). Sleep disorders reduce patients' quality of life, can magnify cognitive impairments and mood dysregulation, contribute to loss of function, are a primary reason for institutionalization, and increase caregivers' burden. The most common sleep disorder associated with AD is irregular sleep-wake rhythm, a circadian rhythm disorder (Roth 2012). Patients with this disorder lack a well-defined sleep period (e.g., they might alternate between sleeping for 2–3 hours and remaining awake for 2–3 hours throughout an entire 24-hour cycle). Other common sleep disorders among individuals with AD include sundowning, nighttime wandering, difficulty with sleep onset or maintenance, and increased diurnal distribution of sleep (as opposed to an overall decreased amount of sleep) (Camargos et al. 2014; Roth 2012). Electroencephalograms (EEGs) of patients with AD show increased stage I sleep, non–rapid eye movement (REM) differentiation in later stages, and reduced REM sleep quantity in late stages. Causes of sleep disorders in AD are multifactorial. Various brain hormones and systems (e.g., suprachiasmatic nucleus, vasopressin, pineal gland, melatonin systems) critical for the regulation of the sleep-wake cycle are affected by the disease. For instance, in some patients with AD, the suprachiasmatic nucleus demonstrates tangles and neuronal cell loss with reactive gliosis (Roth 2012). Individuals with AD who are homozygous *APOE*E4* carriers also have greater reductions in melatonin levels than those who have the *APOE*E3* and *APOE*E4* alleles. On the other hand, persons with AD often have changes in zeitgebers (environmental cues critical for reinforcing circadian rhythm patterns), such as disturbed patterns of light exposure, due to inactivity and inadequate stimulation at home or in nursing homes.

Agitation and psychosis.   Detailed discussions of the causes and the common presentations of psychosis and agitation in dementia appear in Chapter 11, "Schizophrenia Spectrum and Other Psychotic Disorders," and Chapter 19, "Agitation in Older Adults," respectively.

The Predictors Study, a population-based study that recruited individuals mostly in relatively early stages of AD, demonstrated that symptoms such as agitation, restlessness, and wandering were associated with faster cognitive decline (Scarmeas et al. 2007). Agitation and restlessness were also associated with faster functional decline, whereas wandering was associated with faster functional decline and institutionalization. Other studies demonstrated that apathy, depression, and psychosis predict subsequent rapid cognitive decline. In the CCMS, individuals who demonstrated clinically significant symptoms in at least one domain on the Neuropsychiatric Inventory were more likely to progress to severe AD and progressed more rapidly than those with only mild symptoms or no symptoms at all (Rabins et al. 2013). Moreover, in one study, early development of psychosis, agitation/aggression, or any clinically significant NPS was predictive of earlier progression to severe dementia and death (Peters et al. 2015).

Several studies have reported that genetic factors (most notably *APOE*E4*) confer increased risk of NPS in AD, including aggression, depression, and psychosis. However, most studies have not shown a relationship between *APOE* genotype and NPS (Treiber et al. 2008). What is unclear is whether there is a causal relationship between

NPS and disease severity or between treatments targeting symptoms and disease severity, or whether symptoms and treatments interact to influence disease severity. Also, it is unknown whether pharmacological or nonpharmacological interventions targeting NPS influence the rate of progression to severe AD. Whether there is an association between NPS and mortality remains controversial (Rabins et al. 2013; Scarmeas et al. 2007), yet analysis of the CCMS data indicated that specific NPS were predictive of earlier progression to death (Peters et al. 2015).

The Brain in Alzheimer's Disease and the Amyloid Hypothesis

The brain changes in Alzheimer's dementia are well known. Even in early stages of the disease, brain imaging studies show volume reduction in the hippocampus bilaterally, which appears to progress with the illness, and brain imaging using fluorodeoxyglucose PET typically shows bitemporoparietal and often frontal hypoperfusion. This hypoperfusion spreads throughout the brain as the disease progresses. PET or SPECT imaging of neurotransmitters involving the cholinergic, dopaminergic, and serotonergic systems shows neurotransmitter loss even in living patients in the early stages of Alzheimer's dementia (Sabbagh et al. 2006). Researchers and clinicians have been able to image amyloid deposition in the brain using florbetapir, PiB, 2-(1-{6-[(2-[18F]fluoroethyl)(methyl)amino]-2-naphthyl}ethylidene)malononitrile (FDDNP), and other PET or SPECT ligands. Using these ligands, researchers have found that by the time dementia begins, there is already an abundant deposition of amyloid in the brain, which does not necessarily increase over time and is not necessarily specific to Alzheimer's dementia (Engler et al. 2006). Amyloid deposition may be extensive by the time symptoms appear, suggesting a time course of many years, perhaps decades, of brain changes between the pathological onset and clinical expression of dementia (Blennow et al. 2006).

Pathologically, the characteristic lesions of AD include senile or neuritic plaques containing $A\beta$ and neurofibrillary tangles composed of hyperphosphorylated tau proteins, with associated loss of neurons in several neurotransmitter systems: cholinergic, serotonergic, and dopaminergic. These changes typically occur early in the disease and affect both the nuclei and the cortical projections of neurons. Over time, these changes result in synaptic dysfunction. Until recently, the dominant hypothesis about etiopathogenesis suggested an amyloid cascade in which the increased production or decreased clearance of $A\beta$ in the brain causes the disease (Pimplikar 2009). $A\beta_{40}$ and $A\beta_{42}$ peptides accumulate, resulting in the aggregation and formation of insoluble plaques; this triggers a cascade of deleterious changes, resulting in neuronal death (Pimplikar 2009). The amyloid hypothesis, which dominated research for more than 20 years (Selkoe 1991), is now evolving such that $A\beta$ is no longer considered the sole instigator of downstream events (Morelli et al. 2012; Mucke and Selkoe 2012; Pimplikar 2009).

$A\beta$ peptides are derived in the amyloidogenic pathway of APP (Morelli et al. 2012). APP, a transmembrane glycoprotein, is present on most neurons, but its function is unknown. In the nonamyloidogenic APP pathway, α-secretase followed by γ-secretase cleaves APP within the $A\beta$ peptide region, preventing $A\beta$ generation (Morelli et al. 2012). In the amyloidogenic pathway, APP undergoes site-specific sequential proteolysis by β-secretase followed by γ-secretase (the core proteins of which are PSEN1 and PSEN2) (Morelli et al. 2012). APP is rapidly processed (speed > 10 molecules/neuron/second), and the vast majority of its metabolite is deposited in the extracellular space (Moghekar et al. 2011). $A\beta_{40}$ and $A\beta_{42}$ peptides predominate in the fragments released following proteolysis by β-secretase and γ-secretase. Aβ is likewise secreted into the extracellular space at extremely high rates (two to four molecules per neuron per second) (Moghekar et al. 2011). $A\beta_{42}$, a longer form of Aβ, is more prone to aggregate and to form plaques (Pimplikar 2009). It accumulates close to the synaptic cleft and is thought to lead over time to synaptic disconnection, the loss of neurotransmitter systems, and the emergence of symptoms. Plaques contain other proteins, such as APOE. One hypothesis is that some *APOE*E4*, in particular, acts as an amyloid catalyst or "pathological chaperone" (Morelli et al. 2012). Although many mutations in *APP* or *PSEN1* result in increased levels of $A\beta_{42}$, some mutations in *PSEN1* decrease the $A\beta_{40}$ levels, thus effectively changing the ratio of $A\beta_{40}$ to $A\beta_{42}$ (Pimplikar 2009). Evidence suggests that the increase in the ratio of $A\beta_{42}$ to $A\beta_{40}$, rather than the absolute level of $A\beta_{42}$, is pathogenic and triggers events ultimately leading to the disease (Pimplikar 2009). Indeed, some studies suggest that the increased ratio of $A\beta_{42}$ to $A\beta_{40}$ is inversely related to the age at onset of AD (Bentahir et al. 2006).

Patients may develop end-stage dementia despite having no evidence of amyloid plaques (Holmes et al. 2008). Moreover, cognitively healthy individuals may demonstrate substantial amounts of senile plaques (Villemagne et al. 2008). Increasing data support that insoluble plaques are not necessarily the cause of the disease (Pimplikar 2009). Newer research has focused on soluble forms of Aβ, referred to as Aβ oligomers, which are believed to be a particularly biologically active form of Aβ, and evidence indicates that these are the disease-causing pathogenic agent (Walsh and Selkoe 2007). Other data suggest that *PSEN1* mutations alone can trigger the toxic events seen in AD and that the increased concentration of Aβ and senile plaques may only be a secondary effect (Pimplikar 2009).

The manifestation of AD symptomatology probably depends more on the brain location and neurotransmitter systems affected than on the cause of the pathology present (Lyketsos 2006). Neuritic plaques first begin in the frontal cortex before spreading over the entire cortical region; on the other hand, tau and neurofibrillary tangles first appear in the limbic system before spreading to the cortex (Pimplikar 2009). Although Aβ is associated with brain neuronal changes, it may also bind to other brain cells, such as microglia, and cause neuronal injury (Mucke and Selkoe 2012). High levels of Aβ can structurally and functionally alter microglia, astrocytes, and the endothelial and smooth muscle cells of cerebral blood vessels (Mucke and Selkoe 2012). Other downstream factors involved in progression include glutamatergic toxicity, lipid peroxidation products, and the loss of trophic factor. The precise mechanisms by which Aβ contributes to neuronal dysfunction and ultimately to death are still unknown (Mucke and Selkoe 2012).

Alzheimer's pathology likely begins many years and perhaps decades before the onset of symptoms, which will offer an opportunity for prevention once future advances make it possible to diagnose the disease before symptom onset using biomarkers. The distribution of the neuropathology appears to change with the course of the disease; it begins in the mesial temporal lobe and then disseminates widely throughout the brain. The tissue loss that follows can become extensive, so that patients with advanced AD have atrophic brains and significantly enlarged ventricles. These changes may mean that different treatments will have differential efficacy at different phases of the disease.

Dementia Due to Cerebrovascular Disease (Vascular Dementia)

VaD continues to be a controversial nosological entity, in part because of the absence of clear neuropathological agreement about it. Patients who have dementia due to AD are difficult to differentiate on clinical grounds alone from those who have VaD. Further complicating the differentiation, abundant evidence suggests that cerebrovascular risk factors and diseases influence both the progression of dementia due to AD (e.g., Mielke et al. 2007) and the emergence of Alzheimer's pathology in the brain (e.g., Beach et al. 2007). Most patients with VaD who come to autopsy have mixed pathology, often with significant AD pathology (Jellinger and Attems 2006).

VaD, therefore, is best understood as a heterogeneous group of dementias. At one end of the spectrum are patients with pure genetic forms, such as 1) cerebral autosomal dominant arteriopathy with subcortical infarcts and leukoencephalopathy and 2) mitochondrial encephalopathy with lactic acidosis and strokelike episodes. At the other end are patients who develop dementia after multiple strokes in which significant portions of the brain are damaged. Between these two end points are patients with mixed pathologies and clinical presentations that impact one another (e.g., smaller strokes or chronic subcortical hypoxia might both damage brain tissue and lead to the onset and progression of Alzheimer's pathology). Genes and risk factors that predispose individuals to cerebrovascular disorders are also risk factors for VaD, including diseases of the large and small vessels of the brain, diabetes, hypertension, and atrial fibrillation and other cardiac diseases.

The clinical presentation of VaD is variable and very often resembles that of AD. Typically, it presents in fits and spurts, often with acute or subacute onset after a cerebrovascular event. A mix of symptoms is usually present, often including apathy, depression, and motor symptoms. Among patients with VaD or dementia due to AD who have similar MMSE scores, individuals with VaD are usually more functionally impaired. Gait disorders, parkinsonism, and incontinence are early features of VaD.

Diagnosis of VaD is based on a typical clinical history and associated physical examination findings. It requires brain imaging showing completed infarcts or lacunes in brain areas associated with the cognitive changes. One should be able to show a temporal relationship between the brain vascular disease and the cognitive changes, but this may be difficult. Radiological findings of white matter changes alone, with no evidence of completed strokes or associated exam findings (e.g., focal motor symptoms or a gait disorder), do *not* support a VaD diagnosis. White matter changes, as seen on MRI, are common in cognitively healthy older people (Longstreth et al. 2005). The diagnosis becomes more complex when patients with established Alzheimer's dementia develop strokes; many such patients also meet criteria for a diagnosis of VaD. Results from the Nun Study (Snowdon et al. 1997) and the Religious Order Study (Schneider et al. 2004) suggested that, for a given degree of Alzheimer's pathology, dementia is more severe in the presence of comorbid cerebrovascular disease.

Little is known about the progression of clinically diagnosed VaD; therefore, we can only make speculative comments here. Clinical anecdotes suggest that many patients with VaD can have a nonprogressive condition for many years as long as they do not have other strokes. However, other patients decline rather precipitously, and most patients have variably slower rates of progressive decline.

Lewy Body Disorders

In 2007, a consensus panel (Lippa et al. 2007) proposed the term *Lewy body disorders* as an umbrella term for Parkinson's disease (PD), Parkinson's disease dementia (PDD), and dementia with Lewy bodies (DLB). This proposal appropriately recognized the existence of a spectrum of dementias associated with Lewy body disease of the brain whose shared pathology involves impairments in α-synuclein metabolism. In these three conditions, also termed *synucleinopathies*, α-synuclein aggregates to form insoluble fibrils. α-Synuclein, a synaptic protein, is the primary structural component of Lewy body filaments. Lewy bodies, in turn, are cytoplasmic, eosinophilic, round, or oblong neuronal inclusions. Lewy bodies (as well as Lewy neurites, related proteinaceous structures composed of α-synuclein) develop in discrete regions throughout the brain stem, diencephalon, basal ganglia, and neocortex (Ballard et al. 2013). Neuronal degeneration, cognitive impairment, and eventually dementia ensue in all Lewy body disorders. The sequence of events involved is poorly known.

One of the complicating factors in determining a diagnosis is that many patients with Lewy body pathologies have coexisting pathologies, particularly Alzheimer's and vascular pathologies. For instance, approximately half of patients with PDD meet the neuropathological criteria for AD (Sabbagh et al. 2009). Amyloid plaques are typically seen in DLB (although not as dense as in AD), and neurofibrillary tangles can be found in some DLB cases. Parkinsonian features can be seen in AD, although typically late in the disease course. Patients with AD also are often treated with psychotropic medications that cause long-lasting extrapyramidal side effects even after they are discontinued. The clinical presentations of PDD and DLB can be similar. Patients develop a progressive subcortical dementia with the following hallmark features: executive dysfunction, cognitive fluctuations, inattention, visuospatial dysfunction, parkinsonism, visual hallucinations, and sleep disturbances (McKeith et al. 2017).

Dementia With Lewy Bodies

DLB is the second most common type of progressive dementia after AD, accounting for ~20% of late-onset dementia cases (Ballard et al. 2013). It generally affects individuals age 60 years and older and becomes more prevalent with age. The Dementia with Lewy Bodies Consortium continues to systematically update diagnostic and management recommendations for DLB, and the fourth report of the consortium now distinguishes between clinical features and diagnostic biomarkers (McKeith et al. 2017). Clinical signs and symptoms are now labeled as core or supportive, and the category of suggestive features is no longer used. The central feature is a progressive cognitive decline. Whereas AD typically presents with memory loss initially, DLB's early deficits are in attention, executive function, and visuospatial abilities. Core clinical features include fluctuating cognition with variations in attention and levels of alertness, recurrent well-formed visual hallucinations, REM sleep behavior disorder that may precede cognitive decline, and parkinsonian features. Indicative biomarkers are reduced dopamine transporter uptake in basal ganglia as demonstrated by SPECT or PET, abnormal (low-uptake) [123]iodine-MIBG (metaiodobenzylguanidine) myocardial scintigraphy, and polysomnographic confirmation of REM sleep without atonia. The diagnostic criteria for probable DLB require the presence of dementia plus two or more core clinical features, with or without the presence of indicative biomarkers, or the presence of dementia plus only one core clinical feature, but with one or more indicative biomarkers also present. It should not be diagnosed solely on the basis of biomarkers. The diagnostic criteria for possible DLB require one core clinical feature of DLB or one or more indicative biomarkers.

The Dementia with Lewy Bodies Consortium also provided a long list of supportive clinical features that lack diagnostic specificity but can support a clinical diagnosis of DLB, particularly when they occur over time or if several occur simultaneously (McKeith et al. 2017). Examples of such supportive features include repeated falls, syncope, transient and unexplained loss of consciousness, severe autonomic dysfunction such as constipation or orthostatic hypotension, hallucinations (other than visual) or systematized delusions, and depression. Similarly, the consortium listed supportive biomarkers, including relative preservation of medial temporal lobe structures on CT/MRI, generalized low uptake on SPECT/PET with reduced occipital activity, and certain electroencephalographic activity.

Fluctuating cognition occurs in about 60%–80% of people with DLB (McKeith et al. 1996) and is often mistaken for delirium. The symptoms and their duration vary between individuals and even within the same person. Symptoms range widely from episodes resembling blackouts or absence seizures to speech changes seen in strokes. They can last from seconds to days. Recurrent visual hallucinations occur in up to 80% of patients with DLB (McKeith et al. 2017; Simard and van Reekum 2004) and are the most frequently reported psychotic symptom. Hallucinations tend to be well-formed images of people, animals, or objects (Ballard et al. 2013) but can be as simple as shapes in the corner of one's eye. They can occur at any time but are more common at night and are not typically distressing unless accompanied by delusions or occurring in individuals with severe dementia (Ballard et al. 2013). Parkinsonian features are similar to those found in PD (e.g., dyskinesias, rigidity, gait disorders, tremor) and occur in more than 85% of individuals with DLB (McKeith et al. 2017).

If dementia and parkinsonism coexist, the differential diagnosis is sorted out by examining the relative course of the cognitive and motor symptoms. The emergence of dementia after many years of motor symptoms supports a diagnosis of PDD. In contrast, the early presence of dementia in a patient with motor parkinsonism supports a diagnosis of DLB. Researchers use a 1-year interval between onset of PD and onset of dementia to differentiate PDD from DLB.

Many patients with Alzheimer's dementia develop a clinical DLB picture, reflected in the neuropathology, and many patients with DLB have concurrent Alzheimer's dementia pathology. Daytime drowsiness and naps, staring spells, and episodes of disorganized speech have high positive predictive value for a diagnosis of DLB over Alzheimer's dementia (McKeith et al. 2017). Neuroleptic sensitivity is much more common and severe in DLB than in AD. Autonomic dysfunction, such as urinary incontinence, tends to be an early sign in DLB, whereas it often occurs in late stages of AD. Both visual hallucinations and delusions are more common in DLB (as well as in PDD) than in Alzheimer's dementia and have high positive predictive value. In fact, visual hallucinations may be the most clinically useful feature to distinguish DLB from AD (Tiraboschi et al. 2006).

Although the progression of DLB tends to be similar overall to that of Alzheimer's dementia, the course of DLB is more variable. Because many patients have a more fulminant course, some experts believe that DLB has a worse prognosis than Alzheimer's dementia (McKeith et al. 2004). DLB is associated with considerable suffering for patients and families, in part because of common, difficult-to-treat, and persistent NPS (hallucinations, delusions, and affective symptoms). Patients also tend to become affected early with balance, sleep, and motor disorders and to become confined in their mobility.

Parkinson's Disease Dementia

PDD refers to patients who have had PD for many years and then develop dementia, most likely caused by the PD itself. With the advent of the use of L-dopa to help control the motoric symptoms of PD, it has become apparent that some of the most common and impairing symptoms of PD are in the cognitive realm. PDD is associated with excess disability, reduced quality of life, increased risk for psychosis, increased nursing home admission and therefore disease-related costs, increased mortality, and increased caregiver burden (Emre 2003). Patients with PD typically show impairments in executive functioning (e.g., problem solving, set shifting, and planning), deficiencies in attention, and poor fluency. They also have memory impairments affecting working memory and the organization and retrieval of explicit memory. Memory retrieval is often improved by cueing. Some individuals have visuospatial difficulties arising out of problems with set shifting and the need for high executive demand to complete visuospatial tests.

The average time from onset of PD to the development of dementia is ~10 years (Hughes et al. 2000). At least 75% of patients with PD who survive longer than 10 years will develop dementia. Risk factors for the development of dementia in individuals with PD include old age, PD onset after age 60 years, duration of PD, severity of motor symptoms (particularly postural and gait disturbances), REM sleep behavior disorder, visual hallucinations (which increase the risk of developing dementia 20-fold) (Galvin et al. 2006), and MCI. Once individuals with PD begin to demonstrate cognitive impairment, their MMSE scores decline by an average of 2.4 points per year (Kandiah et al. 2009). However, because the MMSE is not very sensitive to detecting executive dysfunction, patients may have significant cognitive impairment even with normal MMSE scores. The MoCA may be a more sensitive tool for identifying early cognitive impairment in PD (Zadikoff et al. 2008).

Classically, neuropathological staging of PD is based in part on a predictable neuroanatomical spread of Lewy body pathology, starting with the olfactory system and lower brain stem and eventually progressing to the cortex (Braak et al. 2004). Although the neuropathological stage of PD generally correlates with the severity of dementia, some patients may develop cognitive decline despite mild cortical pathology, whereas others may have normal cognitive function despite widespread cortical pathology (Braak et al. 2005). Although high rates of Alzheimer's pathology appear to be present in patients with PD and dementia, this linkage remains controversial because of the different findings in various autopsy series. One proposed theory linking PD and AD is that the pathways of Aβ, tau, and α-synuclein aggregation may potentiate each other, leading to neuronal dysfunction and cell death (Shulman and De Jager 2009). For more information, see Metzler-Baddeley (2007) and Figure 8–6 in the previous edition of this textbook (Steffens et al. 2015).

Cognitive impairment in PD has been associated with deficits in several neurotransmitter systems, including dopaminergic, cholinergic, serotonergic, and noradrenergic. Many studies have demonstrated a relationship between frontostriatal dopaminergic pathways and working memory (e.g., Cools and D'Esposito 2011). Although dopaminergic medications may promote mild improvement on short-term memory tests early in the disease course, they are unlikely to be helpful in moderate to severe cases of PDD (Morrison et al. 2004). Cholinergic systems appear to have an important role in the cognitive decline associated with PDD. PET scans have demonstrated cholinergic dysfunction in the cerebral cortex, beginning in early PD and becoming more widespread in PDD (Shimada et al. 2009). Cholinesterase inhibitors modestly improve cognitive function in PDD, leading to the FDA's approval of the cholinesterase inhibitor rivastigmine for the treatment of PDD.

NPS are common in PD both with and without dementia. These symptoms include depression, psychosis, anxiety, impulse-control disorders, disorders of sleep and wakefulness, and apathy (Weintraub and Burn 2011). Depression can be seen in up to 40% of patients. Sleep disorders occur in up to 30% of patients and include REM sleep behavior disorders, nightmares, sleep fragmentation, and daytime sleepiness. Anxiety occurs in about one-third of patients with PD and includes both anxiety syndromes seen in the general population and syndromes unique to PD, such as episodic anxiety associated with weaning off of dopaminergic medications (Pontone et al. 2019). Patients often experience visual hallucinations (e.g., "passage hallucinations" or transient visual hallucinations in the periphery) and persecutory delusions (Mack et al. 2012). Many medications used to treat PD, such as anticholinergic agents, amantadine, dopaminergic agents, and catechol O-methyltransferase inhibitors, can exacerbate visual hallucinations and delusions. Often, prescribers will decrease these medications when psychotic symptoms begin, starting with the medications less likely to affect motor function (Taylor et al. 2016).

Dementia Due to Frontotemporal Lobar Degeneration

FTLD is in many ways the paradigmatic non-Alzheimer's dementia. It has become a major focus of interest because FTLD is the second most common form of dementia in individuals younger than 65 years, with a rate of occurrence close to that of Alzheimer's dementia (Neary et al. 2005). Previously referred to as Pick's disease, FTLD is a clinically and pathologically heterogeneous disorder characterized by a progressive change in personality, behavior, and language and focal degeneration of the frontal and temporal lobes. Less commonly, FTLD can also present with progressive motor decline in addition to behavior and language deficits. As the condition progresses and global dementia ensues, however, symptoms overlap, and it becomes increasingly difficult to group patients into one category of FTLD or another.

The behavioral variant of FTLD (bvFTLD) is the most common presentation (Kertesz et al. 2007). It is characterized by progressive changes in personality and behavior and by cognitive dysfunction. Patients may exhibit an amalgam of executive dysfunction, such as social inappropriateness and disinhibition, poor insight, hyperorality, changes in affect, emotional blunting and apathy, and stereotyped behaviors. Because of the prevalence of apathy in this variant, it is often misdiagnosed as depression (Bertoux et al. 2012). Cognitive tests such as the MMSE may not reveal cognitive deficits early in the course of bvFTLD.

The second most common presentation of FTLD is primary progressive aphasia (PPA) (Kertesz et al. 2007). PPA is characterized by the insidious onset of a prominent progressive impairment in speech and language, with deficits in speech production, naming, grammar, and word comprehension. Behavioral features often develop in individuals with PPA. The three main variants of PPA are progressive nonfluent aphasia (nfvPPA), semantic dementia (svPPA), and logopenic progressive aphasia (lvPPA). Patients with nfvPPA demonstrate anomia, impaired fluency, paraphasic errors, and agrammatism with telegraphic speech. Language comprehension and repetition are spared early in the course; patients ultimately progress to mutism. Those with svPPA present with anomia, impaired single-word comprehension, and semantic paraphasic errors. Semantic memory is affected, but speech production and repetition are spared. The third variant, lvPPA, is characterized by a paucity and slowed rate of speech, impairment in single-word retrieval and repetition, and phonological paraphasias. Episodic memory and calculation are often affected. Speech production, grammar, and single-word comprehension are spared, at least early on.

Approximately 10%–15% of patients with FTLD also have motor neuron disease. Individuals with the bvFTLD type are most often affected, and motor symptoms can either precede or follow changes in behavior and personality. Patients present with progressive lower motor neuron signs of muscular atrophy and fasciculations preferentially affecting bulbar and upper extremity muscles. The progression to death is hastened. One motor impairment syndrome that co-occurs with FTLD is amyotrophic lateral sclerosis (ALS). Some patients with FTLD develop ALS presentations (known as FTLD-ALS) as their disease progresses, whereas some patients with ALS develop FTLD over their disease course.

There is significant clinical, pathological, and genetic overlap between FTLD-ALS and two atypical parkinsonian syndromes: progressive supranuclear palsy and corticobasal syndrome (Seltman and Matthews 2012). Both syndromes have cognitive and behavioral features that overlap with FTLD and are often classified on the spectrum of FTLD clinical syndromes. Clinical features of progressive supranuclear palsy include postural instability, axial rigidity, frequent falls, bradykinesia, dysarthria, supranuclear gaze deficits, progressive cognitive decline, and apathy. Clinical features of corticobasal syndrome include the simultaneous occurrence of asymmetrical cortical signs (e.g., limb apraxia, myoclonus, alien limb phenomenon) and extrapyramidal signs (e.g., bradykinesia, tremor, limb rigidity, dystonia). Although progressive supranuclear palsy is characterized by neuronal loss and atrophy in the basal ganglia with relative sparing of the frontal cortex, the pattern of frontal lobe atrophy in corticobasal syndrome closely resembles the pattern of FTLD. Because some patients with FTLD may manifest both extrapyramidal symptoms and psychosis, they are sometimes diagnosed as having DLB. Individuals with FTLD may also exhibit hypersomnia, fluctuating cognition, and sleep disorders (Claassen et al. 2008), leading to a diagnosis of DLB. Clinicopathological studies can be helpful in understanding the underlying neurodegenerative process in patients who meet criteria for both FTLD and DLB.

A revised consensus of neuropathological criteria considers advances in both genetics and biochemistry and reflects the diversity of pathological pictures (Cairns et al. 2007). Pathologically, FTLD is characterized by knife-edge lobar atrophy, typically in the anterior temporal and posterior inferior areas of the frontal lobes. Microscopically, neurons appear enlarged and vacuolar, with extensive gliosis and loss of myelin. Neurons and glial cells may contain abnormal cytoplasmic or nuclear protein inclusions. Inclusions tend to comprise either hyperphosphorylated tau protein or transactive response DNA binding protein 43 (TDP-43). Inclusions containing tau protein can be seen in various disorders such as FTLD with Pick bodies, corticobasal degeneration, progressive supranuclear palsy, and hippocampal sclerosis, disorders collectively known as *tauopathies*.

FTLD is familial in a considerable number of patients, often in an autosomal dominant pattern of inheritance. Mutations in the tau, progranulin, and ubiquitin genes have been associated with the condition. Familial TDP-43 proteinopathy is associated with defects in multiple genes and several neuropathological types (Cairns et al. 2007). FTLD is a clinical diagnosis; although neuroimaging is not necessary to establish the diagnosis, it may support the diagnosis and is necessary to exclude alternative pathology. FTLD is sometimes misdiagnosed as Alzheimer's dementia, but clinicians can differentiate the diagnoses based on FTLD's early age at onset (average in the late 50s or early 60s), early prominent NPS, and lack of significant memory or visuospatial impairments. Other symptoms that support a diagnosis of FTLD over Alzheimer's dementia include abnormal eating behaviors, social inappropriateness, degree of apathy, and stereotyped behaviors. FTLD is almost invariably progressive, especially if language symptoms occur early on. In clinical settings, the time from an FTLD diagnosis to death is on the order of 3–5 years, which is shorter than the periods associated with Alzheimer's dementia (Chow et al. 2006). However, one meta-analysis suggested that the survival rate of FTLD, with the exception of FTLD-ALS, is longer, on the order of 6–12 years, similar to that of AD (Kansal et al. 2016). Compared with Alzheimer's dementia, FTLD is a greater burden to caregivers given the disinhibited beaviors that are hard to treat and require aggressive supervision to manage.

Less Common Dementias

Dementia Due to Normal-Pressure Hydrocephalus

The dementia of normal-pressure hydrocephalus (NPH) is a subcortical dementia associated with a characteristic magnetic-like gait disorder, incontinence, and cognitive dysfunction. Gait impairment is often more prominent than cognitive impairment. Little is known about its epidemiology and progression. It is estimated to have an annual incidence of 0.5–2 per million individuals (Wilson and Williams 2006). Idiopathic NPH is most common after age 60 years. Cognitive symptoms may include psychomotor slowing, executive dysfunction, personality changes, inattention, impaired recall, and decreased fine motor speed (Finney 2009). The condition is suspected when patients present with the classic triad of findings and brain imaging reveals enlarged ventricles disproportionate to cortical atrophy. The diagnosis is confirmed by a patient's response to either lumbar puncture drainage of a large volume (40–50 mL) of CSF, response to an extended CSF drainage trial through a lumbar spinal catheter, or measurement of resistance to CSF outflow during a lumbar puncture. NPH is difficult to diagnose because gait difficulty, cognitive decline, urinary incontinence, and enlarged ventricles (ventricle size increases with age) are all common in elderly adults and can have many causes; furthermore, no combination of cardinal findings is pathognomonic or specific for NPH (Graff-Radford 2007). Because NPH is often seen in older adults, a factor complicating its diagnosis is that 75% of those with idiopathic NPH also meet clinical criteria for AD or VaD (Bech-Azeddine et al. 2007). Moreover, a significant percentage of patients with idiopathic

NPH show positivity for biomarkers typically found in AD, such as Aβ (Leinonen et al. 2012). A great deal of interest has focused on efforts to diagnose and treat NPH using shunts (discussed in "Disease-Modifying Therapies" later in this chapter). Of note, out of the classic triad of findings, gait impairment is most likely to respond to shunting.

Dementia Due to Prion Diseases and Other Rapidly Progressive Dementias

The rapidly progressive dementias (RPDs) represent a heterogeneous group of disorders that can be categorized by their underlying pathophysiology, including neurodegenerative, inflammatory, vascular, toxic, metabolic, neoplastic, and infectious causes (Woodruff 2007). Although relatively rare, human transmissible spongiform encephalopathies, or prion diseases, are probably foremost in the minds of clinicians when evaluating RPDs (Woodruff 2007). Prion diseases represent a large portion of neurodegenerative causes of RPD (Appleby and Lyketsos 2011; Geschwind et al. 2008). However, in a University of California, San Francisco, cohort of 178 patients with suspected prion disease or other RPD, 38% of patients were diagnosed with a nonprion condition (Geschwind et al. 2008). The largest group of nonprion patients in the cohort had neurodegenerative diseases (14.6% of the entire cohort and 39% of all nonprion cases), including AD, DLB, FTLD, corticobasal syndrome, and progressive supranuclear palsy. The second-largest group had autoimmune conditions (8.4% of the entire cohort and 22% of nonprion cases), including Hashimoto's encephalopathy, antibody-mediated limbic encephalitis associated with cancer (paraneoplastic) or without cancer (nonparaneoplastic), multiple sclerosis, and neurosarcoidosis. The third-largest group had dementia of unknown cause (4.5% of the entire cohort and 12% of nonprion cases). Several patients had encephalitis of presumed viral etiology (enterovirus was confirmed in one patient). Other nonprion causes of RPD included toxic-metabolic causes (e.g., methylmalonic acidemia, encephalopathy secondary to alcohol intoxication, methotrexate toxicity), encephalopathy associated with cancer but without evidence of autoantibodies, and psychiatric conditions, among others.

Recent knowledge regarding prion protein transmission across species has led to concerns about animal-to-human transmission of these proteins through the diet, followed by incurable RPD. In the United States, the annual incidence of CJD, the most common human prion dementia, is ~1.2 per million individuals (Maddox et al. 2020). The incidence peaks between the ages of 65 and 74 years (Holman et al. 2010). Although most cases (75%–85%) of CJD are sporadic, other forms include genetic (10%–22%) and acquired (iatrogenic and variant CJD; <1%–3%) (Appleby and Lyketsos 2011; Geschwind et al. 2008; Uttley et al. 2020).

The basic pathophysiology of CJD, partly worked out by Stanley Prusiner (who won the Nobel Prize in Medicine for this work), is thought to involve abnormal transformation of prion protein (PrP^c) from its α-helical form to a β-sheet form. The pathological prion protein (PrP^{res}) reuses itself as a template (prions do not require nucleic acids to replicate) to convert more PrP^c to PrP^{res}. This leads to a snowball cascade with widespread dissemination of these proteins, which become clumpy and toxic, leading to the classic spongiform appearance of the nervous system. How this is brought about is uncertain. It might occur spontaneously or result from interactions with mutant prion proteins or those of other species that make their way into the human brain. Some cases have resulted from transplanting affected organs. Little is known about factors that initiate or accelerate these transitions, although some of the familial cases appear to have been initiated by biological stress to the brain through stroke, hypoxia, or TBI (Lyketsos 1999). At present, this disease is incurable. The familial forms are a target of genetic counseling.

All mammals, including humans, carry the prion protein gene *PRNP* on the short arm of chromosome 20. Several mutations in this gene have been reported and are associated with a familial progressive dementia (Michalczyk and Ziman 2007), sometimes referred to as Gerstmann-Sträussler-Scheinker syndrome. In 1996, variant CJD was discovered in the United Kingdom. It was linked to bovine spongiform encephalopathy, which was most likely transmitted to humans through ingestion of affected beef. By the end of 2005, ~190 human cases had been identified (Collee et al. 2006). This epidemic appears to have subsided.

CJD and Gerstmann-Sträussler-Scheinker syndrome have variable clinical presentations, although the most characteristic presentation is that of RPD, prominent gait disorder (e.g., ataxic gait), extrapyramidal symptoms, and motor findings (e.g., myoclonus) early on. Early cognitive deficits involve memory, concentration, judgment, and language (e.g., aphasia). Sleep disturbances can also occur, such as insomnia, and visual disturbances that range from field defects to cortical blindness (Puoti et al. 2012). Patients may have an apprehensive or fearful gaze and may be hypersensitive (Puoti et al. 2012). They become disabled rapidly and may have difficulty obtaining a diagnosis because they often present with psychiatric symptoms such as depression, anxiety, apathy, and executive dysfunction. In one-third of individuals, vague complaints of fatigue, headache, sleep disturbance, vertigo, malaise, weight loss, pain, depression, or behavioral changes precede the dementia by weeks to months (Geschwind et al. 2008). However, obvious impairments in gait, behavior, and cognition can become apparent within a matter of days (Puoti et al. 2012). The median survival time is 5 months, and ~85% of patients die within 1 year of symptom onset (Geschwind et al. 2008). Although the time course of CJD is almost invariably rapid, cases in the literature have reported longer courses, sometimes lasting years. Familial cases tend to run longer courses, as long as a decade in younger individuals (Lyketsos 1999).

The only way to definitively confirm a diagnosis of sporadic prion disease in living patients is through brain tissue biopsy. However, the combination of a clinical assessment and either CSF assay or MRI imaging has sufficient sensitivity and specificity to accurately diagnose the disease (Puoti et al. 2012). That said, up to 80% of prion disease cases, including genetic forms, are initially misdiagnosed (Appleby and Lyketsos 2011). The rarity of the disease often delays diagnosis. Furthermore, diagnostic patterns vary by country or clinical center (e.g., community hospital vs. university hospital) (Appleby and Lyketsos 2011). The Centers for Disease Control and Prevention (2018) published criteria for probable sporadic CJD, which are outlined in Table 8–4.

Although neurodegenerative dementias such as AD, DLB, and FTLD are typically characterized by gradual onset and insidious progression, they can sometimes present in a fulminant form, developing over months, with death occurring in <3 years (Geschwind et al. 2008). These neurodegenerative dementias can resemble CJD because of an overlap of motor symptoms (particularly gait disturbances, extrapyramidal signs, and myoclonus) and cognitive, behavioral, and psychiatric manifestations. Electroencephalographic and CSF abnormalities can likewise overlap. For instance, the periodic 1- to 2-Hz triphasic sharp waves characteristically seen on EEG in CJD can also be seen, although rarely, in the end stages of AD or DLB, as well as in toxic-metabolic

TABLE 8–4.   **Centers for Disease Control and Prevention criteria for probable sporadic Creutzfeldt-Jakob disease**

Rapidly progressive dementia *and* at least two of the following four features:
  Myoclonus
  Visual or cerebellar signs
  Extrapyramidal or pyramidal signs
  Akinetic mutism
And a positive result on at least one of the following three laboratory tests:
  Periodic sharp wave complexes on electroencephalogram during an illness of any duration
  Positive 14-3-3 cerebrospinal fluid assay in patients with a disease duration of <2 years
  MRI signal abnormalities in the caudate nucleus and/or putamen on diffusion-weighted imaging or fluid-attenuated inversion recovery
Routine investigations should not suggest an alternative diagnosis

Source.   Adapted from Centers for Disease Control and Prevention 2018.

conditions and in Hashimoto's encephalopathy. Furthermore, this electroencephalographic finding usually appears only in the later stages of CJD. Thus, the EEG lacks sensitivity and specificity and misses many early and some late cases. CSF findings in CJD are likewise neither sensitive nor specific for the disease. False-positive results for CSF 14-3-3 protein can be seen in fulminant AD cases. A more sensitive and specific test for CJD could be the combination of fluid-attenuated inversion recovery and diffusion-weighted imaging MRI sequences (Geschwind et al. 2008).

Autoimmune diseases of the brain causing limbic encephalopathy can also resemble CJD. Symptoms include memory loss, depression, anxiety, personality changes, emotional lability, and seizures. Clinicians should consider a paraneoplastic syndrome when there is a subacute or rapid development of dementia, cancer risk factors, extrapyramidal or cerebellar symptoms, other neurological symptoms, evidence of inflammation in CSF analysis, or a family history of cancer (Geschwind et al. 2008). Detection of paraneoplastic antibodies should prompt clinicians to aggressively investigate for the corresponding tumors. Primary CNS vasculitis often presents with headache, altered mentation, focal neurological signs, and CSF pleocytosis (Geschwind et al. 2008). Vasculitides can be distinguished from CJD and other RPDs by the presence of systemic manifestations or by specific brain MRI abnormalities, such as brain hemorrhage or multiple infarctions of different ages. Even in the absence of gastrointestinal symptoms, celiac disease can cause ataxia, NPS, seizures, headaches, neuropathy, and dementia. Geschwind et al. (2008) and Woodruff (2007) provided further information regarding the various causes of RPD, as well as diagnostic approaches, screening tests, representative imaging abnormalities, and treatment options.

Treatment

Treatment for Milder Cognitive Syndromes

Memory clinics and primary care physicians anecdotally report that the increased public awareness of dementia has led to patients presenting with increasingly milder cognitive symptoms to request diagnosis and treatment. At present, there is little empirical knowledge about how to manage these patients clinically. Most experts recommend continued observation and the use of nonpharmacological therapies, such as controlling vascular risk factors (e.g., healthy diet, exercise, smoking cessation) due to the relationship of cardiovascular health to cognitive health, use of meditation, cognitive stimulation, and cognitive rehabilitation (e.g., using memory cues and organizational aids).

Cooper et al. (2013) reviewed nonpharmacological interventions for MCI to identify which had the best treatment evidence. The only type of nonpharmacological intervention for which they found preliminary evidence was a long-term group program of memory training, reminiscence and cognitive stimulation, recreation, and social interaction, which improved cognition over 6 months. They found limited evidence that individual aerobic exercise programs improve executive functioning and category fluency or that computerized cognitive training programs improve delayed recall. However, a 2017 systematic review and meta-analysis of computerized cognitive training programs in older patients with MCI demonstrated a beneficial therapeutic role in the short-term on most memory and learning domains, although these effects were moderate (Hill et al. 2017). Nonetheless, exercise has been associated with favorable effects on neuronal survivability and function, neuroinflammation, vascularization, neuroendocrine response to stress, and brain amyloid burden (Baker et al. 2010). Cooper and colleagues highlighted the limited generalizability of the nonpharmacological interventions they reviewed, most of which had been underpowered and lacked sufficient evidence of efficacy. A Cochrane review determined that specific neuropsychological ("brain") exercises designed to strengthen memory in people with MCI improved immediate and delayed verbal recall compared with no treatment (Martin et al. 2011); however, these effects were lost when the exercise group was compared with an active control group.

A number of vitamins (e.g., B_6, B_{12}, folate, E), supplements (e.g., *Gingko biloba*), and NSAIDs (e.g., rofecoxib, triflusal) have not been shown to reliably improve cognition in patients with MCI or prevent progression to dementia, although a recent 12-month randomized controlled trial (RCT) of daily oral vitamin D supplementation improved cognitive function in several domains in older Chinese adults with MCI (Yang et al. 2020). Nicotine patches improved attention (and verbal recall as a secondary outcome) but not global functioning over 6 months in a small study of nonsmokers (Newhouse et al. 2012).

Adherence to a Mediterranean diet—consumption of unrefined cereals, fruits, vegetables, and olive oil with low meat consumption and moderate dairy and alcohol consumption—has been linked to a lower risk of chronic illness, as has the Dietary Approach to Systolic Hypertension (DASH) diet. In a systematic review of 32 studies examining the effect of the Mediterranean diet on cognitive function and dementia, most studies showed that the diet may contribute to better cognitive performance and may protect against cognitive impairment and AD (Petersson and Philippou 2016). A specifically designed diet high in green leafy vegetables and berries was associated with slower decline in cognitive abilities in almost 1,000 community-dwelling elders without dementia, even after controlling for physical activity and education (Morris et al. 2015).

Alternatively, researchers are examining the benefits of the ketogenic, or high-fat/low-carbohydrate, diet. This nutritional approach is based on mounting evidence that changes in brain energy metabolism, particularly impaired glucose metabolism, play a role in the development of AD. Preliminary evidence from a very small sample indicated that a modified Atkins diet could enhance episodic memory in very early AD (Brandt et al. 2019). However, implementing a ketogenic or modified ketogenic diet in elderly patients with cognitive impairment can be challenging, as indicated by difficulties in retention and adherence.

At least one randomized trial has suggested that the cholinesterase inhibitor donepezil may delay progression to dementia, especially in patients who are *APOE*E4* carriers (Petersen et al. 2005), but this has not been replicated or supported by other trials (Rosenberg et al. 2006). More recent reviews and meta-analyses (e.g., Cooper et al. 2013; Russ and Morling 2012) found very little evidence that cholinesterase inhibitors either affected progression to dementia or improved cognitive scores in patients with MCI. Furthermore, those who received cholinesterase inhibitors had an increased risk of adverse events, particularly gastrointestinal, and an unexplained increased mortality rate with galantamine specifically (Cooper et al. 2013). Thus, in most cases, cholinesterase inhibitors should not be prescribed for individuals with MCI (Cooper et al. 2013; National Institute for Health and Care Excellence 2011). We recommend initiating pharmacological therapy *only* in cases in which there is strong evidence of likely benefit—for example, when a patient appears to be about to transition to Alzheimer's dementia or when the cognitive impairment is particularly worrisome to the patient. Rosenberg et al. (2006) and Cooper et al. (2013) provide more detailed approaches to this issue.

The Four Pillars of Dementia Care

Dementia care has four basic elements, or pillars (Lyketsos et al. 2006). The first pillar relates to management of key aspects of the disease, with the goal of reversing its effects or delaying its progression in the brain. Although few disease therapies exist at present, several therapies are being developed for different types of dementia that are targeted at underlying pathophysiological mechanisms. The second pillar of dementia care relates to the management of its symptoms, whether they are cognitive, neuropsychiatric, or functional. The final two pillars involve providing supportive care to patients and caregivers in ways that are systematic and evidence-based.

The overall premise of this approach is that an effective, systematic care model exists for patients with dementia resulting from AD (Lyketsos et al. 2006). This care model also has implications for patients with other forms of dementia. Until recently, dementia care interventions were few and provided on faith, with limited evidence of effectiveness. Evidence from randomized trials now indicates that a dementia care "package" provides significant benefits to patients and caregivers. While rigorous, well-controlled trials to evaluate the efficacy of care interventions are sparse, several high-quality trials of care coordination in dementia have shown modest to moderate positive effects on patient quality of life, care quality, NPS, caregiver burden, unmet needs, and depression (Samus et al. 2014). Based on results from a randomized trial, Callahan et al. (2006) reported that in primary care settings, guideline-based dementia care led to better patient and caregiver outcomes, likely due to the more appropriate use of medications and interventions that targeted both caregivers and patients. Long-term follow-up studies (Mittelman et al. 2006) have shown that caregiver-targeted interventions (e.g., counseling and support programs) can prolong the time that patients spend in the community. An observational cohort from the Maryland Assisted Living Study supported these findings (Lyketsos et al. 2007), suggesting that treatment for dementia might delay discharge from assisted living facilities by as long as 7 months.

Multicomponent supportive dementia care programs can improve patients' ability to age in place. In a recent 18-month RCT of 303 community-living elders (Maximizing Independence at Home; Samus et al. 2014), home-based dementia care delivered by community-based nonclinical coordinators and supervised by geriatric clinicians led to delays in transitioning from home, reduced unmet needs, and improved self-reported quality of life. The intervention was considered low risk, with no intervention-related adverse events. Over 18 months, participants in the intervention group had a 51-day mean delay of transition out of their home, with a 228-day median delay over an extended follow-up period (median of 26 months) compared with control participants. Given the positive effect of being able to stay at home versus residing in costly facilities (e.g., nursing homes or assisted living placements), these findings imply a cost savings (Samus et al. 2014). Furthermore, most contacts (72%) between the community-based coordinator and another person (e.g., patient, study partner, health provider, clinician) were phone-based, which implies that benefits can be achieved in a potentially cost-efficient manner (Samus et al. 2014). In a randomized control trial, Tremont et al. (2015) demonstrated that a telephone-delivered dementia intervention resulted in improved depressive symptoms among caregivers and improved reactions to the care recipient's memory and behavior problems. Nevertheless, in-person visits are likely essential to visually identify a wide range of home and personal safety needs (e.g., fall risk, medication use adherence, wander risk) and the physical condition of participants and study partners (Samus et al. 2014).

An optimal dementia care team includes a dementia care specialist, occupational and physical therapists, a nurse, a psychologist, a social worker, and a case manager, all working closely with the primary care physician and caregivers. One of the roles of the dementia care specialist, who is often a gerontologist or geriatric psychiatrist, is to manage, both pharmacologically and nonpharmacologically, the cognitive and neuropsychiatric symptoms that accompany dementia. Nonpharmacological strategies can be very effective and avoid the risks and side effects associated with medications. One such strategy is tailoring activities based on the preserved capabilities and interests of the individual with dementia. A randomized pilot study of 60 caregiver–patient dyads utilized the Tailored Activity Program, which consisted of eight sessions in which occupational therapists trained caregivers to use customized activities for engaging with patients and reducing behavioral disturbances. At 4 months, the frequency of problem behaviors (specifically shadowing and repetitive questioning) and caregivers' appraisal of time that they spent "on duty" were both significantly reduced (Gitlin et al. 2008).

Over time, however, medications often become a necessary and integral part of symptom management. A particularly useful and well-known adage for medication management in geriatric patients is to start low and go slow. When initiating or titrating medications, the care specialist should be mindful of the following:

- Elderly patients have decreased renal clearance and slowed hepatic metabolism.
- Because elderly patients often have multiple medical illnesses and often are taking a number of medications, the clinician must evaluate for potential drug–drug interactions.

- Because geriatric patients are at increased risk of orthostasis and falls, in part due to decreased vascular tone, medications contributing to orthostasis should be used cautiously.
- Deliriogenic medications (e.g., anticholinergics and benzodiazepines) should be used judiciously and sparingly.

Disease-Modifying Therapies

Alzheimer's Disease

As articulated in the principles of care of the American Association for Geriatric Psychiatry (Lyketsos et al. 2006), estrogen, anti-inflammatory agents (e.g., prednisone, NSAIDs), and *Ginkgo biloba* are not effective treatments for Alzheimer's dementia. One large RCT showed that high doses of the antioxidant vitamin E delay progression of Alzheimer's dementia, lengthening the time to onset of the next phase by 2 years (Sano et al. 1997). Given safety concerns about dosing, the AAGP recommended considering vitamin E for Alzheimer's dementia but avoiding doses >400 IU/day. In a study evaluating the use of high-dosage (2,000 IU/day) vitamin E in patients with mild to moderate AD, Dysken et al. (2014) found that vitamin E may slow functional decline and decrease caregiver burden for some patients. However, a Cochrane Database systematic review of a small number of available studies did not find evidence for the use of vitamin E in preventing progression of MCI to dementia or improving cognitive function in people with MCI or AD (Farina et al. 2017).

One of the most effective therapies for AD is the aggressive management of associated vascular risk factors such as high blood pressure (particularly keeping systolic blood pressure below 160 mm Hg), high cholesterol, diabetes, obesity, and sedentary lifestyle (Mielke et al. 2007). Although statins have shown promise as treatments for cognitive decline and dementia in observational studies, several large RCTs (e.g., Trompet et al. 2010) did not show any significant effect on cognition.

A better understanding of the etiopathogenesis of Alzheimer's dementia has led to the development of therapies that target APP metabolism, $A\beta_{1-42}$ deposition or clearance, and ways by which amyloid injures neurons. For example, APP normally is hydrolyzed by α-secretase and then γ-secretase, which does not produce insoluble $A\beta$. Under abnormal processing, APP is hydrolyzed by β-secretase and then γ-secretase, which produces insoluble $A\beta$. In 2021, the FDA approved monoclonal antibody aducanumab for the treatment of mild AD and MCI. Aducanumab was approved using the FDA's accelerated approval pathway, meaning it was approved based on its effect on a surrogate endpoint (reduction of $A\beta$ plaque in the brain, considered reasonably likely to predict a clinical benefit to patients), with a follow-up study under way to verify that the drug provides this clinical benefit. Currently, aducanumab is not widely prescribed due to its risks of amyloid-related imaging abnormalities (ARIA) presenting as swelling; the high costs of the drug and of the accompanying brain scans to monitor for ARIA; and its controversial accelerated approval. Lastly, antitau therapies target tau hyperphosphorylation and the inhibition of tau aggregation. *Nature Reviews Neurology* published a summary of clinical trials of tau-targeting treatments for AD and other tauopathies (Congdon and Sigurdsson 2018).

For the most part, clinical trials have not been successful at producing safe and effective disease-modifying therapies for AD. Given AD's complexity, the central hypothesis of "one protein, one drug, one disease" must be modified (Mangialasche et al. 2010). There are complex interactions at every level of the human body, from genes to organs, as well as interactions between the person and the environment. Few people have "pure" AD; amyloid plaques and Lewy bodies may interact in yet-unknown ways. It is difficult to account for these nonlinear and rather unpredictable interactions in clinical trials. Many clinical trials aim to find a selective compound that acts on a specific disease target (e.g., Aβ) to produce a desired clinical effect. However, some RCTs have shown that even when therapies completely remove amyloid plaques, patients may still develop end-stage dementia, suggesting that clearing amyloid plaques alone cannot repair already damaged neurons or stop the clinical progression of AD (Holmes et al. 2008). Researchers neither completely understand the functions of Aβ nor know its upper and lower safe limits (Carrillo et al. 2013). Many drugs bind to more than one target, increasing the risk of unforeseen and unwanted complications.

Mangialasche et al. (2010) highlighted other barriers to the development of successful disease-modifying therapies, including the following:

- RCT protocols can be costly and time-consuming for the patient and the caregiver, thus increasing withdrawal rates.
- Validated biomarkers with established cutoffs are lacking.
- Studies that have unsuccessful preclinical and clinical results are not always published, leading to repetition of errors.
- Some drugs with positive results in preclinical and early clinical testing fail large Phase III RCTs.
- Designing selective compounds without intolerable and potentially toxic side effects is difficult.
- Some drugs are hindered by the inability to reach a therapeutic dosage, or treatment duration may have been too short to result in an effect.
- There are genetic differences among patients (e.g., *APOE*E4* carriers or cytochrome P450 variability).
- Reliable evaluation of patients requires adequate training and monitoring of RCT raters.
- Even if a drug targets mild to moderate stages of AD, the disease could have already advanced too far for detection of a disease-modifying effect.

Indeed, even by the time MCI develops, the pathological process may have advanced too far for treatments to be preventive, and it may be necessary to target the disease earlier, at the stage of subjective memory impairment (Cooper et al. 2013).

Given that disease-modifying therapies have largely been unsuccessful, that targeting patients even in early stages of dementia may prove too late, and that physicians are increasingly able to diagnose AD in very early stages (i.e., in a presymptomatic phase) using biomarkers, trials have started targeting *prevention* of AD. Carrillo et al. (2013) described various ongoing trials in their early phases. The following are some examples:

- The Anti-Amyloid Treatment for Asymptomatic AD Trial (A4) targets cognitively normal adults ages 65–80 years with PET evidence of Aβ. Because the participants have evidence of Aβ, they are more likely to demonstrate cognitive decline over time during the trial, making them a good target population for prevention. Participants were randomly assigned to receive solanezumab or placebo. The primary outcome measure will be the rate of cognitive decline.

- The Centre for Studies on Prevention of AD at the Douglas Institute in Montreal, Quebec, is testing various preventive interventions in people older than 60 years with a family history of AD. Interventions include medications such as intranasal insulin and lifestyle modifications such as aerobic exercise and dietary changes. A trial of naproxen from this center did not delay progression of presymptomatic AD (Meyer et al. 2019). The goals are to find optimal biomarker end points and to identify interventions that move biomarkers or mitigate their progression.

- The Australian Imaging Biomarkers and Lifestyle Flagship Study of Ageing is investigating the interaction between vascular and AD pathologies and exploring the possibility of delaying AD by reducing vascular risk factors through physical activity. The target population is individuals older than 60 years with subjective memory complaints or a diagnosis of MCI and at least one cardiovascular risk factor. Thus far, they have found that a 24-month moderate-intensity physical activity intervention does not have an effect on white matter hyperintensities or hippocampal volume in participants with subjective memory concerns and MCI with vascular risk factors (Venkatraman et al. 2020).

- The Multidomain Alzheimer Preventive Trial in France tested the protective effects of a multifactorial intervention consisting of nutritional advice, cognitive and physical activity, and omega-3 treatment. The targeted population included frail (because of evidence linking frailty with cognitive decline) or prefrail individuals without dementia, age 70 years and older, with subjective memory complaints and a limitation in at least one IADL. The trial showed no significant effects with any of the three treatment interventions compared with placebo on the primary outcomes and 15 secondary outcomes (Yassine and Schneider 2017).

Many risk factors contributing to the development of late-life dementia are modifiable. Cognitive stimulation, complexity of occupation, an engaged lifestyle, and a reduction of vascular risk factors (e.g., high cholesterol and smoking) may have protective effects (Carrillo et al. 2013). Physical activity has long been a proposed protective mechanism against cognitive decline. The randomized Lifestyle Interventions and Independence for Elders trial examined 24 months of moderate-intensity exercise (including walking, resistance training, and flexibility exercises) versus health education in more than 1,600 participants ages 70–89. No significant differences were found between the treatment groups in incident MCI or dementia at 24 months (Sink et al. 2015). A 2015 systematic review of aerobic exercise trials among individuals with normal cognition concluded that there is limited evidence that aerobic physical activity has cognitive benefit in cognitively healthy older adults (Young et al. 2015). The Finnish Geriatric Intervention Study to Prevent Cognitive Impairment and Disability was a large multidomain intervention trial of elderly adults at risk of cognitive decline (Ngandu et al. 2015). Exercise, in combination with dietary counseling and cognitive training, was part of the intervention. Participants in the intervention arm had improved outcomes on a global cognitive measure, executive functioning, and processing speed. However, the intensity of the intervention makes it hard to generalize, and the benefits were very small. For further review of studies examining lifestyle interventions to prevent cognitive impairment, *Nature Reviews Neurology* summarized the evidence for various preventive interventions (Kivipelto et al. 2018).

Various prevention trials have focused on different populations, such as asymptomatic individuals with AD pathology and presymptomatic individuals with dominant mutations or other risk factors that increase the likelihood of developing AD (Carrillo et al. 2013; Cummings et al. 2018). However, these trials may not necessarily be generalizable because they may represent two different pathological processes that may respond differently to a given treatment. Furthermore, ethical issues arise in prevention studies. At this point in time, we cannot predict whether a person with AD pathology will definitively develop dementia. Both false-positives and false-negatives can have detrimental effects on a patient and family.

Other Diseases

No disease-modifying treatments are yet available for DLB, PDD, FTLD, or CJD. Management of stroke risk, typically with anticoagulants and by mitigating vascular risk factors, is fully indicated when treating patients with VaD or possibly Alzheimer's dementia with relevant vascular comorbidities. L-dopa agonists may be effective for the treatment of PDD. Some patients with DLB may also have a partial response. Although L-dopa can precipitate or exacerbate psychosis and somnolence, this risk is lower than with dopamine agonists (Fernandez et al. 2003).

Although many patients with NPH have favorable outcomes that can endure after shunt insertion, these beneficial effects typically involve gait and continence and not cognition (Klassen and Ahlskog 2011). The response of patients with NPH or AD to shunt insertion is poorer than that of patients without neurodegenerative pathology (Hamilton et al. 2010). Indicators of positive response to shunting include improvement in gait after a high-volume lumbar puncture or high CSF flow pressure on continuous monitoring (Graff-Radford 2007). Other positive prognostic factors include 1) a short duration of cognitive impairment, 2) a mild impairment in cognition, 3) the appearance of gait disturbance prior to the onset of cognitive impairment, and 4) the presence of a secondary cause for NPH (Graff-Radford 2007). Indicators of negative response to shunting include 1) moderate or severe cognitive impairment, 2) the presence of dementia for longer than 2 years, 3) the appearance of cognitive impairment before gait disturbance, 4) the presence of aphasia, and 5) patient abuse of alcohol (Graff-Radford 2007). The size of ventricle or severity of gait disorder is not a good predictor of outcome (Meier et al. 2006). Up to 40%–50% of patients experience complications from shunting. In a Dutch study (Vanneste et al. 1992), the largest outcome study to date, notable mortality was observed after shunt placement, with the risks of shunting outweighing the benefits. No RCT has been conducted to evaluate the long-term benefit of shunting. Although confirmatory diagnostic tests for NPH are available, shunting for patients with NPH remains controversial due to an absence of trials demonstrating long-term benefit (see also Saper 2016).

Several RPDs already have disease-modifying treatments that can potentially halt or reverse their disease process. However, no disease-modifying treatments for prion diseases are yet available (Mahajan and Appleby 2017). Researchers are identifying potential novel approaches to treatment, such as vaccines, RNA interference, and anti-inflammatory agents. One of the most popular approaches is to block neuronal PrP^c, which has been done successfully in animal models. Most treatment studies of human prion diseases have been case reports or series and have been hampered by disease heterogeneity, lack of standardized outcome measures, low prevalence and statistical power, and rapid progression. Furthermore, families may decline noncurative treatments due to the rapid progression and severity of neurocognitive decline seen in prion diseases. Individuals at risk of developing prion diseases (e.g., genetic forms of prion diseases) are most likely to receive the greatest benefit from treatments. Thus, the most important aspect of establishing treatment for RPD is an early and accurate diagnosis. For instance, a brain fluorodeoxyglucose-PET scan study of fatal familial insomnia mutation carriers demonstrated hypometabolism in the thalamus 13–21 months prior to onset of clinical symptoms (Cortelli et al. 2006). Once therapeutics become available, early detection of prion diseases using biomarkers could enable clinicians to administer effective treatments in presymptomatic stages or prior to severe brain damage, allowing for a better quality of life for patients.

Therapies for Cognitive Symptoms Associated With Dementia

The cholinesterase inhibitors donepezil, rivastigmine, galantamine, and tacrine and the NMDA receptor antagonist memantine are all approved by the FDA for the treatment of cognitive symptoms in AD. However, they only modestly and temporarily stabilize the changes to cognition and ADLs associated with the disease. They do not reverse or stop the degenerative process. Data are mixed as to whether these medications improve long-term outcomes, such as the need for nursing home admission.

Cholinesterase inhibitors inhibit the enzymes that degrade acetylcholine (acetyl-cholinesterase and butyrylcholinesterase), effectively increasing the concentration of acetylcholine at synaptic clefts in the brain. Acetylcholine is a neurotransmitter hypothesized to be important in cognition. Donepezil, rivastigmine, and galantamine are all approved for the treatment of mild to moderate AD. Donepezil and the patch preparation of rivastigmine are approved for the treatment of severe AD. Tacrine, the first agent approved for use in AD, is no longer available in the United States because it can cause hepatotoxicity, specifically a transient and reversible transaminitis. These medications are available in a variety of formulations: oral immediate-release tablet or capsule, once-daily dosing tablet (donepezil only), extended-release preparations (memantine and galantamine), orally disintegrating tablet (donepezil only), solution (rivastigmine and galantamine), and transdermal patch form (rivastigmine only).

Researchers have studied another cholinesterase inhibitor, huperzine, an over-the-counter Chinese herb extract whose safety is poorly understood. One meta-analysis (Yang et al. 2013) suggested that huperzine A may have some beneficial effects on cognitive function, ADLs, and global clinical assessment in patients with AD; however, the study acknowledged that its findings should be interpreted with caution due to the poor methodological quality of the trials included.

Memantine, which is hypothesized to work by preventing the excitotoxic effects of glutamate in the brain, is approved for the treatment of moderate to severe AD. It is available in oral immediate-release, extended-release, and solution preparations. A summary of the four FDA-approved medications available in the United States for the treatment of cognitive symptoms is provided in Table 8–5.

TABLE 8–5. FDA-approved medications available in the United States for the treatment of cognitive symptoms in Alzheimer's dementia

Drug	Disease stage	Preparations	Dosing	Common side effects and dosing tips
Donepezil	All stages of AD	Oral tablet; once-daily tablet; oral disintegrating tablet	Initially 5 mg/day; may increase to 10 mg/day after 4–6 weeks.	Nausea, vomiting, diarrhea, anorexia, weight loss, dyspepsia, insomnia, and vagotonic effects leading to bradycardia and heart block. Dosage may have to be reduced in cases of hepatic impairment.
Rivastigmine	Mild to moderate AD; transdermal patch also approved for severe AD. Oral tablet and transdermal patch also approved for mild to moderate PDD.	Oral capsule; oral solution; transdermal patch	Initially 1.5 mg bid. Increase by 3 mg every 2 weeks as tolerated to maximum dosage of 6 mg bid.	Nausea, vomiting, diarrhea, anorexia, abdominal pain, weight loss, dyspepsia, dizziness, headache, EPS, CNS depression, and vagotonic effects leading to bradycardia and heart block. GI side effects may be reduced if taken with food and dosage is titrated slowly. If treatment is stopped for more than several days, start titration over with initial dosage.
Galantamine	Mild to moderate AD	Oral tablet; extended-release capsule; oral solution	Initially 4 mg bid; increase to 8 mg bid after 4 weeks. May increase to 12 mg bid if indicated.	Nausea, vomiting, diarrhea, anorexia, weight loss, dyspepsia, muscle cramps, and vagotonic effects leading to bradycardia and heart block. Associated with increased mortality, mainly due to cardiovascular events, in some placebo-controlled trials. GI side effects may be reduced if taken with food and dosage is titrated slowly. Use caution in patients with renal or hepatic impairments.
Memantine	Moderate to severe AD (monotherapy and in combination with ACE inhibitor)	Oral tablet; extended-release capsule; oral solution	Initially 5 mg/day. May increase by 5 mg weekly to maximum of 20 mg bid. Dosages >5 mg should be divided.	Dizziness, headache, confusion, constipation, and fatigue. Use caution in patients with renal or hepatic impairments. Dosage may have to be reduced in cases of renal impairment.

ACE=acetylcholinesterase; AD=Alzheimer's disease; EPS=extrapyramidal symptoms; GI=gastrointestinal; PDD=Parkinson's disease dementia.
Source. Data from Stahl 2006.

The approved cholinesterase inhibitors appear to have comparable efficacy. However, because each of the medications has individual pharmacological particularities as well as pharmacokinetic and pharmacodynamic properties that make them distinct, a patient may respond to one medication over another (Massoud et al. 2011). Prior to development of the patch delivery form of rivastigmine, approved in the United States in 2007, and the extended-release form of galantamine, there were important differences in their toxicity that entered into the clinical decision as to which medication to use first. Rivastigmine also has biological activity against butyrylcholinesterase, whereas galantamine is also an allosteric modulator of the nicotinic receptors. Despite these differences in biological activity, in the absence of solid relevant clinical data, the choice of agent continues to be driven by ease of use and titration, cost, and physician experience.

There is ample evidence to recommend initiating a cholinesterase inhibitor for the treatment of mild to moderate AD, provided that the agent appears to have a worthwhile effect on cognitive, global, functional, or neuropsychiatric symptoms and that a dementia care specialist initiates and routinely reviews treatment (National Institute for Health and Care Excellence 2011). Although memantine is frequently prescribed off-label for mild AD, independent reviews have found no differences between memantine and placebo on any outcome for patients with mild AD (Schwarz et al. 2012). Furthermore, these reviews detected only small differences on some outcomes in patients with moderate AD taking memantine (Schwarz et al. 2012). Thus, many experts recommend against memantine for mild AD but recommend it as an option for moderate AD only for patients who are intolerant of or have a contraindication to cholinesterase inhibitors (National Institute for Health and Care Excellence 2011).

Several RCTs and withdrawal studies suggest that in patients with moderate or severe AD, cholinesterase inhibitors are associated with clinically relevant cognitive and functional benefits (Birks and Harvey 2018; Birks et al. 2015; Schwarz et al. 2012). Available evidence also supports the use of memantine in patients with severe AD (McShane et al. 2019; National Institute for Health and Care Excellence 2011; Schwarz et al. 2012). There is no consensus, however, on when to switch from cholinesterase inhibitors to memantine in individuals with severe AD (Schwarz et al. 2012).

Most experts recommend and data support initiating and titrating one of these medications to the highest approved and tolerated dosage and assessing response over 6–12 months (Rabins et al. 2016). Cholinesterase inhibitors lead to notable, albeit temporary, symptomatic improvements in 10%–15% of cases. Symptomatic improvements often last for 6–9 months. In clinical practice, the judgment as to the response to treatment relies greatly on the expectations that patients, their families, and their prescribing physicians have for this class of medications (Massoud et al. 2011). Mild improvement or stabilization should be considered an appropriate and realistic goal (Massoud et al. 2011). No consensus has been reached on how to estimate clinical efficacy (Schwarz et al. 2012).

There is debate, however, about whether patients should continue taking a cholinesterase inhibitor for a longer period. In primary care settings in the United States, most patients who start a prescription do not continue taking it for more than a few months. Nevertheless, many experts recommend continuing therapy once it begins because patients may develop rapid cognitive and functional decline when a cholinesterase inhibitor is discontinued (Schwarz et al. 2012). It is unclear whether clinical deterioration following discontinuation of a cholinesterase inhibitor is due to a loss of therapeutic effect or to withdrawal from the medication (Schwarz et al. 2012).

Other experts point out that some patients do well after a discontinuation trial and that many benefit from switching agents. Massoud et al. (2011) reviewed eight open-label or retrospective switching studies involving patients in the mild to moderate stages of AD. In general, >50% of patients who were switched for unsatisfactory response showed stabilization or improvement in global evaluations, cognitive measures, and functional measures. More than 50% of patients switched for intolerance tolerated the second agent. The authors concluded that because cholinesterase inhibitors have individual pharmacological properties, switching is a valid clinical choice for patients with AD who either do not tolerate or have a *lack* of response to the initial agent. They considered significant deterioration within the first 6 months of treatment to represent a *lack* of efficacy and deterioration beyond the first 6 months of treatment to represent *loss* of efficacy (measured by a decline of at least 2 points on the MMSE and a documented deterioration in functional autonomy, global impression, or behavior). The authors suggested that either lack or loss of efficacy was a reasonable justification for switching agents. On the other hand, they did not recommend switching for loss of response with the initial cholinesterase inhibitors beyond 1 year of use, because this is most often due to the natural course of AD (most evident during the transition from mild to moderate or from moderate to severe stages). In these latter cases, the authors recommended adding memantine to the cholinesterase inhibitor. In practice, however, fewer than one-third of patients switch cholinesterase inhibitors. One of the authors of this chapter (C.G.L.) has followed a patient who benefited from the sequential use of four of the cholinesterase agents (huperzine, donepezil, rivastigmine, and galantamine). Although clearly that was an extreme case, which is probably quite rare, it shows that the issue of long-term therapy is not a settled matter.

Although cholinesterase inhibitors and memantine are licensed for monotherapy, combining the two could theoretically potentiate their benefits (Schwarz et al. 2012). Even though it is common practice to combine cholinesterase inhibitors with memantine, many experts do not endorse this practice because of a lack of clinical evidence to support additional benefit (National Institute for Health and Care Excellence 2011; Schwarz et al. 2012). Several randomized trials and observational studies have found no additional (or inconclusive) superiority of combination donepezil and memantine over donepezil alone (National Institute for Health and Care Excellence 2011).

Clinical trials have suggested that cholinesterase inhibitors may be of value in treating VaD; however, none of these drugs has been approved by the FDA for that purpose. One study suggested that donepezil is associated with increased mortality in VaD compared with placebo. The National Institute for Health and Care Excellence (2018) recommended that cholinesterase inhibitors and memantine not be prescribed clinically for the treatment of cognitive decline in patients with VaD.

Both oral and transdermal preparations of rivastigmine have been approved for the treatment of mild to moderate dementia in PDD. In a large, parallel-group RCT in PDD (Emre et al. 2004), patients who received rivastigmine demonstrated an average 1-point advantage on the MMSE over the 24-week treatment period compared with those who received placebo. The treatment group also demonstrated an average advantage of nearly 3 points on the Alzheimer's Disease Assessment Scale–Cognitive subscale, particularly in areas of attention and executive function; 2 points on an ADL scale; and 2 points on the total Neuropsychiatric Inventory score. In a Cochrane review of cholinesterase inhibitors for PDD, DLB, and MCI associated with PD, Rolinski et al. (2012) determined that current evidence supported the use of cholinesterase inhibitors in patients with PDD, with a positive impact on global assessment, cognitive function, NPS, and ADLs. However, evidence from RCTs for cholinesterase inhibitors other than rivastigmine is inconclusive (Ballard et al. 2011). Likewise, although memantine is well tolerated, it does not appear to demonstrate positive effects on nonmotoric symptoms in PDD (Schwarz et al. 2012).

Cholinesterase inhibitors have been effective in treating cognitive impairment in DLB, although this is considered off-label use. Furthermore, they have demonstrated therapeutic benefit in treating hallucinations and are considered first-line therapy for treating psychosis in DLB. Studies on the use of memantine for DLB have been inconclusive (Schwarz et al. 2012). At best, memantine seems to provide modest positive global effects in DLB. However, benefits from memantine treatment are rapidly lost following discontinuation. Although no cholinesterase inhibitors have demonstrated value in treating cognitive deficits in patients with FTLD, a medication trial is reasonable when the underlying cause of dementia is unclear.

Therapies for Neuropsychiatric Symptoms in Dementia

NPS are nearly universal in patients with dementia, affecting up to 98% of individuals across dementia stages and etiologies (Kales et al. 2014; Lyketsos et al. 2011). They are associated with poor patient outcomes, including excess morbidity and mortality, more rapid disease progression, increased health care utilization, and earlier nursing home placement. NPS are also associated with negative caregiver outcomes, including stress, depression, reduced employment, and poorer quality of life. Thirty percent of the cost of caring for community-dwelling patients with dementia can be directly attributed to NPS management. Nevertheless, uncertainty remains regarding how to manage these symptoms. A detailed discussion of the evaluation and management of NPS in dementia is beyond the scope of this chapter. We articulate a few principles here from Kales et al. (2014) and Lyketsos et al. (2011); Rabins et al. (2016) have provided a more in-depth discussion.

A useful mnemonic for the management of NPS is DICE: Describe, Investigate, Create, and Evaluate (Kales et al. 2014). The *describe* phase involves an evaluation in which the patient, caregivers, and other relevant informants accurately characterize what is occurring behaviorally. This phase enables the provider to identify underlying patterns or contributory factors to the behavior. Another important goal of this phase is to determine what aspects of the NPS are most disturbing or problematic for the patient and caregiver, as well as to establish the treatment goal.

In the *investigate* phase, the clinician examines the patient and identifies potential underlying and modifiable etiologies. Contributing factors include undiagnosed medical conditions (e.g., pain, infection, constipation, dehydration), medication side effects and drug–drug interactions, underlying psychiatric comorbidity (e.g., depressive or anxiety disorders), limitations in functional abilities, poor sleep hygiene, boredom, psychological factors (e.g., feelings of inadequacy, helplessness, fear), sensory impairments (e.g., hearing, vision), and environmental factors (e.g., an over- or understimulating environment, lack of a predictable routine, diminished pleasurable activities).

TABLE 8–6.   **Contributing causes of neuropsychiatric symptoms**

Biological stress or delirium that accompanies a recurrent or new medical condition (e.g., constipation, urinary or upper respiratory infection, pain, poor dentition, headaches, hunger, thirst)

Identifiable psychiatric syndrome that is either recurrent or associated with the dementia

Aspects of the cognitive disturbance itself (e.g., a catastrophic reaction due to inability to express oneself vocally)

Environmental stressor (e.g., excessive noise or stimulation, unfamiliar surroundings, not enough heat)

Unmet needs (e.g., hunger, thirst, feeling lonely)

Unsophisticated or intrusive caregiving (e.g., poor communication, being rushed)

Medication side effects, whether from new or previously prescribed medications

---

Table 8–6 lists the major components contributing to NPS. In general, most disturbances are multifactorial, and it is best to address several contributing factors at once. The workup for underlying causes often includes laboratory studies.

In the *create* phase, the person with dementia, the caregiver, and the treatment team (provider, visiting nurse, social worker, occupational therapist) collaborate to design and implement a treatment plan consisting of behavioral, environmental, pharmacological (prescribing new medications and discontinuing any that contribute to NPS), and educational approaches that target the identified causes. For example, a provider might treat a patient's urinary tract infection or constipation while simultaneously teaching the caregiver not to rush the patient during toileting and to use a combination of scheduled and prompted toileting for incontinence. A provider may educate a caregiver about sleep hygiene while simultaneously tapering the patient's daytime sedating medications that contribute to excessive napping. The plan should target physical problems (aggressively managing pain, constipation, dehydration, sleep disturbances, sensory impairments, and infections), underlying psychiatric conditions, safety concerns (e.g., putting safety knobs on stoves, eliminating throw rugs, removing weapons, providing sufficient lighting), and other environmental factors (e.g., establishing structured routines and meaningful activities for the patient). Caregivers provide important insight as to what has worked in the past and what has not. Considering the patient's interests, the team can more effectively tailor a patient-specific treatment plan. Providers can assist caregivers by modeling problem solving, giving constructive feedback, providing emotional support, validating that what the caregivers are doing is important, and ensuring that they are taking care of themselves.

Finally, the *evaluate* phase involves assessing whether an intervention was attempted and whether it was effective. If the caregiver implemented an intervention, it is important to evaluate whether the NPS improved, whether the intervention helped decrease the patient's and caregiver's distress, and whether there were any unintended side effects or consequences. If the caregiver did not implement an intervention, the provider should attempt to understand why not and brainstorm solutions with the caregiver. If the intervention included a psychotropic medication, the provider and caregiver should sequentially monitor behaviors and potential new side effects and consider a trial of tapering the dosage or discontinuing the medication to ensure that the medication continues to be necessary.

Because of the increased risks inherent in using medications to treat NPS in patients with dementia, the clinician should consider using nonpharmacological interventions as first-line therapy. The exception is in emergency situations when NPS could compromise the safety of the patient or others, in which case the standard of care supports psychotropic use (Kales et al. 2014). Small studies have shown modest benefit with aromatherapy, bright light therapy, music therapy, controlled multisensory stimulation (Snoezelen rooms), animal-assisted therapy, exercise programs, physical therapy, occupational therapy, and speech therapy. Some of these therapies are useful during a treatment session but have no longer-term benefits. Behavioral therapy using a behavioral monitoring log can help identify triggers to avoid or manage and can provide sustained improvements in behavior in individuals with dementia. A Cochrane review and meta-analysis (Moniz Cook et al. 2012) suggested that functional analysis (in which a therapist develops an understanding of the function or meaning behind the patient's distress and symptoms) is associated with a decrease in the frequency of challenging behaviors and an improvement in the caregiver's reaction to them. A stable, structured, predictable environment that avoids over- or understimulation can be very beneficial for patients. Distraction, redirection, removing environmental cues for behaviors caregivers want to discourage (e.g., taking car keys to discourage driving), or offering simple choices can be effective in decreasing agitation and anxiety. Educating caregivers and professional staff about how to manage NPS can lead to reductions in patients' behavioral outbursts and less restraint use. As mentioned, tailored activities, outlined by occupational therapists, can be effective in reducing anxiety and motor disturbances, among other NPS (de Oliveira et al. 2019). Psychotherapy can be a useful strategy, particularly in early dementia, with patients who are anxious, depressed, or demoralized. Interventions with the best evidence to support their use are outlined in Table 8–7.

Although extensive effort has been put into developing nonpharmacological approaches, little controlled evidence is available to suggest that they work, and they are often difficult to implement in real-world settings, especially in primary or institutional care (Livingston et al. 2005). A study of newly admitted nursing home residents demonstrated that within the first 3 months of admission, only 12% received nonpharmacological interventions, whereas 71% received at least one psychotropic medication (Molinari et al. 2010). Furthermore, more than 15% were taking four or more psychotropic medications. Of those treated with psychotropics, 64% had not received psychopharmacological treatment for the 6 months preceding admission and 71% had not received a psychiatric diagnosis during the same time frame.

No pharmacotherapy has FDA approval for dementia-related NPS. Despite well-known, significant concerns about the safety and efficacy of psychotropic medications in treating NPS in individuals with dementia, clinicians commonly use these drugs to manage these symptoms. Clinicians often prescribe these medications without first methodically assessing the potential underlying causes of behaviors. They may utilize a "symptom cluster" approach, in which they match a medication to a symptom that resembles a known symptom of an illness (e.g., mood stabilizers for decreased sleep and pressured speech or antidepressants for dysphoria and apathy). Because dementia is usually progressive and NPS can fluctuate over time, clinicians and caregivers may be trying to hit a "moving target" with psychotropics. Caregivers frequently attempt to manage several NPS disturbances concomitantly, often with more than one

TABLE 8–7. General nonpharmacological strategies for managing neuropsychiatric symptoms

Domain	Key strategies
Behavior management	
Memory-related problems (e.g., disorientation or confusion with object recognition)	Identify self and others if patient does not remember names or is aphasic.
	Use memory aids (calendar or whiteboard showing current date).
	Keep all objects for a task in a labeled container (e.g., grooming).
	Supervise medication taking and secure medications.
	Present a single object at a time.
	Paint doors to identify or disguise them.
Falling and poor balance	Remove clutter or unnecessary objects.
	Use a fall alert system if the patient can remember to activate it.
	Consider referral to occupational therapy for home safety evaluation and removal of tripping hazards.
	Consider referral to physical therapy for simple balance exercise.
	Minimize alcohol intake.
Hearing voices or noises (especially at night)	Evaluate hearing and adjust amplification of hearing aids.
	Evaluate quality and severity of auditory disturbances.
	If hallucinations are present, evaluate whether they present an actual threat to safety or function when deciding whether to treat with antipsychotics.
Wandering or inability to respond to emergency (difficulty calling for help)	Educate caregiver about the need to supervise the patient.
	Inform neighbors, fire department, and police of the patient's condition.
	Develop emergency plan involving others if possible.
	Outfit the patient with an identification bracelet (e.g., Alzheimer Safe Return Program).
	Identify potential triggers for elopement and modify them.
Nighttime wakefulness, turning on lights, waking caregiver, feeling insecure at night	Implement good sleep hygiene.
	Evaluate bedroom for disturbances (e.g., temperature, noise, light, shadows, and level of comfort.)

TABLE 8–7.   General nonpharmacological strategies for managing neuropsychiatric symptoms (*continued*)

Domain	Key strategies
Behavior management (*continued*)	
Nighttime wakefulness, turning on lights, waking caregiver, feeling insecure at night (*continued*)	Eliminate caffeinated beverages (starting in the afternoon).
	Create a structured schedule that includes exercise and activities throughout the day.
	Limit daytime napping.
	Use a nightlight.
	Create a quiet routine for bedtime that includes a calming activity and calming music.
	Address daytime loneliness and boredom that may contribute to nighttime insecurities.
	Hire nighttime assistance to enable caregiver to sleep.
Repetitive questioning	Respond using a calm, reassuring voice.
	Use a light touch to reassure, calm, or redirect.
	Inform patient of events as they occur (vs. indicating what will happen in the near or far future).
	Use distraction.
Care management	
Communication	Use a calm, reassuring voice.
	Avoid negative words and tone.
	Use a light touch to reassure, calm, or redirect.
	Allow patient sufficient time to respond to a question.
	Help patient find words to express him- or herself.
	Offer simple choices (no more than two at a time).
Simplifying the environment	Use labeling or other visual cues.
	Remove unnecessary objects to reduce confusion with tasks.
	Eliminate noise and distractions while you are communicating or when patient is engaging in an activity.
	Use simple visual reminders (e.g., arrows pointing to bathroom).

TABLE 8–7. **General nonpharmacological strategies for managing neuropsychiatric symptoms** *(continued)*

Domain	Key strategies
Care management *(continued)*	
Caregiver education and support	Understand that patient behaviors are not intentional.
	Learn to relax the rules (e.g., baths do not have to happen daily; there is no right or wrong in performing activities or tasks as long as patient and caregiver are safe).
	Go along with patient's view of what is true and avoid arguing or trying to reason or convince.
Task structuring	Break each task into very simple steps.
	Provide one- or two-step simple verbal commands.
	Use verbal or tactile prompts for each step.
	Provide structured daily routines that are predictable.
Activities	Engage patient with meaningful activities that tap into preserved capabilities and previous interests.
	Introduce activities involving repetitive motion (washing windows, folding towels, and putting coins in a container).
	Guide and cue patient to initiate, sequence, organize, and complete tasks.

Note. Domains and strategies listed are potential approaches used in randomized clinical trials but are not exhaustive. One strategy may be effective for one patient but not for another. Only consider these strategies following a thorough assessment and diagnostic workup.
Source. Adapted from Gitlin et al. 2012.

medication, contributing to an unpredictable and undecipherable outcome. Even in the few cases in which psychotropics, specifically antipsychotics, demonstrate modest efficacy in improving NPS, the benefits may be negated by significant adverse effects. Psychotropic medications are unlikely to affect poor self-care or refusal of care, memory problems, inattention, unfriendliness, repetitive verbalizations or questioning, shadowing, or wandering (Kales et al. 2014). They are also unlikely to improve behaviors that can ultimately be attributed to apraxia or agnosia (e.g., urinating in a trash can because it resembles a toilet bowl). Gerlach and Kales (2020) presented a concise review of available evidence for the effectiveness and tolerability of pharmacological treatments in addressing behavioral disturbances in dementia. If medication treatments are indicated, it is important to follow guidelines similar to those outlined in Table 8–8. Sink et al. (2005) published a widely employed algorithm for using medications to treat NPS in dementia.

Several different classes of medications have been studied. For some of them, safety concerns exist, and efficacy remains uncertain. The use of both conventional and atypical antipsychotics is controversial because their efficacy is modest and they have been associated with side effects (including rapid cognitive decline), a higher risk of cerebrovascular or cardiovascular events, and mortality in patients with dementia (Schneider et al. 2005). The FDA has issued black box warnings regarding the use of antipsychotics in treating patients with dementia-related psychosis (U.S. Food and Drug Administration 2008). Both conventional and atypical antipsychotics carry this increased mortality risk in dementia, whereas other psychotropic medications, such as antidepressants and anticonvulsants, do not.

Antipsychotics are the core treatments of agitation and psychosis. In the Clinical Antipsychotic Trial of International Effectiveness–Alzheimer's Disease study, risperidone and olanzapine showed the most, albeit modest, benefit of symptom reduction as assessed by various rating scales. Antipsychotics had no effect on other outcomes such as cognition, functioning, or quality of life (Sultzer et al. 2008). While these antipsychotics are not contraindicated in dementia, the risk-benefit ratio is high, and they should be used with caution (Rabins and Lyketsos 2005). Some RCTs have shown that antipsychotics can be discontinued for most patients receiving chronic antipsychotic therapy without a worsening of behavior (Seitz et al. 2013). However, the Antipsychotic Discontinuation in Alzheimer's Disease trial showed that after patients with AD and psychosis or agitation achieved and maintained a treatment response with risperidone (mean dosage 0.97 mg/day) for 4–8 months, a switch from risperidone to placebo in a randomized, double-blind manner was associated with a markedly increased risk of relapse relative to continuing risperidone (Devanand et al. 2012). The predictors of successful discontinuation of antipsychotics included lower baseline severity of NPS and use of lower dosages of antipsychotics to achieve symptom control (Seitz et al. 2013). For a more detailed description of the pharmacological treatment of agitation and psychosis in the context of dementia, see Chapters 11 and 19 in this textbook.

Patients with DLB present an additional challenge to antipsychotic therapy because they are extremely sensitive to the extrapyramidal side effects of all antipsychotics except clozapine. Adverse events range from parkinsonism to acute dystonia to neuroleptic malignant syndrome. Clinicians should avoid use of conventional antipsychotics in patients with DLB. Similarly, although antipsychotics can be useful in

TABLE 8–8.	Guidelines for use of medications to treat neuropsychiatric symptoms

Differentiate which disturbance is present; they are not all the same.

Consider possible contributing causes and the need for medical workup.

Implement nonpharmacological interventions concomitantly.

Use medications cautiously, with defined targets and close monitoring for adverse effects potentially caused by psychotropic medications.

Educate caregivers to notify clinicians immediately should the patient develop an adverse drug reaction.

Routinely review the risk-benefit ratio of treatment.

Avoid knee-jerk prescribing of psychotropics in response to symptoms to better elicit the underlying cause(s).

Be mindful that some isolated disturbances are unlikely to respond to medications.

Use of psychotropics should always be time limited, because symptoms may resolve over time with or without pharmacological treatment.

Have in place a backup plan and a plan to deal with after-hours crises.

Source. Adapted from Gitlin et al. 2012.

treating visual hallucinations and delusions associated with PDD, they must be used with caution due to the inherent risk of exacerbating parkinsonian symptoms. Quetiapine and especially clozapine are the least likely to worsen parkinsonism.

Evidence suggests that selective serotonin reuptake inhibitors (SSRIs) such as citalopram (Leonpacher et al. 2016; Porsteinsson et al. 2014; Seitz et al. 2013), sertraline (Lyketsos et al. 2003), and escitalopram (Seitz et al. 2013) are efficacious in treating agitation and apathy in patients with Alzheimer's dementia. Double-blind trials comparing the serotonin antagonist and reuptake inhibitor trazodone with placebo, however, have not shown benefit in the treatment of NPS (Ballard and Corbett 2010). In contrast to their treatment of agitation and apathy, traditional antidepressants do not appear to have efficacy for depression in AD. In the Depression in Alzheimer's Disease–2 study, sertraline was not associated with clinical improvement of depression in AD (Rosenberg et al. 2010). Similarly, sertraline and mirtazapine were no more efficacious than placebo in treating depression in AD in a double-blind U.K. study (Banerjee et al. 2011).

Moreover, although the rates of adverse events with antidepressants may be lower than those observed with antipsychotics, antidepressants should in no way be considered harmless (Seitz et al. 2013). In older adults, serotonergic agents are associated with adverse events, including injurious falls (evident even at low dosages, but increasing as much as threefold at higher dosages), fractures, bleeding, and hyponatremia (Schwarz et al. 2012; Seitz et al. 2013). There are also reports that SSRIs induce an amotivational or apathy syndrome, which is reversible when the drug is stopped or the dosage is decreased (Berman et al. 2012). Some observational studies have also found an increased risk of stroke and death (Seitz et al. 2013). RCTs have shown that citalopram and escitalopram may be as effective as risperidone or perphenazine and may be more effective than placebo in hospitalized populations with dementia and NPS (Seitz et al. 2013). A randomized, placebo-controlled, double-blind trial, the Citalopram for Agitation in Alzheimer Disease study, evaluated 186 patients with probable AD and clinically significant agitation (Porsteinsson et al. 2014). Over 9 weeks, patients treated with citalopram 30 mg/day showed a clinically relevant, significant reduction of agitation on several rating scales compared with patients given placebo. This improvement is comparable with that of antipsychotic drugs in other trials (Porsteinsson et al. 2014). Adverse events were modest and were consistent with known side effects of SSRIs (e.g., gastrointestinal complaints, respiratory tract infections, falls). Compared with patients given placebo, those who were given citalopram had a 1-point greater decline in MMSE scores over 9 weeks. Although the clinical significance of this effect on cognition is unclear, this decline is less than what experts consider to be a minimum clinically significant change (1.4 points). It is also unclear whether the cognitive effect continues beyond 9 weeks and whether citalopram adversely affects the course of AD.

One limitation of using citalopram is a dosage-dependent risk of QT prolongation, potentially leading to torsades de pointes. This risk generated an FDA advisory warning in 2011 that citalopram should no longer be used at dosages >20 mg/day in individuals older than 60 years because of the potential for cardiac electrical abnormalities (U.S. Food and Drug Administration 2012). There are insufficient data on the efficacy of citalopram for agitation at dosages of <30 mg/day (Porsteinsson et al. 2014). Blood concentration models of citalopram enantiomers suggest that the R-enantiomer (citalopram) accounted for more of the adverse consequences, including cognitive changes, whereas the S-enantiomer (escitalopram) was associated with increased likelihood of improvement in agitation (Ho et al. 2016). Escitalopram for Agitation in Alzheimer's Disease is a randomized, multicenter clinical trial to further assess the effect of escitalopram in treating agitation in AD. Participants will be randomized to escitalopram 15 mg versus matching placebo, in addition to receiving standard-of-care structured psychosocial intervention. The primary outcome measure is the modified AD Cooperative Study Clinical Global Impression of Change (Ehrhardt et al. 2019).

Evidence is limited regarding the efficacy of cholinesterase inhibitors and memantine for NPS, but these drugs may help delay the emergence of symptoms or treat very mild symptoms. In general, they should not be considered first-line agents in managing acute NPS of moderate or greater severity until better evidence of their efficacy emerges (Weintraub and Katz 2005).

Depression

Multiple meta-analyses suggest that evidence supporting the use of antidepressants to treat comorbid depression in AD is weak at best (Schwarz et al. 2012; Sepehry et al. 2012). However, they were limited by the heterogeneity of their included studies, with differing criteria for the diagnosis of depression, the compound tested, and outcome measures for depression. Many clinical trials also excluded patients with more severe depression, likely limiting the apparent treatment benefit in these studies (Ballard and Corbett 2010). Choosing an antidepressant is complicated because of the frailty and susceptibility to side effects of many individuals with dementia (Ballard and Corbett 2010). Tricyclic antidepressants are limited by significant adverse effects (e.g., confusion, falls due to orthostatic hypotension, cardiac arrhythmias).

One small, placebo-controlled, double-blind, randomized study examined venlafaxine, a serotonin-norepinephrine reuptake inhibitor (SNRI), in the treatment of depression in dementia and demonstrated essentially no difference in improvement on a depression rating scale between low-dosage venlafaxine (mean immediate-release dosage 75 mg/day, range 37.5–131.25 mg/day) and placebo at 6 weeks (de Vasconcelos Cunha et al. 2007). There also was no statistically significant difference in the incidence of adverse events between the groups. No clinical studies have been published of either duloxetine, an SNRI, or bupropion, a norepinephrine-dopamine reuptake inhibitor, for depression in dementia. Randomized placebo-controlled trials of sertraline and mirtazapine have found an absence of benefit with antidepressants over placebo after 3 months of treatment (Banerjee et al. 2011; Rosenberg et al. 2010; Weintraub et al. 2010). Patients with AD and depression who received antidepressants did not show improvement in global cognition (Sepehry et al. 2012); moreover, patients treated with antidepressants experienced an increased rate of adverse events. Experts emphasize, however, that the limited evidence of efficacy of antidepressant therapy from clinical trials should *not* be used as a reason to withhold antidepressant treatment from a patient with AD who is severely depressed (Ballard and Corbett 2010). Various international organizations (e.g., British Psychological Society, Royal College of Psychiatrists, Canadian Consensus Conference on Dementia) recommend treating an individual with dementia and depression with antidepressants (giving preference to an SSRI or to avoiding medications with anticholinergic effects) if the patient has had an inadequate response to nonpharmacological interventions (e.g., increasing pleasant activities and social interactions), after carefully assessing the risk-benefit ratio (Sepehry et al. 2012). Although the duration of treatment is unclear, a general rule of thumb is to treat major depression for at least 6 months.

Little is known about treating depression associated with other types of dementia because most studies have focused on AD. SSRIs may be efficacious in treating depression and anxiety associated with DLB. Observational studies have demonstrated some benefit for SSRIs in reducing disinhibition, anxiety, depression, impulsivity, repetitive behaviors, and eating disorders in patients with FTLD. In the absence of any specific evidence guiding the treatment of depression in other non-AD dementias, clinicians should follow the same treatment approaches as they would for depression in AD (Ballard and Corbett 2010).

Apathy

Few studies have examined treatments for apathy in dementia. Even fewer have targeted apathy as a primary outcome. These studies tended to be open-label, were underpowered, involved mixed dementias, and had a wide range of definitions for apathy. Cholinesterase inhibitors have the best evidence for improving or stabilizing apathy, with no clear indication that any one of these drugs is superior to another (Berman et al. 2012). There is some evidence of modest benefit with memantine, mixed evidence of benefit with atypical antipsychotics, and no good evidence to support using antidepressants, antiepileptics, or traditional antipsychotics to treat apathy (Berman et al. 2012). Potential adverse effects limit the use of these classes of medications.

Despite a perception that apathy is treatable with stimulants, only a handful of small eligible trials of methylphenidate since 1975 have shown significant improvement. The Apathy in Dementia Methylphenidate Trial compared methylphenidate 20 mg/day with placebo in a 6-week randomized, double-blind trial (Rosenberg et al. 2013). Methylphenidate treatment was associated with significant improvement in two out of three efficacy outcomes. Global cognition trended toward improvement with methylphenidate but was not statistically significant. Although the methylphenidate group experienced minimal significant adverse events overall, this group trended toward experiencing weight loss and greater anxiety. The investigators recently published results from a larger, longer trial of methylphenidate over 6 months that found a modest reduction in apathy—evident by 2 months of treatment—as measured by the NPI Apathy subscale (Mintzer et al. 2021). A very small trial of modafinil for apathy did not support its effectiveness (Ruthirakuhan et al. 2018).

Apathy tends to be chronic and progressive; for this reason, it is unclear when to initiate treatment and how long to continue treatment. Treatment may be useful if a patient's quality of life can potentially be improved, if the patient has excessive disability, or if a patient's caregiver is significantly distressed or burdened by the repercussions of this symptom (Berman et al. 2012). Long-term therapy may be indicated if a patient demonstrates a positive response to medications.

Sleep Disorders

Comprehensive discussion on the treatment of sleep disorders in dementia is beyond the scope of this chapter. A useful first step is to take an individualized sleep inventory (Roth 2012), such as the Epworth Sleepiness Scale (Johns 1991). After identifying which type of sleep disorder (e.g., difficulty falling asleep at night, excessive daytime sleepiness, restless leg syndrome, obstructive sleep apnea) is present and which symptoms are most concerning to the patient or caregiver, the dementia team can tailor treatments to the specific disorder and symptoms. Medications causing the symptoms should be discontinued and behavioral/nonpharmacological measures (e.g., improving sleep hygiene, hiring nighttime assistants so caregivers can sleep, using continuous positive airway pressure therapy for obstructive sleep apnea) should be implemented. Clinicians should attempt to identify underlying problems and target specific issues before treating general symptoms (Camargos et al. 2014; Roth 2012).

There is a paucity of studies evaluating pharmacological interventions for sleep disorders in patients with dementia. Many of the extant studies have been limited by small sample sizes, retrospective data collection, open-label testing, or the fact that sleep was evaluated as a secondary outcome (Camargos et al. 2014). Trials evaluating the effects of triazolam, haloperidol, and melatonin on sleep have had disappointing results (Camargos et al. 2014). Quetiapine and mirtazapine are sometimes utilized to treat sleep difficulties (e.g., quetiapine may improve REM sleep behavior disorder), but they can worsen restless legs syndrome and periodic limb movements of sleep (Roth 2012). The typical starting dosage of quetiapine is 12.5 mg/day (increasing in increments of 12.5 mg). The typical starting dosage of mirtazapine is 7.5 mg/day, and the dosage can be increased by increments of 7.5 mg; however, it is important to remember that higher dosages tend to be *less* sedating (Roth 2012). A recent double-blind, placebo-controlled study of trazodone in patients with AD and sleep disorders demonstrated promising results (Camargos et al. 2014). Compared with individuals in the placebo group, individuals who received trazodone 50 mg/day slept 42.5 more minutes per night and experienced no drug effect on daytime sleepiness, naps, cognition, or function. More in-depth discussions of the etiology, evaluation, and treatment of sleep disorders in specific dementias are provided in Chapter 16, "Sleep and Circadian Rhythm Sleep-Wake Disorders," and in Roth (2012).

Supportive Care for Patients

An estimated 60%–70% of older adults with AD and other dementias live in the community and are cared for by family members and friends (Theis et al. 2013). Nearly all (up to 99%) of community-residing individuals with dementia have unmet needs for care, services, and support (Black et al. 2013). Unmet dementia-related needs increase the risk of undesirable health outcomes, nursing home placement, and death (Black et al. 2013). It is critical to provide systematic supportive care to patients with dementia. The first step is for patients, caregivers, and team members to collaborate to determine unmet care needs. A needs assessment is an efficient tool to help identify these gaps. Once an assessment is completed, the patient, caregiver, and team can prioritize unmet needs by importance and feasibility and then devise a tailored treatment plan to meet these needs.

The Maximizing Independence at Home study set out to determine the prevalence and correlates of unmet needs in a sample of community-residing individuals with dementia and their informal caregivers (Black et al. 2013). Utilizing a dementia care needs assessment (Black et al. 2008), evaluators were able to determine the proportion of unmet items in six pre-specified need categories: evaluation and treatment of memory symptoms, NPS management, home and personal safety, general health and medical care, daily and meaningful activities, and legal issues and advance care planning. Participants, study partners, and primary care physicians received the written results of the assessment, which included recommendations for each identified unmet need. Coordinators then conducted an in-home visit with each participant and study partner, reviewed and prioritized needs, and developed a care plan. Care components could be individually tailored to unmet needs and updated based on emergent needs of either participants or caregivers. A coordinator helped guide the study partner or participant (when appropriate) in implementing the plan. Ninety percent of participants had unmet home and personal safety needs, particularly for wander and fall risk management and home safety evaluations. More than 60% of participants had unmet general health and medical care needs, including the need to see a primary care provider, medical subspecialist, or a dental, vision, or hearing specialist. More than 50% had unmet meaningful activity needs, including the need for adult day care, senior center involvement, and in-home activities. Forty-eight percent had unmet legal-issue and advance care–planning needs. Almost 33% of participants had not received a prior evaluation or diagnosis of dementia. Higher unmet needs for individuals with dementia were significantly associated with nonwhite race, lower income, early stage dementia and less impairment in ADLs, more symptoms of depression, and caregivers with lower education.

Table 8–9 lists supportive areas that a dementia care team should address in every case (Lyketsos et al. 2006). Teams should educate patients, when appropriate, about their condition, including giving them their diagnosis and anticipated course. Early diagnosis can provide opportunities to initiate treatment for dementia symptoms and to help individuals and families plan for future care (Black et al. 2013). When patients, caregivers, and clinicians recognize medical conditions earlier, the costs of care may be lowered, quality of life improved, and hospitalizations prevented (Black et al. 2013). Supportive care for patients should be aimed at preserving their dignity, maintaining their optimal physical and mental health, encouraging their abilities to persist for longer periods of time, and making their caregivers' lives easier. Teams should work with caregivers to find safe environments that maximize the patient's remaining physical and cognitive abilities, within the restrictions of the environment. Ideally, environments would permit patients to be well nourished and hydrated, receive a certain amount of activity and socialization, receive support for their ADLs and IADLs, and maintain good sleep hygiene. In-home activities customized to the interests and capabilities of individuals with dementia can significantly increase their engagement, reduce NPS, and reduce caregiver burden (Black et al. 2013). An in-home occupational therapy assessment, using a functional assessment method such as the Assessment of Motor and Processing Skills (Fisher 2003), can provide useful data about a patient's level-of-care needs and about home safety. Additional information about providing supportive care for patients is available in the book *The 36-Hour Day* by Mace and Rabins (2011) and from the Alzheimer's Association website (www.alz.org).

Community-dwelling adults with dementia generally receive more care from caregivers as their disease progresses (Theis et al. 2013). The daunting tasks of caregivers include assisting with ADLs, managing the patient's safety or NPS, identifying and navigating a loose network of long-term care support services, facilitating health care visits, advocating for the patient, and making proxy financial and health care decisions (Black et al. 2013). This work occurs within a context of loss—both for the person with dementia and for the caregivers (Black et al. 2013), who often face greater burdens and stress than caregivers of adults with other illnesses. Depression is common (Black et al. 2013). Caregiver burnout affects not only the caregiver but also the patient. Stress, deteriorating mental and physical health, and financial hardships can have deleterious effects on the patient. Caregiver stress is predictive of nursing home admission for older adults with dementia, and unmet caregiver needs are associated with lower quality of life (Black et al. 2013). In the Maximizing Independence at Home study, almost all caregivers (97%) had one or more unmet needs (Black et al. 2013). More than 85% of caregivers had unmet needs for referrals to community resources (e.g., Alzheimer's Association) and education (e.g., developing caregiver skills and learning how dementia impacts their loved ones). More than 40% of caregivers also had unmet needs for mental health care. Nonwhite race, less education, and more symptoms of depression were significantly associated with higher unmet caregiver needs.

Because caregivers are the lifeline of the patient and are greatly affected by dementia, they should be involved intimately in the development and implementation of any dementia care program. As with addressing unmet needs of individuals with dementia, a needs assessment can serve as a useful foundation to gather data on unmet caregiver needs. Table 8–10 lists key intervention areas involving caregivers (Lyketsos

---

TABLE 8–9.   **Supportive care for patients**

Provide comfort and emotional support.

Address safety concerns regarding driving, living alone, environmental hazards (eliminating access to dangerous items), medications, falls, and wandering (using a monitoring device).

Maintain a safe, predictable place to live with graded support (as little help as possible), role modeling, and cueing for activities of daily living and instrumental activities of daily living.

Provide structure, activity, and stimulation in day-to-day life to maximize remaining abilities and function.

Provide environmental cues for behaviors (e.g., laying out clothing for self-care).

Assist with decision making.

Aggressively manage medical comorbidities.

Maintain up-to-date advance directives and advance care planning decisions.

Provide good nursing care in advanced stages.

TABLE 8–10.   **Supportive care for caregivers**

Provide comfort and emotional support.

Educate caregivers about dementia.

Instruct caregivers on the skills of caregiving and support them with problem-solving techniques.

Ensure that an expert clinician is always available for consultation, especially for crisis intervention.

Encourage respite from caregiving.

Encourage caregivers to maintain a social network.

Attend to caregivers' general and mental health, including scheduling preventive health care visits.

---

et al. 2006; Rabins et al. 2016; Selwood et al. 2007). Mittelman et al. (2006) highlighted the importance of the delivery of interventions for caregivers. Their work suggested that caregiver interventions can have effect sizes as large as or larger than medications in delaying out-of-home placement for patients with dementia. Central to good dementia care is making sure that caregivers are educated about dementia, understand the diagnosis, can access resources, use respite appropriately, and have an expert available around the clock to help them in times of crisis.

Conclusion

Dementia is a clinical syndrome of cognitive disturbance with functional neuropsychiatric (behavioral), and neurological impairments, whereas MCI affects cognition and not function. A thorough history and cognitive assessment are essential to the evaluation and diagnosis of dementia and MCI. AD is the most common form of dementia, and other common causes include cerebrovascular disease, Lewy body disease, and FTLD. Dementia care consists of treating the disease (for which we have few therapies at present), managing the symptoms (including cognitive, neuropsychiatric, and functional), and providing supportive care to the patient and caregiver.

Key Points

- Dementia is an epidemic clinical syndrome consisting of global cognitive decline and memory deficits, with at least one other area of cognition affected.

- Dementia can be accurately diagnosed and differentiated from mild cognitive impairment (MCI) and cognitive impairment, no dementia.

- Amnestic MCI is likely the prodrome to Alzheimer's dementia, the most common form of dementia.

- The evaluation and differential diagnosis of dementia and of mild neurocognitive disorders involve an initial focus on defining the phenomenology of the syndrome and its associated features, followed by a workup for a putative cause.

- The four pillars of dementia treatment are disease treatment, symptom treatments, supportive care for the patient, and supportive care for the caregiver. All four areas must be addressed in contemporary dementia care. A needs assessment is an efficient tool to help identify unmet care needs.

- The concept of treatable and nontreatable dementias is no longer relevant; all dementias are treatable, albeit not necessarily curable. One of the most effective therapies for Alzheimer's disease (AD) is aggressively managing associated vascular risk factors.

- The amyloid cascade hypothesis of AD is rapidly evolving, impacting clinical trials. Many prevention trials are ongoing in the field, with results yet to be determined.

- Neuropsychiatric symptoms are nearly universal across dementia stages and etiologies. No pharmacotherapy has FDA approval for dementia-related neuropsychiatric symptoms. Nonpharmacological interventions can be as effective as currently available medications and should be considered first-line therapy except in emergency situations.

- Disease-modifying therapies in AD have largely been unsuccessful, and no such treatments are available for dementia with Lewy bodies, Parkinson's disease dementia, frontotemporal lobar degeneration, or Creutzfeldt-Jakob disease. Cholinesterase inhibitors provide only modest and temporary stabilization of the changes to cognition and activities of daily living associated with the disease. They do not reverse or stop the degenerative process.

Suggested Readings

Blennow K, de Leon MJ, Zetterberg H: Alzheimer's disease. Lancet 368:387–403, 2006
Livingston G, Johnston K, Katona C, et al: Systematic review of psychological approaches to the management of neuropsychiatric symptoms of dementia. Am J Psychiatry 162:1996–2021, 2005

Lyketsos CG: Lessons from neuropsychiatry. J Neuropsychiatry Clin Neurosci 18:445–449, 2006

Mace NL, Rabins PV: The 36-Hour Day: A Family Guide to Caring for People Who Have Alzheimer Disease, Related Dementias, and Memory Loss, 5th Edition. Baltimore, MD, The Johns Hopkins University Press, 2011

Metzler-Baddeley C: A review of cognitive impairments in dementia with Lewy bodies relative to Alzheimer's disease and Parkinson's disease with dementia. Cortex 43:583–600, 2007

Neary D, Snowden J, Mann D: Frontotemporal dementia. Lancet Neurol 4:771–780, 2005

Prince M, Bryce R, Albanese E, et al: The global prevalence of dementia: a systematic review and metaanalysis. Alzheimers Dement 9(1):63–75.e2, 2013

Rabins PV, Lyketsos CG, Steele CD: Practical Dementia Care, 3rd Edition. New York, Oxford University Press, 2016

Rosenberg PB, Johnston D, Lyketsos CG: A clinical approach to mild cognitive impairment. Am J Psychiatry 163:1884–1890, 2006

Sink KM, Holden KF, Yaffe K: Pharmacological treatment of neuropsychiatric symptoms of dementia: a review of the evidence. JAMA 293:596–608, 2005

Steinberg M, Shao H, Zandi P, et al: Point and 5-year period prevalence of neuropsychiatric symptoms in dementia: the Cache County Study. Int J Geriatr Psychiatry 23:170–177, 2008

References

Albert MS, DeKosky ST, Dickson D, et al: The diagnosis of mild cognitive impairment due to Alzheimer's disease: recommendations from the National Institute on Aging-Alzheimer's Association workgroups on diagnostic guidelines for Alzheimer's disease. Alzheimers Dement 7(3):270–279, 2011 21514249

Alzheimer's Association: 2019 Alzheimer's disease facts and figures. Alzheimers Dement 15(3):321–387, 2019

American Psychiatric Association: Diagnostic and Statistical Manual of Mental Disorders, 5th Edition. Arlington, VA, American Psychiatric Association, 2013

Appleby BS, Lyketsos CG: Rapidly progressive dementias and the treatment of human prion diseases. Expert Opin Pharmacother 12(1):1–12, 2011 21091283

Baker LD, Frank LL, Foster-Schubert K, et al: Effects of aerobic exercise on mild cognitive impairment: a controlled trial. Arch Neurol 67(1):71–79, 2010 20065132

Ballard C, Corbett A: Management of neuropsychiatric symptoms in people with dementia. CNS Drugs 24(9):729–739, 2010 20806986

Ballard C, Kahn Z, Corbett A: Treatment of dementia with Lewy bodies and Parkinson's disease dementia. Drugs Aging 28(10):769–777, 2011 21970305

Ballard C, Aarsland D, Francis P, Corbett A: Neuropsychiatric symptoms in patients with dementias associated with cortical Lewy bodies: pathophysiology, clinical features, and pharmacological management. Drugs Aging 30(8):603–611, 2013 23681401

Banerjee S, Hellier J, Dewey M, et al: Sertraline or mirtazapine for depression in dementia (HTA-SADD): a randomised, multicentre, double-blind, placebo-controlled trial. Lancet 378(9789):403–411, 2011 21764118

Barthel H, Sabri O: Clinical use and utility of amyloid imaging. J Nucl Med 58(11):1711–1717, 2017 28818990

Beach TG, Wilson JR, Sue LI, et al: Circle of Willis atherosclerosis: association with Alzheimer's disease, neuritic plaques and neurofibrillary tangles. Acta Neuropathol 113(1):13–21, 2007 17021755

Bech-Azeddine R, Høgh P, Juhler M, et al: Idiopathic normal-pressure hydrocephalus: clinical comorbidity correlated with cerebral biopsy findings and outcome of cerebrospinal fluid shunting. J Neurol Neurosurg Psychiatry 78(2):157–161, 2007 17012342

Bennett DA, Wilson RS, Boyle PA, et al: Relation of neuropathology to cognition in persons without cognitive impairment. Ann Neurol 72(4):599–609, 2012 23109154

Bentahir M, Nyabi O, Verhamme J, et al: Presenilin clinical mutations can affect gamma-secretase activity by different mechanisms. J Neurochem 96(3):732–742, 2006 16405513

Bergvall N, Brinck P, Eek D, et al: Relative importance of patient disease indicators on informal care and caregiver burden in Alzheimer's disease. Int Psychogeriatr 23(1):73–85, 2011 20619068

Berman K, Brodaty H, Withall A, Seeher K: Pharmacologic treatment of apathy in dementia. Am J Geriatr Psychiatry 20(2):104–122, 2012 21841459

Bertoux M, Delavest M, de Souza LC, et al: Social cognition and emotional assessment differentiates frontotemporal dementia from depression. J Neurol Neurosurg Psychiatry 83(4):411–416, 2012 22291219

Birks JS, Harvey RJ: Donepezil for dementia due to Alzheimer's disease. Cochrane Database Syst Rev 6(6):CD001190, 2018

Birks JS, Chong LY, Grimley Evans J: Rivastigmine for Alzheimer's disease. Cochrane Database Syst Rev 9(9):CD001191, 2015

Black BS, Johnston D, Handel S, et al: Manual for the Johns Hopkins Dementia Care Needs Assessment (JHDCNA). Baltimore, MD, self-published, 2008

Black BS, Johnston D, Rabins PV, et al: Unmet needs of community-residing persons with dementia and their informal caregivers: findings from the Maximizing Independence at Home study. J Am Geriatr Soc 61(12):2087–2095, 2013 24479141

Blennow K, de Leon MJ, Zetterberg H: Alzheimer's disease. Lancet 368(9533):387–403, 2006 16876668

Boccardi M, Altomare D, Ferrari C, et al: Assessment of the incremental diagnostic value of florbetapir F18 imaging in patients with cognitive impairment: the Incremental Diagnostic Value of Amyloid PET with [18F]-Florbetapir (INDIA-FBP) Study. JAMA Neurol 73(12):1417–1424, 2016 27802513

Bowler JV, Hachinski V: Vascular cognitive impairment: a new approach to vascular dementia. Baillieres Clin Neurol 4(2):357–376, 1995 7496625

Braak H, Ghebremedhin E, Rüb U, et al: Stages in the development of Parkinson's disease-related pathology. Cell Tissue Res 318(1):121–134, 2004 15338272

Braak H, Rüb U, Jansen Steur EN, et al: Cognitive status correlates with neuropathologic stage in Parkinson disease. Neurology 64(8):1404–1410, 2005 15851731

Brandt J, Buchholz A, Henry-Barron B, et al: Preliminary report on the feasibility and efficacy of the modified Atkins diet for treatment of mild cognitive impairment and early Alzheimer's disease. J Alzheimers Dis 68(3):969–981, 2019 30856112

Breitner JC, Wyse BW, Anthony JC, et al: APOE-ε4 count predicts age when prevalence of AD increases, then declines: the Cache County Study. Neurology 53(2):321–331, 1999 10430421

Cairns NJ, Bigio EH, Mackenzie IR, et al: Neuropathologic diagnostic and nosologic criteria for frontotemporal lobar degeneration: consensus of the Consortium for Frontotemporal Lobar Degeneration. Acta Neuropathol 114(1):5–22, 2007 17579875

Callahan CM, Boustani MA, Unverzagt FW, et al: Effectiveness of collaborative care for older adults with Alzheimer disease in primary care: a randomized controlled trial. JAMA 295(18):2148–2157, 2006 16684985

Camargos EF, Louzada LL, Quintas JL, et al: Trazodone improves sleep parameters in Alzheimer disease patients: a randomized, double-blind, and placebo-controlled study. Am J Geriatr Psychiatry 22(12):1565–1574, 2014 24495406

Canevelli M, Adali N, Voisin T, et al: Behavioral and psychological subsyndromes in Alzheimer's disease using the Neuropsychiatric Inventory. Int J Geriatr Psychiatry 28(8):795–803, 2013 23147419

Carrillo MC, Brashear HR, Logovinsky V, et al: Can we prevent Alzheimer's disease? Secondary "prevention" trials in Alzheimer's disease. Alzheimers Dement 9(2):123–131, 2013 23411394

Ceccaldi M, Jonveaux T, Verger A, et al: Added value of 18F-florbetaben amyloid PET in the diagnostic workup of most complex patients with dementia in France: a naturalistic study. Alzheimers Dement 14(3):293–305, 2018 29107051

Centers for Disease Control and Prevention: Diagnostic Criteria for Creutzfeldt-Jakob Disease (CJD) (online). Atlanta, GA, Centers for Disease Control and Prevention, August 26, 2010. Available at: https://www.cdc.gov/prions/cjd/diagnostic-criteria.html. Accessed November 1, 2021.

Chien DT, Bahri S, Szardenings AK, et al: Early clinical PET imaging results with the novel PHF-tau radioligand [F-18]-T807. J Alzheimers Dis 34(2):457–468, 2013 23234879

Cho H, Choi JY, Hwang MS, et al: Tau PET in Alzheimer disease and mild cognitive impairment. Neurology 87(4):375–383, 2016

Chow TW, Hynan LS, Lipton AM: MMSE scores decline at a greater rate in frontotemporal degeneration than in AD. Dement Geriatr Cogn Disord 22(3):194–199, 2006 16899996

Claassen DO, Parisi JE, Giannini C, et al: Frontotemporal dementia mimicking dementia with Lewy bodies. Cogn Behav Neurol 21(3):157–163, 2008 18797258

Collee JG, Bradley R, Liberski PP: Variant CJD (vCJD) and bovine spongiform encephalopathy (BSE): 10 and 20 years on: part 2. Folia Neuropathol 44(2):102–110, 2006 16823692

Congdon EE, Sigurdsson EM: Tau-targeting therapies for Alzheimer disease. Nat Rev Neurol 14(7):399–415, 2018 29895964

Cools R, D'Esposito M: Inverted-U-shaped dopamine actions on human working memory and cognitive control. Biol Psychiatry 69(12):e113–e125, 2011 21531388

Cooper C, Li R, Lyketsos C, Livingston G: Treatment for mild cognitive impairment: systematic review. Br J Psychiatry 203(3):255–264, 2013 24085737

Cortelli P, Perani D, Montagna P, et al: Pre-symptomatic diagnosis in fatal familial insomnia: serial neurophysiological and 18FDG-PET studies. Brain 129(pt 3):668–675, 2006 16399807

Cummings J, Lee G, Ritter A, Zhong K: Alzheimer's disease drug development pipeline: 2018. Alzheimers Dement (NY) 4:195–214, 2018

Cuyvers E, Sleegers K: Genetic variations underlying Alzheimer's disease: evidence from genome-wide association studies and beyond. Lancet Neurol 15(8):857–868, 2016 27302364

de Medeiros K, Robert P, Gauthier S, et al: The Neuropsychiatric Inventory–Clinician rating scale (NPI-C): reliability and validity of a revised assessment of neuropsychiatric symptoms in dementia. Int Psychogeriatr 22(6):984–994, 2010 20594384

de Oliveira AM, Radanovic M, Homem de Mello PC, et al: An intervention to reduce neuropsychiatric symptoms and caregiver burden in dementia: preliminary results from a randomized trial of the tailored activity program–outpatient version. Int J Geriatr Psychiatry 34(9):1301–1307, 2019 30035341

Devanand DP, Mintzer J, Schultz SK, et al: Relapse risk after discontinuation of risperidone in Alzheimer's disease. N Engl J Med 367(16):1497–1507, 2012 23075176

de Vasconcelos Cunha UG, Lopes Rocha F, Avila de Melo R, et al: A placebo-controlled double-blind randomized study of venlafaxine in the treatment of depression in dementia. Dement Geriatr Cogn Disord 24(1):36–41, 2007 17495474

Dourlen P, Kilinc D, Malmanche N, et al: The new genetic landscape of Alzheimer's disease: from amyloid cascade to genetically driven synaptic failure hypothesis? Acta Neuropathol 138(2):221–236, 2019 30982098

Dowling NM, Tomaszewski Farias S, Reed BR, et al: Neuropathological associates of multiple cognitive functions in two community-based cohorts of older adults. J Int Neuropsychol Soc 17(4):602–614, 2011 21092373

Dubois B, Slachevsky A, Litvan I, Pillon B: The FAB: a frontal assessment battery at bedside. Neurology 55(11):1621–1626, 2000 11113214

Dysken MW, Sano M, Asthana S, et al: Effect of vitamin E and memantine on functional decline in Alzheimer disease: the TEAM-AD VA cooperative randomized trial. JAMA 311(1):33–44, 2014 24381967

Ehrhardt S, Porsteinsson AP, Munro CA, et al: Escitalopram for Agitation in Alzheimer's Disease (S-CitAD): Methods and design of an investigator-initiated, randomized, controlled, multicenter clinical trial. Alzheimers Dement 15(11):1427–1436, 2019 31587995

Emre M: Dementia associated with Parkinson's disease. Lancet Neurol 2(4):229–237, 2003 12849211

Emre M, Aarsland D, Albanese A, et al: Rivastigmine for dementia associated with Parkinson's disease. N Engl J Med 351(24):2509–2518, 2004 15590953

Engler H, Forsberg A, Almkvist O, et al: Two-year follow-up of amyloid deposition in patients with Alzheimer's disease. Brain 129(Pt 11):2856–2866, 2006 16854944

Farina N, Llewellyn D, Isaac MGEKN, Tabet N: Vitamin E for Alzheimer's dementia and mild cognitive impairment. Cochrane Database Syst Rev (4):CD002854, 2017 28418065

Fernandez HH, Wu CK, Ott BR: Pharmacotherapy of dementia with Lewy bodies. Expert Opin Pharmacother 4(11):2027–2037, 2003 14596656

Finney GR: Normal pressure hydrocephalus. Int Rev Neurobiol 84:263–281, 2009 19501723

Fisher A: Assessment of Motor and Process Skills: Development, Standardization, and Administration Manual, Vol 1, 5th Edition. Fort Collins, CO, Three Star Press, 2003

Folstein MF, Folstein SE, McHugh PR: "Mini-Mental State." A practical method for grading the cognitive state of patients for the clinician. J Psychiatr Res 12(3):189–198, 1975 1202204

Galvin JE, Pollack J, Morris JC: Clinical phenotype of Parkinson disease dementia. Neurology 67(9):1605–1611, 2006 17101891

Ganguli M, Chang C-C, Snitz BE, et al: Prevalence of mild cognitive impairment by multiple classifications: the Monongahela-Youghiogheny Healthy Aging Team (MYHAT) project. Am J Geriatr Psychiatry 18(8):674–683, 2010 20220597

Geda YE, Schneider LS, Gitlin LN, et al: Neuropsychiatric symptoms in Alzheimer's disease: past progress and anticipation of the future. Alzheimers Dement 9(5):602–608, 2013 23562430

Gerlach LB, Kales HC: Pharmacological management of neuropsychiatric symptoms of dementia. Curr Treat Options Psychiatry 7(4):489–507, 2020

Geschwind MD, Shu H, Haman A, et al: Rapidly progressive dementia. Ann Neurol 64(1):97–108, 2008 18668637g

Gitlin LN, Winter L, Burke J, et al: Tailored activities to manage neuropsychiatric behaviors in persons with dementia and reduce caregiver burden: a randomized pilot study. Am J Geriatr Psychiatry 16(3):229–239, 2008 18310553

Gitlin LN, Kales HC, Lyketsos CG: Nonpharmacologic management of behavioral symptoms in dementia. JAMA 308(19):2020–2029, 2012

Gordon BA, Blazey TM, Christensen J, et al: Tau PET in autosomal dominant Alzheimer's disease: relationship with cognition, dementia and other biomarkers. Brain 142(4):1063–1076, 2019 30753379

Graff-Radford NR: Normal pressure hydrocephalus. Neurol Clin 25(3):809–832, vii–viii, 2007 17659191

Graham JE, Rockwood K, Beattie BL, et al: Prevalence and severity of cognitive impairment with and without dementia in an elderly population. Lancet 349(9068):1793–1796, 1997 9269213

Hachinski V: Vascular dementia: a radical redefinition. Dementia 5(3–4):130–132, 1994 8087166

Hachinski V: The 2005 Thomas Willis Lecture: stroke and vascular cognitive impairment: a transdisciplinary, translational and transactional approach. Stroke 38(4):1396, 2007 17347469

Hamilton R, Patel S, Lee EB, et al: Lack of shunt response in suspected idiopathic normal pressure hydrocephalus with Alzheimer disease pathology. Ann Neurol 68(4):535–540, 2010 20687117

Hayden KM, Zandi PP, Lyketsos CG, et al: Vascular risk factors for incident Alzheimer disease and vascular dementia: the Cache County study. Alzheimer Dis Assoc Disord 20(2):93–100, 2006 16772744

Heron M: Deaths: Leading Causes for 2016. Natl Vital Stat Rep 67(6):1–77, 2018

Hill NT, Mowszowski L, Naismith SL, et al: Computerized cognitive training in older adults with mild cognitive impairment or dementia: a systematic review and meta-analysis. Am J Psychiatry 174(4):329–340, 2017 27838936

Ho T, Pollock BG, Mulsant BH, et al: R- and S-citalopram concentrations have differential effects on neuropsychiatric scores in elders with dementia and agitation. Br J Clin Pharmacol 82(3):784–792, 2016 27145364

Holman RC, Belay ED, Christensen KY, et al: Human prion diseases in the United States. PLoS One 5(1):e8521, 2010 20049325

Holmes C, Boche D, Wilkinson D, et al: Long-term effects of Aβ42 immunisation in Alzheimer's disease: follow-up of a randomised, placebo-controlled phase I trial. Lancet 372(9634):216–223, 2008 18640458

Hughes TA, Ross HF, Musa S, et al: A 10-year study of the incidence of and factors predicting dementia in Parkinson's disease. Neurology 54(8):1596–1602, 2000 10762499

Ismail Z, Smith EE, Geda Y, et al: Neuropsychiatric symptoms as early manifestations of emergent dementia: provisional diagnostic criteria for mild behavioral impairment. Alzheimers Dement 12(2):195–202, 2016 26096665

Isoniemi H, Tenovuo O, Portin R, et al: Outcome of traumatic brain injury after three decades: relationship to ApoE genotype. J Neurotrauma 23(11):1600–1608, 2006 17115907

Jack CR Jr, Bennett DA, Blennow K, et al: A/T/N: an unbiased descriptive classification scheme for Alzheimer disease biomarkers. Neurology 87(5):539–547, 2016 27371494

Jellinger KA, Attems J: Prevalence and impact of cerebrovascular pathology in Alzheimer's disease and parkinsonism. Acta Neurol Scand 114(1):38–46, 2006 16774626

Johns MW: A new method for measuring daytime sleepiness: the Epworth sleepiness scale. Sleep 14(6):540–545, 1991 1798888

Johnson KA, Schultz A, Betensky RA, et al: Tau positron emission tomographic imaging in aging and early Alzheimer disease. Ann Neurol 79(1):110–119, 2016 26505746

Jones BN, Teng EL, Folstein MF, Harrison KS: A new bedside test of cognition for patients with HIV infection. Ann Intern Med 119(10):1001–1004, 1993 8214976

Kales HC, Gitlin LN, Lyketsos CG: Management of neuropsychiatric symptoms of dementia in clinical settings: recommendations from a multidisciplinary expert panel. J Am Geriatr Soc 62(4):762–769, 2014 24635665

Kandiah N, Narasimhalu K, Lau PN, et al: Cognitive decline in early Parkinson's disease. Mov Disord 24(4):605–608, 2009 19191342

Kansal K, Mareddy M, Sloane KL, et al: Survival in frontotemporal dementia phenotypes: a meta-analysis. Dement Geriatr Cogn Disord 41(1–2):109–122, 2016 26854827

Kemp EC, Ebner MK, Ramanan S, et al: Statin use and risk of cognitive decline in the ADNI cohort. Am J Geriatr Psychiatry 28(5):507–517, 2020 31806426

Kertesz A, Blair M, McMonagle P, Munoz DG: The diagnosis and course of frontotemporal dementia. Alzheimer Dis Assoc Disord 21(2):155–163, 2007 17545742

Kim Y, Rosenberg P, Oh E: A review of diagnostic impact of amyloid positron emission tomography imaging in clinical practice. Dement Geriatr Cogn Disord 46(3–4):154–167, 2018 30199882

Kivipelto M, Mangialasche F, Ngandu T: Lifestyle interventions to prevent cognitive impairment, dementia and Alzheimer disease. Nat Rev Neurol 14(11):653–666, 2018 30291317

Klassen BT, Ahlskog JE: Normal pressure hydrocephalus: how often does the diagnosis hold water? Neurology 77(12):1119–1125, 2011 21849644

Knopman DS, DeKosky ST, Cummings JL, et al: Practice parameter: diagnosis of dementia (an evidence-based review): report of the Quality Standards Subcommittee of the American Academy of Neurology. Neurology 56(9):1143–1153, 2001 11342678

Lambert JC, Ibrahim-Verbaas CA, Harold D, et al: Meta-analysis of 74,046 individuals identifies 11 new susceptibility loci for Alzheimer's disease. Nat Genet 45(12):1452–1458, 2013 24162737

Leinonen V, Koivisto AM, Alafuzoff I, et al: Cortical brain biopsy in long-term prognostication of 468 patients with possible normal pressure hydrocephalus. Neurodegener Dis 10(1–4):166–169, 2012 22343771

Leonpacher AK, Peters ME, Drye LT, et al: Effects of citalopram on neuropsychiatric symptoms in Alzheimer's dementia: evidence from the CitAD Study. Am J Psychiatry 173(5):473–480, 2016 27032628

Leuzy A, Savitcheva I, Chiotis K, et al: Clinical impact of [18F]flutemetamol PET among memory clinic patients with an unclear diagnosis. Eur J Nucl Med Mol Imaging 46(6):1276–1286, 2019 30915522

Levy K, Lanctôt KL, Farber SB, et al: Does pharmacological treatment of neuropsychiatric symptoms in Alzheimer's disease relieve caregiver burden? Drugs Aging 29(3):167–179, 2012 22350526

Lippa CF, Duda JE, Grossman M, et al: DLB and PDD boundary issues: diagnosis, treatment, molecular pathology, and biomarkers. Neurology 68(11):812–819, 2007 17353469

Livingston G, Johnston K, Katona C, et al: Systematic review of psychological approaches to the management of neuropsychiatric symptoms of dementia. Am J Psychiatry 162(11):1996–2021, 2005 16263837

Longstreth WT Jr, Arnold AM, Beauchamp NJ Jr, et al: Incidence, manifestations, and predictors of worsening white matter on serial cranial magnetic resonance imaging in the elderly: the Cardiovascular Health Study. Stroke 36(1):56–61, 2005 15569873

Lopez OL, Jagust WJ, DeKosky ST, et al: Prevalence and classification of mild cognitive impairment in the Cardiovascular Health Study Cognition Study: part 1. Arch Neurol 60(10):1385–1389, 2003 14568808

Lyketsos C: The prion dementias. Maryland Medical Journal 48(1):18–22, 1999 10048280

Lyketsos CG: Lessons from neuropsychiatry. J Neuropsychiatry Clin Neurosci 18(4):445–449, 2006 17135372

Lyketsos CG, DelCampo L, Steinberg M, et al: Treating depression in Alzheimer disease: efficacy and safety of sertraline therapy, and the benefits of depression reduction: the DIADS. Arch Gen Psychiatry 60(7):737–746, 2003 12860778

Lyketsos CG, Rosenblatt A, Rabins P: Forgotten frontal lobe syndrome or "executive dysfunction syndrome." Psychosomatics 45(3):247–255, 2004 15123852

Lyketsos CG, Colenda CC, Beck C, et al: Position statement of the American Association for Geriatric Psychiatry regarding principles of care for patients with dementia resulting from Alzheimer disease. Am J Geriatr Psychiatry 14(7):561–572, 2006 16816009

Lyketsos CG, Samus QM, Baker A, et al: Effect of dementia and treatment of dementia on time to discharge from assisted living facilities: the Maryland assisted living study. J Am Geriatr Soc 55(7):1031–1037, 2007 17608875

Lyketsos CG, Carrillo MC, Ryan JM, et al: Neuropsychiatric symptoms in Alzheimer's disease. Alzheimers Dement 7(5):532–539, 2011 21889116

Mace NL, Rabins PV: The 36-Hour Day: A Family Guide to Caring for People Who Have Alzheimer Disease, Related Dementias, and Memory Loss, 5th Edition. Baltimore, MD, The Johns Hopkins University Press, 2011

Mack J, Rabins P, Anderson K, et al: Prevalence of psychotic symptoms in a community-based Parkinson disease sample. Am J Geriatr Psychiatry 20(2):123–132, 2012 21617521

Maddox RA, Person MK, Blevins JE, et al: Prion disease incidence in the United States: 2003–2015. Neurology 94(2):e153–e157, 2020

Mahajan S, Appleby BS: Comprehensive and methodical: diagnostic and management approaches to rapidly progressive dementia. Curr Treat Options Neurol 19(11):40, 2017

Mangialasche F, Solomon A, Winblad B, et al: Alzheimer's disease: clinical trials and drug development. Lancet Neurol 9(7):702–716, 2010 20610346

Manix M, Kalakoti P, Henry M, et al: Creutzfeldt-Jakob disease: updated diagnostic criteria, treatment algorithm, and the utility of brain biopsy. Neurosurg Focus 39(5):E2, 2015 26646926

Martin M, Clare L, Altgassen AM, et al: Cognition-based interventions for healthy older people and people with mild cognitive impairment. Cochrane Database Syst Rev 1(1):CD006220, 2011 21249675

Massoud F: The role of functional assessment as an outcome measure in antidementia treatment. Can J Neurol Sci 34(suppl 1):S47–S51, 2007 17469682

Massoud F, Desmarais JE, Gauthier S: Switching cholinesterase inhibitors in older adults with dementia. Int Psychogeriatr 23(3):372–378, 2011 21044399

McKeith IG, Galasko D, Kosaka K, et al: Consensus guidelines for the clinical and pathologic diagnosis of dementia with Lewy bodies (DLB): report of the Consortium on DLB International Workshop. Neurology 47(5):1113–1124, 1996 8909416

McKeith I, Mintzer J, Aarsland D, et al: Dementia with Lewy bodies. Lancet Neurol 3(1):19–28, 2004 14693108

McKeith IG, Boeve BF, Dickson DW, et al: Diagnosis and management of dementia with Lewy bodies: fourth consensus report of the DLB Consortium. Neurology 89(1):88–100, 2017 28592453

McShane R, Westby MJ, Roberts E, et al: Memantine for dementia. Cochrane Database Syst Rev 3(3):CD003154, 2019

Medway C, Morgan K: Review: the genetics of Alzheimer's disease; putting flesh on the bones. Neuropathol Appl Neurobiol 40(2):97–105, 2014 24443964

Meier U, Lemcke J, Neumann U: Predictors of outcome in patients with normal-pressure hydrocephalus. Acta Neurochir Suppl (Wien) 96:352–357, 2006 16671484

Metzler-Baddeley C: A review of cognitive impairments in dementia with Lewy bodies relative to Alzheimer's disease and Parkinson's disease with dementia. Cortex 43(5):583–600, 2007 17715794

Meyer PF, Tremblay-Mercier J, Leoutsakos J, et al: A randomized trial of naproxen to slow progress of presymptomatic Alzheimer disease. Neurology 92(18):e2070–e2080, 2019

Michalczyk K, Ziman M: Current concepts in human prion protein (Prp) misfolding, Prnp gene polymorphisms and their contribution to Creutzfeldt-Jakob Disease (CJD). Histol Histopathol 22(10):1149–1159, 2007 17616941

Mielke MM, Rosenberg PB, Tschanz J, et al: Vascular factors predict rate of progression in Alzheimer disease. Neurology 69(19):1850–1858, 2007 17984453

Mintzer J, Lanctôt KL, Scherer RW, et al: Effect of methylphenidate on apathy in patients with Alzheimer disease: the ADMET 2 randomized clinical trial. JAMA Neurol 78(11):1324–1332, 2021

Mittelman MS, Haley WE, Clay OJ, Roth DL: Improving caregiver well-being delays nursing home placement of patients with Alzheimer disease. Neurology 67(9):1592–1599, 2006 17101889

Moghekar A, Rao S, Li M, et al: Large quantities of Aβ peptide are constitutively released during amyloid precursor protein metabolism in vivo and in vitro. J Biol Chem 286(18):15989–15997, 2011 21454701

Molinari V, Chiriboga D, Branch LG, et al: Provision of psychopharmacological services in nursing homes. J Gerontol B Psychol Sci Soc Sci 65B(1):57–60, 2010 19846475

Moniz Cook ED, Swift K, James I, et al: Functional analysis-based interventions for challenging behaviour in dementia. Cochrane Database Syst Rev 2(2):CD006929, 2012 22336826

Morelli L, Perry G, Tagliavini F: The contribution of the amyloid hypothesis to the understanding of Alzheimer's disease: a critical overview. Int J Alzheimers Dis 2012:709613, 2012 22970405

Morris MC, Tangney CC, Wang Y, et al: MIND diet slows cognitive decline with aging. Alzheimers Dement 11(9):1015–1022, 2015 26086182

Morrison CE, Borod JC, Brin MF, et al: Effects of levodopa on cognitive functioning in moderate-to-severe Parkinson's disease (MSPD). J Neural Transm 111(10–11):1333–1341, 2004 15480842

Mucke L, Selkoe DJ: Neurotoxicity of amyloid β-protein: synaptic and network dysfunction. Cold Spring Harb Perspect Med 2(7):a006338, 2012 22762015

Nagaraja D, Jayashree S: Randomized study of the dopamine receptor agonist piribedil in the treatment of mild cognitive impairment. Am J Psychiatry 158(9):1517–1519, 2001 11532743

Nasreddine ZS, Phillips NA, Bédirian V, et al: The Montreal Cognitive Assessment, MoCA: a brief screening tool for mild cognitive impairment. J Am Geriatr Soc 53(4):695–699, 2005 15817019

National Institute for Health and Care Excellence: Donepezil, Galantamine, Rivastigmine and Memantine for the Treatment of Alzheimer's Disease. Review of NICE Technology Appraisal Guidance 117. London, National Institute for Health and Care Excellence, 2011. Available at: http://guidance.nice.org.uk/TA217/Guidance/pdf/English. Accessed February 2014.

National Institute for Health and Care Excellence: Dementia: Assessment, Management, and Support for People Living With Dementia and Their Carers. NICE Guideline 97. London, National Institute for Health and Care Excellence, 2018. Available at: https://www.nice.org.uk/guidance/ng97/chapter/Recommendations#diagnosis. Accessed December 2019.

Neary D, Snowden J, Mann D: Frontotemporal dementia. Lancet Neurol 4(11):771–780, 2005 16239184

Negash S, Bennett DA, Wilson RS, et al: Cognition and neuropathology in aging: multidimensional perspectives from the Rush Religious Orders Study and Rush Memory and Aging Project. Curr Alzheimer Res 8(4):336–340, 2011 21222592

Newhouse P, Kellar K, Aisen P, et al: Nicotine treatment of mild cognitive impairment: a 6-month double-blind pilot clinical trial. Neurology 78(2):91–101, 2012 22232050

Ngandu T, Lehtisalo J, Solomon A, et al: A 2 year multidomain intervention of diet, exercise, cognitive training, and vascular risk monitoring versus control to prevent cognitive decline in at-risk elderly people (FINGER): a randomised controlled trial. Lancet 385(9984):2255–2263, 2015 25771249

Nowrangi MA, Rao V, Lyketsos CG: Epidemiology, assessment, and treatment of dementia. Psychiatr Clin North Am 34(2):275–294, 2011

Okura T, Plassman BL, Steffens DC, et al: Prevalence of neuropsychiatric symptoms and their association with functional limitations in older adults in the United States: the aging, demographics, and memory study. J Am Geriatr Soc 58(2):330–337, 2010 20374406

Ossenkoppele R, Schonhaut DR, Schöll M, et al: Tau PET patterns mirror clinical and neuroanatomical variability in Alzheimer's disease. Brain 139(Pt 5):1551–1567, 2016 26962052

Palmer K, Berger AK, Monastero R, et al: Predictors of progression from mild cognitive impairment to Alzheimer disease. Neurology 68(19):1596–1602, 2007 17485646

Peters ME, Rosenberg PB, Steinberg M, et al: Neuropsychiatric symptoms as risk factors for progression from CIND to dementia: the Cache County Study. Am J Geriatr Psychiatry 21(11):1116–1124, 2013 23567370

Peters ME, Schwartz S, Han D, et al: Neuropsychiatric symptoms as predictors of progression to severe Alzheimer's dementia and death: the Cache County Dementia Progression Study. Am J Psychiatry 172(5):460–465, 2015 25585033

Petersen RC, Thomas RG, Grundman M, et al: Vitamin E and donepezil for the treatment of mild cognitive impairment. N Engl J Med 352(23):2379–2388, 2005 15829527

Petersen RC, Roberts RO, Knopman DS, et al: Mild cognitive impairment: ten years later. Arch Neurol 66(12):1447–1455, 2009 20008648

Petersson SD, Philippou E: Mediterranean diet, cognitive function, and dementia: a systematic review of the evidence. Adv Nutr 7(5):889–904, 2016 27633105

Pimplikar SW: Reassessing the amyloid cascade hypothesis of Alzheimer's disease. Int J Biochem Cell Biol 41(6):1261–1268, 2009 19124085

Pontone GM, Dissanayka N, Apostolova L, et al: Report from a multidisciplinary meeting on anxiety as a non-motor manifestation of Parkinson's disease. NPJ Parkinsons Dis 5:30, 2019 31840044

Porsteinsson AP, Drye LT, Pollock BG, et al: Effect of citalopram on agitation in Alzheimer disease: the CitAD randomized clinical trial. JAMA 311(7):682–691, 2014 24549548

Prince M, Bryce R, Albanese E, et al: The global prevalence of dementia: a systematic review and metaanalysis. Alzheimers Dement 9(1):63–75, 2013 23305823

Puoti G, Bizzi A, Forloni G, et al: Sporadic human prion diseases: molecular insights and diagnosis. Lancet Neurol 11(7):618–628, 2012 22710755

Rabinovici GD, Gatsonis C, Apgar C, et al: Association of amyloid positron emission tomography with subsequent change in clinical management among Medicare beneficiaries with mild cognitive impairment or dementia. JAMA 321(13):1286–1294, 2019 30938796

Rabins PV, Lyketsos CG: Antipsychotic drugs in dementia: what should be made of the risks? JAMA 294(15):1963–1965, 2005 16234504

Rabins PV, Schwartz S, Black BS, et al: Predictors of progression to severe Alzheimer's disease in an incidence sample. Alzheimers Dement 9(2):204–207, 2013 23123228

Rabins PV, Lyketsos CG, Steele CD: Practical Dementia Care, 3rd Edition. New York, Oxford University Press, 2016

Ranginwala NA, Hynan LS, Weiner MF, White CL III: Clinical criteria for the diagnosis of Alzheimer disease: still good after all these years. Am J Geriatr Psychiatry 16(5):384–388, 2008 18448850

Rogaeva E, Meng Y, Lee JH, et al: The neuronal sortilin-related receptor SORL1 is genetically associated with Alzheimer disease. Nat Genet 39(2):168–177, 2007 17220890

Rolinski M, Fox C, Maidment I, McShane R: Cholinesterase inhibitors for dementia with Lewy bodies, Parkinson's disease dementia and cognitive impairment in Parkinson's disease. Cochrane Database Syst Rev 3(3):CD006504, 2012 22419314

Rosenberg PB, Johnston D, Lyketsos CG: A clinical approach to mild cognitive impairment. Am J Psychiatry 163(11):1884–1890, 2006 17074938

Rosenberg PB, Drye LT, Martin BK, et al: Sertraline for the treatment of depression in Alzheimer disease. Am J Geriatr Psychiatry 18(2):136–145, 2010 20087081

Rosenberg PB, Lanctôt KL, Drye LT, et al: Safety and efficacy of methylphenidate for apathy in Alzheimer's disease: a randomized, placebo-controlled trial. J Clin Psychiatry 74(8):810–816, 2013 24021498

Roth HL: Dementia and sleep. Neurol Clin 30(4):1213–1248, 2012 23099135

Royall DR, Lauterbach EC, Kaufer D, et al: The cognitive correlates of functional status: a review from the Committee on Research of the American Neuropsychiatric Association. J Neuropsychiatry Clin Neurosci 19(3):249–265, 2007 17827410

Russ TC, Morling JR: Cholinesterase inhibitors for mild cognitive impairment. Cochrane Database Syst Rev 9(9):CD009132, 2012 22972133

Ruthirakuhan MT, Herrmann N, Abraham EH, et al: Pharmacological interventions for apathy in Alzheimer's disease. Cochrane Database Syst Rev (5):CD012197, 2018 29727467

Sabbagh MN, Shah F, Reid RT, et al: Pathologic and nicotinic receptor binding differences between mild cognitive impairment, Alzheimer disease, and normal aging. Arch Neurol 63(12):1771–1776, 2006 17172618

Sabbagh MN, Adler CH, Lahti TJ, et al: Parkinson disease with dementia: comparing patients with and without Alzheimer pathology. Alzheimer Dis Assoc Disord 23(3):295–297, 2009 19812474

Samus QM, Johnston D, Black BS, et al: A multidimensional home-based care coordination intervention for elders with memory disorders: the Maximizing Independence at Home (MIND) pilot randomized trial. Am J Geriatr Psychiatry 22(4):398–414, 2014 24502822

Sano M, Ernesto C, Thomas RG, et al: A controlled trial of selegiline, alpha-tocopherol, or both as treatment for Alzheimer's disease: the Alzheimer's Disease Cooperative Study. N Engl J Med 336(17):1216–1222, 1997 9110909

Saper CB: The emperor has no clothes. Ann Neurol 79:165–166, 2016

Scarmeas N, Brandt J, Blacker D, et al: Disruptive behavior as a predictor in Alzheimer disease. Arch Neurol 64(12):1755–1761, 2007 18071039

Scherer RW, Drye L, Mintzer J, et al: The Apathy in Dementia Methylphenidate Trial 2 (ADMET 2): study protocol for a randomized controlled trial. Trials 19(1):46, 2018 29347996

Schneider JA, Wilson RS, Bienias JL, et al: Cerebral infarctions and the likelihood of dementia from Alzheimer disease pathology. Neurology 62(7):1148–1155, 2004 15079015

Schneider LS, Dagerman KS, Insel P: Risk of death with atypical antipsychotic drug treatment for dementia: meta-analysis of randomized placebo-controlled trials. JAMA 294(15):1934–1943, 2005 16234500

Schwarz S, Froelich L, Burns A: Pharmacological treatment of dementia. Curr Opin Psychiatry 25(6):542–550, 2012 22992546

Seitz DP, Gill SS, Herrmann N, et al: Pharmacological treatments for neuropsychiatric symptoms of dementia in long-term care: a systematic review. Int Psychogeriatr 25(2):185–203, 2013 23083438

Selkoe DJ: The molecular pathology of Alzheimer's disease. Neuron 6(4):487–498, 1991 1673054

Seltman RE, Matthews BR: Frontotemporal lobar degeneration: epidemiology, pathology, diagnosis and management. CNS Drugs 26(10):841–870, 2012 22950490

Selwood A, Johnston K, Katona C, et al: Systematic review of the effect of psychological interventions on family caregivers of people with dementia. J Affect Disord 101(1–3):75–89, 2007 17173977

Sepehry AA, Lee PE, Hsiung GY, et al: Effect of selective serotonin reuptake inhibitors in Alzheimer's disease with comorbid depression: a meta-analysis of depression and cognitive outcomes. Drugs Aging 29(10):793–806, 2012 23079957

Shimada H, Hirano S, Shinotoh H, et al: Mapping of brain acetylcholinesterase alterations in Lewy body disease by PET. Neurology 73(4):273–278, 2009 19474411

Shulman JM, De Jager PL: Evidence for a common pathway linking neurodegenerative diseases. Nat Genet 41(12):1261–1262, 2009 19935760

Simard M, van Reekum R: The acetylcholinesterase inhibitors for treatment of cognitive and behavioral symptoms in dementia with Lewy bodies. J Neuropsychiatry Clin Neurosci 16(4):409–425, 2004 15616167

Sink KM, Holden KF, Yaffe K: Pharmacological treatment of neuropsychiatric symptoms of dementia: a review of the evidence. JAMA 293(5):596–608, 2005 15687315

Sink KM, Espeland MA, Castro CM, et al: Effect of a 24-month physical activity intervention vs. health education on cognitive outcomes in sedentary older adults: the LIFE randomized trial. JAMA 314(8):781–790, 2015 26305648

Snowdon DA, Greiner LH, Mortimer JA, et al: Brain infarction and the clinical expression of Alzheimer disease: the Nun Study. JAMA 277(10):813–817, 1997 9052711

Steffens DC, Blazer DG, Thakur ME (eds): The American Psychiatric Publishing Textbook of Geriatric Psychiatry, 5th Edition. Washington, DC, American Psychiatric Publishing, 2015

Stahl SM: Essential Psychopharmacology: The Prescriber's Guide, Revised and Updated Edition. New York, Cambridge University Press, 2006

Steinberg M, Shao H, Zandi P, et al: Point and 5-year period prevalence of neuropsychiatric symptoms in dementia: the Cache County Study. Int J Geriatr Psychiatry 23(2):170–177, 2008 17607801

Sultzer DL, Davis SM, Tariot PN, et al: Clinical symptom responses to atypical antipsychotic medications in Alzheimer's disease: phase 1 outcomes from the CATIE-AD effectiveness trial. Am J Psychiatry 165(7):844–854, 2008 18519523

Taylor J, Anderson WS, Brandt J, et al: Neuropsychiatric complications of Parkinson disease treatments: importance of multidisciplinary care. Am J Geriatr Psychiatry 24(12):1171–1180, 2016 27746069

Teng EL, Chui HC: The Modified Mini-Mental State (3MS) examination. J Clin Psychiatry 48(8):314–318, 1987 3611032

Theis W, Bleiler L, Alzheimer's Association: 2013 Alzheimer's disease facts and figures. Alzheimers Dement 9(2):208–245, 2013 23507120

Tiraboschi P, Salmon DP, Hansen LA, et al: What best differentiates Lewy body from Alzheimer's disease in early stage dementia? Brain 129(pt 3):729–735, 2006 16401618

Treiber KA, Lyketsos CG, Corcoran C, et al: Vascular factors and risk for neuropsychiatric symptoms in Alzheimer's disease: the Cache County Study. Int Psychogeriatr 20(3):538–553, 2008 18289451

Tremont G, Davis J, Papandonatos GD, et al: A telephone intervention for dementia caregivers: background, design, and baseline characteristics. Contemp Clin Trials 36(2):338–347, 2013 23916916

Tremont G, Davis J, Papandonatos GD, et al: Psychosocial telephone intervention for dementia caregivers: a randomized, controlled trial. Alzheimers Dement 11(5):541–548, 2015 25074341

Trompet S, van Vliet P, de Craen AJ, et al: Pravastatin and cognitive function in the elderly: results of the PROSPER study. J Neurol 257(1):85–90, 2010 19653027

Tschanz JT, Welsh-Bohmer KA, Lyketsos CG, et al: Conversion to dementia from mild cognitive disorder: the Cache County Study. Neurology 67(2):229–234, 2006 16864813

Tschanz JT, Corcoran CD, Schwartz S, et al: Progression of cognitive, functional, and neuropsychiatric symptom domains in a population cohort with Alzheimer dementia: the Cache County Dementia Progression Study. Am J Geriatr Psychiatry 19(6):532–542, 2011 21606896

Tschanz JT, Norton MC, Zandi PP, Lyketsos CG: The Cache County Study on Memory in Aging: factors affecting risk of Alzheimer's disease and its progression after onset. Int Rev Psychiatry 25(6):673–685, 2013 24423221

U.S. Food and Drug Administration: FDA Drug Safety and Availability: Information for Healthcare Professionals: Conventional Antipsychotics. Silver Spring, MD, U.S. Food and Drug Administration, 2008. Available at: http://www.fda.gov/Drugs/DrugSafety/ucm124830.htm. Accessed March 1, 2013.

U.S. Food and Drug Administration: FDA Drug Safety and Availability: Revised Recommendations for Celexa (Citalopram Hydrobromide) Related to a Potential Risk of Abnormal Heart Rhythms With High Doses. Silver Spring, MD, U.S. Food and Drug Administration, 2012. Available at: http://www.fda.gov/Drugs/DrugSafety/ucm297391.htm. Accessed March 1, 2013.

Uttley L, Carroll C, Wong R, et al: Creutzfeldt-Jakob disease: a systematic review of global incidence, prevalence, infectivity, and incubation. Lancet Infect Dis 20(1):e2–e10, 2020 31876504

van der Burg M, Bouwen A, Stessens J, et al: Scoring clock tests for dementia screening: a comparison of two scoring methods. Int J Geriatr Psychiatry 19(7):685–689, 2004 15254925

Vanneste J, Augustijn P, Dirven C, et al: Shunting normal-pressure hydrocephalus: do the benefits outweigh the risks? A multicenter study and literature review. Neurology 42(1):54–59, 1992 1734324

Venkatraman VK, Sanderson A, Cox KL, et al: Effect of a 24-month physical activity program on brain changes in older adults at risk of Alzheimer's disease: the AIBL active trial. Neurobiol Aging 89:132–141, 2020

Villemagne VL, Fodero-Tavoletti MT, Pike KE, et al: The ART of loss: Abeta imaging in the evaluation of Alzheimer's disease and other dementias. Mol Neurobiol 38(1):1–15, 2008 18690556

Walsh DM, Selkoe DJ: Aβ oligomers: a decade of discovery. J Neurochem 101(5):1172–1184, 2007 17286590

Weintraub D, Burn DJ: Parkinson's disease: the quintessential neuropsychiatric disorder. Mov Disord 26(6):1022–1031, 2011 21626547

Weintraub D, Katz IR: Pharmacologic interventions for psychosis and agitation in neurodegenerative diseases: evidence about efficacy and safety. Psychiatr Clin North Am 28:941–983, ix–x, 2005

Weintraub D, Rosenberg PB, Drye LT, et al: Sertraline for the treatment of depression in Alzheimer disease: week-24 outcomes. Am J Geriatr Psychiatry 18(4):332–340, 2010 20220589

White L: Brain lesions at autopsy in older Japanese-American men as related to cognitive impairment and dementia in the final years of life: a summary report from the Honolulu-Asia aging study. J Alzheimers Dis 18(3):713–725, 2009 19661625

Wilson RK, Williams MA: Normal pressure hydrocephalus. Clin Geriatr Med 22:935–951, 2006

Wolfson C, Wolfson DB, Asgharian M, et al: A reevaluation of the duration of survival after the onset of dementia. N Engl J Med 344(15):1111–1116, 2001 11297701

Wong DF, Rosenberg PB, Zhou Y, et al: In vivo imaging of amyloid deposition in Alzheimer disease using the radioligand 18F-AV-45 (florbetapir [corrected] F 18). J Nucl Med 51(6):913–920, 2010 20501908

Woodruff BK: Evaluation of rapidly progressive dementia. Semin Neurol 27(4):363–375, 2007 17701874

Yang G, Wang Y, Tian J, Liu JP: Huperzine A for Alzheimer's disease: a systematic review and meta-analysis of randomized clinical trials. PLoS One 8(9):e74916, 2013 24086396

Yang T, Wang H, Xiong Y, et al: Vitamin D supplementation improves cognitive function through reducing oxidative stress regulated by telomere length in older adults with mild cognitive impairment: a 12-month randomized controlled trial. J Alzheimers Dis 78(4):1509–1518, 2020 33164936

Yassine HN, Schneider LS: Lessons from the Multidomain Alzheimer Preventive Trial. Lancet Neurol 16(8):585–586, 2017

Young J, Angevaren M, Rusted J, Tabet N: Aerobic exercise to improve cognitive function in older people without known cognitive impairment. Cochrane Database Syst Rev (4):CD005381, 2015 25900537

Yu JT, Li JQ, Suckling J, et al: Frequency and longitudinal clinical outcomes of Alzheimer's AT(N) biomarker profiles: a longitudinal study. Alzheimers Dement 15(9):1208–1217, 2019 31399333

Zadikoff C, Fox SH, Tang-Wai DF, et al: A comparison of the Mini Mental State Exam to the Montreal Cognitive Assessment in identifying cognitive deficits in Parkinson's disease. Mov Disord 23(2):297–299, 2008 18044697

CHAPTER 9

Depressive Disorders

Patricia Andrews, M.D.

Warren D. Taylor, M.D., M.H.Sc.

Depression in later life is heterogeneous. It can present either as a recurrent episode in an elderly person with a personal history of multiple prior episodes or as a first episode in someone with no prior lifetime history. It can occur following loss, such as bereavement or loss of independence, or without obvious precipitating stresses. Depression can develop alongside chronic pain or persistent medical illness or accompany cognitive decline and dementia. Some individuals respond to the first treatment offered, whereas others have treatment-resistant late-life depression (LLD). How can one make sense of this heterogeneity? Answers to this question in part depend on how depression is defined.

The prevailing paradigm is to conceive of depression as phenomenologically homogeneous using a syndrome-based categorical approach, as exemplified in DSM-5 (American Psychiatric Association 2013). If one views mood disorders as a group of distinct entities or independent syndromes, the diagnosis and management of depression are allied with the traditional medical model. Given the availability of effective biological and psychosocial therapies for depressed older adults, this categorical approach is used by most geriatric psychiatrists. Specific therapies are thus targeted to distinct diagnostic entities.

An alternative approach is to view depression as a unitary phenomenon, with its various manifestations forming a continuum. Depression symptom checklist scales, such as the Center for Epidemiologic Studies–Depression Scale (Radloff 1977) and the Geriatric Depression Scale (Yesavage et al. 1982–1983), are useful in determining the degree to which an individual experiences depressive symptoms. Compared with DSM-5's categorical approach, this continuum offers the advantage of identifying mild depressive symptoms that are below the syndrome threshold but may still adversely affect health outcomes. However, it shares a common limitation with categorical diagnoses in that two individuals with a similar diagnosis may exhibit very different symptom profiles.

Another conceptualization of the elder person with depression is to take a functional approach: when the depressive symptoms become so severe that functioning is impaired, the case is considered worthy of clinical attention. Social functioning, especially the performance of role responsibilities, is a key outcome variable when monitoring treatment. Functional capacity is a critical element for family members, who do not view symptom remission alone as an essential marker of improvement but rather emphasize a return to social involvement and improved life satisfaction. An older adult who sleeps better, has a better appetite, and ceases to be suicidal may be considered improved by the clinician but not by the family if the patient's isolation and disinterest in the social environment persist. Functional impairment should thus be considered in any conceptualization of depression. A limitation of relying exclusively on this approach is that less severe symptoms that do not dramatically affect function may be overlooked.

Key depressive disorders included in DSM-5 that are relevant to depression in elderly patients include 1) major depressive disorder (MDD; either with or without psychotic features), 2) persistent depressive disorder (dysthymia), 3) depressive episode with insufficient symptoms (previously called minor or subsyndromal depression), 4) substance/medication-induced depressive disorder, and 5) depressive disorder due to another medical condition. Moving to mood disorders more broadly, we see that bipolar disorders also present with distinct depressive episodes. Depressive symptoms are likewise present in other disorder categories in DSM-5; for example, adjustment disorder with depressed mood is classified with the DSM-5 trauma- and stressor-related disorders, and persistent complex bereavement disorder is listed under "Other Specified Trauma- and Stressor-Related Disorders."

Epidemiology

An overview of the epidemiology of psychiatric disorders in late life is presented in Chapter 1, "Epidemiology of Psychiatric Disorders in Later Life." In this chapter, we discuss information specific to mood disorders. In an early community survey, investigators at Duke University Medical Center attempted to untangle the different subtypes of depression in late life (Blazer et al. 1987). More than 1,300 older adults age 60 years and older were screened for depressive symptoms. Of the 27% who reported such symptoms, 19% had only mild dysphoria. Individuals with more severe symptoms made up 4% of the population. These more severely affected individuals were primarily experiencing stressors such as physical illness and stressful life events. Only 2% had dysthymia, and 0.8% were experiencing a current major depressive episode.

In another study, the frequency of MDD in the community was ~3.7% among subjects ages 75–84 and 2.1% among those age 75 years and older; 1.2% had a mixed depression and anxiety syndrome (Institute of Medicine Committee on Mental Health Workforce for Geriatric Populations 2012). Most studies have found that a DSM-5 diagnosis occurs in 4%–5% of older, community-dwelling adults (Blazer 2003). Surveys have confirmed the lower frequency of MDD in the community (Kessler et al. 2005). These data suggest that the DSM-5 depression categories may not clearly capture the experience of older adults in the community who experience depressive symptoms.

In hospital and long-term care settings, the frequency of MDD among older adults is much higher than in community settings. Up to 21% of hospitalized elder patients meet criteria for a major depressive episode, and an additional 20%–25% have minor (subsyndromal) depression (Koenig et al. 1988). Rates of MDD among elderly nursing home patients exceed 25% in some studies (Parmelee et al. 1992). Depressive symptoms are even more common following critical care hospitalizations and are found in 37% of patients (Jackson et al. 2014).

How does one reconcile these seemingly disparate results? "Depression in late life" remains a generic term that captures many constructs, some of which are well-defined and others ill-defined. The burden of depression in elderly patients, as indicated by the frequency of significant depressive symptoms in community populations just described, is unquestioned. Many older persons with atypical presentations of depression do not meet criteria for MDD yet have clinically significant depressive symptoms (Hybels et al. 2001).

Clinical Course

Depression is a recurrent and, at times, chronic illness. Data from community studies illustrate this chronicity: among subjects with clinically significant depressive symptoms, 23% improved, 44% had an unfavorable but fluctuating course, and 33% had a severe and chronic course (Beekman et al. 2002). A chronic course was observed in 35% of older subjects diagnosed with MDD and 52% of subjects with dysthymic disorder. When compared with younger cohorts, older age is a risk factor for a poor course of MDD, including greater chronicity, longer time to remission, and greater depression severity (Schaakxs et al. 2018).

Studies focused on older adults in clinical settings have found similar courses of illness (Alexopoulos et al. 1996; Deng et al. 2018; Murphy 1983). In a group of elderly subjects with depression followed for more than 1 year, 35% experienced a good outcome, 48% experienced a fluctuating course or remained continuously ill, and 14% died (Murphy 1983). In a group of elderly patients followed for 25 years after experiencing severe depression earlier in life, only 12% fully remitted and experienced no recurrences over the study duration (Brodaty et al. 2001). Comorbid depression is associated with a less favorable prognosis. For example, when MDD is comorbid with persistent depressive disorder (dysthymia), the prognosis is poor. Poor social support and functional limitations increase the risk of not achieving remission or of achieving only partial remission (Hybels et al. 2005).

Depressive symptoms that do not meet criteria for MDD are common in older adult populations. Individuals with a persistent depressive disorder (dysthymia) have a more chronic clinical course than do older adults with MDD. Per DSM-5, a person's depressive symptoms must last at least 2 years for this diagnosis. An undetermined percentage (as high as 4%–8%) of community-dwelling elderly adults experience moderately severe depressive symptoms for more than 2 years, although they describe intermittent periods, not lasting longer than a few days, of relative freedom from their depressive symptoms. The severity of their symptoms is not great enough to meet the criteria for MDD, and the intermittent symptom-free periods disqualify them from the diagnosis of persistent depressive disorder (dysthymia). Such subthreshold depression is two to three times more prevalent than MDD and increases the risk for the development of a full major depressive episode (Meeks et al. 2011).

Acute treatment of depressive episodes in older adults includes the same options as treatment used for younger adults, including psychotherapy, pharmacotherapy, and neurostimulation (and are discussed in detail later in this chapter). Typically, psychotherapy or first-line pharmacotherapy options are used as initial treatments for mild or moderate depression severity, with second- or third-line pharmacotherapy or neurostimulation reserved for severe or treatment-resistant depression. Data clearly support that these treatments are effective in older adults (Huang et al. 2015; Nelson and Devanand 2011; Nelson et al. 2008), with response rates ranging from 40% to 50% or higher for electroconvulsive therapy (ECT). More recent work has focused on non-pharmacological approaches that may enhance resilience to stressors, such as meditation or movement-based exercise interventions (Laird et al. 2019).

Even when remission is achieved, the risk of recurrence remains substantial. Although maintenance antidepressant treatment reduces this risk (Reynolds et al. 1999, 2006), even with continued treatment, recurrence rates can approach 60% over 4 years (Deng et al. 2018). Despite the recurrent nature of LLD, little is known regarding what clinical and biological factors contribute to this recurrence (Andreescu et al. 2019). Although we know that a greater number of past depressive episodes is a strong predictor of future recurrence, other clinical factors that increase the risk for recurrence of LLD include residual depressive symptoms, earlier age at initial depression onset, greater physical disability, less support with activities, and higher perceived stress (Deng et al. 2018).

Complications and Consequences of Late-Life Depression

Cognitive Impairment

Depressive symptoms are associated with both poorer performance on cognitive and neuropsychological testing and outright cognitive impairment. Greater impairment in cognitive performance, particularly executive dysfunction, is associated with a poor acute response to antidepressant medications (Alexopoulos et al. 2005; Baldwin et al. 2004; Sneed et al. 2007). Executive dysfunction is a frontally mediated cognitive domain (Elderkin-Thompson et al. 2003; Nebes et al. 2001) that is characterized by poor performance on measures of verbal fluency, problem solving, cognitive flexibility, and response inhibition. While executive dysfunction is the best studied, deficits in episodic memory and processing speed are also associated with poorer acute antidepressant response (Sheline et al. 2010) and poorer long-term course of depression (Story et al. 2008).

When antidepressant treatment is successful, cognitive performance often improves. However, elder persons with previous depression still may not perform as well as expected, and deficits often persist (Bhalla et al. 2006, 2009; Butters et al. 2000; Koenig et al. 2015; Nebes et al. 2003). Even following remission, LLD is associated with accelerated cognitive decline (Koenig et al. 2015; Riddle et al. 2017). In time, this may evolve into a clear neurocognitive disorder; LLD is associated with an increased risk of dementia, with an odds ratio of ~2.0 (Diniz et al. 2013). Depressive symptoms accompanied by cognitive impairment may thus represent a preclinical sign and should be considered a risk marker for Alzheimer's disease (AD) or vascular dementia (Li et al. 2001). The effects of depression and neuropathology appear additive. When depression is comorbid with mild cognitive impairment or AD, it can worsen cognitive impairment beyond what would be expected based on neuropathology alone (Wilson et al. 2014).

Medical Comorbidity

Depression and medical problems are frequently comorbid, and the causal pathway may be bidirectional (Blazer and Hybels 2005; Taylor 2014). Many chronic medical illnesses, such as cardiovascular disease, diabetes, osteoporosis, back pain, and hip fracture, are associated with a greater frequency of depression, and co-occurring depression may contribute to poorer medical outcomes (Heikkinen et al. 2019; Jiang et al. 2001; Lenze et al. 2007; Moulton et al. 2015). Depression in older adults is similarly associated with frailty (Rutherford et al. 2017), a syndrome defined by weakness, decreased activity, slowed gait, and unintentional weight loss (Fried et al. 2001). Many older adults with severe depression meet frailty criteria, and as with other medical illness, the relationship between depression and frailty is bidirectional (Mezuk et al. 2013). Depression with comorbid frailty is associated with greater functional impairment and a poorer course than that with either illness alone (Brown et al. 2014).

Perhaps the best-established association between depression and physical problems is that between depression and functional impairment (Bruce 2001). Older adults with depression are 67% more likely than those without depression to experience impairment in activities of daily living and 73% more likely to experience mobility restrictions 6 years after the initial evaluation (Penninx et al. 1999). Disability, in turn, increases the risk for depressive symptoms (Kennedy et al. 1990). Functional decline is not inevitable when the older adult becomes depressed, however; for example, instrumental support provided to older adults, such as help in tasks necessary for daily living, can protect against worsening disability and therefore buffer against its effect on the development or perpetuation of depression (Hays et al. 2001).

Mortality

Mortality is a significant adverse outcome resulting from LLD. A large meta-analysis of depression in the community found that, after adjusting for publication bias, the relative risk of mortality in participants with depression relative to participants without depression was 1.52 (95% CI 1.45–1.59) (Cuijpers et al. 2014). This equates to an ~50% increased mortality risk in people with depression. In chronic obstructive pulmonary disease, depression is associated with a higher mortality risk than is seen in other medical disorders; however, there is no indication that the impact of depression on the relative risk of mortality significantly differs across patient samples with heart disease, cerebrovascular disease, cancer, kidney disease, or other illnesses (Cuijpers et al. 2014; Eurelings et al. 2018). Depression's effect on mortality risk may be slightly higher in lower- or middle-income countries (Brandão et al. 2019). Both severity and duration of depressive symptoms predicted mortality in elderly populations (Geerlings et al. 2002), although some have found that apathy may be particularly related to mortality (Eurelings et al. 2018).

Suicide

Suicide is the tenth leading cause of death in the United States, and rates are increasing. Data from the Centers for Disease Control and Prevention indicate that the age-adjusted suicide rate has increased by 35% since 1999, and suicide was responsible for more than 48,000 deaths in 2018 (Hedegaard et al. 2020). Although suicide rates have steadily increased across all age groups, older adults disproportionately contribute to these numbers. Adults age 70 are older have the highest risk for suicide in most regions in the world (Van Orden and Conwell 2016), but risk varies by sex. Suicide rates among males are highest for those age 75 years and older, at 39.9 per 100,000 people. In contrast, suicide rates in females are highest for those age 45–64 years; females age 75 years and older have a *lower* risk compared with all other age groups except early adolescence (Hedegaard et al. 2020). Suicide rates in older adults with dementia may be even higher (Erlangsen et al. 2008). Some of these demographic changes may be related to cohort effects, because members of the Baby Boomer generation have traditionally had higher suicide rates than other birth cohorts (Conwell et al. 2011).

Although there are far more episodes of suicidal ideation or attempts than there are completed suicides, suicidal behavior in older adults is more likely to result in death than in those of younger ages. Although the ratio of suicide attempts to completed suicides in the general population is estimated at 10–20 to 1 (Nock et al. 2008), in older adults as many as 1 in 4 suicide attempts may be successful (Crosby et al. 1999). There may be many reasons for this. Older adults are less likely to report suicidal thoughts (Duberstein et al. 1999), have a greater likelihood of using highly lethal methods such as firearms (Kaplan and Geling 1999), and are less likely to receive care in mental health clinics (Conwell and Thompson 2008). Instead, they may present to primary care, with up to two-thirds of older adults who commit suicide having been seen by their primary care physician within 1 month of their deaths (Conwell et al. 2000). Brief depression screens at primary care visits can identify older adults with suicidal thoughts (Heisel et al. 2010). Less severe suicidal thoughts, such as the presence of passive suicidal ideation or thoughts of death, are also common. In community samples, passive thoughts in the past month are estimated at 6.5% (Ayalon and Litwin 2009), with a frequency of 15% in primary care samples (Raue et al. 2010). Ideation in older adults with depression may range from 25% to almost 60% (Britton et al. 2008; Bruce et al. 2004). While some thoughts of death may be a normal response to nearing the end of life, they should not be discounted. Among older adults, those who endorse passive ideation may switch to active ideation during depressive episodes (Szanto et al. 1996).

Etiology

The etiology of late-life depressive disorders is undoubtedly multifactorial, with a combination of biological and psychological factors influencing vulnerability and risk (Table 9–1). Each person with depression may have a distinct pattern of risk factors. Moreover, some risk factors may be interrelated, such as medical illnesses contributing to cerebrovascular changes or stressful life events influencing endocrine or inflammatory changes.

Although LLD is a heterogeneous disorder with multiple potential contributors or causal factors, a simple assessment of age at depression onset may help parse this het-

Biological risk factors	Psychological risk factors
Genetics	Personality attributes (e.g., hopelessness, ambivalence)
Female sex	
Endocrine changes	Neuroticism
Medical illness	Cognitive distortions (e.g., feelings of abandonment when left alone for brief periods)
Other psychiatric disorders (e.g., long-standing anxiety disorder)	Social origins
Vascular changes (vascular depression)	Stressful life events, including chronic stress or strain
Inflammation	
Neurodegenerative illnesses	Early life stressors or traumas
	Low socioeconomic status

TABLE 9–1. Origins of late-life depression

erogeneity. *Age at onset* is defined as the age when a patient had the first depressive episode or, barring a clear diagnosis, clinically significant depressive symptoms. Past work has defined "late-onset depression" as an initial episode of MDD occurring after age 50–60 years, with no clear consensus on a formal cutoff. In contrast, "early-onset depression" would be an onset of depression occurring earlier in life. Individuals with late-onset depression tend to exhibit greater medical morbidity; more abnormalities on MRI, including evidence of cerebrovascular disease; and more cognitive impairment than those with early onset (Krishnan et al. 1997; Sachs-Ericsson et al. 2013; Salloway et al. 1996; Sheline et al. 1999; Taylor et al. 2004). They also are less likely to report a family history of mood disorders, comorbid anxiety symptoms, or maladaptive personality traits (Baldwin and Tomenson 1995; Brodaty et al. 2001; Hayward et al. 2013). Thus late-onset depression can generally be conceptualized as more likely to have a contribution from vascular or neurodegenerative processes, putting the patient at higher risk for cognitive decline, whereas early-onset depression may have a stronger relationship with psychiatry-related genetic risk factors, family history, or early life stress. However, this is not a uniform distinction, because individuals with early-life onset are aging and may also remain at increased risk for development of both vascular disease and cognitive decline (Park et al. 2015; Riddle et al. 2017).

Biological Origins

Genetics

Genetic contributions appear to play a role in geriatric depression. Twin studies support that depressive symptoms in later life have a low to moderate level of heritability. Genetic contributions may explain between 14% and 55% of the variance, with environmental effects influencing the remaining variability (Carmelli et al. 2000; Gatz et al. 1992; Johnson et al. 2002). Heritability rates may be slightly higher for females than males (Jansson et al. 2004).

Although more than 100 candidate gene studies in LLD have been reported (Tsang et al. 2017), their replicability has been a significant problem. However, meta-analyses support that LLD risk is associated with three genes: apolipoprotein E (*APOE*), brain-derived neurotrophic factor (*BDNF*), and solute carrier family 6 member 4 (*SLC6A4*) (Tsang et al. 2017). Studies examining *APOE* typically focus on the ε4 allele, a risk factor for AD. Individual studies are mixed, but the ε4 allele appears to be associated with LLD, with an odds ratio of 1.49 (95% CI 1.03–2.17) (Tsang et al. 2017). *BDNF* codes for the BDNF protein involved in neurogenesis and implicated in memory function. The *BDNF* Met variant is associated with decreased BDNF secretion (Egan et al. 2003) and LLD risk (Taylor et al. 2007; Tsang et al. 2017) and is associated with poorer memory performance in younger adults (Hariri et al. 2003), although this finding was not replicated in LLD (Benjamin et al. 2010). Finally, *SLC6A4* is involved in serotonin transport. A 44bp deletion/insertion variant in the promoter region (*5-HTTLPR*) was identified (Heils et al. 1996), resulting in a 14-repeat short (S) variant with less transcriptional activity and lower serotonin uptake compared with the 16-repeat long (L) variant. The short variant is associated with reduced hippocampal volume (Taylor et al. 2005b) and a slightly increased risk for LLD (Tsang et al. 2017).

Genome-wide association studies (GWASs) have been challenging for studies of MDD in younger adults, and even more so in older adults with depression; however, progress is being made. A genome-wide meta-analysis of adult depression incorporating data from more than 800,000 cases and control subjects associated depression with 102 independently segregating variants (Howard et al. 2019). When the variants were assessed in a replication sample of 1.3 million individuals, 87 of them remained statistically significant, particularly identifying genes and gene pathways associated with neurotransmission and synaptic structure (Howard et al. 2019). The only GWAS in depressive symptoms in older adults included a sample of more than 34,000 cases and control subjects from 17 population studies (Hek et al. 2013). No loci reached genome-wide significance in this study, but this may have been due to the study being underpowered.

Endocrine Changes

Age-related changes in sex hormones are associated with depressive symptoms. Depressive symptoms in females are linked to ovarian hormone changes. Females with a history of depression are more likely to experience increased depressive symptoms during times of ovarian hormone fluctuation than at other times (Young and Korszun 2010) and are at increased risk for mood disorders during periods of ovarian hormone changes, including premenstrual mood disorder, postpartum depression, and perimenopausal depression (Freeman et al. 2014). Although most females do not develop mood disorders as a result of ovarian hormone changes, risk for depression may be increased because estrogen declines during the late perimenopause (Schmidt and Rubinow 2009), suggesting that some women may be susceptible to mood dysregulation as a result of changing estradiol levels. In some of these females, hormone replacement has resulted in improvement of mood (Schmidt and Rubinow 2009).

Males are not immune to similar changes, because serum testosterone levels also decline with aging (Travison et al. 2007). Testosterone levels are lower in elderly males with dysthymia than in those without depressive symptoms (Seidman et al. 2002). Some studies have examined testosterone treatment for MDD in males, but a systematic review published by the American College of Physicians found that although testosterone therapy was associated with benefits to sexual functioning and overall quality of life, the effect sizes were small and there was no clear benefit for depressive symptoms or cognition (Diem et al. 2020).

Alterations in the hypothalamic-pituitary-adrenal (HPA) axis and hypersecretion of corticotropin-releasing factor (CRF) are associated with depression across the life cycle (Pariante and Lightman 2008). CRF is thought to mediate sleep and appetite disturbances, reduced libido, and psychomotor changes (Arborelius et al. 1999) and is diminished with normal aging (Gottfries 1990). Aging is associated with an increased responsiveness of dehydroepiandrosterone sulfate, an endogenous steroid produced by the adrenal cortex, to CRF (Luisi et al. 1998). Importantly, alterations of the glucocorticoid receptor may play a critical role in the relationship between HPA axis hyperactivity and depression.

Such endocrine dysregulation has been associated with anatomical changes related to late-life depressive symptoms. Depressive symptoms are associated with hippocampal atrophy (Sheline et al. 1996; Steffens et al. 2002; Taylor et al. 2014). Stress that accumulates over the life cycle may lead to a sustained increase in secretion of cortisol, resulting in loss of preexisting neurons in the hippocampus and other brain regions (McEwen et al. 2016) and measurable loss of volume (Zannas et al. 2013). This loss may be potentially prevented with use of antidepressant medications (Czéh et al. 2001).

Medical and Psychiatric Comorbidity

Myocardial infarction and other cardiac conditions frequently are associated with an increased frequency of LLD (Sullivan et al. 1997), as are diabetes (Blazer et al. 2002), hip fracture (Magaziner et al. 1990), and stroke (Robinson et al. 1984). In a survey of community-dwelling Mexican Americans, depressive symptoms were associated with multiple medical comorbidities, including diabetes, arthritis, urinary incontinence, bowel incontinence, kidney disease, and ulcers (Black et al. 1998). Poor functional status secondary to physical illness and dementing disorders is a critical cause of depressive symptoms in older adults (Bruce 2001; Hays et al. 1997). For example, in one longitudinal study conducted over 6 years, depressive symptoms increased the risk for disability in activities of daily living and mobility by 67% and 73%, respectively (Penninx et al. 1999). Depressive symptoms are consistently associated with health status in cross-sectional studies of older adults (Kraaij et al. 2002); however, longitudinal associations are not always as clear. In one study, for example, health status was associated with depressive symptoms, but new illnesses in the previous 3 years did not consistently predict increases in depressive symptoms (Fiske et al. 2003).

The relationship between depression and medical comorbidity in older adults may be bidirectional. Medical problems, such as chronic pain, and their associated functional disability may predispose individuals to depression. However, the presence of depression may also increase the risk of adverse outcomes or complications of medical illnesses, including cardiac disease (Barefoot et al. 1996; Jiang et al. 2001) and diabetes (Nouwen et al. 2019).

LLD is frequently comorbid with other psychiatric disorders, although comorbidity rates are less frequent in late life than earlier in the life cycle. Alcohol use and MDD often co-occur, as would be expected in community studies of older adults (Devanand 2002). Due to legalization and increasing social acceptance, cannabis use is increasing among older adults (Han et al. 2017), and its use will likely become increasingly common in older adults with depression. Anxiety is commonly comorbid with depressive symptoms, regardless of whether those symptoms meet criteria for a depressive disorder. Anxiety may be problematic because it is associated with poor antidepressant treatment responses (Andreescu et al. 2007, 2009). Similarly, insomnia and sleep disruption not only are risk factors for LLD but also increase the risk for suicidality, anxiety, and dementia (Nadorff et al. 2018).

Vascular Depression

For several decades, vascular risk factors have been associated with depressive symptoms (Post 1962). MDD in older adults is common in patients with hypertension (Rabkin et al. 1983) and is a frequent outcome of stroke (Robinson et al. 1984). With the advent of MRI, LLD was further associated with MRI stigmata of cerebral small vessel disease, such as lacunes, microbleeds, leukoencephalopathy, and white matter hyperintensities (WMHs) (Coffey et al. 1990; Krishnan et al. 1988; Rensma et al. 2018; Taylor et al. 2005a), bright regions in the brain parenchyma observed on T_2-weighted or fluid-attenuated inversion recovery MRI.

In the late 1990s, investigators hypothesized that vascular disease contributes to the development or perpetuation of depression in some older individuals, coining the term *vascular depression* (Alexopoulos et al. 1997; Krishnan et al. 1997). Focusing on WMHs as the radiological hallmark, MRI criteria and, later, provisional diagnostic criteria were proposed for the diagnosis of vascular depression (Krishnan et al. 1997, 2004). Among populations of elder persons with depression, vascular depression appears to be common. An epidemiological population-based study from South Korea found that approximately half of older adults with MDD met MRI criteria for vascular depression, whereas 34% of adults with subsyndromal depressive symptoms met those same criteria (Park et al. 2015). In the United States, vascular depression is more prevalent among older Blacks than among white individuals (Reinlieb et al. 2014). WMHs increase with age, and worsening WMH disease is associated with poor longer-term depression outcomes (Taylor et al. 2003). Although negative studies exist, greater WMH severity is also associated with poor acute response to antidepressant medications (Sheline et al. 2010; Taylor et al. 2013a) and with cognitive deficits such as executive dysfunction (Lesser et al. 1996; Respino et al. 2019), which is itself associated with poor antidepressant response (Alexopoulos et al. 2005).

Although WMHs in LLD are typically ischemic in origin (Thomas et al. 2002a, 2002b), the mechanism by which they contribute to the occurrence or persistence of depressive symptoms remains unclear. Although several possible mechanisms have been proposed, a prevailing theory is the disconnection hypothesis (Taylor et al. 2013a), which theorizes that WMHs disrupt neural circuits and intrinsic networks involved in mood regulation, cognitive control, reward processes, or other functions implicated in depressive disorders through damage to white matter fiber bundles and neuronal axons. This theory is supported by work showing that WMHs occur in specific fiber tracts in LLD (Sheline et al. 2008; Taylor et al. 2013b) and that greater WMH burden adversely affects brain function during cognitive and affective tasks (Aizenstein et al. 2011; Venkatraman et al. 2010).

Inflammation

An extensive body of work supports the role of inflammation in the occurrence of depression (Miller and Raison 2016). Patients with depression exhibit multiple signs of an inflammatory response, including increased plasma and cerebrospinal fluid levels of proinflammatory cytokines, acute-phase reactants, and chemokines (Miller et al. 2009). Administration of inflammatory cytokines such as interferon-α to individuals without depression can induce depressive symptoms (Capuron et al. 2002; Reichenberg et al. 2001). Supported by in vitro studies, antidepressant treatment may reduce peripheral proinflammatory markers (Miller et al. 2009). Moreover, blockade of proinflammatory pathways can reduce depressive symptoms in medical illnesses, such as psoriasis and rheumatoid arthritis (Köhler et al. 2014; Tyring et al. 2006), and may potentially have clinical benefit in MDD when accompanied by elevated levels of proinflammatory cytokines (Raison et al. 2013).

These relationships may be even more important in LLD (Alexopoulos and Morimoto 2011; Taylor et al. 2013a). Aging- and disease-related processes disrupt immune function and promote proinflammatory states in older individuals, increasing peripheral immune activity and shifting the CNS into a proinflammatory state (Dilger and Johnson 2008). Increased peripheral cytokine levels in older adults are associated with depressive symptoms (Baune et al. 2012; Sonsin-Diaz et al. 2020; Tiemeier et al. 2003) and cognitive deficits, including poorer global cognition, executive function, and memory performance (Elderkin-Thompson et al. 2012; Schram et al. 2007). Inflammation may also contribute to neurodegenerative processes, with peripheral and central inflammation being associated with risk for dementia (Koyama et al. 2013; Rubio-Perez and Morillas-Ruiz 2012).

Depression Related to Neurodegenerative Disorders

Depression appears to be both a risk factor for and a prodrome of dementia, including AD (Ownby et al. 2006). Depressive symptoms may commonly precede the development of overt cognitive impairment in dementia, occurring in ~10%–15% of AD cases. Depression is additionally associated with an increased risk of all-cause dementia, with an odds ratio of ~2 (Diniz et al. 2013); these odds are slightly lower for AD and are slightly higher for vascular dementia. Moreover, the risk for AD increases with an increasing number of depressive episodes (Dotson et al. 2010). It is not clear what factors contribute to this vulnerability, although many biological mechanisms have been proposed (Byers and Yaffe 2011), including glucocorticoid system abnormalities, proinflammatory processes, or abnormal changes in nerve growth factors. This suggests that, for some individuals, these processes may contribute to the etiology of both depression and dementia. It is also possible that amyloid accumulation in some individuals may predispose them to LLD (Mahgoub and Alexopoulos 2016). This association may be particularly relevant for late-onset depression, which in some patients may be a prodrome of AD. It may also be relevant for individuals with recurrent, early-onset depression, who may also exhibit significant amyloid accumulation in brain regions implicated in mood regulation (Wu et al. 2014).

Psychological Origins

Psychological factors, such as personality attributes, neuroticism, cognitive distortions, and difficulty with emotional control, may contribute to the onset of LLD. Although not specific to the origin of depression in older individuals, the presence of these traits may still affect the presentation and course of depression. When compared with older adults who have depression without comorbid personality disorders, older adults with depression and personality disorders are four times more likely to experience a continuation or reemergence of depression despite treatment (Morse and Lynch 2004). Specific personality traits are not necessarily correlated with clinical features of depression, such as age at onset or number of previous episodes. However, some maladaptive traits were associated with depressive symptoms, such as hopelessness or suicidal ideation (Szücs et al. 2018). Basic personality attributes thus can underlie the origin and expression of depressive symptoms in older adults.

Neuroticism—a construct that is more commonly studied in Europe and Australia than in the United States—is consistently associated with late-life depressive symptoms in cross-sectional and longitudinal studies of community samples (Henderson et al. 1997; Lyness et al. 2002) and older adults in residential homes (Eisses et al. 2004). Characterized by high levels of negative affect in response to minor stressors, neuroticism can be seen in some people with depression who overreact to life events or misinterpret these events and exaggerate their adverse outcome. Neuroticism influences how people cope with stressors. Compared with those with fewer symptoms, elderly persons with more depressive symptoms engage in maladaptive cognitive distortions such as rumination and catastrophizing to a greater extent and expressed positive reappraisal or acceptance to a lesser extent (Kraaij and de Wilde 2001). Neuroticism is associated with a poorer response to acute treatment with selective serotonin reuptake inhibitors (SSRIs), with greater stress vulnerability (a neuroticism subscale) associated with lower likelihood of remission (Steffens et al. 2018). Neuroticism is further associated with poorer longitudinal mood and cognitive outcomes in treated older patients with depression who were followed for up to 10 years (Manning et al. 2017; Steffens et al. 2013).

Several other psychological constructs are similarly associated with the development and persistence of depression. An *external locus of control* is associated with the emergence and continuation of depressive symptoms over 3 years (Beekman et al. 2001). This trait-type marker is defined as the extent to which people consider themselves to be victims of fate or circumstance rather than being in control of their lives. In comorbid insomnia and depression, dysfunctional beliefs about not being able to function and needing to avoid activities after a night of disrupted sleep were related to mental and physical fatigue (Carney et al. 2014). In contrast, a higher level of *mastery*—that is, a perception of being able to accomplish tasks and having control over one's life—has a direct association with fewer depressive symptoms in older individuals and may buffer the adverse impact of disability on depression (Jang et al. 2002). Similarly, *self-efficacy*, or belief in one's capacity to manage one's behavior and social environment, may have a direct effect of reducing risk for depression and may work indirectly to prevent depressive symptoms through its positive effect on social support (Paukert et al. 2010). Low self-efficacy may mediate the effect of maladaptive personality traits on depressive symptoms in older adults (O'Shea et al. 2017).

Social Origins

In addition to biological and psychological origins, LLD also develops from social origins, including stressful life events, bereavement, chronic stress or strain, low socioeconomic status, and impaired social support. The relative contributions of these factors may vary across the life cycle.

Stressful Life Events and Chronic Stress

Decades of research have found a strong association between both stressful life events (e.g., bereavement, life-threatening illness in oneself or someone close) and social difficulties (e.g., difficulties in health of someone close, housing issues, marital and family relationships) and the onset of depressive episodes (Kendler et al. 1999; Kessler 1997). The risk of developing a new depressive episode increases with a greater severity and number of stressful events. These relationships between stressful events and the onset of depression persist into later life (Kraaij et al. 2002; Murphy 1982), and chronic stressors may contribute to the persistence of depression (Zannas et al. 2012). Older individuals who lack a confidant are especially vulnerable to the effects of life stress, whereas social support may buffer the effect of stressful events.

These associations may not be straightforward, and a number of factors may modify them. First, with repeated depressive episodes over the life span, less stress may be required to trigger a new episode (Kendler et al. 2000). This is concordant with some observations that stressful events, particularly ongoing problems, may have a smaller contribution to depression in older adults than in younger adults (Bruce 2002; Karel 1997). Second, some events that can lead to depression, such as divorce, job stress, and legal difficulties, are more frequent early in adulthood than in later life. However, later life carries its own stress, including the effect of chronic medical illnesses, disability, and financial difficulties. Third, stressful events that are predictable or expected often cause less depression in older adults than in younger adults. For example, the death of a spouse is a severe and at times catastrophic event leading to depression. For young or middle-aged adults, this event is usually unexpected, and the adjustment is particularly difficult. Older adults, in contrast, recognize that the death of a spouse is expected (by observing their peers) and in some cases even rehearse the event, such as by considering what they might do if a spouse dies. However, bereavement remains a common cause of depressive symptoms in late life (Clayton 1990; Prigerson et al. 1994). In a study of 1,810 community-dwelling older adults, the death of a partner or other relative predicted the onset of clinically significant depressive symptoms over a 3-year follow-up period (Prigerson et al. 1994). Multiple losses and deaths of family or friends within a short time frame may also have a cumulative effect and increase the risk of depression in some people.

Another common cause of depression in later life is serving as a caregiver to a family member with significant dementia or other disability. The prevalence of depressive symptoms in caregivers of people with dementia ranges from 43% to 47% (Livingston et al. 1996; Waite et al. 2004). Providing support for caregivers and acknowledging their treatment needs is important for preventing the onset and progression of depression in this vulnerable group.

Finally, lower socioeconomic status has been associated with depression across the life span. Both the frequency of depressive symptoms and their persistence over a period of 2–4 years were associated with socioeconomic disadvantage in a sample of community-dwelling older adults who originally met criteria for MDD (Mojtabai and Olfson 2004). In cross-sectional analyses using data from a community study of older

Mexican Americans, financial strain was associated with depressive symptoms (Black et al. 1998). Such financial stresses may be partially related to lower education levels. Although level of education did not predict emergence of depressive symptoms over 1 year, emergence of depression over a 3-year period was predicted by a lower level of education (Beekman et al. 2001).

Social Support

Social support is a multifactorial construct that includes the perception of support, structure of the social network, and tangible help and assistance. Although social support can mitigate the emotional response to negative events (Chou and Chi 2001), in the community, depressive symptoms are associated with a range of impaired social support measures, including a small or insufficient social network, lower social contact frequency, decreased satisfaction with social support, and limited instrumental-emotional support (Chi and Chou 2001; Golden et al. 2009). However, perceived lack of social support is the most robust predictor of LLD symptoms (Bruce 2002). Poor social support and greater feelings of loneliness predict depressive symptoms years later (Henderson et al. 1997; Holvast et al. 2015), whereas loneliness is also associated with accelerated cognitive decline (Donovan et al. 2017).

Do not assume that all older adults experience deficits in social support or loneliness. Social support is perceived as adequate by most older persons, even in clinical samples (Blazer 1982). Most older adults believe they have sufficient contact with both family and friends and feel positively about the relationships they have with their social networks. However, when that social network is depleted, whether through loss of someone close (e.g., a spouse or child), a change in the quality of the relationship (e.g., a dispute within the family), or a move to a different geographical location, this loss of social support may emerge as an important contributor to LLD.

Religion and Faith

Although not limited to geriatric populations, a key source of social support used by recent generations of older adults to help with coping is religious involvement. In a study of middle-aged and elderly adults, one-third of men and nearly two-thirds of women described religious beliefs as helping them cope with a stressful period (Koenig et al. 1988). Several studies report inverse associations between religious coping and depressive symptoms in older adults with or without medical illness (Braam et al. 1997b; Koenig 2007a). Use of religious beliefs as a coping mechanism and religious involvement have been associated with a greater likelihood of experiencing improvement in depressive symptoms and are predictive of a faster recovery in both inpatient and community-dwelling older adults (Braam et al. 1997a; Koenig 2007b).

Multiple Possible Etiologies and Overall Vulnerability

How does one resolve the relatively lower frequency of MDD in older adults, who have increased biological vulnerability and perhaps have only slightly better social resources, compared with younger adults? For example, most older individuals who experience a significant physical illness or even the death of a partner do not become depressed. The answer to this question lies in the conceptualization of depression. Ultimately, the brain guides behavior. The clinical and behavioral expression of LLD is the manifestation of alterations in brain function across brain regions and networks. Age-, disease-, psychology-, and social-related factors all contribute in varying degrees to these functional alterations. Some of these factors, such as personality traits or long-lasting effects of trauma, may have been present since childhood, whereas others develop with aging, stress exposure, or medical infirmity. Any person may have multiple potential "etiological factors" that contribute to LLD vulnerability. Only when these etiological factors affect brain function sufficiently and disrupt neural network homeostasis do depressive symptoms develop (Andreescu et al. 2019). Such a threshold model acknowledges multifactorial contributions to LLD and may also explain why other individuals experience similar stresses and challenges yet do not become depressed (Taylor et al. 2013a).

Aging may also be associated with positive changes that are protective, such as the acquisition of increased wisdom. Wisdom is a nebulous concept, but it can be operationalized (Baltes and Staudinger 2000) as an expert knowledge system about the fundamental pragmatics of life, including knowledge and judgment about the meaning and conduct of life and the orchestration of human development toward excellence while attending conjointly to personal and collective well-being. Wisdom includes rich factual knowledge, rich procedural knowledge (e.g., the ability to develop strategies for addressing problems), life span contextualization (e.g., integrating life experiences), relativism of values and life priorities (e.g., tolerance of differences in society), and recognition and management of uncertainty (accepting that the future cannot be known with certainty and that the ability to assess one's sociocultural environment is inherently constrained). Wisdom is thought to accumulate over the life cycle, if severe physical illness and cognitive impairment do not intervene. Cumulative wisdom over time may protect older persons from depression when confronted with negative experiences and loss.

Differential Diagnosis of Late-Life Mood Disorders

Clinical entities included as mood disorders in DSM-5 that are relevant to depression in elderly patients are discussed in the following subsections. Depressive symptoms are likewise present in other DSM-5 disorder categories, such as persistent complex bereavement disorder and adjustment disorder with depressed mood.

Major Depressive Disorder

The diagnosis of a major depressive episode is made when the person exhibits one or both of two core symptoms—depressed mood and lack of interest or pleasure—as well as four or more of the following symptoms for at least 2 weeks: significant weight loss, insomnia or hypersomnia, psychomotor agitation or retardation, fatigue or loss of energy, feelings of worthlessness or excessive or inappropriate guilt, diminished ability to concentrate or make decisions, and recurrent thoughts of death or suicidal ideation (American Psychiatric Association 2013). First-onset episodes of MDD after age 50–60 years (referred to as *late onset*) are common, making up about one-half of all episodes in older adults. Personality disorders and a family history of psychiatric illness are more common if the depression is *early onset* (i.e., first episode occurs before age 50–60 years), but, for the most part, the phenomenology is no different between early- and late-onset MDD (Brodaty et al. 2001). Please refer to the "Etiology" section earlier in the chapter.

DSM-5 has additional criteria modifiers for an MDD diagnosis (Box 9–1). These include *anxious distress*, when the person also exhibits two of the following symptoms: being tense, feeling restless, having difficulty concentrating because of worry, fearing something awful may happen, or having feelings of losing control. The specifier *with melancholic features* is added when the person has lost pleasure in almost all activities or lacks reactivity to stimuli that usually elicit pleasure and experiences three or more of the following six symptoms during the most severe stage of the depressive episode: despondency or despair, depression that is worse in the morning, early morning awakening, marked psychomotor agitation or retardation, weight loss or anorexia, and excessive or inappropriate guilt. The *mixed features* specifier is added when manic or hypomanic symptoms are present. The *atypical features* specifier can be applied when there is a predominance of mood reactivity and two or more of the following: weight gain or increase in appetite, hypersomnia, leaden paralysis, and a long-standing pattern of interpersonal rejection sensitivity. The specifier *with seasonal pattern* can be applied to a pattern of major depressive episodes that begin in the fall or winter and remit in spring over at least a 2-year period, with no other depressive episodes occurring at other times of the year. There is also a *catatonia* specifier for when catatonia features are present during a depressive episode, and a specifier for *psychotic features* when delusions or hallucinations are present (American Psychiatric Association 2013).

Box 9–1.   DSM-5 Diagnostic Criteria for Major Depressive Disorder

A. Five (or more) of the following symptoms have been present during the same 2-week period and represent a change from previous functioning; at least one of the symptoms is either (1) depressed mood or (2) loss of interest or pleasure.
   Note: Do not include symptoms that are clearly attributable to another medical condition.

   1. Depressed mood most of the day, nearly every day, as indicated by either subjective report (e.g., feels sad, empty, hopeless) or observation made by others (e.g., appears tearful). **(Note:** In children and adolescents, can be irritable mood.)
   2. Markedly diminished interest or pleasure in all, or almost all, activities most of the day, nearly every day (as indicated by either subjective account or observation).
   3. Significant weight loss when not dieting or weight gain (e.g., a change of more than 5% of body weight in a month), or decrease or increase in appetite nearly every day. **(Note:** In children, consider failure to make expected weight gain.)
   4. Insomnia or hypersomnia nearly every day.
   5. Psychomotor agitation or retardation nearly every day (observable by others, not merely subjective feelings of restlessness or being slowed down).
   6. Fatigue or loss of energy nearly every day.
   7. Feelings of worthlessness or excessive or inappropriate guilt (which may be delusional) nearly every day (not merely self-reproach or guilt about being sick).
   8. Diminished ability to think or concentrate, or indecisiveness, nearly every day (either by subjective account or as observed by others).
   9. Recurrent thoughts of death (not just fear of dying), recurrent suicidal ideation without a specific plan, or a suicide attempt or a specific plan for committing suicide.

B. The symptoms cause clinically significant distress or impairment in social, occupational, or other important areas of functioning.

C. The episode is not attributable to the physiological effects of a substance or another medical condition.

Note: Criteria A–C represent a major depressive episode.

Note: Responses to a significant loss (e.g., bereavement, financial ruin, losses from a natural disaster, a serious medical illness or disability) may include the feelings of intense sadness, rumination about the loss, insomnia, poor appetite, and weight loss noted in Criterion A, which may resemble a depressive episode. Although such symptoms may be understandable or considered appropriate to the loss, the presence of a major depressive episode in addition to the normal response to a significant loss should also be carefully considered. This decision inevitably requires the exercise of clinical judgment based on the individual's history and the cultural norms for the expression of distress in the context of loss.

D. The occurrence of the major depressive episode is not better explained by schizoaffective disorder, schizophrenia, schizophreniform disorder, delusional disorder, or other specified and unspecified schizophrenia spectrum and other psychotic disorders.

E. There has never been a manic episode or a hypomanic episode.

Note: This exclusion does not apply if all of the manic-like or hypomanic-like episodes are substance-induced or are attributable to the physiological effects of another medical condition.

Note. Criteria set above contains only the diagnostic criteria and specifiers; refer to DSM-5 for the full criteria set, including specifier descriptions and coding and reporting procedures.

Source. Reprinted from *Diagnostic and Statistical Manual of Mental Disorders*, 5th Edition. Arlington, VA, American Psychiatric Association, 2013, pp. 602–603. Used with permission. Copyright © 2013 American Psychiatric Association.

Major Depressive Disorder With Psychotic Features

Late-onset psychotic depression deserves special attention given the high prevalence of delusions in adults older than 60 years, particularly elderly inpatients with depression (Meyers and Greenberg 1986). The DSM-5 criteria for depressive disorders with psychotic features require that delusions or hallucinations be present at any time during the depressive episode. If the theme of the hallucinations and delusions is consistent with the depressive content, such as being related to personal inadequacy, guilt, disease, death, nihilism, or deserved punishment, then psychotic features are referred to as *mood congruent*. If the psychotic symptoms do not include these depressive themes, then they are considered to be *mood incongruent*. Although psychotic symptoms may occur in cognitively intact elder persons with depression, they can also occur in the context of neurocognitive disorders.

In older adults, delusions of persecution or of having an incurable illness are more common than those associated with guilt. If guilt predominates in the delusional picture, it usually involves some relatively minor episode that occurred many years before the onset of the depressive episode and was forgotten over time but is currently viewed as a major problem. For example, a one-time sexual liaison, forgotten or forgiven by the spouse, is resurrected by a patient who fears an ongoing venereal disease or cancer or is associated with chronic and severe pain. Nihilistic delusions (delusions of nothingness) may occur more commonly in late life. Focus on the abdomen is a common element of somatic delusions. Hallucinations are less common. Individuals with a later-life onset of depression with psychotic features are more likely to exhibit hypochondriacal or nihilistic delusions (Gournellis et al. 2001).

Research has compared the clinical, demographic, and social characteristics of patients with psychotic and nonpsychotic depression. Younger age, greater severity of depression, psychomotor retardation, guilt, feelings of worthlessness, a history of delusions, and increased suicidal ideation and intent are more common in patients with psychotic depression (Gournellis et al. 2001; Thakur et al. 1999). It also tends to be associated with poor social support and, not surprisingly, with bipolar illness. Psychotic depression can be a malignant, dangerous illness. ECT may be needed, and pharmacological treatment typically includes both an antidepressant and an antipsychotic medication. Pharmacological management is discussed later in the chapter.

Bipolar Disorders

Any evaluation for depression should include an assessment for previously unrecognized bipolar disorder, requiring screening for past manic or hypomanic episodes. To meet criteria for a manic episode, a person must exhibit three or more (four or more if the mood is only irritable) of the following symptoms:

- Inflated self-esteem or grandiosity
- Decreased need for sleep
- More talkativeness than usual
- Flight of ideas
- Distractibility
- Increased goal-directed activity (e.g., at work) or psychomotor agitation
- Excessive involvement in pleasurable activities with potential adverse consequences (e.g., unrestricted buying episodes)

Bipolar disorder varies somewhat with aging. Older adults present less often with psychotic manic episodes and more often with depressive symptoms (Sajatovic et al. 2015). It is thus even more important to assess for past episodes of mania to distinguish depression from bipolar disorder. When a person is experiencing a full-blown manic episode, cognitive function is difficult to test, yet perseverative behavior, catatonia-like symptoms, and even negativistic symptoms may emerge. Manic episodes, therefore, must be distinguished (but often with difficulty) from neurocognitive disorders, such as a delirium characterized by hallucinations, delusions, and agitation.

Persistent Depressive Disorder (Dysthymia)

Most clinicians working with elderly patients have observed persistent depression, characterized by significant and unremitting depressive symptoms often associated with chronic psychosocial stressors. Like MDD, persistent depressive disorder is diagnosed across the life cycle and in DSM-5 comprises the DSM-IV (American Psychiatric Association 1994) diagnoses of dysthymia or dysthymic disorder and chronic MDD. Diagnostic criteria require depressed mood for most of the day, for more days than not, plus at least two additional symptoms:

- Poor appetite or overeating
- Insomnia or hypersomnia

- Low energy or fatigue
- Low self-esteem
- Poor concentration or trouble making decisions
- Feelings of hopelessness

Although persistent depressive disorder requires fewer criteria symptoms than MDD, the symptoms must occur most of the day, for more days than not, over 2 years or longer and cannot be absent for more than 2 months at a time. Dysthymia and non-chronic, recurrent MDD may coexist, leading to episodes of "double depression."

Dysthymia in older adults has a prevalence of ~2% (Blazer et al. 1987), but its presentation may differ from that in younger persons. Older adults with dysthymia may present with an initial onset of symptoms in later life, without a prior history of major depressive episodes or other psychiatric illness and with a lower rate of psychiatric family history and, in contrast to younger adults with chronic depression, lower rates of comorbid personality disorders. They often report social stressors, including a loss of social support or loneliness, and may exhibit cerebrovascular or neurodegenerative pathology (Devanand 2014). Although antidepressant medications can help treat dysthymia (Devanand et al. 2005; Kerner et al. 2014), they may have only moderate efficacy in this population.

Depressive Episode With Insufficient Symptoms (Minor or Subsyndromal Depression)

Depressive episodes with insufficient symptoms (previously called minor, subsyndromal, or subthreshold depression) are coded under the DSM-5 category "other specified depressive disorder." This diagnosis is assigned when a person who has never met criteria for a mood disorder experiences depressed affect plus at least one other symptom of a major depressive episode that persists for at least 2 weeks. Although the terms "insufficient," "minor," or "subsyndromal" imply lower severity, the consequences of minor depression are similar to those for MDD, including impaired physical functioning, greater disability, poorer self-rated health, use of psychotropic medications, and perceived low social support (Hybels et al. 2001). Given these outcomes, treatment with psychotherapy or pharmacotherapy can be helpful (Biella et al. 2019). Although the absence of a depressed affect would not qualify patients for this specific DSM-5 diagnosis, some investigators have suggested a syndrome of depression without sadness, thought to be more common in older adults (Gallo et al. 1997).

Depressive Disorder Due to Another Medical Condition

Depressive disorders are common in and associated with various physical illnesses, including cardiovascular disease, endocrine disturbances, autoimmune disorders, and neurological disorders including stroke, Parkinson's disease, and dementia. Controversy continues over the extent to which acute or chronic medical illnesses cause depression through direct physiological effects on the brain or as part of a psychological reaction to the disability, implications for mortality, and other life changes evoked by these illnesses. To meet criteria for "due to another medical condition," there must be evidence that the mood disturbance is "the direct pathophysiological consequence of another medical condition." The disturbance also cannot occur exclusively during a delirium or be better explained by another mental disorder. For example, a new onset of depressive symptoms following a stroke could qualify for this diagnosis. In contrast, distress following a medical diagnosis may be better diagnosed as adjustment disorder with depressed mood, with the medical problem being the stressor. If there is insufficient evidence to determine the likely etiology of the depressive symptoms, a diagnosis of "other specified depressive disorder" or "unspecified depressive disorder" should be considered.

Adjustment Disorder With Depressed Mood

Adjustment disorder with depressed mood is included in the "Trauma- and Stress-Related Disorders" section of DSM-5. This diagnosis is reserved for individuals who exhibit a maladaptive reaction to an identifiable stressor, characterized by distress out of proportion to the situation or significant impairment in function. The relationship of the symptoms to the stressful event must be clear and must occur within 3 months of the stressor. Typical stressors for older adults include life events, such as marital problems; difficulty with children; loss of a social role; or an ill-advised change of residence. Normal bereavement is an exclusion for this diagnosis. Retirement is usually not a source of excessive stress for the older adult. Therefore, the onset of significant depressive symptoms and withdrawal from activities after retirement may not indicate a true adjustment disorder. Of much greater frequency is the development of depressive symptoms secondary to a physical illness. When an episode of depression accompanies a physical illness and the level of symptoms dramatically exceeds the expected level, a diagnosis of either adjustment disorder or depression due to medical illness is indicated.

Diagnostic Workup of the Older Adult With Depression

At its core, the diagnosis of a mood disorder in older adults is made on the basis of a history, augmented with a physical examination and fine-tuned by laboratory studies (Taylor 2014) (Table 9–2). No biological markers or tests are available to confirm the diagnosis of depression or to inform prognosis, yet some tests may assist in identifying comorbid conditions that contribute to depressive symptoms, such as polysomnography for any underlying sleep disturbances. Critical elements of the psychiatric history to evaluate in an older patient with depression include the duration of the current depressive episode; the history of previous episodes and age of initial depression onset; the history of drug and alcohol abuse; response to and side effects from previous antidepressant interventions; a family history of depression, suicide, or alcohol abuse; and the severity of the depressive symptoms.

Reviewing thoughts of and risk factors for suicide is essential. Discussions about suicidal thoughts are not always easy, but talking openly about it is crucial to ensure patients' safety and determine the best course of treatment. The discussion can begin by asking patients about thoughts of death or wishes to be dead, then progressing to questions about a desire to die or an intent or plan to harm themselves. A history of suicide attempts should always be evaluated because it is a strong predictor of future

TABLE 9–2.   **Workup of patients with late-life depression**

Routine clinical evaluations

Screening (particularly in primary care settings)	Standard symptom checklists such as the Patient Health Questionnaire–9 or Geriatric Depression Scale
Psychiatric history	Present and past depressive episodes, family history, antidepressant treatment history, and assessment of psychological function and social stressors, as well as a review of medical history, current medications, nutritional status, and functional status.
Suicide risk	Current ideation and any preparations, past preparations or attempts, and past psychiatric hospitalizations
Screening for cognitive impairment	Screening scale such as the Mini-Mental State Examination or Montreal Cognitive Assessment
Medical history	Medical problems and surgical history, evaluating functional limitations and chronic pain syndromes
Physical examination	Neurological examination in particular

Laboratory evaluations (as indicated based on clinical evaluation)

Vitamin deficiencies	Folate, vitamins B_{12} and D
Thyroid dysfunction	Triiodothyronine, thyroxine, thyroid-stimulating hormone levels
Polysomnography for underlying sleep disorders	

behavior. One should also evaluate factors that modify suicide risk, including both protective factors, such as social support, religious involvement, and engagement in treatment, and risk factors, including substance use, isolation, and access to lethal methods such as firearms.

Given the frequent comorbidity between depression and cognitive impairment, screening for cognitive impairment and assessment of cognitive status are critical to the evaluation of older patients with depression. Use of a screening scale such as the Mini-Mental State Examination (Folstein et al. 1975) or Montreal Cognitive Assessment (Nasreddine et al. 2005) is a good adjunct to the diagnostic workup. Patients' medical and surgical histories should be reviewed, focusing on disability, pain, or other conditions that they associate with the perpetuation of their depressive symptoms. The physical examination should include a neurological examination to determine if soft neurological signs (e.g., frontal release signs) or laterality is present. Psychomotor retardation, in conjunction with tremor or subtle rigidity, may also detect early parkinsonism symptoms.

The diagnostic interview should include a careful assessment of potential underlying sleep disturbances. Sleep disorders, such as restless leg syndrome and obstructive sleep apnea, are more common in older adults with depression than in the general population (Koo et al. 2016). Moreover, sleep apnea may contribute to poor cognitive performance (Kerner and Roose 2016). If a careful history indicates the possibility of such diagnoses, the full workup of these issues should include polysomnography.

The laboratory workup of the older adult with depression is important. It should include a thyroid panel (triiodothyronine, thyroxine) and a determination of thyroid-stimulating hormone levels. A blood screening enables the clinician to detect the presence of anemia. Because both depressive and cognitive symptoms can be caused by deficits in vitamin B_{12} or folate, it is important to obtain levels of these vitamins and to measure vitamin D levels because vitamin D deficiency is common in depression (Anglin et al. 2013). Such deficiencies may require supplementation, although it is unclear whether supplementation alone will improve depressive symptoms (Okereke et al. 2018).

Screening for depression is helpful, using standardized scales such as the Patient Health Questionnaire–9 (Kroenke et al. 2001) or Geriatric Depression Scale. Although Medicare now reimburses for depression screening in primary care settings, the clinical effectiveness of screening is mixed. A positive screening must be accompanied by a careful clinical evaluation and followed by treatment as needed. Although internists often accept responsibility for treating LLD, they may perceive their clinical skills to be inadequate and become frustrated with their practice environment (Callahan et al. 1992).

Treatment of Depression in Older Adults

Treatment options for LLD include psychotherapy, pharmacotherapy, and neurostimulation. These approaches are discussed in the sections that follow.

Psychotherapy

Depression-specific psychotherapy should be considered an initial treatment choice for older individuals with mild or moderate depression severity. In this population, psychotherapy has efficacy comparable with that of antidepressant medications, with an overall effect size of ~0.64 and number needed to treat of 3 (Kirkham et al. 2016; Pinquart et al. 2006). Available evidence supports several types of structured psychotherapies in LLD.

Cognitive-behavioral therapy (CBT) was designed specifically to treat depression and is the best-studied psychotherapy. The goal of CBT is to change patients' behavior and modes of thinking. This is accomplished through behavioral interventions such as weekly activity schedules, mastery and pleasure logs, and graded task assignments. Cognitive approaches to restructuring negative cognitions or automatic thoughts include subjecting these cognitions to empirical reality testing, examining distortions (e.g., overgeneralizations, catastrophizing, dichotomous thinking), and generating new ways of viewing one's life. Several meta-analyses support CBT's efficacy in older adults, with effect sizes ranging from 0.70 to 1.34 (Gould et al. 2012; Wilson et al. 2008). CBT is similarly effective in elderly patients with depression and chronic medical illnesses, such as diabetes and heart disease (Kohn et al. 2000; Lustman et al. 1998). An advantage of CBT in treating older adults is that the therapy is directive and time limited, usually involving between 10 and 25 sessions. However, the benefit of CBT in older adults with cognitive impairment is less clear.

Interpersonal psychotherapy (IPT) was developed from psychodynamic theory and focuses on interpersonal relationships that may contribute to depression. IPT is a structured treatment that includes psychoeducation, goal setting, and identification of and focus on interpersonal issues. Interpersonal problems in older adults may include issues of grief and loss, difficulties with role transitions, and interpersonal conflicts or deficits (Renn and Areán 2017). IPT has clear efficacy for depression, with effect sizes comparable with those of other psychological treatments (Cuijpers et al. 2016). There is relatively less evidence of IPT's effectiveness in treating LLD, although this literature is notable for positive trials and the potential benefit of reducing suicidal ideation (Heisel et al. 2015; Reynolds et al. 1999; van Schaik et al. 2007).

Problem-solving therapy (PST) is based on the premise that helping patients become better managers of their lives can reduce stress and depression. PST teaches patients to identify the problems that adversely affect their well-being and provides a method for selecting and implementing plans to solve those problems (Renn and Areán 2017). PST is structured and time limited and exhibits efficacy in older adults with depression and medical problems and even in those with depression and cognitive impairment, including executive dysfunction (Areán et al. 1993, 2008, 2010). Meta-analyses suggest that PST may be more effective in older adults than in younger adults with depression (Kirkham et al. 2016). Notably, PST in LLD demonstrates superior efficacy relative to supportive therapy (Areán et al. 2010) and to CBT in medically ill older adults (Sharpe et al. 2012).

"Engage" is a neurobiologically informed intervention designed to streamline psychotherapy for LLD (Alexopoulos and Areán 2014). It is a structured, stepwise, personalized treatment that focuses on "reward exposure" (exposure to meaningful and rewarding activities) in order to retrain the reward system. Treatment also includes evaluation and a focus on barriers to reward exposure, such as apathy, negativity bias, or emotional dysregulation. Although the literature supporting its use is still in the early stages, Engage appears to improve behavioral activation and depressive symptoms in older adults, with efficacy comparable with that seen with PST (Alexopoulos et al. 2015, 2016).

Although psychotherapy is effective for older adults with depression, access to trained, skilled providers is a significant challenge. This barrier may be particularly challenging in rural areas or for older adults with limited financial resources. However, older adults with minor depression or adjustment disorders, or those who experience dysphoria because of losses of various types, often require less intensive forms of psychotherapy. Active listening and simple support may be sufficient to help distressed elder persons cope with their situation. Because religion is an important factor in the lives of many older adults, referral to a pastoral counselor may be helpful and acceptable (Koenig et al. 2004).

Pharmacotherapy

Antidepressant medications can effectively treat depression in older adults and are overall superior to placebo. A large meta-analysis of 51 randomized trials in adults age 55 years and older reported a response rate of 48%, compared with 38% in those given placebo (Kok et al. 2012). However, despite the availability of a wide range of effective antidepressant medications, patients with LLD are often inadequately treated, being prescribed medications at lower than recommended dosages, treated for too brief a time, or not treated at all (Barry et al. 2012; Wang et al. 2005). Only one-third of older patients with depression appear to receive at least some antidepressant treatment (Cole et al. 1999).

As in younger adults, SSRIs are commonly used for depression in older adults. These agents are the first-line choice for treating mild to moderate forms of depression. Important advantages of SSRIs when treating elderly patients are their lack of anticholinergic, orthostatic, and cardiac side effects; lack of sedation; and safety in overdose. Nevertheless, for a significant number of older adults, SSRIs cause other unacceptable effects, including excessive activation and disturbance of sleep, tremor, headache, gastrointestinal side effects, and, rarely, hyponatremia. With these safety considerations, escitalopram and sertraline could be considered first. Fluoxetine has a longer half-life, so it could be reserved for individuals with poor medication adherence. In contrast, paroxetine has some anticholinergic effects, and citalopram has concerns for QTc prolongation, so it may not be considered as a first-line SSRI.

There are several options for second-line agents, but data in geriatric populations are more limited. These include medications affecting both the serotonergic and noradrenergic systems (serotonin-norepinephrine reuptake inhibitors [SNRIs]), with duloxetine (Raskin et al. 2008) and venlafaxine (Staab and Evans 2000) demonstrating efficacy in geriatric depression trials. Second-line options include novel agents such as bupropion and mirtazapine. Despite a lack of high-quality clinical trial data, these agents are often used in older adults. Bupropion may be used in the context of fatigue or persistent anhedonia due to its effects at the norepinephrine and dopamine transporters. Mirtazapine's tendency to increase appetite and sedation may be useful in older adults with insomnia and weight loss. Due to their unique mechanisms of action, bupropion or mirtazapine can be used to augment an SSRI, with data from the Sequenced Treatment Alternatives to Relieve Depression (STAR*D) trial in a general adult population supporting this option (Warden et al. 2007). Two newer agents, vilazodone and vortioxetine, have limited data in elderly patients despite evidence that vortioxetine may benefit cognitive performance in depression (Mahableshwarkar et al. 2015).

Tricyclic antidepressants (TCAs) are a reasonable choice for some patients with more severe forms of MDD who can tolerate the side effects and do not respond to the medications just mentioned. Medications that are effective yet carry a lower risk of side effects (especially cardiovascular effects) are preferred. In recent years, nortriptyline and desipramine have become the more popular medications for treating older adults with endogenous or melancholic MDD. However, doxepin remains a favorite among many practitioners. It is recommended that all elderly patients have an electrocardiogram (ECG) before initiation of treatment and again after therapeutic blood levels have been achieved. If the ECG shows a second-degree (or higher) block, a bifascicular bundle branch block, a left bundle branch block, or a QTc interval >480 ms, treatment with TCAs should not be initiated or should be stopped (Caravati and Bossart 1991). TCAs, specifically amitriptyline, may occasionally be used for pain syndromes, but at lower dosages than those used to treat depression.

Initial antidepressant dosages prescribed for persons in late life should be case specific but are generally lower than those prescribed for persons in midlife. However, if well tolerated, the medication may need to be titrated to a higher dosage to provide efficacy. Thus, the geriatric mantra of "start low, go slow" does not necessarily mean "stop at a lower dosage." Table 9–3 provides guidance on initial starting dosages for geriatric patients and FDA-approved maximum dosages. Plasma levels of TCAs are important for determining dosing: desipramine levels >125 ng/mL and nortriptyline levels of 50–150 ng/mL have been found to be therapeutic.

TABLE 9–3. **Pharmacological treatment of late-life depression: antidepressant dosing**

Medication	Initial daily dosage, *mg*	Maximum daily dosage, *mg*
Selective serotonin reuptake inhibitors		
Citalopram	10	20–40
Escitalopram	10	20
Fluoxetine	10–20	80
Paroxetine	10–20 (IR); 12.5–25 (ER)	50 (IR); 62.5 (ER)
Sertraline	25–50	200
Serotonin-norepinephrine reuptake inhibitors		
Desvenlafaxine	25–50	100
Duloxetine	20–30	120
Levomilnacipran	20	120
Venlafaxine (ER)	37.5–75	225
Tricyclic antidepressants*		
Desipramine	25 bid	150–300
Nortriptyline	25–50	150
Other agents		
Bupropion (ER)	150	450
Mirtazapine	7.5–15	45
Vilazodone	10	40
Vortioxetine	5–10	20

ER=extended-release formulation; IR=immediate-release formulation.
*Use blood levels to inform dosing decisions.

Monoamine oxidase inhibitors (MAOIs) are a pharmacological alternative to these antidepressants. Although effective for depression, MAOIs are less commonly used due to their risks, side effects, potentially dangerous drug–drug interactions, and need for dietary restrictions to maintain a low-tyramine diet. Notably, if MAOIs are being considered because of an intolerance to the side effects of other antidepressants, older adults usually do not tolerate MAOIs any better. If treatment with an MAOI is to follow treatment with an SSRI, a minimum washout period of 1–2 weeks (or 2–4 weeks following fluoxetine) must elapse after the SSRI is discontinued before the MAOI can be initiated, to avoid a serotonin syndrome. A similar 2-week window is needed when stopping an MAOI and starting another antidepressant medication. If a patient's depression is severe and ECT is contemplated, use of an MAOI also precludes initiation of ECT until 10–14 days after the drug is discontinued. Such a delay may seriously impede clinical management of the suicidal elder person.

Finally, an additional augmentation approach used by some clinicians is to prescribe morning doses of stimulant medications, such as methylphenidate. Clinical trial data support that when using a flexible dosage titration of methylphenidate ranging from 5 mg to 40 mg daily, augmentation of an SSRI with methylphenidate results in greater improvement than using an SSRI alone (Lavretsky et al. 2015). In this study, methylphenidate was well tolerated, although caution should be used in patients with past addictions, high levels of anxiety, or comorbid cardiac disease. Only rarely does the clinician encounter an elder person with a propensity to abuse stimulants or to become addicted when these drugs are given once daily.

Treatment-Resistant Late-Life Depression

Unfortunately, depression in a sizable proportion of older adults may fail to remit with SSRI or SNRI treatment. Although there is limited literature guiding next steps, studies examining adults with treatment-resistant depression may also inform treatment for older individuals. A placebo-controlled multisite study found that aripiprazole provided clinical benefit to elders with depression whose illness did not remit with venlafaxine monotherapy (Lenze et al. 2015). Aripiprazole was well tolerated in this study, although its use was associated with akathisia and parkinsonism. In contrast, a small placebo-controlled trial of intranasal esketamine in treatment-resistant geriatric depression did not observe a statistically significant drug effect (Ochs-Ross et al. 2020). However, secondary analyses observed that individuals ages 65–75 years exhibited a greater reduction in depression severity than did those older than 75 years, whereas individuals with an earlier-life initial onset of depression exhibited greater improvement than those with a later-life onset. Thus, esketamine may have a role for some patients.

Another subtype of treatment-resistant LLD may be depression that occurs in the context of dementia. Major depressive episodes or clinically significant depressive syndromes occur in 20%–30% or more of patients with dementia (Lyketsos et al. 2000). Unfortunately, evidence does not indicate that conventional antidepressant medications are effective in this population (Banerjee et al. 2011; Nelson and Devanand 2011; Rosenberg et al. 2010). Although further work is needed to identify effective antidepressant medications for use in patients with depression and dementia, other interventions such as behavioral therapy or caregiver education may provide some benefit (Kok and Reynolds 2017).

Psychotic Depression

MDD with psychotic features is a malignant illness and, compared with nonpsychotic depression, is associated with poorer acute treatment outcomes, longer recovery time, and greater disability and mortality (Coryell et al. 1996; Maj et al. 2007; Vythilingam et al. 2003). Meta-analyses have clearly shown that psychotic depression can be effectively treated with either ECT or with pharmacotherapy using a combination of antipsychotic and antidepressant medications (Farahani and Correll 2012; Wijkstra et al. 2015). This combination is more effective than monotherapy with an antipsychotic in younger and older adults (Meyers et al. 2009). Several clinical factors may predict a poorer response to pharmacotherapy, including impaired insight, suicidality, and cerebrovascular risk factors (Bingham et al. 2015, 2017; Gerretsen et al. 2015). Although cognitive performance deficits are associated with poor response to treatment in nonpsychotic depression, they do not appear to predict treatment response during psychotic depression (Bingham et al. 2015). Once a patient with psychotic depression has stabilized, both the antidepressant and antipsychotic medications should be continued because withdrawal of the antipsychotic is associated with a higher risk of relapse (Flint et al. 2019). However, this benefit must be balanced against the metabolic risks of second-generation antipsychotic medications.

Neurostimulation

Electroconvulsive Therapy

ECT continues to be the most effective form of treatment for patients with more severe major depressive episodes (Haq et al. 2015). ECT was first established as a treatment in 1938, but it is used less often now than immediately after its development. ECT has been shown to be effective in selected individuals, especially older adults with more severe depression, those at high risk for suicide, and individuals who have MDD with psychotic symptoms. Historically, it has also been indicated for melancholic depression, although more recent evidence questions that lore (van Diermen et al. 2018). Despite its effectiveness, ECT is not the first-line treatment of choice for patients with MDD and is often considered only after other therapeutic modalities have been ineffective. The presence of self-destructive behavior, such as a suicide attempt or refusal to eat, increases the necessity for intervening effectively; in such situations, ECT may be the treatment of choice.

If ECT is selected as an intervention, the clinician must first discuss in detail with the patient and family the nature of the treatment, its risks, and the reasons for the recommendation. It is important to explain why ECT is necessary, what procedures the patient will undergo during a course of ECT, how many treatments can be expected, how long hospitalization will continue, whether ECT can be performed on an outpatient basis, what the risks and side effects of ECT are, and what results, both immediate and long term, can be expected. Even when an elderly patient is severely depressed and reluctant to proceed, careful and thoughtful discussion with the patient and family will often result in the patient (often with encouragement from the family) becoming willing to undergo the course of ECT treatments. Once treatment begins, fears about ECT usually remit.

The medical workup before ECT includes a complete psychiatric and medical history, a physical examination, and consultation with a cardiologist if any cardiac abnormalities are recognized. Knowledge of any family history of psychiatric disorders, suicide, or treatment with ECT is helpful in predicting a patient's response to treatment. Laboratory examination includes a complete blood count, urinalysis, routine chemistries, chest and spinal X-rays (the latter to document previous compression fractures), ECG, and consideration of the need for neuroimaging such as a CT scan or MRI. However, the presence of most age-associated abnormalities seen on MRI does not necessarily serve as a contraindication to ECT.

Before an older patient undergoes ECT treatment, all of the patient's medications should be reviewed for safety. Some psychotropic medications may need to be withdrawn, whereas other medications are continued. For those being continued, the dosages should not be titrated so ECT's effects are not confounded by multiple treatment changes. As noted earlier, any MAOIs must be withdrawn 10–14 days before the procedure to prevent any toxic interactions with the anesthetic used during ECT. Lithium, antipsychotics, and antianxiety agents (including sedative-hypnotics) are not absolutely contraindicated in older patients who undergo ECT; however, benzodiazepines increase the seizure threshold and should be avoided as much as possible.

The basic techniques for ECT are well described. Thirty minutes before treatment, an anticholinergic agent is administered to prevent complications of cardiac arrhythmias and aspiration. Directly before treatment, a short-acting anesthetic, such as thiopental or methohexital, is administered until an eyelash response is no longer present. Then a muscle relaxant, such as succinylcholine, is administered along with airway management to prevent severe muscle contractions.

Initial clinical treatment commonly uses right unilateral electrode placement, often using an ultrabrief pulse (defined as ≤0.5 ms). Such an approach, when combined with an antidepressant, has clear efficacy in treatment-resistant LLD, with almost two-thirds of patients achieving remission (Kellner et al. 2016b). Although unilateral ECT has a favorable risk profile with a lower risk of cognitive side effects, in some cases, bilateral electrode placement may be required. Bilateral treatment may be more effective for some patients, although it increases the risk of confusion and cognitive side effects. After lead placement, the electrical stimulus is applied and the seizure is monitored, either by applying a tourniquet to one arm and observing the tonic and clonic movements in the extremity peripheral to the tourniquet or by using direct electroencephalographic monitoring. The latter is preferred, and a seizure lasting ≥25 seconds is required for optimal results. ECT treatments are generally administered three times per week, and usually 6–12 treatments are necessary for adequate therapeutic response. Depression severity should be monitored using a rating scale to document improvement and to assess when the treatment effect has hit a plateau. Two or three treatments are generally given after the patient's improvement appears to stabilize.

The risks and side effects of ECT in elderly patients are similar to those in younger adults but may be complicated by comorbid conditions. Cardiovascular effects are of greatest concern and include premature ventricular contractions, ventricular arrhythmias, and transient systolic hypertension. Frequent monitoring during treatment decreases the (already low) risk that one of these side effects will lead to permanent problems. Confusion and amnesia often result after an ECT session, but the duration of this episode is typically brief. However, even with unilateral electrode placement, some patients have prolonged anterograde memory difficulties; these typically resolve with cessation of ECT. Headaches are common with ECT and usually respond to nonnarcotic analgesics or premedication with nonsteroidal anti-inflammatory drugs. Status epilepticus and vertebral compression fractures are some of the rare but more serious adverse effects. Compression fractures are a particular risk in older women because of the high incidence of osteoporosis in the postmenopausal population.

The overall success rate of ECT in patients who have not responded to drug therapy is ~70% (Kellner et al. 2006, 2010), with good efficacy in older adults (Kellner et al. 2016b; Spaans et al. 2015). Older age is not a marker of treatment resistance to ECT but, in fact, has been positively associated with speed and likelihood of response (Kellner et al. 2016b). There is also evidence that ECT may be more effective and have fewer side effects than antidepressants when used to treat depression in older geriatric patients, or those older than 75 years of age (Manly et al. 2000). Although not extensively studied, it appears that ECT may also be an effective treatment for depression in the context of dementia (Oudman 2012). Moreover, ECT may reduce agitation in dementia, although robust clinical trials are needed to fully determine benefits and potential risks (Glass et al. 2017).

Unfortunately, once a patient has completed an index course of ECT, the relapse rate with no prophylactic intervention may exceed 50% in the next year. This can be decreased if antidepressants or lithium carbonate is prescribed following the index course. Maintenance ECT may be necessary for some patients who exhibit a high likelihood of recurrence despite use of prophylactic medication or who experience high toxicity and therefore cannot tolerate prophylactic medications. For such patients, weekly or monthly treatments (usually on an outpatient basis) are prescribed, with careful monitoring of response and side effects. Maintenance ECT in combination with antidepressant treatment is clearly superior to maintenance treatment with antidepressant medications alone (Kellner et al. 2016a).

Transcranial Magnetic Stimulation

Repetitive transcranial magnetic stimulation (rTMS) was FDA approved for treating depression in 2008 and involves the generation of a time-varying magnetic field by a current pulse through a simulator coil placed over the scalp, inducing electric current intracranially and, thus, neural activation. The intensity of stimulation is set at a fixed percentage of the individual's motor threshold, measured as the output required to produce movement of the thumb or fingers. Using standard guidelines, rTMS is a safe and well-tolerated treatment, with minimal risk of inducing an epileptic seizure. Although there is much interest in alternative placements of the delivery coil, when rTMS is utilized to treat depression, the stimulus is typically placed over the left dorsolateral prefrontal cortex. A treatment course typically involves 40-minute sessions 5 days a week for 4–6 weeks.

rTMS treatment for MDD in adult populations is clearly effective (Lefaucheur et al. 2014; Perera et al. 2016). Meta-analyses of sham-controlled trials in MDD have shown response rates of 30%–40% and remission rates of 18%–38% (Berlim et al. 2013, 2014). Although these rates are not as robust as those seen for ECT, they are encouraging because most individuals receiving rTMS have exhibited treatment resistance to antidepressants. Moreover, rTMS is better tolerated than both ECT and antidepressants. It does not have risks for cardiac events, anesthesia, or memory impairment and does not contribute to polypharmacy. The most common side effects experienced with rTMS are typically mild and include headaches, muscle twitching, and slight pain at the stimulation site.

In contrast to the broader literature on rTMS, studies of its use in geriatric depression are limited. A small blinded, sham-controlled trial in LLD found that active rTMS was superior to sham administration, with a response rate of 40.0% compared with 14.8% and a number needed to treat of 4.0 (95% CI 2.1–56.5) (Kaster et al. 2018). Moreover, rTMS has demonstrated efficacy in MRI-defined vascular depression in older adults (Jorge et al. 2008). However, its safety profile and tolerability make rTMS a reasonable choice for elder persons with depression who have not responded to or cannot take antidepressant medication.

Conclusion

Depressive disorders are among the most frequent mental health problems encountered by those who care for older adults. We perhaps know more about these disorders in older adults, particularly how to successfully treat them, than about any other late-life psychiatric disorders. In addition, we have improved diagnostic capabilities and many treatment options. It is not an understatement to suggest that despite how bleak the world may seem when one is depressed, hope yet remains.

Key Points

- Late-life depression (LLD) in the community may be less frequent than depression at other stages of the life cycle, yet its frequency increases with physical illness and cognitive impairment.

- The relationship between depression and medical comorbidity is often reciprocal, with one illness contributing to poor outcomes in the other.

- The biopsychosocial model works well in placing the origins of LLD in context. Most cases derive from a variety of causes.

- Several physiological changes seen with aging may contribute to the development or perpetuation of depression in older adults, including subclinical vascular brain disease or proinflammatory processes.

- Older adults who are cognitively intact may experience a buffering of depression because of a lifetime of cumulative wisdom coupled with a different view of events given their age.

- Diagnostic workup of the older adult with depression centers on a detailed history, ideally from both the patient and family, including an assessment of suicide risk.

- For moderately severe depression, a combination of antidepressant therapy and psychotherapy is optimal.

- Electroconvulsive therapy is indicated for more severe and treatment-resistant depressive disorders in late life and is generally well tolerated.

Suggested Readings

Byers AL, Yaffe K: Depression and risk of developing dementia. Nat Rev Neurol 7(6):323–331, 2011 21537355

Conwell Y, Van Orden K, Caine ED: Suicide in older adults. Psychiatr Clin North Am 34(2):451–468, 2011 21536168

Haq AU, Sitzmann AF, Goldman ML, et al: Response of depression to electroconvulsive therapy: a meta-analysis of clinical predictors. J Clin Psychiatry 76(10):1374–1384, 2015 26528644

Kok RM, Reynolds CF 3rd: Management of depression in older adults: a review. JAMA 317(20):2114–2122, 2017 28535241

Nelson JC, Delucchi K, Schneider LS: Efficacy of second generation antidepressants in late-life depression: a meta-analysis of the evidence. Am J Geriatr Psychiatry 16(7):558–567, 2008 18591576

Taylor WD: Clinical practice: depression in the elderly. N Engl J Med 371(13):1228–1236, 2014 25251617

Taylor WD, Aizenstein HJ, Alexopoulos GS: The vascular depression hypothesis: mechanisms linking vascular disease with depression. Mol Psychiatry 18(9):963–974, 2013 23439482

References

Aizenstein HJ, Andreescu C, Edelman KL, et al: fMRI correlates of white matter hyperintensities in late-life depression. Am J Psychiatry 168(10):1075–1082, 2011 21799066

Alexopoulos GS, Areán P: A model for streamlining psychotherapy in the RDoC era: the example of "Engage." Mol Psychiatry 19(1):14–19, 2014 24280983

Alexopoulos GS, Morimoto SS: The inflammation hypothesis in geriatric depression. Int J Geriatr Psychiatry 26(11):1109–1118, 2011 21370276

Alexopoulos GS, Meyers BS, Young RC, et al: Recovery in geriatric depression. Arch Gen Psychiatry 53(4):305–312, 1996 8634008

Alexopoulos GS, Meyers BS, Young RC, et al: "Vascular depression" hypothesis. Arch Gen Psychiatry 54(10):915–922, 1997 9337771

Alexopoulos GS, Kiosses DN, Heo M, et al: Executive dysfunction and the course of geriatric depression. Biol Psychiatry 58(3):204–210, 2005 16018984

Alexopoulos GS, Raue PJ, Kiosses DN, et al: Comparing engage with PST in late-life major depression: a preliminary report. Am J Geriatr Psychiatry 23(5):506–513, 2015 25081818

Alexopoulos GS, Raue PJ, Gunning F, et al: "Engage" therapy: behavioral activation and improvement of late-life major depression. Am J Geriatr Psychiatry 24(4):320–326, 2016 26905044

American Psychiatric Association: Diagnostic and Statistical Manual of Mental Disorders, 4th Edition. Washington, DC, American Psychiatric Association, 1994

American Psychiatric Association: Diagnostic and Statistical Manual of Mental Disorders, 5th Edition. Arlington, VA, American Psychiatric Association, 2013

Andreescu C, Lenze EJ, Dew MA, et al: Effect of comorbid anxiety on treatment response and relapse risk in late-life depression: controlled study. Br J Psychiatry 190:344–349, 2007 17401042

Andreescu C, Lenze EJ, Mulsant BH, et al: High worry severity is associated with poorer acute and maintenance efficacy of antidepressants in late-life depression. Depress Anxiety 26(3):266–272, 2009 19212971

Andreescu C, Ajilore O, Aizenstein HJ, et al: Disruption of neural homeostasis as a model of relapse and recurrence in late-life depression. Am J Geriatr Psychiatry 27(12):1316–1330, 2019 31477459

Anglin RE, Samaan Z, Walter SD, McDonald SD: Vitamin D deficiency and depression in adults: systematic review and meta-analysis. Br J Psychiatry 202:100–107, 2013 23377209

Arborelius L, Owens MJ, Plotsky PM, Nemeroff CB: The role of corticotropin-releasing factor in depression and anxiety disorders. J Endocrinol 160(1):1–12, 1999 9854171

Areán PA, Perri MG, Nezu AM, et al: Comparative effectiveness of social problem-solving therapy and reminiscence therapy as treatments for depression in older adults. J Consult Clin Psychol 61(6):1003–1010, 1993 8113478

Areán P, Hegel M, Vannoy S, et al: Effectiveness of problem-solving therapy for older, primary care patients with depression: results from the IMPACT project. Gerontologist 48(3):311–323, 2008 18591356

Areán PA, Raue P, Mackin RS, et al: Problem-solving therapy and supportive therapy in older adults with major depression and executive dysfunction. Am J Psychiatry 167(11):1391–1398, 2010 20516155

Ayalon L, Litwin H: What cognitive functions are associated with passive suicidal ideation? Findings from a national sample of community dwelling Israelis. Int J Geriatr Psychiatry 24(5):472–478, 2009 18837056

Baldwin R, Tomenson B: Depression in later life: a comparison of symptoms and risk factors in early and late onset cases. Br J Psychiatry 167(5):649–652, 1995 8564322

Baldwin R, Jeffries S, Jackson A, et al: Treatment response in late-onset depression: relationship to neuropsychological, neuroradiological and vascular risk factors. Psychol Med 34(1):125–136, 2004 14971633

Baltes PB, Staudinger UM: Wisdom: a metaheuristic (pragmatic) to orchestrate mind and virtue toward excellence. Am Psychol 55(1):122–136, 2000 11392856

Banerjee S, Hellier J, Dewey M, et al: Sertraline or mirtazapine for depression in dementia (HTA-SADD): a randomised, multicentre, double-blind, placebo-controlled trial. Lancet 378(9789):403–411, 2011 21764118

Barefoot JC, Helms MJ, Mark DB, et al: Depression and long-term mortality risk in patients with coronary artery disease. Am J Cardiol 78(6):613–617, 1996 8831391

Barry LC, Abou JJ, Simen AA, Gill TM: Under-treatment of depression in older persons. J Affect Disord 136(3):789–796, 2012 22030136

Baune BT, Smith E, Reppermund S, et al: Inflammatory biomarkers predict depressive, but not anxiety symptoms during aging: the prospective Sydney Memory and Aging Study. Psychoneuroendocrinology 37(9):1521–1530, 2012 22406002

Beekman AT, Deeg DJ, Geerlings SW, et al: Emergence and persistence of late life depression: a 3-year follow-up of the Longitudinal Aging Study Amsterdam. J Affect Disord 65(2):131–138, 2001 11356236

Beekman AT, Geerlings SW, Deeg DJ, et al: The natural history of late-life depression: a 6-year prospective study in the community. Arch Gen Psychiatry 59(7):605–611, 2002 12090813

Benjamin S, McQuoid DR, Potter GG, et al: The brain-derived neurotrophic factor Val66Met polymorphism, hippocampal volume, and cognitive function in geriatric depression. Am J Geriatr Psychiatry 18(4):323–331, 2010 20220593

Berlim MT, Van den Eynde F, Jeff Daskalakis Z: Clinically meaningful efficacy and acceptability of low-frequency repetitive transcranial magnetic stimulation (rTMS) for treating primary major depression: a meta-analysis of randomized, double-blind and sham-controlled trials. Neuropsychopharmacology 38(4):543–551, 2013 23249815

Berlim MT, van den Eynde F, Tovar-Perdomo S, Daskalakis ZJ: Response, remission and drop-out rates following high-frequency repetitive transcranial magnetic stimulation (rTMS) for treating major depression: a systematic review and meta-analysis of randomized, double-blind and sham-controlled trials. Psychol Med 44(2):225–239, 2014 23507264

Bhalla RK, Butters MA, Mulsant BH, et al: Persistence of neuropsychologic deficits in the remitted state of late-life depression. Am J Geriatr Psychiatry 14(5):419–427, 2006 16670246

Bhalla RK, Butters MA, Becker JT, et al: Patterns of mild cognitive impairment after treatment of depression in the elderly. Am J Geriatr Psychiatry 17(4):308–316, 2009 19307859

Biella MM, Borges MK, Strauss J, et al: Subthreshold depression needs a prime time in old age psychiatry? A narrative review of current evidence. Neuropsychiatr Dis Treat 15:2763–2772, 2019 31576131

Bingham KS, Whyte EM, Meyers BS, et al: Relationship between cerebrovascular risk, cognition, and treatment outcome in late-life psychotic depression. Am J Geriatr Psychiatry 23(12):1270–1275, 2015 26560512

Bingham KS, Rothschild AJ, Mulsant BH, et al: The association of baseline suicidality with treatment outcome in psychotic depression. J Clin Psychiatry 78(8):1149–1154, 2017 28445632

Black SA, Goodwin JS, Markides KS: The association between chronic diseases and depressive symptomatology in older Mexican Americans. J Gerontol A Biol Sci Med Sci 53(3):M188–M194, 1998 9597050

Blazer DG: Social support and mortality in an elderly community population. Am J Epidemiol 115(5):684–694, 1982 7081200

Blazer DG: Depression in late life: review and commentary. J Gerontol A Biol Sci Med Sci 58(3):249–265, 2003 12634292

Blazer DG, Hughes DC, George LK: The epidemiology of depression in an elderly community population. Gerontologist 27(3):281–287, 1987 3609795

Blazer DG, Moody-Ayers S, Craft-Morgan J, Burchett B: Depression in diabetes and obesity: racial/ethnic/gender issues in older adults. J Psychosom Res 53(4):913–916, 2002 12377303

Blazer DG II, Hybels CF: Origins of depression in later life. Psychol Med 35(9):1241–1252, 2005 16168147

Braam AW, Beekman AT, Deeg DJ, et al: Religiosity as a protective or prognostic factor of depression in later life; results from a community survey in The Netherlands. Acta Psychiatr Scand 96(3):199–205, 1997a 9296551

Braam AW, Beekman AT, van Tilburg TG, et al: Religious involvement and depression in older Dutch citizens. Soc Psychiatry Psychiatr Epidemiol 32(5):284–291, 1997b 9257519

Brandão DJ, Fontenelle LF, da Silva SA, et al: Depression and excess mortality in the elderly living in low- and middle-income countries: Systematic review and meta-analysis. Int J Geriatr Psychiatry 34(1):22–30, 2019 30306638

Britton PC, Duberstein PR, Conner KR, et al: Reasons for living, hopelessness, and suicide ideation among depressed adults 50 years or older. Am J Geriatr Psychiatry 16(9):736–741, 2008 18757767

Brodaty H, Luscombe G, Parker G, et al: Early and late onset depression in old age: different aetiologies, same phenomenology. J Affect Disord 66(2–3):225–236, 2001 11578676

Brown PJ, Roose SP, Fieo R, et al: Frailty and depression in older adults: a high-risk clinical population. Am J Geriatr Psychiatry 22(11):1083–1095, 2014 23973252

Bruce ML: Depression and disability in late life: directions for future research. Am J Geriatr Psychiatry 9(2):102–112, 2001 11316615

Bruce ML: Psychosocial risk factors for depressive disorders in late life. Biol Psychiatry 52(3):175–184, 2002 12182924

Bruce ML, Ten Have TR, Reynolds CF III, et al: Reducing suicidal ideation and depressive symptoms in depressed older primary care patients: a randomized controlled trial. JAMA 291(9):1081–1091, 2004 14996777

Butters MA, Becker JT, Nebes RD, et al: Changes in cognitive functioning following treatment of late-life depression. Am J Psychiatry 157(12):1949–1954, 2000 11097959

Byers AL, Yaffe K: Depression and risk of developing dementia. Nat Rev Neurol 7(6):323–331, 2011 21537355

Callahan CM, Nienaber NA, Hendrie HC, Tierney WM: Depression of elderly outpatients: primary care physicians' attitudes and practice patterns. J Gen Intern Med 7(1):26–31, 1992 1548545

Capuron L, Gumnick JF, Musselman DL, et al: Neurobehavioral effects of interferon-alpha in cancer patients: phenomenology and paroxetine responsiveness of symptom dimensions. Neuropsychopharmacology 26(5):643–652, 2002 11927189

Caravati EM, Bossart PJ: Demographic and electrocardiographic factors associated with severe tricyclic antidepressant toxicity. J Toxicol Clin Toxicol 29(1):31–43, 1991 2005664

Carmelli D, Swan GE, Kelly Hayes M, et al: Longitudinal changes in the contribution of genetic and environmental influences to symptoms of depression in older male twins. Psychol Aging 15(3):505–510, 2000 11014713

Carney CE, Moss TG, Lachowski AM, Atwood ME: Understanding mental and physical fatigue complaints in those with depression and insomnia. Behav Sleep Med 12(4):272–289, 2014 24128300

Chi I, Chou KL: Social support and depression among elderly Chinese people in Hong Kong. Int J Aging Hum Dev 52(3):231–252, 2001 11407488

Chou KL, Chi I: Stressful life events and depressive symptoms: social support and sense of control as mediators or moderators? Int J Aging Hum Dev 52(2):155–171, 2001 11352200

Clayton PJ: Bereavement and depression. J Clin Psychiatry 51(suppl):34–38, discussion 39–40, 1990

Coffey CE, Figiel GS, Djang WT, Weiner RD: Subcortical hyperintensity on magnetic resonance imaging: a comparison of normal and depressed elderly subjects. Am J Psychiatry 147(2):187–189, 1990 2301657

Cole MG, Bellavance F, Mansour A: Prognosis of depression in elderly community and primary care populations: a systematic review and meta-analysis. Am J Psychiatry 156(8):1182–1189, 1999 10450258

Conwell Y, Thompson C: Suicidal behavior in elders. Psychiatr Clin North Am 31(2):333–356, 2008 18439452

Conwell Y, Lyness JM, Duberstein P, et al: Completed suicide among older patients in primary care practices: a controlled study. J Am Geriatr Soc 48(1):23–29, 2000 10642017

Conwell Y, Van Orden K, Caine ED: Suicide in older adults. Psychiatr Clin North Am 34(2):451–468, 2011 21536168

Coryell W, Leon A, Winokur G, et al: Importance of psychotic features to long-term course in major depressive disorder. Am J Psychiatry 153(4):483–489, 1996 8599395

Crosby AE, Cheltenham MP, Sacks JJ: Incidence of suicidal ideation and behavior in the United States, 1994. Suicide Life Threat Behav 29(2):131–140, 1999 10407966

Cuijpers P, Vogelzangs N, Twisk J, et al: Comprehensive meta-analysis of excess mortality in depression in the general community versus patients with specific illnesses. Am J Psychiatry 171(4):453–462, 2014 24434956

Cuijpers P, Donker T, Weissman MM, et al: Interpersonal psychotherapy for mental health problems: a comprehensive meta-analysis. Am J Psychiatry 173(7):680–687, 2016 27032627

Czéh B, Michaelis T, Watanabe T, et al: Stress-induced changes in cerebral metabolites, hippo-campal volume, and cell proliferation are prevented by antidepressant treatment with tianeptine. Proc Natl Acad Sci USA 98(22):12796–12801, 2001 11675510

Deng Y, McQuoid DR, Potter GG, et al: Predictors of recurrence in remitted late-life depression. Depress Anxiety 35(7):658–667, 2018 29749006

Devanand DP: Comorbid psychiatric disorders in late life depression. Biol Psychiatry 52(3):236–242, 2002 12182929

Devanand DP: Dysthymic disorder in the elderly population. Int Psychogeriatr 26(1):39–48, 2014 24152873

Devanand DP, Nobler MS, Cheng J, et al: Randomized, double-blind, placebo-controlled trial of fluoxetine treatment for elderly patients with dysthymic disorder. Am J Geriatr Psychiatry 13(1):59–68, 2005 15653941

Diem SJ, Greer NL, MacDonald R, et al: Efficacy and safety of testosterone treatment in men: an evidence report for a clinical practice guideline by the American College of Physicians. Ann Intern Med 172(2):105–118, 2020 31905375

Dilger RN, Johnson RW: Aging, microglial cell priming, and the discordant central inflamma-tory response to signals from the peripheral immune system. J Leukoc Biol 84(4):932–939, 2008 18495785

Diniz BS, Butters MA, Albert SM, et al: Late-life depression and risk of vascular dementia and Alzheimer's disease: systematic review and meta-analysis of community-based cohort studies. Br J Psychiatry 202(5):329–335, 2013 23637108

Donovan NJ, Wu Q, Rentz DM, et al: Loneliness, depression and cognitive function in older U.S. adults. Int J Geriatr Psychiatry 32(5):564–573, 2017 27162047

Dotson VM, Beydoun MA, Zonderman AB: Recurrent depressive symptoms and the incidence of dementia and mild cognitive impairment. Neurology 75(1):27–34, 2010 20603482

Duberstein PR, Conwell Y, Seidlitz L, et al: Age and suicidal ideation in older depressed inpa-tients. Am J Geriatr Psychiatry 7(4):289–296, 1999 10521160

Egan MF, Kojima M, Callicott JH, et al: The BDNF val66met polymorphism affects activity-dependent secretion of BDNF and human memory and hippocampal function. Cell 112(2):257–269, 2003 12553913

Eisses AM, Kluiter H, Jongenelis K, et al: Risk indicators of depression in residential homes. Int J Geriatr Psychiatry 19(7):634–640, 2004 15254919

Elderkin-Thompson V, Kumar A, Bilker WB, et al: Neuropsychological deficits among patients with late-onset minor and major depression. Arch Clin Neuropsychol 18(5):529–549, 2003 14591448

Elderkin-Thompson V, Irwin MR, Hellemann G, Kumar A: Interleukin-6 and memory functions of encoding and recall in healthy and depressed elderly adults. Am J Geriatr Psychiatry 20(9):753–763, 2012 22892560

Erlangsen A, Zarit SH, Conwell Y: Hospital-diagnosed dementia and suicide: a longitudinal study using prospective, nationwide register data. Am J Geriatr Psychiatry 16(3):220–228, 2008 18310552

Eurelings LS, van Dalen JW, Ter Riet G, et al: Apathy and depressive symptoms in older people and incident myocardial infarction, stroke, and mortality: a systematic review and meta-analysis of individual participant data. Clin Epidemiol 10:363–379, 2018 29670402

Farahani A, Correll CU: Are antipsychotics or antidepressants needed for psychotic depression? A systematic review and meta-analysis of trials comparing antidepressant or antipsychotic monotherapy with combination treatment. J Clin Psychiatry 73(4):486–496, 2012 22579147

Fiske A, Gatz M, Pedersen NL: Depressive symptoms and aging: the effects of illness and non-health-related events. J Gerontol B Psychol Sci Soc Sci 58(6):320–328, 2003 14614116

Flint AJ, Meyers BS, Rothschild AJ, et al: Effect of continuing olanzapine vs placebo on relapse among patients with psychotic depression in remission: the STOP-PD II randomized clin-ical trial. JAMA 322(7):622–631, 2019 31429896

Folstein MF, Folstein SE, McHugh PR: "Mini-Mental State": a practical method for grading the cognitive state of patients for the clinician. J Psychiatr Res 12(3):189–198, 1975 1202204

Freeman EW, Sammel MD, Boorman DW, Zhang R: Longitudinal pattern of depressive symptoms around natural menopause. JAMA Psychiatry 71(1):36–43, 2014 24227182

Fried LP, Tangen CM, Walston J, et al: Frailty in older adults: evidence for a phenotype. J Gerontol A Biol Sci Med Sci 56(3):M146–M156, 2001 11253156

Gallo JJ, Rabins PV, Lyketsos CG, et al: Depression without sadness: functional outcomes of nondysphoric depression in later life. J Am Geriatr Soc 45(5):570–578, 1997 9158577

Gatz M, Pedersen NL, Plomin R, et al: Importance of shared genes and shared environments for symptoms of depression in older adults. J Abnorm Psychol 101(4):701–708, 1992 1430610

Geerlings SW, Beekman AT, Deeg DJ, et al: Duration and severity of depression predict mortality in older adults in the community. Psychol Med 32(4):609–618, 2002 12102375

Gerretsen P, Flint AJ, Whyte EM, et al: Impaired insight into delusions predicts treatment outcome during a randomized controlled trial for psychotic depression (STOP-PD study). J Clin Psychiatry 76(4):427–433, 2015 25919834

Glass OM, Forester BP, Hermida AP: Electroconvulsive therapy (ECT) for treating agitation in dementia (major neurocognitive disorder): a promising option. Int Psychogeriatr 29(5):717–726, 2017 28095946

Golden J, Conroy RM, Bruce I, et al: Loneliness, social support networks, mood and wellbeing in community-dwelling elderly. Int J Geriatr Psychiatry 24(7):694–700, 2009 19274642

Gottfries CG: Neurochemical aspects on aging and diseases with cognitive impairment. J Neurosci Res 27(4):541–547, 1990 2079715

Gould RL, Coulson MC, Howard RJ: Cognitive behavioral therapy for depression in older people: a meta-analysis and meta-regression of randomized controlled trials. J Am Geriatr Soc 60(10):1817–1830, 2012 23003115

Gournellis R, Lykouras L, Fortos A, et al: Psychotic (delusional) major depression in late life: a clinical study. Int J Geriatr Psychiatry 16(11):1085–1091, 2001 11746655

Han BH, Sherman S, Mauro PM, et al: Demographic trends among older cannabis users in the United States, 2006–13. Addiction 112(3):516–525, 2017 27767235

Haq AU, Sitzmann AF, Goldman ML, et al: Response of depression to electroconvulsive therapy: a meta-analysis of clinical predictors. J Clin Psychiatry 76(10):1374–1384, 2015 26528644

Hariri AR, Goldberg TE, Mattay VS, et al: Brain-derived neurotrophic factor val66met polymorphism affects human memory-related hippocampal activity and predicts memory performance. J Neurosci 23(17):6690–6694, 2003 12890761

Hays JC, Krishnan KR, George LK, et al: Psychosocial and physical correlates of chronic depression. Psychiatry Res 72(3):149–159, 1997 9406904

Hays JC, Steffens DC, Flint EP, et al: Does social support buffer functional decline in elderly patients with unipolar depression? Am J Psychiatry 158(11):1850–1855, 2001 11691691

Hayward RD, Taylor WD, Smoski MJ, et al: Association of five-factor model personality domains and facets with presence, onset, and treatment outcomes of major depression in older adults. Am J Geriatr Psychiatry 21(1):88–96, 2013 23290206

Hedegaard H, Curtin SC, Warner M: Increase in Suicide Mortality in the United States, 1999–2018. NCHS Data Brief, no 362. Hyattsville, MD, National Center for Health Statistics, 2020

Heikkinen J, Honkanen R, Williams L, et al: Depressive disorders, anxiety disorders and subjective mental health in common musculoskeletal diseases: a review. Maturitas 127:18–25, 2019 31351516

Heils A, Teufel A, Petri S, et al: Allelic variation of human serotonin transporter gene expression. J Neurochem 66(6):2621–2624, 1996 8632190

Heisel MJ, Duberstein PR, Lyness JM, Feldman MD: Screening for suicide ideation among older primary care patients. J Am Board Fam Med 23(2):260–269, 2010 20207936

Heisel MJ, Talbot NL, King DA, et al: Adapting interpersonal psychotherapy for older adults at risk for suicide. Am J Geriatr Psychiatry 23(1):87–98, 2015 24840611

Hek K, Demirkan A, Lahti J, et al: A genome-wide association study of depressive symptoms. Biol Psychiatry 73(7):667–678, 2013 23290196

Henderson AS, Korten AE, Jacomb PA, et al: The course of depression in the elderly: a longitudinal community-based study in Australia. Psychol Med 27(1):119–129, 1997 9122292

Holvast F, Burger H, de Waal MM, et al: Loneliness is associated with poor prognosis in late-life depression: longitudinal analysis of the Netherlands Study of Depression in Older Persons. J Affect Disord 185:1–7, 2015 26142687

Howard DM, Adams MJ, Clarke TK, et al: Genome-wide meta-analysis of depression identifies 102 independent variants and highlights the importance of the prefrontal brain regions. Nat Neurosci 22(3):343–352, 2019 30718901

Huang AX, Delucchi K, Dunn LB, Nelson JC: A systematic review and meta-analysis of psychotherapy for late-life depression. Am J Geriatr Psychiatry 23(3):261–273, 2015 24856580

Hybels CF, Blazer DG, Pieper CF: Toward a threshold for subthreshold depression: an analysis of correlates of depression by severity of symptoms using data from an elderly community sample. Gerontologist 41(3):357–365, 2001 11405433

Hybels CF, Blazer DG, Steffens DC: Predictors of partial remission in older patients treated for major depression: the role of comorbid dysthymia. Am J Geriatr Psychiatry 13(8):713–721, 2005 16085788

Institute of Medicine Committee on Mental Health Workforce for Geriatric Populations: The Mental Health and Substance Use Workforce for Older Adults: In Whose Hands? Washington, DC, National Academies Press, 2012

Jackson JC, Pandharipande PP, Girard TD, et al: Depression, post-traumatic stress disorder, and functional disability in survivors of critical illness in the BRAIN-ICU study: a longitudinal cohort study. Lancet Respir Med 2(5):369–379, 2014 24815803

Jang Y, Haley WE, Small BJ, Mortimer JA: The role of mastery and social resources in the associations between disability and depression in later life. Gerontologist 42(6):807–813, 2002 12451162

Jansson M, Gatz M, Berg S, et al: Gender differences in heritability of depressive symptoms in the elderly. Psychol Med 34(3):471–479, 2004 15259832

Jiang W, Alexander J, Christopher E, et al: Relationship of depression to increased risk of mortality and rehospitalization in patients with congestive heart failure. Arch Intern Med 161(15):1849–1856, 2001 11493126

Johnson W, McGue M, Gaist D, et al: Frequency and heritability of depression symptomatology in the second half of life: evidence from Danish twins over 45. Psychol Med 32(7):1175–1185, 2002 12420887

Jorge RE, Moser DJ, Acion L, Robinson RG: Treatment of vascular depression using repetitive transcranial magnetic stimulation. Arch Gen Psychiatry 65(3):268–276, 2008 18316673

Kaplan MS, Geling O: Sociodemographic and geographic patterns of firearm suicide in the United States, 1989–1993. Health Place 5(2):179–185, 1999 10670999

Karel MJ: Aging and depression: vulnerability and stress across adulthood. Clin Psychol Rev 17(8):847–879, 1997 9439871

Kaster TS, Daskalakis ZJ, Noda Y, et al: Efficacy, tolerability, and cognitive effects of deep transcranial magnetic stimulation for late-life depression: a prospective randomized controlled trial. Neuropsychopharmacology 43(11):2231–2238, 2018 29946106

Kellner CH, Knapp RG, Petrides G, et al: Continuation electroconvulsive therapy vs pharmacotherapy for relapse prevention in major depression: a multisite study from the Consortium for Research in Electroconvulsive Therapy (CORE). Arch Gen Psychiatry 63(12):1337–1344, 2006 17146008

Kellner CH, Knapp R, Husain MM, et al: Bifrontal, bitemporal and right unilateral electrode placement in ECT: randomised trial. Br J Psychiatry 196(3):226–234, 2010 20194546

Kellner CH, Husain MM, Knapp RG, et al: A novel strategy for continuation ECT in geriatric depression: phase 2 of the PRIDE Study. Am J Psychiatry 173(11):1110–1118, 2016a 27418381

Kellner CH, Husain MM, Knapp RG, et al: Right unilateral ultrabrief pulse ECT in geriatric depression: phase 1 of the PRIDE Study. Am J Psychiatry 173(11):1101–1109, 2016b 27418379

Kendler KS, Karkowski LM, Prescott CA: Causal relationship between stressful life events and the onset of major depression. Am J Psychiatry 156(6):837–841, 1999 10360120

Kendler KS, Thornton LM, Gardner CO: Stressful life events and previous episodes in the etiology of major depression in women: an evaluation of the "kindling" hypothesis. Am J Psychiatry 157(8):1243–1251, 2000 10910786

Kennedy GJ, Kelman HR, Thomas C: The emergence of depressive symptoms in late life: the importance of declining health and increasing disability. J Community Health 15(2):93–104, 1990 2141337

Kerner N, Roose SP: Obstructive sleep apnea is linked to depression and cognitive impairment: evidence and potential mechanisms. Am J Geriatr Psychiatry 24(6):496–508, 2016 27139243

Kerner N, D'Antonio K, Pelton GH, et al: An open treatment trial of duloxetine in elderly patients with dysthymic disorder. SAGE Open Med 2, 2014 25177490

Kessler RC: The effects of stressful life events on depression. Annu Rev Psychol 48:191–214, 1997 9046559

Kessler RC, Chiu WT, Demler O, et al: Prevalence, severity, and comorbidity of 12-month DSM-IV disorders in the National Comorbidity Survey Replication. Arch Gen Psychiatry 62(6):617–627, 2005 15939839

Kirkham JG, Choi N, Seitz DP: Meta-analysis of problem solving therapy for the treatment of major depressive disorder in older adults. Int J Geriatr Psychiatry 31(5):526–535, 2016 26437368

Koenig HG: Religion and depression in older medical inpatients. Am J Geriatr Psychiatry 15(4):282–291, 2007a 17384313

Koenig HG: Religion and remission of depression in medical inpatients with heart failure/pulmonary disease. J Nerv Ment Dis 195(5):389–395, 2007b 17502804

Koenig AM, DeLozier IJ, Zmuda MD, et al: Neuropsychological functioning in the acute and remitted states of late-life depression. J Alzheimers Dis 45(1):175–185, 2015 25471193

Koenig HG, Meador KG, Cohen HJ, Blazer DG: Depression in elderly hospitalized patients with medical illness. Arch Intern Med 148(9):1929–1936, 1988 3415405

Koenig HG, George LK, Titus P: Religion, spirituality, and health in medically ill hospitalized older patients. J Am Geriatr Soc 52(4):554–562, 2004 15066070

Köhler O, Benros ME, Nordentoft M, et al: Effect of anti-inflammatory treatment on depression, depressive symptoms, and adverse effects: a systematic review and meta-analysis of randomized clinical trials. JAMA Psychiatry 71(12):1381–1391, 2014 25322082

Kohn CS, Petrucci RJ, Baessler C, et al: The effect of psychological intervention on patients' long-term adjustment to the ICD: a prospective study. Pacing Clin Electrophysiol 23(4 pt 1):450–456, 2000 10793433

Kok RM, Reynolds CF III: Management of depression in older adults: a review. JAMA 317(20):2114–2122, 2017 28535241

Kok RM, Nolen WA, Heeren TJ: Efficacy of treatment in older depressed patients: a systematic review and meta-analysis of double-blind randomized controlled trials with antidepressants. J Affect Disord 141(2–3):103–115, 2012 22480823

Koo BB, Blackwell T, Lee HB, et al: Restless legs syndrome and depression: effect mediation by disturbed sleep and periodic limb movements. Am J Geriatr Psychiatry 24(11):1105–1116, 2016 27526989

Koyama A, O'Brien J, Weuve J, et al: The role of peripheral inflammatory markers in dementia and Alzheimer's disease: a meta-analysis. J Gerontol A Biol Sci Med Sci 68(4):433–440, 2013 22982688

Kraaij V, de Wilde EJ: Negative life events and depressive symptoms in the elderly: a life span perspective. Aging Ment Health 5(1):84–91, 2001 11513018

Kraaij V, Arensman E, Spinhoven P: Negative life events and depression in elderly persons: a meta-analysis. J Gerontol B Psychol Sci Soc Sci 57(1):87–94, 2002 11773227

Krishnan KR, Goli V, Ellinwood EH, et al: Leukoencephalopathy in patients diagnosed as major depressive. Biol Psychiatry 23(5):519–522, 1988 3345325

Krishnan KR, Hays JC, Blazer DG: MRI-defined vascular depression. Am J Psychiatry 154(4):497–501, 1997 9090336

Krishnan KR, Taylor WD, McQuoid DR, et al: Clinical characteristics of magnetic resonance imaging-defined subcortical ischemic depression. Biol Psychiatry 55(4):390–397, 2004 14960292

Kroenke K, Spitzer RL, Williams JB: The PHQ-9: validity of a brief depression severity measure. J Gen Intern Med 16(9):606–613, 2001 11556941

Laird KT, Krause B, Funes C, Lavretsky H: Psychobiological factors of resilience and depression in late life. Transl Psychiatry 9(1):88, 2019 30765686

Lavretsky H, Reinlieb M, St Cyr N, et al: Citalopram, methylphenidate, or their combination in geriatric depression: a randomized, double-blind, placebo-controlled trial. Am J Psychiatry 172(6):561–569, 2015 25677354

Lefaucheur JP, André-Obadia N, Antal A, et al: Evidence-based guidelines on the therapeutic use of repetitive transcranial magnetic stimulation (rTMS). Clin Neurophysiol 125(11):2150–2206, 2014 25034472

Lenze EJ, Munin MC, Skidmore ER, et al: Onset of depression in elderly persons after hip fracture: implications for prevention and early intervention of late-life depression. J Am Geriatr Soc 55(1):81–86, 2007 17233689

Lenze EJ, Mulsant BH, Blumberger DM, et al: Efficacy, safety, and tolerability of augmentation pharmacotherapy with aripiprazole for treatment-resistant depression in late life: a randomised, double-blind, placebo-controlled trial. Lancet 386(10011):2404–2412, 2015 26423182

Lesser IM, Boone KB, Mehringer CM, et al: Cognition and white matter hyperintensities in older depressed patients. Am J Psychiatry 153(10):1280–1287, 1996 8831435

Li YS, Meyer JS, Thornby J: Longitudinal follow-up of depressive symptoms among normal versus cognitively impaired elderly. Int J Geriatr Psychiatry 16(7):718–727, 2001 11466752

Livingston G, Manela M, Katona C: Depression and other psychiatric morbidity in carers of elderly people living at home. BMJ 312(7024):153–156, 1996 8563534

Luisi S, Tonetti A, Bernardi F, et al: Effect of acute corticotropin releasing factor on pituitary-adrenocortical responsiveness in elderly women and men. J Endocrinol Invest 21(7):449–453, 1998 9766260

Lustman PJ, Griffith LS, Freedland KE, et al: Cognitive behavior therapy for depression in type 2 diabetes mellitus: a randomized, controlled trial. Ann Intern Med 129(8):613–621, 1998 9786808

Lyketsos CG, Steinberg M, Tschanz JT, et al: Mental and behavioral disturbances in dementia: findings from the Cache County Study on Memory in Aging. Am J Psychiatry 157(5):708–714, 2000 10784462

Lyness JM, Caine ED, King DA, et al: Depressive disorders and symptoms in older primary care patients: one-year outcomes. Am J Geriatr Psychiatry 10(3):275–282, 2002 11994214

Magaziner J, Simonsick EM, Kashner TM, et al: Predictors of functional recovery one year following hospital discharge for hip fracture: a prospective study. J Gerontol 45(3):M101–M107, 1990 2335719

Mahableshwarkar AR, Zajecka J, Jacobson W, et al: A randomized, placebo-controlled, active-reference, double-blind, flexible-dose study of the efficacy of vortioxetine on cognitive function in major depressive disorder. Neuropsychopharmacology 40(8):2025–2037, 2015 25687662

Mahgoub N, Alexopoulos GS: Amyloid hypothesis: is there a role for antiamyloid treatment in late-life depression? Am J Geriatr Psychiatry 24(3):239–247, 2016 26946981

Maj M, Pirozzi R, Magliano L, et al: Phenomenology and prognostic significance of delusions in major depressive disorder: a 10-year prospective follow-up study. J Clin Psychiatry 68(9):1411–1417, 2007 17915981

Manly DT, Oakley SP Jr, Bloch RM: Electroconvulsive therapy in old-old patients. Am J Geriatr Psychiatry 8(3):232–236, 2000 10910422

Manning KJ, Chan G, Steffens DC: Neuroticism traits selectively impact long term illness course and cognitive decline in late-life depression. Am J Geriatr Psychiatry 25(3):220–229, 2017 27825555

McEwen BS, Nasca C, Gray JD: Stress effects on neuronal structure: hippocampus, amygdala, and prefrontal cortex. Neuropsychopharmacology 41(1):3–23, 2016 26076834

Meeks TW, Vahia IV, Lavretsky H, et al: A tune in "a minor" can "b major": a review of epidemiology, illness course, and public health implications of subthreshold depression in older adults. J Affect Disord 129(1–3):126–142, 2011 20926139

Meyers BS, Greenberg R: Late-life delusional depression. J Affect Disord 11(2):133–137, 1986 2948986

Meyers BS, Flint AJ, Rothschild AJ, et al: A double-blind randomized controlled trial of olanzapine plus sertraline vs olanzapine plus placebo for psychotic depression: the Study of Pharmacotherapy of Psychotic Depression (STOP-PD). Arch Gen Psychiatry 66(8):838–847, 2009 19652123

Mezuk B, Lohman M, Dumenci L, Lapane KL: Are depression and frailty overlapping syndromes in mid- and late-life? A latent variable analysis. Am J Geriatr Psychiatry 21(6):560–569, 2013 23567406

Miller AH, Raison CL: The role of inflammation in depression: from evolutionary imperative to modern treatment target. Nat Rev Immunol 16(1):22–34, 2016 26711676

Miller AH, Maletic V, Raison CL: Inflammation and its discontents: the role of cytokines in the pathophysiology of major depression. Biol Psychiatry 65(9):732–741, 2009 19150053

Mojtabai R, Olfson M: Major depression in community-dwelling middle-aged and older adults: prevalence and 2- and 4-year follow-up symptoms. Psychol Med 34(4):623–634, 2004 15099417

Morse JQ, Lynch TR: A preliminary investigation of self-reported personality disorders in late life: prevalence, predictors of depressive severity, and clinical correlates. Aging Ment Health 8(4):307–315, 2004 15370047

Moulton CD, Pickup JC, Ismail K: The link between depression and diabetes: the search for shared mechanisms. Lancet Diabetes Endocrinol 3(6):461–471, 2015 25995124

Murphy E: Social origins of depression in old age. Br J Psychiatry 141:135–142, 1982 7116052

Murphy E: The prognosis of depression in old age. Br J Psychiatry 142:111–119, 1983 6839065

Nadorff MR, Drapeau CW, Pigeon WR: Psychiatric illness and sleep in older adults: comorbidity and opportunities for intervention. Sleep Med Clin 13(1):81–91, 2018 29412986

Nasreddine ZS, Phillips NA, Bédirian V, et al: The Montreal Cognitive Assessment, MoCA: a brief screening tool for mild cognitive impairment. J Am Geriatr Soc 53(4):695–699, 2005 15817019

Nebes RD, Butters MA, Houck PR, et al: Dual-task performance in depressed geriatric patients. Psychiatry Res 102(2):139–151, 2001 11408053

Nebes RD, Pollock BG, Houck PR, et al: Persistence of cognitive impairment in geriatric patients following antidepressant treatment: a randomized, double-blind clinical trial with nortriptyline and paroxetine. J Psychiatr Res 37(2):99–108, 2003 12842163

Nelson JC, Devanand DP: A systematic review and meta-analysis of placebo-controlled antidepressant studies in people with depression and dementia. J Am Geriatr Soc 59(4):577–585, 2011 21453380

Nelson JC, Delucchi K, Schneider LS: Efficacy of second generation antidepressants in late-life depression: a meta-analysis of the evidence. Am J Geriatr Psychiatry 16(7):558–567, 2008 18591576

Nock MK, Borges G, Bromet EJ, et al: Suicide and suicidal behavior. Epidemiol Rev 30:133–154, 2008 18653727

Nouwen A, Adriaanse MC, van Dam K, et al: Longitudinal associations between depression and diabetes complications: a systematic review and meta-analysis. Diabet Med 36(12):1562–1572, 2019 31215077

Ochs-Ross R, Daly EJ, Zhang Y, et al: Efficacy and safety of esketamine nasal spray plus an oral antidepressant in elderly patients with treatment-resistant depression–TRANSFORM-3. Am J Geriatr Psychiatry 28(2):121–141, 2020 31734084

Okereke OI, Reynolds CF III, Mischoulon D, et al: The VITamin D and OmegA-3 TriaL-Depression Endpoint Prevention (VITAL-DEP): rationale and design of a large-scale ancillary study evaluating vitamin D and marine omega-3 fatty acid supplements for prevention of late-life depression. Contemp Clin Trials 68:133–145, 2018 29526608

O'Shea DM, Dotson VM, Fieo RA: Aging perceptions and self-efficacy mediate the association between personality traits and depressive symptoms in older adults. Int J Geriatr Psychiatry 32(12):1217–1225, 2017 27653811

Oudman E: Is electroconvulsive therapy (ECT) effective and safe for treatment of depression in dementia? A short review. J ECT 28(1):34–38, 2012 22330702

Ownby RL, Crocco E, Acevedo A, et al: Depression and risk for Alzheimer disease: systematic review, meta-analysis, and metaregression analysis. Arch Gen Psychiatry 63(5):530–538, 2006 16651510

Pariante CM, Lightman SL: The HPA axis in major depression: classical theories and new developments. Trends Neurosci 31(9):464–468, 2008 18675469

Park JH, Lee SB, Lee JJ, et al: Epidemiology of MRI-defined vascular depression: a longitudinal, community-based study in Korean elders. J Affect Disord 180:200–206, 2015 25913805

Parmelee PA, Katz IR, Lawton MP: Incidence of depression in long-term care settings. J Gerontol 47(6):M189–M196, 1992 1430853

Paukert AL, Pettit JW, Kunik ME, et al: The roles of social support and self-efficacy in physical health's impact on depressive and anxiety symptoms in older adults. J Clin Psychol Med Settings 17(4):387–400, 2010 21110074

Penninx BW, Leveille S, Ferrucci L, et al: Exploring the effect of depression on physical disability: longitudinal evidence from the established populations for epidemiologic studies of the elderly. Am J Public Health 89(9):1346–1352, 1999 10474551

Perera T, George MS, Grammer G, et al: The Clinical TMS Society consensus review and treatment recommendations for TMS therapy for major depressive disorder. Brain Stimul 9(3):336–346, 2016 27090022

Pinquart M, Duberstein PR, Lyness JM: Treatments for later-life depressive conditions: a meta-analytic comparison of pharmacotherapy and psychotherapy. Am J Psychiatry 163(9):1493–1501, 2006 16946172

Post F: The Significance of Affective Symptoms in Old Age: A Follow-Up Study of One Hundred Patients. Institute of Psychiatry, Mudsley Monographs No 10. London, Oxford University Press, 1962

Prigerson HG, Reynolds CF III, Frank E, et al: Stressful life events, social rhythms, and depressive symptoms among the elderly: an examination of hypothesized causal linkages. Psychiatry Res 51(1):33–49, 1994 8197270

Rabkin JG, Charles E, Kass F: Hypertension and DSM-III depression in psychiatric outpatients. Am J Psychiatry 140(8):1072–1074, 1983 6869595

Radloff LS: The CES-D scale: a self-report depression scale for research in the general population. Appl Psychol Meas 1:385–401, 1977

Raison CL, Rutherford RE, Woolwine BJ, et al: A randomized controlled trial of the tumor necrosis factor antagonist infliximab for treatment-resistant depression: the role of baseline inflammatory biomarkers. JAMA Psychiatry 70(1):31–41, 2013 22945416

Raskin J, Wiltse CG, Dinkel JJ, et al: Safety and tolerability of duloxetine at 60 mg once daily in elderly patients with major depressive disorder. J Clin Psychopharmacol 28(1):32–38, 2008 18204338

Raue PJ, Morales KH, Post EP, et al: The wish to die and 5-year mortality in elderly primary care patients. Am J Geriatr Psychiatry 18(4):341–350, 2010 19910882

Reichenberg A, Yirmiya R, Schuld A, et al: Cytokine-associated emotional and cognitive disturbances in humans. Arch Gen Psychiatry 58(5):445–452, 2001 11343523

Reinlieb ME, Persaud A, Singh D, et al: Vascular depression: overrepresented among African Americans? Int J Geriatr Psychiatry 29(5):470–477, 2014 24123266

Renn BN, Areán PA: Psychosocial treatment options for major depressive disorder in older adults. Curr Treat Options Psychiatry 4(1):1–12, 2017 28932652

Rensma SP, van Sloten TT, Launer LJ, Stehouwer CDA: Cerebral small vessel disease and risk of incident stroke, dementia and depression, and all-cause mortality: a systematic review and meta-analysis. Neurosci Biobehav Rev 90:164–173, 2018 29656031

Respino M, Jaywant A, Kuceyeski A, et al: The impact of white matter hyperintensities on the structural connectome in late-life depression: relationship to executive functions. Neuroimage Clin 23:101852, 2019 31077981

Reynolds CF III, Frank E, Perel JM, et al: Nortriptyline and interpersonal psychotherapy as maintenance therapies for recurrent major depression: a randomized controlled trial in patients older than 59 years. JAMA 281(1):39–45, 1999 9892449

Reynolds CF III, Dew MA, Pollock BG, et al: Maintenance treatment of major depression in old age. N Engl J Med 354(11):1130–1138, 2006 16540613

Riddle M, Potter GG, McQuoid DR, et al: Longitudinal cognitive outcomes of clinical phenotypes of late-life depression. Am J Geriatr Psychiatry 25(10):1123–1134, 2017 28479153

Robinson RG, Kubos KL, Starr LB, et al: Mood disorders in stroke patients: importance of location of lesion. Brain 107(pt 1):81–93, 1984 6697163

Rosenberg PB, Drye LT, Martin BK, et al: Sertraline for the treatment of depression in Alzheimer disease. Am J Geriatr Psychiatry 18(2):136–145, 2010 20087081

Rubio-Perez JM, Morillas-Ruiz JM: A review: inflammatory process in Alzheimer's disease, role of cytokines. ScientificWorldJournal 2012:756357, 2012 22566778

Rutherford BR, Taylor WD, Brown PJ, et al: Biological aging and the future of geriatric psychiatry. J Gerontol A Biol Sci Med Sci 72(3):343–352, 2017 27994004

Sachs-Ericsson N, Corsentino E, Moxley J, et al: A longitudinal study of differences in late- and early-onset geriatric depression: depressive symptoms and psychosocial, cognitive, and neurological functioning. Aging Ment Health 17(1):1–11, 2013 22934752

Sajatovic M, Strejilevich SA, Gildengers AG, et al: A report on older-age bipolar disorder from the International Society for Bipolar Disorders Task Force. Bipolar Disord 17(7):689–704, 2015 26384588

Salloway S, Malloy P, Kohn R, et al: MRI and neuropsychological differences in early and late-life-onset geriatric depression. Neurology 46(6):1567–1574, 1996 8649550

Schaakxs R, Comijs HC, Lamers F, et al: Associations between age and the course of major depressive disorder: a 2-year longitudinal cohort study. Lancet Psychiatry 5(7):581–590, 2018 29887519

Schmidt PJ, Rubinow DR: Sex hormones and mood in the perimenopause. Ann N Y Acad Sci 1179:70–85, 2009 19906233

Schram MT, Euser SM, de Craen AJ, et al: Systemic markers of inflammation and cognitive decline in old age. J Am Geriatr Soc 55(5):708–716, 2007 17493190

Seidman SN, Araujo AB, Roose SP, et al: Low testosterone levels in elderly men with dysthymic disorder. Am J Psychiatry 159(3):456–459, 2002 11870011

Sharpe L, Gittins CB, Correia HM, et al: Problem-solving versus cognitive restructuring of medically ill seniors with depression (PROMISE-D trial): study protocol and design. BMC Psychiatry 12:207, 2012 23173830

Sheline YI, Wang PW, Gado MH, et al: Hippocampal atrophy in recurrent major depression. Proc Natl Acad Sci USA 93(9):3908–3913, 1996 8632988

Sheline YI, Sanghavi M, Mintun MA, Gado MH: Depression duration but not age predicts hippocampal volume loss in medically healthy women with recurrent major depression. J Neurosci 19(12):5034–5043, 1999 10366636

Sheline YI, Price JL, Vaishnavi SN, et al: Regional white matter hyperintensity burden in automated segmentation distinguishes late-life depressed subjects from comparison subjects matched for vascular risk factors. Am J Psychiatry 165(4):524–532, 2008 18281408

Sheline YI, Pieper CF, Barch DM, et al: Support for the vascular depression hypothesis in late-life depression: results of a 2-site, prospective, antidepressant treatment trial. Arch Gen Psychiatry 67(3):277–285, 2010 20194828

Sneed JR, Roose SP, Keilp JG, et al: Response inhibition predicts poor antidepressant treatment response in very old depressed patients. Am J Geriatr Psychiatry 15(7):553–563, 2007 17586780

Sonsin-Diaz N, Gottesman RF, Fracica E, et al: Chronic systemic inflammation is associated with symptoms of late-life depression: the ARIC study. Am J Geriatr Psychiatry 28(1):87–98, 2020 31182350

Spaans HP, Sienaert P, Bouckaert F, et al: Speed of remission in elderly patients with depression: electroconvulsive therapy v. medication. Br J Psychiatry 206(1):67–71, 2015 25323140

Staab JP, Evans DL: Efficacy of venlafaxine in geriatric depression. Depress Anxiety 12(suppl 1):63–68, 2000 11098416

Steffens DC, Payne ME, Greenberg DL, et al: Hippocampal volume and incident dementia in geriatric depression. Am J Geriatr Psychiatry 10(1):62–71, 2002 11790636

Steffens DC, McQuoid DR, Smoski MJ, Potter GG: Clinical outcomes of older depressed patients with and without comorbid neuroticism. Int Psychogeriatr 25(12):1985–1990, 2013 23941723

Steffens DC, Wu R, Grady JJ, Manning KJ: Presence of neuroticism and antidepressant remission rates in late-life depression: results from the Neurobiology of Late-Life Depression (NBOLD) study. Int Psychogeriatr 30(7):1069–1074, 2018 29198213

Story TJ, Potter GG, Attix DK, et al: Neurocognitive correlates of response to treatment in late-life depression. Am J Geriatr Psychiatry 16(9):752–759, 2008 18697883

Sullivan MD, LaCroix AZ, Baum C, et al: Functional status in coronary artery disease: a one-year prospective study of the role of anxiety and depression. Am J Med 103(5):348–356, 1997 9375701

Szanto K, Reynolds CF III, Frank E, et al: Suicide in elderly depressed patients: is active vs. passive suicidal ideation a clinically valid distinction? Am J Geriatr Psychiatry 4(3):197–207, 1996 28531078

Szücs A, Szanto K, Aubry JM, Dombrovski AY: Personality and suicidal behavior in old age: a systematic literature review. Front Psychiatry 9:128, 2018 29867594

Taylor WD: Clinical practice: depression in the elderly. N Engl J Med 371(13):1228–1236, 2014 25251617

Taylor WD, Steffens DC, MacFall JR, et al: White matter hyperintensity progression and late-life depression outcomes. Arch Gen Psychiatry 60(11):1090–1096, 2003 14609884

Taylor WD, McQuoid DR, Krishnan KR: Medical comorbidity in late-life depression. Int J Geriatr Psychiatry 19(10):935–943, 2004 15449369

Taylor WD, MacFall JR, Payne ME, et al: Greater MRI lesion volumes in elderly depressed subjects than in control subjects. Psychiatry Res 139(1):1–7, 2005a 15927454

Taylor WD, Steffens DC, Payne ME, et al: Influence of serotonin transporter promoter region polymorphisms on hippocampal volumes in late-life depression. Arch Gen Psychiatry 62(5):537–544, 2005b 15867107

Taylor WD, Zuchner S, Mcquoid DR, et al: Allelic differences in the brain-derived neurotrophic factor Val66Met polymorphism in late-life depression. Am J Geriatr Psychiatry 15:850–857, 2007 17911362

Taylor WD, Aizenstein HJ, Alexopoulos GS: The vascular depression hypothesis: mechanisms linking vascular disease with depression. Mol Psychiatry 18(9):963–974, 2013a 23439482

Taylor WD, Zhao Z, Ashley-Koch A, et al: Fiber tract-specific white matter lesion severity: findings in late-life depression and by AGTR1 A1166C genotype. Hum Brain Mapp 34(2):295–303, 2013b 22021115

Taylor WD, McQuoid DR, Payne ME, et al: Hippocampus atrophy and the longitudinal course of late-life depression. Am J Geriatr Psychiatry 22(12):1504–1512, 2014 24378256

Thakur M, Hays J, Krishnan KR: Clinical, demographic and social characteristics of psychotic depression. Psychiatry Res 86(2):99–106, 1999 10397412

Thomas AJ, O'Brien JT, Davis S, et al: Ischemic basis for deep white matter hyperintensities in major depression: a neuropathological study. Arch Gen Psychiatry 59(9):785–792, 2002a 12215077

Thomas AJ, Perry R, Barber R, et al: Pathologies and pathological mechanisms for white matter hyperintensities in depression. Ann N Y Acad Sci 977:333–339, 2002b 12480770

Tiemeier H, Hofman A, van Tuijl HR, et al: Inflammatory proteins and depression in the elderly. Epidemiology 14(1):103–107, 2003 12500057

Travison TG, Araujo AB, Kupelian V, et al: The relative contributions of aging, health, and lifestyle factors to serum testosterone decline in men. J Clin Endocrinol Metab 92(2):549–555, 2007 17148559

Tsang RS, Mather KA, Sachdev PS, Reppermund S: Systematic review and meta-analysis of genetic studies of late-life depression. Neurosci Biobehav Rev 75:129–139, 2017 28137459

Tyring S, Gottlieb A, Papp K, et al: Etanercept and clinical outcomes, fatigue, and depression in psoriasis: double-blind placebo-controlled randomised phase III trial. Lancet 367(9504):29–35, 2006 16399150

van Diermen L, van den Ameele S, Kamperman AM, et al: Prediction of electroconvulsive therapy response and remission in major depression: meta-analysis. Br J Psychiatry 212(2):71–80, 2018 29436330

Van Orden KA, Conwell Y: Issues in research on aging and suicide. Aging Ment Health 20(2):240–251, 2016 26179380

van Schaik DJ, van Marwijk HW, Beekman AT, et al: Interpersonal psychotherapy (IPT) for late-life depression in general practice: uptake and satisfaction by patients, therapists and physicians. BMC Fam Pract 8:52, 2007 17854480

Venkatraman VK, Aizenstein H, Guralnik J, et al: Executive control function, brain activation and white matter hyperintensities in older adults. Neuroimage 49(4):3436–3442, 2010 19922803

Vythilingam M, Chen J, Bremner JD, et al: Psychotic depression and mortality. Am J Psychiatry 160(3):574–576, 2003 12611843

Waite A, Bebbington P, Skelton-Robinson M, Orrell M: Social factors and depression in carers of people with dementia. Int J Geriatr Psychiatry 19(6):582–587, 2004 15211540

Wang PS, Schneeweiss S, Brookhart MA, et al: Suboptimal antidepressant use in the elderly. J Clin Psychopharmacol 25(2):118–126, 2005 15738742

Warden D, Rush AJ, Trivedi MH, et al: The STAR*D project results: a comprehensive review of findings. Curr Psychiatry Rep 9(6):449–459, 2007 18221624

Wijkstra J, Lijmer J, Burger H, et al: Pharmacological treatment for psychotic depression. Cochrane Database Syst Rev (7):CD004044, 2015 26225902

Wilson KC, Mottram PG, Vassilas CA: Psychotherapeutic treatments for older depressed people. Cochrane Database Syst Rev (1):CD004853, 2008 18254062

Wilson RS, Capuano AW, Boyle PA, et al: Clinical-pathologic study of depressive symptoms and cognitive decline in old age. Neurology 83(8):702–709, 2014 25080520

Wu KY, Hsiao IT, Chen CS, et al: Increased brain amyloid deposition in patients with a lifetime history of major depression: evidenced on 18F-florbetapir (AV-45/Amyvid) positron emission tomography. Eur J Nucl Med Mol Imaging 41(4):714–722, 2014 24233127

Yesavage JA, Brink TL, Rose TL, et al: Development and validation of a geriatric depression screening scale: a preliminary report. J Psychiatr Res 17(1):37–49, 1982–1983 7183759

Young E, Korszun A: Sex, trauma, stress hormones and depression. Mol Psychiatry 15(1):23–28, 2010 19773810

Zannas AS, McQuoid DR, Steffens DC, et al: Stressful life events, perceived stress, and 12-month course of geriatric depression: direct effects and moderation by the 5-HTTLPR and COMT Val158Met polymorphisms. Stress 15(4):425–434, 2012 22044241

Zannas AS, McQuoid DR, Payne ME, et al: Negative life stress and longitudinal hippocampal volume changes in older adults with and without depression. J Psychiatr Res 47(6):829–834, 2013 23478048

CHAPTER 10

Bipolar and Related Disorders

John L. Beyer, M.D.

Bipolar disorders can be severe, relapsing mental illnesses that share characteristics with both the major depressive disorders and the psychotic disorders. Like the depressive disorders, bipolar disorders feature recurrent episodes of altered mood. Like schizophrenia, they may cause altered cognition and perceptions (often involving psychotic episodes). However, bipolar disorders are not part of a continuum between schizophrenia and depressive disorders. Rather, they are a group of distinct psychiatric disorders with their own pattern of clinical presentation, prevalence, genetic history, and treatment response. Although often difficult to discriminate from other mental illnesses early in presentation, a better understanding of bipolar disorders, especially in late life, can lead to improved recognition and treatment.

Diagnosis

Bipolar disorders are cycling illnesses that affect a person's ability to regulate moods. At the extreme, abnormal moods can become episodes of mania or depression. DSM-5 (American Psychiatric Association 2013) lists six diagnoses in the bipolar disorder category: bipolar I disorder, bipolar II disorder, cyclothymic disorder, substance/medication-induced bipolar disorder, bipolar due to another medical condition, and other specified or unspecified bipolar and related disorders.

Bipolar I Disorder

The bipolar I disorder criteria represent the current understanding of what had traditionally been referred to as "manic-depressive disorder." To meet the diagnostic criteria for bipolar I disorder, the patient must have experienced at least one manic episode—that is, an alteration in mood that is euphoric, expansive, or irritable and is

TABLE 10–1.   Manic episode

1. Mood change—A distinct period of abnormal and persistent elevated, expansive or irritable mood

2. Energy change—Abnormal and persistent increased activity or energy

3. Duration—1 week or more in which symptoms are present for most of the day

4. Other symptoms (must have at least three of the following; four if mood is predominantly irritable):

    a. Inflated self-esteem/grandiosity

    b. Decreased need for sleep

    c. More talkative or pressured conversation

    d. Flight of ideas or racing thoughts

    e. Distractibility

    f. Increased goal-directed activity or psychomotor agitation

    g. Increased activities with high risk for painful outcomes

5. Severity of mood disturbance causes impairment or hospitalization (or involves psychosis)

associated with increased energy (Table 10–1). These changes must last for at least 1 week and must be accompanied by three of the seven associated symptoms (e.g., decreased need for sleep, racing thoughts, pressured speech, increased behaviors that may have high likelihood for bad outcome). It is not necessary for a patient to have experienced a depressive episode to be diagnosed with a bipolar disorder, although the vast majority of patients with bipolar disorders have experienced depression, and many report it to be the most commonly experienced mood problem.

Bipolar II Disorder

For a diagnosis of bipolar II disorder, the patient must have experienced one or more major depressive episodes and at least one hypomanic episode. A hypomanic episode is defined as at least 4 days of altered mood (e.g., expansive, euphoric, irritable) occurring with at least three of the seven associated symptoms listed in DSM-5 (Table 10–2).

Cyclothymic Disorder

Cyclothymic disorder is characterized by the presence of hypomanic symptoms (that do not meet criteria for a hypomanic episode) and depressive symptoms (that do not meet criteria for a major depressive episode) that occur over a 2-year period. During this period, the person has not been without these hypomanic or depressive symptoms for more than 2 months at a time. It is unclear whether cyclothymia is a separate disease process or represents either a temperament variation or a premorbid state for bipolar II disorder (Baldessarini et al. 2011), given that there is a 15%–50% risk that a person with cyclothymic disorder will later meet criteria for bipolar I or bipolar II disorder (American Psychiatric Association 2013).

Other Related Disorders

Bipolar I and bipolar II are the most recognized and most common bipolar conditions. They are defined by symptom presentation and intensity. The following two diagno-

TABLE 10–2.	**Hypomanic episode**

1. Mood change—Distinct period of abnormal and persistent elevated, expansive, or irritable mood
2. Energy change—Abnormal and persistent increased activity or energy
3. Duration—4 days or more in which symptoms are present for most of the day
4. Other symptoms (must have at least three of the following; four if mood is predominantly irritable):
   a. Inflated self-esteem/grandiosity
   b. Decreased need for sleep
   c. More talkative or pressured conversation
   d. Flight of ideas or racing thoughts
   e. Distractibility
   f. Increased goal-directed activity or psychomotor agitation
   g. Increased activities with high risk for painful outcomes
5. Severity of mood disturbance causes a change in functioning, but not to the degree that social and/or occupational functioning is severely affected
6. Observability—Others notice the change in the affected individual

ses have similar symptoms and intensity, but are defined by the causes for the altered mood: 1) *substance/medication-induced bipolar disorder* refers to an episode of altered mood that meets criteria for a manic episode but occurs during or soon after substance intoxication or withdrawal or after exposure to a medication, and 2) *bipolar disorder due to another medical condition* refers to an episode of altered mood that meets criteria for a manic episode but is caused by a known medical condition.

The last two categories of bipolar disorders refer to episodes of altered mood that interfere with functioning but that do not completely meet criteria for any disorder in the bipolar and related disorders diagnostic class. *Other specified bipolar and related disorders* may include hypomanic episodes that last only 2–3 days, hypomanic episodes without a history of major depressive episodes, or cyclothymia lasting longer than 24 months. The diagnosis of *unspecified bipolar and related disorder* applies to presentations in which symptoms characteristic of a bipolar disorder cause clinical distress or impairment but do not meet the full criteria for any of the specified disorders.

For the most part, the current research literature is relatively sparse for information about bipolar II, cyclothymia, and the other related disorders in late life; therefore, this chapter focuses on bipolar I disorder and substance-induced and medication-related illnesses, unless otherwise noted.

Epidemiology and Clinical Presentation

Prevalence

The exact prevalence of bipolar disorder in late life is uncertain. Based on five large-scale studies that used very different sampling methods (Table 10–3), the prevalence of bipolar disorder in late life in the community has been reported to range from 0.08% to 1.0%. This is much lower than the prevalence rates noted for young and middle-

TABLE 10–3.   Epidemiological surveys of bipolar prevalence in the United States

Study	Survey type	Diagnostic criteria	Sample	Prevalence results	
				Age <65 years	Age >65 years
Weissman et al. 1988	Epidemiologic Catchment Area— five sites across the United States	DSM-III	18,263 interviews of community-dwelling adults	1.4% 18–44; 0.4% 45–64	0.1%
Unützer et al. 1998	Health maintenance organization (HMO) in Washington state	DSM-III-R	294,284 adults enrolled in HMO	0.45% 18–39; 0.46% 40–64	0.25%
Hirschfeld et al. 2003	Mailed survey to U.S. households selected from a database maintained by National Family Opinion, Inc., a marketing firm	DSM-IV	85,358 adult responders	3.9% 18–24; 3.9% 25–34; 3.2% 35–44; 2.5% 45–54; 1.5% 55–64 (3.4% total sample)	0.5%
Klap et al. 2003	HealthCare for Communities Household Telephone Survey	DSM-IV	9,585 households	1.13% 18–29; 1.17% 30–64	0.08%
Kessler et al. 2005	National Comorbidity Study–Replication	DSM-IV	9,282 interviews of community-dwelling adults	5.9% 18–29; 4.5% 30–44; 3.5% 45–59; (3.9% total sample)	1.0%

aged adults. The reason for this decreased prevalence is unclear. Winokur (1975) proposed that patients with mania may "burn out" after a number of episodes. Initially, this appeared to be supported by a major retrospective study (Angst et al. 1973) that described a finite number of episodes in patients with mania, thus suggesting that the illness may be self-limiting. However, a later prospective longitudinal study (Angst and Preisig 1995) followed 209 patients with bipolar disorder over a period of 40 years until a median age of 68 years. They found that manic episodes did not decrease with age and that many patients continued to have episodes into their 60s.

Other hypotheses for the observed decline in prevalence with age have been proposed. Some have suggested that cognitive and emotional maturation (along with improved coping skills) allows patients with bipolar disorder to better compensate for the disease's emotional dysregulation, thus minimizing symptoms that may lead to an episode (and subsequent diagnosis). Alternatively, some have suggested that the observed decline in prevalence with age may be due to the increased mortality associated with bipolar illness. Kessing et al. (2015) recently calculated that young adults (ages 25–40 years) with bipolar disorder had a life expectancy decrease of 8–12 years. However, even this large decline in life expectancy does not completely explain the decrease in overall prevalence with age. It should be noted that the decline in prevalence rates of bipolar disorder with age is consistent with findings for other mental illnesses, such as depression and schizophrenia (Depp and Jeste 2004).

Because most large-scale prevalence surveys have excluded patients who were institutionalized in hospitals, nursing homes, or other residential treatment centers, critics have suggested that the prevalence data may underrepresent the true prevalence because older patients with mental illness are more likely to require institutionalized care. Two surveys of mental illness in nursing homes found a prevalence of bipolar disorder of 3%–10% (Koenig and Blazer 1992; Tariot et al. 1993), whereas Speer (1992) reported a prevalence rate of 17.4% in residential psychiatric programs for older adults.

In contrast to the relatively low rates of bipolar disorder in the community, the use of psychiatric services among patients with bipolar disorder in later life is relatively high. Bipolar disorder in late life accounts for 6%–8.7% of inpatient admissions (see Depp and Jeste 2004; Dols et al. 2014a), although some have argued that this may be an underestimation because many of the inpatient surveys did not include subjects with bipolar depression or reported prevalence only for those whose bipolar disorder began after age 60 years. Bipolar disorder in late life also accounts for 6% of geriatric outpatient visits and 17% of elderly patients in psychiatric emergency departments.

In summary, the prevalence of bipolar disorder may depend in part on the diagnostic criteria or measurement used and population sampled. Community surveys show that bipolar disorder appears to decrease with age, a change consistent with declines seen in other mental disorders. Nevertheless, the proportion of older patients using services (either inpatient or outpatient) appears to be the same as in younger populations. Furthermore, there may be increasing use of institutional care with age.

Sex

Epidemiological studies in the United States have indicated that bipolar disorder is approximately equally common in males and females (American Psychiatric Association 2013). Depp and Jeste (2004) pooled 17 studies reporting various samples of late-life bipolar disorder and found that the weighted mean of elderly females with bipolar disorder was 69% (range 45%–89%). However, they noted that this percentage was similar to the sex ratio among older adults in the general population.

Comorbidity

Psychiatric Comorbidity

Psychiatric comorbidity is frequently seen in bipolar disorder and has been a major point of discussion in the literature, yet there is very little information about its presence in late-life bipolar disorder. Most reporting has been limited to small data groups.

Sajatovic et al. (2006) reviewed the national Veterans Health Administration database to examine the prevalence of three comorbid psychiatric conditions (i.e., anxiety, PTSD, and dementia) in older patients with bipolar disorder. Of the 4,668 subjects with bipolar disorder (mean age 70 years), 9.4% had an anxiety disorder, 5.4% had PTSD, and 4.5% had dementia. As noted, each of these prevalences was lower than that seen in younger adults with bipolar disorder. Similarly, Dols et al. (2014b) studied comorbid anxiety disorders in The Netherlands and found them to be relatively rare (1-month panic disorder, 2%; 1-month social anxiety, 3%; 6-month generalized anxiety disorder,

5%) in later-life bipolar disorder. There are no published reports on comorbid eating disorders or attention disorders, although these conditions are noted to be frequently comorbid in younger subjects with bipolar disorder.

The best evidence for the prevalence of comorbid substance abuse and bipolar disorders comes from the National Comorbidity Survey, in which 61% of individuals with bipolar disorder also had a substance use disorder (Kessler et al. 1997). Unfortunately, this survey excluded adults older than 55 years. Cassidy et al. (2001) reviewed rates of substance abuse in 392 patients hospitalized for bipolar disorder at a state psychiatric facility. Nearly 60% had some history of lifetime substance abuse (consistent with the finding of the National Comorbidity Survey), but of the 51 patients older than 60 years, only 29% had a history of lifetime substance abuse. Supporting this finding of lower-than-expected substance abuse disorders in older patients with bipolar disorder are a small inpatient retrospective study (Ponce et al. 1999), a review of elderly adults with bipolar disorder using mental health system outpatient services (Depp et al. 2005), the database from The Netherlands (Dols et al. 2014b), and a large review of the Veterans Health Administration database (Sajatovic et al. 2006). The reason for this unexpected finding is unclear.

Only one study has reviewed the presence of personality disorders together with co-occurring late-life mental disorders. Molinari and Marmion (1995) studied 27 geriatric outpatients and inpatients with bipolar disorder and found that 70% had a personality disorder. The authors suggested that the unusually high rate of personality disorders may be due in part to the difficult and chronic patterns of affective disorders.

Medical Comorbidity

The evaluation of medical comorbidities in older adults with bipolar disorder is important for several reasons. First, understanding common medical problems helps guide treatment recommendations. Older adults are much more likely than younger adults to have illness and to take larger numbers of concomitant medications. Lala and Sajatovic (2012) reported that most elderly patients with bipolar disorder have at least three or four significant medical conditions. Second, medical comorbidities may be caused by either the bipolar disorder diagnosis or its treatments over the years (e.g., hypercholesterolemia with chronic antipsychotic use, kidney disease with lithium use). Finally, medical comorbidities may help guide understanding of the potential causes of bipolar disorder. It has been well known that many illnesses may induce a manic episode (e.g., hyperthyroidism, multiple sclerosis, Parkinson's disease). This may be especially applicable in late-life bipolar disorder because of the high association that secondary mania has with late-onset manic episodes (see "Age at Onset" later). Because medical illnesses may suggest the cause of an episode or a limitation on treatment options, the presence of comorbid medical problems—the most common being neurological illnesses—has been extensively studied in late-life bipolar disorder.

Depp and Jeste (2004) reviewed eight studies that reported the presence of illness and noted that despite a variety in reporting strategies, the sample-weighted prevalence for neurological illnesses was 23.1%. Shulman et al. (1992) compared 50 geriatric patients hospitalized for mania with 50 age-matched patients hospitalized for unipolar depression. They found that the rates of neurological illness in patients with mania were significantly higher (36% vs. 8%), suggesting that neurological disease is associated with mania in late life.

Other comorbid medical disorders are also common in bipolar disorder, especially in late-life bipolar disorder. Regenold et al. (2002) found that type II diabetes was present in 26% of older adult inpatients with bipolar disorder. This was a much higher rate than in older patients with unipolar depression or schizophrenia. In a study of 101 older adults with bipolar disorder, Dols et al. (2014b) found that they frequently also had hypertension (27.8%), arthrosis (29.1%), allergies (25.6%), and peripheral atherosclerotic disease (18.8%). Only 21.8% had no somatic illnesses. Interestingly, metabolic syndrome was found in 28.7% of patients.

Dementia

Dementia has become an increasing concern for older adults in general and possibly a special concern for older adults with bipolar disorder. Studies of four inpatient samples found that the rate of comorbid dementia was highly variable, ranging from 3% to 25% (Broadhead and Jacoby 1990; Himmelhoch et al. 1980; Ponce et al. 1999; Stone 1989), although this finding is probably more related to the catchment areas of the individual hospitals. Sajatovic et al. (2006) reported dementia in 4.5% of veterans treated for bipolar disorder through the Veterans Health Administration system, although a comparison rate was not reported for other psychiatric illnesses.

Comorbidity does not necessarily imply an association, although this has been a particular concern in late-life bipolar disorder. Tsai et al. (2003) reported that 30.7% of the early onset patients they followed had Mini-Mental State Examination (MMSE) scores of <24, a percentage higher than expected. Furthermore, Dhingra and Rabins (1991) reviewed a group of elderly patients who had been hospitalized 5–7 years previously for manic episodes and found that 32% demonstrated a significant decline in their MMSE scores. Kocsis et al. (1993) followed 38 elderly patients with bipolar disorder treated with lithium and found that rates of cognitive and functional impairment were much higher than in the general population. This concern about cognition and bipolar disorder is further discussed later in the chapter.

Mortality

People with mental illness at any age have higher mortality rates, from both natural and unnatural causes, than the general population (Laursen et al. 2007). This is especially true for those with bipolar disorder. As noted, the presence of bipolar disorder in an adult (ages 25–40) is associated with an 8- to 12-year decrease in life expectancy (Kessing et al. 2015). Ramsey et al. (2013) reported on the 26-year follow-up data from participants in the Epidemiologic Catchment Area Survey. They found that the odds of mortality for patients with lifetime manic spectrum episodes (either full manic, hypomanic, or subthreshold manic symptoms) were much higher (OR 1.4) than for those with no lifetime manic spectrum episodes. Furthermore, this mortality rate for bipolar disorder appears to be significantly increased over those for other affective disorders. Shulman et al. (1992) found that the mortality rate over a 10- to 15-year follow-up for elderly hospitalized patients with bipolar disorder was significantly higher than that of elderly hospitalized patients with unipolar depression (50% vs. 20%), suggesting that mania appears to have a poorer prognosis and to be a more severe form of affective illness than unipolar depression.

In summary, psychiatric comorbidity is frequent in patients with bipolar disorder, but the exact prevalence of these comorbidities in older patients with bipolar disorder is unclear given the limited data available. Substance abuse, the most common and best-reported comorbid condition in the literature, appears to be less common in older than in younger patients with bipolar disorder. A lifetime prevalence of substance abuse is also less likely to be seen in older patients with bipolar disorder. Dementia and poorer cognitive performance on neurological testing (see "Neurocognitive Testing" later) are possibly increased, or apparent earlier, in older adults with bipolar disorder. Medical comorbidity is also higher in older adults with bipolar disorder (Beyer et al. 2005), and there is a special concern for neurological illness and diabetes. All of these problems may contribute to higher mortality rates for patients with bipolar disorder.

Course

After reviewing studies that retrospectively looked at the course of bipolar disorder prior to hospitalization, Goodwin and Jamison (1990) reported that depression was more often the initial episode in older adults than in younger patients. Kessing (2006), in a study of Denmark's health care utilization, found that first psychiatric hospitalizations for older adults with bipolar disorder were much more likely to be for depressive episodes than for manic episodes. Various investigators have described a latency period of 10–20 years between the first depressed episode and the onset of mania (Broadhead and Jacoby 1990; Shulman and Post 1980; Shulman et al. 1992; Snowdon 1991; Stone 1989).

Only minor differences have been found in the symptom presentation between older and younger adults with bipolar disorder (Almeida and Fenner 2002; Kessing 2006) and between those who had an earlier versus later onset of the illness (Depp and Jeste 2004). A review from the Systematic Treatment Enhancement Program for Bipolar Disorder (STEP-BD) found no significant association between age and symptom presentation of acute depression or mood elevation or psychosis (Al Jurdi et al. 2012).

Angst and Preisig (1995) followed 209 psychiatrically hospitalized patients with bipolar disorder over a 40-year period, until a median age of 68 years. Of these patients, only 16% fully recovered (defined as no episodes in the previous 5 years and a Global Assessment of Functioning [GAF] Scale score >60), whereas 26% had no episodes but had GAF scores <60. The largest group (36%) had experienced episodes within the previous 5 years, and another 16% demonstrated a chronic course. Seven percent had committed suicide.

A study comparing health-related quality of life and functioning in elderly adults with bipolar disorder ($n=54$) with that in a group without psychiatric illness ($n=38$) found that even patients in remission from bipolar disorder had quality-of-life scores that were lower than those of the healthy comparison group. Overall, bipolar disorder was associated with substantial disability, comparable with schizophrenia, and incomplete improvement in functioning even among those classified as remitters (Depp et al. 2006).

Interestingly, despite the greater risk of suicide reported with aging and among individuals with bipolar disorder, the risk of suicide in late-life bipolar disorder appears lower than expected. Tsai et al. (2002) studied suicide rates in Taiwan among patients with bipolar disorder and found that the highest risk was during the first 7–12 years after the onset of the illness and for individuals younger than 35 years. Depp and Jeste (2004) suggested that older patients with early-onset bipolar disorder may constitute a "survivor cohort."

Age at Onset

The mean age at onset for bipolar disorder is in the late teens to early 20s (Weissman et al. 1996). Although most studies have found bipolar disorder to be unimodal in distribution, a few studies have noted two peaks for the onset of mania, with the first occurring in the mid-20s and a second, smaller peak occurring closer to middle age, in the late 40s (Angst 1978; Goodwin and Jamison 1984; Petterson 1977).

An estimated 5%–10% of individuals with bipolar disorder will be 50 years of age or older at the time of their first manic or hypomanic episode (Depp and Jeste 2004; Hirschfeld et al. 2003; Prabhakar and Balon 2010; Yassa et al. 1988). Despite being phenotypically similar to the other age-at-onset subtypes, the late-onset subtype has historically been viewed as an "organic" variant of bipolar disorder. This may be due in part to the relatively small number of new-onset cases in older adults compared with younger adults, as well as the known physical changes associated with age. For example, females may be at risk for a first episode around the time of menopause (Angst 1978; Petterson 1977; Sibisi 1990; Zis et al. 1979), and males may have increased risk in their 70s and 80s (Sibisi 1990; Spicer et al. 1973), possibly due to neurological causes. In a large multicenter study of bipolar disorder in Spain, a higher frequency of males was observed in the late-onset subgroup (Montes et al. 2013). The definition of neurological illness varied in eight studies that examined this issue, but six of the studies showed significantly higher rates in patients with late-onset illness (Almeida and Fenner 2002; Huang et al. 2012; Snowdon 1991; Subramaniam et al. 2007; Tohen et al. 1994; Wylie et al. 1999), and the other two studies showed a trend toward increased levels (Broadhead and Jacoby 1990; Hays et al. 1998).

Cognitive function also appears to be different between patients with early-onset and those with later-onset bipolar disorder. Late-onset patients have more extensive neurocognitive impairments, despite the difference in chronicity (Gildengers et al. 2013; Martino et al. 2013a; Schouws et al. 2007; Torrent et al. 2013). Because of the association of neurological illness and late-onset bipolar disorder, it has been hypothesized that the late-onset subtype may often have underlying cerebral changes due to aging that convert them to mania. Similarly, there is general support for the tentative association between mania and vascular risk factors and between mania and cerebrovascular disease. The term *vascular mania* has been proposed to describe a possible mechanism for late-onset bipolar disorder. The proposed diagnostic criteria have defined a subtype of mania with late age at onset (≥50 years) and associated neuroimaging and neuropsychological changes not specific to this age group (Wijeratne and Malhi 2007).

In a European longitudinal study of bipolar disorder, 88 older adults (≥60 years) were followed for up to 7.7 years. The researchers (García-López et al. 2017) noted that patients with later-onset bipolar disorder were more likely to have a bipolar II disorder. This finding supported studies noting that hypomanic episodes occur more frequently than mania when bipolar disorder emerges in later years (Vasudev and Thomas 2010). The authors suggested that this observation is due to the different pathophysiology of late-onset bipolar disorder—in that it is related to more medical and neurological conditions.

Many researchers have noted the utility of dividing bipolar disorder into early- and late-onset subtypes, suggesting that they represent different forms of bipolar disorder

(Sajatovic et al. 2015b). Early-onset illness may have greater genetic loading because it is more often associated with a family history of mood disorders, whereas late-onset illness is associated with neurological diseases (i.e., cerebrovascular factors), higher risk of cognitive deterioration, mortality, and possibly a different treatment response. DSM-5 does not make a distinction based on age at onset, but given the functional differences noted, researchers have suggested that the age of 50 years appears to be a reasonable working cut point for late-onset bipolar disorder research (Sajatovic et al. 2015b).

Neurocognitive Testing

Cognitive dysfunctions are increasingly recognized as a core feature of bipolar disorder even though there is great cognitive heterogeneity among patients. Affected abilities are most often noted in assessments of executive function, verbal memory, and processing speed. Cluster analytic cross-sectional studies suggest that there may be identifiable subgroups of patients with bipolar disorder that express different cognitive profiles at various stages of the illness (Van Rheenen et al. 2020). Longitudinal evidence suggests that the specific cognitive path of individuals with bipolar disorder may be set early on. Some of the cognitive changes noted to be inherent in bipolar disorder may also be apparent in first-degree nonaffected relatives, suggesting a genetic basis for these paths.

Individuals with bipolar disorder exhibit a range of cognitive deficits that persist across illness stages and during symptom remission, the severity of which may rival those described in schizophrenia (Balanzá-Martínez et al. 2005; Depp et al. 2007). Studies of older patients with bipolar disorder have found patterns similar to those of younger adults with bipolar disorder: deficits in executive functioning, working memory, verbal memory, attention, construction, and processing speed (Aprahamian et al. 2014; Delaloye et al. 2011; Gildengers et al. 2010; Gunning-Dixon et al. 2008; Lewandowski et al. 2014; Samamé et al. 2013; Young et al. 2006). Both older and younger adults with bipolar disorder tend to score lower than healthy age-matched comparators (Schouws et al. 2007). Martino et al. (2013a) noted that adults with late-onset bipolar disorder had more extensive and severe cognitive impairments than their peers with earlier onset. Furthermore, the presence of psychotic symptoms was associated with poorer cognitive functioning and more rapid cognitive decline over a 6-year follow-up (Köhler et al. 2013).

The course of cognitive functioning over the life span in adults with bipolar disorder has been less clear. Some research has suggested that, compared with mentally healthy individuals of similar age and education, older adults with bipolar disorder not only had worse performance but also appeared to have a faster decline (Dhingra and Rabins 1991; Gildengers et al. 2004, 2009, 2013). These findings would seem to support the hypothesis that bipolar disorder may be related to a neurodegenerative process, because the dysfunctions could not be counted as solely related to residual mood effects, drug effects, or other confounding factors. However, others have suggested that the cognitive impairment and associated functional disability of older individuals with bipolar disorder appear to be due to long-standing neuroprogressive processes (e.g., glutamatergic excitotoxicity, neuroinflammation, oxidative stress, mitochondrial dysfunction) compounded by normal cognitive aging, rather than a neurodegenerative process. For the late-onset group, the presence of a higher incidence of neurological diseases suggests a different pathway for cognitive challenge.

Neuroimaging

Neuroimaging has been increasingly used to identify structural brain abnormalities that may be associated with clinical manifestations of bipolar disorder in late life. These abnormalities may be well-identified clinical syndromes (e.g., strokes, tumors, hydrocephalus), macro changes (e.g., cerebral vascular disease across the brain or changes in gray and white matter volumes), or micro changes (e.g., white matter tract integrity or volumetric changes in certain brain substructures). MRI, magnetic resonance spectroscopy, CT, and PET have been increasingly used in both clinical assessments and research to better understand bipolar illnesses and their relationship to the brain's function, structure, age-related changes, or diseases.

As discussed earlier, neurological illnesses have been found to be present more often in older adults with bipolar disorder. Using primarily CT and MRI technologies, researchers have evaluated the location of strokes and associated mood regulation difficulties. Compared with unipolar depression, mania following a stroke is relatively uncommon. However, a controlled study of patients with secondary mania showed that when manic symptoms are present, the right hemisphere of the brain (both cortical and subcortical areas) is more frequently the site of the lesion (Starkstein et al. 1987, 1991). This is especially true when the basal region of the right temporal lobe is involved (Starkstein et al. 1990).

Researchers have observed that cerebral infarctions are frequently found in older adults with bipolar disorder, regardless of age at onset. Most of these are "silent strokes" not noted to have been associated with any physical function change (Huang et al. 2012). Possibly related to strokes, "hyperintense" signals viewed on T_2-weighted MRIs have been one of the earliest and most consistent neuroimaging findings in the study of bipolar disorder. Hyperintensities represent areas of neuronal cell death, although the mechanism by which this occurs is unclear. Pathological examination has found that hyperintensities could characterize areas of arteriosclerotic disease, demyelination, loss of axons, arteriolar hyalinization, rarefaction, infarctions, and necrosis. Fujikawa et al. (1997) used the term *silent cerebral ischemia* to refer to these hyperintensities. Electroencephalographic studies in patients with dementia suggest that white matter hyperintensities may result in a functional brain disconnection. Therefore, some researchers have suggested that for patients with mood disorders, hyperintensities may "disconnect" different pathways in the mood regulation circuits.

Three meta-analyses strongly support the relationship between hyperintensities and bipolar disorder (Altshuler et al. 1995; Beyer et al. 2009; Videbech 1997), even when controlling for medical risk factors. In studies of mixed- and older-age patients with bipolar disorder, hyperintensities were more often found in the subependymal region, subcortical gray nuclei, and deep white matter (de Asis et al. 2006; McDonald et al. 1999). Older adults with bipolar disorder tended to have both more lesions and larger lesion sizes, which were especially prominent on the right side of the brain in the late-onset group. The presence of hyperintensities may be especially important in late-life bipolar disorder because of their impact on treatment response and severity of illness. MRI hyperintensities have been found to be associated with longer hospital stays and more frequent rehospitalizations (Dupont et al. 1990; McDonald et al. 1999).

Over the past two decades, further neuroimaging studies have supported emerging hypotheses about how lesion location may disrupt brain function in mood regulation circuitry (Phillips 2006). Functional studies have found increased activity in the subcortical and limbic regions that make an initial assessment of "emotional stimulus" (i.e., amygdala, anterior insula). This results in increased activity in the regions associated with mood generation and decision processing of the emotional material (i.e., ventromedial and ventrolateral prefrontal cortices, ventral anterior cingulate gyrus). Finally, there is reduced activity in regions that regulate these responses and attentional processes (i.e., dorsomedial prefrontal cortices), causing the mood lability. Neuroimaging results specific to late-life bipolar disorders have been relatively limited, but the published studies have supported significant volumetric abnormalities in certain areas that are consistent with this theory. Findings note that, in contrast to younger patients with bipolar disorder, those with late-life bipolar disorder have reduced volume in the caudate (Beyer et al. 2004b). Patients with late-onset illness may also have a decreased total brain volume size compared with those with early-onset illness (Beyer et al. 2004a). In addition, MRI studies using diffusion tensor imaging, a technique that evaluates white matter tract integrity, found potentially impaired connectivity in the prefrontal corticolimbic mood regulation circuits of the orbitomedial prefrontal cortex (Vederine et al. 2011). Finally, gray matter concentration changes and microstructural alterations in white matter in neocortical regions and the corpus callosum have also been documented (Haller et al. 2011), in addition to gray matter changes in the right anterior insula, head of the caudate, nucleus accumbens, ventral putamen, and frontal orbital cortex.

Some researchers have suggested that many of these observed changes may indicate that bipolar disorder is a neuroprogressive disorder. *Neuroprogression* refers to functional and cognitive decline that may occur over time, caused by developmental or progressive neurophysiological alterations. Several pathways have been suggested for this, including neurochemical dysregulation (e.g., excessive dopamine and glutamate neurotransmission), neuroinflammation, oxidative stress, mitochondrial dysfunction, changes in brain-derived neurotrophic factor, or epigenetics (Berk et al. 2011; Yildiz-Yesiloglu and Ankerst 2006).

For example, the association of the structural changes noted earlier with cognitive capabilities is unclear. Some researchers (Bearden et al. 2001) have noted that hyperintensities appear to be associated with cognitive impairment with increasing age and chronicity of the disorder. This suggests that it is the overall medical burden (and its impact on brain structure) that contributes to the cognitive declines noted. However, Rej et al. (2014) disputed this, noting that in their studies, cognitive dysfunction was not associated with white matter hyperintensity burden or gray matter volume. They suggested that other potential neuroprogressive pathways, such as inflammation, mitochondrial dysfunction, serum anticholinergic burden, and altered neurogenesis, may play a role. This has been supported by a study evaluating the allostatic load and its impact on cognitive function in bipolar disorder (Vaccarino et al. 2018). *Allostasis* is the process by which the body responds to stressors to regain homeostasis. The allostatic load measures the "wear and tear" on the system from bipolar illness processes. The authors found that the allostatic score, rather than just medical burden, was associated with poorer cognitive performance in older adults with bipolar disorder (Vaccarino et al. 2018).

Similarly, studies that demonstrate volumetric difference as a function of age suggest that increased activity of the stress hormone cortisol during episodes of bipolar depression may drive cumulative excitotoxicity in specific brain regions (Doty et al. 2008). Recently, Tsai et al. (2019) noted that persistent inflammation is associated with reduction of hippocampal and gray matter volume in older patients with bipolar disorder. This phenomenon was supported by increases in soluble tumor necrosis factor receptor 1, soluble interleukin-2 receptor, and interleukin-1β levels. This neuroprogressive/neurodegenerative model of bipolar disorder continues to be actively researched. Currently, there are not enough data from neuroimaging and other studies to make a conclusive assessment of its role in bipolar disorder (Sajatovic et al. 2015b). What we may discover is that the disparate results noted in cognitive progression, structural changes, medical burden, and so on suggest that different subtypes of bipolar illness exist, some of which are more influenced by genetic, environmental, or internal neuroprogressive pathways or a combination of these processes (Martino et al. 2013b).

Differential Diagnosis

There are five potential presentations of patients with late-life bipolar disorder:

1. Those who had early onset of bipolar disease and have now reached old age
2. Those who previously experienced only episodes of depression but have now switched to a manic episode
3. Those who have never had an affective illness but develop mania because of a specific medical or neurological event (e.g., head trauma, cerebrovascular accident, hyperthyroidism)
4. Those who have never been recognized as having bipolar symptoms or who have been misdiagnosed with another disorder
5. Those who have never had an affective illness but develop mania for unknown reasons

It is unknown how common each presentation may be, especially because it is not uncommon for the diagnosis to have been missed earlier in life (Hirschfeld et al. 2003). Because the onset of bipolar disorder in late life is relatively uncommon, every patient who presents with a new onset of mania should undergo a thorough medical evaluation, with special emphasis on the neurological examination. Because older adults may be taking a higher number of medications, these should be reviewed for possible temporal association with symptom onset. A laboratory workup consisting of a thyroid panel and basic tests should also be completed. Finally, consideration should be given to neuroimaging, especially if the presentation is associated with psychosis.

Treatment

Treatment of bipolar disorder is frequently challenging for a variety of reasons. In addition to the challenge of medication management in older adults, elderly patients with bipolar disorder often have an incomplete response, recurrent episodes, potentially severe psychopathology, and higher mortality rates. Furthermore, the disease itself tends to cause poor insight and subsequent poor compliance with treatment. Finally, data are limited on the use of medications and psychotherapies for older patients with bipolar disorder compared with younger and middle-aged patients. Many treatment practices are based on results from clinical trials in younger populations that have been adapted for geriatric use. In a review of 34 identified guidelines for the treatment of bipolar disorder, most gave no separate recommendations for treatment in older adults (Dols et al. 2016).

Lithium

Lithium has traditionally been identified as the gold standard for treatment of bipolar disorder and has been widely prescribed to older patients with the disorder (Shulman et al. 2003; Umapathy et al. 2000). Because of the need to better understand treatment in this vulnerable population, the National Institute for Mental Health (NIMH) commissioned a study to evaluate the efficacy and tolerability of lithium and valproate in late-life mania. Young et al. (2017) conducted a blinded trial of 224 patients older than 60 years with mania who were administered either lithium or valproate. They found that both lithium and valproate were well tolerated and efficacious, but lithium was associated with a greater reduction in mania scores.

The recommended lithium level for acute mania in geriatric patients is unclear. In the study by Young et al. (2017), the mean dosage of lithium was 780±315 mg/day, with a mean serum concentration of 0.76±0.35 mEq/L. However, some case series have suggested that elderly patients may respond to lower lithium levels (0.5–0.8 mEq/L) than those recommended for younger adults (0.6–1.2 mEq/L) (Chen et al. 1999; Prien et al. 1972; Roose et al. 1979), whereas other studies have not found a difference (DeBattista and Schatzberg 2006; Young et al. 1992).

Special care must be taken when dosing geriatric patients with lithium. With aging, the renal clearance of lithium decreases and elimination half-life increases (Foster 1992; Shulman et al. 1987; Sproule et al. 2000). Furthermore, medications commonly prescribed to elderly patients, such as thiazide diuretics, nonsteroidal anti-inflammatory agents, and angiotensin-converting enzyme inhibitors, can increase lithium concentrations, whereas other medications, such as theophylline, can decrease lithium concentrations. Finally, because lithium use can contribute to hypothyroidism and a decline in renal clearance, it should be used with caution in patients with kidney problems or thyroid disorders.

Lithium toxicity in elderly patients is not uncommon (De Fazio et al. 2017; Foster 1992; Fotso Soh et al. 2019). Commonly reported adverse effects of lithium in elderly persons include cognitive impairment, ataxia, urinary frequency, weight gain, edema, tremor, and worsening of psoriasis and arthritis. Because of adverse effects (including neurotoxicity) that can occur even at therapeutic levels, appropriate serum lithium levels in elderly patients are largely determined by medical status, frailty, and conservative dosing (Sajatovic et al. 2005b; Young et al. 2004).

Anticonvulsants

Anticonvulsants have been accepted as the "standard" baseline treatment in bipolar disorder. Since 1993, four anticonvulsants have been approved by the FDA to treat bipolar disorder: valproate, carbamazepine, oxcarbazepine, and lamotrigine. Information on this use of anticonvulsants in older patients with bipolar disorder is limited primarily to case reports and post hoc subanalyses of data from mixed-age Phase III clinical trials.

Valproate

Since 2000, the prescription of valproate for bipolar disorder has increased markedly, especially for elderly patients. In 1999, Oshima and Higuchi proposed that lithium be the first choice in treatment guidelines for geriatric bipolar disorder. However, Shulman et al. (2003) noted that, by the early 2000s, prescriptions of valproate for elderly patients with bipolar disorder had increased, whereas prescriptions of lithium had decreased, so that valproate became the most prescribed medication for treating older persons with bipolar disorder.

In the NIMH study on the tolerability and efficacy of lithium and valproate in late-life mania (Young et al. 2017), both drugs were noted as well tolerated and efficacious (although lithium showed a greater reduction in mania scores overall). The mean daily dosage was 1,200±550 mg/day and mean serum concentration was 74±21 µg/mL. The recommended blood level concentration for valproate in adults is 50–120 µg/mL (Bowden et al. 2002), although Chen et al. (1999) found that elderly patients with mania who had a blood level concentration from 65 µg/mL to 90 µg/mL improved more than patients with lower concentrations.

As patients age, the elimination half-life of valproate may be prolonged, and the free fraction of plasma valproate increases. The clinical significance of this is unknown, although it should be noted that usual laboratory tests measure the total valproate level. Thus, the reported level may underrepresent the actual quantity available to the brain in geriatric patients (Sajatovic et al. 2005b; Young et al. 2004). Common medications taken concurrently may also influence the level of valproate: aspirin can increase the valproate free fraction, and phenytoin and carbamazepine may decrease the valproate level. In turn, valproate may affect other medications' effects. It can inhibit the metabolism of lamotrigine so that the dosage of lamotrigine may need to be lowered to minimize side effects. It also may increase the unbound fraction of warfarin; coagulation parameters should therefore be monitored in patients undergoing anticoagulation therapy (Panjehshahin et al. 1991).

The most common side effects associated with valproate are nausea, somnolence, and weight gain. Less common side effects that may be particularly important to geriatric patients are hair thinning, thrombocytopenia, hepatotoxicity, and pancreatitis (the latter two are less likely to occur with age) (Bowden et al. 2002). Valproate is available in sprinkle and liquid formulations for patients who have difficulty swallowing. In addition, Regenold and Prasad (2001) have reported on the intravenous use of valproate in three geriatric patients.

Carbamazepine

Carbamazepine was FDA approved for the treatment of bipolar mania in 1996, and its extended-release formulation was approved in 2005. Researchers have suggested that carbamazepine may be the preferred mood-stabilizing agent, rather than lithium, for patients with secondary mania (Evans et al. 1995; Sajatovic 2002); however, very little information is available on the use of carbamazepine (in either preparation) for elderly patients with bipolar disorder. Okuma et al. (1990) noted that seven elderly patients with mania were included in a larger sample of 50 patients treated with carbamazepine in a double-blind study that showed good efficacy.

Before initiating carbamazepine, physicians should check patients' liver enzymes, electrolytes, and complete blood cell count. Because carbamazepine can also affect the heart's rhythm, an electrocardiogram should be considered. In elderly patients, carbamazepine may be started at 100 mg either once or twice daily and gradually increased every 3–5 days to 400–800 mg/day (McDonald 2000). Target serum levels are between 6 and 12 µg/L.

Carbamazepine is metabolized in the liver by cytochrome P450 enzyme 3A4/5. Because carbamazepine can induce its own metabolism, dosage increases may need to be adjusted during the first 1–2 months. Furthermore, carbamazepine clearance is decreased in an age-dependent manner, presumably due to a reduction in CYP3A4/5 metabolism, suggesting that elderly patients may require lower dosages than younger patients in order to achieve similar blood levels (Battino et al. 2003). Notably, carbamazepine also may alter the pharmacokinetics of other medications, including oral hormones, calcium channel blockers, cimetidine, terfenadine, and erythromycin (Sajatovic 2002).

Possible adverse effects associated with carbamazepine include sedation, ataxia, nystagmus/blurred vision, leukopenia, hyponatremia (secondary to the syndrome of inappropriate antidiuretic hormone secretion), and agranulocytosis. The FDA has recommended that patients of Asian ancestry have a genetic blood test to identify an inherited variant of the human leukocyte antigen allele *HLA-B*1502* (found almost exclusively in people of Asian ancestry) before starting therapy (U.S. Food and Drug Administration 2007). Patients testing positive should not be given carbamazepine.

Lamotrigine

Lamotrigine was approved by the FDA in 2003 for the maintenance phase of bipolar disorder. Sajatovic et al. (2005a) conducted a retrospective analysis of two placebo-controlled, double-blind clinical trials for maintenance therapy in bipolar disorder, focusing on 98 subjects who were age 55 years or older. They found that, similar to the parent study, lamotrigine significantly delayed the time to intervention for any mood episode, whereas lithium and placebo did not. In a subanalysis of the type of mood episode that was more likely to recur (Sajatovic et al. 2007), the authors found that lamotrigine was significantly more effective than lithium and placebo at increasing the time to intervention for depressive recurrences, but lithium performed much better in increasing the time to intervention for manic episodes. Overall, the authors found that lamotrigine was well tolerated (compared with lithium) by older patients with bipolar disorder, and no increased incidence of rash was noted (Sajatovic et al. 2007).

In a multisite 12-week, open-label trial, 57 older patients with bipolar type I or II (mean age 66.5 years) received add-on lamotrigine therapy (mean dosage 150.9 mg/day) (Sajatovic et al. 2011). Response and remission rates were 64.8% and 57.4%, respectively. In a follow-up analysis evaluating clinical correlates of treatment response, Gildengers et al. (2012) noted that lamotrigine worked best in patients with depression who had more cardiometabolic risk factors and a low level of manic symptoms.

Lamotrigine is metabolized in the liver and eliminated through hepatic glucuronide conjugation. Minor decreases in hepatic glucuronidation occur with aging, although the impact on lamotrigine dosing in elderly patients is not thought to be significant (Hussein and Posner 1997; Posner et al. 1991). Serious skin rashes (Stevens-Johnson syndrome) have been reported, so dosage should be titrated slowly. Lamotrigine may have fewer negative effects on cognition than other anticonvulsant medications, which may be important for some geriatric patients (Aldenkamp et al. 2003).

Antidepressants

Antidepressants are frequently prescribed for the treatment of bipolar depression in elderly patients (Beyer et al. 2008; Rej et al. 2017), although the use of antidepressants in bipolar disorder is a point of continued concern among psychiatrists (Dols et al. 2016; Ghaemi 2012). Three issues highlight the controversy: 1) the literature is ambiguous as to the efficacy of antidepressants in bipolar depression, 2) antidepressants have the potential to induce a manic episode, and 3) antidepressants may also induce a rapid-cycling course. Given these concerns, most consensus guidelines have recommended that primary treatment of bipolar depression be with a mood stabilizer or atypical antipsychotic, while antidepressant augmentation may be considered if there is limited or no response (Dols et al. 2016; Yatham et al. 2018).

There are no specific studies of the use of antidepressants in geriatric populations. In a retrospective study of elderly inpatients who had antidepressant-induced mania, Young et al. (2003) found that tricyclic antidepressants were more likely than other antidepressants to induce mania in late life, suggesting that the use of selective serotonin reuptake inhibitors may be preferable in elderly patients.

Antipsychotic Agents

The atypical antipsychotic agents are increasingly being utilized for treatment of the various phases of bipolar disorder. Aripiprazole, asenapine, cariprazine, olanzapine, quetiapine and quetiapine XR (extended release), risperidone, and ziprasidone are currently approved by the FDA for the treatment of acute mania; cariprazine, lurasidone, olanzapine-fluoxetine combination, and quetiapine and quetiapine XR are approved for the treatment of acute bipolar depression; and aripiprazole, olanzapine, quetiapine and quetiapine XR, risperidone, and ziprasidone are approved for maintenance-phase treatment. Despite the increasing number of FDA-approved options for the treatment of bipolar manic and depressed episodes and for maintenance treatment, the information regarding their use in older adults (especially those older than 65 years) is limited.

Antipsychotic Use in Mania

Beyer et al. (2001) reported on a pooled subanalysis of three double-blind, placebo-controlled clinical trials of olanzapine in acute bipolar mania, focusing on subjects older than 50 years. In comparison with placebo, olanzapine was found to be efficacious for the treatment of acute mania without any significant change in the side effect profile. A post hoc secondary analysis of two double-blind, placebo-controlled studies of quetiapine monotherapy (440–800 mg/day) in bipolar mania found that both older (≥55 years) and younger subjects had an improvement in symptoms from baseline compared with placebo. Clinically significant improvement was noted as early as day 4 of treatment (Sajatovic et al. 2008a). The mean modal dosage was 550 mg/day for older participants compared with 643 mg/day for younger participants. Case reports and open-label studies of the treatment of older adults in a manic episode have been published for risperidone (Madhusoodanan et al. 1995, 1999), clozapine (Frye et al. 1996; Shulman et al. 1997), and asenapine (Baruch et al. 2013).

Antipsychotic Use in Bipolar Depression

Sajatovic and Paulsson (2007) conducted a post hoc secondary analysis of two 8-week double-blind, placebo-controlled studies of quetiapine monotherapy (300 mg/day and 600 mg/day) in patients with bipolar depression. They found that in the subgroup of 72 older patients (ages 55–65 years), remission occurred more often with both quetiapine dosages compared with placebo (45%, 48%, and 28%, respectively). Sajatovic et al. (2016) also conducted a post hoc analysis of a subgroup of 142 older adults with bipolar I depression who had participated in two large clinical trials evaluating the efficacy of lurasidone monotherapy or lurasidone adjunctive treatment. In the lurasidone monotherapy study, the older subgroup had significantly greater improvement with lurasidone compared with placebo; however, in the adjunctive therapy study, mean change for lurasidone was not significantly different from placebo. Uncontrolled studies have noted improvement with aripiprazole (mean dosage 10.3 mg/day) (Sajatovic et al. 2008b) and asenapine (mean dosage 11.2 mg/day) (Sajatovic et al. 2015a) in older adults with bipolar depression.

Antipsychotics in Bipolar Maintenance

Forester et al. (2018) evaluated the safety and effectiveness of 6 months of lurasidone treatment in older adults who completed a clinical trial for treatment of bipolar depression. They noted that antidepressant effectiveness was maintained over the 6-month period and that minimal effects were noted on weight and metabolic parameters during this time. Overall, maintenance lurasidone therapy was noted to be well tolerated, with low rates of mood-emergent switching. However, they also noted that the proportion of adults who met relapse criteria during the 6-month follow-up was much higher in the older group than in the younger group.

In general, a lower-dosage strategy in elderly patients has been recommended for most atypical antipsychotics (Alexopoulos et al. 2004), although this may be less of a concern in the acute state and not necessarily supported by the clinical trials noted earlier. A major concern regarding atypical antipsychotic use is the potential risk of metabolic abnormalities, such as obesity, diabetes, and dyslipidemia. This risk may be less of a concern for elderly patients because they have less propensity for weight gain and other metabolic effects associated with atypical antipsychotics (Meyer 2002).

In 2006, a black box warning was added to each of the atypical antipsychotic agents indicating that their use in elderly adults with dementia may be associated with a higher incidence of death. The exact mechanism of this increased mortality risk is unknown, although it may be due to increased infections and cardiovascular causes. Information on the mortality risk in patients with late-life bipolar disorder is limited. A review of the U.S. Department of Veterans Affairs registries for older patients with bipolar disorders showed differences in mortality risk for various atypical antipsychotics; patients who were given risperidone had the highest mortality rate, whereas those given quetiapine had the lowest rate (Bhalerao et al. 2012). Although Bhalerao et al. (2012) noted that data could not be translated to recommendations for use of one agent over another, they proposed that these findings suggested a cautious approach to the use of any atypical antipsychotics in older adults and recommended using them judiciously when traditional mood stabilizers and psychotherapies do not fully address patients' needs.

Electroconvulsive Therapy

Electroconvulsive therapy (ECT) has long been known to be effective for the treatment of bipolar disorder. However, very limited data are available on its use in elderly patients with bipolar disorder, especially when compared with the quantity of literature on ECT for unipolar depression. McDonald and Thompson (2001) reported on a case series of three elderly patients with mania who also had some dementia and whose illness was resistant to pharmacotherapy but did respond to ECT treatment. Little et al. (2004) reported on a case series of elderly patients with depression that included five patients with bipolar depression who were treated with bifrontal ECT.

Conclusion

Bipolar disorders are common illnesses seen in older adults. Although less prevalent than in younger adults, bipolar episodes in older patients most often are continuations of this chronic cycling illness that first onset in young adulthood. However, there is also a significant proportion of late-onset cases. When these occur, the psychiatric provider should be attentive to the possibility that the new-onset episode may be associated with physical illness (e.g., neurological disease, reaction to medications, hormonal changes). Treatment of bipolar disorders in older individuals poses particular challenges for several reasons. First, most recommended therapies for bipolar disorder have only limited information for use in older patients. Furthermore, age-related physical changes and drug–drug interactions with patients' total medication regimens must be considered when dosing for elderly patients. Also, because bipolar disorder is a chronic cycling condition, it is not uncommon to find that older adults have failed or not tolerated many of the limited options approved for treatment. Finally, comorbid medical conditions may limit the applicability of treatment options. Despite their vulnerability to early mortality, more physical comorbidities, and increased neurocognitive disorders, older adults with bipolar disorder may also show marked resiliencies. Closer observation of the disease process in older adults may be key to improved understanding of all bipolar disorders and successful treatment interventions.

Key Points

- The prevalence of bipolar disorder, like that of other mental illnesses, decreases with age. However, bipolar disorder in late life continues to be a frequent cause of admission to psychiatric inpatient facilities and disruption of patients' lives.

- The mortality rate for older adults with bipolar disorder is significantly higher than that for the general population and for patients with unipolar depression.

- The onset of bipolar disorder at a later age may be associated with fewer genetic associations and more neurological illnesses.

- Treatment guidelines for late-life bipolar disorder are based primarily on case reports and extrapolation from bipolar treatment in younger adults. As in other geriatric treatment recommendations, the maxim "start low and go slow" is applicable to late-life bipolar treatment.

- Elderly patients may require lower dosages of lithium because of decreased renal clearance.

Suggested Readings

Beyer JL, Burchitt B, Gersing K, et al: Patterns of pharmacotherapy and treatment response in elderly adults with bipolar disorder. Psychopharmacol Bull 41:102–114, 2008
Depp CA, Jeste DV: Bipolar disorder in older adults: a critical review. Bipolar Disord 6:343–367, 2004
Sajatovic M, Strejilevich SA, Gildengers AG, et al: A report on older-age bipolar disorder from the International Society for Bipolar Disorders Task Force. Bipolar Disord 17(7):689–704, 2015
Young RC, Mulsant BH, Sajatovic M, et al: A randomized double-blind controlled trial of lithium and divalproex in the treatment of mania in older patients with bipolar disorder. Am J Psychiatry 174(11):1086–1093, 2017

References

Aldenkamp AP, De Krom M, Reijs R: Newer antiepileptic drugs and cognitive issues. Epilepsia 44(suppl 4):21–29, 2003 12823566
Alexopoulos GS, Streim J, Carpenter D, et al: Using antipsychotic agents in older patients. J Clin Psychiatry 65(suppl 2):5–99, discussion 100–102, quiz 103–104, 2004
Al Jurdi RK, Nguyen QX, Petersen NJ, et al: Acute bipolar I affective episode presentation across life span. J Geriatr Psychiatry Neurol 25(1):6–14, 2012 22467840
Almeida OP, Fenner S: Bipolar disorder: similarities and differences between patients with illness onset before and after 65 years of age. Int Psychogeriatr 14(3):311–322, 2002 12475092
Altshuler LL, Curran JG, Hauser P, et al: T2 hyperintensities in bipolar disorder: magnetic resonance imaging comparison and literature meta-analysis. Am J Psychiatry 152(8):1139–1144, 1995 7625460
American Psychiatric Association: Diagnostic and Statistical Manual of Mental Disorders, 5th Edition. Arlington, VA, American Psychiatric Association, 2013
Angst J: The course of affective disorders, II: typology of bipolar manic-depressive illness. Arch Psychiatr Nervenkr 226(1):65–73, 1978 708228
Angst J, Preisig M: Course of a clinical cohort of unipolar, bipolar and schizoaffective patients: results of a prospective study from 1959 to 1985. Schweiz Arch Neurol Psychiatr 146(1):5–16, 1995 7792568
Angst J, Baastrup P, Grof P, et al: The course of monopolar depression and bipolar psychoses. Psychiatr Neurol Neurochir 76(6):489–500, 1973 4781526
Aprahamian I, Ladeira RB, Diniz BS, et al: Cognitive impairment in euthymic older adults with bipolar disorder: a controlled study using cognitive screening tests. Am J Geriatr Psychiatry 22(4):389–397, 2014 23567429
Balanzá-Martínez V, Tabarés-Seisdedos R, Selva-Vera G, et al: Persistent cognitive dysfunctions in bipolar I disorder and schizophrenic patients: a 3-year follow-up study. Psychother Psychosom 74(2):113–119, 2005 15741761
Baldessarini RJ, Vázquez G, Tondo L: Treatment of cyclothymic disorder: commentary. Psychother Psychosom 80(3):131–135, 2011 21372620
Baruch Y, Tadger S, Plopski I, Barak Y: Asenapine for elderly bipolar manic patients. J Affect Disord 145(1):130–132, 2013 22877962

Battino D, Croci D, Rossini A, et al: Serum carbamazepine concentrations in elderly patients: a case-matched pharmacokinetic evaluation based on therapeutic drug monitoring data. Epilepsia 44(7):923–929, 2003 12823575

Bearden CE, Hoffman KM, Cannon TD: The neuropsychology and neuroanatomy of bipolar affective disorder: a critical review. Bipolar Disord 3(3):106–150, discussion 151–153, 2001 11465675

Berk M, Kapczinski F, Andreazza AC, et al: Pathways underlying neuroprogression in bipolar disorder: focus on inflammation, oxidative stress and neurotrophic factors. Neurosci Biobehav Rev 35(3):804–817, 2011 20934453

Beyer JL, Siegal A, Kennedy JS, et al: Olanzapine, divalproex, and placebo treatment non-head-to-head comparisons of older adult acute mania. Presented at the annual meeting of the International Psychogeriatric Association, Nice, France, September 2001

Beyer JL, Kuchibhatla M, Payne M, et al: Caudate volume measurement in older adults with bipolar disorder. Int J Geriatr Psychiatry 19(2):109–114, 2004a 14758576

Beyer JL, Kuchibhatla M, Payne ME, et al: Hippocampal volume measurement in older adults with bipolar disorder. Am J Geriatr Psychiatry 12(6):613–620, 2004b 15545329

Beyer J, Kuchibhatla M, Gersing K, Krishnan KR: Medical comorbidity in a bipolar outpatient clinical population. Neuropsychopharmacology 30(2):401–404, 2005 15536492

Beyer JL, Burchitt B, Gersing K, Krishnan KR: Patterns of pharmacotherapy and treatment response in elderly adults with bipolar disorder. Psychopharmacol Bull 41(1):102–114, 2008

Beyer JL, Young R, Kuchibhatla M, Krishnan KR: Hyperintense MRI lesions in bipolar disorder: a meta-analysis and review. Int Rev Psychiatry 21(4):394–409, 2009 20374153

Bhalerao S, Seyfried LS, Kim HM, et al: Mortality risk with the use of atypical antipsychotics in later-life bipolar disorder. J Geriatr Psychiatry Neurol 25(1):29–36, 2012 22467844

Bowden CL, Lawson DM, Cunningham M, et al: The role of divalproex in the treatment of bipolar disorder. Psychiatr Ann 32:742–750, 2002

Broadhead J, Jacoby R: Mania in old age: a first prospective study. Int J Geriatr Psychiatry 5:215–222, 1990

Cassidy F, Ahearn EP, Carroll BJ: Substance abuse in bipolar disorder. Bipolar Disord 3(4):181–188, 2001 11552957

Chen ST, Altshuler LL, Melnyk KA, et al: Efficacy of lithium vs. valproate in the treatment of mania in the elderly: a retrospective study. J Clin Psychiatry 60(3):181–186, 1999 10192594

de Asis JM, Greenwald BS, Alexopoulos GS, et al: Frontal signal hyperintensities in mania in old age. Am J Geriatr Psychiatry 14(7):598–604, 2006 16816013

DeBattista C, Schatzberg AF: Current psychotropic dosing and monitoring guidelines. Prim Psychiatry 13(6):61–81, 2006

De Fazio P, Gaetano R, Caroleo M, et al: Lithium in late-life mania: a systematic review. Neuropsychiatr Dis Treat 13:755–766, 2017 28331326

Delaloye C, Moy G, de Bilbao F, et al: Longitudinal analysis of cognitive performances and structural brain changes in late-life bipolar disorder. Int J Geriatr Psychiatry 26(12):1309–1318, 2011 21394788

Depp CA, Jeste DV: Bipolar disorder in older adults: a critical review. Bipolar Disord 6(5):343–367, 2004 15383127

Depp CA, Lindamer LA, Folsom DP, et al: Differences in clinical features and mental health service use in bipolar disorder across the lifespan. Am J Geriatr Psychiatry 13(4):290–298, 2005

Depp CA, Davis CE, Mittal D, et al: Health-related quality of life and functioning of middle-aged and elderly adults with bipolar disorder. J Clin Psychiatry 67(2):215–221, 2006 16566616

Depp CA, Moore DJ, Sitzer D, et al: Neurocognitive impairment in middle-aged and older adults with bipolar disorder: comparison to schizophrenia and normal comparison subjects. J Affect Disord 101(1–3):201–209, 2007 17224185

Dhingra U, Rabins PV: Mania in the elderly: a 5–7 year follow-up. J Am Geriatr Soc 39(6):581–583, 1991 2037748

Dols A, Kupka RW, van Lammeren A, et al: The prevalence of late-life mania: a review. Bipolar Disord 16(2):113–118, 2014a 23919307

Dols A, Rhebergen D, Beekman A, et al: Psychiatric and medical comorbidities: results from a bipolar elderly cohort study. Am J Geriatr Psychiatry 22(11):1066–1074, 2014b 24495405

Dols A, Kessing LV, Strejilevich SA, et al: Do current national and international guidelines have specific recommendations for older adults with bipolar disorder? A brief report. Int J Geriatr Psychiatry 31(12):1295–1300, 2016 27442023

Doty TJ, Payne ME, Steffens DC, et al: Age-dependent reduction of amygdala volume in bipolar disorder. Psychiatry Res 163(1):84–94, 2008 18407469

Dupont RM, Jernigan TL, Butters N, et al: Subcortical abnormalities detected in bipolar affective disorder using magnetic resonance imaging. Clinical and neuropsychological significance. Arch Gen Psychiatry 47(1):55–59, 1990 2294856

Evans DL, Byerly MJ, Greer RA: Secondary mania: diagnosis and treatment. J Clin Psychiatry 56(suppl 3):31–37, 1995 7883741

Forester BP, Sajatovic M, Tsai J, et al: Safety and effectiveness of long-term treatment with lurasidone in older adults with bipolar depression: post-hoc analysis of a 6-month, open-label study. Am J Geriatr Psychiatry 26(2):150–159, 2018 29146409

Foster JR: Use of lithium in elderly psychiatric patients: a review of the literature. Lithium 3:77–93, 1992

Fotso Soh J, Klil-Drori S, Rej S: Using lithium in older age bipolar disorder: special considerations. Drugs Aging 36(2):147–154, 2019 30613911

Frye MA, Altshuler LL, Bitran JA: Clozapine in rapid cycling bipolar disorder. J Clin Psychopharmacol 16(1):87–90, 1996 8834431

Fujikawa T, Yanai I, Yamawaki S: Psychosocial stressors in patients with major depression and silent cerebral infarction. Stroke 28(6):1123–1125, 1997 9183336

García-López A, Ezquiaga E, De Dios C, Agud JL: Depressive symptoms in early and late-onset older bipolar patients compared with younger ones. Int J Geriatr Psychiatry 32(2):201–207, 2017 27017999

Ghaemi SN: Antidepressants in bipolar depression: the clinical debate. Aust N Z J Psychiatry 46(4):298–301, 2012 22508588

Gildengers AG, Butters MA, Seligman K, et al: Cognitive functioning in late-life bipolar disorder. Am J Psychiatry 161(4):736–738, 2004 15056521

Gildengers AG, Mulsant BH, Begley A, et al: The longitudinal course of cognition in older adults with bipolar disorder. Bipolar Disord 11(7):744–752, 2009 19719787

Gildengers AG, Mulsant BH, Al Jurdi RK, et al: The relationship of bipolar disorder lifetime duration and vascular burden to cognition in older adults. Bipolar Disord 12(8):851–858, 2010

Gildengers A, Tatsuoka C, Bialko C, et al: Correlates of treatment response in depressed older adults with bipolar disorder. J Geriatr Psychiatry Neurol 25(1):37–42, 2012 22467845

Gildengers AG, Chisholm D, Butters MA, et al: Two-year course of cognitive function and instrumental activities of daily living in older adults with bipolar disorder: evidence for neuroprogression? Psychol Med 43(4):801–811, 2013 22846332

Goodwin FK, Jamison KR: The natural course of manic depressive illness, in Neurobiology of Mood Disorders. Edited by Post RM, Ballenger JC. Baltimore, MD, Williams and Wilkins, 1984, pp 20–37

Goodwin FK, Jamison KR: Manic-Depressive Illness. New York, Oxford University Press, 1990

Gunning-Dixon FM, Murphy CF, Alexopoulos GS, et al: Executive dysfunction in elderly bipolar manic patients. Am J Geriatr Psychiatry 16(6):506–512, 2008 18515695

Haller S, Xekardaki A, Delaloye C, et al: Combined analysis of grey matter voxel-based morphometry and white matter tract-based spatial statistics in late-life bipolar disorder. J Psychiatry Neurosci 36(6):391–401, 2011 21284917

Hays JC, Krishnan KR, George LK, Blazer DG: Age of first onset of bipolar disorder: demographic, family history, and psychosocial correlates. Depress Anxiety 7(2):76–82, 1998 9614596

Himmelhoch JM, Neil JF, May SJ, et al: Age, dementia, dyskinesias, and lithium response. Am J Psychiatry 137(8):941–945, 1980 7416295

Hirschfeld RM, Lewis L, Vornik LA: Perceptions and impact of bipolar disorder: how far have we really come? Results of the national depressive and manic-depressive association 2000 survey of individuals with bipolar disorder. J Clin Psychiatry 64(2):161–174, 2003 12633125

Huang SH, Chung KH, Hsu JL, et al: The risk factors for elderly patients with bipolar disorder having cerebral infarction. J Geriatr Psychiatry Neurol 25(1):15–19, 2012 22467841

Hussein Z, Posner J: Population pharmacokinetics of lamotrigine monotherapy in patients with epilepsy: retrospective analysis of routine monitoring data. Br J Clin Pharmacol 43(5):457–465, 1997 9159559

Kessing LV: Diagnostic subtypes of bipolar disorder in older versus younger adults. Bipolar Disord 8(1):56–64, 2006 16411981

Kessing LV, Vradi E, Andersen PK: Life expectancy in bipolar disorder. Bipolar Disord 17(5):543–548, 2015 25846854

Kessler RC, Rubinow DR, Holmes C, et al: The epidemiology of DSM-III-R bipolar I disorder in a general population survey. Psychol Med 27(5):1079–1089, 1997 9300513

Kessler RC, Berglund P, Demler O, et al: Lifetime prevalence and age-of-onset distributions of DSM-IV disorders in the National Comorbidity Survey Replication. Arch Gen Psychiatry 62(6):593–602, 2005 15939837

Klap R, Unroe KT, Unützer J: Caring for mental illness in the United States: a focus on older adults. Am J Geriatr Psychiatry 11(5):517–524, 2003 14506085

Kocsis JH, Shaw ED, Stokes PE, et al: Neuropsychologic effects of lithium discontinuation. J Clin Psychopharmacol 13(4):268–275, 1993 8376614

Koenig HG, Blazer DG: Epidemiology of geriatric affective disorders. Clin Geriatr Med 8(2):235–251, 1992 1600475

Köhler S, Allardyce J, Verhey FR, et al: Cognitive decline and dementia risk in older adults with psychotic symptoms: a prospective cohort study. Am J Geriatr Psychiatry 21(2):119–128, 2013 23343485

Lala SV, Sajatovic M: Medical and psychiatric comorbidities among elderly individuals with bipolar disorder: a literature review. J Geriatr Psychiatry Neurol 25(1):20–25, 2012 22467842

Laursen TM, Munk-Olsen T, Nordentoft M, Mortensen PB: Increased mortality among patients admitted with major psychiatric disorders: a register-based study comparing mortality in unipolar depressive disorder, bipolar affective disorder, schizoaffective disorder, and schizophrenia. J Clin Psychiatry 68(6):899–907, 2007 17592915

Lewandowski KE, Sperry SH, Malloy MC, Forester BP: Age as a predictor of cognitive decline in bipolar disorder. Am J Geriatr Psychiatry 22(12):1462–1468, 2014 24262287

Little JD, Atkins MR, Munday J, et al: Bifrontal electroconvulsive therapy in the elderly: a 2-year retrospective. J ECT 20(3):139–141, 2004 15342996

Madhusoodanan S, Brenner R, Araujo L, Abaza A: Efficacy of risperidone treatment for psychoses associated with schizophrenia, schizoaffective disorder, bipolar disorder, or senile dementia in 11 geriatric patients: a case series. J Clin Psychiatry 56(11):514–518, 1995 7592504

Madhusoodanan S, Brecher M, Brenner R, et al: Risperidone in the treatment of elderly patients with psychotic disorders. Am J Geriatr Psychiatry 7(2):132–138, 1999 10322240

Martino DJ, Strejilevich SA, Manes F: Neurocognitive functioning in early-onset and late-onset older patients with euthymic bipolar disorder. Int J Geriatr Psychiatry 28(2):142–148, 2013a 22451354

Martino DJ, Strejilevich SA, Marengo E, et al: Relationship between neurocognitive functioning and episode recurrences in bipolar disorder. J Affect Disord 147(1–3):345–351, 2013b 23232419

McDonald WM: Epidemiology, etiology, and treatment of geriatric mania. J Clin Psychiatry 61(supp 13):3–11, 2000 11153809

McDonald WM, Thompson TR: Treatment of mania in dementia with electroconvulsive therapy. Psychopharmacol Bull 35(2):72–82, 2001 12397888

McDonald WM, Tupler LA, Marsteller FA, et al: Hyperintense lesions on magnetic resonance images in bipolar disorder. Biol Psychiatry 45(8):965–971, 1999 10386178

Meyer JM: A retrospective comparison of weight, lipid, and glucose changes between risperidone- and olanzapine-treated inpatients: metabolic outcomes after 1 year. J Clin Psychiatry 63(5):425–433, 2002 12019668

Molinari V, Marmion J: Relationship between affective disorders and Axis II diagnoses in geropsychiatric patients. J Geriatr Psychiatry Neurol 8(1):61–64, 1995 7710650

Montes JM, Alegria A, Garcia-Lopez A, et al: Understanding bipolar disorder in late life: clinical and treatment correlates of a sample of elderly outpatients. J Nerv Ment Dis 201(8):674–679, 2013 23896848

Okuma T, Yamashita I, Takahashi R, et al: Comparison of the antimanic efficacy of carbamazepine and lithium carbonate by double-blind controlled study. Pharmacopsychiatry 23(3):143–150, 1990 1973844

Oshima A, Higuchi T: Treatment guidelines for geriatric mood disorders. Psychiatry Clin Neurosci 53(suppl):S55–S59, 1999 10560900

Panjehshahin MR, Bowmer CJ, Yates MS: Effect of valproic acid, its unsaturated metabolites and some structurally related fatty acids on the binding of warfarin and dansylsarcosine to human albumin. Biochem Pharmacol 41(8):1227–1233, 1991 1706921

Petterson U: Manic-depressive illness: a clinical, social and genetic study. Acta Psychiatr Scand 56(suppl 269):1–93, 1977 343505

Phillips ML: The neural basis of mood dysregulation in bipolar disorder. Cogn Neuropsychiatry 11(3):233–249, 2006 17354070

Ponce H, Kunik M, Molinari V, et al: Divalproex sodium treatment in elderly male bipolar patients. Journal of Geriatric Drug Therapy 12:55–63, 1999

Posner J, Holdrich T, Crome P: Comparison of lamotrigine pharmacokinetics in young and elderly healthy volunteers. J Pharm Med 1:121–128, 1991

Prabhakar D, Balon R: Late-onset bipolar disorder: a case for careful appraisal. Psychiatry 7(1):34–37, 2010 20386635

Prien RF, Caffey EM Jr, Klett CJ: Relationship between serum lithium level and clinical response in acute mania treated with lithium. Br J Psychiatry 120(557):409–414, 1972 4557271

Ramsey CM, Spira AP, Mojtabai R, et al: Lifetime manic spectrum episodes and all-cause mortality: 26-year follow-up of the NIMH Epidemiologic Catchment Area Study. J Affect Disord 151(1):337–142, 2013

Regenold WT, Prasad M: Uses of intravenous valproate in geriatric psychiatry. Am J Geriatr Psychiatry 9(3):306–308, 2001 11481141

Regenold WT, Thapar RK, Marano C, et al: Increased prevalence of type 2 diabetes mellitus among psychiatric inpatients with bipolar I affective and schizoaffective disorders independent of psychotropic drug use. J Affect Disord 70(1):19–26, 2002 12113916

Rej S, Butters MA, Aizenstein HJ, et al: Neuroimaging and neurocognitive abnormalities associated with bipolar disorder in old age. Int J Geriatr Psychiatry 29(4):421–427, 2014 24006234

Rej S, Herrmann N, Shulman K, et al: Current psychotropic medication prescribing patterns in late-life bipolar disorder. Int J Geriatr Psychiatry 32(12):1459–1465, 2017 27911003

Roose SP, Bone S, Haidorfer C, et al: Lithium treatment in older patients. Am J Psychiatry 136(6):843–844, 1979 443475

Sajatovic M: Treatment of bipolar disorder in older adults. Int J Geriatr Psychiatry 17(9):865–873, 2002 12221662

Sajatovic M, Paulsson B: Quetiapine for the treatment of depressive episodes in adults aged 55 to 65 years with bipolar disorder. Presented at the American Association of Geriatric Psychiatry Annual Meeting, New Orleans, LA, 2007

Sajatovic M, Gyulai L, Calabrese JR, et al: Maintenance treatment outcomes in older patients with bipolar I disorder. Am J Geriatr Psychiatry 13(4):305–311, 2005a 15845756

Sajatovic M, Madhusoodanan S, Coconcea N: Managing bipolar disorder in the elderly: defining the role of the newer agents. Drugs Aging 22(1):39–54, 2005b 15663348

Sajatovic M, Blow FC, Ignacio RV: Psychiatric comorbidity in older adults with bipolar disorder. Int J Geriatr Psychiatry 21(6):582–587, 2006 16783798

Sajatovic M, Ramsay E, Nanry K, Thompson T: Lamotrigine therapy in elderly patients with epilepsy, bipolar disorder or dementia. Int J Geriatr Psychiatry 22(10):945–950, 2007 17326238

Sajatovic M, Calabrese JR, Mullen J: Quetiapine for the treatment of bipolar mania in older adults. Bipolar Disord 10(6):662–671, 2008a 18837860

Sajatovic M, Coconcea N, Ignacio RV, et al: Aripiprazole therapy in 20 older adults with bipolar disorder: a 12-week, open-label trial. J Clin Psychiatry 69(1):41–46, 2008b 18312036

Sajatovic M, Gildengers A, Al Jurdi RK, et al: Multisite, open-label, prospective trial of lamotrigine for geriatric bipolar depression: a preliminary report. Bipolar Disord 13(3):294–302, 2011 21676132

Sajatovic M, Dines P, Fuentes-Casiano E, et al: Asenapine in the treatment of older adults with bipolar disorder. Int J Geriatr Psychiatry 30(7):710–719, 2015a 25335125

Sajatovic M, Strejilevich SA, Gildengers AG, et al: A report on older-age bipolar disorder from the International Society for Bipolar Disorders Task Force. Bipolar Disord 17(7):689–704, 2015b 26384588

Sajatovic M, Forester BP, Tsai J, et al: Efficacy of lurasidone in adults aged 55 years and older with bipolar depression: post hoc analysis of 2 double-blind, placebo-controlled studies. J Clin Psychiatry 77(10):e1324–e1331, 2016 27529375

Samamé C, Martino DJ, Strejilevich SA: A quantitative review of neurocognition in euthymic late-life bipolar disorder. Bipolar Disord 15(6):633–644, 2013 23651122

Schouws SN, Zoeteman JB, Comijs HC, et al: Cognitive functioning in elderly patients with early onset bipolar disorder. Int J Geriatr Psychiatry 22(9):856–861, 2007 17262882

Shulman K, Post F: Bipolar affective disorder in old age. Br J Psychiatry 136:26–32, 1980 7357218

Shulman KI, Mackenzie S, Hardy B: The clinical use of lithium carbonate in old age: a review. Prog Neuropsychopharmacol Biol Psychiatry 11(2–3):159–164, 1987 3114827

Shulman KI, Tohen M, Satlin A, et al: Mania compared with unipolar depression in old age. Am J Psychiatry 149(3):341–345, 1992 1536272

Shulman RW, Singh A, Shulman KI: Treatment of elderly institutionalized bipolar patients with clozapine. Psychopharmacol Bull 33(1):113–118, 1997 9133761

Shulman KI, Rochon P, Sykora K, et al: Changing prescription patterns for lithium and valproic acid in old age: shifting practice without evidence. BMJ 326(7396):960–961, 2003 12727769

Sibisi CDT: Sex differences in the age of onset of bipolar affective illness. Br J Psychiatry 156:842–845, 1990 2207514

Snowdon J: A retrospective case-note study of bipolar disorder in old age. Br J Psychiatry 158:485–490, 1991 2054563

Speer DC: Differences in social resources and treatment history among diagnostic groups of older adults. Hosp Community Psychiatry 43(3):270–274, 1992 1555823

Spicer CC, Hare EH, Slater E: Neurotic and psychotic forms of depressive illness: evidence from age-incidence in a national sample. Br J Psychiatry 123(576):535–541, 1973 4766651

Sproule BA, Hardy BG, Shulman KI: Differential pharmacokinetics of lithium in elderly patients. Drugs Aging 16(3):165–177, 2000 10803857

Starkstein SE, Robinson RG, Price TR: Comparison of cortical and subcortical lesions in the production of poststroke mood disorders. Brain 110(Pt 4):1045–1059, 1987 3651794

Starkstein SE, Mayberg HS, Berthier ML, et al: Mania after brain injury: neuroradiological and metabolic findings. Ann Neurol 27(6):652–659, 1990 2360802

Starkstein SE, Fedoroff P, Berthier ML, Robinson RG: Manic-depressive and pure manic states after brain lesions. Biol Psychiatry 29(2):149–158, 1991 1995084

Stone K: Mania in the elderly. Br J Psychiatry 155:220–224, 1989 2597918

Subramaniam H, Dennis MS, Byrne EJ: The role of vascular risk factors in late onset bipolar disorder. Int J Geriatr Psychiatry 22(8):733–737, 2007 17146839

Tariot PN, Podgorski CA, Blazina L, Leibovici A: Mental disorders in the nursing home: another perspective. Am J Psychiatry 150(7):1063–1069, 1993 8317577

Tohen M, Shulman KI, Satlin A: First-episode mania in late life. Am J Psychiatry 151(1):130–132, 1994 8267112

Torrent C, Bonnin CdM, Martínez-Arán A, et al: Efficacy of functional remediation in bipolar disorder: a multicenter randomized controlled study. Am J Psychiatry 170(8):852–859, 2013 23511717

Tsai SY, Kuo CJ, Chen CC, Lee HC: Risk factors for completed suicide in bipolar disorder. J Clin Psychiatry 63(6):469–476, 2002 12088157

Tsai S, Lee H, Shang C, et al: The correlates of cognitive dysfunction in early onset elderly bipolar patients. Presented at the International Congress of the International Psychogeriatrics Association, Chicago, IL, August 2003

Tsai SY, Gildengers AG, Hsu JL, et al: Inflammation associated with volume reduction in the gray matter and hippocampus of older patients with bipolar disorder. J Affect Disord 244:60–66, 2019 30317016

Umapathy C, Mulsant BH, Pollock BG: Bipolar disorder in the elderly. Psychiatr Ann 30:473–480, 2000

Unützer J, Simon G, Pabiniak C, et al: The treated prevalence of bipolar disorder in a large staff-model HMO. Psychiatr Serv 49(8):1072–1078, 1998 9712215

U.S. Food and Drug Administration: Carbamazepine prescribing information to include recommendation of genetic test for patients with Asian ancestry. FDA News, December 12, 2007. Available at http://www.fda.gov/bbs/topics/NEWS/2007/NEW01755.html. Accessed February 17, 2008.

Vaccarino SR, Rajji TK, Gildengers AG, et al: Allostatic load but not medical burden predicts memory performance in late-life bipolar disorder. Int J Geriatr Psychiatry 33(3):546–552, 2018 29235143

Van Rheenen TE, Lewandowski KE, Bauer IE, et al: Current understandings of the trajectory and emerging correlates of cognitive impairment in bipolar disorder: an overview of evidence. Bipolar Disord 22(1):13–27, 2020 31408230

Vasudev A, Thomas A: "Bipolar disorder" in the elderly: what's in a name? Maturitas 66(3):231–235, 2010

Vederine FE, Wessa M, Leboyer M, Houenou J: A meta-analysis of whole-brain diffusion tensor imaging studies in bipolar disorder. Prog Neuropsychopharmacol Biol Psychiatry 35(8):1820–1826, 2011 21624424

Videbech P: MRI findings in patients with affective disorder: a meta-analysis. Acta Psychiatr Scand 96(3):157–168, 1997 9296545

Weissman MM, Leaf PJ, Tischler GL, et al: Affective disorders in five United States communities. Psychol Med 18(1):141–153, 1988 3363034

Weissman MM, Bland RC, Canino GJ, et al: Cross-national epidemiology of major depression and bipolar disorder. JAMA 276(4):293–299, 1996 8656541

Wijeratne C, Malhi GS: Vascular mania: an old concept in danger of sclerosing? A clinical overview. Acta Psychiatr Scand Suppl (434):35–40, 2007 17688461

Winokur G: The Iowa 500: heterogeneity and course in manic-depressive illness (bipolar). Compr Psychiatry 16(2):125–131, 1975 1120412

Wylie ME, Mulsant BH, Pollock BG, et al: Age at onset in geriatric bipolar disorder: effects on clinical presentation and treatment outcomes in an inpatient sample. Am J Geriatr Psychiatry 7(1):77–83, 1999 9919324

Yassa R, Nair NP, Iskandar H: Late-onset bipolar disorder. Psychiatr Clin North Am 11(1):117–131, 1988 3288976

Yatham LN, Kennedy SH, Parikh SV, et al: Canadian Network for Mood and Anxiety Treatments (CANMAT) and International Society for Bipolar Disorders (ISBD) 2018 guidelines for the management of patients with bipolar disorder. Bipolar Disord 20(2):97–170, 2018 29536616

Yildiz-Yesiloglu A, Ankerst DP: Neurochemical alterations of the brain in bipolar disorder and their implications for pathophysiology: a systematic review of the in vivo proton magnetic resonance spectroscopy findings. Prog Neuropsychopharmacol Biol Psychiatry 30(6):969–995, 2006 16677749

Young RC, Kalayam B, Tsuboyama G, et al: Mania: response to lithium across the age spectrum (abstract). Society for Neuroscience Abstracts 18:669, 1992

Young RC, Jain H, Kiosses DN, Meyers BS: Antidepressant-associated mania in late life. Int J Geriatr Psychiatry 18(5):421–424, 2003 12766919

Young RC, Gyulai L, Mulsant BH, et al: Pharmacotherapy of bipolar disorder in old age: review and recommendations. Am J Geriatr Psychiatry 12(4):342–357, 2004 15249272

Young RC, Murphy CF, Heo M, et al: Cognitive impairment in bipolar disorder in old age: literature review and findings in manic patients. J Affect Disord 92(1):125–131, 2006 16469389

Young RC, Mulsant BH, Sajatovic M, et al: GERI-BD: a randomized double-blind controlled trial of lithium and divalproex in the treatment of mania in older patients with bipolar disorder. Am J Psychiatry 174(11):1086–1093, 2017 29088928

Zis AP, Grof P, Goodwin FK: The natural course of affective disorders: implications for lithium prophylaxis, in Lithium: Controversies and Unsolved Issues. Edited by Cooper TB, Gershon S, Kline NS, Shou M. Amsterdam, The Netherlands, Excerpta Medica, 1979, pp 381–398

CHAPTER 11

Schizophrenia Spectrum and Other Psychotic Disorders

Sarah A. Graham, Ph.D.

David H. Adamowicz, M.D., Ph.D.

Dilip V. Jeste, M.D.

Ellen E. Lee, M.D.

Delusions, hallucinations, and other psychotic symptoms can accompany a variety of conditions in late life. These symptoms may be more common than previously thought; Swedish investigators found that in a sample of individuals age 85 years, the prevalence of psychotic symptoms was 10.1%, with 6.9% of subjects having hallucinations, 5.5% having delusions, and 6.9% having paranoid ideation (Östling and Skoog 2002). Conditions causing acute psychotic symptoms that tend to resolve when the underlying condition is treated are discussed elsewhere in this textbook (e.g., delirium in Chapter 7, "Delirium," and drug-induced psychosis in Chapter 20, "Psychopharmacology"). In this chapter, we review the epidemiology, presentation, and treatment of chronic late-life psychotic disorders that are not secondary to a mood disorder or a general medical condition other than a neurocognitive disorder. These include early-onset schizophrenia, late-onset schizophrenia, very-late-onset schizophrenia-like psychosis (VLOSLP; onset after age 60 years), delusional disorder, and psychosis related to a major neurocognitive disorder such as Alzheimer's disease (AD).

Schizophrenia

Early-Onset Schizophrenia

Typically, individuals with schizophrenia develop the disorder in the second or third decade of life (American Psychiatric Association 2000). Although mortality rates in general, and suicide and homicide rates in particular, are higher among individuals with schizophrenia than in the general population (Hannerz et al. 2001; Hiroeh et al. 2001; Joukamaa et al. 2001), many people with early-onset schizophrenia are now living into older adulthood. Therefore, most of the older adults with schizophrenia have had an early onset followed by a chronic course of illness spanning several decades. The prevalence of schizophrenia is ~0.6% among adults ages 45–64 and 0.1%–0.5% among elderly adults (Castle and Murray 1993; Copeland et al. 1998; Keith et al. 1991).

Longitudinal follow-up of patients with schizophrenia indicates considerable heterogeneity of outcomes. A minority of patients experience remission of both positive and negative symptoms (Ciompi 1980; Harding et al. 1987; Huber 1997). Auslander and Jeste (2004) reported that nearly 10% of community-dwelling older patients with schizophrenia met strict research criteria for sustained remission. Although a small proportion of patients experience deterioration of symptoms, the course in most patients is largely unchanged over time (Belitsky and McGlashan 1993; Cohen 1990; Harvey et al. 1999). However, there is generally an improvement in positive symptoms (Jeste et al. 2003). A possibility of survivor bias—that is, that the sickest patients die young, and the hardier ones survive into older age—should be kept in mind when studying older patients with early-onset illness.

Factors associated with poor prognosis for early-onset schizophrenia include chronicity, insidious onset, premorbid psychosocial or functional deficits, and prominent negative symptoms (Ram et al. 1992). In one sample of chronically institutionalized patients with schizophrenia, older age was associated with lower levels of positive symptoms and higher levels of negative symptoms (Davidson et al. 1995). However, Harding (2002) noted that the strength of the association between the predictors of outcome and the actual outcome in patients with schizophrenia weakens over time. The increased physical comorbidity and premature mortality in schizophrenia have resulted in a 15- to 20-year longevity gap relative to the general population (Laursen et al. 2014), and that gap has been growing since the 1970s (Lee et al. 2018). Studies of inflammation, oxidative stress, and other aging biomarkers and of aging-related diseases have supported a theory of accelerated biological aging in schizophrenia (Hong et al. 2017; Kirkpatrick et al. 2008; Lee et al. 2016, 2017; Wolkowitz et al. 2017). Although biomarker abnormalities (e.g., inflammation, oxidative stress, telomeres, metabolic dysfunction) are present in high-risk and first-episode patients, lifestyle factors such as smoking and exposure to antipsychotic medications contribute to these physical health outcomes (S. Chen et al. 2013; Chen et al. 2016; Steiner et al. 2017, 2019; Zhang et al. 2015). Thus, aging with schizophrenia greatly impacts physical health and functioning.

Cognition in Older Patients With Schizophrenia

The pattern of cognitive deficits in schizophrenia differs significantly from that in AD; patients with AD have less efficient learning and more rapid forgetting than those with schizophrenia (Heaton et al. 2001). Among community-dwelling older outpatients with schizophrenia, cognitive functioning seems to remain relatively stable, other than the changes expected from normal aging (Heaton et al. 2001). A small proportion of chronically institutionalized older patients with schizophrenia have cognitive decline greater than that expected for their age (Putnam and Harvey 2000).

Depression in Older Patients With Schizophrenia

Depression is a common source of comorbidity in older patients with schizophrenia. Studies have shown depressive symptoms to be distinct from negative symptoms (Baynes et al. 2000). Depression is also a major predictor of suicidality in this population (Montross et al. 2006). Subsyndromal depression has been found to be associated with greater morbidity (Diwan et al. 2007; Zisook et al. 2007). Detection and management of subsyndromal depression may have an important role to play in the management of this population.

Functional Capacity

The level of functional impairment varies considerably older adults with schizophrenia. In a study of middle-aged and older outpatients with schizophrenia, Palmer et al. (2002b) found that 30% had been employed at least part-time since the onset of psychosis, 43% were current drivers, and 73% were living independently. In general, worse neuropsychological test performance, lower educational level, and negative symptoms but not positive symptoms are associated with poorer functional capacity in older outpatients with schizophrenia (Evans et al. 2003).

Quality of Life

Self-appraisal is considered essential in studies of quality of life for patients with schizophrenia. A number of studies have found poorer self-assessed quality of life to be associated with depression, positive and negative symptoms, cognitive deficits, financial strain, poor social support, and poor social skills (Vahia et al. 2007). These findings suggest that a multimodal approach to management of these patients is necessary to improve their quality of life.

Late-Onset Schizophrenia

Historically, schizophrenia has been considered a disease of younger adulthood. Kraepelin (1921) termed schizophrenia *dementia praecox* to distinguish it from organic disorders arising in late life and to indicate a poor prognosis with a course of progressive deterioration. However, in later years, Kraepelin himself observed that some cases arose for the first time in older patients and that progressive decline was not a universal feature of the disease. Bleuler (1943) and Roth (1955) developed this concept further, with studies demonstrating the late-onset phenotype to be a distinct entity from the early-onset form. A literature review found that ~23% of patients with schizophrenia had onset after age 40, with 3% being older than 60 years (Harris and Jeste 1988). An investigation involving first-contact patients reported that 29% had an onset after age 44, with 12% having onset after age 64 (Howard et al. 1993). The consensus statement by the International Late-Onset Schizophrenia Group suggested that schizophrenia with an onset after age 40 should be called "late-onset schizophrenia" and should be considered to be a subtype of schizophrenia rather than a related disorder (Howard et al. 2000).

DSM has changed its stance on distinguishing late-onset from earlier-onset schizophrenia over the past several editions. Whereas DSM-III (American Psychiatric Association 1980) did not allow for the diagnosis of schizophrenia if the patient's symptoms emerged after age 45, the late-onset specifier was introduced for such cases in the revised edition (DSM-III-R; American Psychiatric Association 1987). However, the term was eliminated from DSM-IV (American Psychiatric Association 1994) and kept out of DSM-5 (American Psychiatric Association 2013). DSM-5 states that "late-onset cases can still meet the diagnostic criteria for schizophrenia, but it is not yet clear whether this is the same condition as schizophrenia diagnosed prior to mid-life (e.g., prior to age 55 years)" (p. 103). It also mentions that these cases are overrepresented by females and are characterized by predominant psychotic symptoms with relative preservation of affect and social functioning.

The risk factors and clinical presentation associated with late-onset schizophrenia are similar to those associated with early-onset schizophrenia (Brodaty et al. 1999; Jeste et al. 1995). Similar proportions of individuals with early-onset or late-onset schizophrenia reported a family history of schizophrenia (10%–15%) (Jeste et al. 1997). Levels of childhood maladjustment, measured retrospectively, were also similar in both groups and higher than in healthy subjects (Jeste et al. 1997). Patients with early- and late-onset schizophrenia have increased rates of minor physical anomalies relative to healthy subjects (Lohr et al. 1997).

Females predominate among individuals with onset of schizophrenia in middle to late life (Häfner et al. 1998; Jeste et al. 1997). It has been speculated that estrogen may serve as an endogenous antipsychotic, masking schizophrenic symptoms in vulnerable females until after menopause (Seeman 1996). However, investigations on the efficacy of hormone replacement therapy as an adjunct treatment for postmenopausal females with psychosis have not had promising results (Kulkarni et al. 1996, 2001; Lindamer et al. 2001).

Neuroimaging studies show that, compared with patients with early-onset schizophrenia, patients with late-onset schizophrenia have more nonspecific structural abnormalities, such as enlarged ventricles and increased white matter hyperintensities (Sachdev et al. 1999) and larger thalamus volume on MRI (Corey-Bloom et al. 1995). A single small study employing diffusion tensor imaging recently found evidence of abnormal white matter integrity in the left parietal lobe and right posterior cingulum in patients with late-onset schizophrenia ($n=20$) compared with age-matched healthy control subjects ($n=17$), although no associations were found between these abnormalities and symptom levels (L. Chen et al. 2013). Other imaging studies have ruled out strokes, tumors, and other abnormalities as potential causes of schizophrenia in late life (Rivkin et al. 2000). Finally, long-term neuropsychological follow-up of patients with late-onset schizophrenia revealed no evidence of cognitive decline, suggesting a neurodevelopmental rather than a neurodegenerative process (Palmer et al. 2003).

Most studies have found that patients with late-onset schizophrenia have lower levels of positive symptoms and a lower daily antipsychotic dosage requirement than patients with early-onset disease (Vahia et al. 2010). Patients with late-onset schizophrenia tend to have more organized delusions, auditory hallucinations or those with a running commentary, and persecutory delusions with and without hallucinations (Howard et al. 2000). Data from initial smaller studies suggested a higher prevalence of the paranoid subtype and lower levels of negative symptoms on average among patients with late-onset schizophrenia (~75%) than among patients with early-onset schizophrenia (~50%) (Jeste et al. 1997). However, a more recent larger study from our center, including data collected over 20 years comparing 744 patients with early-onset schizophrenia and 110 patients with late-onset schizophrenia, found that the two groups had similar relative proportions of patients with the paranoid subtype and no differences in severity of negative symptoms (Vahia et al. 2010).

On neuropsychological testing, after correction for age, education, and sex, patients with late-onset schizophrenia tend to have less impairment in learning, abstraction, and flexibility in thinking than those with early-onset schizophrenia (Jeste et al. 1997). Compared with patients with early-onset schizophrenia, a greater proportion of those with late-onset schizophrenia have successful occupational and marital histories and generally higher premorbid functioning. Sensory deficits, particularly hearing loss, are associated with psychotic symptoms in late life and have been proposed as a risk factor for late-onset schizophrenia (Howard et al. 1994; Raghuram et al. 1980). However, other data suggest that patients with either early- or late-onset schizophrenia may be less likely than healthy older adults to receive appropriate correction for vision and hearing impairments (Prager and Jeste 1993). Thus, uncorrected sensory deficits may reflect generally poorer health care utilization by older patients with psychosis and may not be a potential cause of psychosis in the elderly population.

Several studies have reported elevated levels of inflammatory markers and oxidative stress markers in schizophrenia, although few studies have examined these specifically in late-onset cases (Joseph et al. 2015; Lee et al. 2016, 2017). These studies were expanded to include a number of chemokines and vascular endothelial biomarkers (Hong et al. 2017; Nguyen et al. 2018). A 20-year longitudinal Danish cohort study of more than 78,000 individuals demonstrated that an elevated level of C-reactive protein (CRP), a biomarker of systemic inflammation, was associated with a 6- to 11-fold increased risk for late-onset schizophrenia (Wium-Andersen et al. 2014). Mean CRP levels were higher for persons with schizophrenia (both early- and late-onset) than for those without schizophrenia, even when adjusting for age and sex. This was the first study examining a large cohort for late-onset schizophrenia with regard to inflammatory markers.

In summary, early- and late-onset schizophrenia share similarities in many key clinical characteristics. However, there are important differences, including the greater proportion of females, lower average severity of positive symptoms, and lower average antipsychotic dosage requirement in late-onset schizophrenia. More analyses of large data sets and studies designed to elucidate the pathophysiological pathways underlying early- and late-onset schizophrenia are needed to better understand how these two groups differ (Jeste et al. 2005).

Very-Late-Onset Schizophrenia-Like Psychosis

In its consensus statement, the International Late-Onset Schizophrenia Group proposed the diagnostic term *very-late-onset schizophrenia-like psychosis* for patients whose psychosis begins after age 60 years (Howard et al. 2000). Table 11–1 compares risk factors for and clinical features of early-onset schizophrenia, late-onset schizophrenia, and VLOSLP. VLOSLP may be difficult to diagnose clinically because its clinical picture can be confused with other conditions (e.g., delirium, psychosis due to underly-

TABLE 11–1.   Comparison of early-onset schizophrenia, late-onset schizophrenia, and very-late-onset schizophrenia-like psychosis (VLOSLP)

Feature	Early-onset schizophrenia	Late-onset schizophrenia	VLOSLP
Age at onset, *years*	Before age 40	Middle age (~40–60)	Late life (60+)
Female preponderance	–	+	++
Negative symptoms	++	+	–
Minor physical anomalies	+	+	–
Neuropsychological impairment			
Impairment in learning	++	+	?++
Impairment in retention	–	–	?++
Progressive cognitive deterioration	–	–	++
Brain structure abnormalities (e.g., strokes, tumors)	–	–	++
Family history of schizophrenia	+	+	–
Early childhood maladjustment	+	+	–
Daily neuroleptic dose	++	+	+
Risk of tardive dyskinesia	+	+	++

+=mildly present; ++=strongly present; ?++=probably strongly present, but limited data exist; –=absent.
Source.   Adapted from Palmer et al. 2001.

ing medical illness). Nevertheless, new-onset primary psychotic symptoms have been described in older adults. Indeed, Cervantes et al. (2006) described a clinical case of primary-onset psychosis in a 100-year-old patient.

Factors that distinguish patients with VLOSLP from those with "true" schizophrenia include a smaller genetic load, less evidence of early childhood maladjustment, relative lack of thought disorder and negative symptoms (including blunted affect), greater risk of tardive dyskinesia (TD), and evidence of a neurodegenerative rather than a neurodevelopmental process (Andreasen 1999; Howard et al. 1997). Although the term was initially considered a catchall phrase for a number of different entities, research has since suggested that VLOSLP may be a distinct entity. It has been noted to be more common among immigrant populations, suggesting that psychosocial factors may play a role (Mitter et al. 2005). Imaging studies have shown underlying focal white matter abnormalities in cerebral tracts (Jones et al. 2005). One study suggested that the cognitive biases common in younger individuals with delusions are absent in patients with VLOSLP (Moore et al. 2006). A study by Mazeh et al. (2005) suggested that individuals with VLOSLP may have somewhat more stable cognitive and everyday functioning than do chronically institutionalized elderly patients with schizophrenia. In summary, clinical vigilance must be exercised when treating apparent primary-onset psychotic symptoms in older patients, and "organic" causes should be meticulously ruled out.

Delusional Disorder

At least 6% of older individuals have paranoid symptoms such as persecutory delusions, but most of these individuals have a neurocognitive disorder (Christenson and

Blazer 1984; Forsell and Henderson 1998; Henderson et al. 1998). The essential feature of a delusional disorder is a nonbizarre delusion (e.g., persecutory, somatic, erotomanic, grandiose, or jealous delusion) without prominent auditory or visual hallucinations. The symptoms must be present for at least 1 month. When delusional disorder arises in late life, basic personality features, intellectual performance, and occupational functioning are preserved, but social functioning is compromised. To diagnose delusional disorder, the clinician must rule out delirium, major neurocognitive disorder, psychotic disorder due to another medical condition or to substance or medication use, schizophrenia, and mood disorders with psychotic features. The course of persecutory delusional disorder is typically chronic, but individuals with other types of delusions may have partial remissions and relapses.

According to DSM-5, the lifetime prevalence of delusional disorder is estimated to be 0.2%, and the most common subtype is persecutory. There are no significant sex differences in the prevalence of delusional disorder, although the jealous subtype may be more frequent in males than in females (American Psychiatric Association 2013). The disorder typically first appears in middle to late adulthood, with an average age at onset of 40–49 years for males and 60–69 years for females.

The risk factors for delusional disorder include a family history of schizophrenia or avoidant, paranoid, or schizoid personality disorder (Kendler and Davis 1981). Evidence supporting hearing loss as a risk factor for paranoia is mixed (Cooper and Curry 1976; Moore 1981). In one neuroimaging study, brain atrophy and white matter hyperintensities did not distinguish older patients with psychosis and somatic delusions from patients without such delusions (Rockwell et al. 1994). According to Maher (2005), a subset of the population that is prone to primary perceptual abnormalities may be prone to developing delusions as a result, and "normal" persons may demonstrate "delusional" behavior as a result of sensory disturbances. Evans et al. (1996) compared middle-aged and older patients with schizophrenia or delusional disorder and found no differences in neuropsychological impairment but more severe psychopathology associated with delusional disorder. Finally, immigration and low socioeconomic status may be risk factors for delusional disorder (American Psychiatric Association 2000).

Psychosis of Alzheimer's Disease

Based on a review of 55 studies, Ropacki and Jeste (2005) estimated the median prevalence of psychosis in AD to be about 41% (range 12.2%–74.1%). Psychosis is associated with more rapid cognitive decline. Some studies found a significant association between psychosis and age, age at onset of AD, and illness duration; however, sex, education, and family history of dementia or psychiatric illness showed weak or inconsistent relationships with psychosis. In a large sample of patients with probable AD, Paulsen et al. (2000) found a cumulative incidence of psychotic symptoms of 20% at 1 year, 36% at 2 years, 50% at 3 years, and 51% at 4 years. Delusions, especially of a persecutory nature, tend to be the most common symptom (median prevalence 36%); visual hallucinations (median prevalence 18.7%) and auditory hallucinations (median prevalence 9.2%) are less common (Ropacki and Jeste 2005). These symptoms often must be inferred from the patient's behavior, because he or she may be unable to verbalize thoughts or perceptions due to cognitive impairment, particularly in the later stages of the disease. In one large naturalistic study of the course of psychotic symptoms in dementia, Devanand et al. (1997) found that hallucinations and paranoid delusions were more persistent than depressive symptoms over time but less prevalent and less persistent than behavioral disturbances, particularly agitation.

In Table 11–2, characteristics associated with psychosis of AD are compared with characteristics of schizophrenia in elderly patients (Jeste and Finkel 2000). Two common psychotic symptoms in AD are misidentification of caregivers and delusions of theft (Jeste et al. 2006). Schneiderian first-rank symptoms, such as hearing multiple voices talking to one another or a running commentary on one's actions, are rare (Burns et al. 1990a, 1990b). Disorganization of speech and behavior and negative symptoms are also uncommon (Jeste et al. 2006). Active suicidal ideation and past history of psychosis are rare. Because psychotic symptoms in patients with dementia tend to remit in the late stages of the disease, very-long-term maintenance therapy with antipsychotics is typically unnecessary.

Patients with psychosis of AD and patients with AD without psychosis differ in several important ways. Neuropsychologically, patients who have psychosis of AD have demonstrated greater impairment in executive functioning, more rapid cognitive decline (Jeste et al. 1992; Stern et al. 1994), and greater prevalence of extrapyramidal symptoms (EPS) (Stern et al. 1994) than those without psychosis. Delusions in dementia have been associated with dysfunction in paralimbic areas of the frontotemporal cortex (Sultzer 1996). Neuropathologically, patients with psychosis related to a neurocognitive disorder have shown increased neurodegenerative changes in the cortex, increased norepinephrine in subcortical regions, and reduced serotonin levels in both cortical and subcortical areas (Zubenko et al. 1991). In one study, participants with psychosis of AD had much higher levels of tau protein in the entorhinal and temporal cortices than did those without psychosis (Mukaetova-Ladinska et al. 1995). Furthermore, Wilkosz et al. (2006) suggested that the misidentification subtype and the paranoid subtype of psychosis of AD may be distinct.

Jeste and Finkel (2000) recommended specific diagnostic criteria for psychosis of AD to facilitate epidemiological, clinical, and therapeutic research. These include the presence of visual or auditory hallucinations or delusions, a primary diagnosis of AD, a duration of at least 1 month, and a chronology indicating that symptoms of AD preceded those of psychosis. Alternative causes of psychosis must be excluded, and sufficient functional impairment should be present for this diagnosis to be made. There is evidence for good interrater and test-retest reliability of these criteria (Jeste et al. 2006).

Psychosis in Mild Cognitive Impairment

Over the past several years, mild cognitive impairment (MCI) has increasingly been viewed as a distinct construct rather than simply as a prodrome for dementia. Reports of psychotic symptoms in this population have emerged, and the prevalence has been estimated to be lower than that in AD (10%–14%). Van Der Mussele et al. (2015) found that patients with MCI and psychosis tend to display more frontal lobe symptoms (based on the Middleheim Frontality Score) and physically nonaggressive agitated behavior (based on the Cohen-Mansfield Agitation Inventory) than those without psycho-

TABLE 11–2. Comparison of psychosis of AD with schizophrenia in older patients

Feature	Psychosis of AD	Schizophrenia
Prevalence	35%–50% of patients with AD	<1% of general population
Bizarre or complex delusions	Rare	Frequent
Misidentification of caregivers	Frequent	Rare
Common form of hallucinations	Visual	Auditory
Schneiderian first-rank symptoms	Rare	Frequent
Active suicidal ideation	Rare	Frequent
Past history of psychosis	Rare	Very common
Eventual remission of psychosis	Frequent	Uncommon
Need for years of maintenance on antipsychotic medication	Uncommon	Very common
Usual optimal daily dosages of commonly used atypical antipsychotics		
Risperidone	0.75–1.5 mg	1.5–2.5 mg
Olanzapine	2.5–7.5 mg	7.5–12.5 mg
Recommended adjunctive psychosocial treatment	Sensory enhancement, structured activities, social contact, behavior therapy[a]	CBT, social skills training[b]

AD=Alzheimer's disease; CBT=cognitive-behavioral therapy.
[a]Cohen-Mansfield 2001.
[b]Granholm et al. 2002; McQuaid et al. 2000.
Source. Adapted from Jeste DV, Finkel SI: "Psychosis of Alzheimer's Disease and Related Dementias: Diagnostic Criteria for a Distinct Syndrome." *American Journal of Geriatric Psychiatry* 8:29–34, 2000. Used with permission.

sis; however, these symptoms are not as severe as those in AD. The concept of mild behavioral impairment, or MBI, has also been proposed recently as an entity distinct from MCI, with abnormal perception or thought content (e.g., hallucinations and delusions) as a diagnostic criterion in addition to decreased motivation, affective dysregulation, impulse dyscontrol, and social inappropriateness (Ismail et al. 2016). Per these criteria, MBI does not require concurrent MCI, but the two can coexist. Taragano et al. (2018) estimated that more than 70% of patients with MBI convert to dementia, which is almost twice as many as those with MCI, with the overlap group in between. A study by Dietlin et al. (2019) found that delusions, aggression, agitation, and aberrant motor behavior in MCI were predictive of conversion to dementia. More research is needed, however, on this newly proposed category of MBI.

Psychosis in Parkinson's Disease

The view on psychotic symptoms in Parkinson's disease (PD) has evolved to comprise a spectrum characterized in its early stages by the presence of hallucinations and illusions, with preserved insight, whereas the late stages have the addition of delusions and hallucinations in other, nonvisual modalities (Ffytche et al. 2017). The early phenomena have been described as a "feeling of presence," in some cases with concurrent unformed visual hallucinations; in one study, more than 75% of patients did not find them distressing (Fénelon et al. 2011). Their overall prevalence has been estimated to be as high as 50%, or threefold higher than well-formed visual hallucinations (Wood et al. 2015). As the diseases progresses, multidomain hallucinations may become the norm; one study reported 60% of patients experiencing them after a 10-year follow-up (Goetz et al. 2011). Delusions also become more common and have been estimated at 16% in a cohort excluding patients with dementia (Factor et al. 2014). Although delusions have not been directly linked to cognitive decline, the development of hallucinations over a 6.5-year follow-up period was associated with cognitive impairment in a study by Uc et al. (2009). Visual hallucinations are a characteristic feature of Lewy body disease, which includes both dementia with Lewy bodies (DLB) and Parkinson's disease dementia (PDD), with the nomenclature depending on the timing of symptom onset (Lippa et al. 2007). In one DLB cohort of 102 patients, 70% had visual hallucinations, 10% had auditory hallucinations, and 41% had delusions (Snowden et al. 2012).

Psychosis in Other Major Neurocognitive Disorders

Psychosis is also common in other neurocognitive disorders. Visual hallucinations and secondary delusions are common in Lewy body disease, and vascular neurocognitive disorder may also be accompanied by delusions or hallucinations (Schneider 1999). Naimark et al. (1996) found psychotic symptoms in approximately one-third of a sample of patients with PD, with hallucinations being more common than delusions. Psychosis in frontotemporal lobar degeneration is poorly characterized but may be as common as psychosis in AD (Srikanth et al. 2005).

In a review of 122 studies, Shinagawa et al. (2014) found a prevalence of ~10% for psychosis in frontotemporal dementia (FTD), with certain pathologies such as transactive response DNA-binding protein 43 (TDP-43) and fused in sarcoma (FUS) mutations likely having higher frequencies. Certain mutations such as progranulin (PGRN) and C9Orf72 have been associated with hallucinations in patients with FTD (Le Ber et al. 2008; Snowden et al. 2012). Galimberti et al. (2015) noted that neurodegenerative disease is often misdiagnosed as psychiatric disease and that patients with FTD are at the highest risk, leading to delayed or inappropriate treatment. Some studies have shown that up to 30% of patients with an ultimate diagnosis of FTD were initially diagnosed with psychotic disorder, with an eventual diagnosis of dementia an average of 5 years later (Hall and Finger 2015). While it is possible for late-onset psychiatric disorders to be comorbid with FTD, this is much less likely than FTD developing in the context of preexisting psychiatric disorders that have been ongoing for decades. These cases can appear to be treatment resistant when really it is the diagnosis that has changed.

Treatment

The modern era of pharmacological treatment for schizophrenia and other psychotic disorders began with the introduction of chlorpromazine in the early 1950s. Although this and other conventional agents substantially improved the positive symptoms of schizophrenia (e.g., hallucinations and delusions), a number of treatment liabilities have been recognized over the years, such as movement disorders, sedation, orthostatic hypotension, and increased prolactin concentrations. In addition, older adults have a significantly higher risk for developing TD than do younger adults, making use of conventional antipsychotics in this population highly problematic.

Thus, when the atypical antipsychotics—which are associated with a significantly lower incidence of TD—were introduced, they were hailed as the drugs of choice for older patients with psychotic disorders. However, these agents have since been linked to an increased risk of metabolic dysfunction, including diabetes, dyslipidemia, and obesity, leading to a worsened cardiovascular risk profile. In elderly patients with dementia, atypical antipsychotics have been associated with an increased risk of cerebrovascular adverse events and mortality compared with placebo; therefore, leading pharmaceutical regulatory agencies have issued warnings regarding their use in this population (Meeks and Jeste 2008). At the same time, because of the dearth of evidence-based pharmacological alternatives to antipsychotics for patients with dementia, clinicians are restricted to off-label treatments, which must be used with caution and close monitoring. Psychosocial treatments for older adults with psychosis have been developed and tested in randomized controlled trials (RCTs) and show promise as primary or adjunctive treatments.

Schizophrenia, VLOSLP, and Delusional Disorder

Pharmacological Treatments

Pharmacotherapy for older adults with chronic psychotic disorders can be challenging. Although few randomized, placebo-controlled, double-blind clinical trials have been conducted in this population, some information has become available. Maintenance pharmacotherapy is usually required for older patients with schizophrenia due to risk of relapse. Because older patients are at higher risk of adverse antipsychotic effects due to age-related pharmacokinetic and pharmacodynamic factors (Hämmerlein et al. 1998), coexisting medical illnesses, and concomitant medications, the recommended starting and maintenance dosages of antipsychotics in older adults are much lower than the usual dosages in younger adults (Lehman et al. 2004). Patients with late-onset schizophrenia respond well to low-dosage antipsychotic medication, requiring about 50% of the dosage typically taken by older patients with early-onset schizophrenia and 25%–33% of the dosage used in younger patients with schizophrenia.

The use of conventional or typical antipsychotics in older adults is problematic because of the higher incidence of TD in older patients. Aging appears to be the most important risk factor for the development of TD (American Psychiatric Association 2000; Yassa and Jeste 1992). The cumulative 1-year incidence of TD is 29% in older adults (mean age 65 years) despite low dosing (Jeste et al. 1999b), whereas the annual cumulative incidence in young adults is 4%–5% (Kane et al. 1993). The risk of severe TD is also higher in older patients (Caligiuri et al. 1997). Other side effects of conventional neuroleptics include sedation, anticholinergic effects, cardiovascular effects (including orthostatic hypotension), parkinsonian reactions, and neuroleptic malignant syndrome. Despite these side effects, a conventional antipsychotic occasionally may be the most reasonable treatment option for a given patient, and these agents can be used at flexible, individualized low dosages to minimize side effects (Jeste et al. 1999b).

Valbenazine, a selective vesicular monoamine transporter 2 (VMAT2) inhibitor, was approved by the FDA in 2017 for the treatment of TD in adults. Unlike tetrabenazine, a VMAT2 inhibitor approved for Huntington's chorea, valbenazine had few side effects related to monoamine depletion (Huntington Study Group 2006). The once-daily medication was shown to significantly improve motor symptoms as rated by the Abnormal Involuntary Movement Scale and the Clinical Global Impression of Change–Tardive Dyskinesia over a 6-week trial and was well tolerated by participants (Hauser et al. 2017; O'Brien et al. 2015). These trials were conducted in patients ages 18–85 years (average age 55–57 years). More than half of the patients were diagnosed with schizophrenia or schizoaffective disorder, although some patients with mood disorders and gastrointestinal disorders were also included. It was not specified what proportion of the patients had late-onset schizophrenia or VLOSLP. Further studies on the effects of this new TD treatment in older patients are warranted to fine-tune its use.

Few efficacy comparisons have been done of conventional antipsychotics versus atypical antipsychotics in patients older than 65 years with schizophrenia. In a study of 42 elderly inpatients, Howanitz et al. (1999) found that clozapine (≤300 mg/day) and chlorpromazine (≤600 mg/day) had similar efficacy. Kennedy et al. (2003) compared olanzapine (5–20 mg/day) and haloperidol (5–20 mg/day) in a 6-week trial of 117 patients age 60 years and older who had schizophrenia and related disorders. Olanzapine (mean modal dosage 11.9 mg/day) produced significantly greater symptomatic improvement and was associated with fewer motor side effects than haloperidol (mean modal dosage 9.4 mg/day) (Kennedy et al. 2003). The National Institute of Mental Health's Clinical Antipsychotic Trials of Intervention Effectiveness (CATIE) study (Lieberman et al. 2005), which included adults ages 18–65, found no significant differences in effectiveness between the conventional antipsychotic perphenazine and the atypical antipsychotics risperidone, olanzapine, quetiapine, or ziprasidone, but it is unknown how these findings would translate to patients older than 65 years.

Generally, atypical antipsychotics carry a much lower risk of TD than conventional neuroleptics, even when taken by very-high-risk patients such as middle-aged and older adults with borderline TD (Dolder and Jeste 2003; Jeste et al. 1999a). Clozapine has demonstrated efficacy in reducing TD in patients who develop it (Kane et al. 1993; Lieberman et al. 1991; Simpson et al. 1978; Small et al. 1987); however, other side effects limit clozapine's use, particularly in elderly patients. A beneficial effect of other atypical agents, specifically risperidone and olanzapine, on preexisting TD has also been reported (Jeste et al. 1999a; Kinon et al. 2004; Littrell et al. 1998; Street et al. 2000).

Atypical antipsychotics have a less favorable side effect profile, however, in terms of metabolic function. Common metabolic side effects include excessive weight gain and obesity, glucose intolerance, new-onset type II diabetes mellitus, diabetic ketoacidosis, and dyslipidemia (Allison et al. 1999; Jin et al. 2002, 2004; Wirshing et al. 1998). Although there are no guidelines for management of these side effects specifically in older patients with schizophrenia, the monitoring recommendations developed by the American Diabetes Association et al. (2004) are potentially applicable. Because elderly patients tend to be at higher risk for cardiovascular disease than younger patients, closer monitoring is necessary for older adults.

The short-term benefit of risperidone and olanzapine for treatment of psychotic symptoms in middle-aged and older adults with schizophrenia has been supported in several double-blind trials (Feldman et al. 2003; Jeste et al. 2003; Riedel et al. 2009;

Suzuki et al. 2011), and one short-term trial suggested that paliperidone might be of benefit (Tzimos et al. 2008). Data supporting the short-term benefit of other atypical antipsychotics come only from open-label or retrospectively designed studies. Although clozapine has been shown to have superior effectiveness over other antipsychotics in younger adults (Jones et al. 2006; Lieberman et al. 2005), it is difficult to use in elderly persons due to the risk of leukopenia and agranulocytosis, as well as other side effects such as orthostasis, sedation, and anticholinergic effects. The necessity of weekly blood draws also may pose a problem for older patients.

Data from a study by Jin et al. (2013) raised serious concerns about the longer-term safety and effectiveness of atypical antipsychotics in middle-aged and older adults. Use of aripiprazole, olanzapine, quetiapine, and risperidone was studied in 332 outpatients older than 40 years who had psychotic symptoms related to various diagnoses, including schizophrenia, mood disorders, PTSD, and neurocognitive disorder. The patients were followed for up to 2 years. The high 1-year cumulative incidence of metabolic syndrome (36% in 1 year) and high rates of both serious (23.7%) and nonserious (50.8%) adverse events were particularly concerning given that no significant improvement in psychopathology was detected. More than half of the study participants discontinued their medication within 6 months, often due to side effects (51.6%) or lack of efficacy (26%), and the quetiapine arm of the study was discontinued early because the incidence of serious adverse events was found to be twice that of the other three atypical antipsychotics.

The concerns about the long-term safety and efficacy of atypical antipsychotics in middle-aged and older adults, combined with the data on the increased risk of strokes and mortality in elderly patients with dementia treated with these drugs and the consequent FDA black box warnings (discussed in "Psychosis of Alzheimer's Disease and Other Neurocognitive Disorders" later), underscore the need for clinicians to exercise caution when prescribing these drugs for older patients with schizophrenia. We strongly recommend educating patients and caregivers about the potential risks and benefits of medications and encouraging shared decision-making. If the decision is made to use an antipsychotic medication, it is generally best to start with a low initial dosage (25%–50% of that used in a younger patient) and titrate slowly. In patients who have been on stable dosages of antipsychotic medications for long periods of time, clinicians should consider gradual and incremental decreases to determine the lowest effective dosage. Patients should be monitored closely for medication effectiveness and possible side effects.

Certain newer antipsychotics have limited data supporting their use in older patients with schizophrenia, without making an explicit distinction for late-onset cases (Khan et al. 2015). Based on data from four 6-week controlled studies, lurasidone in patients ages 65–85 years had medication blood levels similar to those in younger patients, indicating that dosage adjustment may not be necessary unless hepatic or renal impairment occurs. Its side effect profile is attractive given the lower risk of metabolic changes or hypotension. In contrast, ziprasidone has the greatest QTc prolongation among atypical antipsychotics, despite a similar side effect profile, which is why it is not often used in older adults, and current data are insufficient to recommend its use. Trials for iloperidone have also failed to include enough patients older than 65 years to make meaningful conclusions about its use in this population at this stage. Asenapine is another newer antipsychotic with insufficient large-scale data in older adults;

however, one small study showed the drug was well tolerated in its sublingual formulation in patients older than 65 years, with no dosage adjustment necessary (Dubovsky et al. 2012).

Few data are available regarding the safety and effectiveness of pharmacological treatment specifically of VLOSLP or delusional disorder in older individuals. A 2012 Cochrane review of antipsychotic treatments for older adults with late-onset schizophrenia reported that only one study of risperidone and olanzapine met criteria and showed the medications to be well tolerated (Essali and Ali 2012). A recent randomized, controlled, double-blind trial conducted in the United Kingdom found that low-dosage amisulpride was effective and well tolerated in VLOSLP (Howard et al. 2018); however, the drug has not been approved by the FDA for this particular indication. In the realm of herbal remedies, an open-label trial of yokukansan, a standardized combination of herbs with serotonergic, dopaminergic, and glutamatergic actions that has been studied in patients with treatment-resistant schizophrenia and those with dementia with agitation (Matsuda et al. 2013), found significant improvement in psychotic symptoms in patients with VLOSLP versus placebo (Miyaoka et al. 2013).

Alexopoulos et al. (2004) surveyed 48 experts in geriatric care and found antipsychotics to be the only recommended treatment for delusional disorder in older adults. Risperidone (0.75–2.5 mg/day) was the most favored recommendation for older adults with delusional disorder , followed by olanzapine (5–10 mg/day) and quetiapine (50–200 mg/day). More research is required regarding the pharmacological treatment of these conditions in older adults.

Psychosocial Treatments

Since the early part of the 21st century, effective psychosocial interventions for older adults with chronic psychotic disorders have been developed. Granholm et al. (2005) conducted an RCT to examine the effects of adding cognitive-behavioral social skills training (CBSST) to treatment as usual for 76 middle-aged and elderly stable outpatients with schizophrenia. This training intervention teaches cognitive and behavioral coping techniques, social functioning skills, problem-solving techniques, and compensatory aids for neurocognitive impairments. The authors found that CBSST led to significantly increased frequency of social functioning activities, greater cognitive insight (more objectivity in reappraising psychotic symptoms), and greater skill mastery. At 12-month follow-up, the CBSST group had maintained their greater skill acquisition and performance of everyday living skills; however, the greater cognitive insight seen in this group at the end of the treatment was not maintained at 12-month follow-up, suggesting a possible need for booster sessions (Granholm et al. 2007).

Patterson et al. (2006) conducted an RCT to compare a behavioral group intervention called Functional Adaptation Skills Training (FAST) with a time-equivalent attention control condition. FAST is a manualized behavioral intervention that is designed to improve everyday living skills (e.g., medication management, social and communication skills, organization and planning, transportation, financial management) of middle-aged and older adults with schizophrenia or schizoaffective disorder. Compared with participants randomized to the attention control, the FAST group showed significant improvement in daily living and social skills but not in medication management. FAST has also been culturally adapted and pilot-tested in middle-aged and older Spanish-speaking Mexican American patients with schizophrenia or schizoaffective disorder. This intervention, called *Programa de Entrenamiento para el Desarrollo de Aptitudes para Latinos* (PEDAL), was compared with a time-equivalent friendly support group in a randomized controlled pilot study (Patterson et al. 2005). The PEDAL group demonstrated a significant improvement in everyday living skills that was maintained at 12-month follow-up.

Helping Older People Experience Success (HOPES), a 12-month program combining social skills training and a nurse-administered preventive health care program, was associated with improved community living skills and functioning, greater self-efficacy, and lower levels of negative symptoms in adults older than 50 years with serious mental illness, including schizophrenia. Improvement in their community living skills was maintained at 3-year follow-up (Bartels et al. 2014; Mueser et al. 2010).

Following an examination of employment outcomes among middle-aged and older adults with schizophrenia who each participated in one of three types of work rehabilitation programs, Twamley et al. (2005) reported that the highest rates of volunteer or paid work (81%) and competitive/paid work (69%) occurred for patients who were placed in a job chosen with a vocational counselor and who then received individualized on-site support. The less successful programs (achieving at best a 44% rate of volunteer or paid work) employed a train-then-place approach.

Psychosis of Alzheimer's Disease and Other Neurocognitive Disorders

Atypical antipsychotics have for the most part replaced conventional antipsychotics in treating psychosis, aggression, and agitation in patients with neurocognitive disorders because of their greater perceived tolerability, lower risk for acute EPS, and comparatively lower risk of TD. Most antipsychotics prescribed for older adults are for behavioral disturbances associated with neurocognitive disorders, despite their lacking this FDA-approved indication (Weiss et al. 2000).

Atypical antipsychotics seem to have modest short-term efficacy for treating psychosis of AD (Ballard et al. 2006; Sink et al. 2005); however, studies have not always found a significant advantage for atypical antipsychotics over placebo in treating psychotic symptoms (Kindermann et al. 2002; Schneider et al. 2006a). In the CATIE-AD trial—the largest ($N=421$) non-industry-sponsored trial of atypical antipsychotics for psychosis or agitation/aggression in people with dementia—olanzapine, quetiapine, and risperidone were no better than placebo for the primary outcome (time to discontinuation for any reason) (Schneider et al. 2006b). Time to discontinuation due to lack of efficacy favored olanzapine and risperidone, whereas time to discontinuation due to adverse events favored placebo. A meta-analysis of RCTs of atypical antipsychotics in dementia reported that the number needed to treat ranged from 5 to 14, depending on the outcome measure, criteria for improvement, and methodology used (Schneider et al. 2006a). The authors found that the overall average treatment effect was ~18%, which is remarkably similar to that reported in a meta-analysis of conventional antipsychotics in this population (Schneider et al. 1990). In a more recent review, Ballard and Corbett (2013) identified 18 RCTs of atypical antipsychotic treatment of agitation and aggression in AD over periods of 6–12 weeks. They identified five clinical trials reporting statistically significant but clinically modest improvement in aggression with risperidone at total dosages of ≤2 mg/day compared with placebo. The evidence to support the benefit of risperidone for nonaggressive symptoms was less consistent, and evidence to support the value of other atypical antipsychotics was limited and conflicting.

Only a few RCTs have compared atypical and conventional antipsychotics for the treatment of neurocognitive disorders: three trials compared risperidone with haloperidol (Chan et al. 2001; De Deyn et al. 1999; Suh et al. 2004), and one compared quetiapine with haloperidol (Tariot et al. 2006). One of these found superior efficacy for the atypical over the typical agent, and the others reported no significant differences between the two types. In all four studies, haloperidol was associated with more EPS. In addition, the use of atypical antipsychotics in elderly patients with dementia has been associated with both cerebrovascular adverse events (CVAEs) and death, leading to black box warnings by the FDA. Currently, risperidone, olanzapine, and aripiprazole carry these warnings for stroke risk in older patients with neurocognitive disorders. The data for quetiapine in this population are more limited than for risperidone, olanzapine, and aripiprazole. The attribution of risk of CVAEs to atypical antipsychotics is limited, however, in that these studies were not designed to determine a cause-and-effect relationship between atypical antipsychotics and CVAEs, and serious CVAEs were not operationally defined in the trials. Additionally, retrospective database reviews (Gill et al. 2005; Herrmann et al. 2004) did not find any difference in incidence of CVAEs for typical versus atypical antipsychotic use, although these studies were not originally designed to examine CVAE risk.

In May 2004, the FDA issued a black box warning that elderly patients with dementia treated with atypical antipsychotic drugs are at increased risk for death compared with those treated with placebo. A 2005 meta-analysis of 15 RCTs reported a mortality risk of 3.5% for patients treated with atypical antipsychotics compared with a risk of 2.5% for patients given placebo (OR 1.5; 95% CI 1.1–2.2) (Schneider et al. 2005). The causes of death were most commonly cardiac or infectious, the two most common causes of death in patients with dementia (Kammoun et al. 2000; Keene et al. 2001). The data on mortality risk associated with typical versus atypical antipsychotics have been mixed (Jeste et al. 2008).

Patients with Lewy body or parkinsonian dementia are especially sensitive to side effects such as EPS and anticholinergic effects; therefore, very low dosages and slow titration schedules should be used to avoid worsening of motor symptoms (Stoppe et al. 1999). Low-dosage clozapine has demonstrated efficacy in reducing the symptoms of psychosis, and the drug does not worsen and can even improve the parkinsonian tremor (Bonuccelli et al. 1997; Masand 2000; Parkinson Study Group 1999; Pollak et al. 2004). Several trials of olanzapine in patients with PD have found worsened motor function without demonstrable efficacy in treating psychosis (Chou et al. 2007; Miyasaki et al. 2006). Quetiapine does not appear to worsen motor functioning, but data regarding its efficacy for psychosis in PD are mixed (Chou et al. 2007; Yeung et al. 2000). The limited data (generally from small, open-label studies) on ziprasidone and aripiprazole do not clearly support their use in patients with movement disorders; however, no large RCTs have yet been published (Chou et al. 2007). One double-blind, placebo-controlled trial that addressed the treatment of psychosis in DLB ($N=120$) found that twice as many patients treated with rivastigmine (≤12 mg/day) (63%) versus those given placebo (30%) had at least 30% improvement in delusions and hallucinations without worsening of motor symptoms (McKeith et al. 2000).

Pimavanserin, a selective serotonin 5-HT$_{2A}$ receptor inverse agonist, was approved by the FDA in 2016 for the treatment of PD psychosis. The once-daily medication was shown to significantly improve psychotic symptoms as rated on the Scale for Assessment of Positive Symptoms Adapted for Parkinson's Disease over a 6-week trial and was well tolerated by participants, with no significant worsening of motor function (Cummings et al. 2014). Subjects were older than 40 years (average age 72–73 years), their PD had been diagnosed at least 1 year prior, and the psychotic symptoms had developed afterward and lasted for at least 1 month. Patients with dementia or delirium were excluded.

Nonuse of active treatment may be a reasonable option for some mild to moderate cases, but in many clinical scenarios, this would be an unacceptably risky alternative. Because of the concerns about the safety and effectiveness of antipsychotic medications discussed earlier and the lack of alternative FDA-approved pharmacotherapies for treating psychosis in patients with dementia, most current treatment guidelines recommend nonpharmacological treatments as a first-line approach to management of these symptoms unless more aggressive management is deemed necessary to preserve safety. Accordingly, several studies have tested promising nonpharmacological interventions, although when strict inclusion criteria are used, very few of these studies can be considered evidence-based because the results are often inconclusive (Ayalon et al. 2006; Livingston et al. 2005). Recent reviews have highlighted several promising psychosocial therapies (e.g., individualized daily social interactions and caregiver training) (Ballard and Corbett 2013).

Nonpharmacological Treatments

Functional capacity. The level of functional impairment varies considerably among older adults with schizophrenia. As mentioned earlier, in a study of a group of middle-aged and older outpatients with schizophrenia, Palmer et al. (2002a) found that 30% had been employed at least part-time since the onset of psychosis, 43% were current drivers, and 73% were living independently. In general, worse neuropsychological test performance, lower educational level, and presence of negative symptoms but not positive symptoms are associated with poorer functional capacity in older outpatients with schizophrenia (Evans et al. 2003). In older adults with schizophrenia, female participants had better neurocognition and less severe experiential deficits, and older age was associated with greater expressive deficits among males, but there were no sex differences in social skills (Muralidharan et al. 2018). Older adults with schizophrenia show modest worsening in their everyday functioning, and Reichenberg et al. (2014) found that these changes were predicted by worsening in functional capacity, a history of institutionalization, and worsening of negative symptoms. Czaja et al. (2017) showed that adults with schizophrenia (mean age 54 years) underperformed nonpsychiatric comparison subjects (mean age 65 years) in functional capacity and on computerized tests of automated teller machine use, telephone voice menu use, and computerized form completion. Global cognition has been shown to be a strong predictor of functional competence across the life span (19–79 years) in functional performance skills, including comprehension and planning of recreational activities, financial management, communication, and use of transportation (Kalache et al. 2015). Kumar et al. (2016) also demonstrated that neurocognitive performance was strongly associated with functional capacity in older patients (>50 years) with schizophrenia. Reducing anticholinergic burden may represent a target for intervention to improve functional capacity; Khan et al. (2021) found that anticholinergic burden, age, education, and cognition independently predicted functional capacity and that anticholinergic burden predicted cognition among those older than 55 years.

Limited interventions have been developed and empirically evaluated to improve functioning in older adults with serious mental illnesses (Bartels et al. 2018). Cognitive remediation shows some positive effects in improving aspects of cognition such as working memory; however, the benefits of this behavioral intervention technique appear more pronounced for patients with early- rather than late-stage chronic schizophrenia (Corbera et al. 2017). HOPES, a combined psychosocial skills training and preventive health care intervention for older adults (≥50 years) with serious mental illnesses, demonstrated improvements in functioning, symptoms, self-efficacy, preventive health care screening, and advance care planning following 12 months of weekly skills training classes, twice-monthly community practice trips, and monthly nurse preventive health care visits (Bartels et al. 2014). Given the high occurrence of physical comorbidity in older adults with severe mental illnesses, interventions designed to address both mental and physical health conditions simultaneously may be of greater benefit in improving everyday functioning (Bartels et al. 2018).

Physical exercise interventions.   Physical exercise has shown potential as a non-pharmacological complementary treatment option primarily for improving cognitive functioning, metabolic syndrome, negative symptoms, and lifestyle factors in patients with chronic severe mental illnesses. In a meta-analysis of exercise interventions, Firth et al. (2017) found that aerobic exercise improved global cognition, with a medium effect size for people with schizophrenia, and that interventions that involved greater amounts of exercise and supervision by fitness professionals were more effective. The proposed neural correlates of exercise training in patients with schizophrenia include maintenance of or increases in hippocampal volume; increased volume of the left superior, middle, and inferior anterior temporal gyri; thickening of cortices; and improved white matter tract integrity (van der Stouwe et al. 2018). The importance of professional supervision in helping participants with schizophrenia reap the benefits of physical exercise was also supported in a review by Vancampfort et al. (2016), which demonstrated that the qualification of the professional delivering the intervention moderated treatment dropout rates.

Older age predicted better physical activity–related outcomes in a systematic review of longitudinal studies (Hassan et al. 2019), suggesting that this age group may be more receptive to physical activity–related behavior modifications. Improved cardiometabolic risk profiles including reduced weight, BMI, waist circumference, and blood glucose levels have been observed following interventions addressing physical health aspects such as dietary modification, physical activity, or exercise and psychoeducation (Gurusamy et al. 2018). A review by Dauwan et al. (2016) found beneficial effects of exercise on improving total symptom severity (positive and negative), quality of life, global functioning, and depressive symptoms. The positive effects of exercise on positive and negative symptoms were confirmed in a subsequent review by Sabe et al. (2020) and driven by aerobic exercise specifically.

Technology for the mental health care of older adults with serious mental illnesses.   Between 2015 and 2020, a notable increase was seen in the use of artificial intelligence (AI) and digital technologies for the mental health care of patients aging with mental illnesses (Depp et al. 2019; Graham et al. 2019). AI in psychiatry refers to the use of computers and algorithms to identify patterns in data for the diagnosis, prevention, and treatment of mental illnesses. Such intelligent systems are increasingly being used to support clinical decision-making (Topol 2019). Data streams used for AI predictions include sociodemographics, clinical and psychometric assessments, neuroimaging and neurophysiology, electronic health records and claims, genomics and other omics, and those derived from digital technologies such as smartphones, wearable devices, video, and ambient sensors (Depp et al. 2019; Graham et al. 2019; Granholm et al. 2020). Digital tools and mobile and wireless technologies for health care offer opportunities to serve large numbers of adults despite the shortage of mental health practitioners, to remotely monitor symptoms and comorbid health conditions, to remotely deliver treatment/interventions, and to aid older adults with cognitive and physical tasks such as those required for activities of daily living (Fortuna et al. 2019). Fortuna et al. (2019) outlined important considerations for making digital mental health care accessible for older adults, including different rates of technology adoption, appropriate design principles, and the unique preferences and concerns of older adults. Few AI or digital technology studies in the literature focus on older adults with psychoses, and most are still in the early proof-of-concept stage.

Motion technologies have demonstrated a potential for revealing objective patterns of everyday behavior in older adults with serious mental illnesses. These technologies include wearable sensors such as Fitbits, smartphones with global positioning systems (GPS), passive-motion sensors (e.g., video, Wi-Fi, radio signals), or a blend of body-worn and passive sensors often found in smart home models (Collier et al. 2018). For example, motion tracking via wearable accelerometer devices has shown that individuals with schizophrenia engage in higher levels of sedentary behavior (~12.5 hours/day) than those without mental illness (Stubbs et al. 2016) and that the increased sedentary time is associated with increased cardiometabolic risk (Stubbs et al. 2017). Fitbits or similar wearables may also support behavioral weight loss among people with serious mental illnesses by encouraging wearers to take more steps per day (Naslund et al. 2016). Wearables and smartphones also enable tracking of sleep behaviors, such as duration of sleep, bed and wake times, and disruptions, which are increasingly emerging as important features in mental illnesses (Aledavood et al. 2019). Poor sleep quality in patients with psychiatric diagnoses is associated with increased risk of suicide (Malik et al. 2014), and sleep abnormalities may serve as an early sign of relapse and decompensation in patients with psychotic disorders (Kaskie et al. 2017).

In addition to physical activity and sleep behaviors, geolocation data provided by GPS trackers are increasingly being used in digital phenotyping to monitor daily behaviors such as independence, withdrawal, and social and recreational activities that may be indicative of imminent psychotic relapse (Fraccaro et al. 2019). Reduced GPS mobility has also been related to greater negative symptom severity in schizophrenia, particularly diminished motivation, and greater mobility is associated with more community functioning (Depp et al. 2019). In addition to being used for motion tracking, smartphones also serve as tools to regularly query individuals with serious mental illnesses about their social interactions and functioning via ecological momentary assessment (EMA) and can deliver interventions through mobile applications. Granholm et al. (2020) found excellent adherence to EMA among both control participants and those with schizophrenia, with both groups completing an average of 85% of surveys and only 3% of participants with schizophrenia excluded for poor adherence. Relative to control subjects, participants with schizophrenia reported less total productive activity, fewer social interactions, more nonproductive behaviors, and more time at home over a 1-week period. Also, using a smartphone, Fortuna et al. (2018) tested the feasibility of a peer-delivered and technology-supported self-management intervention called PeerTECH for 10 older adults with serious mental illnesses. They observed significant improvements in psychiatric self-management among older adults with a diagnosis of schizophrenia, schizoaffective disorder, bipolar disorder, or major depressive disorder and demonstrated that individuals in this age group were willing and able to use a smartphone application to manage their illness.

Chivilgina et al. (2020) reviewed mobile health, big data, and technology applications for schizophrenia spectrum disorders and discussed the potential of such tools to empower patients to initiate, participate in, and guide their own health care and manage their medical data. The authors also advised caution unique to the use of mobile health in serious mental illnesses because of potential limitations in patients' decision-making capacity, cognition, affect, and perceptions. A diverse community of experts from multiple disciplines (e.g., clinicians, engineers, patients) must communicate and collaborate to address such concerns as the adoption of AI and digital technologies continues to increase in the coming years. Psychiatrists will require training and should remain up to date in technological advances in these areas.

Conclusion

Chronic psychotic disorders of late life may include early-onset schizophrenia (onset before age 40), late-onset schizophrenia (onset between ages 40 and 60), VLOSLP (onset after age 60), delusional disorder, and psychosis related to AD or other neurocognitive disorders. Psychosocial treatments have an important place as adjunctive treatments for older adults with psychosis. Aging is associated with increased risk for antipsychotic-related adverse reactions. Older adults have a much higher risk of developing TD compared with younger patients, and atypical antipsychotics are associated with metabolic liabilities. There are also concerns about the long-term safety and effectiveness of atypical antipsychotics in older patients. No FDA-approved treatments are currently available for psychosis and agitation in neurocognitive disorders, and atypical antipsychotic use in this population has been associated with an increased risk of CVAEs and mortality. Use of pharmacological treatments for older adults with psychosis therefore requires careful consideration of the potential risks and benefits and shared decision-making with patients and their caregivers.

Key Points

- Schizophrenia may be classified by age at onset into early-onset schizophrenia (onset before age 40), late-onset schizophrenia (onset between ages 40 and 60), and very-late-onset schizophrenia-like psychosis (VLOSLP; onset after age 60).

- There is considerable heterogeneity in course and outcome with aging in patients with early-onset schizophrenia, although positive symptoms generally improve.

- Patients with late-onset schizophrenia are similar to those with early-onset schizophrenia with regard to risk factors, clinical presentation, family history of schizophrenia, and medication response. However, females are overrepresented among the late-onset patients. Also, late-onset schizophrenia is characterized by lower average severity of positive symptoms and a lower average antipsychotic dosage requirement.

- VLOSLP is a heterogeneous entity with varied etiology.

- Patients with psychosis of Alzheimer's disease tend to have paranoid delusions and visual or auditory hallucinations, a greater risk of agitation, faster cognitive decline, and a greater likelihood of being institutionalized than patients with Alzheimer's disease without psychosis.

- Patients with mild behavioral impairment display abnormal perceptions or delusional thoughts, low motivation, affect dysregulation, impulsivity, and social inappropriateness; they are also more likely to convert to dementia.

- Patients with Parkinson's disease psychosis tend to have presence hallucinations, which often progress to broader hallucinations and delusions. Pimavanserin is a recently approved pharmacotherapy for Parkinson's disease psychosis.

- Compared with younger patients, older adults have a much higher risk of developing tardive dyskinesia (TD). Although the atypical antipsychotics are associated with a significantly lower risk of TD than conventional agents, they have problematic metabolic liabilities.

- Valbenazine is a recently approved pharmacotherapy for TD, although its effects on older adults with schizophrenia have not been explicitly reported.

- Psychosocial treatments have an important place as an adjunctive treatment for older adults with schizophrenia. Cognitive remediation, psychosocial skills training, and physical activity interventions have been shown to improve functional and health outcomes in older adults with serious mental illnesses.

- There are concerns about the longer-term safety and effectiveness of the atypical antipsychotics in older patients with psychotic disorders. Additionally, atypical antipsychotic use in patients with dementia has been associated with an increased risk of cerebrovascular adverse events and mortality, leading the FDA to issue black box warnings for this population.

- Principles of pharmacotherapy for older adults with psychosis include careful consideration of indications, shared decision-making, and use of the lowest effective dosages for the shortest possible time periods.

- Technologically based assessments and interventions have great potential to better track behaviors and improve functioning and outcomes for older adults with schizophrenia. However, interdisciplinary teams are needed to build such tools and ensure ethical usage.

Suggested Readings

Auslander LA, Jeste DV: Sustained remission of schizophrenia among community-dwelling older outpatients. Am J Psychiatry 161:1490–1493, 2004

Chou KL, Borek LL, Friedman JH: The management of psychosis in movement disorder patients. Expert Opin Pharmacother 8:935–943, 2007

Granholm E, McQuaid JR, McClure FS, et al: A randomized, controlled trial of cognitive behavioral social skills training for middle-aged and older outpatients with chronic schizophrenia. Am J Psychiatry 162:520–529, 2005

Howard R, Rabins PV, Seeman MV, et al: Late-onset schizophrenia and very-late-onset schizophrenia-like psychosis: an international consensus. Am J Psychiatry 157:172–178, 2000

Jeste DV, Harris MJ, Krull A, et al: Clinical and neuropsychological characteristics of patients with late-onset schizophrenia. Am J Psychiatry 152:722–730, 1995

Jeste DV, Blazer D, Casey D, et al: ACNP white paper: update on the use of antipsychotic drugs in elderly persons with dementia. Neuropsychopharmacology 33:957–970, 2008

Kendler KS, Tsuang MT, Hays P: Age at onset in schizophrenia: a familial perspective. Arch Gen Psychiatry 44:881–890, 1987

Ropacki SA, Jeste DV: Epidemiology of and risk factors for psychosis of Alzheimer's disease: a review of 55 studies published from 1990 to 2003. Am J Psychiatry 162(11):2022–2030, 2005

Vahia I, Bankole AO, Reyes P, et al: Schizophrenia in later life. Aging Health 3:383–396, 2007

References

Aledavood T, Torous J, Triana Hoyos AM, et al: Smartphone-based tracking of sleep in depression, anxiety, and psychotic disorders. Curr Psychiatry Rep 21(7):49, 2019 31161412

Alexopoulos GS, Streim J, Carpenter D, Docherty JP: Using antipsychotic agents in older patients. J Clin Psychiatry 65(suppl 2):5–99, discussion 100–102, quiz 103–104, 2004

Allison DB, Mentore JL, Heo M, et al: Antipsychotic-induced weight gain: a comprehensive research synthesis. Am J Psychiatry 156(11):1686–1696, 1999 10553730

American Diabetes Association, American Psychiatric Association, American Association of Clinical Endocrinologists, North American Association for the Study of Obesity: Consensus development conference on antipsychotic drugs and obesity and diabetes. Obes Res 12(2):362–368, 2004 14981231

American Psychiatric Association: Diagnostic and Statistical Manual of Mental Disorders, 3rd Edition. Washington, DC, American Psychiatric Association, 1980

American Psychiatric Association: Diagnostic and Statistical Manual of Mental Disorders, 3rd Edition Revised. Washington, DC, American Psychiatric Association, 1987

American Psychiatric Association: Diagnostic and Statistical Manual of Mental Disorders, 4th Edition. Washington, DC, American Psychiatric Association, 1994

American Psychiatric Association: Diagnostic and Statistical Manual of Mental Disorders, 4th Edition, Text Revision. Washington, DC, American Psychiatric Association, 2000

American Psychiatric Association: Diagnostic and Statistical Manual of Mental Disorders, 5th Edition. Arlington, VA, American Psychiatric Association, 2013

Andreasen N: I don't believe in late onset schizophrenia, in Late-Onset Schizophrenia. Edited by Howard R, Rabins PV, Castle DJ. Philadelphia, PA, Wrightson Biomedical, 1999, pp 111–123

Auslander LA, Jeste DV: Sustained remission of schizophrenia among community-dwelling older outpatients. Am J Psychiatry 161(8):1490–1493, 2004 15285980

Ayalon L, Gum AM, Feliciano L, Areán PA: Effectiveness of nonpharmacological interventions for the management of neuropsychiatric symptoms in patients with dementia: a systematic review. Arch Intern Med 166(20):2182–2188, 2006 17101935

Ballard C, Corbett A: Agitation and aggression in people with Alzheimer's disease. Curr Opin Psychiatry 26(3):252–259, 2013 23528917

Ballard CG, Waite J, Birks J: The effectiveness of atypical antipsychotics for the treatment of aggression and psychosis in Alzheimer's disease. Cochrane Database Syst Rev (1):CD003476, 2006 16437455

Bartels SJ, Pratt SI, Mueser KT, et al: Long-term outcomes of a randomized trial of integrated skills training and preventive healthcare for older adults with serious mental illness. Am J Geriatr Psychiatry 22(11):1251–1261, 2014

Bartels SJ, DiMilia PR, Fortuna KL, Naslund JA: Integrated care for older adults with serious mental illness and medical comorbidity: evidence-based models and future research directions. Psychiatr Clin North Am 41(1):153–164, 2018 29412843

Baynes D, Mulholland C, Cooper SJ, et al: Depressive symptoms in stable chronic schizophrenia: prevalence and relationship to psychopathology and treatment. Schizophr Res 45(1–2):47–56, 2000 10978872

Belitsky R, McGlashan TH: The manifestations of schizophrenia in late life: a dearth of data. Schizophr Bull 19(4):683–685, 1993 8303218

Bleuler M: Die spatschizophrenen Krankheitsbilder. Fortschr Neurol Psychiatr 15:259–290, 1943

Bonuccelli U, Ceravolo R, Salvetti S, et al: Clozapine in Parkinson's disease tremor: effects of acute and chronic administration. Neurology 49(6):1587–1590, 1997 9409351

Brodaty H, Sachdev P, Rose N, et al: Schizophrenia with onset after age 50 years, I: phenomenology and risk factors. Br J Psychiatry 175(5):410–415, 1999 10789270

Burns A, Jacoby R, Levy R: Psychiatric phenomena in Alzheimer's disease, I: disorders of thought content. Br J Psychiatry 157(1):72–76, 92–94, 1990a 2397365

Burns A, Jacoby R, Levy R: Psychiatric phenomena in Alzheimer's disease, II: disorders of perception. Br J Psychiatry 157(1):76–81, 92–94, 1990b 2397366

Caligiuri MP, Lacro JP, Rockwell E, et al: Incidence and risk factors for severe tardive dyskinesia in older patients. Br J Psychiatry 171(2):148–153, 1997 9337951

Castle DJ, Murray RM: The epidemiology of late-onset schizophrenia. Schizophr Bull 19(4):691–700, 1993 8303220

Cervantes AN, Rabins PV, Slavney PR: Onset of schizophrenia at age 100. Psychosomatics 47(4):356–359, 2006 16844897

Chan WC, Lam LC, Choy CN, et al: A double-blind randomised comparison of risperidone and haloperidol in the treatment of behavioural and psychological symptoms in Chinese dementia patients. Int J Geriatr Psychiatry 16(12):1156–1162, 2001 11748775

Chen DC, Du XD, Yin GZ, et al: Impaired glucose tolerance in first-episode drug-naïve patients with schizophrenia: relationships with clinical phenotypes and cognitive deficits. Psychol Med 46(15):3219–3230, 2016 27604840

Chen L, Chen X, Liu W, et al: White matter microstructural abnormalities in patients with late-onset schizophrenia identified by a voxel-based diffusion tensor imaging. Psychiatry Res 212(3):201–207, 2013 23146248

Chen S, Broqueres-You D, Yang G, et al: Relationship between insulin resistance, dyslipidaemia and positive symptom in Chinese antipsychotic-naive first-episode patients with schizophrenia. Psychiatry Res 210(3):825–829, 2013 24113122

Chivilgina O, Wangmo T, Elger BS, et al: mHealth for schizophrenia spectrum disorders management: a systematic review. Int J Soc Psychiatry 66(7):642–665, 2020 32571123

Chou KL, Borek LL, Friedman JH: The management of psychosis in movement disorder patients. Expert Opin Pharmacother 8(7):935–943, 2007 17472539

Christenson R, Blazer D: Epidemiology of persecutory ideation in an elderly population in the community. Am J Psychiatry 141(9):1088–1091, 1984 6235752

Ciompi L: Catamnestic long-term study on the course of life and aging of schizophrenics. Schizophr Bull 6(4):606–618, 1980 7444392

Cohen CI: Outcome of schizophrenia into later life: an overview. Gerontologist 30(6):790–797, 1990 2286338

Cohen-Mansfield J: Nonpharmacologic interventions for inappropriate behaviors in dementia: a review, summary, and critique. Am J Geriatr Psychiatry 9(4):361–381, 2001 11739063

Collier S, Monette P, Hobbs K, et al: Mapping movement: applying motion measurement technologies to the psychiatric care of older adults. Curr Psychiatry Rep 20(8):64, 2018 30043234

Cooper AF, Curry AR: The pathology of deafness in the paranoid and affective psychoses of later life. J Psychosom Res 20(2):97–105, 1976 1271318

Copeland JRM, Dewey ME, Scott A, et al: Schizophrenia and delusional disorder in older age: community prevalence, incidence, comorbidity, and outcome. Schizophr Bull 24(1):153–161, 1998 9502553

Corbera S, Wexler BE, Poltorak A, et al: Cognitive remediation for adults with schizophrenia: does age matter? Psychiatry Res 247:21–27, 2017 27863314

Corey-Bloom J, Jernigan T, Archibald S, et al: Quantitative magnetic resonance imaging of the brain in late-life schizophrenia. Am J Psychiatry 152(3):447–449, 1995 7864275

Cummings J, Isaacson S, Mills R, et al: Pimavanserin for patients with Parkinson's disease psychosis: a randomised, placebo-controlled phase 3 trial. Lancet 383(9916):533–540, 2014 24183563

Czaja SJ, Loewenstein DA, Lee CC, et al: Assessing functional performance using computer-based simulations of everyday activities. Schizophr Res 183:130–136, 2017 27913159

Dauwan M, Begemann MJ, Heringa SM, Sommer IE: Exercise improves clinical symptoms, quality of life, global functioning, and depression in schizophrenia: a systematic review and meta-analysis. Schizophr Bull 42(3):588–599, 2016 26547223

Davidson M, Harvey PD, Powchik P, et al: Severity of symptoms in chronically institutionalized geriatric schizophrenic patients. Am J Psychiatry 152(2):197–207, 1995 7840352

De Deyn PP, Rabheru K, Rasmussen A, et al: A randomized trial of risperidone, placebo, and haloperidol for behavioral symptoms of dementia. Neurology 53(5):946–955, 1999 10496251

Depp CA, Bashem J, Moore RC, et al: GPS mobility as a digital biomarker of negative symptoms in schizophrenia: a case control study. NPJ Digit Med 2:108, 2019 31728415

Devanand DP, Jacobs DM, Tang MX, et al: The course of psychopathologic features in mild to moderate Alzheimer disease. Arch Gen Psychiatry 54(3):257–263, 1997 9075466

Dietlin S, Soto M, Kiyasova V, et al: Neuropsychiatric symptoms and risk of progression to Alzheimer's disease among mild cognitive impairment subjects. J Alzheimers Dis 70(1):25–34, 2019 31127783

Diwan S, Cohen CI, Bankole AO, et al: Depression in older adults with schizophrenia spectrum disorders: prevalence and associated factors. Am J Geriatr Psychiatry 15(12):991–998, 2007 18056817

Dolder CR, Jeste DV: Incidence of tardive dyskinesia with typical versus atypical antipsychotics in very high risk patients. Biol Psychiatry 53(12):1142–1145, 2003 12814866

Dubovsky SL, Frobose C, Phiri P, et al: Short-term safety and pharmacokinetic profile of asenapine in older patients with psychosis. Int J Geriatr Psychiatry 27(5):472–482, 2012 21755540

Essali A, Ali G: Antipsychotic drug treatment for elderly people with late-onset schizophrenia. Cochrane Database Syst Rev 2012(2):CD004162, 2012 22336800

Evans JD, Paulsen JS, Harris MJ, et al: A clinical and neuropsychological comparison of delusional disorder and schizophrenia. J Neuropsychiatry Clin Neurosci 8(3):281–286, 1996 8854299

Evans JD, Heaton RK, Paulsen JS, et al: The relationship of neuropsychological abilities to specific domains of functional capacity in older schizophrenia patients. Biol Psychiatry 53(5):422–430, 2003 12614995

Factor SA, Scullin MK, Sollinger AB, et al: Cognitive correlates of hallucinations and delusions in Parkinson's disease. J Neurol Sci 347(1–2):316–321, 2014 25466695

Feldman PD, Kaiser CJ, Kennedy JS, et al: Comparison of risperidone and olanzapine in the control of negative symptoms of chronic schizophrenia and related psychotic disorders in patients aged 50 to 65 years. J Clin Psychiatry 64(9):998–1004, 2003 14628974

Fénelon G, Soulas T, Cleret de Langavant L, et al: Feeling of presence in Parkinson's disease. J Neurol Neurosurg Psychiatry 82(11):1219–1224, 2011 21551471

Ffytche DH, Pereira JB, Ballard C, et al: Risk factors for early psychosis in PD: insights from the Parkinson's Progression Markers Initiative. J Neurol Neurosurg Psychiatry 88(4):325–331, 2017 28315846

Firth J, Stubbs B, Rosenbaum S, et al: Aerobic exercise improves cognitive functioning in people with schizophrenia: a systematic review and meta-analysis. Schizophr Bull 43(3):546–556, 2017 27521348

Forsell Y, Henderson AS: Epidemiology of paranoid symptoms in an elderly population. Br J Psychiatry 172(5):429–432, 1998 9747406

Fortuna KL, DiMilia PR, Lohman MC, et al: Feasibility, acceptability, and preliminary effectiveness of a peer-delivered and technology supported self-management intervention for older adults with serious mental illness. Psychiatr Q 89(2):293–305, 2018 28948424

Fortuna KL, Torous J, Depp CA, et al: A future research agenda for digital geriatric mental healthcare. Am J Geriatr Psychiatry 27(11):1277–1285, 2019

Fraccaro P, Beukenhorst A, Sperrin M, et al: Digital biomarkers from geolocation data in bipolar disorder and schizophrenia: a systematic review. J Am Med Inform Assoc 26(11):1412–1420, 2019 31260049

Galimberti D, Dell'Osso B, Altamura AC, Scarpini E: Psychiatric symptoms in frontotemporal dementia: epidemiology, phenotypes, and differential diagnosis. Biol Psychiatry 78(10):684–692, 2015 25958088

Gill SS, Rochon PA, Herrmann N, et al: Atypical antipsychotic drugs and risk of ischaemic stroke: population based retrospective cohort study. BMJ 330(7489):445, 2005 15668211

Goetz CG, Stebbins GT, Ouyang B: Visual plus nonvisual hallucinations in Parkinson's disease: development and evolution over 10 years. Mov Disord 26(12):2196–2200, 2011 21755536

Graham S, Depp C, Lee EE, et al: Artificial intelligence for mental health and mental illnesses: an overview. Curr Psychiatry Rep 21(11):116, 2019 31701320

Granholm E, McQuaid JR, McClure FS, et al: A randomized controlled pilot study of cognitive behavioral social skills training for older patients with schizophrenia (letter). Schizophr Res 53(1–2):167–169, 2002 11728848

Granholm E, McQuaid JR, McClure FS, et al: A randomized, controlled trial of cognitive behavioral social skills training for middle-aged and older outpatients with chronic schizophrenia. Am J Psychiatry 162(3):520–529, 2005 15741469

Granholm E, McQuaid JR, McClure FS, et al: Randomized controlled trial of cognitive behavioral social skills training for older people with schizophrenia: 12-month follow-up. J Clin Psychiatry 68(5):730–737, 2007 17503982

Granholm E, Holden JL, Mikhael T, et al: What do people with schizophrenia do all day? Ecological momentary assessment of real-world functioning in schizophrenia. Schizophr Bull 46(2):242–251, 2020 31504955

Gurusamy J, Gandhi S, Damodharan D, et al: Exercise, diet and educational interventions for metabolic syndrome in persons with schizophrenia: a systematic review. Asian J Psychiatr 36:73–85, 2018 29990631

Häfner H, an der Heiden W, Behrens S, et al: Causes and consequences of the gender difference in age at onset of schizophrenia. Schizophr Bull 24(1):99–113, 1998 9502549

Hall D, Finger EC: Psychotic symptoms in frontotemporal dementia. Curr Neurol Neurosci Rep 15(7):46, 2015 26008815

Hämmerlein A, Derendorf H, Lowenthal DT: Pharmacokinetic and pharmacodynamic changes in the elderly: clinical implications. Clin Pharmacokinet 35(1):49–64, 1998 9673834

Hannerz H, Borgå P, Borritz M: Life expectancies for individuals with psychiatric diagnoses. Public Health 115(5):328–337, 2001 11593442

Harding CM: Changes in schizophrenia across time, in Schizophrenia Into Later Life. Edited by Cohen C. Washington, DC, American Psychiatric Publishing, 2002, pp 19–42

Harding CM, Brooks GW, Ashikaga T, et al: Aging and social functioning in once-chronic schizophrenic patients 22–62 years after first admission: the Vermont story, in Schizophrenia and Aging: Schizophrenia, Paranoia, and Schizophreniform Disorders in Later Life. Edited by Miller NE, Cohen GD. New York, Guilford, 1987, pp 74–82

Harris MJ, Jeste DV: Late-onset schizophrenia: an overview. Schizophr Bull 14(1):39–55, 1988 3291094

Harvey PD, Silverman JM, Mohs RC, et al: Cognitive decline in late-life schizophrenia: a longitudinal study of geriatric chronically hospitalized patients. Biol Psychiatry 45(1):32–40, 1999 9894573

Hassan S, Ross J, Marston L, et al: Factors prospectively associated with physical activity and dietary related outcomes in people with severe mental illness: a systematic review of longitudinal studies. Psychiatry Res 273:181–191, 2019 30654303

Hauser RA, Factor SA, Marder SR, et al: KINECT 3: a phase 3 randomized, double-blind, placebo-controlled trial of valbenazine for tardive dyskinesia. Am J Psychiatry 174(5):476–484, 2017 28320223

Heaton RK, Gladsjo JA, Palmer BW, et al: Stability and course of neuropsychological deficits in schizophrenia. Arch Gen Psychiatry 58(1):24–32, 2001 11146755

Henderson AS, Korten AE, Levings C, et al: Psychotic symptoms in the elderly: a prospective study in a population sample. Int J Geriatr Psychiatry 13(7):484–492, 1998 9695039

Herrmann N, Mamdani M, Lanctôt KL: Atypical antipsychotics and risk of cerebrovascular accidents. Am J Psychiatry 161(6):1113–1115, 2004 15169702

Hiroeh U, Appleby L, Mortensen PB, Dunn G: Death by homicide, suicide, and other unnatural causes in people with mental illness: a population-based study. Lancet 358(9299):2110–2112, 2001 11784624

Hong S, Lee EE, Martin AS, et al: Abnormalities in chemokine levels in schizophrenia and their clinical correlates. Schizophr Res 181:63–69, 2017 27650194

Howanitz E, Pardo M, Smelson DA, et al: The efficacy and safety of clozapine versus chlorpromazine in geriatric schizophrenia. J Clin Psychiatry 60(1):41–44, 1999 10074877

Howard R, Castle D, Wessely S, Murray R: A comparative study of 470 cases of early onset and late-onset schizophrenia. Br J Psychiatry 163(3):352–357, 1993 8401965

Howard R, Almeida O, Levy R: Phenomenology, demography and diagnosis in late paraphrenia. Psychol Med 24(2):397–410, 1994 8084935

Howard R, Graham C, Sham P, et al: A controlled family study of late-onset non-affective psychosis (late paraphrenia). Br J Psychiatry 170(6):511–514, 1997 9330015

Howard R, Rabins PV, Seeman MV, et al: Late-onset schizophrenia and very-late-onset schizophrenia-like psychosis: an international consensus. Am J Psychiatry 157(2):172–178, 2000 10671383

Howard R, Cort E, Bradley R, et al: Antipsychotic treatment of very late-onset schizophrenia-like psychosis (ATLAS): a randomised, controlled, double-blind trial. Lancet Psychiatry 5(7):553–563, 2018 29880238

Huber G: The heterogeneous course of schizophrenia. Schizophr Res 28(2–3):177–185, 1997 9468352

Huntington Study Group: Tetrabenazine as antichorea therapy in Huntington disease: a randomized controlled trial. Neurology 66(3):366–372, 2006 16476934

Ismail Z, Smith EE, Geda Y, et al: Neuropsychiatric symptoms as early manifestations of emergent dementia: provisional diagnostic criteria for mild behavioral impairment. Alzheimers Dement 12(2):195–202, 2016 26096665

Jeste DV, Finkel SI: Psychosis of Alzheimer's disease and related dementias: diagnostic criteria for a distinct syndrome. Am J Geriatr Psychiatry 8(1):29–34, 2000 10648292

Jeste DV, Wragg RE, Salmon DP, et al: Cognitive deficits of patients with Alzheimer's disease with and without delusions. Am J Psychiatry 149(2):184–189, 1992 1734737

Jeste DV, Harris MJ, Krull A, et al: Clinical and neuropsychological characteristics of patients with late-onset schizophrenia. Am J Psychiatry 152(5):722–730, 1995 7726312

Jeste DV, Symonds LL, Harris MJ, et al: Nondementia nonpraecox dementia praecox? Late-onset schizophrenia. Am J Geriatr Psychiatry 5(4):302–317, 1997 9363287

Jeste DV, Lacro JP, Bailey A, et al: Lower incidence of tardive dyskinesia with risperidone compared with haloperidol in older patients. J Am Geriatr Soc 47(6):716–719, 1999a 10366172

Jeste DV, Rockwell E, Harris MJ, et al: Conventional vs. newer antipsychotics in elderly patients. Am J Geriatr Psychiatry 7(1):70–76, 1999b 9919323

Jeste DV, Barak Y, Madhusoodanan S, et al: International multisite double-blind trial of the atypical antipsychotics risperidone and olanzapine in 175 elderly patients with chronic schizophrenia. Am J Geriatr Psychiatry 11(6):638–647, 2003 14609804

Jeste DV, Blazer DG, First M: Aging-related diagnostic variations: need for diagnostic criteria appropriate for elderly psychiatric patients. Biol Psychiatry 58(4):265–271, 2005 16102544

Jeste DV, Meeks TW, Kim DS, Zubenko GS: Research agenda for DSM-V: diagnostic categories and criteria for neuropsychiatric syndromes in dementia. J Geriatr Psychiatry Neurol 19(3):160–171, 2006 16880358

Jeste DV, Blazer D, Casey D, et al: ACNP white paper: update on use of antipsychotic drugs in elderly persons with dementia. Neuropsychopharmacology 33(5):957–970, 2008 17637610

Jin H, Meyer JM, Jeste DV: Phenomenology of and risk factors for new-onset diabetes mellitus and diabetic ketoacidosis associated with atypical antipsychotics: an analysis of 45 published cases. Ann Clin Psychiatry 14(1):59–64, 2002 12046641

Jin H, Meyer JM, Jeste DV: Atypical antipsychotics and glucose dysregulation: a systematic review. Schizophr Res 71(2–3):195–212, 2004 15474892

Jin H, Shih PA, Golshan S, et al: Comparison of longer-term safety and effectiveness of 4 atypical antipsychotics in patients over age 40: a trial using equipoise-stratified randomization. J Clin Psychiatry 74(1):10–18, 2013 23218100

Jones DK, Catani M, Pierpaoli C, et al: A diffusion tensor magnetic resonance imaging study of frontal cortex connections in very-late-onset schizophrenia-like psychosis. Am J Geriatr Psychiatry 13(12):1092–1099, 2005 16319302

Jones PB, Barnes TRE, Davies L, et al: Randomized controlled trial of the effect on quality of life of second- vs first-generation antipsychotic drugs in schizophrenia: Cost Utility of the Latest Antipsychotic Drugs in Schizophrenia Study (CUtLASS 1). Arch Gen Psychiatry 63(10):1079–1087, 2006 17015810

Joseph J, Depp C, Martin AS, et al: Associations of high sensitivity C-reactive protein levels in schizophrenia and comparison groups. Schizophr Res 168(1–2):456–460, 2015 26341579

Joukamaa M, Heliövaara M, Knekt P, et al: Mental disorders and cause-specific mortality. Br J Psychiatry 179(6):498–502, 2001 11731351

Kalache SM, Mulsant BH, Davies SJ, et al: The impact of aging, cognition, and symptoms on functional competence in individuals with schizophrenia across the lifespan. Schizophr Bull 41(2):374–381, 2015 25103208

Kammoun S, Gold G, Bouras C, et al: Immediate causes of death of demented and non-demented elderly. Acta Neurol Scand Suppl 176:96–99, 2000 11261812

Kane JM, Woerner MG, Pollack S, et al: Does clozapine cause tardive dyskinesia? J Clin Psychiatry 54(9):327–330, 1993 8104929

Kaskie RE, Graziano B, Ferrarelli F: Schizophrenia and sleep disorders: links, risks, and management challenges. Nat Sci Sleep 9:227–239, 2017 29033618

Keene J, Hope T, Fairburn CG, Jacoby R: Death and dementia. Int J Geriatr Psychiatry 16(10):969–974, 2001 11607941

Keith SJ, Regier DA, Rae DS: Schizophrenic disorders, in Psychiatric Disorders in America: The Epidemiologic Catchment Area Study. New York, Oxford, 1991, pp 33–52

Kendler KS, Davis KL: The genetics and biochemistry of paranoid schizophrenia and other paranoid psychoses. Schizophr Bull 7(4):689–709, 1981 7034192

Kennedy JS, Jeste D, Kaiser CJ, et al: Olanzapine vs haloperidol in geriatric schizophrenia: analysis of data from a double-blind controlled trial. Int J Geriatr Psychiatry 18(11):1013–1020, 2003 14618553

Khan AY, Redden W, Ovais M, Grossberg GT: Current concepts in the diagnosis and treatment of schizophrenia in later life. Curr Geriatr Rep 4(4):290–300, 2015

Khan WU, Ghazala Z, Brooks HJ, et al: The impact of anticholinergic burden on functional capacity in persons with schizophrenia across the adult life span. Schizophr Bull 47(1):249–257, 2021 32619225

Kindermann SS, Dolder CR, Bailey A, et al: Pharmacological treatment of psychosis and agitation in elderly patients with dementia: four decades of experience. Drugs Aging 19(4):257–276, 2002 12038878

Kinon BJ, Jeste DV, Kollack-Walker S, et al: Olanzapine treatment for tardive dyskinesia in schizophrenia patients: a prospective clinical trial with patients randomized to blinded dose reduction periods. Prog Neuropsychopharmacol Biol Psychiatry 28(6):985–996, 2004 15380859

Kirkpatrick B, Messias E, Harvey PD, et al: Is schizophrenia a syndrome of accelerated aging? Schizophr Bull 34(6):1024–1032, 2008 18156637

Kraepelin E: Dementia praecox and paraphrenia. J Nerv Ment Dis 54(4):384, 1921

Kulkarni J, de Castella A, Smith D, et al: A clinical trial of the effects of estrogen in acutely psychotic women. Schizophr Res 20(3):247–252, 1996 8827850

Kulkarni J, Riedel A, de Castella AR, et al: Estrogen: a potential treatment for schizophrenia. Schizophr Res 48(1):137–144, 2001 11278160

Kumar M, Babaei P, Ji B, Nielsen J: Human gut microbiota and healthy aging: recent developments and future prospective. Nutr Healthy Aging 4(1):3–16, 2016 28035338

Laursen TM, Nordentoft M, Mortensen PB: Excess early mortality in schizophrenia. Annu Rev Clin Psychol 10:425–448, 2014 24313570

Le Ber I, Camuzat A, Hannequin D, et al: Phenotype variability in progranulin mutation carriers: a clinical, neuropsychological, imaging and genetic study. Brain 131(pt 3):732–746, 2008 18245784

Lee EE, Eyler LT, Wolkowitz OM, et al: Elevated plasma F2-isoprostane levels in schizophrenia. Schizophr Res 176(2–3):320–326, 2016 27318521

Lee EE, Hong S, Martin AS, et al: Inflammation in schizophrenia: cytokine levels and their relationships to demographic and clinical variables. Am J Geriatr Psychiatry 25(1):50–61, 2017 27840055

Lee EE, Liu J, Tu X, et al: A widening longevity gap between people with schizophrenia and general population: a literature review and call for action. Schizophr Res 196:9–13, 2018 28964652

Lehman AF, Lieberman JA, Dixon LB, et al: Practice guideline for the treatment of patients with schizophrenia. Am J Psychiatry 161(2 suppl):i–iv, 1–56, 2004

Lieberman JA, Saltz BL, Johns CA, et al: The effects of clozapine on tardive dyskinesia. Br J Psychiatry 158(4):503–510, 1991 1675900

Lieberman JA, Stroup TS, McEvoy JP, et al: Effectiveness of antipsychotic drugs in patients with chronic schizophrenia. N Engl J Med 353(12):1209–1223, 2005 16172203

Lindamer LA, Buse DC, Lohr JB, Jeste DV: Hormone replacement therapy in postmenopausal women with schizophrenia: positive effect on negative symptoms? Biol Psychiatry 49(1):47–51, 2001 11163779

Lippa CF, Boeve BF, Parisi JE, Keegan BM: A 75-year-old man with cognitive impairment and gait changes. Neurology 69(11):1183–1189, 2007 17846418

Littrell KH, Johnson CG, Littrell S, Peabody CD: Marked reduction of tardive dyskinesia with olanzapine. Arch Gen Psychiatry 55(3):279–280, 1998 9510225

Livingston G, Johnston K, Katona C, et al: Systematic review of psychological approaches to the management of neuropsychiatric symptoms of dementia. Am J Psychiatry 162(11):1996–2021, 2005 16263837

Lohr JB, Alder M, Flynn K, et al: Minor physical anomalies in older patients with late-onset schizophrenia, early onset schizophrenia, depression, and Alzheimer's disease. Am J Geriatr Psychiatry 5(4):318–323, 1997 9363288

Maher B: Delusional thinking and cognitive disorder. Integr Physiol Behav Sci 40(3):136–146, 2005 17477206

Malik S, Kanwar A, Sim LA, et al: The association between sleep disturbances and suicidal behaviors in patients with psychiatric diagnoses: a systematic review and meta-analysis. Syst Rev 3:18, 2014 24568642

Masand PS: Atypical antipsychotics for elderly patients with neurodegenerative disorders and medical conditions. Psychiatr Ann 30(3):202–208, 2000

Matsuda Y, Kishi T, Shibayama H, Iwata N: Yokukansan in the treatment of behavioral and psychological symptoms of dementia: a systematic review and meta-analysis of randomized controlled trials. Hum Psychopharmacol 28(1):80–86, 2013 23359469

Mazeh D, Zemishlani C, Aizenberg D, Barak Y: Patients with very-late-onset schizophrenia-like psychosis: a follow-up study. Am J Geriatr Psychiatry 13(5):417–419, 2005 15879591

McKeith I, Del Ser T, Spano P, et al: Efficacy of rivastigmine in dementia with Lewy bodies: a randomised, double-blind, placebo-controlled international study. Lancet 356(9247):2031–2036, 2000 11145488

McQuaid JR, Granholm E, McClure FS, et al: Development of an integrated cognitive-behavioral and social skills training intervention for older patients with schizophrenia. J Psychother Pract Res 9(3):149–156, 2000 10896740

Meeks TW, Jeste DV: Medication-induced movement disorders, in Psychiatry. Hoboken, NJ, John Wiley and Sons, 2008, pp 1773–1793

Mitter P, Reeves S, Romero-Rubiales F, et al: Migrant status, age, gender and social isolation in very late-onset schizophrenia-like psychosis. Int J Geriatr Psychiatry 20(11):1046–1051, 2005 16250076

Miyaoka T, Wake R, Furuya M, et al: Yokukansan (TJ-54) for treatment of very-late-onset schizophrenia-like psychosis: an open-label study. Phytomedicine 20(7):654–658, 2013 23453830

Miyasaki JM, Shannon K, Voon V, et al: Practice parameter: evaluation and treatment of depression, psychosis, and dementia in Parkinson disease (an evidence-based review): report of the Quality Standards Subcommittee of the American Academy of Neurology. Neurology 66(7):996–1002, 2006 16606910

Montross LP, Depp C, Daly J, et al: Correlates of self-rated successful aging among community-dwelling older adults. Am J Geriatr Psychiatry 14(1):43–51, 2006

Moore NC: Is paranoid illness associated with sensory defects in the elderly? J Psychosom Res 25(2):69–74, 1981 7277274

Moore R, Blackwood N, Corcoran R, et al: Misunderstanding the intentions of others: an exploratory study of the cognitive etiology of persecutory delusions in very late-onset schizophrenia-like psychosis. Am J Geriatr Psychiatry 14(5):410–418, 2006 16670245

Mueser KT, Pratt SI, Bartels SJ, et al: Randomized trial of social rehabilitation and integrated health care for older people with severe mental illness. J Consult Clin Psychol 78(4):561–573, 2010 20658812

Mukaetova-Ladinska E, Harrington C, Xuereb J, et al: Biochemical, neuropathological, and clinical correlations of neurofibrillary degeneration in Alzheimer's disease, in Treating Alzheimer's and Other Dementias: Clinical Application of Recent Research Advances. New York, Springer, 1995, pp 57–80

Muralidharan A, Finch A, Bowie CR, Harvey PD: Thought, language, and communication deficits and association with everyday functional outcomes among community-dwelling middle-aged and older adults with schizophrenia. Schizophr Res 196:29–34, 2018 28778553

Naimark D, Jackson E, Rockwell E, Jeste DV: Psychotic symptoms in Parkinson's disease patients with dementia. J Am Geriatr Soc 44(3):296–299, 1996 8600200

Naslund JA, Aschbrenner KA, Scherer EA, et al: Wearable devices and mobile technologies for supporting behavioral weight loss among people with serious mental illness. Psychiatry Res 244:139–144, 2016 27479104

Nguyen TT, Eyler LT, Jeste DV: Systemic biomarkers of accelerated aging in schizophrenia: a critical review and future directions. Schizophr Bull 44(2):398–408, 2018 29462455

O'Brien CF, Jimenez R, Hauser RA, et al: NBI-98854, a selective monoamine transport inhibitor for the treatment of tardive dyskinesia: a randomized, double-blind, placebo-controlled study. Mov Disord 30(12):1681–1687, 2015 26346941

Östling S, Skoog I: Psychotic symptoms and paranoid ideation in a nondemented population-based sample of the very old. Arch Gen Psychiatry 59(1):53–59, 2002 11779282

Palmer BW, McClure FS, Jeste DV: Schizophrenia in late life: findings challenge traditional concepts. Harv Rev Psychiatry 9(2):51–58, 2001 11266402

Palmer BW, Heaton RK, Gladsjo JA, et al: Heterogeneity in functional status among older outpatients with schizophrenia: employment history, living situation, and driving. Schizophr Res 55(3):205–215, 2002a 12048144

Palmer BW, Nayak GV, Jeste D: A comparison of early- and late-onset schizophrenia, in Schizophrenia Into Later Life: Treatment, Research, and Policy. Washington, DC, American Psychiatric Publishing, 2002b, pp 43–55

Palmer BW, Bondi MW, Twamley EW, et al: Are late-onset schizophrenia spectrum disorders neurodegenerative conditions? Annual rates of change on two dementia measures. J Neuropsychiatry Clin Neurosci 15(1):45–52, 2003 12556570

Parkinson Study Group: Low-dose clozapine for the treatment of drug-induced psychosis in Parkinson's disease. N Engl J Med 340(10):757–763, 1999 10072410

Patterson TL, Bucardo J, McKibbin CL, et al: Development and pilot testing of a new psychosocial intervention for older Latinos with chronic psychosis. Schizophr Bull 31(4):922–930, 2005 16037481

Patterson TL, Mausbach BT, McKibbin C, et al: Functional adaptation skills training (FAST): a randomized trial of a psychosocial intervention for middle-aged and older patients with chronic psychotic disorders. Schizophr Res 86(1–3):291–299, 2006 16814526

Paulsen JS, Salmon DP, Thal LJ, et al: Incidence of and risk factors for hallucinations and delusions in patients with probable AD. Neurology 54(10):1965–1971, 2000 10822438

Pollak P, Tison F, Rascol O, et al: Clozapine in drug induced psychosis in Parkinson's disease: a randomised, placebo controlled study with open follow up. J Neurol Neurosurg Psychiatry 75(5):689–695, 2004 15090561

Prager S, Jeste DV: Sensory impairment in late-life schizophrenia. Schizophr Bull 19(4):755–772, 1993 8303225

Putnam KM, Harvey PD: Cognitive impairment and enduring negative symptoms: a comparative study of geriatric and nongeriatric schizophrenia patients. Schizophr Bull 26(4):867–878, 2000 11087019

Raghuram R, Keshavan MD, Channabasavanna SM: Musical hallucinations in a deaf middle-aged patient. J Clin Psychiatry 41(10):357, 1980 7430079

Ram R, Bromet EJ, Eaton WW, et al: The natural course of schizophrenia: a review of first-admission studies. Schizophr Bull 18(2):185–207, 1992 1621068

Reichenberg A, Feo C, Prestia D, et al: The course and correlates of everyday functioning in schizophrenia. Schizophr Res Cogn 1(1):e47–e52, 2014 25045625

Riedel M, Eich FX, Möller HJ: A pilot study of the safety and efficacy of amisulpride and risperidone in elderly psychotic patients. Eur Psychiatry 24(3):149–153, 2009 19070995

Rivkin P, Kraut M, Barta P, et al: White matter hyperintensity volume in late-onset and early onset schizophrenia. Int J Geriatr Psychiatry 15(12):1085–1089, 2000 11180463

Rockwell E, Krull AJ, Dimsdale J, Jeste DV: Late-onset psychosis with somatic delusions. Psychosomatics 35(1):66–72, 1994 8134531

Ropacki SA, Jeste DV: Epidemiology of and risk factors for psychosis of Alzheimer's disease: a review of 55 studies published from 1990 to 2003. Am J Psychiatry 162(11):2022–2030, 2005 16263838

Roth M: The natural history of mental disorder in old age. J Ment Sci 101(423):281–301, 1955 13243044

Sabe M, Kaiser S, Sentissi O: Physical exercise for negative symptoms of schizophrenia: systematic review of randomized controlled trials and meta-analysis. Gen Hosp Psychiatry 62:13–20, 2020 31751931

Sachdev P, Brodaty H, Rose N, Cathcart S: Schizophrenia with onset after age 50 years, 2: neurological, neuropsychological and MRI investigation. Br J Psychiatry 175(5):416–421, 1999 10789271

Schneider LS: Pharmacologic management of psychosis in dementia. J Clin Psychiatry 60(suppl 8):54–60, 1999 10335671

Schneider LS, Pollock VE, Lyness SA: A metaanalysis of controlled trials of neuroleptic treatment in dementia. J Am Geriatr Soc 38(5):553–563, 1990 1970586

Schneider LS, Dagerman KS, Insel P: Risk of death with atypical antipsychotic drug treatment for dementia: meta-analysis of randomized placebo-controlled trials. JAMA 294(15):1934–1943, 2005 16234500

Schneider LS, Dagerman K, Insel PS: Efficacy and adverse effects of atypical antipsychotics for dementia: meta-analysis of randomized, placebo-controlled trials. Am J Geriatr Psychiatry 14(3):191–210, 2006a 16505124

Schneider LS, Tariot PN, Dagerman KS, et al: Effectiveness of atypical antipsychotic drugs in patients with Alzheimer's disease. N Engl J Med 355(15):1525–1538, 2006b 17035647

Seeman MV: The role of estrogen in schizophrenia. J Psychiatry Neurosci 21(2):123–127, 1996 8820178

Shinagawa S, Nakajima S, Plitman E, et al: Psychosis in frontotemporal dementia. J Alzheimers Dis 42(2):485–499, 2014 24898651

Simpson GM, Lee JH, Shrivastava RK: Clozapine in tardive dyskinesia. Psychopharmacology (Berl) 56(1):75–80, 1978 415329

Sink KM, Holden KF, Yaffe K: Pharmacological treatment of neuropsychiatric symptoms of dementia: a review of the evidence. JAMA 293(5):596–608, 2005 15687315

Small JG, Milstein V, Marhenke JD, et al: Treatment outcome with clozapine in tardive dyskinesia, neuroleptic sensitivity, and treatment-resistant psychosis. J Clin Psychiatry 48(7):263–267, 1987 2885310

Snowden JS, Rollinson S, Thompson JC, et al: Distinct clinical and pathological characteristics of frontotemporal dementia associated with C9ORF72 mutations. Brain 135(pt 3):693–708, 2012 22300873

Srikanth S, Nagaraja AV, Ratnavalli E: Neuropsychiatric symptoms in dementia-frequency, relationship to dementia severity and comparison in Alzheimer's disease, vascular dementia and frontotemporal dementia. J Neurol Sci 236(1–2):43–48, 2005 15964021

Steiner J, Berger M, Guest PC, et al: Assessment of insulin resistance among drug-naive patients with first-episode schizophrenia in the context of hormonal stress axis activation. JAMA Psychiatry 74(9):968–970, 2017 28724123

Steiner J, Fernandes BS, Guest PC, et al: Glucose homeostasis in major depression and schizophrenia: a comparison among drug-naive first-episode patients. Eur Arch Psychiatry Clin Neurosci 269(4):373–377, 2019 29352386

Stern Y, Albert M, Brandt J, et al: Utility of extrapyramidal signs and psychosis as predictors of cognitive and functional decline, nursing home admission, and death in Alzheimer's disease: prospective analyses from the Predictors Study. Neurology 44(12):2300–2307, 1994 7991116

Stoppe G, Brandt CA, Staedt JH: Behavioural problems associated with dementia: the role of newer antipsychotics. Drugs Aging 14(1):41–54, 1999 10069407

Street JS, Tollefson GD, Tohen M, et al: Olanzapine for psychotic conditions in the elderly. Psychiatr Ann 30(3):191–196, 2000

Stubbs B, Williams J, Gaughran F, Craig T: How sedentary are people with psychosis? A systematic review and meta-analysis. Schizophr Res 171(1–3):103–109, 2016 26805414

Stubbs B, Chen L-J, Chung M-S, Ku P-W: Physical activity ameliorates the association between sedentary behavior and cardiometabolic risk among inpatients with schizophrenia: a comparison versus controls using accelerometry. Compr Psychiatry 74:144–150, 2017 28167327

Suh G-H, Son HG, Ju Y-S, et al: A randomized, double-blind, crossover comparison of risperidone and haloperidol in Korean dementia patients with behavioral disturbances. Am J Geriatr Psychiatry 12(5):509–516, 2004 15353389

Sultzer DL: Neuroimaging and the origin of psychiatric symptoms in dementia. Int Psychogeriatr 8(suppl 3):239–243, discussion 269–272, 1996 9154570

Suzuki T, Remington G, Uchida H, et al: Management of schizophrenia in late life with antipsychotic medications: a qualitative review. Drugs Aging 28(12):961–980, 2011 22117095

Taragano FE, Allegri RF, Heisecke SL, et al: Risk of conversion to dementia in a mild behavioral impairment group compared to a psychiatric group and to a mild cognitive impairment group. J Alzheimers Dis 62(1):227–238, 2018 29439333

Tariot PN, Schneider L, Katz IR, et al: Quetiapine treatment of psychosis associated with dementia: a double-blind, randomized, placebo-controlled clinical trial. Am J Geriatr Psychiatry 14(9):767–776, 2006 16905684

Topol EJ: High-performance medicine: the convergence of human and artificial intelligence. Nat Med 25(1):44–56, 2019 30617339

Twamley EW, Padin DS, Bayne KS, et al: Work rehabilitation for middle-aged and older people with schizophrenia: a comparison of three approaches. J Nerv Ment Dis 193(9):596–601, 2005 16131942

Tzimos A, Samokhvalov V, Kramer M, et al: Safety and tolerability of oral paliperidone extended-release tablets in elderly patients with schizophrenia: a double-blind, placebo-controlled study with six-month open-label extension. Am J Geriatr Psychiatry 16(1):31–43, 2008 18165460

Uc EY, McDermott MP, Marder KS, et al: Incidence of and risk factors for cognitive impairment in an early Parkinson disease clinical trial cohort. Neurology 73(18):1469–1477, 2009 19884574

Vahia I, Bankole AO, Reyes P, et al: Schizophrenia in later life. Aging Health 3(3):383–396, 2007

Vahia IV, Palmer BW, Depp C, et al: Is late-onset schizophrenia a subtype of schizophrenia? Acta Psychiatr Scand 122(5):414–426, 2010 20199491

Vancampfort D, Rosenbaum S, Schuch FB, et al: Prevalence and predictors of treatment dropout from physical activity interventions in schizophrenia: a meta-analysis. Gen Hosp Psychiatry 39:15–23, 2016 26719106

Van der Mussele S, Mariën P, Saerens J, et al: Psychosis associated behavioral and psychological signs and symptoms in mild cognitive impairment and Alzheimer's dementia. Aging Ment Health 19(9):818–828, 2015 25323000

van der Stouwe ECD, van Busschbach JT, de Vries B, et al: Neural correlates of exercise training in individuals with schizophrenia and in healthy individuals: a systematic review. Neuroimage Clin 19:287–301, 2018 30023171

Weiss E, Hummer M, Koller D, et al: Off-label use of antipsychotic drugs. J Clin Psychopharmacol 20(6):695–698, 2000 11106144

Wilkosz PA, Miyahara S, Lopez OL, et al: Prediction of psychosis onset in Alzheimer disease: the role of cognitive impairment, depressive symptoms, and further evidence for psychosis subtypes. Am J Geriatr Psychiatry 14(4):352–360, 2006 16582044

Wirshing DA, Spellberg BJ, Erhart SM, et al: Novel antipsychotics and new onset diabetes. Biol Psychiatry 44(8):778–783, 1998 9798083

Wium-Andersen MK, Ørsted DD, Nordestgaard BG: Elevated C-reactive protein associated with late- and very-late-onset schizophrenia in the general population: a prospective study. Schizophr Bull 40(5):1117–1127, 2014 23996346

Wolkowitz OM, Jeste DV, Martin AS, et al: Leukocyte telomere length: effects of schizophrenia, age, and gender. J Psychiatr Res 85:42–48, 2017 27835738

Wood RA, Hopkins SA, Moodley KK, Chan D: Fifty percent prevalence of extracampine hallucinations in Parkinson's disease patients. Front Neurol 6:263, 2015 26733937

Yassa R, Jeste DV: Gender differences in tardive dyskinesia: a critical review of the literature. Schizophr Bull 18(4):701–715, 1992 1359633

Yeung PP, Tariot PN, Schneider LS, et al: Quetiapine for elderly patients with psychotic disorders. Psychiatr Ann 30(3):197–201, 2000

Zhang XY, Chen DC, Tan YL, et al: Glucose disturbances in first-episode drug-naïve schizophrenia: relationship to psychopathology. Psychoneuroendocrinology 62:376–380, 2015 26385108

Zisook S, Montross L, Kasckow J, et al: Subsyndromal depressive symptoms in middle-aged and older persons with schizophrenia. Am J Geriatr Psychiatry 15(12):1005–1014, 2007 18056819

Zubenko GS, Moossy J, Martinez AJ, et al: Neuropathologic and neurochemical correlates of psychosis in primary dementia. Arch Neurol 48(6):619–624, 1991 1710105

CHAPTER 12

Anxiety, Obsessive-Compulsive, and Trauma-Related Disorders

Michelle L. Conroy, M.D.

Phelan E. Maruca-Sullivan, M.D.

Chadrick E. Lane, M.D.

Joan M. Cook, Ph.D.

Developments in clinical neuroscience have resulted in a rapid expansion in how brain disorders are understood. Included in this seemingly exponential growth in knowledge is a deepening insight into the biology and clinical phenotypes inherent to late-life neuropsychiatric syndromes. This chapter explores a subset of these syndromes: anxiety, obsessive-compulsive, and trauma-related disorders in older adults. Important to highlight in the beginning is a shift in how these three entities are now conceptualized, which is in part due to advances in basic and translational neuroscience. With the publication of DSM-5 (American Psychiatric Association 2013), trauma-related and obsessive-compulsive disorders were given their own respective sections, acknowledging that, although all three most assuredly contain some facet of anxious symptomatology, several key features warrant their being separated. Doing so allows for more valid diagnostic constructs, lessens heterogeneity in clinical research, and is more in line with neuronal network dysfunction corresponding to illness presentations. By characterizing the relevant epidemiology, biological underpinnings, clinical phenomenology, and evidence-based treatments, this chapter summarizes the current state of the field.

Epidemiology

Historically, two large, multicity epidemiological studies attempted to capture statistics as they pertained to mental health and substance use disorders: the Epidemiologic Catchment Area (ECA) study, conducted between 1980 and 1985 (Regier et al. 1988), and the National Comorbidity Survey (NCS), conducted between 1990 and 1992 (Kessler et al. 1994). Limitations exist for each of these studies in the modern era: the ECA used a diagnostic interview that was based on DSM-III (American Psychiatric Association 1980; Regier et al. 1988), and the NCS was based on DSM-III-R and omitted older adults (American Psychiatric Association 1987; Kessler et al. 1994). Between 2001 and 2003, the National Comorbidity Survey Replication (NCS-R) collected epidemiological data incorporating DSM-IV (American Psychiatric Association 1994; Kessler and Merikangas 2004) and included participants older than 60 years. The National Epidemiological Survey on Alcohol and Related Conditions (NESARC), one of the strongest psychiatric epidemiological studies to date, was divided into Wave 1 (2001–2002) and Wave 2 (2004–2005). These, as well as several other studies, provide data on the prevalence of neuropsychiatric disorders in the aging population.

The ECA study demonstrated a 1-month prevalence rate of 5.5% for individuals age 65 years and older meeting criteria for an anxiety disorder, which at that time included phobias, panic disorder, and OCD (Regier et al. 1990). This is lower than the 1-month prevalence rates in younger populations: 6.6% of those between the ages of 45 and 64 and 8.3% between the ages of 25 and 44 years met criteria for anxiety disorders (Regier et al. 1990). The NCS-R found lifetime prevalence rates in older adults (age ≥60 years) for panic disorder (2.0%), agoraphobia without panic (1.0%), specific phobia (7.5%), social phobia (6.6%), PTSD (2.5%), generalized anxiety disorder (GAD; 3.6%), and OCD (0.7%), as well as the "any anxiety disorder group" (15.3%) (Kessler et al. 2005). Each of these NCS-R lifetime prevalence rates was lower in older adults when compared with each younger cohort.

Wave 1 of the NESARC described the following weighted 12-month prevalence rates in those age 55 years and older: panic disorder (1.1%), social phobia (2.1%), specific phobia (5.3%), and GAD (1.2%) (Mackenzie et al. 2014). By Wave 2, a substantial majority of older adults were in remission from each of these diagnoses (Mackenzie et al. 2014). The Longitudinal Aging Study Amsterdam analyzed risk factors and their correlation to the experience of anxiety disorders, finding associations with the loss of a partner, recent stressful life events, chronic physical illness, functional limitations, and one's subjective sense of health (Beekman et al. 1998). Anxiety disorders were fairly frequent among older, community-dwelling adults living in The Netherlands, with an overall prevalence of 10.2% and individual disorder prevalence rates of 7.3% for GAD, 1.0% for panic disorder, 0.6% for OCD (0.6%), and 3.1% for phobias (Beekman et al. 1998).

Additional epidemiological data have described rates of specific syndromes in older adulthood. Using a sample from the 2007 Australian National Survey of Mental Health and Well-Being, Gonçalves et al. (2011) found a 12-month prevalence rate of 2.8% for GAD in community-dwelling adults ages 55–85 years. Significant predictors for anxiety included functional limitations, a family history of anxiety or depression, worries about having a serious illness, depression, and older age. A study of the prevalence of GAD in French residents age 65 and older demonstrated a lifetime prevalence of

11%, with nearly one-quarter of those reporting onset after age 50 (Zhang et al. 2015a). In the same cohort, agoraphobia had a 1-month prevalence of 10.4%, with roughly one-tenth of subjects reporting a first episode at age 65 or older (Ritchie et al. 2013).

Analysis of data from Wave 2 of the NESARC revealed that older adults had a lower 1-year prevalence of PTSD (2.6%) compared with middle-aged adults (5.2%) and young adults (4.3%) (Reynolds et al. 2016). The lifetime prevalence of PTSD and partial PTSD symptomatology was 4.5% and 5.5%, respectively, in those age 60 and older (Pietrzak et al. 2012). Disorders more typically associated with aging, including hoarding disorder, fear of falling (FOF), and anxiety in the presence of a neurocognitive disorder (NCD), present nuanced challenges for epidemiological description. Criteria for hoarding disorder were established with the release of DSM-5, which complicated attempts to describe prevalence rates preceding the establishment of an operationalized syndrome (Ayers et al. 2015). A similar caveat can be made for FOF and anxiety as they relate to major NCD. Considerable heterogeneity is likely in all of the syndromes when they are comorbid with major NCD, including whether the underlying etiology is neurodegenerative versus due to another cause and any premorbid personality dimensions. It is unclear the extent to which one can extrapolate public health information using criteria specific to idiopathic syndromes delineated in DSM-5.

Recognizing these concerns, a body of literature has attempted to describe the rates of these disorders. One group demonstrated a notable increase in the weighted point prevalence of hoarding behavior from 2.3% in the youngest demographic (age 34–44 years) to 6.2% in the oldest (age 55–94 years) (Samuels et al. 2008). In another study, 15% of nursing home residents and 25% of community-dwelling adult day program participants exhibited hoarding behaviors at least several times per week (Marx and Cohen-Mansfield 2003). Of 133 patients living with major NCD who were admitted to an inpatient geriatric psychiatry unit, 22.6% evidenced hoarding behavior; the authors further noted that those who engaged in hoarding also engaged in repetitive dysfunctional behaviors, hyperphagia, and stealing (Hwang et al. 1998).

The literature regarding FOF is mixed, with some reporting a prevalence of 41.5% in one cohort age 75 and older (Lavedán et al. 2018). A systematic review from 2008 suggested rates ranging from 3% to 85% (Scheffer et al. 2008). Such a wide range highlights concerns about study methodology and validity. A cross-sectional analysis from the Cardiovascular Health Study found rates of anxiety in mild and major NCD to be 10.3% and 25.4%, respectively (Lyketsos et al. 2002). In a large 2016 meta-analysis, the pooled prevalence of anxiety in those with possible or probable Alzheimer's disease was 39%, although there was a wide range across individual studies (Zhao et al. 2016).

Fear, Phobias, and Panic

Phobias and panic disorder are defined by discrete episodes of anxiety confined to specific situations, avoidance of those triggers, and autonomic arousal. In general, across epidemiological studies, older adults are less likely to have these illnesses than younger adults, but the presentation and evaluation of these conditions in older adults can differ in important ways (Beekman et al. 1998; Byers et al. 2010; Regier et al. 1990; Schoevers et al. 2003; Streiner et al. 2006; Trollor et al. 2007). Indeed, one recent study suggested that the drop in prevalence of these disorders as people enter their eighth decade may be as high as 40%–47% (Canuto et al. 2018). That said, late-onset anxiety disorders are not uncommon and may reflect the complexity of biological, psychological, and social factors at play in the aging process.

Anxiogenic factors, including loss of function, grief, or changes in social roles, may contribute to anxiety in older adults. For others, however, aging may bring the opportunity to build resilience, withstand crises, or gain new skills, such as improved emotional regulation. Biologically, the degeneration of certain brain regions, such as the prefrontal cortex, could impair one's ability to manage normal anxiety, while degeneration of others, such as the locus coeruleus, might even decrease one's ability to experience anxiety (Aström 1996; Flint 1994).

Specific Phobia

Specific phobias seem to present similarly regardless of age, with marked and usually immediate fear or anxiety when presented with a specific object or situation. This fear is out of proportion to the actual danger posed, leads to either avoidance of the trigger or endurance of it with intense fear and anxiety, is present for a minimum of 6 months, and causes significant distress and impairment in functioning (Box 12–1). Generally, specific phobias decrease with age, but this does not mean that these disorders are rare in those older than 65. A recent study found a 4.51% prevalence of social phobia in those age 65 and older as well as an association with features of major depressive disorder (MDD) and reduced quality of life (Chou 2009).

Specific phobias may be less obvious in older adults if the patient has avoided the trigger for years, resulting in reduced intensity of the fear over time. The overall prevalence of specific phobia in one recent study in subjects older than 65 was 2%, but this increased to 8.7% when subthreshold fears were included (Grenier et al. 2011). It may be prudent to consider specific phobia as a disorder that fluctuates with age and often manifests as chronic subthreshold fears. Therefore, although older patients might be less likely to meet full DSM-5 criteria, fears may still cause important impairments in function (Sigström et al. 2016).

Box 12–1.   DSM-5 Diagnostic Criteria for Specific Phobia

A. Marked fear or anxiety about a specific object or situation (e.g., flying, heights, animals, receiving an injection, seeing blood).

   Note: In children, the fear or anxiety may be expressed by crying, tantrums, freezing, or clinging.

B. The phobic object or situation almost always provokes immediate fear or anxiety.

C. The phobic object or situation is actively avoided or endured with intense fear or anxiety.

D. The fear or anxiety is out of proportion to the actual danger posed by the specific object or situation and to the sociocultural context.

E. The fear, anxiety, or avoidance is persistent, typically lasting for 6 months or more.

F. The fear, anxiety, or avoidance causes clinically significant distress or impairment in social, occupational, or other important areas of functioning.

G. The disturbance is not better explained by the symptoms of another mental disorder, including fear, anxiety, and avoidance of situations associated with panic-like symptoms or other incapacitating symptoms (as in agoraphobia); objects or situations related to obsessions (as in obsessive-compulsive disorder); reminders of traumatic events (as in posttraumatic stress disorder); separation from home or attachment figures (as in separation anxiety disorder); or social situations (as in social anxiety disorder).

Specify if:

Code based on the phobic stimulus:

300.29 (F40.218) Animal (e.g., spiders, insects, dogs).

300.29 (F40.228) Natural environment (e.g., heights, storms, water).

300.29 (F40.23x) Blood-injection-injury (e.g., needles, invasive medical procedures).

> **Coding note:** Select specific ICD-10-CM code as follows: **F40.230** fear of blood; **F40.231** fear of injections and transfusions; **F40.232** fear of other medical care; or **F40.233** fear of injury.

300.29 (F40.248) Situational (e.g., airplanes, elevators, enclosed places).

300.29 (F40.298) Other (e.g., situations that may lead to choking or vomiting; in children, e.g., loud sounds or costumed characters).

Coding note: When more than one phobic stimulus is present, code all ICD-10-CM codes that apply (e.g., for fear of snakes and flying, F40.218 specific phobia, animal, and F40.248 specific phobia, situational).

Source. Reprinted from American Psychiatric Association: *Diagnostic and Statistical Manual of Mental Disorders*, 5th Edition. Arlington, VA, American Psychiatric Association, 2013, pp. 197–198. Copyright © 2013 American Psychiatric Association. Used with permission.

Social Phobia (Social Anxiety Disorder)

As in specific phobia, social phobias produce intense fear and anxiety; however, these arise only in the context of social situations, such as engaging in conversation, being observed by others, or performing in front of others. Individuals with social anxiety fear being negatively evaluated, humiliated, or rejected (Box 12–2). Although the presentation in older adults is typically similar in nature to that experienced by younger people, the number and severity of symptoms appear to decrease with age (Cairney et al. 2007; Kessler et al. 2005; Miloyan et al. 2014). The aging process poses several biological, psychological, and social challenges that may contribute to anxiety in social settings. For example, age-related sensory deficits, cognitive impairment, physical limitations, or other medical conditions can impact social functioning. Additionally, socially relevant role changes are common in later life, such as those caused by retirement or the death of a partner, and might impact one's confidence in social situations, thus reigniting previously latent or not easily identifiable symptoms of social phobia.

In older adults, social phobia may be long-standing or may develop in later life, but the prevalence and severity of symptoms do appear to decrease over time (Kessler et al. 2005; Miloyan et al. 2014). Furthermore, the recent change in diagnostic criteria in DSM-5—specifically the change to Criterion E that now allows the clinician to judge unreasonableness of fear rather than requiring that the patient find the fear unreasonable—may allow for a more accurate and inclusive diagnosis, perhaps especially for older adults. A recent study investigating the outcome of this change in criteria shows that cases of social phobia diagnosed in adults age 75 years and older may nearly double when DSM-5 criteria are used (Karlsson et al. 2016). Unfortunately, social phobia has been well correlated with significant depressive symptoms and MDD in the older adult population (Chou 2009; Karlsson et al. 2016).

Box 12–2. DSM-5 Diagnostic Criteria for Social Anxiety Disorder (Social Phobia)

A. Marked fear or anxiety about one or more social situations in which the individual is exposed to possible scrutiny by others. Examples include social interactions (e.g., having a conversation, meeting unfamiliar people), being observed (e.g., eating or drinking), and performing in front of others (e.g., giving a speech).

   Note: In children, the anxiety must occur in peer settings and not just during interactions with adults.

B. The individual fears that he or she will act in a way or show anxiety symptoms that will be negatively evaluated (i.e., will be humiliating or embarrassing; will lead to rejection or offend others).

C. The social situations almost always provoke fear or anxiety.

   Note: In children, the fear or anxiety may be expressed by crying, tantrums, freezing, clinging, shrinking, or failing to speak in social situations.

D. The social situations are avoided or endured with intense fear or anxiety.

E. The fear or anxiety is out of proportion to the actual threat posed by the social situation and to the sociocultural context.

F. The fear, anxiety, or avoidance is persistent, typically lasting for 6 months or more.

G. The fear, anxiety, or avoidance causes clinically significant distress or impairment in social, occupational, or other important areas of functioning.

H. The fear, anxiety, or avoidance is not attributable to the physiological effects of a substance (e.g., a drug of abuse, a medication) or another medical condition.

I. The fear, anxiety, or avoidance is not better explained by the symptoms of another mental disorder, such as panic disorder, body dysmorphic disorder, or autism spectrum disorder.

J. If another medical condition (e.g., Parkinson's disease, obesity, disfigurement from burns or injury) is present, the fear, anxiety, or avoidance is clearly unrelated or is excessive.

Specify if:

   Performance only: If the fear is restricted to speaking or performing in public.

Source. Reprinted from American Psychiatric Association: *Diagnostic and Statistical Manual of Mental Disorders*, 5th Edition. Arlington, VA, American Psychiatric Association, 2013, pp. 202–203. Copyright © 2013 American Psychiatric Association. Used with permission.

Agoraphobia

Agoraphobia, like specific and social phobia, causes intense fear that is out of proportion to the danger posed in reality. It is triggered only by specific environments in which the patient fears escape would be difficult and help might be unavailable. To meet DSM-5 criteria, patients must fear two of the following specific environments/situations: public transportation, open spaces, enclosed spaces such as stores or theaters, crowds or lines, or being outside the home alone (Box 12–3). Agoraphobia can exist with or without concurrent panic attacks, but in either scenario patients fear the development of panic-like symptoms. The prevalence of agoraphobia ranges from 0.4% to 7.9% in adults older than 65 years, with some studies suggesting that it is more common in elderly adults and others suggesting that it is less so (Krasucki et al. 1998; McCabe et al. 2006).

   Agoraphobia may be more difficult to detect in older adults because this population is also more likely to be homebound. Mental health practitioners should assess thoroughly for agoraphobia in homebound older adults rather than solely attributing their homebound "status" to limited mobility or other physical or social factors (Gum et al. 2009; Jayasinghe et al. 2013). Studies suggest that older adults with agoraphobia are more likely to be female, to be on the younger end of the included population, and to be widowed or divorced and to have had onset before age 55; however, concurrent panic appears less common in this population (McCabe et al. 2006). The absence of panic symptoms raises questions regarding whether the experience of agoraphobia is qualitatively different for older adults than for their younger counterparts (McCabe et al. 2006). Indeed, recent studies have shown that age, later onset, and a shorter duration of symptoms may impart a better prognosis with respect to agoraphobic avoidance (Hendriks et al. 2014). Age also does not appear to affect patients' response to cognitive-behavioral therapy (CBT) and has been correlated with greater improvement on certain symptom domains (Hendriks et al. 2014).

Box 12–3. DSM-5 Diagnostic Criteria for Agoraphobia

A. Marked fear or anxiety about two (or more) of the following five situations:
   1. Using public transportation (e.g., automobiles, buses, trains, ships, planes).
   2. Being in open spaces (e.g., parking lots, marketplaces, bridges).
   3. Being in enclosed places (e.g., shops, theaters, cinemas).
   4. Standing in line or being in a crowd.
   5. Being outside of the home alone.
B. The individual fears or avoids these situations because of thoughts that escape might be difficult or help might not be available in the event of developing panic-like symptoms or other incapacitating or embarrassing symptoms (e.g., fear of falling in the elderly; fear of incontinence).
C. The agoraphobic situations almost always provoke fear or anxiety.
D. The agoraphobic situations are actively avoided, require the presence of a companion, or are endured with intense fear or anxiety.
E. The fear or anxiety is out of proportion to the actual danger posed by the agoraphobic situations and to the sociocultural context.
F. The fear, anxiety, or avoidance is persistent, typically lasting for 6 months or more.
G. The fear, anxiety, or avoidance causes clinically significant distress or impairment in social, occupational, or other important areas of functioning.
H. If another medical condition (e.g., inflammatory bowel disease, Parkinson's disease) is present, the fear, anxiety, or avoidance is clearly excessive.
I. The fear, anxiety, or avoidance is not better explained by the symptoms of another mental disorder—for example, the symptoms are not confined to specific phobia, situational type; do not involve only social situations (as in social anxiety disorder); and are not related exclusively to obsessions (as in obsessive-compulsive disorder), perceived defects or flaws in physical appearance (as in body dysmorphic disorder), reminders of traumatic events (as in posttraumatic stress disorder), or fear of separation (as in separation anxiety disorder).

Note: Agoraphobia is diagnosed irrespective of the presence of panic disorder. If an individual's presentation meets criteria for panic disorder and agoraphobia, both diagnoses should be assigned.

Panic Disorder

Panic disorder is defined by recurrent and unexpected panic attacks leading to at least 1 month of persistent concerns regarding future attacks or maladaptive behaviors (Box 12–4). A panic attack is the abrupt onset of severe fear with concurrent, intense physiological reactivity that leads to an array of cardiovascular, pulmonary, neurological, and psychological symptoms. The prevalence of panic disorder in older adults ranges from 0.1% to 1.0% (Beekman et al. 1998; Byers et al. 2010; Regier et al. 1990; Schoevers et al. 2003; Streiner et al. 2006; Trollor et al. 2007). When present, panic symptoms tend to be less frequent and severe in older adults than in younger adults (Corna et al. 2007; Sheikh et al. 2004). One possibility is that older individuals may have a less robust autonomic response to anxiety (Flint et al. 2002). However, the avoidance that is associated with panic disorder may be no less disabling, regardless of the severity or the frequency of attacks, and it has been associated with a lower quality of life in those with panic disorder as compared with those without it (Chou 2010; Corna et al. 2007). Although no clear consensus has been found in the scientific literature, childhood trauma may not correlate with panic disorder in older adults as it does in younger adults, but heavier alcohol consumption may be more likely in older adults with panic (Chou 2010; Olaya et al. 2018).

The development of late-onset panic disorder is rare. Therefore, new panic-like symptoms in this age group should prompt a thorough workup of possible medical causes that can produce similar symptoms, of which there are many. Cardiovascular, pulmonary, or neurological diseases common in this age range can all present with panic-like symptoms, and the medical workup should exclude myocardial or cerebral infarction, arrhythmias, chronic obstructive pulmonary disease or asthma, and hypoglycemic states. Panic-like symptoms have also been associated with several endocrinopathies, including thyroid dysfunction, hyperparathyroidism, carcinoid syndrome, and pheochromocytomas. Other possibilities include vestibular dysfunction, seizure disorders, CNS neoplasms, and vitamin B_{12} deficiency. One must also consider substance abuse or withdrawal and a long list of prescribed medications that can lead to panic-like symptoms. Most commonly, but not exhaustively, this could include alcohol, anticholinergics, nicotine, opioids, antihypertensives, sedative-hypnotics, cannabis, hypoglycemics, cocaine, or theophylline. Complicating this workup is the fact that older adults with panic disorder have an increased number of medical comorbidities and increased health care utilization (Chou 2010).

Box 12–4.   DSM-5 Diagnostic Criteria for Panic Disorder

A. Recurrent unexpected panic attacks. A panic attack is an abrupt surge of intense fear or intense discomfort that reaches a peak within minutes, and during which time four (or more) of the following symptoms occur:

Note: The abrupt surge can occur from a calm state or an anxious state.

   1. Palpitations, pounding heart, or accelerated heart rate.
   2. Sweating.
   3. Trembling or shaking.
   4. Sensations of shortness of breath or smothering.

5. Feelings of choking.
6. Chest pain or discomfort.
7. Nausea or abdominal distress.
8. Feeling dizzy, unsteady, light-headed, or faint.
9. Chills or heat sensations.
10. Paresthesias (numbness or tingling sensations).
11. Derealization (feelings of unreality) or depersonalization (being detached from oneself).
12. Fear of losing control or "going crazy."
13. Fear of dying.

Note: Culture-specific symptoms (e.g., tinnitus, neck soreness, headache, uncontrollable screaming or crying) may be seen. Such symptoms should not count as one of the four required symptoms.

B. At least one of the attacks has been followed by 1 month (or more) of one or both of the following:

1. Persistent concern or worry about additional panic attacks or their consequences (e.g., losing control, having a heart attack, "going crazy").
2. A significant maladaptive change in behavior related to the attacks (e.g., behaviors designed to avoid having panic attacks, such as avoidance of exercise or unfamiliar situations).

C. The disturbance is not attributable to the physiological effects of a substance (e.g., a drug of abuse, a medication) or another medical condition (e.g., hyperthyroidism, cardiopulmonary disorders).

D. The disturbance is not better explained by another mental disorder (e.g., the panic attacks do not occur only in response to feared social situations, as in social anxiety disorder; in response to circumscribed phobic objects or situations, as in specific phobia; in response to obsessions, as in obsessive-compulsive disorder; in response to reminders of traumatic events, as in posttraumatic stress disorder; or in response to separation from attachment figures, as in separation anxiety disorder).

Source. Reprinted from American Psychiatric Association: *Diagnostic and Statistical Manual of Mental Disorders*, 5th Edition. Arlington, VA, American Psychiatric Association, 2013, pp. 208–209. Copyright © 2013 American Psychiatric Association. Used with permission.

Generalized Anxiety Disorder

GAD is defined by excessive worry about various topics that is difficult to control, is distressing to the person, and impairs function. It often involves physiological manifestations such as muscle tension, restlessness, problems with sleep and concentration, fatigue, or irritability (Box 12–5). Although prevalence rates vary in the available studies, GAD is generally thought to be one of the most common late-life anxiety disorders, along with specific phobias. A recent study proposed a past-year prevalence of 2.8% for adults age 55 years and older that decreased to 1.88% in those age 75 years and older (Mackenzie et al. 2011).

The assumption that GAD in older adults represents the continuation of a chronic or recurrent form of the disorder that began earlier in the person's life is not entirely accurate. Lifelong GAD is common, and symptoms of GAD in older adults may have been present for decades. However, as many as 24%–46% of cases develop in late life (variably defined in these studies as onset after age 50 or 60) (Mackenzie et al. 2011; Zhang et al. 2015a).

Regardless of age at onset, GAD in those older than 65 years is associated with the conversion of mild NCD to Alzheimer's disease and an increased risk of stroke and other cardiovascular events (Lambiase et al. 2014; Rosenberg et al. 2013). Other correlates include female sex, cognitive impairment, low BMI, recent adverse life events, chronic medical comorbidity, psychiatric comorbidity (especially MDD and other anxiety disorders), and limited emotional support in childhood (Lenze et al. 2005a; Tully et al. 2013; Zhang et al. 2015a, 2015b). Older adults with GAD are nearly 2 times as likely as those without GAD to have a concurrent substance use disorder, 9 times as likely to have an additional anxiety disorder, and 15–16 times as likely to have concurrent MDD (Mackenzie et al. 2011). For most, GAD in late life represents a chronic condition that lasts years to decades, with poor rates of spontaneous remission and a likely need for long-term treatment (Lenze et al. 2005a).

Although the presentation of GAD in older adults is similar to that in their younger peers, there may be a few significant differences. Older adults with GAD are likely to have significantly more sleep disturbance, fewer reassurance-seeking behaviors, greater severity of co-occurring depressive symptoms, and a greater degree of disability in self-reported measures of impairment in social and familial functioning (Altunoz et al. 2018; Brenes et al. 2009). They may also be more likely to focus their worry on their own health, the well-being of their families, and world affairs as compared with younger adults, who more often worry about their future, work, social events, or others' health (Altunoz et al. 2018; Correa and Brown 2019). Although the severity or intensity of worry may diminish with age, its continued presence may be more indicative of a diagnosable anxiety disorder as one ages, and the resultant disability and decline in quality of life may remain substantial (Altunoz et al. 2018; Golden et al. 2011; Lindesay et al. 2006; Porensky et al. 2009; Wetherell et al. 2004).

Box 12–5.   DSM-5 Diagnostic Criteria for Generalized Anxiety Disorder

A. Excessive anxiety and worry (apprehensive expectation), occurring more days than not for at least 6 months, about a number of events or activities (such as work or school performance).

B. The individual finds it difficult to control the worry.

C. The anxiety and worry are associated with three (or more) of the following six symptoms (with at least some symptoms having been present for more days than not for the past 6 months):

Note: Only one item is required in children.

1. Restlessness or feeling keyed up or on edge.
2. Being easily fatigued.
3. Difficulty concentrating or mind going blank.
4. Irritability.
5. Muscle tension.
6. Sleep disturbance (difficulty falling or staying asleep, or restless, unsatisfying sleep).

D. The anxiety, worry, or physical symptoms cause clinically significant distress or impairment in social, occupational, or other important areas of functioning.

E. The disturbance is not attributable to the physiological effects of a substance (e.g., a drug of abuse, a medication) or another medical condition (e.g., hyperthyroidism).

F. The disturbance is not better explained by another mental disorder (e.g., anxiety or worry about having panic attacks in panic disorder, negative evaluation in social anxiety disorder [social phobia], contamination or other obsessions in obsessive-compulsive disorder, separation from attachment figures in separation anxiety disorder, reminders of traumatic events in posttraumatic stress disorder, gaining weight in anorexia nervosa, physical complaints in somatic symptom disorder, perceived appearance flaws in body dysmorphic disorder, having a serious illness in illness anxiety disorder, or the content of delusional beliefs in schizophrenia or delusional disorder).

Source.   Reprinted from American Psychiatric Association: *Diagnostic and Statistical Manual of Mental Disorders*, 5th Edition. Arlington, VA, American Psychiatric Association, 2013, pp. 222. Copyright © 2013 American Psychiatric Association. Used with permission.

Fear of Falling

Falls are relatively common among community-dwelling older adults and can lead to moderate to severe injuries, including head injuries, broken hips, and even death. In addition to serious physical health difficulties, falls are related to losses in mobility, confidence, and functional independence. If FOF is excessive relative to objective risk and leads to a restriction of normal activities and social engagements, DSM-5 can be used to diagnose it as a type of phobia. FOF is present in both those who have fallen and those who have not. Due to the use of different definitions and measurement instruments, the prevalence of FOF in older people varies greatly. However, a systematic review of 28 studies indicated that FOF is a relatively common syndrome among community-dwelling older adults (Scheffer et al. 2008). Older adults with FOF fear not only the feeling experienced when falling but also the potential consequences of falling, including physical injury, becoming infirm or a burden, losing independence, being institutionalized, and being confined to a wheelchair or losing the ability to walk (Tischler and Hobson 2005).

Female sex, physical function, the use of a walking aid, a history of falls, and poor self-rated health are significant factors related to FOF among community-dwelling older individuals (Denkinger et al. 2015). Results are inconsistent regarding the relationship between FOF and depression, anxiety, quantity of medications, and use of psychotropic drugs. In a recent small sample of older adults, GAD and anxiety symptoms were significantly and independently associated with FOF (Payette et al. 2017). However, in another examination of the association between anxiety and falls in a large sample of older adults enrolled in an osteoporosis study, differential relationships were found for males and females (Holloway et al. 2016). Even after accounting for patients' psychotropic medication use, mobility, and blood pressure, lifetime anxiety disorder was associated with a threefold increase in the likelihood of reported falls and high fall risk in males. However, in females, the association between lifetime anxiety disorder and falls was explained by psychotropic medication use, poor mobility, and socioeconomic status.

Obsessive-Compulsive Disorder

OCD is characterized by the combination of obsessions (intrusive thoughts, images, or impulses) and compulsions (behaviors to mitigate the obsessions or avoidance of stimuli) that cause significant distress for the patient (Box 12–6). Typical cases of OCD involve individuals who have fears, such as contamination, and who engage in behaviors as a result of those fears, such as washing their hands an innumerable quantity of times each day. However, many patients with OCD have intrusive, obsessive, and persistent thoughts without obvious compulsive behaviors such as checking, counting, or hand washing.

The lifetime prevalence of OCD is 2.3%, with a mean age of 19.5 years at onset (Ruscio et al. 2010). In a national community sample of more than 2,000 adults ages 60–74, the 1-month prevalence of OCD was 0.4%; those with obsessive or compulsive symptoms who did not meet full criteria had a prevalence of 4.7% and 2.2%, respectively (Pulular et al. 2013). In a second study of adults age 70 years and older, the 1-month prevalence of OCD was 2.9% and was higher in females (Klenfeldt et al. 2014). Those with OCD had high rates of depression (34.6%) and lower Global Assessment of Functioning scores compared with those without OCD (Klenfeldt et al. 2014). In a study of 416 outpatients with OCD, 6% were age 65 or older. Older adults had a later age at onset (29.4±15.1 vs. 18.7±9.2 years) and were less likely to participate in CBT compared with younger participants (Dell'Osso et al. 2017). Members of both groups were more likely to be female (75% vs. 56.4%).

The diagnosis of late-onset OCD is rare. Often, older adults present with obsessive or compulsive symptoms as opposed to meeting the full DSM-5 criteria. Late-onset presentations may manifest because of neurodegenerative disease or cerebral vascular lesions (often in the basal ganglia) (Chacko et al. 2000; Slachevsky et al. 2011). A case series of more than 1,000 patients revealed new-onset OCD after the age of 50 in five individuals; four of these patients had intracerebral lesions in their frontal lobes and caudate nuclei, prompting the recommendation that all patients with new-onset OCD symptoms later in life undergo a comprehensive neurological evaluation (Weiss and Jenike 2000).

Box 12–6.　DSM-5 Diagnostic Criteria for Obsessive-Compulsive Disorder

A. Presence of obsessions, compulsions, or both:

Obsessions are defined by (1) and (2):

1. Recurrent and persistent thoughts, urges, or images that are experienced, at some time during the disturbance, as intrusive and unwanted, and that in most individuals cause marked anxiety or distress.
2. The individual attempts to ignore or suppress such thoughts, urges, or images, or to neutralize them with some other thought or action (i.e., by performing a compulsion).

Compulsions are defined by (1) and (2):

1. Repetitive behaviors (e.g., hand washing, ordering, checking) or mental acts (e.g., praying, counting, repeating words silently) that the individual feels driven to perform in response to an obsession or according to rules that must be applied rigidly.
2. The behaviors or mental acts are aimed at preventing or reducing anxiety or dis-

tress, or preventing some dreaded event or situation; however, these behaviors or mental acts are not connected in a realistic way with what they are designed to neutralize or prevent, or are clearly excessive.

Note: Young children may not be able to articulate the aims of these behaviors or mental acts.

B. The obsessions or compulsions are time-consuming (e.g., take more than 1 hour per day) or cause clinically significant distress or impairment in social, occupational, or other important areas of functioning.

C. The obsessive-compulsive symptoms are not attributable to the physiological effects of a substance (e.g., a drug of abuse, a medication) or another medical condition.

D. The disturbance is not better explained by the symptoms of another mental disorder (e.g., excessive worries, as in generalized anxiety disorder; preoccupation with appearance, as in body dysmorphic disorder; difficulty discarding or parting with possessions, as in hoarding disorder; hair pulling, as in trichotillomania [hair-pulling disorder]; skin picking, as in excoriation [skin-picking] disorder; stereotypies, as in stereotypic movement disorder; ritualized eating behavior, as in eating disorders; preoccupation with substances or gambling, as in substance-related and addictive disorders; preoccupation with having an illness, as in illness anxiety disorder; sexual urges or fantasies, as in paraphilic disorders; impulses, as in disruptive, impulse-control, and conduct disorders; guilty ruminations, as in major depressive disorder; thought insertion or delusional preoccupations, as in schizophrenia spectrum and other psychotic disorders; or repetitive patterns of behavior, as in autism spectrum disorder).

Specify if:

With good or fair insight: The individual recognizes that obsessive-compulsive disorder beliefs are definitely or probably not true or that they may or may not be true.

With poor insight: The individual thinks obsessive-compulsive disorder beliefs are probably true.

With absent insight/delusional beliefs: The individual is completely convinced that obsessive-compulsive disorder beliefs are true.

Specify if:

Tic-related: The individual has a current or past history of a tic disorder.

Source. Reprinted from American Psychiatric Association: *Diagnostic and Statistical Manual of Mental Disorders*, 5th Edition. Arlington, VA, American Psychiatric Association, 2013, pp. 237. Copyright © 2013 American Psychiatric Association. Used with permission.

Hoarding Disorder

Hoarding disorder is characterized by an ongoing difficulty with discarding items and a perceived need to save items regardless of their value. Removal of these items results in significant distress. This results in the accumulation of vast amounts of clutter, which significantly impacts living areas. In elderly populations, hoarding behaviors can result in public health and safety concerns, including falls, impaired personal hygiene, food contamination, medication mismanagement, structural issues in the home, rodent infestation, and mold exposure (Ayers et al. 2014b; Diefenbach et al. 2013; Kim et al. 2001; Steketee et al. 2012). These risks are amplified by low rates of physical and mental health care, high medical comorbidity, and diminished access to the home by emergency personnel and in-home service professionals (Ayers et al. 2014a). Social isolation is also common in this population (Ayers et al. 2010) (Box 12–7).

Hoarding affects ~5.8% of the population (Timpano et al. 2011). In a community-based sample, the rate of hoarding in those ages 55–94 years was 6.2%, compared with <3% in the younger age group (Samuels et al. 2008). Studies indicate that most people develop hoarding disorder before the age of 40; however, one study (Steketee et al. 2012) indicated a bimodal distribution with a second spike after age 50 (Ayers et al. 2010; Tolin et al. 2010).

Hoarding disorder often co-occurs in those older than 60 years who also have other psychiatric disorders, including GAD (23.3%), MDD (28%–51.4%), PTSD (3.5%–11%), and OCD (16%–18.1%) (Ayers et al. 2010; Diefenbach et al. 2013; Samuels et al. 2008). A recent literature review revealed that those with late-life hoarding had significant memory deficits, executive dysfunction, and attention problems (Roane et al. 2017). In one study, the rates of dementia were 26% and 46% in those older than 65 years who were living in squalor and in those who had mild to moderate hoarding, respectively (Snowdon and Halliday 2011). In another study, older adults with hoarding disorder performed worse than age-matched control subjects on tasks involving working memory, mental control, inhibition, and set shifting, indicating executive dysfunction (Ayers et al. 2013). Taken together, these studies suggest that those with a late-life hoarding disorder have high rates of comorbid cognitive dysfunction.

Box 12–7.   DSM-5 Diagnostic Criteria for Hoarding Disorder

A. Persistent difficulty discarding or parting with possessions, regardless of their actual value.

B. This difficulty is due to a perceived need to save the items and to distress associated with discarding them.

C. The difficulty discarding possessions results in the accumulation of possessions that congest and clutter active living areas and substantially compromises their intended use. If living areas are uncluttered, it is only because of the interventions of third parties (e.g., family members, cleaners, authorities).

D. The hoarding causes clinically significant distress or impairment in social, occupational, or other important areas of functioning (including maintaining a safe environment for self and others).

E. The hoarding is not attributable to another medical condition (e.g., brain injury, cerebrovascular disease, Prader-Willi syndrome).

F. The hoarding is not better explained by the symptoms of another mental disorder (e.g., obsessions in obsessive-compulsive disorder, decreased energy in major depressive disorder, delusions in schizophrenia or another psychotic disorder, cognitive deficits in major neurocognitive disorder, restricted interests in autism spectrum disorder).

Specify if:

With excessive acquisition: If difficulty discarding possessions is accompanied by excessive acquisition of items that are not needed or for which there is no available space.

Specify if:

With good or fair insight: The individual recognizes that hoarding-related beliefs and behaviors (pertaining to difficulty discarding items, clutter, or excessive acquisition) are problematic.

With poor insight: The individual is mostly convinced that hoarding-related beliefs and behaviors (pertaining to difficulty discarding items, clutter, or excessive acquisition) are not problematic despite evidence to the contrary.

With absent insight/delusional beliefs: The individual is completely convinced that hoarding-related beliefs and behaviors (pertaining to difficulty discarding items, clutter, or excessive acquisition) are not problematic despite evidence to the contrary.

Source.   Reprinted from American Psychiatric Association: *Diagnostic and Statistical Manual of Mental Disorders*, 5th Edition. Arlington, VA, American Psychiatric Association, 2013, pp. 247. Copyright © 2013 American Psychiatric Association. Used with permission.

PTSD and Acute Stress Disorder

PTSD can be a chronic disorder that waxes and wanes across the life span. It is related to impaired social functioning and poor quality of life and appears to be a risk factor for dementia (Kang et al. 2019). In DSM-5, PTSD was recategorized from an anxiety disorder to one of the disorders in a new section entitled "Trauma- and Stressor-Related Disorders." PTSD is precipitated by exposure to a potentially traumatic event (e.g., combat, sexual assault, domestic violence, childhood physical and sexual abuse, motor vehicle and other accidents, natural or manmade disasters). The event must have produced at least 1 month of symptoms in each of four clusters: 1) intrusion (re-experiencing of the event through thoughts, flashbacks, or nightmares), 2) avoidance (avoiding thoughts of or situations that are reminders of the event), 3) negative alterations in cognitions or mood (detachment, diminished interest in or responsiveness to activities, difficultly experiencing positive emotions), and 4) heightened arousal/reactivity (sleep disturbances, exaggerated startle, irritability) (Box 12–8). If an older individual meets these criteria within the first month after the event, a diagnosis of acute stress disorder is given (Box 12–9).

PTSD has received relatively less empirical investigation in older adults than it has in younger and middle-aged adults, and some clinicians are concerned that it may be underdiagnosed and undertreated in this population. General population surveys in 24 countries across six continents found that, compared with younger age cohorts, subjects age 65 years and older reported higher rates of exposure to collective violence but lower rates of interpersonal violence, sexual violence, accidents/injuries, and being mugged (Benjet et al. 2016). Adults between the ages of 18 and 59 years were more likely to develop PTSD than were those age 60 years and older (Koenen et al. 2017). In a large epidemiological study in the United States, Pietrzak et al. (2012) estimated a 6.5% rate for PTSD in persons age 60 years and older. However, some evidence suggests that older adults may have clinically important PTSD symptoms that do not meet the full diagnostic criteria. Indeed, the rate for subthreshold/partial PTSD in this large investigation was 3.6%. The occurrence or reactivation of PTSD symptoms may be due in part to aging-related life events, such as illness, decrements in functional status, bereavement and loss of social networks, and changes in occupational, social, and familial roles.

In general, acute stress disorder and PTSD prevalence rates are relatively lower in older adults than in other adult age groups. However, specific subsamples within the older adult population may be particularly vulnerable to the effects of traumatic stress (e.g., older adult survivors of extreme and prolonged stress). Typically, epidemiological studies do not include the least healthy and perhaps most vulnerable (e.g., physically or emotionally impaired, homebound, or long-term care residents). Thus, any overarching statements that older individuals are the least likely to experience psychiatric distress following a trauma can be potentially misleading and could keep scarce resources from those most in need.

Box 12–8.   DSM-5 Diagnostic Criteria for Posttraumatic Stress Disorder

A. Exposure to actual or threatened death, serious injury, or sexual violence in one (or more) of the following ways:

   1. Directly experiencing the traumatic event(s).

   2. Witnessing, in person, the event(s) as it occurred to others.

   3. Learning that the traumatic event(s) occurred to a close family member or close friend. In cases of actual or threatened death of a family member or friend, the event(s) must have been violent or accidental.

   4. Experiencing repeated or extreme exposure to aversive details of the traumatic event(s) (e.g., first responders collecting human remains; police officers repeatedly exposed to details of child abuse).

   Note: Criterion A4 does not apply to exposure through electronic media, television, movies, or pictures, unless this exposure is work related.

B. Presence of one (or more) of the following intrusion symptoms associated with the traumatic event(s), beginning after the traumatic event(s) occurred:

   1. Recurrent, involuntary, and intrusive distressing memories of the traumatic event(s).

   Note: In children older than 6 years, repetitive play may occur in which themes or aspects of the traumatic event(s) are expressed.

   2. Recurrent distressing dreams in which the content and/or affect of the dream are related to the traumatic event(s).

   Note: In children, there may be frightening dreams without recognizable content.

   3. Dissociative reactions (e.g., flashbacks) in which the individual feels or acts as if the traumatic event(s) were recurring. (Such reactions may occur on a continuum, with the most extreme expression being a complete loss of awareness of present surroundings.)

   Note: In children, trauma-specific reenactment may occur in play.

   4. Intense or prolonged psychological distress at exposure to internal or external cues that symbolize or resemble an aspect of the traumatic event(s).

   5. Marked physiological reactions to internal or external cues that symbolize or resemble an aspect of the traumatic event(s).

C. Persistent avoidance of stimuli associated with the traumatic event(s), beginning after the traumatic event(s) occurred, as evidenced by one or both of the following:

   1. Avoidance of or efforts to avoid distressing memories, thoughts, or feelings about or closely associated with the traumatic event(s).

   2. Avoidance of or efforts to avoid external reminders (people, places, conversations, activities, objects, situations) that arouse distressing memories, thoughts, or feelings about or closely associated with the traumatic event(s).

D. Negative alterations in cognitions and mood associated with the traumatic event(s), beginning or worsening after the traumatic event(s) occurred, as evidenced by two (or more) of the following:

   1. Inability to remember an important aspect of the traumatic event(s) (typically due to dissociative amnesia and not to other factors such as head injury, alcohol, or drugs).

2. Persistent and exaggerated negative beliefs or expectations about oneself, others, or the world (e.g., "I am bad," "No one can be trusted," "The world is completely dangerous," "My whole nervous system is permanently ruined").
3. Persistent, distorted cognitions about the cause or consequences of the traumatic event(s) that lead the individual to blame himself/herself or others.
4. Persistent negative emotional state (e.g., fear, horror, anger, guilt, or shame).
5. Markedly diminished interest or participation in significant activities.
6. Feelings of detachment or estrangement from others.
7. Persistent inability to experience positive emotions (e.g., inability to experience happiness, satisfaction, or loving feelings).

E. Marked alterations in arousal and reactivity associated with the traumatic event(s), beginning or worsening after the traumatic event(s) occurred, as evidenced by two (or more) of the following:

1. Irritable behavior and angry outbursts (with little or no provocation) typically expressed as verbal or physical aggression toward people or objects.
2. Reckless or self-destructive behavior.
3. Hypervigilance.
4. Exaggerated startle response.
5. Problems with concentration.
6. Sleep disturbance (e.g., difficulty falling or staying asleep or restless sleep).

F. Duration of the disturbance (Criteria B, C, D, and E) is more than 1 month.
G. The disturbance causes clinically significant distress or impairment in social, occupational, or other important areas of functioning.
H. The disturbance is not attributable to the physiological effects of a substance (e.g., medication, alcohol) or another medical condition.

Specify whether:

With dissociative symptoms: The individual's symptoms meet the criteria for posttraumatic stress disorder, and in addition, in response to the stressor, the individual experiences persistent or recurrent symptoms of either of the following:

1. **Depersonalization:** Persistent or recurrent experiences of feeling detached from, and as if one were an outside observer of, one's mental processes or body (e.g., feeling as though one were in a dream; feeling a sense of unreality of self or body or of time moving slowly).
2. **Derealization:** Persistent or recurrent experiences of unreality of surroundings (e.g., the world around the individual is experienced as unreal, dreamlike, distant, or distorted).

Note: To use this subtype, the dissociative symptoms must not be attributable to the physiological effects of a substance (e.g., blackouts, behavior during alcohol intoxication) or another medical condition (e.g., complex partial seizures).

Specify if:

With delayed expression: If the full diagnostic criteria are not met until at least 6 months after the event (although the onset and expression of some symptoms may be immediate).

Source. Reprinted from American Psychiatric Association: *Diagnostic and Statistical Manual of Mental Disorders*, 5th Edition. Arlington, VA, American Psychiatric Association, 2013, pp. 271–272. Copyright © 2013 American Psychiatric Association. Used with permission.

Box 12–9.   DSM-5 Diagnostic Criteria for Acute Stress Disorder
---

A. Exposure to actual or threatened death, serious injury, or sexual violence in one (or more) of the following ways:

   1. Directly experiencing the traumatic event(s).

   2. Witnessing, in person, the event(s) as it occurred to others.

   3. Learning that the event(s) occurred to a close family member or close friend.

     Note: In cases of actual or threatened death of a family member or friend, the event(s) must have been violent or accidental.

   4. Experiencing repeated or extreme exposure to aversive details of the traumatic event(s) (e.g., first responders collecting human remains, police officers repeatedly exposed to details of child abuse).

     Note: This does not apply to exposure through electronic media, television, movies, or pictures, unless this exposure is work related.

B. Presence of nine (or more) of the following symptoms from any of the five categories of intrusion, negative mood, dissociation, avoidance, and arousal, beginning or worsening after the traumatic event(s) occurred:

Intrusion Symptoms

   1. Recurrent, involuntary, and intrusive distressing memories of the traumatic event(s). **Note:** In children, repetitive play may occur in which themes or aspects of the traumatic event(s) are expressed.

   2. Recurrent distressing dreams in which the content and/or affect of the dream are related to the event(s). **Note:** In children, there may be frightening dreams without recognizable content.

   3. Dissociative reactions (e.g., flashbacks) in which the individual feels or acts as though the traumatic event(s) were recurring. (Such reactions may occur on a continuum, with the most extreme expression being a complete loss of awareness of present surroundings.) **Note:** In children, trauma-specific reenactment may occur in play.

   4. Intense or prolonged psychological distress or marked physiological reactions in response to internal or external cues that symbolize or resemble an aspect of the traumatic event(s).

Negative Mood

   5. Persistent inability to experience positive emotions (e.g., inability to experience happiness, satisfaction, or loving feelings).

Dissociative Symptoms

   6. An altered sense of the reality of one's surroundings or oneself (e.g., seeing oneself from another's perspective, being in a daze, time slowing).

   7. Inability to remember an important aspect of the traumatic event(s) (typically due to dissociative amnesia and not to other factors such as head injury, alcohol, or drugs).

Avoidance Symptoms

   8. Efforts to avoid distressing memories, thoughts, or feelings about or closely associated with the traumatic event(s).

   9. Efforts to avoid external reminders (people, places, conversations, activities, objects, situations) that arouse distressing memories, thoughts, or feelings about or closely associated with the traumatic event(s).

Arousal Symptoms

10. Sleep disturbance (e.g., difficulty falling or staying asleep, restless sleep).
11. Irritable behavior and angry outbursts (with little or no provocation), typically expressed as verbal or physical aggression toward people or objects.
12. Hypervigilance.
13. Problems with concentration.
14. Exaggerated startle response.

C. Duration of the disturbance (symptoms in Criterion B) is 3 days to 1 month after trauma exposure.
   Note: Symptoms typically begin immediately after the trauma, but persistence for at least 3 days and up to a month is needed to meet disorder criteria.
D. The disturbance causes clinically significant distress or impairment in social, occupational, or other important areas of functioning.
E. The disturbance is not attributable to the physiological effects of a substance (e.g., medication or alcohol) or another medical condition (e.g., mild traumatic brain injury) and is not better explained by brief psychotic disorder.

Note. These criteria have been shortened and apply to adults, adolescents, and children older than 6 years. For children age 6 years and younger, see full criteria in DSM-5.
Source. Reprinted from American Psychiatric Association: *Diagnostic and Statistical Manual of Mental Disorders*, 5th Edition. Arlington, VA, American Psychiatric Association, 2013, pp. 280–281. Copyright © 2013 American Psychiatric Association. Used with permission.

Anxiety in Comorbid Medical Illness

Several medical conditions can mimic anxiety disorders or precipitate concurrent anxiety. In these instances, mental health practitioners must target treatment to the underlying etiology and not diagnose a primary mental health condition where one is not present. Older adults may be more likely to present with somatic complaints such as sleep disturbance, muscle tension, or pain or to somaticize their psychiatric symptoms, even if GAD symptoms have waned in severity over time (Katon et al. 2007; Rubio and López-Ibor 2007). This is an important consideration when treating older adults for whom potentially unnecessary medical interventions can pose increased risk. Unnecessary prescriptions for sedatives, pain medication, or other agents can substantially increase their risk of adverse outcomes, including falls and fractures, delirium, bleeding, and hospitalization (2019 American Geriatrics Society Beers Criteria Update Expert Panel 2019).

As detailed earlier, several medical conditions may cause symptoms that are easily confused with a primary anxiety disorder. Guidance exists to help clinicians differentiate between anxiety that is of psychological origin and anxiety that is the product of a concurrent medical illness (Mohlman et al. 2012). Namely, anxiety that arises in the absence of any psychiatric history, following the onset of a recent physical illness, concurrently with the initiation of a medication with anxiogenic effects, following discontinuation of a medication capable of inducing withdrawal, in the context of known medical conditions that can mimic anxiety (e.g., cardiac or thyroid disease), or in the absence of other life events should raise suspicion for a possible physiological rather than psychological etiology (Mohlman et al. 2012). In these instances, the diagnosis of anxiety disorder due to another medical condition is most appropriate.

For many older adults, their chronic medical condition is not the cause of their anxiety but exists concurrently alongside another diagnosable anxiety disorder. A recent study characterizing this relationship revealed that patients with chronic medical illnesses, particularly persistently painful conditions, were more likely to experience concurrent anxiety disorders. They were also more likely to report poorer overall health than patients with the same medical conditions or the same anxiety disorders alone (El-Gabalawy et al. 2011). Indeed, this relationship is likely bidirectional; a subsequent study by the same group of investigators found that past-year arthritis in patients age 55 years and older increased the likelihood of developing incident GAD within the next 4 years, and any lifetime anxiety disorder was associated with the development of incident gastrointestinal disease (El-Gabalawy et al. 2014). Other studies have demonstrated a significant increase in the prevalence of anxiety disorders in visually impaired older adults and patients with Parkinson's disease (Dissanayaka et al. 2010; van der Aa et al. 2015). In fact, although particular medical conditions may be more likely to precipitate anxiety, multimorbidity itself may be an important risk factor for anxiety in older adults (Gould et al. 2016). For patients age 65 years and older, the presence of three or more medical conditions imparts a 2.3-fold increase in the likelihood of scoring 12 or higher on the Beck Anxiety Inventory (Gould et al. 2016). Multimorbidity also appeared to be more strongly associated with anxiety than depression, a finding that raises the question of whether mental health screening specifically for anxiety would be of high yield in older, multimorbid populations (Gould et al. 2016). This may be especially true because, as evidence suggests, older adults with anxiety may be less likely to seek care for their symptoms (Scott et al. 2010).

Evidence is mixed regarding the overall burden to the health care system of comorbid anxiety in older adults. For those older than 85 years, concurrent anxiety may increase costs by as much as 31%, but this correlation disappears when adjusted for other covariates such as medical comorbidity, cognitive decline, or functional impairment (Hohls et al. 2019). In a recent systematic review, most studies found an increase in health care utilization and costs for adults older than 65 with anxiety compared with their nonanxious peers (Hohls et al. 2018). Redirection of services, namely to identify those in need of mental health care and to integrate mental health services into the primary care setting, has been an area of interest in recent years. Unfortunately, only about 20% of older adults with anxiety disorders seek care for their symptoms (Scott et al. 2010). Identifying those in need and providing services in the settings where they are likely to seek care may help address not only the underuse of mental health services in older adults but also perhaps the costs of health care use overall.

Anxiety and Late-Life Depression

Studies have demonstrated that the prevalence of comorbid anxiety and late-life depression ranges from 26.1% to 52% (Beekman et al. 2000; King-Kallimanis et al. 2009; van der Veen et al. 2015). The presence of comorbid anxiety amplifies the burden of depression, resulting in greater distress, poorer functioning, and increased somatic symptoms (Braam et al. 2014; Cairney et al. 2008; Lenze et al. 2000; Simning and Seplaki 2020). One study revealed a greater decline in memory, whereas another demonstrated no additive impact on cognitive dysfunction in the presence of both anxiety and depression symptoms (DeLuca et al. 2005; Martinussen et al. 2019). Although some studies indicate higher rates of suicidality and suicidal ideation in this subpopulation, a survey in the United Kingdom revealed that older adults with comorbid anxiety and depression died from suicide at lower rates than those with depression alone, despite having more risk factors for suicide (Allgulander and Lavori 1993; Bartels et al. 2002; Lenze et al. 2000; Oude Voshaar et al. 2016).

In one investigation, patients age 70 years and older with high levels of pretreatment comorbid anxiety and depression had an increased risk of nonresponse acutely and of recurrence during the first 2 years following response to treatment (Andreescu et al. 2007). In contrast, in a meta-analysis, data from eight trials demonstrated no evidence to suggest that the presence of anxiety impacted response to antidepressant intervention in those with late-life depression (Nelson et al. 2009). Additionally, the presence of MDD and comorbid anxiety in older adults who participated in a protocolized intervention with venlafaxine was not a predictor of treatment resistance: remission of depression was similar in patients with anxiety to that in patients with depression but without anxiety (Saade et al. 2019).

In the Prevention of Suicide in Primary Care Elderly: Collaborative Trial (PROSPECT), older primary care patients with depression were randomized to usual care or the PROSPECT intervention, which consisted of trained care managers providing algorithm-based recommendations to primary care providers and assistance to patients over an 18-month time frame with treatment adherence (Alexopoulos et al. 2005). In patients with depression but without anxiety, participants in the intervention group achieved first remission earlier than those in the usual-care group; in the subgroup with comorbid anxiety and depressive symptoms, those with high anxiety did not fare any better in the intervention versus the usual-care group, prompting the recommendation that primary care providers consider a referral to psychiatry for older adults with combined depressive and high anxiety symptoms.

In terms of psychotherapeutic interventions for late-life depression and anxiety, a randomized controlled trial (RCT) of older adults with comorbid anxiety and depression found that 54% of those who participated in group CBT demonstrated recovery from their primary disorder versus 24% in the discussion group. Although improvements were sustained at 6 months, the superiority of the CBT group over the discussion group was no longer significant at that time (Wuthrich et al. 2016).

Two neuroimaging studies revealed a distinct set of findings in patients with comorbid anxiety and depression. In the first, older adults with combined depression and anxiety had less cortical thickness in the amygdala, anterior cingulate cortex, orbitofrontal cortex, insula, and temporal cortex compared with those with anxiety but no history of depression (Potvin et al. 2015). In the second, a sample of adults older than 60 years with depression alone had smaller insular cortex volumes, and those with comorbid depression and anxiety symptoms had both smaller insular cortex and orbitofrontal cortex volumes. These findings suggest lower orbitofrontal cortex volumes may serve as a potential biomarker of anxiety in late-life depression (Laird et al. 2019).

Neurobiological and Neuropsychological Findings

A neurobiological perspective is paramount to accurately diagnose, prognosticate, and treat anxiety and related disorders. Symptoms, signs, and the entire spectrum of mental life are fundamentally emergent properties of the brain. Hippocrates is widely credited as one of the earliest scholars to declare the brain the physical seat of the human psyche, which at the time represented a major shift (Breitenfeld et al. 2014; Green 1973). This critical evolution in thinking sustained repeated assaults for centuries to come, from the Cartesian model of mind-body dualism to the 20th-century behaviorist theories that labeled the brain a "black box" that was irrelevant to understanding mental processes. Physicians, neuropsychologists, and neuroscientists throughout history have written extensively on the neural correlates of cognition, emotion, and behavior. Widely accepted models have moved from conceptualizing the brain as solely a modular organ, with individual cortical areas subserving specific cognitive functions, to one of neural networks that vary in their degree of distribution and overlap. This section touches on some of the pertinent neural substrates, as well as relevant findings in the neuropsychological literature.

Anxiety Disorders

The umbrella of anxiety disorders includes several separate categorical diagnoses, including GAD, panic disorder, specific phobias, and social anxiety disorder. What follows is not an exhaustive review of the neuroscience of each of these to date but a look at the core systems that are affected in states of worry, panic, rumination, and fear and can negatively impact a patient's quality of life. Methods of peering into the brain and its machinations include structural neuroimaging, most commonly MRI and functional MRI, which uses varying states of oxygenated blood as a surrogate for neural activity to elucidate patterns of brain dysfunction.

A limbic structure tucked within the more anterior portions of the temporal lobe is the amygdala. Although posited in years past as the "fear center" of the brain, contemporary thought is that the amygdala assigns motivational salience to sensory input, be it positive or negative in value (O'Neill et al. 2018). In GAD, multiple studies demonstrate abnormal patterns of activity across areas of the prefrontal cortex and the amygdala, as well as diminished connectivity between the amygdala, areas of the prefrontal cortex, and subcortical structures, all of which share reciprocal projections (Hilbert et al. 2014). The amygdala may have larger volumes of gray matter in nonelderly adults with GAD (Schienle et al. 2011), but this finding was not replicated in older individuals (Mohlman et al. 2009). On a neurochemical level, the serotonergic and noradrenergic systems projecting from the dorsal raphe and locus coeruleus brainstem nuclei, respectively, likely contribute to the manifestation of anxiety, although evidence has not convincingly demonstrated consistent dysfunction in GAD (Graeff and Zangrossi 2010; Hernández et al. 2002; Hilbert et al. 2014). Dysregulation in the hypothalamic-pituitary-adrenal (HPA) axis may also contribute to the development of late-life anxiety disorders, with evidence showing older adults with GAD have higher basal and peak salivary cortisol levels (Hellwig and Domschke 2019; Mantella et al. 2008). A course of escitalopram, commonly used to treat anxiety disorders, found a decrease in salivary cortisol levels, further lending support to the HPA axis and endogenous stress response playing a role (Lenze et al. 2012).

In the appropriate context, fear and anxiety serve a valuable purpose. It is evolutionarily adaptive to experience a sense of fear when faced with potentially dangerous consequences. A classic example of this is the lion charging toward an unsuspecting prey. If the prey does not manifest a fight-or-flight response, then the odds of propagating its species decline considerably. The Klüver-Bucy syndrome, thought to be the result of bilateral damage to the amygdala, includes an inappropriate placid response to potentially threatening stimuli (Klüver and Bucy 1937). Again, in the correct context, anxiety, fear, and worry may all be appropriate emotions that assist the person in shaping behaviors. It is when the brain overgeneralizes fear and resists the natural unlearning of associations, known as *extinction*, that anxiety and trauma-related symptoms materialize (Dunsmoor and Paz 2015).

Anxiety is more common among those diagnosed with NCDs, which are explored in more detail later in the chapter. In older adults without NCDs, anxiety has detrimental effects on attention, working memory, and performance on tests of learning and recall (Deptula et al. 1993; Hogan 2003; Mantella et al. 2007). The relationship between anxiety and cognitive deficits is likely bidirectional, at least in a subset of cases (Andreescu and Varon 2015).

Obsessive-Compulsive Disorder

The neurocircuitry of OCD has been the subject of intensive research. The pathogenesis of OCD underscores the importance of cortico-striato-thalamo-cortical circuits. These parallel loops, with varying connections to other networks, roughly follow a course from the frontal cortex to the basal ganglia, the thalamus, and ultimately back to the cortex. Circuits spanning from the frontal lobe to limbic and cerebellar structures are also implicated in OCD (Kwon et al. 2009). When compared that of with healthy control subjects, structural imaging in subjects with OCD supports, on average, a loss of gray matter volume in several frontal lobe regions in conjunction with larger striatal volumes (van den Heuvel et al. 2016; van Velzen et al. 2014). Serotonergic, dopaminergic, and glutamatergic neurotransmitter systems may also contribute to the development of OCD, an idea supported by trials showing benefit from pharmacological agents modulating each of these systems (Bandelow et al. 2017; Ducasse et al. 2014; Kariuki-Nyuthe et al. 2014; Nikolaus et al. 2010; Stein et al. 2019; Taylor 2013). Neuropsychological deficits were detected in multiple domains, including attention, mental flexibility, inhibitory processes, verbal fluency, planning, and memory, although inconsistencies believed to be secondary to methodological matters do exist (Benzina et al. 2016).

Trauma-Related Disorders

Two psychological processes are key to the development and perpetuation of PTSD: fear conditioning and memory reconsolidation (Ross et al. 2017). To again take an evolutionary perspective, it behooves a species to associate cues in its environment with possible threats. For example, if a rustling bush foreshadowed the ominous reveal of a lion to early hominids, then it would have been adaptive to learn the association between a shaking bush and a dangerous creature. The pairing of a natural response—that is, the autonomic arousal and fear at the sight of an approaching lion—with a neutral cue, the rustling bush, is a type of learning known as *classical conditioning*. In PTSD, a traumatic event and the resultant emotional and physiological response become paired with environmental cues; patients often avoid these cues, thus negatively reinforcing the ongoing learned association. Traumatic memories can be recalled and, if left unchallenged, may further reinforce maladaptive beliefs and cognitive distortions, resulting in memory reconsolidation (Ross et al. 2017).

Circuit activity in PTSD reveals a pattern not entirely dissimilar to that in anxiety disorders, namely, overactivity of the amygdala and loss of inhibitory control from the prefrontal cortex (Lang et al. 2009; Seeley et al. 2007). Given that PTSD is partially a disorder of stress response, it makes sense that the HPA axis, a marker of stress resilience, is believed to be overly sensitized (de Kloet et al. 2006). A meta-analysis of late-life PTSD and neuropsychological profiles found the largest detrimental effect size on memory, although the authors acknowledged that a number of the included studies failed to account for the effects of attention and learning (Schuitevoerder et al. 2013).

Anxiety and Related Disorders in the Context of Neurocognitive Impairment

Mild and major NCDs are quintessential neuropsychiatric syndromes that commonly present with affective and behavioral changes along with requisite cognitive decline. Whether due to a neurodegenerative proteinopathy, vascular disease, traumatic injury, or some other means, NCDs are a window through which research may illuminate the pathogenesis of idiopathic psychiatric disorders. Those circuits mediating executive function, complex attention, memory, social cognition, and other domains classically considered cognitive are either directly part of or heavily connected to networks supporting emotion and behavior. The degree to which anxiety may be part of an NCD prodrome and a risk factor for later cognitive decline is an active area of research. Anxiety may predict progression from mild to major NCD; this association is strongest with increasing age, which is consistent with a prodrome (Gallagher et al. 2011; Gulpers et al. 2016; Mah et al. 2015). A large retrospective cohort study of U.S. veterans supports this association: those previously diagnosed with PTSD were approximately twice as likely to develop major NCD over a 7-year period (Yaffe et al. 2010). In civilians, PTSD may increase the risk of major NCD by more than 70% (Flatt et al. 2018). On the other hand, several other studies did not find that anxiety predicted later cognitive impairment (de Bruijn et al. 2014; Devier et al. 2009).

Anxiety often co-occurs in patients diagnosed with major NCD (Lyketsos et al. 2002; Tschanz et al. 2011). A greater burden of anxiety is associated with more severe global functional impairment in those with mild or major NCD (Wadsworth et al. 2012). Anxiety is a feature measured on the Neuropsychiatric Inventory (Cummings 1997), and modified criteria for GAD were validated in the clinical syndrome of Alzheimer's disease (Starkstein et al. 2007). Neuropsychiatric symptoms, including anxiety, agitation, and psychosis, increase caregiver burden (Okura and Langa 2011) and put patients at higher risk of needing long-term care placement (Steele et al. 1990; Yaffe et al. 2002).

Clinicians must be vigilant when assessing late-life anxiety because it may portend the insidious onset of a progressive cognitive disorder. Given how common anxiety is among individuals with established mild NCD and the impact that neuropsychiatric symptoms have on patient distress, caregiver burden, and time to long-term care placement, clinicians must employ early, creative behavioral interventions and, when appropriate, pharmacological strategies to target symptoms of anxiety and improve quality of life.

TABLE 12–1.	Guidelines for assessment of anxiety in older adults

Some older adults may minimize their experiences of distress or assign the symptoms solely to physical causes. Throughout assessment, provide education and understanding of anxiety symptoms to encourage discussion and reduce stigma.

Reflect and use the words endorsed by the patient to describe anxious symptoms (e.g., "nerves," "knots or butterflies in stomach").

When available, use standardized anxiety assessments with established, strong psychometric properties in older adults. According to a systematic review (Therrien and Hunsley 2012), three measures have strong psychometric properties when assessing anxiety in older adults: the Beck Anxiety Inventory, Penn State Worry Questionnaire, and Geriatric Mental Status Examination. In addition, two measures developed specifically for older adults (Worry Scale and Geriatric Anxiety Inventory) were also found to be appropriate.

Avoid using self-report measures with complicated response formats, such as response options (e.g., Strongly Agree, Agree, Undecided/Neutral, Disagree, Strongly Disagree), shifting order, and wording.

Font, spacing, and shading of self-report questionnaires should be altered for easier reading.

Consider using lower cutoffs on symptom measures for meeting full diagnostic criteria and a lower number of symptoms to meet cutoff or diagnostic criteria compared with younger adults.

Single measures are known to underestimate the prevalence of anxiety disorders in older adults. Using more than one method of assessment (e.g., self-report, observation, structured interviews, collateral/caregiver reports, physician and other health care professional consultation, and review of existing medical records) is important for accurate diagnosis and appropriate treatment planning. This is particularly important for older adults with limited cognitive abilities or the presence of aphasias.

Symptoms of medical conditions associated with age (e.g., cardiovascular disease) and side effects of medications (e.g., steroids) can overlap with anxiety symptoms.

Assess the age at onset, severity, duration, and course of anxiety symptoms. Ask questions and look for patterns in how symptoms are associated with changes in social support, mobility, self-care, employment, activity level, living situation, and health status.

Consider patients' level of motivation for treatment, prior treatment experiences (including psychotherapy and pharmacotherapy), and expectations for current treatment.

Assessment Instruments for Anxiety in Older Adults

Traditional assessment measures appear to have less sensitivity for detecting anxiety in older adults for several reasons, including understanding and difficulty with recollection. Table 12–1 provides several recommendations for health care professionals to improve the accuracy of diagnosis, conceptualization, and treatment. These recommendations are based on empirical investigation and clinical experience. Importantly, in a sample of older adults with comorbid anxiety and unipolar mood disorders, the greatest barriers to help-seeking were related to difficulty identifying the need for assistance, with 50% reporting that they believed their symptoms were normal (Wuthrich and Frei 2015). Thus, although health care providers assess for anxiety and other mental health–related disorders, they must also actively educate older adults about the need for, and effectiveness of, psychological therapies for anxiety.

Treatment of Late-Life Anxiety Disorders

Psychotherapy

There is less empirical investigation of psychotherapy in older adults compared with that in younger adults. In addition, there are limits in the methodological rigor (e.g., lack of placebo/control/comparison groups, limited sample size, and lack of generalizability) of available studies. CBT is the most widely studied intervention for older adults with anxiety disorders. It typically involves teaching patients to recognize their anxiety symptoms, followed by teaching relaxation skills, cognitive restructuring and use of coping statements, problem solving, worry control, behavioral activation, exposure therapy, and relapse prevention. Often considered the first-line psychotherapeutic option for GAD, CBT is superior to no treatment (Hall et al. 2016). Even when delivered by telephone, CBT is superior to nonsupportive therapy in reducing worry, GAD, and depressive symptoms at short-term follow-up in older adults with GAD (Brenes et al. 2015). However, no long-term differences were found between the groups (Brenes et al. 2017).

There seem to be feasibility and initial efficacy in GAD for guided self-help treatment based on CBT principles (Landreville et al. 2016) and for lay providers delivering CBT under the supervision of licensed providers (Stanley et al. 2014). A structured review indicated other potentially efficacious options for GAD in older adults, including relaxation, psychodynamic approaches, and mindfulness techniques (Bolognesi et al. 2014). Helping older adults with anxiety disorders learn to self-monitor, work through, and emotionally soothe their intolerance of uncertainty is crucial.

There is little research on the efficacy of psychotherapy for panic, specific or social phobia, OCD, hoarding, or FOF in older adults. Although several studies have included patients with these diagnoses, the published outcomes have not been disorder specific. A few recent studies are worth highlighting. Some data indicate that CBT is feasible for older patients with panic disorder with agoraphobia, with outcomes similar to and sometimes even better than those found in younger individuals (Hendriks et al. 2014). Wetherell et al. (2018) evaluated the safety and acceptability of an intervention integrating a home safety evaluation, physical exercise, and elements of CBT in reducing disproportionate FOF (i.e., high fear, low to moderate objective fall risk). Although the intervention reduced FOF and activity avoidance, these effects were diminished by 6-month follow-up.

A systematic review of psychotherapy for PTSD in older adults (Dinnen et al. 2015) found only case studies and a few small outcome studies. Preliminary evidence indicates that exposure-based treatments appear feasible and efficacious in older adults with varied trauma histories and a sizable span of time since traumatic exposure. A number of these studies also indicated that although older adults experienced a reduction of PTSD, depression, and anxiety symptoms, few experienced a full remission. Thus, although valuable, these treatments alone may not be sufficient or may not have been delivered in ample quantity to significantly reduce PTSD symptoms. Thus, booster sessions and a longer duration of treatment may be needed in older populations who experience trauma (Thorp et al. 2019).

In general, psychotherapy in older adults with anxiety disorders can be flexible and customized to the needs, preferences, capabilities, and treatment goals of individual patients. If older adults with anxiety also have mild to moderate cognitive impairments, adaptations to psychotherapy may be needed (Rehm et al. 2017). These may include changes to the structure of and strategies used in therapy, such as providing sessions in older adults' home environments, as-needed telephone sessions, repeated instructions, increased in-session practice of new skills, simplified session summaries and homework instructions, external memory aids (e.g., cue cards, calendars), caregiver support, and cognitive rehabilitation strategies. A meta-analysis of the few RCTs that investigated the efficacy of CBT in older adults with comorbid anxiety and mild to moderate dementia indicated that the effects of treatment are seen in clinician ratings but not in older adult or caregiver reports (Orgeta et al. 2015).

Pharmacotherapy

Antidepressants (the selective serotonin reuptake inhibitors [SSRIs] and the serotonin-norepinephrine reuptake inhibitors [SNRIs]) are the first-line pharmacological intervention for anxiety disorders in older adults. One systematic review included 12 RCTs of antidepressant interventions for elderly patients with anxiety disorders: eight SSRIs, three SNRIs, and one tricyclic antidepressant (TCA) (Alaka et al. 2014; Balasubramaniam et al. 2019; Blank et al. 2006; Davidson et al. 2008; Hendriks et al. 2010; Katz et al. 2002; Lenze et al. 2005b, 2009; Mokhber et al. 2010; Schuurmans et al. 2006, 2009; Sheikh and Swales 1999; Wetherell et al. 2013). There were no RCTs with outcomes for mirtazapine, fluvoxamine, or fluoxetine. Across studies, anxiety symptoms were reduced with the use of antidepressants, and the medications were generally well tolerated; however, most of the studies focused on GAD as opposed to other anxiety disorders. All trials excluded patients with unstable medical issues and cognitive impairment, limiting the generalizability of the findings to the population often treated by geriatric psychiatrists.

Mirtazapine, a commonly used antidepressant in elderly patients, lacks evidence for its use in older adults with anxiety disorders (Crocco et al. 2017). However, it is generally considered a safe, well-tolerated medication with limited drug–drug interactions and a side effect profile (e.g., sedation, weight gain) that may be favorable in subpopulations of older adults with anxiety disorders. Trazodone is also commonly used as a standing or as-needed medication for the treatment of anxiety disorders in older patients; like mirtazapine, data supporting its use in this subpopulation are limited. Buspirone may have some benefit for the treatment of anxiety disorders but likewise lacks data for its use in older adult populations (Crocco et al. 2017). Alternate pharmacotherapies, such as TCAs/tetracyclic antidepressants, monoamine oxidase inhibitors, mood stabilizers, atypical antipsychotics, benzodiazepines, and β-blockers, lack data for their use in older adults. Due to their side effect profiles, they are typically avoided in elderly patients with primary anxiety disorders (Crocco et al. 2017).

In the management of OCD, SSRIs are considered the first-line treatment, often at higher-than-typical dosages. To date, no known randomized, placebo-controlled trials have been done in older adult populations; however, a 2016 meta-analysis of adults with mean ages ranging from 30 to 42 years revealed improved outcomes with SSRIs compared with placebo (Skapinakis et al. 2016). Participants with OCD without hoarding disorder had a better treatment response than those with hoarding disorder (Bloch et al. 2014).

There are also no known randomized, placebo-controlled trials for PTSD in older adults. In a 2016 meta-analysis (mean age range 28–60 years), fluoxetine, sertraline, paroxetine, and mirtazapine outperformed placebo (Gu et al. 2016). In a study of older adult male veterans, prazosin, a central-acting α_1-adrenergic receptor antagonist that decreases noradrenergic outflow, was effective in the management of nightmares at a mean dosage of 5.1 mg/day (Khaw and Argo 2020). In older adults, noradrenergic outflow is often increased, which may necessitate higher-than-typical dosages of prazosin to target symptoms. However, given the risk of developing hypotension, older adults taking prazosin require blood pressure monitoring at both initiation and during dosage titration.

In January 2019, the American Geriatrics Society published its third iteration of the Beers criteria for potentially inappropriate medication use in older adults (2019 American Geriatrics Society Beers Criteria Update Expert Panel 2019). These criteria are intended to provide pharmacological guidance for the treatment of adults older than 65 years in various settings, including those in ambulatory, institutionalized, and acute care settings. Benzodiazepines, which were traditionally used to manage anxiety disorders in older adults, received a "strong avoid" recommendation because of the risk of cognitive impairment, falls, fractures, delirium, and motor vehicle accidents associated with their use. Additionally, paroxetine has been cited as a highly anticholinergic antidepressant that can cause orthostatic hypotension and sedation. In patients with a history of falls and fractures, all SSRIs, SNRIs, and TCAs were noted to elevate the risk of future falls, with a strong recommendation to avoid their use or, in cases in which their use is necessary, to consider reducing other CNS medications and implementing additional strategies to reduce fall risk. Antihistamines, including diphenhydramine, which are often prescribed for insomnia and anxiety, carry a heightened risk of constipation, dry mouth, and confusion and thereby also received a "strong avoid" recommendation in older adults.

Few studies have compared the efficacy of psychotherapy with that of medication for anxiety in older adults. Health care providers should engage in shared decision-making with older adult patients to determine whether medications, psychotherapy, or stepped or collaborative care is the optimal strategy for treatment.

Clinical Management

The initial approach to caring for older patients with anxiety disorders is like that for other mental health disorders. First, clinicians should strive to create a therapeutic alliance with patients by asking open-ended questions and listening intently, using both verbal and nonverbal cues to indicate active engagement. Clinicians should assess the duration and severity of the anxiety symptoms, their impact on daily functioning, triggers for symptoms, and factors that may mitigate against symptoms. It can be helpful to ask patients, "Why now?" to determine the reason for making the appointment at this time versus some other point in the past. As always, a complete psychiatric review of systems is paramount to determine if comorbid mental health issues are present that may impact therapeutic and pharmacological intervention. Once this information has been collected from the patient, any collateral history from the patient's loved ones, nursing home staff, neighbors, providers, and other close contacts may contribute to the story. Contiguous with data collection, clinicians should complete a thorough chart review, including identifying medical issues that may contribute to their patient's presentation, medications that could cause or exacerbate the presentation (with a focus on the temporal relationship of the anxiety to medication changes), and a history of prior medical trials (if relevant) for mental health disorders. Review of prior medication trials should include both dosage and duration of pharmacological interventions, as well as the reason for discontinuation (e.g., side effects, compliance, cost).

Treatment interventions for older patients with anxiety disorders often involve a multimodal approach that includes psychotherapy, psychopharmacology, and an increase in psychosocial support. Psychosocial support may include recommendations to attend senior centers or adult day care, engagement in an exercise or mindfulness regimen, suggestions for volunteer opportunities, participation in support groups, or a myriad of other opportunities available in the local community.

Conclusion

Some older adults with anxiety disorders do not receive full benefit from or do not have access to evidence-based psychotherapy and pharmacotherapy. Thus, innovative approaches, including adapting or augmenting content, and flexibility in administration (e.g., home visits, telehealth, brief, high-intensity CBT) or alternative delivery options (e.g., brief, low-intensity self-help such as bibliotherapy, internet-delivered CBT bibliotherapy, or e-health) are needed. There is some enthusiasm regarding mindfulness or third-wave behavior therapies, which usually combine elements of meditation, yoga, and acceptance. A recent review (Hazlett-Stevens et al. 2019) found seven RCTs of either mindfulness-based stress reduction or mindfulness-based cognitive therapy conducted entirely with older adults (e.g., Lenze et al. 2014). This work indicated that mindfulness is a promising intervention for older adults experiencing various health concerns (e.g., low back pain, insomnia) and possibly even memory and executive functioning concerns. One trial in this review found that mindfulness-based cognitive therapy effectively reduced symptoms of anxiety, but not depression, in older individuals. Furthermore, preliminary findings from a small pilot study indicated that mindfulness-based stress reduction may be effective in older adults with clinical worry symptoms and co-occurring cognitive dysfunction (Lenze et al. 2014).

Being flexible in how and where the interventions are administered and finding alternative delivery options as needed appear to be wonderful approaches to assisting older adults with anxiety in late life. For example, in an ethnically diverse, medically frail sample of rural, older adults, home-delivered CBT for depression resulted in significantly greater improvements in symptoms of anxiety and phobic anxiety (DiNapoli et al. 2017). Early e-health approaches, such as computerized therapies, and newer methods, including smartphone applications and virtual reality interventions, hold promise (Firth et al. 2018). Mental health interventions for people with mild cognitive impairment or dementia have also become a growing focus of research. Several studies have indicated a positive impact on depression in older adults with early dementia using problem solving and modified CBT as well as other as environmental strategies (Regan and Varanelli 2013). Relatively little of this work has focused on older adults with significant levels of anxiety.

Advances are needed for older adults who do not have access to evidence-based interventions delivered in person or who do not respond to or fail to achieve remission with standard care. Due to the limited number of available studies and their small sample sizes, nonstandardization of interventions, short-term follow-ups, and high risk of bias, future investigations are needed to test the efficacy of these innovations for older adults. In addition, studies should be conducted to identify the predictors and moderators of response and mechanisms of action.

Key Points

- Anxiety disorders in older adults are relatively common and may go undetected, with resultant negative medical, psychological, and psychosocial consequences.

- A thorough evaluation for anxiety, obsessive-compulsive, and trauma-related disorders should be incorporated into mental health evaluations for all older adults.

- Late-life anxiety is frequently comorbid with other psychiatric, medical, and cognitive disorders. Pharmacological and psychotherapeutic interventions for these disorders in older adults are effective and should be implemented to manage symptoms. Health care providers should engage in shared decision-making with older adult patients when determining optimal strategies for care.

- Future research is indicated to better understand the underlying neurocircuitry associated with anxiety disorders in older populations, with the goal of more targeted and successful interventions.

References

Alaka KJ, Noble W, Montejo A, et al: Efficacy and safety of duloxetine in the treatment of older adult patients with generalized anxiety disorder: a randomized, double-blind, placebo-controlled trial. Int J Geriatr Psychiatry 29(9):978–986, 2014 24644106

Alexopoulos GS, Katz IR, Bruce ML, et al: Remission in depressed geriatric primary care patients: a report from the PROSPECT study. Am J Psychiatry 162(4):718–724, 2005 15800144

Allgulander C, Lavori PW: Causes of death among 936 elderly patients with 'pure' anxiety neurosis in Stockholm County, Sweden, and in patients with depressive neurosis or both diagnoses. Compr Psychiatry 34(5):299–302, 1993 8306638

Altunoz U, Kokurcan A, Kirici S, et al: Clinical characteristics of generalized anxiety disorder: older vs. young adults. Nord J Psychiatry 72(2):97–102, 2018 29065768

American Psychiatric Association: Diagnostic and Statistical Manual of Mental Disorders, 3rd Edition. Washington, DC, American Psychiatric Association, 1980

American Psychiatric Association: Diagnostic and Statistical Manual of Mental Disorders, 3rd Edition, Revised. Washington, DC, American Psychiatric Association, 1987

American Psychiatric Association: Diagnostic and Statistical Manual of Mental Disorders, 4th Edition. Washington, DC, American Psychiatric Association, 1994

American Psychiatric Association: Diagnostic and Statistical Manual of Mental Disorders, 5th Edition. Arlington, VA, American Psychiatric Association, 2013

Andreescu C, Varon D: New research on anxiety disorders in the elderly and an update on evidence-based treatments. Curr Psychiatry Rep 17(7):53, 2015 25980510

Andreescu C, Lenze EJ, Dew MA, et al: Effect of comorbid anxiety on treatment response and relapse risk in late-life depression: controlled study. Br J Psychiatry 190:344–349, 2007 17401042

Aström M: Generalized anxiety disorder in stroke patients: a 3-year longitudinal study. Stroke 27(2):270–275, 1996 8571422

Ayers CR, Saxena S, Golshan S, Wetherell JL: Age at onset and clinical features of late life compulsive hoarding. Int J Geriatr Psychiatry 25(2):142–149, 2010 19548272

Ayers CR, Wetherell JL, Schiehser D, et al: Executive functioning in older adults with hoarding disorder. Int J Geriatr Psychiatry 28(11):1175–1181, 2013 23440720

Ayers CR, Iqbal Y, Strickland K: Medical conditions in geriatric hoarding disorder patients. Aging Ment Health 18(2):148–151, 2014a 23863040

Ayers CR, Ly P, Howard I, et al: Hoarding severity predicts functional disability in late-life hoarding disorder patients. Int J Geriatr Psychiatry 29(7):741–746, 2014b 24343998

Ayers CR, Najmi S, Mayes TL, Dozier ME: Hoarding disorder in older adulthood. Am J Geriatr Psychiatry 23(4):416–422, 2015 24953872

Balasubramaniam M, Joshi P, Alag P, et al: Antidepressants for anxiety disorders in late-life: a systematic review. Ann Clin Psychiatry 31(4):277–291, 2019 31369663

Bandelow B, Baldwin D, Abelli M, et al: Biological markers for anxiety disorders, OCD and PTSD: a consensus statement, part II: neurochemistry, neurophysiology and neurocognition. World J Biol Psychiatry 18(3):162–214, 2017 27419272

Bartels SJ, Coakley E, Oxman TE, et al: Suicidal and death ideation in older primary care patients with depression, anxiety, and at-risk alcohol use. Am J Geriatr Psychiatry 10(4):417–427, 2002 12095901

Beekman AT, Bremmer MA, Deeg DJ, et al: Anxiety disorders in later life: a report from the Longitudinal Aging Study Amsterdam. Int J Geriatr Psychiatry 13(10):717–726, 1998 9818308

Beekman AT, de Beurs E, van Balkom AJ, et al: Anxiety and depression in later life: co-occurrence and communality of risk factors. Am J Psychiatry 157(1):89–95, 2000 10618018

Benjet C, Bromet E, Karam EG, et al: The epidemiology of traumatic event exposure worldwide: results from the World Mental Health Survey Consortium. Psychol Med 46(2):327–343, 2016 26511595

Benzina N, Mallet L, Burguière E, et al: Cognitive dysfunction in obsessive-compulsive disorder. Curr Psychiatry Rep 18(9):80, 2016 27423459

Blank S, Lenze EJ, Mulsant BH, et al: Outcomes of late-life anxiety disorders during 32 weeks of citalopram treatment. J Clin Psychiatry 67(3):468–472, 2006 16649835

Bloch MH, Bartley CA, Zipperer L, et al: Meta-analysis: hoarding symptoms associated with poor treatment outcome in obsessive-compulsive disorder. Mol Psychiatry 19(9):1025–1030, 2014 24912494

Bolognesi F, Baldwin DS, Ruini C: Psychological interventions in the treatment of generalized anxiety disorder: a structured review. Ital J Psychopath 20:111–126, 2014

Braam AW, Copeland JRM, Delespaul PAEG, et al: Depression, subthreshold depression and comorbid anxiety symptoms in older Europeans: results from the EURODEP concerted action. J Affect Disord 155:266–272, 2014

Breitenfeld T, Jurasic MJ, Breitenfeld D: Hippocrates: the forefather of neurology. Neurol Sci 35(9):1349–1352, 2014 25027011

Brenes GA, Miller ME, Stanley MA, et al: Insomnia in older adults with generalized anxiety disorder. Am J Geriatr Psychiatry 17(6):465–472, 2009 19472436

Brenes GA, Danhauer SC, Lyles MF, et al: Telephone-delivered cognitive behavioral therapy and telephone-delivered nondirective supportive therapy for rural older adults with generalized anxiety disorder: a randomized clinical trial. JAMA Psychiatry 72(10):1012–1020, 2015 26244854

Brenes GA, Danhauer SC, Lyles MF, et al: Long-term effects of telephone-delivered psychotherapy for late-life GAD. Am J Geriatr Psychiatry 25(11):1249–1257, 2017 28673741

Byers AL, Yaffe K, Covinsky KE, et al: High occurrence of mood and anxiety disorders among older adults: the National Comorbidity Survey Replication. Arch Gen Psychiatry 67(5):489–496, 2010 20439830

Cairney J, McCabe L, Veldhuizen S, et al: Epidemiology of social phobia in later life. Am J Geriatr Psychiatry 15(3):224–233, 2007 17213375

Cairney J, Corna LM, Veldhuizen S, et al: Comorbid depression and anxiety in later life: patterns of association, subjective well-being, and impairment. Am J Geriatr Psychiatry 16(3):201–208, 2008 18310551

Canuto A, Weber K, Baertschi M, et al: Anxiety disorders in old age: psychiatric comorbidities, quality of life, and prevalence according to age, gender, and country. Am J Geriatr Psychiatry 26(2):174–185, 2018 29031568

Chacko RC, Corbin MA, Harper RG: Acquired obsessive-compulsive disorder associated with basal ganglia lesions. J Neuropsychiatry Clin Neurosci 12(2):269–272, 2000 11001608

Chou KL: Specific phobia in older adults: evidence from the national epidemiologic survey on alcohol and related conditions. Am J Geriatr Psychiatry 17(5):376–386, 2009 19390295

Chou KL: Panic disorder in older adults: evidence from the National Epidemiologic Survey on Alcohol and Related Conditions. Int J Geriatr Psychiatry 25(8):822–832, 2010 19946867

Corna LM, Cairney J, Herrmann N, et al: Panic disorder in later life: results from a national survey of Canadians. Int Psychogeriatr 19(6):1084–1096, 2007 17367554

Correa JK, Brown TA: Expression of generalized anxiety disorder across the lifespan. J Psychopathol Behav Assess 41(1):53–59, 2019 31938010

Crocco EA, Jaramillo S, Cruz-Ortiz C, Camfield K: Pharmacological management of anxiety disorders in the elderly. Curr Treat Options Psychiatry 4(1):33–46, 2017 28948135

Cummings JL: The Neuropsychiatric Inventory: assessing psychopathology in dementia patients. Neurology 48(5 suppl 6):S10–S16, 1997 9153155

Davidson J, Allgulander C, Pollack MH, et al: Efficacy and tolerability of duloxetine in elderly patients with generalized anxiety disorder: a pooled analysis of four randomized, double-blind, placebo-controlled studies. Hum Psychopharmacol 23(6):519–526, 2008 18478624

de Bruijn RFAG, Direk N, Mirza SS, et al: Anxiety is not associated with the risk of dementia or cognitive decline: the Rotterdam Study. Am J Geriatr Psychiatry 22(12):1382–1390, 2014 24745561

de Kloet CS, Vermetten E, Geuze E, et al: Assessment of HPA-axis function in posttraumatic stress disorder: pharmacological and non-pharmacological challenge tests, a review. J Psychiatr Res 40(6):550–567, 2006 16214171

Dell'Osso B, Benatti B, Rodriguez CI, et al: Obsessive-compulsive disorder in the elderly: a report from the International College of Obsessive-Compulsive Spectrum Disorders (ICOCS). Eur Psychiatry 45:36–40, 2017 28728093

DeLuca AK, Lenze EJ, Mulsant BH, et al: Comorbid anxiety disorder in late life depression: association with memory decline over four years. Int J Geriatr Psychiatry 20(9):848–854, 2005 16116585

Denkinger MD, Lukas A, Nikolaus T, Hauer K: Factors associated with fear of falling and associated activity restriction in community-dwelling older adults: a systematic review. Am J Geriatr Psychiatry 23(1):72–86, 2015 24745560

Deptula D, Singh R, Pomara N: Aging, emotional states, and memory. Am J Psychiatry 150(3):429–434, 1993 8434658

Devier DJ, Pelton GH, Tabert MH, et al: The impact of anxiety on conversion from mild cognitive impairment to Alzheimer's disease. Int J Geriatr Psychiatry 24(12):1335–1342, 2009 19319929

Diefenbach GJ, DiMauro J, Frost R, et al: Characteristics of hoarding in older adults. Am J Geriatr Psychiatry 21(10):1043–1047, 2013 23567383

DiNapoli EA, Pierpaoli CM, Shah A, et al: Effects of home-delivered cognitive behavioral therapy (CBT) for depression on anxiety symptoms among rural, ethnically diverse older adults. Clin Gerontol 40(3):181–190, 2017 28452665

Dinnen S, Simiola V, Cook JM: Post-traumatic stress disorder in older adults: a systematic review of the psychotherapy treatment literature. Aging Ment Health 19(2):144–150, 2015 24898218

Dissanayaka NN, Sellbach A, Matheson S, et al: Anxiety disorders in Parkinson's disease: prevalence and risk factors. Mov Disord 25(7):838–845, 2010 20461800

Ducasse D, Boyer L, Michel P, et al: D2 and D3 dopamine receptor affinity predicts effectiveness of antipsychotic drugs in obsessive-compulsive disorders: a metaregression analysis. Psychopharmacology (Berl) 231(18):3765–3770, 2014 24599398

Dunsmoor JE, Paz R: Fear generalization and anxiety: behavioral and neural mechanisms. Biol Psychiatry 78(5):336–343, 2015 25981173

El-Gabalawy R, Mackenzie CS, Shooshtari S, Sareen J: Comorbid physical health conditions and anxiety disorders: a population-based exploration of prevalence and health outcomes among older adults. Gen Hosp Psychiatry 33(6):556–564, 2011 21908055

El-Gabalawy R, Mackenzie CS, Pietrzak RH, Sareen J: A longitudinal examination of anxiety disorders and physical health conditions in a nationally representative sample of U.S. older adults. Exp Gerontol 60:46–56, 2014 25245888

Firth J, Torous J, Carney R, et al: Digital technologies in the treatment of anxiety: recent innovations and future directions. Curr Psychiatry Rep 20(6):44, 2018 29779065

Flatt JD, Gilsanz P, Quesenberry CP Jr, et al: Post-traumatic stress disorder and risk of dementia among members of a health care delivery system. Alzheimers Dement 14(1):28–34, 2018 28627380

Flint AJ: Epidemiology and comorbidity of anxiety disorders in the elderly. Am J Psychiatry 151:5, 1994

Flint A, Bradwejn J, Vaccarino F, et al: Aging and panicogenic response to cholecystokinin tetrapeptide: an examination of the cholecystokinin system. Neuropsychopharmacology 27(4):663–671, 2002 12377403

Gallagher D, Coen R, Kilroy D, et al: Anxiety and behavioural disturbance as markers of prodromal Alzheimer's disease in patients with mild cognitive impairment. Int J Geriatr Psychiatry 26(2):166–172, 2011 21229599

Golden J, Conroy RM, Bruce I, et al: The spectrum of worry in the community-dwelling elderly. Aging Ment Health 15(8):985–994, 2011 21749221

Gonçalves DC, Pachana NA, Byrne GJ: Prevalence and correlates of generalized anxiety disorder among older adults in the Australian National Survey of Mental Health and Well-Being. J Affect Disord 132(1–2):223–230, 2011 21429587

Gould CE, O'Hara R, Goldstein MK, Beaudreau SA: Multimorbidity is associated with anxiety in older adults in the Health and Retirement Study. Int J Geriatr Psychiatry 31(10):1105–1115, 2016 27441851

Graeff FG, Zangrossi H Jr: The dual role of serotonin in defense and the mode of action of antidepressants on generalized anxiety and panic disorders. Cent Nerv Syst Agents Med Chem 10(3):207–217, 2010 20528764

Green D: Hippocrates, Plato and neurology. NY State J Med 73(8):957–967, 1973 4511924

Grenier S, Schuurmans J, Goldfarb M, et al: The epidemiology of specific phobia and subthreshold fear subtypes in a community-based sample of older adults. Depress Anxiety 28(6):456–463, 2011 21400642

Gu W, Wang C, Li Z, et al: Pharmacotherapies for posttraumatic stress disorder: a meta-analysis. J Nerv Ment Dis 204(5):331–338, 2016 26894318

Gulpers B, Ramakers I, Hamel R, et al: Anxiety as a predictor for cognitive decline and dementia: a systematic review and meta-analysis. Am J Geriatr Psychiatry 24(10):823–842, 2016 27591161

Gum AM, Petkus A, McDougal SJ, et al: Behavioral health needs and problem recognition by older adults receiving home-based aging services. Int J Geriatr Psychiatry 24(4):400–408, 2009 18836987

Hall J, Kellett S, Berrios R, et al: Efficacy of cognitive behavioral therapy for generalized anxiety disorder in older adults: systematic review, meta-analysis, and meta-regression. Am J Geriatr Psychiatry 24(11):1063–1073, 2016 27687212

Hazlett-Stevens H, Singer J, Chong A: Mindfulness-based stress reduction and mindfulness-based cognitive therapy with older adults: a qualitative review of randomized controlled outcome research. Clin Gerontol 42(4):347–358, 2019 30204557

Hellwig S, Domschke K: Anxiety in late life: an update on pathomechanisms. Gerontology 65(5):465–473, 2019 31212285

Hendriks GJ, Keijsers GP, Kampman M, et al: A randomized controlled study of paroxetine and cognitive-behavioural therapy for late-life panic disorder. Acta Psychiatr Scand 122(1):11–19, 2010 19958308

Hendriks GJ, Kampman M, Keijsers GPJ, et al: Cognitive-behavioral therapy for panic disorder with agoraphobia in older people: a comparison with younger patients. Depress Anxiety 31(8):669–677, 2014 24867666

Hernández E, Lastra S, Urbina M, et al: Serotonin, 5-hydroxyindoleacetic acid and serotonin transporter in blood peripheral lymphocytes of patients with generalized anxiety disorder. Int Immunopharmacol 2(7):893–900, 2002 12188031

Hilbert K, Lueken U, Beesdo-Baum K: Neural structures, functioning and connectivity in generalized anxiety disorder and interaction with neuroendocrine systems: a systematic review. J Affect Disord 158:114–126, 2014 24655775

Hogan MJ: Divided attention in older but not younger adults is impaired by anxiety. Exp Aging Res 29(2):111–136, 2003 12623724

Hohls JK, König HH, Raynik YI, Hajek A: A systematic review of the association of anxiety with health care utilization and costs in people aged 65 years and older. J Affect Disord 232:163–176, 2018 29494900

Hohls JK, Wild B, Heider D, et al: Association of generalized anxiety symptoms and panic with health care costs in older age: results from the ESTHER cohort study. J Affect Disord 245:978–986, 2019 30562680

Holloway KL, Williams LJ, Brennan-Olsen SL, et al: Anxiety disorders and falls among older adults. J Affect Disord 205:20–27, 2016 27391268

Hwang JP, Tsai SJ, Yang CH, et al: Hoarding behavior in dementia: a preliminary report. Am J Geriatr Psychiatry 6(4):285–289, 1998 9793576

Jayasinghe N, Rocha LP, Sheeran T, et al: Anxiety symptoms in older home health care recipients: prevalence and associates. Home Health Care Serv Q 32(3):163–177, 2013 23937710

Kang B, Xu H, McConnell ES: Neurocognitive and psychiatric comorbidities of posttraumatic stress disorder among older veterans: a systematic review. Int J Geriatr Psychiatry 34(4):522–538, 2019 30588665

Kariuki-Nyuthe C, Gomez-Mancilla B, Stein DJ: Obsessive compulsive disorder and the glutamatergic system. Curr Opin Psychiatry 27(1):32–37, 2014 24270485

Karlsson B, Sigström R, Östling S, et al: DSM-IV and DSM-5 prevalence of social anxiety disorder in a population sample of older people. Am J Geriatr Psychiatry 24(12):1237–1245, 2016 27720603

Katon W, Lin EH, Kroenke K: The association of depression and anxiety with medical symptom burden in patients with chronic medical illness. Gen Hosp Psychiatry 29(2):147–155, 2007 17336664

Katz IR, Reynolds CF III, Alexopoulos GS, Hackett D: Venlafaxine ER as a treatment for generalized anxiety disorder in older adults: pooled analysis of five randomized placebo-controlled clinical trials. J Am Geriatr Soc 50(1):18–25, 2002 12028242

Kessler RC, Merikangas KR: The National Comorbidity Survey Replication (NCS-R): background and aims. Int J Methods Psychiatr Res 13(2):60–68, 2004 15297904

Kessler RC, McGonagle KA, Zhao S, et al: Lifetime and 12-month prevalence of DSM-III-R psychiatric disorders in the United States: results from the National Comorbidity Survey. Arch Gen Psychiatry 51(1):8–19, 1994 8279933

Kessler RC, Berglund P, Demler O, et al: Lifetime prevalence and age-of-onset distributions of DSM-IV disorders in the National Comorbidity Survey Replication. Arch Gen Psychiatry 62(6):593–602, 2005 15939837

Khaw C, Argo T: Prazosin outcomes in older veterans with posttraumatic stress disorder. Fed Pract 37(2):72–78, 2020 32269469

Kim HJ, Steketee G, Frost RO: Hoarding by elderly people. Health Soc Work 26(3):176–184, 2001 11531193

King-Kallimanis B, Gum AM, Kohn R: Comorbidity of depressive and anxiety disorders for older Americans in the National Comorbidity Survey–Replication. Am J Geriatr Psychiatry 17(9):782–792, 2009 19700950

Klenfeldt IF, Karlsson B, Sigström R, et al: Prevalence of obsessive-compulsive disorder in relation to depression and cognition in an elderly population. Am J Geriatr Psychiatry 22(3):301–308, 2014 23567423

Klüver H, Bucy PC: "Psychic blindness" and other symptoms following bilateral temporal lobectomy in Rhesus monkeys. Am J Physiol 119:352–353, 1937

Koenen KC, Ratanatharathorn A, Ng L, et al: Posttraumatic stress disorder in the World Mental Health Surveys. Psychol Med 47(13):2260–2274, 2017 28385165

Krasucki C, Howard R, Mann A: The relationship between anxiety disorders and age. Int J Geriatr Psychiatry 13(2):79–99, 1998 9526178

Kwon JS, Jang JH, Choi J-S, Kang D-H: Neuroimaging in obsessive-compulsive disorder. Expert Rev Neurother 9(2):255–269, 2009 19210199

Laird KT, Siddarth P, Krause-Sorio B, et al: Anxiety symptoms are associated with smaller insular and orbitofrontal cortex volumes in late-life depression. J Affect Disord 256:282–287, 2019 31200165

Lambiase MJ, Kubzansky LD, Thurston RC: Prospective study of anxiety and incident stroke. Stroke 45(2):438–443, 2014 24357656

Landreville P, Gosselin P, Grenier S, et al: Guided self-help for generalized anxiety disorder in older adults. Aging Ment Health 20(10):1070–1083, 2016 26158374

Lang S, Kroll A, Lipinski SJ, et al: Context conditioning and extinction in humans: differential contribution of the hippocampus, amygdala and prefrontal cortex. Eur J Neurosci 29(4):823–832, 2009 19200075

Lavedán A, Viladrosa M, Jürschik P, et al: Fear of falling in community-dwelling older adults: a cause of falls, a consequence, or both? PLoS One 13(3):e0194967, 2018 29596521

Lenze EJ, Mulsant BH, Shear MK, et al: Comorbid anxiety disorders in depressed elderly patients. Am J Psychiatry 157(5):722–728, 2000 10784464

Lenze EJ, Mulsant BH, Mohlman J, et al: Generalized anxiety disorder in late life: lifetime course and comorbidity with major depressive disorder. Am J Geriatr Psychiatry 13(1):77–80, 2005a 15653943

Lenze EJ, Mulsant BH, Shear MK, et al: Efficacy and tolerability of citalopram in the treatment of late-life anxiety disorders: results from an 8-week randomized, placebo-controlled trial. Am J Psychiatry 162(1):146–150, 2005b 15625213

Lenze EJ, Rollman BL, Shear MK, et al: Escitalopram for older adults with generalized anxiety disorder: a randomized controlled trial. JAMA 301(3):295–303, 2009 19155456

Lenze EJ, Dixon D, Mantella RC, et al: Treatment-related alteration of cortisol predicts change in neuropsychological function during acute treatment of late-life anxiety disorder. Int J Geriatr Psychiatry 27(5):454–462, 2012 21681817

Lenze EJ, Hickman S, Hershey T, et al: Mindfulness-based stress reduction for older adults with worry symptoms and co-occurring cognitive dysfunction. Int J Geriatr Psychiatry 29(10):991–1000, 2014 24677282

Lindesay J, Baillon S, Brugha T, et al: Worry content across the lifespan: an analysis of 16- to 74-year-old participants in the British National Survey of Psychiatric Morbidity 2000. Psychol Med 36(11):1625–1633, 2006 16863599

Lyketsos CG, Lopez O, Jones B, et al: Prevalence of neuropsychiatric symptoms in dementia and mild cognitive impairment: results from the cardiovascular health study. JAMA 288(12):1475–1483, 2002 12243634

Mackenzie CS, Reynolds K, Chou KL, et al: Prevalence and correlates of generalized anxiety disorder in a national sample of older adults. Am J Geriatr Psychiatry 19(4):305–315, 2011 21427639

Mackenzie CS, El-Gabalawy R, Chou K-L, Sareen J: Prevalence and predictors of persistent versus remitting mood, anxiety, and substance disorders in a national sample of older adults. Am J Geriatr Psychiatry 22(9):854–865, 2014 23800537

Mah L, Binns MA, Steffens DC: Anxiety symptoms in amnestic mild cognitive impairment are associated with medial temporal atrophy and predict conversion to Alzheimer disease. Am J Geriatr Psychiatry 23(5):466–476, 2015 25500120

Mantella RC, Butters MA, Dew MA, et al: Cognitive impairment in late-life generalized anxiety disorder. Am J Geriatr Psychiatry 15(8):673–679, 2007 17426260

Mantella RC, Butters MA, Amico JA, et al: Salivary cortisol is associated with diagnosis and severity of late-life generalized anxiety disorder. Psychoneuroendocrinology 33(6):773–781, 2008 18407426

Martinussen LJ, Šaltyte Benth J, Almdahl IS, et al: The effect of anxiety on cognition in older adult inpatients with depression: results from a multicenter observational study. Heliyon 5(8):e02235, 2019 31497664

Marx MS, Cohen-Mansfield J: Hoarding behavior in the elderly: a comparison between community-dwelling persons and nursing home residents. Int Psychogeriatr 15(3):289–306, 2003 14756164

McCabe L, Cairney J, Veldhuizen S, et al: Prevalence and correlates of agoraphobia in older adults. Am J Geriatr Psychiatry 14(6):515–522, 2006 16731720

Miloyan B, Bulley A, Pachana NA, Byrne GJ: Social phobia symptoms across the adult lifespan. J Affect Disord 168:86–90, 2014 25043319

Mohlman J, Price RB, Eldreth DA, et al: The relation of worry to prefrontal cortex volume in older adults with and without generalized anxiety disorder. Psychiatry Res 173(2):121–127, 2009 19559575

Mohlman J, Bryant C, Lenze EJ, et al: Improving recognition of late life anxiety disorders in Diagnostic and Statistical Manual of Mental Disorders, Fifth Edition: observations and recommendations of the Advisory Committee to the Lifespan Disorders Work Group. Int J Geriatr Psychiatry 27(6):549–556, 2012 21773996

Mokhber N, Azarpazhooh MR, Khajehdaluee M, et al: Randomized, single-blind, trial of sertraline and buspirone for treatment of elderly patients with generalized anxiety disorder. Psychiatry Clin Neurosci 64(2):128–133, 2010 20132529

Nelson JC, Delucchi K, Schneider LS: Anxiety does not predict response to antidepressant treatment in late life depression: results of a meta-analysis. Int J Geriatr Psychiatry 24(5):539–544, 2009 19334041

Nikolaus S, Antke C, Beu M, Müller H-W: Cortical GABA, striatal dopamine and midbrain serotonin as the key players in compulsive and anxiety disorders: results from in vivo imaging studies. Rev Neurosci 21(2):119–139, 2010 20614802

Okura T, Langa KM: Caregiver burden and neuropsychiatric symptoms in older adults with cognitive impairment: the Aging, Demographics, and Memory Study (ADAMS). Alzheimer Dis Assoc Disord 25(2):116–121, 2011 21192239

Olaya B, Moneta MV, Miret M, Ayuso-Mateos JL, Haro JM: Epidemiology of panic attacks, panic disorder and the moderating role of age: results from a population-based study. J Affect Disord 241:627–633, 2018

O'Neill P-K, Gore F, Salzman CD: Basolateral amygdala circuitry in positive and negative valence. Curr Opin Neurobiol 49:175–183, 2018 29525574

Orgeta V, Qazi A, Spector A, Orrell M: Psychological treatments for depression and anxiety in dementia and mild cognitive impairment: systematic review and meta-analysis. Br J Psychiatry 207(4):293–298, 2015 26429684

Oude Voshaar RC, van der Veen DC, Hunt I, Kapur N: Suicide in late-life depression with and without comorbid anxiety disorders. Int J Geriatr Psychiatry 31(2):146–152, 2016 26095418

Payette MC, Bélanger C, Benyebdri F, et al: The association between generalized anxiety disorder, subthreshold anxiety symptoms and fear of falling among older adults: preliminary results from a pilot study. Clin Gerontol 40(3):197–206, 2017 28452660

Pietrzak RH, Goldstein RB, Southwick SM, Grant BF: Psychiatric comorbidity of full and partial posttraumatic stress disorder among older adults in the United States: results from wave 2 of the National Epidemiologic Survey on Alcohol and Related Conditions. Am J Geriatr Psychiatry 20(5):380–390, 2012 22522959

Porensky EK, Dew MA, Karp JF, et al: The burden of late-life generalized anxiety disorder: effects on disability, health-related quality of life, and healthcare utilization. Am J Geriatr Psychiatry 17(6):473–482, 2009 19472438

Potvin O, Catheline G, Bernard C, et al: Gray matter characteristics associated with trait anxiety in older adults are moderated by depression. Int Psychogeriatr 27(11):1813–1824, 2015 26059837

Pulular A, Levy R, Stewart R: Obsessive and compulsive symptoms in a national sample of older people: prevalence, comorbidity, and associations with cognitive function. Am J Geriatr Psychiatry 21(3):263–271, 2013 23395193

Regan B, Varanelli L: Adjustment, depression, and anxiety in mild cognitive impairment and early dementia: a systematic review of psychological intervention studies. Int Psychogeriatr 25(12):1963–1984, 2013 24125507

Regier DA, Boyd JH, Burke JD Jr, et al: One-month prevalence of mental disorders in the United States: based on five Epidemiologic Catchment Area sites. Arch Gen Psychiatry 45(11):977–986, 1988 3263101

Regier DA, Narrow WE, Rae DS: The epidemiology of anxiety disorders: the Epidemiologic Catchment Area (ECA) experience. J Psychiatr Res 24(suppl 2):3–14, 1990b 2280373

Rehm IC, Stargatt J, Willison AT, et al: Cognitive behavioral therapy for older adults with anxiety and cognitive impairment: adaptations and illustrative case study. J Cogn Psychother 31(1):72–88, 2017 32755919

Reynolds K, Pietrzak RH, Mackenzie CS, et al: Post-traumatic stress disorder across the adult lifespan: findings from a nationally representative survey. Am J Geriatr Psychiatry 24(1):81–93, 2016 26706912

Ritchie K, Norton J, Mann A, et al: Late-onset agoraphobia: general population incidence and evidence for a clinical subtype. Am J Psychiatry 170(7):790–798, 2013 23820832

Roane DM, Landers A, Sherratt J, Wilson GS: Hoarding in the elderly: a critical review of the recent literature. Int Psychogeriatr 29(7):1077–1084, 2017 28162112

Rosenberg PB, Mielke MM, Appleby BS, et al: The association of neuropsychiatric symptoms in MCI with incident dementia and Alzheimer disease. Am J Geriatr Psychiatry 21(7):685–695, 2013 23567400

Ross DA, Arbuckle MR, Travis MJ, et al: An integrated neuroscience perspective on formulation and treatment planning for posttraumatic stress disorder: an educational review. JAMA Psychiatry 74(4):407–415, 2017 28273291

Rubio G, López-Ibor JJ: Generalized anxiety disorder: a 40-year follow-up study. Acta Psychiatr Scand 115(5):372–379, 2007 17430415

Ruscio AM, Stein DJ, Chiu WT, Kessler RC: The epidemiology of obsessive-compulsive disorder in the National Comorbidity Survey Replication. Mol Psychiatry 15(1):53–63, 2010 18725912

Saade YM, Nicol G, Lenze EJ, et al: Comorbid anxiety in late-life depression: relationship with remission and suicidal ideation on venlafaxine treatment. Depress Anxiety 36(12):1125–1134, 2019 31682328

Samuels JF, Bienvenu OJ, Grados MA, et al: Prevalence and correlates of hoarding behavior in a community-based sample. Behav Res Ther 46(7):836–844, 2008 18495084

Scheffer AC, Schuurmans MJ, van Dijk N, et al: Fear of falling: measurement strategy, prevalence, risk factors and consequences among older persons. Age Ageing 37(1):19–24, 2008 18194967

Schienle A, Ebner F, Schäfer A: Localized gray matter volume abnormalities in generalized anxiety disorder. Eur Arch Psychiatry Clin Neurosci 261(4):303–307, 2011 20820793

Schoevers RA, Beekman AT, Deeg DJ, et al: Comorbidity and risk-patterns of depression, generalised anxiety disorder and mixed anxiety-depression in later life: results from the AMSTEL study. Int J Geriatr Psychiatry 18(11):994–1001, 2003 14618550

Schuitevoerder S, Rosen JW, Twamley EW, et al: A meta-analysis of cognitive functioning in older adults with PTSD. J Anxiety Disord 27(6):550–558, 2013 23422492

Schuurmans J, Comijs H, Emmelkamp PM, et al: A randomized, controlled trial of the effectiveness of cognitive-behavioral therapy and sertraline versus a waitlist control group for anxiety disorders in older adults. Am J Geriatr Psychiatry 14(3):255–263, 2006 16505130

Schuurmans J, Comijs H, Emmelkamp PM, et al: Long-term effectiveness and prediction of treatment outcome in cognitive behavioral therapy and sertraline for late-life anxiety disorders. Int Psychogeriatr 21(6):1148–1159, 2009 19860993

Scott T, Mackenzie CS, Chipperfield JG, Sareen J: Mental health service use among Canadian older adults with anxiety disorders and clinically significant anxiety symptoms. Aging Ment Health 14(7):790–800, 2010 20635231

Seeley WW, Menon V, Schatzberg AF, et al: Dissociable intrinsic connectivity networks for sa-lience processing and executive control. J Neurosci 27(9):2349–2356, 2007 17329432

Sheikh JI, Swales PJ: Treatment of panic disorder in older adults: a pilot study comparison of alprazolam, imipramine, and placebo. Int J Psychiatry Med 29(1):107–117, 1999 10376237

Sheikh JI, Swales PJ, Carlson EB, Lindley SE: Aging and panic disorder: phenomenology, co-morbidity, and risk factors. Am J Geriatr Psychiatry 12(1):102–109, 2004 14729565

Sigström R, Skoog I, Karlsson B, et al: Nine-year follow-up of specific phobia in a population sample of older people. Depress Anxiety 33(4):339–346, 2016 26645153

Simning A, Seplaki CL: Association of the cumulative burden of late-life anxiety and depressive symptoms with functional impairment. Int J Geriatr Psychiatry 35(1):80–90, 2020 31650615

Skapinakis P, Caldwell DM, Hollingworth W, et al: Pharmacological and psychotherapeutic in-terventions for management of obsessive-compulsive disorder in adults: a systematic re-view and network meta-analysis. Lancet Psychiatry 3(8):730–739, 2016 27318812

Slachevsky A, Muñoz-Neira C, Nuñez-Huasaf J, et al: Late-onset cinephilia and compulsive be-haviors: harbingers of frontotemporal dementia. Prim Care Companion CNS Disord 13(3):e1–e7, 2011 21977365

Snowdon J, Halliday G: A study of severe domestic squalor: 173 cases referred to an old age psychiatry service. Int Psychogeriatr 23(2):308–314, 2011 20678298

Stanley MA, Wilson NL, Amspoker AB, et al: Lay providers can deliver effective cognitive be-havior therapy for older adults with generalized anxiety disorder: a randomized trial. De-press Anxiety 31(5):391–401, 2014 24577847

Starkstein SE, Jorge R, Petracca G, Robinson RG: The construct of generalized anxiety disorder in Alzheimer disease. Am J Geriatr Psychiatry 15(1):42–49, 2007 17194814

Steele C, Rovner B, Chase GA, Folstein M: Psychiatric symptoms and nursing home placement of patients with Alzheimer's disease. Am J Psychiatry 147(8):1049–1051, 1990 2375439

Stein DJ, Costa DLC, Lochner C, et al: Obsessive-compulsive disorder. Nat Rev Dis Primers 5(1):52, 2019 31371720

Steketee G, Schmalisch CS, Dierberger A, et al: Symptoms and history of hoarding in older adults. J Obsessive Compuls Relat Disord 1(1):1–7, 2012

Streiner DL, Cairney J, Veldhuizen S: The epidemiology of psychological problems in the el-derly. Can J Psychiatry 51(3):185–191, 2006 16618010

Taylor S: Molecular genetics of obsessive-compulsive disorder: a comprehensive meta-analysis of genetic association studies. Mol Psychiatry 18(7):799–805, 2013 22665263

Therrien Z, Hunsley J: Assessment of anxiety in older adults: a systematic review of commonly used measures. Aging Ment Health 16(1):1–16, 2012 21838650

Thorp SR, Glassman LH, Wells SY, et al: A randomized controlled trial of prolonged exposure therapy versus relaxation training for older veterans with military-related PTSD. J Anxiety Disord 64:45–54, 2019 30978622

Timpano KR, Exner C, Glaesmer H, et al: The epidemiology of the proposed DSM-5 hoarding disorder: exploration of the acquisition specifier, associated features, and distress. J Clin Psychiatry 72(6):780–786, quiz 878–879, 2011 21733479

Tischler L, Hobson S: Fear of falling: a qualitative study among community-dwelling older adults. Phys Occup Ther Geriatr 23:37–53, 2005

Tolin DF, Meunier SA, Frost RO, Steketee G: Course of compulsive hoarding and its relation-ship to life events. Depress Anxiety 27(9):829–838, 2010 20336803

Trollor JN, Anderson TM, Sachdev PS, et al: Prevalence of mental disorders in the elderly: the Australian National Mental Health and Well-Being Survey. Am J Geriatr Psychiatry 15(6):455–466, 2007 17545446

Tschanz JT, Corcoran CD, Schwartz S, et al: Progression of cognitive, functional, and neuropsy-chiatric symptom domains in a population cohort with Alzheimer dementia: the Cache County Dementia Progression study. Am J Geriatr Psychiatry 19(6):532–542, 2011 21606896

Tully PJ, Cosh SM, Baune BT: A review of the affects of worry and generalized anxiety disorder upon cardiovascular health and coronary heart disease. Psychol Health Med 18(6):627–644, 2013 23324073

2019 American Geriatrics Society Beers Criteria Update Expert Panel: American Geriatrics Society 2019 updated AGS Beers criteria for potentially inappropriate medication use in older adults. J Am Geriatr Soc 67(4):674–694, 2019 30693946

van den Heuvel OA, van Wingen G, Soriano-Mas C, et al: Brain circuitry of compulsivity. Eur Neuropsychopharmacol 26(5):810–827, 2016 26711687

van der Aa HP, Comijs HC, Penninx BW, et al: Major depressive and anxiety disorders in visually impaired older adults. Invest Ophthalmol Vis Sci 56(2):849–854, 2015 25604690

van der Veen DC, van Zelst WH, Schoevers RA, et al: Comorbid anxiety disorders in late-life depression: results of a cohort study. Int Psychogeriatr 27(7):1157–1165, 2015 25370017

van Velzen LS, Vriend C, de Wit SJ, van den Heuvel OA: Response inhibition and interference control in obsessive-compulsive spectrum disorders. Front Hum Neurosci 8:419, 2014 24966828

Wadsworth LP, Lorius N, Donovan NJ, et al: Neuropsychiatric symptoms and global functional impairment along the Alzheimer's continuum. Dement Geriatr Cogn Disord 34(2):96–111, 2012 22922821

Weiss AP, Jenike MA: Late-onset obsessive-compulsive disorder: a case series. J Neuropsychiatry Clin Neurosci 12(2):265–268, 2000 11001607

Wetherell JL, Thorp SR, Patterson TL, et al: Quality of life in geriatric generalized anxiety disorder: a preliminary investigation. J Psychiatr Res 38(3):305–312, 2004 15003436

Wetherell JL, Petkus AJ, White KS, et al: Antidepressant medication augmented with cognitive-behavioral therapy for generalized anxiety disorder in older adults. Am J Psychiatry 170(7):782–789, 2013 23680817

Wetherell JL, Bower ES, Johnson K, et al: Integrated exposure therapy and exercise reduces fear of falling and avoidance in older adults: a randomized pilot study. Am J Geriatr Psychiatry 26(8):849–859, 2018 29754811

Wuthrich VM, Frei J: Barriers to treatment for older adults seeking psychological therapy. Int Psychogeriatr 27(7):1227–1236, 2015 25739459

Wuthrich VM, Rapee RM, Kangas M, Perini S: Randomized controlled trial of group cognitive behavioral therapy compared to a discussion group for co-morbid anxiety and depression in older adults. Psychol Med 46(4):785–795, 2016 26498268

Yaffe K, Fox P, Newcomer R, et al: Patient and caregiver characteristics and nursing home placement in patients with dementia. JAMA 287(16):2090–2097, 2002 11966383

Yaffe K, Vittinghoff E, Lindquist K, et al: Posttraumatic stress disorder and risk of dementia among US veterans. Arch Gen Psychiatry 67(6):608–613, 2010 20530010

Zhang X, Norton J, Carrière I, et al: Generalized anxiety in community-dwelling elderly: prevalence and clinical characteristics. J Affect Disord 172:24–29, 2015a 25451391

Zhang X, Norton J, Carrière I, et al: Risk factors for late-onset generalized anxiety disorder: results from a 12-year prospective cohort (the ESPRIT study). Transl Psychiatry 5(3):e536, 2015b 25826111

Zhao Q-F, Tan L, Wang H-F, et al: The prevalence of neuropsychiatric symptoms in Alzheimer's disease: systematic review and meta-analysis. J Affect Disord 190:264–271, 2016 26540080

CHAPTER 13

Somatic Symptom and Related Disorders

Marc Agronin, M.D.

The somatic symptom and related disorders comprise a heterogeneous group of psychiatric illnesses characterized by prominent physical symptoms or complaints associated with significant distress and impairment. Their conceptualization under the category of somatoform disorders in DSM-IV and DSM-IV-TR (American Psychiatric Association 1994, 2000) required that these presentations lack objective organic causes, often labeled in the literature as "medically unexplained symptoms." This requirement was deleted in DSM-5 (American Psychiatric Association 2013), largely because somatic symptoms often do have related medical conditions. Even when such associations have not been established, the belief that they are not present has often led to patients being labeled in pejorative ways, as though they are faking symptoms or are somehow responsible for their own suffering.

The seven disorders encompassed in the DSM-5 category of somatic symptom and related disorders are somatic symptom disorder, illness anxiety disorder, conversion disorder (functional neurological symptom disorder), psychological factors affecting other medical conditions, factitious disorder, other specified somatic symptom and related disorder, and unspecified somatic symptom and related disorder. DSM-IV disorders that are subsumed under this new nomenclature include somatization disorder, undifferentiated somatoform disorder, hypochondriasis, pain disorder, and factitious disorders (which appeared in their own separate category in DSM-IV). Body dysmorphic disorder is not included in the DSM-5 somatic symptom disorder category and is now classified with the obsessive-compulsive and related disorders.

Prevalence rates in the literature for what were previously labeled somatoform disorders vary by diagnosis, but in general and across ages these disorders have been seen in 16% of primary care outpatients and in 23% of outpatients with medically unexplained symptoms (de Waal et al. 2004; Smith et al. 2005). One review found that the prevalence of DSM-IV somatoform disorders decreased from a range of 10.7%–26.8%

(median 15.3%) in patients younger than 65 years to 1.5%–13% (median 5.4%) in those older than 65 years (Hilderink et al. 2013). Medical symptoms in general that elude diagnosis are common, seen in up to 36% of patients in one study (Rosendal et al. 2015). A comparison of DSM-IV and DSM-5 diagnoses in a sample of patients suggested that prevalence rates are similar across the old and new nomenclatures (Voigt et al. 2012).

Older individuals with the somatic symptom and related disorders are seen in all health care settings, where they frequently overuse medical services and overburden general practitioners (de Waal et al. 2008; Puri and Dimsdale 2011). They often come to the attention of a geriatric psychiatrist after another clinician has attempted unsuccessfully to resolve their physical symptoms. To date, these disorders have not been well studied in late life, in part because many of them tend to begin during early adulthood. In addition, research involving older cohorts has usually focused on reported somatic symptoms rather than on specific diagnoses. A complicating factor is that somatoform symptoms in late life are often obscured by comorbid physical and psychiatric illnesses. These disorders have been seen in association with depression, anxiety, psychological trauma, substance use disorder, and personality disorders (de Waal et al. 2004; Haftgoli et al. 2010; Hanssen et al. 2016; Hasin and Katz 2007; Sack et al. 2007; Tomenson et al. 2012).

Clinical Features

Prominent somatic symptoms that cause significant distress and impairment are commonly seen in outpatient settings. A somatic symptom disorder is more likely when these symptoms shift from transient expressions of somatic concern to more serious bodily preoccupation and impairment and begin to cause excessive emotional or behavioral responses that are out of proportion to what would be expected. Somatic symptoms are experienced by the affected individual as real physical sensations, pain, or discomfort, usually indistinguishable from symptoms of actual medical disorders and frequently coexisting with them. Associated psychological factors are presumed but not always apparent, and patients vary in their degree of insight into such factors. In many but not all cases, no clear organic causes emerge from appropriate workup. Three important factors associated with all of the disorders in this class are high sensitivity to somatic sensations and pain; catastrophizing, in which there are excessive and unrealistic fears regarding one's health status; and excess functional disability associated with the symptoms (Bortz 2008; Egloff et al. 2014).

Patients with somatic symptom and related disorders are often able to accept that their symptoms may be functional and have psychological roots. Unlike malingering, however, the disorders in this class do not represent intentional, conscious attempts by patients to present physical symptoms to achieve a specific goal (e.g., to get out of work). In DSM-IV, somatoform disorders were classified separately from factitious disorders such as Munchausen syndrome because the etiologies of the former were considered wholly unconscious and not always aimed at assuming the sick role. (As noted in the introduction to this chapter, factitious disorder now falls under that somatic symptom and related disorders.) Somatic symptom and related disorders are not characterized by delusional thinking as found in psychotic states. They differ from psychosomatic disorders, which are characterized by actual disease states with presumed psychological triggers.

Specific Somatic Symptom and Related Disorders

The somatic symptom and related disorder diagnoses of primary relevance to older patients that are described in this section are somatic symptom disorder, illness anxiety disorder, and conversion disorder. The DSM-IV diagnoses of pain disorder and undifferentiated somatoform disorder are subsumed under the DSM-5 diagnosis of somatic symptom disorder (with the specifier "with predominant pain" appended in the case of pain disorder). Body dysmorphic disorder is no longer considered a somatic symptom disorder and, like factitious disorder, is rare in elderly patients. Neither is discussed in this chapter.

Somatic Symptom Disorder

Somatic symptom disorder in DSM-5 (Box 13–1) replaces somatization disorder, which was characterized by multiple physical complaints in excess of what would be expected given the patient's history and examination findings. In somatization disorder, the patient's complaints could not be fully explained by medical workup and had to include pain at four or more sites, two gastrointestinal symptoms, one sexual symptom, and one pseudoneurological symptom (other than pain). A term previously used in the literature for this disorder was *Briquet's syndrome* (Liskow et al. 1986). In contrast, DSM-5 somatic symptom disorder is characterized by one or more somatic symptoms that are distressing or significantly disruptive to daily life and are accompanied by excessive thoughts, feelings, or behaviors related to the symptoms. In an older person, localized pain or diffuse discomfort may be the main physical symptom but must be accompanied by persistent high levels of anxiety and excessive time and energy devoted to it.

Box 13–1.   DSM-5 Diagnostic Criteria for Somatic Symptom Disorder

A. One or more somatic symptoms that are distressing or result in significant disruption of daily life.
B. Excessive thoughts, feelings, or behaviors related to the somatic symptoms or associated health concerns as manifested by at least one of the following:

1. Disproportionate and persistent thoughts about the seriousness of one's symptoms.
2. Persistently high level of anxiety about health or symptoms.
3. Excessive time and energy devoted to these symptoms or health concerns.

C. Although any one somatic symptom may not be continuously present, the state of being symptomatic is persistent (typically more than 6 months).

Specify if:
   With predominant pain (previously pain disorder): This specifier is for individuals whose somatic symptoms predominantly involve pain.

Specify if:
   Persistent: A persistent course is characterized by severe symptoms, marked impairment, and long duration (more than 6 months).

Specify current severity:
   Mild: Only one of the symptoms specified in Criterion B is fulfilled.
   Moderate: Two or more of the symptoms specified in Criterion B are fulfilled.

Severe: Two or more of the symptoms specified in Criterion B are fulfilled, plus there are multiple somatic complaints (or one very severe somatic symptom).

Source. Reprinted from American Psychiatric Association: *Diagnostic and Statistical Manual of Mental Disorders*, 5th Edition. Arlington, VA, American Psychiatric Association, 2013, p. 311. Used with permission. Copyright © 2013 American Psychiatric Association.

Symptoms of DSM-IV somatization disorder were postulated to begin before age 30 and to persist for years by the time of diagnosis. The disorder was diagnosed almost exclusively in females, with prevalence rates ranging from <1% to 3% (Faravelli et al. 1997; Rabinowitz et al. 2011). High rates of the disorder have been noted in first-degree female relatives of affected individuals and in certain medical conditions. For example, definite or probable somatization disorder was diagnosed in 42% of a sample of 50 medical outpatients with irritable bowel disease (Miller et al. 2001). Associated problems include drug abuse and dependence, depression and suicidality, disability, and multiple and unnecessary medical treatments, including surgeries (Klengel et al. 2011; Kushwaha et al. 2014; Rabinowitz et al. 2011; Yoshimasu 2012).

With somatization disorder, the most difficult diagnostic feature to establish in elderly patients was the onset of symptoms before age 30 years, because such history can rarely be accurately determined. This is no longer a factor with the new classification. However, determining what would be considered an excessive reaction to somatic symptoms can be difficult in late life given the high incidence of comorbid illnesses and the lack of appreciation for "normal" reactions. Somatization disorder tends to run a chronic course, with most patients demonstrating consistent symptom patterns as they age, even into later life (Pribor et al. 1994). Rabinowitz et al. (2011) found that older individuals with somatization were more lonely, isolated, and dissatisfied with the support they received from others.

The DSM-IV diagnosis of undifferentiated somatoform disorder now falls under the DSM-5 diagnosis of somatic symptom disorder. It was previously defined by the presence of one or more physical complaints, lasting at least 6 months, that could not be fully explained by appropriate medical workup and that resulted in considerable social, occupational, or functional impairment. This diagnosis is complicated in late life by the frequency of comorbid medical disorders. Determining whether the impairment is due to somatoform symptoms rather than comorbid medical disorders is difficult and may be nearly impossible in the case of many debilitated elderly individuals. Prevalence rates for undifferentiated somatoform disorder were not well established for any age group, although one community study in Italy found a rate of 13.8%, significantly higher than rates for every other somatoform disorder (Faravelli et al. 1997). Patients with chronic pain were found to have quite high rates of DSM-IV undifferentiated somatoform disorder (Aigner and Bach 1999).

Pain is the most common medical complaint in elderly individuals, with pain due to musculoskeletal disease (e.g., osteoarthritis, back pain, headache) being the most common type (Deen 2008; Paladini et al. 2015; Zis et al. 2017). Between one-half and two-thirds of elderly individuals have chronic pain (Cheung et al. 2017; Zis et al. 2017), and the percentage may be slightly higher than 80% for those in long-term care (Zanocchi et al. 2008). Up to 17% have substantial daily pain (Sawyer et al. 2007). Persistent pain is associated with significant functional and social impairment as well as comorbid psychiatric symptoms, including depression, insomnia, and substance abuse (Karp and Weiner 2011; Paladini et al. 2015). Pain assessment is often limited because of its dependence on subjective patient reports, which can be influenced by a number of confounding factors in late life, including dementia. Dementia may limit a person's ability to verbalize pain, with the result that caregivers must rely on nonverbal behaviors such as facial expressions, agitation or inactivity, or autonomic responses (Achterberg et al. 2019; Scherder and Plooij 2012). It has also been proposed that the pathological process in Alzheimer's disease may alter pain perception, perhaps by increasing the pain threshold (Scherder et al. 2008). Pharmacological treatment of pain, however, can lead to additional problems resulting from medication side effects and drug–drug interactions.

In the DSM-IV category of pain disorder, pain was the major focus of the clinical presentation, and psychological factors were believed to play critical roles in the onset, severity, exacerbation, or continuation of the pain. Pain disorder would now be classified as a somatic symptom disorder with predominant pain. Even when there are specific causes of pain, diagnosis hinges on identifying an overwhelming preoccupation with pain, sometimes involving a pattern of treatment resistance.

Illness Anxiety Disorder

The DSM-5 category of illness anxiety disorder (Box 13–2) incorporates the essence of what was previously labeled hypochondriasis. It is characterized by an excessive preoccupation with having or acquiring a serious illness, despite the fact that somatic symptoms either are not present or, if present, are mild in intensity. Key to this preoccupation is a high level of anxiety regarding one's health, associated with excessive health-related behaviors such as checking one's body for signs of illness or maladaptive avoidance of medical appointments or settings (American Psychiatric Association 2013). Misinterpretation of normal bodily sensations as indicating severe illness is thought to be the main dynamic underlying this disorder (Krautwurst et al. 2014).

Hypochondriasis has been seen in 3% of medical inpatients and in up to 8.5% of outpatients, equally among both sexes (Barsky 2001; Creed and Barsky 2004; Faravelli et al. 1997; Fink et al. 2004), and there is some debate regarding whether factors such as low education level, low socioeconomic status, and old age increase these rates (El-Gabalawy et al. 2013; Rief et al. 2001). Comorbid psychiatric disorders are common, with up to one-third of individuals with hypochondriasis having major depression and generalized anxiety disorder and more than one-tenth having panic disorder and OCD (Scarella et al. 2016). Personality disorders may be seen in upward of three-fourths of patients with hypochondriasis (Fallon et al. 2012; Sakai et al. 2010).

Box 13–2. DSM-5 Diagnostic Criteria for Illness Anxiety Disorder

A. Preoccupation with having or acquiring a serious illness.

B. Somatic symptoms are not present or, if present, are only mild in intensity. If another medical condition is present or there is a high risk for developing a medical condition (e.g., strong family history is present), the preoccupation is clearly excessive or disproportionate.

C. There is a high level of anxiety about health, and the individual is easily alarmed about personal health status.

D. The individual performs excessive health-related behaviors (e.g., repeatedly checks his or her body for signs of illness) or exhibits maladaptive avoidance (e.g., avoids doctor appointments and hospitals).

E. Illness preoccupation has been present for at least 6 months, but the specific illness that is feared may change over that period of time.

F. The illness-related preoccupation is not better explained by another mental disorder, such as somatic symptom disorder, panic disorder, generalized anxiety disorder, body dysmorphic disorder, obsessive-compulsive disorder, or delusional disorder, somatic type.

Specify whether:

Care-seeking type: Medical care, including physician visits or undergoing tests and procedures, is frequently used.

Care-avoidant type: Medical care is rarely used.

Source. Reprinted from American Psychiatric Association: *Diagnostic and Statistical Manual of Mental Disorders*, 5th Edition. Arlington, VA, American Psychiatric Association, 2013, p. 315. Used with permission. Copyright © 2013 American Psychiatric Association.

Conversion Disorder

Conversion disorder, also called functional neurological symptom disorder in DSM-5 (Box 13–3), is characterized by one or more symptoms of altered voluntary motor or sensory function that do not appear compatible with recognized neurological or medical conditions. The symptoms cause significant distress or impairment in important areas of functioning and may involve weakness or paralysis, abnormal movements (e.g., tremor), swallowing or speech symptoms, pseudoseizures, or sensory loss. As with other somatic symptoms, however, the presence of true medical comorbidity can cloud the picture. Some researchers have argued that conversion disorder is a form of dissociative disorder (Brown et al. 2007). Previous DSM nomenclature for conversion symptoms was rooted in psychodynamic theory and assumed the presence of a psychological conflict that was prompting the symptom.

There are no clear prevalence figures for conversion disorder in older patients, but rates range from 1% to 4% in general medical populations (Rabinowitz and Laek 2005). Comorbid conditions include substance abuse, chronic illness, head trauma, and previous conversion symptoms. Psychogenic nonepileptic seizures (PNESs), sometimes referred to as "pseudoseizures," represent one type of conversion symptom. They are characterized by behavioral spells that mimic various forms of seizures but are not associated with electroencephalographic findings and have a presumed psychological etiology (D'Alessio et al. 2006; Mari et al. 2006). PNESs are more frequent in young adult females, and they are seen in 5%–20% of outpatients with epilepsy, and in combination with an actual seizure disorder in up to 10% of patients (Chabolla et al. 1996; Devinsky et al. 2011). They have also been diagnosed in individuals older than 60 years (Behrouz et al. 2006).

Risk factors for conversion disorder include physical and sexual abuse, trauma, depression, major life stress, personality disorder, and other neurological illnesses (Jankovic et al. 2006; O'Sullivan et al. 2007; Roelofs et al. 2002; Sar et al. 2004; Steffen et al. 2015). Conversion disorder in late life may be even more likely to be associated with an actual comorbid neurological disorder. The prognosis is variable and depends on several factors, including the type of symptoms and the degree of functional impairment and psychiatric comorbidity. Recovery is variable but common (Jankovic et al. 2006; Ness 2007). According to a review by Krem (2004), affected individuals who have more acute, quickly diagnosed conversion symptoms with minimal comorbidity tend to do better over time compared with those who are older or who have symptoms of longer duration and more severe disability, especially seizures and paralysis.

Box 13–3.   DSM-5 Diagnostic Criteria for Conversion Disorder (Functional Neurological Symptom Disorder)

A. One or more symptoms of altered voluntary motor or sensory function.

B. Clinical findings provide evidence of incompatibility between the symptom and recognized neurological or medical conditions.

C. The symptom or deficit is not better explained by another medical or mental disorder.

D. The symptom or deficit causes clinically significant distress or impairment in social, occupational, or other important areas of functioning or warrants medical evaluation.

Coding note: The ICD-9-CM code for conversion disorder is **300.11,** which is assigned regardless of the symptom type. The ICD-10-CM code depends on the symptom type (see below).

Specify symptom type:

(F44.4) With weakness or paralysis

(F44.4) With abnormal movement (e.g., tremor, dystonic movement, myoclonus, gait disorder)

(F44.4) With swallowing symptoms

(F44.4) With speech symptom (e.g., dysphonia, slurred speech)

(F44.5) With attacks or seizures

(F44.6) With anesthesia or sensory loss

(F44.6) With special sensory symptom (e.g., visual, olfactory, or hearing disturbance)

(F44.7) With mixed symptoms

Specify if:

Acute episode: Symptoms present for less than 6 months.

Persistent: Symptoms occurring for 6 months or more.

Specify if:

With psychological stressor *(specify stressor)*

Without psychological stressor

Source.   Reprinted from American Psychiatric Association: *Diagnostic and Statistical Manual of Mental Disorders*, 5th Edition. Arlington, VA, American Psychiatric Association, 2013, pp. 318–319. Used with permission. Copyright © 2013 American Psychiatric Association.

Etiology

The causes of somatic symptom and related disorders are usually multifactorial and often rooted in both early developmental experiences and personality traits. For example, these disorders have been associated with the experience of serious illness early in life (Stuart and Noyes 1999), childhood abuse (Roelofs et al. 2002; Samelius et al. 2007; Waldinger et al. 2006), dissociative amnesia (Brown et al. 2005), significant psychological stress (Hollifield et al. 1999; Ritsner et al. 2000; Steffen et al. 2015), and the personality traits of alexithymia and neuroticism (Bailey and Henry 2007; Duquette 2020; Steffen et al. 2015). As noted throughout the chapter, the somatic symptom and related disorders are also highly associated with comorbid depression, anxiety and panic disorders, substance use disorders, and personality disorders, especially paranoid, avoidant, and obsessive-compulsive personality disorders (Fallon et al. 2012; Noyes et al. 2001; Rabinowitz and Laek 2005; Sar et al. 2004).

Somatization may be more common in females and in older individuals, although the prevalence of actual somatic symptom and related disorders has not been associated with increased age, with the exception of hypochondriasis. When present in late life, especially with late onset, these disorders may be associated with neuropsychological impairment or comorbid neurological illness (Sheehan and Banerjee 1999). Functional magnetic resonance imaging scans have found distinctive patterns of increased cerebral activation in the left inferior frontal lobe and in the left limbic structures associated with somatoform symptoms (Stone et al. 2007; Vuilleumier 2005). Specific neuroimaging studies of patients with conversion symptoms have found altered activity in the motor or somatosensory cortex and emotion processing centers such as the amygdala, along with increased activation in the orbitofrontal and anterior cingulate cortices (Aybek et al. 2015; Hassa et al. 2017; Vuilleumier et al. 2001). Nonetheless, there is not yet sufficient evidence to accurately identify any somatic symptom disorder using neuroimaging (Browning et al. 2011). Overall factors associated with somatic symptom and related disorders are summarized in Table 13–1.

Psychodynamic approaches suggest that somatic symptom and related disorders result from unconscious conflict in which intolerable impulses or affects are believed to be expressed via more tolerable somatic symptoms or complaints. The classic example of this phenomenon is found in conversion disorder, in which intolerable, unconscious impulses are believed to be converted into motor or sensory dysfunction. Freud wrote about such a mechanism based on his studies of young females who had what was then termed "hysteria" (Breuer and Freud 1893–1895/1955). Specifically, psychodynamic theory suggests that excessive and intolerable guilt or hostility is the psychological source of somatization, particularly hypochondriasis (Barsky and Klerman 1983). In such cases, physical symptoms serve as a means of self-punishment for unacceptable unconscious impulses. Anger directed at caregivers is indirectly expressed through distrust of and dissatisfaction with multiple physicians. Some researchers have suggested that underlying and complicating this psychodynamic redirection of anger or guilt is alexithymia, in which a person has a relative inability to identify and express emotional states (Bailey and Henry 2007; Waller and Scheidt 2004). The experiencing and reporting of bodily sensations thus substitute for emotional expression. While alexithymia has long been postulated to play a role in both somatoform and psychosomatic illnesses, not all empirical research has supported the correlation of alexithymia with somatic complaints (Lundh and Simonsson-Sarnecki 2001).

In late life, somatoform disorders may represent a dysfunctional attempt to cope with accumulating physical and psychosocial losses, especially when these losses are associated with functional disability, anxiety, and depression. These include loss of or isolation from family, friends, and caregivers; loss of beauty and strength; financial setbacks; loss of independence; and loss of social role (e.g., as a result of retirement, loss of a spouse, or occupational disability). The psychological distress and anxiety

TABLE 13–1.	Factors associated with somatic symptom and related disorders	
Alexithymia	Low socioeconomic status
Anxiety disorders	Lower educational level
Childhood physical and/or sexual abuse	Neuroticism
Chronic medical illness	Other somatoform disorder
Chronic pain	Personality disorders
Depressive disorders	Psychiatric illness
Dissociative amnesia	Severe, persistent psychological stress or trauma
Female sex	Substance use disorders
Frontal lobe, anterior cingulate, and limbic dysfunction	

over such losses may be less threatening and more controllable when they are shifted to somatic complaints or symptoms. In turn, a sick role might be reinforced by increased social contacts and support. The presence of comorbid medical problems and the use of multiple medications may provide somatic symptoms around which psychological conflict can center. In long-term care, older individuals are faced with many additional overwhelming losses, and their own bodies often serve as the last bastion of control. Somatic preoccupation thus serves as a means of coping with stress, even though it is maladaptive and can result in excessive and unnecessary disability. It may also serve to mobilize and control resources and staff attention within the long-term-care environment.

Treatment

Patients with somatic symptom and related disorders present to clinicians with what appear to be legitimate somatic complaints. It is only after repeated but fruitless workups, multiple and persistent complaints and requests, and sometimes angry and inappropriate reactions to treatment that clinicians begin to suspect a somatic symptom disorder. In some cases, the manner of presentation and the symptom complex are more immediately suggestive of a particular disorder. In any event, it is important for clinicians to remember that the reported symptoms and complaints are quite real and disturbing for the patient. Even after workups have indicated that psychological factors are involved, it is never wise for clinicians to challenge patients or to suggest that the symptoms are "all in your mind." The typical response to such a suggestion is for the patient to seek additional opinions and medical tests, which in turn can perpetuate a cycle of somatization in which the underlying issues are never addressed.

Instead, the clinician's role must be to foster a supportive, consistent, and professional relationship with the affected person. Such a relationship will provide reassurance as well as protect the patient from excessive and unnecessary medical visits and procedures. Clinicians should focus on responding to individual complaints, perhaps with periodic but regularly scheduled appointments, and should set limits on workup and treatment in a firm but empathic manner. This can be difficult to do when patients become demanding and attempt to consume excessive clinic time, but clinicians must endeavor to remain professional and to not personalize the situation or feel as though they are failing the patient. Clinicians should focus on symptom reduction and rehabilitation and not attempt to force patients to gain insight into the potential psychological nature of their symptoms (Houwen et al. 2017).

Clinicians should not attempt to diagnose a somatic symptom disorder prematurely because underlying organic pathology might have eluded diagnosis. For example, multiple sclerosis, systemic lupus erythematosus, and acute intermittent porphyria often have complex presentations that elude initial diagnostic workup (Kellner 1987). The somatic symptom and related disorders may coexist with actual disease states; for example, many individuals with pseudoseizures also have a seizure disorder (D'Alessio et al. 2006; Mari et al. 2006). Moene et al. (2000) found that slightly more than 10% of patients given an initial diagnosis of conversion disorder had a true neurological disorder. At the same time, it is important for clinicians to set limits on what they can offer and to make appropriate referrals to specialists or mental health clinicians.

In contrast to a primary care practitioner or a medical specialist, the geriatric psychiatrist will play a more active role in addressing the disorder itself rather than the actual physical complaints. Because many presentations of somatic symptom and related disorders are chronic, the goal of treatment is often to control symptoms rather than to cure the patient (Henningsen 2018; Houwen et al. 2017). To facilitate this, clinicians must form a therapeutic alliance through empathic listening and acknowledging physical discomfort without trivializing the patient's somatic complaints. An offer to review all available medical records can sometimes be a tangible way of conveying one's seriousness to the patient. Educating patients about various symptom complexes and involving them in part of the decision-making can be empowering, especially for patients with chronic pain.

Individual therapy using a psychodynamic approach will help patients identify and discuss psychological conflict and associated emotions. Cognitive-behavioral therapy (CBT) focuses on identifying distorted thought patterns and anxiety triggers and replacing them with more realistic and adaptive strategies, as well as integrating behavioral techniques to desensitize anxious reactions. An impressive body of research supports the efficacy of psychotherapy, particularly CBT, for treating somatoform disorders, both alone and in combination with antidepressants (Fallon et al. 2017; Kroenke 2007; Thomson and Page 2007; Tyrer et al. 2014; van Dessel et al. 2014).

Pharmacotherapy is a central component of treatment for somatic symptom and related disorders. It can be targeted at a specific disorder or at underlying anxiety and depression. One meta-analysis of 26 randomized controlled trials, however, did not find strong evidence for antidepressant effects (Kleinstäuber et al. 2014). On the other hand, some studies have documented successful treatment of somatization disorder with either antidepressants or mood stabilizers (García-Campayo and Sanz-Carrillo 2001). Hypochondriacal symptoms were found to respond to a variety of antidepressant medications—in particular, selective serotonin reuptake inhibitors (Barsky 2001; Fallon 2004; Fallon et al. 2017; Oosterbaan et al. 2001; Somashekar et al. 2013). Antidepressants and anticonvulsants have long been a mainstay of treatment for pain disorder (Eisenberg et al. 2007; Karp and Weiner 2011; Kroenke 2007; Somashekar et al. 2013).

The tendency of many psychiatrists to focus primarily on pharmacotherapy can become a trap with the somatic symptom and related disorders because the therapeutic relationship is such a key element. Given the chronic nature of somatoform symptoms, it is unlikely that pharmacotherapy will be a quick fix. When this narrow focus on treatment with medications fails to result in rapid symptom control, patients may abandon the therapist for alternative treatment. Other patients may welcome such a focus because it keeps them from having to face underlying psychological issues. Instead, clinicians must be prepared for the long haul and strike a balance between reasonable pharmacotherapy that targets specific symptoms of anxiety or depression and a supportive alliance in which the most appropriate psychotherapy for the patient is used.

Conclusion

For older patients with a somatic symptom disorder, the greatest challenge is always trying to separate out the actual medical disease from the somatic symptoms. The two are sometimes so intertwined that the line between them cannot be reasonably discerned without the successful response of a discrete symptom to either a medical or a psychiatric intervention. Moreover, many patients are quite resistant to psychiatric care because they feel it delegitimizes their physical suffering. Teamwork between internist and psychiatrist is key, allowing both to identify the most important symptoms of concern to the patient, provide appropriate attention and workup, and coordinate medical and psychiatric interventions.

Key Points

- Somatic symptom and related disorders comprise a heterogeneous group of disorders characterized by prominent physical symptoms or complaints that are associated with significant distress and impairment in excess of what would be expected.

- The high degree of both medical and psychiatric comorbidity in late life poses a unique diagnostic challenge for disorders with prominent somatic symptoms.

- The main somatic symptom and related disorders seen in elderly patients are somatic symptom disorder, illness anxiety disorder, and conversion disorder. Previous categories of pain disorder and undifferentiated somatoform disorder are now subsumed within somatic symptom disorder.

- Somatic symptom and related disorders are most commonly diagnosed in younger individuals. Major risk factors include childhood abuse, female sex, chronic illness or pain, lower education and socioeconomic status, and comorbid anxiety, depression, personality disorders, and substance use disorders.

- Management of somatic symptom and related disorders requires a consistent, empathic approach that focuses on symptomatic improvement and rehabilitation, does not challenge the veracity of the patient's reports, and provides efficacious cognitive-behavioral therapy and appropriate pharmacotherapy.

Suggested Readings

Egloff N, Cámara RJ, von Känel R, et al: Hypersensitivity and hyperalgesia in somatoform pain disorders. Gen Hosp Psychiatry 36(3):284–290, 2014 24650586
El-Gabalawy R, Mackenzie CS, Thibodeau MA, et al: Health anxiety disorders in older adults: conceptualizing complex conditions in late life. Clin Psychol Rev 33(8):1096–1105, 2013
Kroenke K: Efficacy of treatment for somatoform disorders: a review of randomized controlled trials. Psychosom Med 69(9):881–888, 2007
Paladini A, Fusco M, Coaccioli S, et al: Chronic pain in the elderly: the case for new therapeutic strategies. Pain Physician 18(5):E863–E876, 2015
Rabinowitz T, Laek J: An approach to the patient with physical complaints or irrational anxiety about an illness or their appearance, in The 10-Minute Guide to Psychiatric Diagnosis and Treatment. Edited by Stern TA. New York, Professional Publishing Group, 2005, pp 225–238
van Dessel N, den Boeft M, van der Wouden JC, et al: Non-pharmacological interventions for somatoform disorders and medically unexplained physical symptoms (MUPS) in adults. Cochrane Database Syst Rev (11):CD011142, 2014

References

Achterberg W, Lautenbacher S, Husebo B, et al: Pain in dementia. Pain Rep 5(1):e803, 2019 32072098
Aigner M, Bach M: Clinical utility of DSM-IV pain disorder. Compr Psychiatry 40(5):353–357, 1999 10509617
American Psychiatric Association: Diagnostic and Statistical Manual of Mental Disorders, 4th Edition. Washington, DC, American Psychiatric Association, 1994
American Psychiatric Association: Diagnostic and Statistical Manual of Mental Disorders, 4th Edition, Text Revision. Washington, DC, American Psychiatric Association, 2000
American Psychiatric Association: Diagnostic and Statistical Manual of Mental Disorders, 5th Edition. Arlington, VA, American Psychiatric Association, 2013
Aybek S, Nicholson TR, O'Daly O, et al: Emotion-motion interactions in conversion disorder: an fMRI study. PLoS One 10(4):e0123273, 2015 25859660
Bailey PE, Henry JD: Alexithymia, somatization and negative affect in a community sample. Psychiatry Res 150(1):13–20, 2007 17258817
Barsky AJ: Clinical practice: the patient with hypochondriasis. N Engl J Med 345(19):1395–1399, 2001 11794173
Barsky AJ, Klerman GL: Overview: hypochondriasis, bodily complaints, and somatic styles. Am J Psychiatry 140(3):273–283, 1983 6338747
Behrouz R, Heriaud L, Benbadis SR: Late-onset psychogenic nonepileptic seizures. Epilepsy Behav 8(3):649–650, 2006 16531122
Bortz JJ: Medically unexplained symptoms in older adults, in Clinical Neurology of the Older Adult. Edited by Sirven JI, Malamut BL. Philadelphia, PA, Lippincott Williams and Wilkins, 2008, pp 561–573
Breuer J, Freud S: Studies on hysteria (1893–1895), in The Standard Edition of the Complete Psychological Works of Sigmund Freud, Vol 2. Translated and edited by Strachey J. London, Hogarth, 1955, pp 1–319
Brown RJ, Schrag A, Trimble MR: Dissociation, childhood interpersonal trauma, and family functioning in patients with somatization disorder. Am J Psychiatry 162(5):899–905, 2005 15863791
Brown RJ, Cardeña E, Nijenhuis E, et al: Should conversion disorder be reclassified as a dissociative disorder in DSM V? Psychosomatics 48(5):369–378, 2007 17878494
Browning M, Fletcher P, Sharpe M: Can neuroimaging help us to understand and classify somatoform disorders? A systematic and critical review. Psychosom Med 73(2):173–184, 2011 21217095

Chabolla DR, Krahn LE, So EL, Rummans TA: Psychogenic nonepileptic seizures. Mayo Clin Proc 71(5):493–500, 1996 8628032

Cheung CW, Choi SW, Wong SSC, et al: Changes in prevalence, outcomes, and help-seeking behavior of chronic pain in an aging population over the last decade. Pain Pract 17(5):643–654, 2017 27735140

Creed F, Barsky A: A systematic review of the epidemiology of somatisation disorder and hypochondriasis. J Psychosom Res 56(4):391–408, 2004 15094023

D'Alessio L, Giagante B, Oddo S, et al: Psychiatric disorders in patients with psychogenic nonepileptic seizures, with and without comorbid epilepsy. Seizure 15(5):333–339, 2006 16720097

Deen HG: Back and neck pain, in Clinical Neurology of the Older Adult. Edited by Sirven JI, Malamut BL. Philadelphia, PA, Lippincott Williams and Wilkins, 2008, pp 213–221

Devinsky O, Gazzola D, LaFrance WC Jr: Differentiating between nonepileptic and epileptic seizures. Nat Rev Neurol 7(4):210–220, 2011 21386814

de Waal MWM, Arnold IA, Eekhof JAH, van Hemert AM: Somatoform disorders in general practice: prevalence, functional impairment and comorbidity with anxiety and depressive disorders. Br J Psychiatry 184(6):470–476, 2004 15172939

de Waal MWM, Arnold IA, Eekhof JA, et al: Follow-up study on health care use of patients with somatoform, anxiety and depressive disorders in primary care. BMC Fam Pract 9:5, 2008 18218070

Duquette P: More than words can say: a multi-disciplinary consideration of the psychotherapeutic evaluation and treatment of alexithymia. Front Psychiatry 11:433, 2020 32523552

Egloff N, Cámara RJ, von Känel R, et al: Hypersensitivity and hyperalgesia in somatoform pain disorders. Gen Hosp Psychiatry 36(3):284–290, 2014 24650586

Eisenberg E, River Y, Shifrin A, Krivoy N: Antiepileptic drugs in the treatment of neuropathic pain. Drugs 67(9):1265–1289, 2007 17547471

El-Gabalawy R, Mackenzie CS, Thibodeau MA, et al: Health anxiety disorders in older adults: conceptualizing complex conditions in late life. Clin Psychol Rev 33(8):1096–1105, 2013 24091001

Fallon BA: Pharmacotherapy of somatoform disorders. J Psychosom Res 56(4):455–460, 2004 15094032

Fallon BA, Harper KM, Landa A, et al: Personality disorders in hypochondriasis: prevalence and comparison with two anxiety disorders. Psychosomatics 53(6):566–574, 2012 22658329

Fallon BA, Ahern DK, Pavlicova M, et al: A randomized controlled trial of medication and cognitive-behavioral therapy for hypochondriasis. Am J Psychiatry 174(8):756–764, 2017 28659038

Faravelli C, Salvatori S, Galassi F, et al: Epidemiology of somatoform disorders: a community survey in Florence. Soc Psychiatry Psychiatr Epidemiol 32(1):24–29, 1997 9029984

Fink P, Hansen MS, Oxhøj ML: The prevalence of somatoform disorders among internal medical inpatients. J Psychosom Res 56(4):413–418, 2004 15094025

García-Campayo J, Sanz-Carrillo C: Gabapentin for the treatment of patients with somatization disorder (letter). J Clin Psychiatry 62(6):474, 2001 11465526

Haftgoli N, Favrat B, Verdon F, et al: Patients presenting with somatic complaints in general practice: depression, anxiety and somatoform disorders are frequent and associated with psychosocial stressors. BMC Fam Pract 11:67, 2010 20843358

Hanssen DJC, Lucassen PLBJ, Hilderink PH, et al: Health-related quality of life in older persons with medically unexplained symptoms. Am J Geriatr Psychiatry 24(11):1117–1127, 2016 27618643

Hasin D, Katz H: Somatoform and substance use disorders. Psychosom Med 69(9):870–875, 2007 18040097

Hassa T, Sebastian A, Liepert J, et al: Symptom-specific amygdala hyperactivity modulates motor control network in conversion disorder. Neuroimage Clin 15:143–150, 2017 28529870

Henningsen P: Management of somatic symptom disorder. Dialogues Clin Neurosci 20(1):23–31, 2018 29946208

Hilderink PH, Collard R, Rosmalen JG, Oude Voshaar RC: Prevalence of somatoform disorders and medically unexplained symptoms in old age populations in comparison with younger age groups: a systematic review. Ageing Res Rev 12(1):151–156, 2013 22575906

Hollifield M, Tuttle L, Paine S, Kellner R: Hypochondriasis and somatization related to personality and attitudes toward self. Psychosomatics 40(5):387–395, 1999 10479943

Houwen J, Lucassen PL, Stappers HW, et al: Improving GP communication in consultations on medically unexplained symptoms: a qualitative interview study with patients in primary care. Br J Gen Pract 67(663):e716–e723, 2017 28847774

Jankovic J, Vuong KD, Thomas M: Psychogenic tremor: long-term outcome. CNS Spectr 11(7):501–508, 2006 16816790

Karp JF, Weiner DK: Persistent pain and older adults, in Principles and Practice of Geriatric Psychiatry, 2nd Edition. Edited by Agronin ME, Maletta G. Philadelphia, PA, Lippincott Williams and Wilkins, 2011, pp 763–782

Kellner R: Hypochondriasis and somatization. JAMA 258(19):2718–2722, 1987 3312664

Kleinstäuber M, Witthöft M, Steffanowski A, et al: Pharmacological interventions for somatoform disorders in adults. Cochrane Database Syst Rev (11):CD010628, 2014 25379990

Klengel T, Heck A, Pfister H, et al: Somatization in major depression: clinical features and genetic associations. Acta Psychiatr Scand 124(4):317–328, 2011 21838737

Krautwurst S, Gerlach AL, Gomille L, et al: Health anxiety: an indicator of higher interoceptive sensitivity? J Behav Ther Exp Psychiatry 45(2):303–309, 2014 24584036

Krem MM: Motor conversion disorders reviewed from a neuropsychiatric perspective. J Clin Psychiatry 65(6):783–790, 2004 15291655

Kroenke K: Efficacy of treatment for somatoform disorders: a review of randomized controlled trials. Psychosom Med 69(9):881–888, 2007 18040099

Kushwaha V, Sinha Deb K, Chadda RK, Mehta M: A study of disability and its correlates in somatization disorder. Asian J Psychiatr 8:56–58, 2014 24655628

Liskow B, Othmer E, Penick EC, et al: Is Briquet's syndrome a heterogeneous disorder? Am J Psychiatry 143(5):626–629, 1986 3963251

Lundh LG, Simonsson-Sarnecki M: Alexithymia, emotion, and somatic complaints. J Pers 69(3):483–510, 2001 11478734

Mari F, Di Bonaventura C, Vanacore N, et al: Video-EEG study of psychogenic nonepileptic seizures: differential characteristics in patients with and without epilepsy. Epilepsia 47(suppl 5):64–67, 2006 17239109

Miller AR, North CS, Clouse RE, et al: The association of irritable bowel syndrome and somatization disorder. Ann Clin Psychiatry 13(1):25–30, 2001 11465682

Moene FC, Landberg EH, Hoogduin KA, et al: Organic syndromes diagnosed as conversion disorder: identification and frequency in a study of 85 patients. J Psychosom Res 49(1):7–12, 2000 11053598

Ness D: Physical therapy management for conversion disorder: case series. J Neurol Phys Ther 31(1):30–39, 2007 17419887

Noyes R Jr, Langbehn DR, Happel RL, et al: Personality dysfunction among somatizing patients. Psychosomatics 42(4):320–329, 2001 11496021

Oosterbaan DB, van Balkom AJ, van Boeijen CA, et al: An open study of paroxetine in hypochondriasis. Prog Neuropsychopharmacol Biol Psychiatry 25(5):1023–1033, 2001 11444675

O'Sullivan SS, Spillane JE, McMahon EM, et al: Clinical characteristics and outcome of patients diagnosed with psychogenic nonepileptic seizures: a 5-year review. Epilepsy Behav 11(1):77–84, 2007 17517535

Paladini A, Fusco M, Coaccioli S, et al: Chronic pain in the elderly: the case for new therapeutic strategies. Pain Physician 18(5):E863–E876, 2015 26431140

Pribor EF, Smith DS, Yutzy SH: Somatization disorder in elderly patients. Am J Geriatr Psychiatry 2(2):109–117, 1994 28530990

Puri PR, Dimsdale JE: Health care utilization and poor reassurance: potential predictors of somatoform disorders. Psychiatr Clin North Am 34(3):525–544, 2011 21889677

Rabinowitz T, Laek J: An approach to the patient with physical complaints or irrational anxiety about an illness or their appearance, in The 10-Minute Guide to Psychiatric Diagnosis and Treatment. Edited by Stern TA. New York, Professional Publishing Group, 2005, pp 225–238

Rabinowitz T, Hirdes JP, Desjardins I: Somatoform disorders in late life, in Principles and Practice of Geriatric Psychiatry, 2nd Edition. Edited by Agronin ME, Maletta G. Philadelphia, PA, Lippincott Williams and Wilkins, 2011, pp 565–581

Rief W, Hessel A, Braehler E: Somatization symptoms and hypochondriacal features in the general population. Psychosom Med 63(4):595–602, 2001 11485113

Ritsner M, Ponizovsky A, Kurs R, Modai I: Somatization in an immigrant population in Israel: a community survey of prevalence, risk factors, and help-seeking behavior. Am J Psychiatry 157(3):385–392, 2000 10698814

Roelofs K, Keijsers GP, Hoogduin KA, et al: Childhood abuse in patients with conversion disorder. Am J Psychiatry 159(11):1908–1913, 2002 12411227

Rosendal M, Carlsen AH, Rask MT, Moth G: Symptoms as the main problem in primary care: a cross-sectional study of frequency and characteristics. Scand J Prim Health Care 33(2):91–99, 2015 25961812

Sack M, Lahmann C, Jaeger B, Henningsen P: Trauma prevalence and somatoform symptoms: are there specific somatoform symptoms related to traumatic experiences? J Nerv Ment Dis 195(11):928–933, 2007 18000455

Sakai R, Nestoriuc Y, Nolido NV, Barsky AJ: The prevalence of personality disorders in hypochondriasis. J Clin Psychiatry 71(1):41–47, 2010 20129004

Samelius L, Wijma B, Wingren G, Wijma K: Somatization in abused women. J Womens Health (Larchmt) 16(6):909–918, 2007 17678462

Sar V, Akyüz G, Kundakçi T, et al: Childhood trauma, dissociation, and psychiatric comorbidity in patients with conversion disorder. Am J Psychiatry 161(12):2271–2276, 2004 15569899

Sawyer P, Lillis JP, Bodner EV, Allman RM: Substantial daily pain among nursing home residents. J Am Med Dir Assoc 8(3):158–165, 2007 17349944

Scarella TM, Laferton JA, Ahern DK, et al: The relationship of hypochondriasis to anxiety, depressive, and somatoform disorders. Psychosomatics 57(2):200–207, 2016 26785798

Scherder EJ, Plooij B: Assessment and management of pain, with particular emphasis on central neuropathic pain, in moderate to severe dementia. Drugs Aging 29(9):701–706, 2012 23018606

Scherder EJ, Eggermont L, Plooij B, et al: Relationship between chronic pain and cognition in cognitively intact older persons and in patients with Alzheimer's disease: the need to control for mood. Gerontology 54(1):50–58, 2008 18185014

Sheehan B, Banerjee S: Review: somatization in the elderly. Int J Geriatr Psychiatry 14(12):1044–1049, 1999 10607972

Smith RC, Gardiner JC, Lyles JS, et al: Exploration of DSM-IV criteria in primary care patients with medically unexplained symptoms. Psychosom Med 67(1):123–129, 2005 15673634

Somashekar B, Jainer A, Wuntakal B: Psychopharmacotherapy of somatic symptoms disorders. Int Rev Psychiatry 25(1):107–115, 2013 23383672

Steffen A, Fiess J, Schmidt R, Rockstroh B: "That pulled the rug out from under my feet!": adverse experiences and altered emotion processing in patients with functional neurological symptoms compared to healthy comparison subjects. BMC Psychiatry 15:133, 2015 26103961

Stone J, Zeman A, Simonotto E, et al: FMRI in patients with motor conversion symptoms and controls with simulated weakness. Psychosom Med 69(9):961–969, 2007 17991812

Stuart S, Noyes R Jr: Attachment and interpersonal communication in somatization. Psychosomatics 40(1):34–43, 1999 9989119

Thomson AB, Page LA: Psychotherapies for hypochondriasis. Cochrane Database Syst Rev (4):CD006520, 2007 17943915

Tomenson B, McBeth J, Chew-Graham CA, et al: Somatization and health anxiety as predictors of health care use. Psychosom Med 74(6):656–664, 2012 22753632

Tyrer P, Cooper S, Salkovskis P, et al: Clinical and cost-effectiveness of cognitive behaviour therapy for health anxiety in medical patients: a multicentre randomised controlled trial. Lancet 383(9913):219–225, 2014 24139977

van Dessel N, den Boeft M, van der Wouden JC, et al: Non-pharmacological interventions for somatoform disorders and medically unexplained physical symptoms (MUPS) in adults. Cochrane Database Syst Rev (11):CD011142, 2014 25362239

Voigt K, Wollburg E, Weinmann N, et al: Predictive validity and clinical utility of DSM-5 so-
    matic symptom disorder: comparison with DSM-IV somatoform disorders and additional
    criteria for consideration. J Psychosom Res 73(5):345–350, 2012 23062807
Vuilleumier P: Hysterical conversion and brain function. Prog Brain Res 150:309–329, 2005
    16186033
Vuilleumier P, Chicherio C, Assal F, et al: Functional neuroanatomical correlates of hysterical
    sensorimotor loss. Brain 124(pt 6):1077–1090, 2001 11353724
Waldinger RJ, Schulz MS, Barsky AJ, Ahern DK: Mapping the road from childhood trauma to
    adult somatization: the role of attachment. Psychosom Med 68(1):129–135, 2006 16449423
Waller E, Scheidt CE: Somatoform disorders as disorders of affect regulation: a study compar-
    ing the TAS-20 with non-self-report measures of alexithymia. J Psychosom Res 57(3):239–
    247, 2004 15507250
Yoshimasu K: Substance-related disorders and somatic symptoms: how should clinicians un-
    derstand the associations? Curr Drug Abuse Rev 5(4):291–303, 2012 23244342
Zanocchi M, Maero B, Nicola E, et al: Chronic pain in a sample of nursing home residents: prev-
    alence, characteristics, influence on quality of life (QoL). Arch Gerontol Geriatr 47(1):121–
    128, 2008 18006088
Zis P, Daskalaki A, Bountouni I, et al: Depression and chronic pain in the elderly: links and
    management challenges. Clin Interv Aging 12:709–720, 2017 28461745

CHAPTER 14

Sexuality and Aging

Marc Agronin, M.D.

People are living longer and healthier lives, and many expect sexuality to play an ongoing, important role. As a result, sexual issues and disorders are an important part of assessment and treatment by the geriatric psychiatrist in both outpatient and long-term care settings. The idea of sexuality in late life, once regarded with denial, humor, or even disgust, too often led clinicians to view sexual dysfunction as a normal and untreatable part of aging. Such distorted attitudes have changed widely, however, starting with the sexual and feminist revolutions in the 1960s and 1970s and buoyed by the widespread use of hormone replacement therapy and the advent of oral erectogenic agents for erectile dysfunction. In recent years, attitudes toward sexual orientation have also changed for the better, even among older generations who grew up during eras in which gay or lesbian issues were taboo. This widespread openness toward late-life sexuality, coupled with reliable treatments for sexual dysfunction, has made sexuality a more common and comfortable topic of conversation among older patients and their clinicians and can now ensure the persistence of enjoyable sexual function in later years. In addition, the destigmatization of sexual dysfunction has no doubt encouraged many older couples to seek treatment who otherwise might have suffered in silence and shame.

Sexual Behaviors in Late Life

Several major studies over the past 25 years have shown that most middle-aged and older individuals continue to be sexually active, although with modest decreases in activity, determined in part by gender and the availability of partners. These studies have indicated that older men are more sexually active than older women and that individuals with steady partners are more active than single individuals. In general, sexual interest and activity in late life depend on the previous level of sexual activity; the availability, health, and sexual interest of the partner; and the individual's overall physical health (Bell et al. 2017; Graham et al. 2017; Schick et al. 2010). Physical health appears to be the most important factor for older men, whereas the quality of the relationship is most influential for older women (Schick et al. 2010). Having one or more health conditions has been associated with a lower frequency of sexual activity but has not been shown to reduce the level of satisfaction, regardless of sexual orientation (Erens et al. 2019).

Starting in 1999, a series of studies of late-life sexuality conducted by AARP showed that most middle-aged and older individuals remain sexually active, with men being more sexually active and overall rates generally declining with increased age. In their original 1999 mail survey, researchers gathered responses from 1,384 men and women age 45 years and older (Jacoby 1999), and found that three-quarters of both men and women in the sample remained sexually active. Eighty-four percent of men and 78% of women ages 45–59 years had steady sexual partners, compared with 58% of men and 21% of women older than age 75. In terms of frequency, 50% of individuals ages 45–59 years reported having sex at least once a week, compared with 30% of men and 24% of women ages 60–74 years. Of the respondents, most men without partners said they masturbated, whereas more than 77% of women did not. The study also examined attitudes toward specific aspects of sexuality; 60% of men and 35% of women said that sexual activity was important to their overall quality of life. Two-thirds of all respondents were extremely or somewhat satisfied with sex. Attitudes toward partners were generally favorable, with most of both sexes describing their partners with terms that included "best friend," "kind and gentle," and "physically attractive." The study also found several generational differences in attitudes toward sex. Individuals older than 60 were less likely than younger respondents to approve of oral sex, masturbation, and sex between unmarried partners.

A 2004 update of the AARP late-life sexuality study surveyed 2,930 men and women in the United States age 45 and older and included respondents with Black, Asian, and Hispanic ethnicities (AARP 2005). Of this group, approximately two-thirds were married or living with a partner, and 5% identified themselves as gay or lesbian. Attitudes toward sexuality were remarkably similar to those seen in the 1999 survey, with only a few new findings. As before, the vast majority of individuals had positive attitudes toward sex, and those with partners described themselves as more satisfied, optimistic, and tolerant than those without partners. Blacks and Hispanics were more likely to be extremely satisfied with their partners. Those who engaged in physical exercise on a regular basis had greater degrees of sexual satisfaction. An increasing number of individuals were seeking information on sex from the internet and from health care providers. Compared with the 1999 survey, the 2004 survey found less opposition to sex between unmarried partners.

The 2004 AARP survey found no major changes in sexual behaviors, with 86% of respondents continuing to be sexually active. Men were more active than women, and rates of sexual activity declined with age. The percentage of men seeking erectogenic medications doubled from 10% to 22%, with 68% of these respondents saying that the treatment helped. The number of women undergoing hormone replacement therapy (HRT) dropped by 50%, no doubt related to warnings about potentially increased cancer risks. More individuals reported engaging in masturbation and oral sex in 2004 than in 1999. Sixty percent of men and 50% of women reported engaging in masturbation at least once in the 6 months prior to the survey.

AARP conducted another survey in 2009 using a probability sample of 1,670 individuals age 45 years and older, which included 630 Hispanic respondents (AARP 2010). In contrast to previous surveys, the overall percentage of individuals having sexual intercourse at least once a week dropped about 10 points to 41% of those with a steady partner (and 28% overall), and there were similar drops in levels of sexual satisfaction. Approximately 50% of men and 26% of women ages 45–49 years reported having sexual intercourse at least once a week, which dropped to 15% of men and 5% of women age 70 years and older. Levels of both sexual activity and satisfaction were higher among individuals who were single than among those who were married. Although all of these findings suggest important changes from previous surveys, it is important to keep in mind that the methodology of the 2009 survey was different, using telephone versus mail surveys.

In their most recent survey in 2017, AARP sponsored the National Poll on Healthy Aging, which focused on sex and was conducted by the University of Michigan Institute for Healthcare Policy and Innovation (University of Michigan 2018). The survey covered a national sample of 1,002 individuals ages 65–80. Several interesting findings emerged. Approximately 76% of respondents felt that sex was an important part of a relationship (84% of men vs. 69% of women), and 65% were interested in sex (50% of men were extremely or very interested vs. 12% of women). At the same time, only 40% of the sample was currently sexually active, dropping from 46% of those ages 65–70 years to 39% of those ages 71–75 and 25% of those ages 76–80 years. Overall, more men (51%) than women (31%) were sexually active. Health status was a clear predictor, with 45% of individuals who reported good health being sexually active versus 22% of those who reported fair or poor health. Most sexually active individuals (73%) were satisfied with their sex life, with more women (43%) reporting being extremely or very satisfied than men (31%). One in five men reported using medications to improve sexual function, and three-quarters of them found it helpful. Of note, although 62% of respondents said they would speak to a health care provider about sexual issues, only 17% had done so in the prior 2 years.

Aging Lesbian, Gay, and Bisexual Individuals

Lesbian, gay, and bisexual (LGB) individuals represent 2%–8% of the population older than age 60 in the United States, representing ~1–3 million individuals (Fredriksen-Goldsen and Muraco 2010). The 2009 AARP survey found that 8% of male and 2% of female respondents reported having same-sex relationships; 3% of males described themselves as gay, <0.5% of females reported being lesbian, and 1% of respondents described themselves as bisexual (AARP 2010). Several studies have documented the many challenges faced by aging LGB individuals, including lower self-esteem, poorer mental health, discrimination, and victimization (Brotman et al. 2003; D'Augelli and Grossman 2001; Srinivasan et al. 2019). On the other hand, most LGB individuals have a rich network of social supports from family, friends, partners, and community resources (Grossman et al. 2001). A small but growing literature indicates that most older gay and lesbian individuals continue to be sexually active. In one study of 100 gay men ages 40–77 years, 80% were sexually active, with 34% reporting having sex more than once a week and 69% reporting the same amount of sexual enjoyment as when they were younger (Pope and Schulz 1990). Gay men experience significant satisfaction with both their lifestyle and their sex lives and higher levels of sexual desire compared with heterosexual men (Adelman 1990; Manuela Peixoto 2019).

Sexuality in Long-Term Care Settings

Residents in long-term care settings face multiple barriers to sexual expression, including loss of interest, chronic illness, cognitive impairment, sexual dysfunction, and negative attitudes among themselves and staff (Mahieu and Gastmans 2015; Roelofs et al. 2015; Villar et al. 2014). Residents may perceive themselves as unattractive or incapable of sex. Staff members might acknowledge the need for affection and sexual expression but not see it as a priority (Mroczek et al. 2013). Given these widespread attitudes, it is important to educate both residents and long-term care staff about residents' need for and right to sexual expression and to dispel stereotypes (Roach 2004). One way to facilitate these educational goals is to develop and promote a policy on sexuality. Of note, about two-thirds of facilities in one survey had a written policy, with a small number requiring a physician to approve or restrict residents' sexual activity (Lester et al. 2016). A key element of such policies is the requirement that a sexual history be obtained during intake and during routine nursing, medical, and mental health evaluations. These evaluations can also be used to assess residents' concerns about and capacities for sexual function and relationships. Policies should also ensure that the facility provides adequate opportunities, spaces, and privacy for couples wishing to be intimate.

Sexual Response Cycle and Aging

The effects of aging on sexual function must be viewed against the backdrop of normal adult sexual response. A four-stage model of the normal sexual response cycle was developed by sex researchers Masters and Johnson (1966) from their pioneering work in human sexuality. The four-stage cycle illustrates the physiological changes that take place in the body during sexual activity. These four stages are excitement or arousal, plateau, orgasm, and resolution. Kaplan (1974) and others added a fifth stage, desire, to account for a psychological and physiological component of sexuality that underlies sexual response (Snarch 1991; Zilbergeld and Ellison 1980). In this later model, sexual response is not a linear process but rather a waxing and waning pattern of sexual arousal that may culminate in orgasm, depending on a host of factors. All these factors can be influenced by age-related changes in sexual function.

The first stage of the five-stage model, desire, involves physical and psychological urges to seek out and respond to sexual interaction. This drive is centered in the limbic system of the brain, particularly in the hypothalamus, and is stimulated in both sexes by testosterone. Desire is intimately linked to the physiological process of sexual excitement or arousal (the second stage); it is difficult for one to exist without the other. In both sexes, sexual arousal can be triggered by thoughts and fantasies or by direct physical stimulation. Stimulation of the autonomic nervous system leads to predictable physiological responses, including increased muscle tone, heart and respiratory

TABLE 14–1.   Normal age-related changes in sexual function

Men	Women
Testosterone production modestly decreases, with unpredictable effect on sexual function.	During menopause, estrogen production decreases and eventually stops.
	Blood supply to pelvic region is reduced.
Sperm count changes minimally, but amount of functional sperm and rate of conception decrease.	Sexual desire (libido) may decrease due in part to decreased testosterone levels.
There are no predictable changes in sexual desire (libido).	Vagina shortens and narrows. Vaginal mucosa is thinner and less lubricated.
Increased tactile stimulation is needed for sexual arousal.	Sexual arousal may take longer and may require increased stimulation.
Erections take longer to achieve and are more difficult to sustain.	During arousal, vaginal lubrication and swelling occur more slowly and are decreased.
Penile rigidity decreases because of decreases in blood flow and smooth muscle relaxation.	During orgasm, strength and amount of vaginal contractions decrease.
Sensation of urgency during plateau stage is diminished.	
Ejaculation is less forceful, with decreased ejaculate volume.	
Refractory period increases by hours to days.	

rates, and blood flow to the genitals (vasocongestion). In men, these responses result in penile erection, whereas in women, they result in vaginal lubrication and swelling of the breast and genital tissues, especially the clitoris. The relatively brief plateau stage is characterized by a sense of impending orgasm and is followed by orgasm and then a refractory period of relaxation called resolution. In both sexes, orgasm is characterized by euphoria associated with rhythmic contractions of genital muscles. In men, orgasm is brief and accompanied by ejaculation. In women, orgasm tends to last longer, and there may be multiple successive occurrences.

Normal aging produces several changes in the sexual response cycle (Table 14–1). In females, the most significant changes occur during menopause, a 2- to 10-year period that usually ends in the early 50s. The decline and eventual cessation of ovarian estrogen production during menopause leads to important changes in sexual function, including atrophy of urogenital tissue; a decrease in vaginal size; and diminished vaginal lubrication, vasocongestion, and erotic sensitivity of nipple, clitoral, and vulvar tissue. Many menopausal females also experience symptoms such as hot flashes, headaches and neck aches, mood changes, and excess fatigue (El Khoudary et al. 2019). As a result, sexual desire may decrease, sexual arousal may require more time, sexual intercourse may be more uncomfortable because of reduced lubrication of vaginal and clitoral tissue, and orgasms may feel less intense (Harder et al. 2019). During menopause, women also experience decreases in testosterone production that may lead to diminished sensitivity of erogenous tissue and reduced libido (Vegunta et al. 2020).

In most women, HRT largely reverses menopause-associated changes in sexual function. Estrogen is often prescribed with synthetic progesterone, called *progestin*, to replicate previous hormone levels. It can be administered orally or via slow-release transdermal patch, and estrogen cream can be applied directly to genital tissues to relieve irritation and enhance lubrication (Marjoribanks et al. 2012; Minkin et al. 2014). There has been a great deal of controversy about HRT due to concern about increased risks of coronary heart disease and breast cancer associated with long-term use, largely driven by data from the 2002 Women's Health Initiative studies (Lacey et al. 2002). However, current thinking supports the benefits of HRT in the years right after menopause (ages 50–60), with cited risks emerging after age 60 (Lobo 2017; Thaung Zaw et al. 2018).

Compared with women, the sexual changes in aging men occur more gradually with a less predictable time frame (Morley 2003; Westheimer and Lopater 2002). As men age, desire may involve less anticipatory physical arousal, and sexual arousal and orgasm may take longer to achieve. Older men require more physical stimulation to achieve erections, which tend to be less frequent, less durable, and less reliable. The volume of ejaculate during orgasm is decreased. The resolution or refractory stage is much longer, lasting hours to days instead of minutes to hours, as in younger men. With increasing age, the total testosterone level in men drops by an average of 1.6% per year. Symptoms of low testosterone or hypogonadism (< 250 ng/dL) may include loss of libido, erectile dysfunction, loss of bone and muscle mass, loss of strength, fatigue, and even poor concentration and depression. By age 60, 20% of men have low testosterone levels, and this rises to 50% of men over age 80 (Jia et al. 2015; Stanworth and Jones 2008). Some researchers have suggested the existence of a male menopause or andropause resulting from declining testosterone levels and involving a symptom complex that includes decreased libido and sexual function; diminished bone and muscle mass, muscle power, and body hair; and decreased lean body mass (Haider et al. 2014; Pines 2011). Research has suggested that testosterone replacement therapy may improve many of these symptoms along with the overall quality of life (Bassil and Morley 2010; Rosen et al. 2017).

In both sexes, the effects of physiological changes in sexual function are mediated by a number of psychosocial factors. The more a person knows about what constitutes normal age-associated changes in sexual function, the easier it may be for that person to accept these changes. For example, a man who does not understand the normal changes in erectile function may misinterpret them and believe that he has a sexual problem. Similarly, a woman may misinterpret vaginal dryness as an indication that she does not want to have sex. Such overreactions to normal changes can lead to less frequent or more limited sexual activity.

In addition, some older adults may accept ageist stereotypes about sexuality and view their behaviors as inappropriate or potentially harmful, despite their relatively normal sexual desire and capacity. Others may lose self-confidence and feel less sexy, especially as they struggle to cope with age-associated changes in physical appearance, strength, and endurance. Such attitudinal barriers may be more damaging to sexuality than actual physiological changes. The quality of a person's relationship with a partner is also influential. Couples often must adapt sexual techniques and spend more time on foreplay to preserve previous levels of sexual function and enjoyment. Partners who are unable to work together may have difficulty with sex and perhaps even sexual dysfunction. On the other hand, aging can bring new possibilities for sexuality in later life. Partners may have more time to spend with each other once children have left home or during retirement. For postmenopausal females, sex may be associated with a reduced level of anxiety because of the impossibility of pregnancy.

Sexually Transmitted Diseases

According to surveillance data from the Centers for Disease Control and Prevention (2017), the rates of sexually transmitted diseases (STDs), including chlamydia, gonorrhea, and syphilis, are increasing across all age groups, including those 65 years and older, even though in comparison they have the lowest rates. These rises in prevalence are concerning and have been seen in other surveys as well. For example, rates of all STDs in individuals 60 and older increased by 23% between 2014 and 2017, compared with 11% overall for all age groups (Pereto 2018). With respect to HIV, data from 2018 indicated that 51% of affected individuals were 50 years or older, and 17% of new diagnoses were being made in this age group (Centers for Disease Control and Prevention 2018). The good news is that HIV-infected individuals are living longer and healthier lives because of current treatment options.

The increased prevalence of STDs in older individuals reflects the significant risks faced by sexually active adults who neglect safe sex practices, perhaps because of lack of knowledge, the absence of pregnancy risk, or a false sense of safety from knowing that STDs are more prevalent in younger people. One survey of a representative sample of 1,670 individuals 45 years and older found that <20% of participants who were single and dating reported using a condom or any other form of protection on a regular basis during sexual intercourse (AARP 2010).

Sexual Dysfunction in Late Life

Although most older individuals continue to engage in sexual activity, the prevalence of sexual dysfunction does increase with age (Lindau et al. 2007; Mulligan et al. 2003). The DSM-5 (American Psychiatric Association 2013) classification of sexual disorders is provided in Table 14–2. Erectile dysfunction (ED) is the most common form of sexual dysfunction among older men, affecting 20%–40% of men in their 60s and 50%–70% of men in their 70s and 80s (Laumann and Waite 2008; Lewis et al. 2004). In older women, the most common forms of sexual dysfunction are hypoactive sexual desire, female orgasmic disorder, and dyspareunia (Bitzer et al. 2008; Lindau et al. 2007). One study found that 44%–49% of women ages 57–85 years reported low desire, 35%–44% reported having difficulty with lubrication, and 34%–38% reported having anorgasmia (Lindau et al. 2007). In the same study, 31%–44% of men reported ED, and 14% were taking medication for it.

Although medical and psychiatric problems and medication effects are usually the main causes of sexual dysfunction in late life, numerous psychological factors must be considered, including performance anxiety, the presence of another sexual disorder in one or both partners, fears of self-injury or death due to medical conditions (e.g., a history of myocardial infarction, shortness of breath), sensitivity to loss of personal appearance or control of bodily functions (e.g., incontinence), relationship problems, and life stress. Psychogenic sexual dysfunction often first occurs after a stressful event,

TABLE 14–2.   DSM-5 classification of sexual dysfunctions

Female sexual interest/ arousal disorder	Absent or reduced sexual interest, thoughts or fantasies, initiated behaviors, excitement or pleasure, or genital or nongenital sensations during sexual activity or in response to sexual stimulation
Male hypoactive sexual desire disorder	Persistent or recurrent deficiency in or absence of sexual thoughts, fantasies, or desire
Erectile disorder	Marked difficulty in attaining an erection during sexual activity, or marked difficulty in maintaining an erection until the completion of sexual activity, or marked decrease in erectile rigidity
Delayed ejaculation	Marked delay in ejaculation or marked infrequency or absence of ejaculation
Female orgasmic disorder	Marked delay in, infrequency of, or absence of orgasm, or markedly reduced intensity of orgasmic sensations
Premature (early) ejaculation	Persistent or recurrent pattern of ejaculation during partnered sexual activity within ~1 minute following vaginal penetration
Substance/medication- induced sexual dysfunction	Significant disturbance in sexual function during substance intoxication or withdrawal or after exposure to a medication
Genito-pelvic pain/ penetration disorder	Persistent or recurrent difficulties during intercourse with vaginal penetration, pelvic pain, fear or anxiety about pain, or tensing and tightening of pelvic floor muscles

Note.   Symptoms of each of these sexual disorders occur on almost all or all occasions of sexual activity.

such as the loss of a loved one, a divorce, a financial or occupational strain, or a major health scare. Such major stresses may break sexual patterns and lead to uncertainty about how to resume sexual activity. As noted, the availability of partners is an acute issue for women, who outnumber men by more than two to one by age 85 years.

Medical and psychiatric disorders that are the most common causes of sexual dysfunction in geriatric patients are listed in Table 14–3. In both sexes, major risk factors for sexual dysfunction include diabetes mellitus, peripheral vascular disease, cancer, pulmonary disease, anxiety disorders, depression, stroke, dementia, Parkinson's disease, and substance abuse (Basson and Gilks 2018; Margolesky et al. 2020; McCabe et al. 2016; Shivananda and Rao 2016). These and other medical disorders exert both primary and secondary effects on sexual function. Examples of primary effects include impaired sexual arousal due to diabetic neuropathy and impaired genital vasocongestion due to peripheral vascular disease. Secondary effects such as fatigue, pain, sensory loss, and physical disability due to medical illness can make individuals feel less sexy and less confident in their sexual ability, which in turn can lead to hypoactive desire. Medications can also cause sexual dysfunction in both sexes at any point in the sexual response cycle (Ludwig and Phillips 2014; Thomas 2003). The most common problematic medications include antihypertensives (e.g., β-blockers, diuretics), anti-androgens, and many psychotropic medications (Nicolai et al. 2014; Segraves and Balon 2014). Some of the medications most commonly associated with sexual dysfunction in late life are listed in Table 14–4.

TABLE 14–3. **Medical and psychiatric conditions commonly associated with sexual dysfunction in late life**

Anxiety disorders (generalized anxiety disorder, panic disorder)

Arthritis and other degenerative joint diseases

Atherosclerosis (peripheral vascular disease, stroke)

Cancer (especially urological and genital cancers and their treatments)

Cardiac disease (coronary artery disease, congestive heart failure, myocardial infarction)

Chronic obstructive pulmonary disease

Chronic organ failure (renal, hepatic)

Diabetes mellitus

Mood disorders (major depressive disorder, bipolar disorder)

Multiple sclerosis

Neurocognitive disorders (Alzheimer's disease, vascular dementia, Lewy body dementia)

Obsessive-compulsive disorder

Parkinson's disease

Prostate disease and prostate surgery

Schizophrenia and other chronic psychotic disorders

Substance use disorders

Sexual dysfunction in late life is often comorbid with other psychiatric disorders. Symptoms range from transient dysfunction, present only during episodes of illness, to full-blown sexual disorders independent of the primary psychiatric disorder. Major depression often features loss of libido but may also be associated with inhibited arousal and ED. Symptomatic anxiety as well as anxiety and panic disorders are frequently associated with sexual dysfunction, including sexual phobias and sexual aversion (Kaplan 1987; Rajkumar and Kumaran 2015). Unfortunately, many of the antidepressants used to treat mood or anxiety disorders can cause or exacerbate sexual dysfunction, including hypoactive desire, delayed orgasm, and ED (see Table 14–4). Among these agents, selective serotonin reuptake inhibitors (SSRIs) tend to cause the greatest degree of sexual dysfunction, whereas bupropion and vilazodone have a significantly lower risk (Lorenz et al. 2016; Reichenpfader et al. 2014). All antipsychotic medications can cause sexual dysfunction, usually in proportion to the dosage, with higher rates of dysfunction seen with prolactin-raising agents such as risperidone, haloperidol, olanzapine, and clozapine than with prolactin-sparing agents such as quetiapine, aripiprazole, and ziprasidone (Baggaley 2008; Serretti and Chiesa 2011).

Assessment

Assessment of sexual dysfunction in late life involves identifying the specific problem and then obtaining a comprehensive medical, psychiatric, and sexual history to determine potential causes. A comprehensive sexual history involves asking patients about prior sexual experiences, current sexual functioning, and attitudes toward sexuality and toward any current partner. With older couples, interviewers must be able to identify relevant age-appropriate issues (Agronin 2014; Agronin and Westheimer

TABLE 14–4.   Medications associated with sexual dysfunction in late life

α-Adrenergic blockers (prazosin, phentolamine)

Antiandrogens (leuprolide, ketoconazole)

Antidepressants (monoamine oxidase inhibitors, tricyclic antidepressants, selective serotonin reuptake inhibitors, venlafaxine)

Antihistamines

Antihypertensives (thiazide diuretics, β-blockers, acetylcholinesterase inhibitors, clonidine, spironolactone, calcium channel blockers)

Antipsychotics (conventional and atypical)

Benzodiazepines

Cancer chemotherapeutic agents

Cardiac medications (e.g., digoxin, amiodarone)

Corticosteroids

Disopyramide

L-dopa

Histamine subtype 2 (H_2) receptor blockers

Mood stabilizers (lithium, valproic acid, carbamazepine)

2011). It is important to balance the need to gather sexual history with sensitivity to the fact that this is often the most personal information a patient will ever divulge. Ultimately, an accurate assessment of sexual dysfunction will benefit from a comfortable and productive doctor–patient relationship in which the right questions are asked, sufficient testing is performed, and partner cooperation is engaged.

The medical workup for sexual dysfunction may involve a physical examination, laboratory testing, and specialized diagnostic testing. The focus of the physical examination is on genital and urological anatomy and function, including underlying vascular and neurological function. Laboratory testing typically involves examination of routine blood chemistry (e.g., blood count, electrolyte levels, glucose levels, lipid profile), testosterone and prolactin levels, thyroid function, and, in males, prostate-specific antigen levels. Specialized diagnostic tests for ED may include nocturnal penile tumescence and rigidity testing (to determine whether natural erections occur during sleep) and penile duplex ultrasonography (to assess blood flow in the penis). This workup is typically conducted by a urologist.

Treatment

Preservation and enhancement of sexual activity in older patients is predicated on the fact that they want and intend to continue having sex, despite changes in physical and sexual function. Once an evaluation is complete, both partners should be educated about normal and dysfunctional sexuality (Bitzer et al. 2008). This information helps to reassure the affected individuals that they are not the only ones with the problem and that there are specific causes that can be treated. In addition, clinicians can help patients recognize sexuality as a form of physical and psychological intimacy and not solely as sexual intercourse. This discussion will build trust between the patient and

TABLE 14–5.   **Ten ways to enhance sexual function in late life**

1. Cultivate a positive attitude toward sexuality in later life.
2. Maintain optimal health and fitness. Avoid use of tobacco and excessive use of alcohol.
3. Maintain open and honest communication with your partner about how your sexual responsiveness has changed over time.
4. Focus on foreplay as much as on intercourse. Be open-minded about adapting sexual practices to your needs.
5. Maximize treatment of medical problems or disabilities that are interfering with sexual function. Consult a physician about any concerns regarding excess exertion during sex. To achieve adequate stamina, use appropriate exercise to build up strength and self-confidence.
6. Before sex, maximize treatment of symptoms that affect sex. For pain, consider taking a warm shower or bath, having a relaxing massage, or taking analgesics before sex. For shortness of breath, adapt sexual activity to minimize exertion and use prescribed inhalers ahead of time. Choose times of day for sex when pain is at a minimum.
7. For females, consider the use of estrogen cream to relieve vaginal dryness and improve vasocongestion in peri- or postmenopause. Tender genital or breast tissue may require more gentle stimulation, sometimes along with the use of an external lubricant.
8. Identify problematic medications and investigate alternative agents or strategies.
9. Avoid unrealistic expectations that sex must be the same as when you were younger.
10. Explore sexual positions that decrease exertion or account for equipment such as oxygen tanks or ostomy bags. Suggested positions for intercourse include lying side by side or sitting face-to-face.

Source.   Agronin and Westheimer 2011; Bitzer et al. 2008; Goodwin and Agronin 2015.

the clinician and will help the patient feel comfortable about seeking follow-up and being open about emotional reactions to the problem. Many treatments fail at this point because the patient and clinician never establish a solid working relationship. Treatment can also fail when one partner refuses to cooperate or when problems within the couple's entire relationship become insurmountable. Some ways in which an older couple can enhance sexual function and cope with disability are outlined in Table 14–5.

Unique challenges are faced by couples in which one or both partners have a chronic medical illness or disability. These couples often need to shift their focus from intercourse to foreplay and to adapt sexual practices to account for physical limitations such as fatigue, loss of muscle strength, and pain (Agronin and Westheimer 2011; Bronner 2011; Enzlin 2014; Schover and Jensen 1988). Physicians should work to maximize both rehabilitative and palliative treatments—for example, prescribing analgesics for pain, inhalers for shortness of breath, or physical therapy for joint immobility and muscle weakness. In addition, the appropriate treatment of depression, anxiety, or psychosis can often lead to significant improvement in sexual function, assuming the medications used to treat these disorders do not themselves cause problems. When medications do appear to be the culprit, initial strategies include reducing the dosage or replacing the medication with an equally effective alternative (Baggaley 2008; Clayton et al. 2014; Serretti and Chiesa 2011; Reichenpfader et al. 2014). Another strategy is to add an antidote to either override or reverse the medication's sexual effects, such as prescribing oral erectogenic medications for ED in males or bupropion for low desire in females (Taylor et al. 2013).

Sex Therapy

In some older couples, sexual dysfunction has clear psychological roots; for example, sexual dysfunction often occurs within the context of a dysfunctional relationship. Sex therapy is always best done conjointly, where both partners participate because both are an integral part of the problem and the solution. Historically, a psychodynamic model was used in sex therapy to uncover underlying unconscious conflicts, but that approach is now viewed as less successful, and cognitive-behavioral techniques are utilized in current treatment models (Brotto and Luria 2014; Kaplan 1983, 1974). Brief supportive and educational counseling is a first step in treatment and can help dispel distorted and uninformed attitudes toward sexuality in general and toward a sexual problem in particular. Counseling can also help a person or couple change their sexual practices to resolve a problem. In other cases, more intensive couples therapy is needed to resolve long-standing relationship issues before work on a sexual problem can begin. Sex therapy involves both cognitive and behavioral techniques, with an overall goal of building an association between relaxed and sensual physical intimacy and sexual relations. The same principles can be applied across the life span, with several refinements in later life. Using cognitive therapy techniques, therapists attempt to change patients' distorted cognitive attitudes toward sexual activity into more practical attitudes. They help patients to gain insight into the negative effects of their distorted thoughts and then to practice replacing these thoughts with more realistic and hopeful ones, sometimes even with positive assertions or affirmations of success (Goodwin and Agronin 2015).

Behavioral techniques used during sex therapy begin with exercises called *sensate focus*, in which the couple practices physical relaxation techniques during nonpressured sensual touching. Sensate focus helps reduce performance anxiety and restore the natural flow of the sexual response cycle. Once the partners feel relaxed and physically intimate together without sexual stimulation, they gradually progress to genital stimulation and then to intercourse. A number of adjustments in these exercises may be required for the older couple. For example, older patients who have physical problems that involve some degree of disability may express concerns about their ability to exert themselves adequately during sexual activity. In this case, the therapist might recommend one of several positions that minimize exertion, such as lying side by side or having one partner kneel on pillows and support him- or herself on a low bed. Other suggestions outlined in Table 14–5 might also apply. Such simple suggestions may remove some of the most anxiety-provoking barriers for an older couple, especially the common but unfounded belief that they lack the stamina or the dexterity for sexual activity.

During sex therapy, the therapist continues to work with the couple on their relationship and tries to identify and confront the resistance that inevitably arises during treatment. Such resistance to these seemingly innocuous exercises often reveals key problems in the relationship that are either causing the sexual dysfunction or impeding its treatment. Regardless of age, many couples find that sexual interest and pleasure reemerge and that sexual function improves during sex therapy, allowing them to once again enjoy such a fundamental component of their relationship. In addition to sex therapy, other approaches can be used for specific sexual disorders (Table 14–6).

TABLE 14–6.   **Treatment for specific sexual disorders**

Sexual disorder	Treatment approaches
Female sexual interest/ arousal disorder	Sexual education and counseling
	Hormone therapy with estrogens and/or androgens (Brotto and Luria 2014; Cappelletti and Wallen 2016)
	Bremelanotide (Kingsberg et al. 2019)
Erectile disorder	Sexual education and counseling
	Treatment of underlying problems with erectile physiology (Ludwig and Phillips 2014)
	Testosterone replacement for hypogonadism (Jacob 2011)
	Oral erectogenic medications/selective inhibitors of phosphodiesterase type 5 (PDE-5): sildenafil, tadalafil, and vardenafil (Ciocanel et al. 2019)
Female orgasmic disorder	Sexual education and counseling
	Guided masturbation/Use of vibrators (Graham 2014)
	Sildenafil (Akbarzadeh et al. 2014)
Premature (early) ejaculation	Sexual education and counseling
	Behavioral therapy with partner (Althof 2014)
	Topical anesthetic agents
	PDE-5 inhibitors (Aversa et al. 2011; Wang et al. 2007)
	Selective serotonin reuptake inhibitors (Waldinger 2007)

Sexual Function and Dysfunction in Dementia

Sexuality continues to play an important role in the lives of many adults with dementia, often by providing a nonverbal means of communication and intimacy (Davies et al. 2010). As the dementia progresses, however, the cognitively intact partner may become concerned about whether the affected partner is truly consenting to the sexual activity. Unaffected partners may also feel frustrated with a partner who does not always recognize them or who requests sex repeatedly because they cannot remember when they last had it (Redinbaugh et al. 1997). Sexual dysfunction is common, with more than three-quarters of affected individuals reporting at least one sexual problem, including lack of interest (reported by 40% of men and 65% of women) (Lindau et al. 2018). Neurocognitive changes can impair capacity for paying attention during sex as well as the ability to initiate and perform components of lovemaking (Rosen et al. 2010). Agitation, disinhibition, and psychosis associated with dementia may give rise to sexually aggressive or inappropriate behaviors.

These changes can prompt caregivers to have conflicting feelings of love and fidelity for their spouses with dementia alongside drops in libido and even desires for extramarital intimacy. It is not surprising, then, that these couples face a high degree of stress and an overall decrease in sexual activity (Bronner et al. 2015; Davies et al. 2012). For example, one study found that although 46% of couples remained sexually active 3 years after the initial diagnosis of dementia, this rate dropped to 41% at the 5-year mark and to 28% after 7 years (Eloniemi-Sulkava et al. 2002). Unfortunately, health care professionals often fail to inquire about such issues, despite the frequency with which they affect couples (Agronin 2014; Robinson and Davis 2013).

Although the percentage of adults with dementia who exhibit sexually aggressive or inappropriate behaviors is relatively small, these behaviors tend to generate a disproportionate amount of anxiety for caregivers and require a disproportionate amount of clinical attention (Joller et al. 2013). Problematic behaviors associated with dementia include inappropriate sexual comments or demands, hypersexual behaviors (e.g., repeated requests for sexual gratification, compulsive masturbation), disinhibition (e.g., exposing oneself, disrobing, masturbating in public), and sexually aggressive behaviors (e.g., attempts to grope, fondle, or force sex on another person) (Torrisi et al. 2017). In various studies, these behaviors were seen in <2% to nearly 25% of individuals with dementia (Chapman and Spitznagel 2019). Because frontal and temporal regions of the brain are involved in behavioral control and inhibition, individuals with dementia that affects these areas of the brain may be particularly vulnerable to developing such inappropriate behaviors (Mendez and Shapira 2013). Other factors associated with inappropriate or hyperactive sexual behaviors include mania, psychosis, medication effects, alcohol or drug abuse, stroke, and head trauma (Guay 2008; Wallace and Safer 2009). These behaviors raise concerns in long-term care settings when they are aggressively directed toward other residents (Rosen et al. 2010).

When the clinician is assessing a patient who has allegedly exhibited problematic behaviors, it is critical to identify the context of the behaviors. For example, public disrobing or touching of genitals in public may not be related to sexual urges but may instead reflect underlying confusion, delirium, motor restlessness, or stereotypy associated with dementia. Grabbing out toward others may be a means of getting attention when the individual cannot verbally express a need for attention. Caregivers and long-term care staff sometimes misinterpret these relatively innocuous behaviors as evidence of sexual disinhibition (Kamel and Hajjar 2004; Redinbaugh et al. 1997). It is also important to recognize that even individuals with severe dementia have legitimate needs for physical stimulation and intimacy but often lack the means to communicate them and obtain some form of gratification.

Regardless of the setting, adults with dementia have a right to engage in sexual relationships if they retain the capacity to understand the nature of the relationship and to provide reasonable consent. If cognitively intact partners are concerned about the capacity of their affected partners to engage in sexual activity, a psychiatric or psychological consultation may shed light on the affected person's understanding of the relationship. Lichtenberg and Strzepek (1990) proposed several questions to answer in any interview to determine a person's capacity to consent to a sexual relationship: Does the individual know who is initiating sexual contact? Can the person describe their preferred degree of intimacy? Is the sexual activity consistent with the person's previous beliefs and values? Can the person say "no" to unwanted activity? Does the person understand that a sexual relationship with someone other than their life partner may be temporary? Can the person describe how they would react if the sexual relationship were to end? Responses to these questions will help determine the affected partner's awareness of the relationship, ability to avoid coercion and exploitation, and awareness of the possible risks. One main purpose of psychological or psychiatric intervention is to provide education about sexuality to caregivers in the community and to staff in long-term care settings. Such education will improve interpretation of and response to apparent inappropriate sexual behaviors. In addition, educational programs for long-term care staff may foster attitudes that are more open-minded.

Behavioral approaches for inappropriate sexual comments include setting verbal limits and redirecting the individual to a different topic. Staff and caregivers must be careful to avoid reinforcing inappropriate comments, such as by laughing at off-color jokes or teasing patients in a seductive manner in response to sexual comments. In the case of inappropriate or aggressive sexual advances, staff may need to physically remove the patient from the situation or keep him or her away from vulnerable individuals. Because sexual advances may reflect unmet sexual needs, existing spouses or romantic partners can consider providing some appropriate form of physical intimacy, with the hope that it may attenuate the individual's drive to engage in inappropriate behaviors.

When behavioral approaches are insufficient to curtail aggressive or inappropriate sexual behaviors, there are several pharmacological strategies that might help, depending on any known or presumed underlying psychopathology (Tucker 2010). Antidepressants and antipsychotics have been used to treat more general aggressive behaviors and can be considered in these situations (Joller et al. 2013; Ozkan et al. 2008). For example, an antidepressant with sexual side effects such as an SSRI may reduce impulsive or intrusive sexual behaviors that reflect an overactive libido. Mood stabilizers, including antipsychotics, may treat sexual behaviors that reflect underlying mania or mood instability. When prescribing antipsychotics, clinicians should be mindful of potential side effects, such as sedation, falls, and metabolic changes, and black box warnings about increased mortality associated with their use in the setting of dementia. Although both estrogen and medroxyprogesterone have been shown to reduce libido and sexual aggression in men with dementia (Kyomen et al. 1999; Light and Holroyd 2006), the potential side effects such as weight gain, glucose intolerance, and liver dysfunction might outweigh the benefits.

Conclusion

Sexual function and behavior change in significant ways with age but continue to be important and vital parts of overall wellness. One of the most important components to healthy sexual functioning in later life is the maintenance of good underlying physical health, with a focus on specific disease states and medications that can be problematic. Sexual dysfunction is increasingly common but can be readily identified and treated with psychotherapeutic and, when necessary, pharmacological approaches.

Key Points

- Sexuality continues to play an important role in the lives of aging adults who are increasingly living longer, healthier lives. It is facilitated by increasingly positive attitudes and newer and more effective treatments for sexual dysfunction.

- Sexual surveys indicate that although most individuals age 65 years and older continue to be sexually active, there are declines in both the rate and the frequency of sexual activity, particularly in older single women.

- The main predictors of sexual activity in late life are previous sexual behaviors; the availability, health, and interest of a partner; and the individual's overall physical health.

- Rates of sexual dysfunction increase with age, with erectile disorder being the most common disorder in older men and sexual interest/arousal disorder being the most common disorder in older women.

- Depending on its form, sexual dysfunction in late life can be treated with a variety of approaches, including the treatment of any causative medical or medication-related factors, psychoeducation, individual or couples counseling, sex therapy, and the use of disorder-specific medications, such as oral erectogenic agents for erectile dysfunction.

- Dementia can affect sexuality in several ways, including increasing the rate of sexual dysfunction and causing sexually inappropriate behaviors. Still, sexual expression is both a need and a right for individuals with dementia and should be included as part of assessment, education, and management strategies.

Suggested Readings

Agronin ME: Sexuality and aging, in Principles and Practice of Sex Therapy, 5th Edition. Edited by Binik YM, Hall KSK. New York, Guilford, 2014, pp 525–539

Bitzer J, Platano G, Tschudin S, et al: Sexual counselling in elderly couples. J Sex Med 5(9):2027–2043, 2008

Eloniemi-Sulkava U, Notkola IL, Hämä-läinen K, et al: Spouse caregivers' perceptions of influence of dementia on marriage. Psychogeriatrics 14(1):47–58, 2002

Mroczek B, Kurpas D, Gronowska M, et a: Psychosexual needs and sexual behaviors of nursing care home residents. Arch Gerontol Geriatr 57(1):32–38, 2013

Nelson HD, Walker M, Zakher B, et al: Menopausal hormone therapy for the primary prevention of chronic conditions: a systematic review to update the U.S. Preventive Services Task Force recommendations. Ann Intern Med 157(2):104–113, 2012

Robinson KM, Davis SJ: Influence of cognitive decline on sexuality in individuals with dementia and their caregivers. J Gerontol Nurs 39(11):30–36, 2013

Rosen T, Lachs MS, Pillemer K: Sexual aggression between residents in nursing homes: literature synthesis of an underrecognized problem. J Am Geriatr Soc 58(10):1970–1979, 2010

Tucker I: Management of inappropriate sexual behaviors in dementia: a literature review. Int Psychogeriatr 22(5):683–692, 2010

University of Michigan: National Poll on Healthy Aging: Let's Talk About Sex. Available at: https://www.healthyagingpoll.org/sites/default/files/2018–05/NPHA-Sexual-Health-Report_050118_final2.pdf. 2018. Accessed October 6, 2020.

Vegunta S, Kling JM, Kapoor E. Androgen therapy in women. J Womens Health 29(1):57–64, 2020

References

AARP: Sexuality at Midlife and Beyond: 2004 Update of Attitudes and Behaviors. Washington, DC, AARP, 2005. Available at: https://assets.aarp.org/rgcenter/general/2004_sexuality.pdf. Accessed October 6, 2020.

AARP: Sex, Romance, and Relationships: AARP Survey of Midlife and Older Adults (Publ D19234). Washington, DC, AARP, April 2010. Available at: https://assets.aarp.org/rgcenter/general/srr_09.pdf. Accessed October 6, 2020.

Adelman M: Stigma, gay lifestyles, and adjustment to aging: a study of later-life gay men and lesbians. J Homosex 20(3–4):7–32, 1990 2086652

Agronin ME: Sexuality and aging, in Principles and Practice of Sex Therapy, 5th Edition. Edited by Binik YM, Hall KSK. New York, Guilford, 2014, pp 525–539

Agronin ME, Westheimer RK: Sexuality and sexual disorders in late life, in Principles and Practice of Geriatric Psychiatry, 2nd Edition. Edited by Agronin ME, Maletta G. Philadelphia, PA, Lippincott, Williams and Wilkins, 2011, pp 603–625

Akbarzadeh M, Zeinalzadeh S, Zolghadri J, et al: Comparison of Elaeagnus angustifolia extract and sildenafil citrate on female orgasmic disorders: a randomized clinical tial. J Reprod Infertil 15(4):190–198, 2014 25473627

Althof SE: Treatment of premature ejaculation: psychotherapy, pharmacotherapy and combined therapy, in Principles and Practice of Sex Therapy, 5th Edition. Edited by Binik YM, Hall KSK. New York, Guilford, 2014, pp 112–137

American Psychiatric Association: Diagnostic and Statistical Manual of Mental Disorders, 5th Edition. Arlington, VA, American Psychiatric Association, 2013

Aversa A, Francomano D, Bruzziches R, et al: Is there a role for phosphodiesterase type-5 inhibitors in the treatment of premature ejaculation? Int J Impot Res 23(1):17–23, 2011 21270821

Baggaley M: Sexual dysfunction in schizophrenia: focus on recent evidence. Hum Psychopharmacol 23(3):201–209, 2008 18338766

Bassil N, Morley JE: Late-life onset hypogonadism: a review. Clin Geriatr Med 26(2):197–222, 2010 20497841

Basson R, Gilks T: Women's sexual dysfunction associated with psychiatric disorders and their treatment. Womens Health 14:1745506518762664, 2018

Bell S, Reissing ED, Henry LA, VanZuylen H: Sexual activity after 60: a systematic review of associated factors. Sex Med Rev 5(1):52–80, 2017

Bitzer J, Platano G, Tschudin S, Alder J: Sexual counseling in elderly couples. J Sex Med 5(9):2027–2043, 2008 18637999

Bronner G: Sexual problems in Parkinson's disease: the multidimensional nature of the problem and of the intervention. J Neurol Sci 310(1–2):139–143, 2011 21723568

Bronner G, Aharon-Peretz J, Hassin-Baer S: Sexuality in patients with Parkinson's disease, Alzheimer's disease, and other dementias. Handb Clin Neurol 130:297–323, 2015 26003251

Brotman S, Ryan B, Cormier R: The health and social service needs of gay and lesbian elders and their families in Canada. Gerontologist 43(2):192–202, 2003 12677076

Brotto L, Luria M: Sexual interest/arousal disorder in woman, in Principles and Practice of Sex Therapy, 5th Edition. Edited by Binik YM, Hall KSK. New York, Guilford, 2014, pp 17–41

Cappelletti M, Wallen K: Increasing women's sexual desire: the comparative effectiveness of estrogens and androgens. Horm Behav 78:178–193, 2016 26589379

Centers for Disease Control and Prevention: HIV and Older Americans. Atlanta, GA, Centers for Disease Control and Prevention, 2018. Available at: https://www.cdc.gov/hiv/group/age/olderamericans/index.html. Accessed October 18, 2020.

Centers for Disease Control and Prevention: Sexually Transmitted Disease Surveillance. Atlanta, GA, Centers for Disease Control and Prevention, 2017. Available at: https://www.cdc.gov/std/stats17/2017-STD-Surveillance-Report_CDC-clearance-9.10.18.pdf. Accessed October 18, 2020.

Chapman KR, Spitznagel MB: Measurement of sexual disinhibition in dementia: a systematic review. Int J Geriatr Psychiatry 34(12):1747–1757, 2019 31489715

Ciocanel O, Power K, Eriksen A: Interventions to treat erectile dysfunction and premature ejaculation: an overview of systematic reviews. Sex Med 7(3):251–269, 2019 31300388

Clayton AH, Croft HA, Handiwala L: Antidepressants and sexual dysfunction: mechanisms and clinical implications. Postgrad Med 126(2):91–99, 2014 24685972

D'Augelli AR, Grossman AH: Disclosure of sexual orientation, victimization, and mental health among lesbian, gay, and bisexual older adults. J Interpers Violence 16:1008–1027, 2001

Davies HD, Newkirk LA, Pitts CB, et al: The impact of dementia and mild memory impairment (MMI) on intimacy and sexuality in spousal relationships. Int Psychogeriatr 22(4):618–628, 2010 20226112

Davies HD, Sridhar SB, Newkirk LA, et al: Gender differences in sexual behaviors of AD patients and their relationship to spousal caregiver well-being. Aging Ment Health 16(1):89–101, 2012 21999712

El Khoudary SR, Greendale G, Crawford SL, et al: The menopause transition and women's health at midlife: a progress report from the Study of Women's Health Across the Nation (SWAN). Menopause 26(10):1213–1227, 2019 31568098

Eloniemi-Sulkava U, Notkola IL, Hämäläinen K, et al: Spouse caregivers' perceptions of influence of dementia on marriage. Int Psychogeriatr 14(1):47–58, 2002 12094907

Enzlin P: Sexuality in the context of chronic illness, in Principles and Practice of Sex Therapy, 5th Edition. Edited by Binik YM, Hall KSK. New York, Guilford, 2014, pp 436–456

Erens B, Mitchell KR, Gibson L, et al: Health status, sexual activity and satisfaction among older people in Britain: a mixed methods study. PLoS One 14(3):e0213835, 2019 30917152

Fredriksen-Goldsen KI, Muraco A: Aging and sexual orientation: a 25-year review of the literature. Res Aging 32(3):372–413, 2010 24098063

Goodwin AJ, Agronin ME: A Women's Guide to Overcoming Sexual Fear and Pain. Brattleboro, VT, Echo Point Books and Media, 2015

Graham CA: Orgasm disorders in women, in Principles and Practice of Sex Therapy, 5th Edition. Edited by Binik YM, Hall KSK. New York, Guilford, 2014, pp 89–111

Graham CA, Mercer CH, Tanton C, et al: What factors are associated with reporting lacking interest in sex and how do these vary by gender? Findings from the third British national survey of sexual attitudes and lifestyles. BMJ Open 7(9):e016942, 2017

Grossman AH, D'Augelli AR, O'Connell TS: Being lesbian, gay, bisexual and 60 or older in North America. J Gay Lesbian Soc Serv 13(4):23–40, 2001

Guay DR: Inappropriate sexual behaviors in cognitively impaired older individuals. Am J Geriatr Pharmacother 6(5):269–288, 2008 19161930

Haider A, Meergans U, Traish A, et al: Progressive improvement of T-scores in men with osteoporosis and subnormal serum testosterone levels upon treatment with testosterone over six years. Int J Endocrinol 2014:496948, 2014 24688541

Harder H, Starkings RML, Fallowfield LJ, et al: Sexual functioning in 4,418 postmenopausal women participating in UKCTOCS: a qualitative free-text analysis. Menopause 26(10):1100–1009, 2019 31290761

Jacob BC: Testosterone replacement therapy in males with erectile dysfunction. J Pharm Pract 24(3):298–306, 2011 21676853

Jacoby S: Great sex: what's age got to do with it? Modern Maturity (Sept/Oct):43–48, 1999

Jia H, Sullivan CT, McCoy SC, et al: Review of health risks of low testosterone and testosterone administration. World J Clin Cases 3(4):338–344, 2015 25879005

Joller P, Gupta N, Seitz DP, et al: Approach to inappropriate sexual behaviour in people with dementia. Can Fam Physician 59(3):255–260, 2013 23486794

Kamel HK, Hajjar RR: Sexuality in the nursing home, part 2: managing abnormal behavior: legal and ethical issues. J Am Med Dir Assoc 5(2 suppl):S48–S52, 2004 14984611

Kaplan HS: The New Sex Therapy. New York, Brunner/Mazel, 1974

Kaplan HS: The Evaluation of Sexual Disorders: Psychological and Medical Aspects. New York, Brunner/Mazel, 1983

Kaplan HS: Sexual Aversion, Sexual Phobias, and Panic Disorder. New York, Brunner/Mazel, 1987

Kingsberg SA, Clayton AH, Portman D, et al: Bremelanotide for the treatment of hypoactive sexual desire disorder: two randomized phase 3 trials. Obstet Gynecol 134(5):899–908, 2019 31599840

Kyomen HH, Satlin A, Hennen J, Wei JY: Estrogen therapy and aggressive behavior in elderly patients with moderate-to-severe dementia: results from a short-term, randomized, double-blind trial. Am J Geriatr Psychiatry 7(4):339–348, 1999 10521168

Lacey JV Jr, Mink PJ, Lubin JH, et al: Menopausal hormone replacement therapy and risk of ovarian cancer. JAMA 288(3):334–341, 2002 12117398

Laumann EO, Waite LJ: Sexual dysfunction among older adults: prevalence and risk factors from a nationally representative U.S. probability sample of men and women 57–85 years of age. J Sex Med 5(10):2300–2311, 2008 18702640

Lester PE, Kohen I, Stefanacci RG, Feuerman M: Sex in nursing homes: a survey of nursing home policies governing resident sexual activity. J Am Med Dir Assoc 17(1):71–74, 2016 26441358

Lewis RW, Fugl-Meyer KS, Bosch R, et al: Epidemiology/risk factors of sexual dysfunction. J Sex Med 1(1):35–39, 2004 16422981

Lichtenberg PA, Strzepek DM: Assessments of institutionalized dementia patients' competencies to participate in intimate relationships. Gerontologist 30(1):117–120, 1990 2311954

Light SA, Holroyd S: The use of medroxyprogesterone acetate for the treatment of sexually inappropriate behaviour in patients with dementia. J Psychiatry Neurosci 31(2):132–134, 2006 16575429

Lindau ST, Schumm LP, Laumann EO, et al: A study of sexuality and health among older adults in the United States. N Engl J Med 357(8):762–774, 2007 17715410

Lindau ST, Dale W, Feldmeth G, et al: Sexuality and cognitive status: A U.S. nationally representative study of home-dwelling older adults. J Am Geriatr Soc 66(10):1902–1910, 2018 30207599

Lobo RA: Hormone-replacement therapy: current thinking. Nat Rev Endocrinol 13(4):220–231, 2017 27716751

Lorenz T, Rullo J, Faubion S: Antidepressant-induced female sexual dysfunction. Mayo Clin Proc 91(9):1280–1286, 2016 27594188

Ludwig W, Phillips M: Organic causes of erectile dysfunction in men under 40. Urol Int 92(1):1–6, 2014 24281298

Mahieu L, Gastmans C: Older residents' perspectives on aged sexuality in institutionalized elderly care: a systematic literature review. Int J Nurs Stud 52(12):1891–1905, 2015 26296654

Manuela Peixoto M: Sexual satisfaction, solitary, and dyadic sexual desire in men according to sexual orientation. J Homosex 66(6):769–779, 2019 29863980

Margolesky J, Betté S, Singer C: Management of urologic and sexual dysfunction in Parkinson disease. Clin Geriatr Med 36(1):69–80, 2020 31733703

Marjoribanks J, Farquhar C, Roberts H, Lethaby A: Long term hormone therapy for perimenopausal and postmenopausal women. Cochrane Database Syst Rev 7(7):CD004143, 2012 22786488

Masters WH, Johnson VE: Human Sexual Response. Boston, MA, Little, Brown, 1966

McCabe MP, Sharlip ID, Lewis R, et al: Risk factors for sexual dysfunction among women and men: a consensus statement from the fourth international consultation on sexual medicine 2015. J Sex Med 13(2):153–167, 2016 26953830

Mendez MF, Shapira JS: Hypersexual behavior in frontotemporal dementia: a comparison with early onset Alzheimer's disease. Arch Sex Behav 42(3):501–509, 2013 23297146

Minkin MJ, Maamari R, Reiter S: Postmenopausal vaginal atrophy: evaluation of treatment with local estrogen therapy. Int J Womens Health 6(6):281–288, 2014 24648772

Morley JE: Testosterone and behavior. Clin Geriatr Med 19(3):605–616, 2003 14567011

Mroczek B, Kurpas D, Gronowska M, et al: Psychosexual needs and sexual behaviors of nursing care home residents. Arch Gerontol Geriatr 57(1):32–38, 2013 23478162

Mulligan T, Reddy S, Gulur PV, Godschalk M: Disorders of male sexual function. Clin Geriatr Med 19(3):473–481, v, 2003 14567002

Nicolai MP, Liem SS, Both S, et al: A review of the positive and negative effects of cardiovascular drugs on sexual function: a proposed table for use in clinical practice. Neth Heart J 22(1):11–19, 2014 24155101

Ozkan B, Wilkins K, Muralee S, Tampi RR: Pharmacotherapy for inappropriate sexual behaviors in dementia: a systematic review of literature. Am J Alzheimers Dis Other Demen 23(4):344–354, 2008 18509106

Pereto A: Patients over 60? Screen for STIs. Athena Health, May 16, 2018. Available at: https://www.athenahealth.com/knowledge-hub/clinical-trends/over-60-stis-may-not-be-done-you. Accessed October 18, 2020.

Pines A: Male menopause: is it a real clinical syndrome? Climacteric 14(1):15–17, 2011 20670200

Pope M, Schulz R: Sexual attitudes and behavior in midlife and aging homosexual males. J Homosex 20(3–4):169–177, 1990 2086646

Rajkumar RP, Kumaran AK: Depression and anxiety in men with sexual dysfunction: a retrospective study. Compr Psychiatry 60:114–118, 2015 25818906

Redinbaugh EM, Zeiss AM, Davies HD, et al: Sexual behavior in men with dementing illnesses. Clin Geriatr 5:45–50, 1997

Reichenpfader U, Gartlehner G, Morgan LC, et al: Sexual dysfunction associated with second-generation antidepressants in patients with major depressive disorder: results from a systematic review with network meta-analysis. Drug Saf 37(1):19–31, 2014 24338044

Roach SM: Sexual behaviour of nursing home residents: staff perceptions and responses. J Adv Nurs 48(4):371–379, 2004 15500531

Robinson KM, Davis SJ: Influence of cognitive decline on sexuality in individuals with dementia and their caregivers. J Gerontol Nurs 39(11):30–36, 2013 24066786

Roelofs TS, Luijkx KG, Embregts PJ: Intimacy and sexuality of nursing home residents with dementia: a systematic review. Int Psychogeriatr 27(3):367–384, 2015 25381794

Rosen RC, Wu F, Behre HM, et al: Quality of life and sexual function benefits of long-term testosterone treatment: longitudinal results from the Registry of Hypogonadism in Men (RHYME). J Sex Med 14(9):1104–1115, 2017 28781213

Rosen T, Lachs MS, Pillemer K: Sexual aggression between residents in nursing homes: literature synthesis of an underrecognized problem. J Am Geriatr Soc 58(10):1970–1979, 2010 20840462

Schick V, Herbenick D, Reece M, et al: Sexual behaviors, condom use, and sexual health of Americans over 50: implications for sexual health promotion for older adults. J Sex Med 7(suppl 5):315–329, 2010 21029388

Schover LR, Jensen SB: Sexuality and Chronic Illness. New York, Guilford, 1988

Segraves RT, Balon R: Antidepressant-induced sexual dysfunction in men. Pharmacol Biochem Behav 121:132–137, 2014 24239785

Serretti A, Chiesa A: A meta-analysis of sexual dysfunction in psychiatric patients taking antipsychotics. Int Clin Psychopharmacol 26(3):130–140, 2011 21191308

Shivananda MJ, Rao TS: Sexual dysfunction in medical practice. Curr Opin Psychiatry 29(6):331–335, 2016 27636599

Snarch D: Constructing the Sexual Crucible: An Integration of Sexual and Marital Therapy. New York, WW Norton, 1991

Srinivasan S, Glover J, Tampi RR, et al: Sexuality and the older adult. Curr Psychiatry Rep 21(10):97–105, 2019 31522296

Stanworth RD, Jones TH: Testosterone for the aging male; current evidence and recommended practice. Clin Interv Aging 3(1):25–44, 2008 18488876

Taylor MJ, Rudkin L, Bullemor-Day P, et al: Strategies for managing sexual dysfunction induced by antidepressant medication. Cochrane Database Syst Rev 5(5):CD003382, 2013 23728643

Thaung Zaw JJ, Howe PRC, Wong RHX: Postmenopausal health interventions: time to move on from the Women's Health Initiative? Ageing Res Rev 48:79–86, 2018 30355506

Thomas DR: Medications and sexual function. Clin Geriatr Med 19(3):553–562, 2003 14567007

Torrisi M, Cacciola A, Marra A, et al: Inappropriate behaviors and hypersexuality in individuals with dementia: an overview of a neglected issue. Geriatr Gerontol Int 17(6):865–874, 2017 27489168

Tucker I: Management of inappropriate sexual behaviors in dementia: a literature review. Int Psychogeriatr 22(5):683–692, 2010 20226113

University of Michigan: National Poll on Healthy Aging: Let's Talk About Sex. Available at: https://www.healthyagingpoll.org/reports-more/report/lets-talk-about-sex. 2018. Accessed October 6, 2020.

Vegunta S, Kling JM, Kapoor E: Androgen therapy in women. J Womens Health 29(1):57–64, 2020 31687883

Villar F, Celdrán M, Fabà J, Serrat R: Barriers to sexual expression in residential aged care facilities (RACFs): comparison of staff and residents' views. J Adv Nurs 70(11):2518–2527, 2014 24655133

Waldinger MD: Premature ejaculation: state of the art. Urol Clin North Am 34(4):591–599, 2007 17983899

Wallace M, Safer M: Hypersexuality among cognitively impaired older adults. Geriatr Nurs 30(4):230–237, 2009 19665665

Wang WF, Wang Y, Minhas S, Ralph DJ: Can sildenafil treat primary premature ejaculation? A prospective clinical study. Int J Urol 14(4):331–335, 2007 17470165

Westheimer RK, Lopater S: Human Sexuality: A Psychosocial Perspective. Philadelphia, PA, Lippincott Williams and Wilkins, 2002

Zilbergeld B, Ellison C: Desire discrepancies and arousal problems in sex therapy, in Principles and Practice of Sex Therapy. Edited by Leiblum S, Pervin L. New York, Guilford, 1980, pp 65–101

CHAPTER 15

Bereavement

Moria J. Smoski, Ph.D.
Stephanie A. Schuette, M.A.
Larry W. Thompson, Ph.D.

As the Baby Boomer population ages, increasing numbers of adults are confronting late-life bereavement. In this chapter, we examine the current research on bereavement in elderly persons and explore the following salient areas: the demographics of bereavement, theoretical and empirical perspectives on adjustment to the loss of a loved one, and therapeutic considerations in the diagnosis and treatment of complicated grief.

Late-Life Bereavement

The terms *bereavement* and *grief reaction* have been used to refer to any number of losses, including (but not limited to) the death of a spouse, an adult child, another family member, or a close personal friend; divorce (Cain 1988); predeath grief associated with providing care for a severely impaired loved one (Meichsner et al. 2020); and a significant decline in one's own health, attractiveness, capabilities, opportunities, and so forth (Kalish 1987). When used in its narrowest sense, however, *bereavement* refers to the reaction or process that results after the death of someone close. Indeed, the death of a spouse is generally accepted as the most common and traumatic life event in late life (Jacobs and Ostfeld 1977).

In the United States, 34% of women and 12% of men older than 65 years have lost a spouse (Federal Interagency Forum on Aging-Related Statistics 2016). The mean duration of widow- or widowerhood is ~14 years for women versus only 7 years for men (U.S. Census Bureau 2001). These data, plus the fact that widowers are more likely than widows to remarry after losing their spouses, have often led to the interpretation that bereavement is a "women's issue." Although older women may live without a spouse longer than their male peers, they also have lower mortality rates. For example, in a University of Southern California longitudinal study of spousal bereavement, the first year after a bereavement saw a mortality rate of 12% in men but only ~1% in women (Gallagher-Thompson et al. 1993; Thompson et al. 1991). Thus, the loss of a spouse is an important issue regardless of gender or sex.

Theories About Adjustment to Permanent Losses

Numerous theoretical perspectives on the function and process of bereavement have been developed over the years. We provide here only a brief review; more comprehensive reviews are available elsewhere (Neimeyer et al. 2011; Osterweis et al. 1984; Stroebe and Schut 1999; Stroebe et al. 2001a).

Early work emphasized that mourning was a process whereby the bereaved gradually "surrendered" attachment to the lost loved one by engaging in certain specific psychological and behavioral tasks at appropriate time points during the bereavement (Freud 1917[1915]/1957; Lindemann 1944). This process was thought to be necessary for people to develop constructive new attachments to others entering their lives. Failure to complete these tasks would result in the development of a psychiatric disorder. Bowlby (1961) offered a somewhat different interpretation of grief behaviors. He posited that any involuntary separation, including bereavement, gives rise to many forms of attachment behavior (e.g., separation anxiety and pining) that reflect the person's desire to reunite with the lost person. In his view, the function of bereavement is not surrendering attachment but attempting to regain a sense of connection with the lost object of attachment. With time, these behaviors were thought to dissipate through a series of stages, including shock, protest, despair, and finally breakage of the bond and adjustment to a new self.

Parkes (1972) and Horowitz (1976) proposed models that involve phases or stages of reaction to the death of a loved one, similar to Kübler-Ross's (1969) seminal stage model of the reactions of individuals facing a terminal illness. The initial period is characterized by shock and disbelief, combined with emotional numbness and cognitive confusion, with intense free-floating anxiety and sharp mood fluctuations. The second phase generally begins as the numbness and anxiety start to decrease. During this period, family and friends gradually become less available and often convey the message that the bereaved person should be getting over the grief and moving on with life, although the individual is far from ready to do so. Specific symptoms such as frequent crying, chronic sleep disturbance, blue mood, poor appetite, low energy, feelings of fatigue, loss of interest in daily living, and problems with attention and concentration are common. Even though these symptoms can also be indicative of depression, most grieving individuals do not develop major depression; the sadness that accompanies bereavement is specific to the loss of the loved person, rather than the more global dejection that characterizes major depression. This second phase is described as a time of "yearning and protest," during which the bereaved may actively or implicitly search for the deceased (Parkes 1972). Even though these seeking experiences may be startling to an outside observer (e.g., believing one has seen or heard the lost loved one), they are common. In one study, approximately half of bereaved individuals reported seeing, hearing, or sensing their deceased spouse within 13 months of their death, an experience that is sometimes reported as positive or comforting (Carlsson and Nilsson 2007). Although many bereaved individuals report a profound sense of connection to and an ongoing presence of the deceased, others note no such experiences and seem mystified by the idea of such a phenomenon. Such polarity in bereavement experiences further complicates any attempts to describe a "typical" bereavement scenario (Bonanno 2009).

The final phase of the stage model is referred to as "identity reconstruction" (Lopata 1996). During this period, the bereaved person gradually reinvests the psychic energy that had been completely focused on the lost loved one into forming new relationships and participating in activities. Lopata (1996) estimated that identity reconstruction takes a year or longer, depending on what she referred to as the "centrality of roles" involved and the complexity of new learning that must occur in developing a new sense of self.

Stage theories of adaptation have been widely accepted by health care professionals, yet little empirical evidence exists to support them. For example, although stage theories would predict an eventual end stage at which grieving ceases, grief symptoms often do not abate in elderly widows and widowers (Aoun et al. 2021). To expect that grief will resolve or end is now considered erroneous by some theorists (Stroebe et al. 2001a). Bereavement, as Rosenblatt (1996) contended, is a dynamic process that may continue for many years and even for the remainder of one's life. Also, bereaved individuals do not proceed from one clearly identifiable phase to another in an orderly fashion, a fact particularly true of older adults. Maciejewski et al. (2007) provide one of the few empirical attempts to test a stage theory: they examined Jacobs's (1993) stage theory, which posits that bereaved persons pass through stages of disbelief, yearning, anger, depression, and acceptance. The results were mixed: Across indicators, acceptance was the most frequent response given and yearning the second most frequent response at all time points across 2 years after the loss. However, when the researchers examined the peak frequency within each indicator, peaks occurred in the predicted order. Disbelief was at its highest immediately after loss and declined over time; yearning peaked at ~4 months post loss and then declined; all other indicators peaked in the predicted order (Maciejewski et al. 2007). Even though participants did not complete a stage before moving to a new one, the stage model did provide potentially useful information regarding the ebb and flow of a given characteristic of grief. Although the specific process of moving through stages has not been supported, stage models may provide a useful descriptive overview of many commonly recognized facets of the bereavement process.

Another trend in bereavement theory has been to consider environmental changes and role adaptation along with individual emotional and psychological adjustments. Whereas earlier positions had focused solely on intrapsychic processes (e.g., Bowlby 1961), more recently theorists have incorporated interpersonal and social processes into their models (see, e.g., Neimeyer 1998). Grieving is not only a process involving preoccupation with the deceased individual, accepting the loss, trying to make sense of what has happened, and so on; it is also an attempt to construct meaning from the loss and to reduce the chaos associated with such traumatic events. As Stroebe and Schut (1999, 2010) addressed with their dual process model, the bereaved oscillate between dealing with *loss-oriented stressors* and *restoration-oriented stressors*. The former relate to the specific components of the loss leading to emotional, behavioral, and cognitive symptoms and how to deal with these; the latter pertain to how one must interact constructively with social/environmental systems in order to maintain adaptive functioning in social, vocational, and avocational activities. Grief-related tasks usually include confronting the loss, restructuring thoughts and memories about the deceased person, and emotionally withdrawing from (but not forgetting) the deceased person. Restoration tasks include accepting the changed world, spending time away from grieving, and developing new relationships and identities. In keeping with T.S. Eliot's contention that "humankind cannot bear very much reality," Stroebe and Schut (1999) argued that alternation or oscillation in dealing with these two types of stressors is critical in the adjustment process. Provided that they are not persistently implemented and are not the only coping efforts employed, psychological mechanisms that allow the bereaved person to avoid or minimize the massive impact of the loss can help that person adapt. Balance in dealing with the two types of stressors as a result of oscillation thus precludes the preoccupation with one or the other that may lead to prolonged and complicated bereavement. Limited empirical support for this model is emerging, with individuals who report actively dealing with both loss-oriented stressors and restoration-oriented stressors showing the best psychological outcomes (Bennett et al. 2010).

Course of Bereavement Symptoms and Clinical Definitions

Several longitudinal studies have had consistent findings regarding the course of depressed mood, anxiety, well-being, and level of grief following a loss. Grief is separable from depression and can include components of nonacceptance of, emotional responses to, and thoughts about the loss (Futterman et al. 2010). Generally, significant differences between bereaved and nonbereaved individuals are readily apparent during the first 6 months following the loss. However, at ~12 months post loss, levels of reported distress by the bereaved are substantially reduced, and the difference between bereaved and nonbereaved control subjects is often difficult to detect (Harlow et al. 1991; Thompson et al. 1991). While considerable recovery has occurred and the bereaved person is successfully handling tasks of daily living, many symptoms are still present (Harlow et al. 1991; Thompson et al. 1984), and some sadness may persist (Bonanno 2009). As described by Zisook and DeVaul (1984), "In uncomplicated bereavement, acute grief is gradually replaced by slow resolution" (p. 175).

Although a period of distress followed by gradual abatement may be the most common course following a loss, it is not the only pattern. Several prospective and retrospective studies have identified other common patterns, including *resilience, relief,* and *chronic grief.* Individuals identified as resilient demonstrate consistently low levels of depression or negative affect across the post-loss period. This pattern is perhaps surprisingly common, with estimates of the percentage of bereaved individuals following the resilient pattern ranging from 34% (Nielsen et al. 2019; Ott et al. 2007) to 46% (Bonanno et al. 2004). The resilient individuals did not differ from the common or chronic grief groups in either relationship quality or interviewer ratings of interpersonal skill or warmth (Bonanno et al. 2004; Ott et al. 2007), but they were more likely than the other groups to utilize religious coping (Ott et al. 2007). Follow-up analyses found that the resilient group reported the most comfort from positive memories of their spouse and the least search for meaning in the death (Bonanno et al. 2004). Identifying the characteristics of individuals following a resilient course is an active area of current research (Coifman et al. 2007a, 2007b). Promising in this regard is a Malaysian study of elderly widowed Muslim adults that found that personal religiosity (i.e., viewing religion as important and engaging in private prayer) decreased the negative psychological effects of losing a spouse (Momtaz et al. 2010).

Individuals who have witnessed a loved one's steady decline, and in many cases have functioned as caregivers for their dying loved one, often manifest a relief pattern. Observing the illness transforms both the loved partner and the relationship, and dealing with the preparatory grief accompanying that transformation often leaves caregivers physically and psychologically spent. Rather than being shaken by their loss, they may discover a sense of freedom, both for the deceased person who has been liberated from suffering and for themselves because they can recover the life they relinquished to attend to the needs of the significant other (Bonanno 2009).

Chronic grief is characterized by unremitting distress that lasts for an extended period following a loss. Awareness of the impact of chronic grief and an interest in better understanding chronic grief as a mental disorder have grown in recent years. Maciejewski et al. (2016) focused on a conceptualization of prolonged grief disorder (PGD), whereas Shear et al. (2011) focused on one of complicated grief. These conceptualizations differ in how they view grief-related pathology, with the intensity and duration of grief indicating pathology in prolonged grief, and associated complications of grief indicating pathology in complicated grief (Maciejewski et al. 2016). They also differ in the specific symptom constellations within their proposed diagnostic criteria (Maciejewski et al. 2016; Shear et al. 2011). However, both converge on a conceptualization characterized by intense, prolonged grief and functional impairment that continues for longer than 6–12 months following a loss. Symptoms may include yearning, longing, or preoccupation with the deceased accompanied by emotional pain, difficulty with acceptance, or emotional numbness (Meichsner et al. 2020). PGD was included in ICD-11 (World Health Organization 2019) and recently has been incorporated in Section II of the text revision of DSM-5 (DSM-5-TR; American Psychiatric Association 2022). Prolonged grief occurs in 10%–30% of individuals (Bonanno et al. 2002; Maciejewski et al. 2016; Ott et al. 2007), with higher rates estimated in older adults (Meichsner et al. 2020).

Diverse cultural norms further complicate the distinction between adaptive and abnormal grieving practices. Although the Western consciousness typically encourages bereaved individuals to move through the grieving process in a timely manner by disengaging from the deceased and returning to the business of living, more studies are demonstrating the potentially positive effects of maintaining a meaningful connection with the lost loved one. A qualitative analysis of "sense of presence experiences" among 12 bereaved individuals revealed that continued bonds facilitated meaning-making during the grieving process (Steffen and Coyle 2011). Chinese bereavement rituals both underscore this point and provide a distinctive perspective. In contrast to the Western focus on the emotional experience of the grieving person, the Chinese focus on the behavior of the bereaved and the importance of demonstrating proper respect and love for the deceased by carrying out mourning rituals in an appropriate manner. Conducting funeral observances correctly is viewed as a way of helping the deceased complete the transition, both moving successfully into the land of the dead and establishing a good afterlife. Sending clear messages of love and support through meaningful rituals is a manifestation of the Chinese belief in the importance of an ongoing connection with the deceased (Bonanno 2009). Rather than dichotomously categorizing ongoing attachment to a deceased loved one as optimal or maladaptive, current research indicates a more complex picture in which variables such as quality of the relationship with the deceased person, personal religious beliefs, and the cultural context surrounding the bereaved contribute to the meaning of such a connection and its potential for good or harm (Bonanno 2009).

Although no consensus is yet apparent, the groundwork is being laid for specific criteria to distinguish abnormal (i.e., complicated or traumatic) from healthy grief reactions. Continued research is needed to help refine and solidify what cognitive, affective, and behavioral features characterize these two forms. One study compared neurocognitive task performance among spousally bereaved older adults with complicated grief, those with noncomplicated grief, and nonbereaved control participants (O'Connor and Arizmendi 2014). Individuals with major depressive disorder (MDD) were excluded. There were no differences in working memory or set shifting between the three groups. However, individuals with complicated grief demonstrated longer reaction times to grief-related (but not neutral) words. These findings demonstrate that complicated grief impacts cognitive functioning in ways distinct from the ways that uncomplicated grief does and independent of MDD. As data accumulate, theories and therapies will continue to be modified. For example, as noted earlier in this section, it is becoming increasingly apparent that continued attachment often can be comforting (Stroebe et al. 2010; Wortman and Silver 1987). Variations in grief practices across cultures have also emphasized the impact that cultural traditions and beliefs can have on bereavement practices and have widened the scope of what can be defined as "normal" grief reactions. Thus, one might wonder whether it is necessary to minimize one's attachment to a deceased individual to resolve one's grief or whether grief resolution itself should be the goal. Other issues include what constitutes a reasonable period for a "normal" grief reaction and what reactions constitute the indisputable signs of abnormal bereavement patterns predictive of poor adjustment. Until such time as these issues are resolved, clinicians are encouraged to exercise sensitivity when eliciting the meaning that the bereaved person ascribes to events, recognize the cultural norms relevant to the person's experience, and use currently available guidelines, as noted in this chapter, to help evaluate and assist the individual patient.

DSM-5 and ICD-11 Definitions

To differentiate normative grief from disorders such as depression, DSM-5 (American Psychiatric Association 2013) provides a clear distinction between the feelings of loss and emptiness that typically characterize bereavement and the persistent depressed mood and global inability to experience pleasure indicative of a major depressive episode. The manual notes that the sadness accompanying grief tends to come in waves, and when it abates, feelings of joy and the ability for humor often manifest; in contrast, the "down" state of a major depressive episode offers no respite. DSM-5 eliminated the "bereavement exclusion" that disallowed a diagnosis of MDD in the context of bereavement, noting that bereaved individuals whose symptoms meet the criteria for a major depressive episode should not be denied this diagnosis because of their bereaved status (Pies 2013).

Both the DSM and ICD diagnostic systems have taken recent steps to acknowledge chronic grief as a separable mental disorder. PGD was recently included in the ICD-11 (World Health Organization 2019) under the "Disorders Specifically Associated With Stress." The ICD-11 specifies that PGD is a persistent and pervasive grief response more than 6 months after the loss that both is outside the norm for the person's cultural context and includes significant functional impairment. DSM-5 includes persistent complex bereavement disorder as a condition for further study, also specifying a prolonged grief response of more than 6 months that involves intense yearning or longing for the deceased person and a minimum number of psychological symptoms that can include intense emotional pain, numbness, loneliness/detachment, and identity disturbance, among others. PGD has been approved for inclusion in Section II (full diagnostic status) of DSM-5-TR under the "Trauma- and Stressor-Related Disorders." The revised criteria set requires a longer period post loss than does ICD-11 or prior persistent complex bereavement disorder criteria (minimum 12 months post loss) and specifies that at least three Criterion C psychological symptoms be present along with the persistent grief response (Prigerson et al. 2021).

Adaptation to Late-Life Bereavement: Risk Factors for Intensification of Grief

Grief has been characterized by many not only as a highly charged emotional state but also as a significant risk factor for a wide range of negative outcomes, including mortality and major physical and mental health disturbances. In contrast, some clinicians and researchers have been struck by the ability of many older adults to survive and cope quite well overall with the profound losses of old age. In their 10-year follow-up study of a national sample of bereaved men and women, McCrae and Costa (1993) found that the great majority of individuals showed considerable ability to adapt to this major life stress (although the length of recovery seemed to vary considerably), and this finding was echoed in the resilience demonstrated by the majority of grieving individuals (Bonanno 2009). Nevertheless, identifying elder persons at risk for negative outcomes after the loss of a partner is an important mental health objective (for a thorough review, see Sanders 1993 and Stroebe et al. 2001a). Variables that are often associated with prolonged or complicated bereavement include the 1) age and sex of the surviving partner, 2) mode of death, 3) presence of significant depression shortly after the death, 4) ability to accept the loss, 5) prior relationship satisfaction, and 6) social support available. Strength of religious commitment and involvement, participation in culturally appropriate mourning rituals, and redistribution of roles within the family after the death may also affect the grief process to some degree.

Gender differences in bereavement are complex. Stroebe et al. (2001b) concluded that "widowers are indeed at relatively higher risk [of death] than widows, and, given that death is the most extreme consequence of bereavement, much weight may be attached to this finding" (p. 69). Bowling (1988–1989) followed up with 500 elderly widows and widowers for 6 years following their loss and found that men age 75 years and older had excessive mortality compared with men of the same age in the general population. Gallagher-Thompson et al. (1993) found that widowers who died within the first year of spousal bereavement had reported more often than survivors that their wives were their main confidants and that they had minimal involvement in activities with other persons after their wives' deaths. The differential psychological impact of bereavement on men and women may also be unbalanced.

Some studies have found that bereavement has a greater impact on depression scores in men than in women (van Grootheest et al. 1999; Williams 2003), although more recent findings show no difference according to gender (Sasson and Umberson 2014). Elevated depression scores for men may indicate that they begin to experience greater depression before the loss of their wives and that this level of comorbid depression is maintained in bereavement (Lee and DeMaris 2007). Women have been found to have less life satisfaction than men following the loss of a spouse (Lichtenstein et al. 1996; Williams 2003; see also Bratt et al. 2017), but they may also experience more personal growth after the loss (Carr 2004). Referring to their dual process model, Stroebe et al. (2001b) hypothesized that women are more focused on psychological aspects of coping with the loss, whereas men are more focused on restoring their life pattern without the loved one. However, societal and structural demands may prompt flexible coping in women who have followed more traditional gender roles (e.g., in addition to loss-focused coping, they must adjust to new financial and domestic circumstances), whereas less pressure exists for men to engage with their nonpreferred coping focus. Further research is needed to determine whether less flexibility in coping focus mediates the relationship between gender and psychological outcomes.

Violent, stigmatized (as in the case of AIDS), or unexpected deaths generally are associated with poorer adaptation (Farberow et al. 1987; Osterweis et al. 1984; Parkes and Weiss 1983; van der Houwen et al. 2010; Worden 2002), although comparisons of the impact of long-term illness versus that of unexpected loss have been inconsistent (Burton et al. 2006; Kitson 2000). Clinically significant depression occurring within the first 2 months following the loss is a significant risk factor for poor outcome over time. Lund et al. (1993) found that intense negative emotions at 2 months post loss—such as a desire to die and frequent crying—were associated with poor coping 2 years later. Wortman and Silver (1989) reviewed several studies indicating that depression confounds successful resolution of grief. Both pre-loss depression and depression early in bereavement may play a significant role in adjustment. In a prospective longitudinal study of the course of bereavement outcomes, a higher proportion of individuals with pre-loss depression remained depressed at 18 months post loss (43%) than of those without pre-loss depression (21%) (Bonanno et al. 2002). In work investigating the relationship between depression and later bereavement outcome, Gilewski et al. (1991) found that individuals with self-reported moderate to severe depression were at greatest risk for all other psychopathological symptoms, such as increased anxiety, hostility, and interpersonal sensitivity. This result occurred whether their spouses had died from suicide or from natural causes. However, subjects whose spouses had committed suicide and who had moderate to severely depression at the outset had the highest mean score of any subgroup on the depression measure used. Individuals in this group also maintained higher mean levels of depression over time and were more likely to score high on other distress measures. These data suggest that, again, the interaction of one or more risk factors may contribute to the greatest distress.

An important psychological factor in predicting poor clinical outcomes is the ability of bereaved partners to accept the loss. Feelings of acceptance after a loss can vary widely, from a sense that "it was time" or a feeling of relief at the resolution of the deceased partner's pain and suffering to a profound sense of unfairness and lack of resolution at the loss. Analyses of the Texas Revised Inventory of Grief–Present scale (TRIG-Present; Zisook et al. 1982), a well-supported and validated measure of grief symptoms, identified nonacceptance as a key dimension of grief symptoms that remains stable over time (Futterman et al. 2010). Importantly, heightened nonacceptance, but not the other TRIG-Present factors of grief-related thoughts or emotional response, predicted more intense grief 12 months post loss (Holland et al. 2013). By including "marked sense of disbelief about the death" as a Criterion C symptom for PGD, DSM-5-TR highlights its importance in the clinical picture of bereavement.

The association between pre-loss relationship characteristics and clinical symptoms of bereavement is complex (Itzhar-Nabarro and Smoski 2012). More positive ratings of relationship satisfaction were associated with more severe depression initially, but this correspondence was lower at 30 months post loss. Bonanno et al. (2002) found that a poor relationship quality rating pre-loss was most strongly associated with a pattern either of pre-loss depression followed by an improvement in symptoms post loss or of chronic depression beginning pre-loss and continuing throughout bereavement. Follow-up analyses found increased idealization of the relationship in bereaved individuals, but the degree of idealization did not differ based on level of adjustment (Bonanno et al. 2004). Relationship dependency was associated with risk of chronic grief (Ott et al. 2007). These studies indicate that relationship variables may interact with several other variables, including general psychological health and a change in perspective on the relationship over the course of the bereavement process.

The role of social support is less ambiguous overall. Since the publication of Cobb's (1976) seminal paper on its stress-buffering effects, social support has been widely recognized as a moderator of many kinds of life stress. Across bereavement types (e.g., spousal, parental) and ages, social support is predictive of positive mood as well as the nature of grief and depressive symptoms (van der Houwen et al. 2010). In a comprehensive review of the role of social support in mitigating the effects of late-life spousal bereavement, Dimond et al. (1987) found in their longitudinal study that the total size of the reported support network at baseline was positively correlated with perceived coping skills and life satisfaction at later times of measurement. They also found that the quality of the network was inversely related to later depression and was positively correlated with later measures of life satisfaction. Finally, through a series of multiple regression analyses, they found that several baseline social network factors contributed independently to the variance accounted for in predicting depression at later times of measurement. This finding suggests that social support mitigates severe negative reactions to the loss of a spouse in older individuals.

Based on these data, several risk factors appear to be associated with a more difficult subsequent grief process in elderly adults. However, the available research was conducted using volunteer subjects who typically enjoyed higher educational and socioeconomic levels compared with average members of the general population. Furthermore, the response rate in survey studies of bereavement tends to be low (around 30%–40%), and this clearly limits the ability to generalize findings. Greater efforts should be made to engage elderly persons who are economically disadvantaged, who are in poor health, and who have low social support systems and low community involvement. In addition, more studies are needed not only to explore the interactive effect of several of these risk factors (particularly because they may change over time in relative salience to the individual) but also to determine whether the intensity or the same risk factors apply to bereavement due to other causes, such as divorce and the death of a parent or an adult child. Clearly, more research also is needed on risk factors among ethnically and culturally diverse elder adults.

Interventions for Late-Life Bereavement

Clinical comments throughout the bereavement literature indicate that treatment can be immensely helpful to some individuals. The extent to which a treatment might be effective depends in large measure on the intensity and pattern of symptoms present. In some situations, intervention beyond the usual family and community support is not called for and may even be counterproductive. In other cases, however, medication, psychotherapy, or a combination of both may be indicated. Decisions regarding treatment strategy are facilitated by knowing whether the symptom pattern is consistent a "normal grief reaction" for the cultural group with which the person identifies or whether the severity, type of symptoms present, and risk factor profile appear to suggest a prolonged course. It is important to determine whether the symptom picture is consistent with the diagnostic criteria for some other psychiatric disorder, such as MDD or PTSD. This distinction is critical for making appropriate intervention choices (Raphael et al. 2001).

Treatment of Complicated Bereavement (Prolonged Grief Disorder)

A thorough assessment for any comorbid psychological condition should be conducted before beginning treatment for bereavement. This is especially important for conditions whose symptoms are similar to those of bereavement, such as MDD. Clinical levels of depression should be treated with medication, psychotherapy, or both before the focus of treatment can effectively shift to bereavement (National Institutes of Health Consensus Conference 1992; Parkes and Weiss 1983; Raphael et al. 2001; Reynolds 1992). On the issue of when to begin treatment of depression after a loss, Reynolds (1992) stated, "Our clinical practice has been to intervene as early as 2 months, and certainly by 4 months, in the presence of clear syndromal major depression" (p. 50). Remission of depression will enable the focus of treatment to return to the bereavement. Careful attention to the grief process can often then determine whether additional interventions are required. Risk factors may become an important focus for remediation. For example, considerable evidence indicates that older widowers may not thrive if they do not have a constructive support system. Isolation is a documented risk factor, and men undergoing stress may not have the requisite skills to build or implement a nourishing social network. It may become necessary to provide specific assistance with this problem. Once this is accomplished, other interventions may not be necessary.

Other common complications that are particularly significant in older bereaved persons (Rozenzweig et al. 1997) and that require treatment include PTSD, anxiety disorders (that may or may not be related to the bereavement), and subsyndromal depression (Reynolds et al. 1999). A series of empirical studies focused on the efficacy of specific psychotropic treatment programs during bereavement for these conditions. Open-label trials of bupropion (Zisook et al. 2001), nortriptyline (Pasternak et al. 1991), either nortriptyline or sertraline (Oakley et al. 2002), and paroxetine (Zygmont et al. 1998) for bereavement-related MDD in older adults have shown promise. A review of pharmacotherapy for complicated grief concluded that tricyclic antidepressants (TCAs) appear to address only depressive symptoms, whereas selective serotonin reuptake inhibitors (SSRIs) may have efficacy for both depressive and grief symptoms (Bui et al. 2012). However, a recent randomized controlled trial did not confirm efficacy of an SSRI for grief symptoms (Shear et al. 2016). Citalopram in addition to complicated grief treatment helped reduce depressive symptoms but did not alter grief outcomes. A combination of medication and psychotherapy appears to be more effective than either alone when attempting to reduce the psychiatric symptoms that occur with bereavement (Miller et al. 1997; Reynolds et al. 1999; Shear et al. 2016; Simon et al. 2008).

Some older individuals either cannot or will not use psychotropic medications. Although data have suggested that counseling of various kinds may not be particularly helpful for individuals undergoing a normal grief reaction (discussed later), there is evidence that various psychological treatments can have a positive effect in treating complicated bereavement (Currier et al. 2008; Neimeyer 2000; Shear et al. 2005). A growing number of psychological interventions have been developed specifically to target symptoms of complicated grief. A meta-analysis found a medium effect size favoring these targeted interventions, especially those grounded in cognitive-behavioral therapy (CBT), as more effective than other supportive therapies, interpersonal psychotherapy, or wait-list control conditions (Wittouck et al. 2011). Cognitive therapy and CBTs of various forms are effective in treating patients with complex bereavement reactions (Currier et al. 2010).

One treatment for complicated grief, known as complicated grief treatment (CGT), integrates attachment theory via interpersonal therapy with CBT (Shear et al. 2005; Wetherell 2012). CGT includes a series of cognitive-behavioral techniques such as revisiting the story of the death, including recording the narrative of finding out about the death and its aftermath; using in vivo, graded exposure to avoided death-related circumstances; mindful breathing; sharing positive and negative memories of the loved one; and building connections with current important relationships. Also integral to the treatment are homework assignments involving listening to tapes of imaginal exposure. Following the dual process model (discussed earlier; see "Theories About Adjustment to Permanent Losses"), CGT also involves motivational enhancement and goal setting to facilitate restorative goals. The results of this treatment have been encouraging: complicated grief, anxiety, and depressive symptoms were significantly reduced. In a randomized controlled trial, individuals undergoing CGT showed a greater response than did those undergoing interpersonal psychotherapy (Shear et al. 2005), and CGT has gone on to show efficacy across several clinical trials, including a trial specifically in older adults (Shear and Bloom 2017).

One of the more common psychodynamic therapies used with complicated bereavement is Horowitz's (1976) time-limited psychodynamic therapy. This 12-session phase-oriented strategy is designed to help individuals work through emotional reactions to traumatic life events. Careful attention is also paid to tailoring treatment to the patient's particular personality type. Abreaction, clarification, and interpretation of defenses and affects are used to facilitate realistic appraisals of the implications of a death and to explore the effect of the loss of a relationship on the bereaved person's self-concept. Empirical data showing the effectiveness of this treatment are available (Horowitz et al. 1981, 1984).

To assist practitioners in assessing the efficacy of their bereavement treatment, Wilson (2011) developed the Assimilation of Problematic Experiences Sequence model, which describes the psychosocial changes demonstrated by individuals as they deal with a challenging experience such as grief. The complete assimilation sequence includes eight developmental levels, from 0 to 7, and describes a person's progression from warding off/being dissociated from the experience, to developing a vague awareness of the painful situation, to gaining understanding/insight, and eventually to a movement toward problem solution and ultimately integration/mastery.

Finally, several interventions have targeted caregivers in an attempt to both reduce distress during caregiving and prevent complications during bereavement. A support intervention targeting caregivers of persons with Alzheimer's disease reduced depressive symptoms both pre- and post loss compared with caregivers in the no-treatment control condition (Haley et al. 2008). Another intervention for caregivers of patients with Alzheimer's disease was found to reduce grief symptoms, but its impact on depression symptoms was less clear (Holland et al. 2009). Given that pre-loss psychopathology, including depression, is a predictor of chronic grief, interventions for at-risk groups such as caregivers hold promise for altering the course of symptoms post loss.

Treatment of Normal Grief Reactions

There is a long history of formal and informal interventions for normal grief reactions, including self-help groups and individual and group counseling. Most bereaved persons (particularly elders) do not seek professional assistance for their grief. Self-help support groups for bereaved persons are often used by those who find the experience too painful and the loneliness overwhelming. Despite conceptual and anecdotal support for the effectiveness of these programs, relatively little empirical support has been found. Several reviews have examined the literature on counseling for normal grief reactions and concluded that, by and large, these interventions neither reduce grief or depressive symptoms above and beyond the effects of time nor facilitate better adjustment post intervention (Currier et al. 2008; Jordan and Neimeyer 2003; Schut et al. 2001). A recent meta-analysis tested baseline symptom severity and duration since loss (minimum of 6 months based on PGD diagnostic criteria) as moderators of treatment effects on grief symptoms. Intervention effect sizes were larger in studies in which participants were more than 6 months past their loss. However, higher baseline symptoms were not associated with larger effects after adjustment for other moderators (i.e., the measure used to assess grief) (Johannsen et al. 2019). Of note, certain studies have in fact found that individuals experiencing uncomplicated bereavement may experience an iatrogenic effect of treatment, appearing to be worse off at the end of the treatment than if they had not participated (García et al. 2013; Neimeyer 2000). Bonanno's (2009) research on the inherent resilience of a person to cope with, adjust to, and assimilate the loss of a loved one further substantiates these findings. World Health Organization (WHO) guidelines now specifically recommend against the routine use of structured psychological interventions in uncomplicated bereavement (Tol et al. 2013). As an alternative, Aoun et al. (2018) advocated for a "compassionate communities" approach involving supportive family, friends, and community members who most frequently care for the bereaved, rather than an overreliance on professional services.

Using medication to treat uncomplicated grief (other than for specific symptoms such as insomnia) has also been questioned. Many clinicians think that medication, if used at all, should be minimal and used only briefly. For example, Raphael et al. (2001) argued that if depression is not evident, antidepressants should not be prescribed to reduce symptoms of grief. There are concerns that medication may impede recovery by masking the full experience of bereavement (Parkes 1972; Worden 2002) and that prescribing medication pathologizes a natural human process. Other clinicians believe that providers should intervene sooner rather than later given the tendency of depressive symptoms to persist throughout the first year of spousal bereavement (Reynolds 1992). Given that there is limited empirical evidence indicating that one must go through a difficult grieving process in order to resume one's life effectively (Bonanno et al. 2002), it has been argued that pharmacological (and other) treatments for pain and suffering should be available to those who request them (Wortman and Silver 1987). The empirical literature is equivocal regarding the effectiveness of medication use in uncomplicated grief in the absence of clinical depression symptoms. There is some indication that antidepressants, including TCAs and SSRIs, are effective for reducing symptoms that are also present in depression. A small randomized controlled trial comparing benzodiazepine use with placebo noted no significant differences between groups in bereavement symptoms, although there was a trend for a negative impact of benzodiazepine use on sleep initiation and bad dreams (Warner et al. 2001). Also, WHO guidelines on the management of stress- and trauma-related disorders specifically recommend against the use of benzodiazepines in the management of bereavement (Tol et al. 2013). Psychotropic medication use following bereavement is common; a study in the United Kingdom noted that almost one in five individuals age 60 years and older received a new prescription for a psychotropic drug (most commonly an anxiolytic, hypnotic, or antidepressant) in the year following bereavement (Shah et al. 2013). Given the added concern of polypharmacy in older adults, Das et al. (2016) encouraged clinicians to consider watchful waiting in the first few weeks after an initial visit with a bereaved person (pending no immediate safety concerns). They recommended treating with CBT if symptoms persist and reserving pharmacotherapy for more serious cases. Further research is necessary to determine the optimum level of pharmacological intervention (including none) both to ease suffering and to allow the natural process of bereavement to take its course.

Conclusion

Bereavement is a common and life-altering occurrence in late life. There is no single common course of bereavement or "right" way to grieve, and bereavement may not follow a linear course from loss to recovery. However, over time, many individuals follow a path of resilience as they mourn their loss and build a new way of living without their loved one, with no intervention required. When complicated grief persistently interferes with a person's functioning over a long period, psychological interventions are available, and pharmacological interventions may be appropriate to address specific symptoms.

Key Points

- *Bereavement* can refer to a person's reactions to any set of significant losses but typically refers to the loss of a loved one, such as a spouse.

- Among persons age 65 years and older, 40% of women and 13% of men have experienced the loss of a spouse.

- The dual process model of bereavement focuses on the interplay of loss-oriented stressors related to losing the presence of the loved one in a person's life (e.g., loneliness, loss of support) and restoration-oriented stressors related to building a new life without the presence of the loved one (e.g., taking on roles previously performed by the spouse, changing one's identity from that of wife to widow). Bereaved persons' oscillation of their focus between these two stressors is thought to promote healthy adjustment.

- Culture can play a key role in the expected course of grief, and clinicians should take culture into consideration when assessing or designing interventions for complicated grief.

- Although many individuals demonstrate resilience to or recovery from depressive symptoms within 18 months after the loss of a spouse, symptoms of grief such as missing the deceased person and engaging in fond remembrances of the lost loved one may continue indefinitely, even in individuals who show minimal depressive symptoms.

- Post-loss adjustment among bereaved individuals can vary widely. Several risk factors are predictive of poor adjustment. These include male sex; loss through a violent, stigmatized, or unexpected death; the presence of significant depressive symptoms early in the loss; poor coping skills and low self-esteem; and poor breadth and quality of social support.

- Bereavement reactions can be categorized as normal or chronic. Most people experience "normal" grief, which can include the experience of sadness, loneliness, or longing for the deceased; experiencing the "presence" of the deceased; or disruptions in sleep and appetite. Although it is early in the development of consensus criteria for complicated or persistent grief, typical definitions include the following concerns: marked distress, prolonged duration of symptoms, and avoidance of or failure to adapt to new life roles.

- Several empirically validated treatments are available for complicated bereavement. In addition to standard cognitive-behavioral therapy, complicated grief therapy is a promising intervention based on principles used in the treatment of PTSD.

- Normal bereavement typically resolves without the need for treatment beyond targeted interventions for specific symptoms (e.g., disturbed sleep). In fact, some common interventions for normal bereavement have been found to lead to a worsening of symptoms and are not recommended.

Suggested Readings

Aoun EG, Porta G, Melhem NM, Brent DA: Prospective evaluation of the DSM-5 persistent complex bereavement disorder criteria in adults: dimensional and diagnostic approaches. Psychol Med 51(5):825–834, 2021

Bonanno GA: The Other Side of Sadness: What the New Science of Bereavement Tells Us About Life After Loss. New York, Basic Books, 2009

Currier JM, Neimeyer RA, Berman JS: The effectiveness of psychotherapeutic interventions for bereaved persons: a comprehensive quantitative review. Psychol Bull 134:648–661, 2008

Johannsen M, Damholdt MF, Zachariae R, et al: Psychological interventions for grief in adults: a systematic review and meta-analysis of randomized controlled trials. J Affect Disord 253:69–86, 2019

Maciejewski PK, Zhang B, Block SD, et al: An empirical examination of the stage theory of grief. JAMA 297:716–723, 2007

Neimeyer R: Searching for the meaning of meaning: grief therapy and the process of reconstruction. Death Stud 24:531–558, 2000

Ott CH, Lueger RJ, Kelber ST, et al: Spousal bereavement in older adults: common, resilient, and chronic grief with defining characteristics. J Nerv Ment Dis 195:332–341, 2007

Shear MK, Reynolds CF, Simon NM, et al: Optimizing treatment of complicated grief: a randomized clinical trial. JAMA Psychiatry 73(7):685–694, 2016

Stroebe M, Schut H: The dual process model of coping with bereavement: rationale and description. Death Stud 23:197–224, 1999

References

American Psychiatric Association: Diagnostic and Statistical Manual of Mental Disorders, 5th Edition. Arlington, VA, American Psychiatric Association, 2013

American Psychiatric Association: Diagnostic and Statistical Manual of Mental Disorders, 5th Edition, Text Revision. Washington, DC, American Psychiatric Association, 2022

Aoun SM, Breen LJ, White I, et al: What sources of bereavement support are perceived helpful by bereaved people and why? Empirical evidence for the compassionate communities approach. Palliat Med 32(8):1378–1388, 2018 29754514

Aoun EG, Porta G, Melhem NM, Brent DA: Prospective evaluation of the DSM-5 persistent complex bereavement disorder criteria in adults: dimensional and diagnostic approaches. Psychol Med 51:825–834, 2021 31941562

Bennett KM, Gibbons K, Mackenzie-Smith S: Loss and restoration in later life: an examination of dual process model of coping with bereavement. Omega (Westport) 61(4):315–332, 2010 21058612

Bonanno GA: The Other Side of Sadness: What the New Science of Bereavement Tells Us about Life After Loss. New York, Basic Books, 2009

Bonanno GA, Wortman CB, Lehman DR, et al: Resilience to loss and chronic grief: a prospective study from preloss to 18-months postloss. J Pers Soc Psychol 83(5):1150–1164, 2002 12416919

Bonanno GA, Wortman CB, Nesse RM: Prospective patterns of resilience and maladjustment during widowhood. Psychol Aging 19(2):260–271, 2004 15222819

Bowlby J: Processes of mourning. Int J Psychoanal 42:317–340, 1961 13872076

Bowling A: Who dies after widow(er)hood? A discriminant analysis. Omega 19:135–153, 1988–1989

Bratt AS, Stenström U, Rennemark M: Effects on life satisfaction of older adults after child and spouse bereavement. Aging Ment Health 21(6):602–608, 2017 26768164

Bui E, Nadal-Vicens M, Simon NM: Pharmacological approaches to the treatment of complicated grief: rationale and a brief review of the literature. Dialogues Clin Neurosci
14(2):149–157, 2012 22754287

Burton AM, Haley WE, Small BJ: Bereavement after caregiving or unexpected death: effects on
elderly spouses. Aging Ment Health 10(3):319–326, 2006 16777661

Cain BS: Divorce among elderly women: a growing social phenomenon. Soc Casework 69:563–
568, 1988

Carlsson ME, Nilsson IM: Bereaved spouses' adjustment after the patients' death in palliative
care. Palliat Support Care 5(4):397–404, 2007 18044417

Carr D: Gender, preloss marital dependence, and older adults' adjustment to widowhood.
J Marriage Fam 66:220–235, 2004

Cobb S: Presidential address–1976: social support as a moderator of life stress. Psychosom Med
38(5):300–314, 1976 981490

Coifman KG, Bonanno G, Rafaeli E: Affect dynamics, bereavement and resilience to loss. J Happiness Stud 8:371–392, 2007a

Coifman KG, Bonanno GA, Ray RD, Gross JJ: Does repressive coping promote resilience? Af-
fective-autonomic response discrepancy during bereavement. J Pers Soc Psychol
92(4):745–758, 2007b 17469956

Currier JM, Neimeyer RA, Berman JS: The effectiveness of psychotherapeutic interventions for
bereaved persons: a comprehensive quantitative review. Psychol Bull 134(5):648–661, 2008
18729566

Currier JM, Holland JM, Neimeyer RA: Do CBT-based interventions alleviate distress following bereavement? A review of the current evidence. Int J Cogn Ther 3:77–93, 2010

Das A, Maiti A, Sinha S: Antidepressant prescription in the geriatric population: a teachable
moment. JAMA Intern Med 176(11):1608–1609, 2016 27668672

Dimond M, Lund DA, Caserta MS: The role of social support in the first two years of bereavement in an elderly sample. Gerontologist 27(5):599–604, 1987 3678899

Farberow NL, Gallagher DE, Gilewski MJ, Thompson LW: An examination of the early impact
of bereavement on psychological distress in survivors of suicide. Gerontologist 27(5):592–
598, 1987 3678898

Federal Interagency Forum on Aging-Related Statistics: Older Americans 2016: Key Indicators
of Well-Being. Washington, DC, Federal Interagency Forum on Aging-Related Statistics,
August 2016

Freud S: Mourning and melancholia (1917 [1915]), in The Standard Edition of the Complete
Psychological Works of Sigmund Freud, Vol 14. Translated and edited by Strachey J. London, Hogarth, 1957, pp 237–260

Futterman A, Holland JM, Brown PJ, et al: Factorial validity of the Texas Revised Inventory of
Grief–Present scale among bereaved older adults. Psychol Assess 22(3):675–687, 2010
20822280

Gallagher-Thompson D, Futterman A, Farberow N, et al: The impact of spousal bereavement
on older widows and widowers, in Handbook of Bereavement. Edited by Stroebe MS,
Stroebe W, Hansson R. Cambridge, UK, Cambridge University Press, 1993, pp 227–239

García JA, Landa V, Grandes G, et al: Effectiveness of "primary bereavement care" for widows:
a cluster randomized controlled trial involving family physicians. Death Stud 37(4):287–
310, 2013 24520889

Gilewski MJ, Farberow NL, Gallagher DE, Thompson LW: Interaction of depression and bereavement on mental health in the elderly. Psychol Aging 6(1):67–75, 1991 2029370

Haley WE, Bergman EJ, Roth DL, et al: Long-term effects of bereavement and caregiver intervention
on dementia caregiver depressive symptoms. Gerontologist 48(6):732–740, 2008 19139247

Harlow SD, Goldberg EL, Comstock GW: A longitudinal study of the prevalence of depressive
symptomatology in elderly widowed and married women. Arch Gen Psychiatry
48(12):1065–1068, 1991 1845223

Holland JM, Currier JM, Gallagher-Thompson D: Outcomes from the Resources for Enhancing
Alzheimer's Caregiver Health (REACH) program for bereaved caregivers. Psychol Aging
24(1):190–202, 2009 19290751

Holland JM, Futterman A, Thompson LW, et al: Difficulties accepting the loss of a spouse: a precursor for intensified grieving among widowed older adults. Death Stud 37(2):126–144, 2013 24520845

Horowitz MJ: Stress Response Syndromes. New York, Jason Aronson, 1976

Horowitz MJ, Krupnick J, Kaltreider N, et al: Initial psychological response to parental death. Arch Gen Psychiatry 38(3):316–323, 1981 7212963

Horowitz MJ, Weiss DS, Kaltreider N, et al: Reactions to the death of a parent: results from patients and field subjects. J Nerv Ment Dis 172(7):383–392, 1984 6726208

Itzhar-Nabarro Z, Smoski MJ: A review of theoretical and empirical perspectives on marital satisfaction and bereavement outcomes: implications for working with older adults. Clin Gerontol 35:257–269, 2012

Jacobs S: Pathologic Grief: Maladaptation to Loss. Washington, DC, American Psychiatric Press, 1993

Jacobs S, Ostfeld A: An epidemiological review of the mortality of bereavement. Psychosom Med 39(5):344–357, 1977 333498

Johannsen M, Damholdt MF, Zachariae R, et al: Psychological interventions for grief in adults: a systematic review and meta-analysis of randomized controlled trials. J Affect Disord 253:69–86, 2019 31029856

Jordan JR, Neimeyer RA: Does grief counseling work? Death Stud 27(9):765–786, 2003 14577426

Kalish RA: Older people and grief. Generations 11:33–38, 1987

Kitson GC: Adjustment to violent and natural deaths in later and earlier life for black and white widows. J Gerontol B Psychol Sci Soc Sci 55(6):S341–S351, 2000 11078111

Kübler-Ross E: On Death and Dying. New York, Simon and Schuster, 1969

Lee GR, DeMaris A: Widowhood, gender, and depression: a longitudinal analysis. Res Aging 29:56–72, 2007

Lichtenstein P, Gatz M, Pedersen NL, et al: A co-twin–control study of response to widowhood. J Gerontol B Psychol Sci Soc Sci 51(5):279–289, 1996 8809004

Lindemann E: Symptomatology and management of acute grief. Am J Psychiatry 101:141–148, 1944 8192191

Lopata HZ: Current Widowhood: Myths and Realities. Thousand Oaks, CA, Sage, 1996

Lund DA, Caserta M, Dimond M: The course of spousal bereavement in later life, in Handbook of Bereavement. Edited by Stroebe MS, Stroebe W, Hansson R. Cambridge, UK, Cambridge University Press, 1993, pp 240–254

Maciejewski PK, Zhang B, Block SD, Prigerson HG: An empirical examination of the stage theory of grief. JAMA 297(7):716–723, 2007 17312291

Maciejewski PK, Maercker A, Boelen PA, Prigerson HG: "Prolonged grief disorder" and "persistent complex bereavement disorder", but not "complicated grief", are one and the same diagnostic entity: an analysis of data from the Yale Bereavement Study. World Psychiatry 15(3):266–275, 2016 27717273

McCrae RR, Costa PT: Psychological resilience among widowed men and women: a 10-year follow-up of a national sample, in Handbook of Bereavement. Edited by Stroebe MS, Stroebe W, Hansson R. Cambridge, UK, Cambridge University Press, 1993, pp 196–207

Meichsner F, O'Connor M, Skritskaya N, Shear MK: Grief before and after bereavement in the elderly: an approach to care. Am J Geriatr Psychiatry 28(5):560–569, 2020 32037292

Miller MD, Wolfson L, Frank E, et al: Using interpersonal psychotherapy (IPT) in a combined psychotherapy/medication research protocol with depressed elders: a descriptive report with case vignettes. J Psychother Pract Res 7(1):47–55, 1997 9407475

Momtaz YA, Ibrahim R, Hamid TA, Yahaya N: Mediating effects of social and personal religiosity on the psychological well being of widowed elderly people. Omega (Westport) 61(2):145–162, 2010 20712141

National Institutes of Health Consensus Conference: Diagnosis and treatment of depression in late life. JAMA 268:1018–1024, 1992 1501308

Neimeyer RA: The Lessons of Loss: A Guide to Coping. Raleigh, NC, McGraw-Hill, 1998

Neimeyer RA: Searching for the meaning of meaning: grief therapy and the process of reconstruction. Death Stud 24(6):541–558, 2000 11503667

Neimeyer RA, Harris DL, Winokuer HR, et al (eds): Grief and Bereavement in Contemporary Society: Bridging Research and Practice. New York, Routledge, 2011

Nielsen MK, Carlsen AH, Neergaard MA, et al: Looking beyond the mean in grief trajectories: a prospective, population-based cohort study. Soc Sci Med 232:460–469, 2019 31230666

Oakley F, Khin NA, Parks R, et al: Improvement in activities of daily living in elderly following treatment for post-bereavement depression. Acta Psychiatr Scand 105(3):231–234, 2002 11939978

O'Connor MF, Arizmendi BJ: Neuropsychological correlates of complicated grief in older spousally bereaved adults. J Gerontol B Psychol Sci Soc Sci 69(1):12–18, 2014 23551907

Osterweis M, Solomon F, Green M: Bereavement: Reactions, Consequences, and Care: A Report of the Institute of Medicine, National Academy of Sciences. Washington, DC, National Academy Press, 1984

Ott CH, Lueger RJ, Kelber ST, Prigerson HG: Spousal bereavement in older adults: common, resilient, and chronic grief with defining characteristics. J Nerv Ment Dis 195(4):332–341, 2007 17435484

Parkes CM: Bereavement: Studies of Grief in Adult Life. New York, International Universities Press, 1972

Parkes CM, Weiss RS: Recovery From Bereavement. New York, Basic Books, 1983

Pasternak RE, Reynolds CF III, Schlernitzauer M, et al: Acute open-trial nortriptyline therapy of bereavement-related depression in late life. J Clin Psychiatry 52(7):307–310, 1991 2071562

Pies R: How the DSM-5 got grief, bereavement right. Psych Central, 2013. Available at: https://psychcentral.com/blog/how-the-dsm-5-got-grief-bereavement-right#1. Accessed November 15, 2013.

Prigerson HG, Shear MK, Jacobs SC, et al: Consensus criteria for traumatic grief: a preliminary empirical test. Br J Psychiatry 174:67–73, 1999 10211154

Prigerson HG, Boelen PA, Xu J, et al: Validation of the new DSM-5-TR criteria for prolonged grief disorder and the PG-13-Revised (PG-13-R) scale. World Psychiatry 20(1):96–106, 2021 33432758

Raphael B, Minkov C, Dobson M: Psychotherapeutic and pharmacological intervention for bereaved persons, in Handbook of Bereavement Research: Consequences, Coping, and Care. Edited by Stroebe MS, Hansson RO, Stroebe W, et al. Washington, DC, American Psychological Association, 2001, pp 587–612

Reynolds CF III: Treatment of depression in special populations. J Clin Psychiatry 53(suppl):45–53, 1992 1522079

Reynolds CF III, Miller MD, Pasternak RE, et al: Treatment of bereavement-related major depressive episodes in later life: a controlled study of acute and continuation treatment with nortriptyline and interpersonal psychotherapy. Am J Psychiatry 156(2):202–208, 1999 9989555

Rosenblatt PC: Grief that does not end, in Continuing Bonds: New Understandings of Grief (Series in Death Education, Aging, and Health Care). Edited by Klass D, Silverman PR, Nickman SL. Washington, DC, Taylor and Francis, 1996, pp 45–58

Rozenzweig A, Prigerson H, Miller MD, Reynolds CF 3rd: Bereavement and late-life depression: grief and its complications in the elderly. Annu Rev Med 48:421–428, 1997 9046973

Sanders CM: Risk factors in bereavement outcome, in Handbook of Bereavement. Edited by Stroebe MS, Stroebe W, Hansson R. Cambridge, UK, Cambridge University Press, 1993, pp 255–267

Sasson I, Umberson DJ: Widowhood and depression: new light on gender differences, selection, and psychological adjustment. J Gerontol B Psychol Sci Soc Sci 69(1):135–145, 2014 23811294

Schut H, Stroebe MS, van den Bout J, et al: The efficacy of bereavement interventions: determining who benefits, in Handbook of Bereavement Research: Consequences, Coping, and Care. Edited by Stroebe MS, Hansson RO, Stroebe W, et al. Washington, DC, American Psychological Association, 2001, pp 705–737

Shah SM, Carey IM, Harris T, et al: Initiation of psychotropic medication after partner bereavement: a matched cohort study. PLoS One 8(11):e77734, 2013 24223722

Shear MK, Bloom CG: Complicated grief treatment: an evidence-based approach to grief therapy. J Ration Emot Cogn Behav Ther 35:6–25, 2017

Shear K, Frank E, Houck PR, Reynolds CF III: Treatment of complicated grief: a randomized controlled trial. JAMA 293(21):2601–2608, 2005 15928281

Shear MK, Simon N, Wall M, et al: Complicated grief and related bereavement issues for DSM-5. Depress Anxiety 28(2):103–117, 2011 21284063

Shear MK, Reynolds CF III, Simon NM, et al: Optimizing treatment of complicated grief: a randomized clinical trial. JAMA Psychiatry 73(7):685–694, 2016 27276373

Simon NM, Shear MK, Fagiolini A, et al: Impact of concurrent naturalistic pharmacotherapy on psychotherapy of complicated grief. Psychiatry Res 159(1–2):31–36, 2008 18336918

Steffen E, Coyle A: Sense of presence experiences and meaning-making in bereavement: a qualitative analysis. Death Stud 35(7):579–609, 2011 24501839

Stroebe M, Schut H: The dual process model of coping with bereavement: rationale and description. Death Stud 23(3):197–224, 1999 10848151

Stroebe M, Schut H: The dual process model of coping with bereavement: a decade on. Omega (Westport) 61(4):273–289, 2010 21058610

Stroebe M, Hansson RO, Stroebe W, et al: Introduction: concepts and issues in contemporary research on bereavement, in Handbook of Bereavement Research: Consequences, Coping, and Care. Edited by Stroebe MS, Hansson RO, Stroebe W, et al. Washington, DC, American Psychological Association, 2001a, pp 3–22

Stroebe MS, Stroebe W, Schut H: Gender differences in adjustment to bereavement: an empirical and theoretical review. Rev Gen Psychol 5:62–83, 2001b

Stroebe M, Schut H, Boerner K: Continuing bonds in adaptation to bereavement: toward theoretical integration. Clin Psychol Rev 30(2):259–268, 2010 20034720

Thompson LW, Breckenridge JN, Gallagher D, Peterson J: Effects of bereavement on self-perceptions of physical health in elderly widows and widowers. J Gerontol 39(3):309–314, 1984 6715808

Thompson LW, Gallagher-Thompson D, Futterman A, et al: The effects of late-life spousal bereavement over a 30-month interval. Psychol Aging 6(3):434–441, 1991 1930760

Tol WA, Barbui C, van Ommeren M: Management of acute stress, PTSD, and bereavement: WHO recommendations. JAMA 310(5):477–478, 2013 23925613

U.S. Census Bureau: Marital Status of People 15 Years and Over, By Age, Sex, Personal Earnings, Race, and Hispanic Origin, March 2000. Washington, DC, U.S. Census Bureau, June 29, 2001

van der Houwen K, Stroebe M, Stroebe W, et al: Risk factors for bereavement outcome: a multivariate approach. Death Stud 34(3):195–220, 2010 24479181

van Grootheest DS, Beekman ATF, Broese van Groenou MI, Deeg DJ: Sex differences in depression after widowhood: do men suffer more? Soc Psychiatry Psychiatr Epidemiol 34(7):391–398, 1999 10477960

Warner J, Metcalfe C, King M: Evaluating the use of benzodiazepines following recent bereavement. Br J Psychiatry 178(1):36–41, 2001 11136208

Wetherell JL: Complicated grief therapy as a new treatment approach. Dialogues Clin Neurosci 14(2):159–166, 2012 22754288

Williams K: Has the future of marriage arrived? A contemporary examination of gender, marriage, and psychological well-being. J Health Soc Behav 44(4):470–487, 2003 15038144

Wilson J: The assimilation of problematic experiences sequence: an approach to evidence-based practice in bereavement counseling. J Soc Work End Life Palliat Care 7(4):350–362, 2011 22150179

Wittouck C, Van Autreve S, De Jaegere E, et al: The prevention and treatment of complicated grief: a meta-analysis. Clin Psychol Rev 31(1):69–78, 2011 21130937

Worden JW: Grief Counseling and Grief Therapy, 3rd Edition. New York, Springer, 2002

World Health Organization: International Statistical Classification of Diseases and Related Health Problems, 11th Revision. Geneva, World Health Organization, 2019

Wortman C, Silver RC: Coping with irrevocable loss, in Cataclysms, Crises, and Catastrophes: Psychology in Action (The Master Lectures). Edited by Van den Bos G, Bryant BK. Washington, DC, American Psychological Association, 1987, pp 185–235

Wortman CB, Silver RC: The myths of coping with loss. J Consult Clin Psychol 57(3):349–357, 1989 2661609

Zisook S, DeVaul R: Measuring acute grief. Psychiatr Med 2(2):169–176, 1984 6571620

Zisook S, Devaul RA, Click MA Jr: Measuring symptoms of grief and bereavement. Am J Psychiatry 139(12):1590–1593, 1982 7149059

Zisook S, Shuchter SR, Pedrelli P, et al: Bupropion sustained release for bereavement: results of an open trial. J Clin Psychiatry 62(4):227–230, 2001 11379835

Zygmont M, Prigerson HG, Houck PR, et al: A post hoc comparison of paroxetine and nortriptyline for symptoms of traumatic grief. J Clin Psychiatry 59(5):241–245, 1998 9632035

CHAPTER 16

Sleep and Circadian Rhythm Sleep-Wake Disorders

Meredith E. Rumble, Ph.D.
David T. Plante, M.D., Ph.D.

More than half of persons age 65 years and older report some type of sleep disturbance (Foley et al. 1995), and sleep disturbance is associated with increased risk of significant health consequences in older adults such as increased emergency department use, hospitalization, falls, nursing home placement, and mortality (Spira et al. 2012; Stone et al. 2008; Tzuang et al. 2021; Wallace et al. 2019). Unfortunately, a widespread misconception is that increased sleep disturbance is a normal function of aging. Although some normative changes in sleep are related to aging (Ohayon et al. 2004), sleep disturbance in older adults is not normative and is more likely to occur when common medical and psychiatric issues are present (Foley et al. 1995). Moreover, historically, sleep disturbance has been considered a secondary symptom of medical and psychiatric issues (e.g., chronic pain, depression). However, epidemiological data have supported a comorbid model in which sleep disturbance and medical and psychiatric issues have bidirectional relationships (Afolalu et al. 2018; Bao et al. 2017; Finan et al. 2013). This model supports the idea that all issues may warrant clinical attention, including the often-ignored issue of sleep disturbance. Thus, sleep disturbance is a key area to consider within geriatric psychiatry. In this chapter, we review normative age-related changes in sleep and the most common sleep disorders, medical and psychiatric comorbidities, medications and substances, and psychosocial stressors associated with sleep disturbance in older adults (Table 16–1). We also consider sleep assessment and treatment approaches in older adults.

TABLE 16–1.   Common areas to consider in older adults with sleep disturbance

Sleep-wake disorders	**Medications**
Circadian rhythm sleep-wake disorder	Antihypertensives
Advanced phase type	Cholinesterase inhibitors
Irregular sleep-wake type	Corticosteroids
Insomnia disorder	Decongestants
Obstructive sleep apnea	Dopamine agonists
Periodic limb movement disorder	Diuretics
Restless legs syndrome	Lipid-lowering agents
	Psychiatric medications
Psychiatric comorbidities	Second-generation antihistamines
Anxiety	Stimulants
Bereavement	
Depression	**Behaviors**
Suicidal ideation and behavior	Alcohol
	Caffeine
Medical comorbidities	Cannabis
Alzheimer's disease	Nicotine
Chronic obstructive pulmonary disease	Routines
Delirium	
Nocturia	
Pain	
Parkinson's disease	

Normal Age-Related Changes

Sleep is made up of two different states: rapid eye movement (REM) and non-REM (NREM) sleep (American Academy of Sleep Medicine 2007; Rechtschaffen and Kales 1968). NREM is further divided into N1 and N2 (lighter sleep) and N3 stages (deep or slow-wave sleep [SWS]). Sleep is usually composed of ~90-minute cycles, with more deep sleep occurring in the first half of the night and more REM sleep in the second half of the night. Sleep timing and structure are regulated by a two-part process: the circadian rhythm (i.e., the physiological process regulating the sleep-wake cycle and other bodily processes such as temperature, heart rate, and hormonal release) and the homeostatic mechanism (i.e., the body's sleep pressure as a function of time awake) (Borbély 1982).

A meta-analysis of quantitative sleep parameters across the life span of 3,577 participants ages 5–102 years revealed some consistent age-related changes in sleep, including decreased total sleep time, sleep efficiency (percentage of time spent asleep during the period set aside for sleep), SWS, and REM sleep and increased wake time after sleep onset and N1 and N2 sleep (Ohayon et al. 2004). More specifically, for changes with a large effect size, total sleep time, sleep efficiency, and percentage of SWS are estimated to decrease by about 10 minutes, 3%, and 2%, respectively, per decade, and wake time after sleep onset is estimated to increase by 10 minutes per decade. However, most of these changes were found in subjects between the ages of 18 and 60 years, with one exception of decreased sleep efficiency starting at age 40 and continuing past age 60 (Ohayon et al. 2004). A potential explanation for these age-related changes is a decline in the homeostatic mechanism (Li et al. 2018).

There is also evidence for changes in the sleep-wake cycle with aging. A review of the literature on aging and circadian rhythms demonstrated that the foremost age-related change in this domain is the phase advance of sleep (Duffy et al. 2015). There is also evidence that the amplitudes of both the sleep-wake cycle and the 24-hour body temperature rhythm appear to decrease with aging (Duffy et al. 2015). Other changes to the sleep-wake cycle include older adults reporting greater excessive daytime sleepiness and more frequent napping than younger adults (Bixler et al. 2005; Buysse et al. 1992; Miner et al. 2019).

Sleep Disorders

Insomnia Disorder

Insomnia symptoms include difficulty initiating sleep, difficulty maintaining sleep, and waking up too early, and epidemiological studies demonstrate that ~33% of the general population endorses at least one such symptom (Ohayon 2002). Insomnia disorder is defined as at least one insomnia symptom with daytime consequences occurring at least 3 nights a week for at least 3 months, despite adequate opportunity for sleep (American Psychiatric Association 2013). Most commonly, individuals have symptoms that meet criteria for comorbid insomnia (Ohayon 2002). Epidemiological studies have demonstrated that about 6%–10% of the adult population has an insomnia disorder, impacting functioning in several areas. Although epidemiological research shows an increase in insomnia symptoms with age, evidence is mixed as to whether insomnia disorder is more prevalent with age. Regardless, insomnia symptoms and insomnia disorder are common issues among older adults (Ohayon 2002).

Obstructive Sleep Apnea

The most common sleep-related breathing disorder diagnosed in older adults is obstructive sleep apnea (OSA). OSA is characterized by breathing cessation due to oropharyngeal collapse for periods of 10 seconds or longer (Benca 2012). Breathing events can either be defined as *apnea* (complete breathing cessation) or *hypopnea* (partial decrease in breathing) (American Academy of Sleep Medicine 2014; American Psychiatric Association 2013). To meet the diagnostic criteria for OSA, the apnea-hypopnea index (AHI) derived from polysomnography or other overnight monitoring needs to be 5 or higher per hour with symptoms of nocturnal breathing disturbance, daytime sleepiness, or fatigue or an AHI of 15 or more per hour without accompanying symptoms (American Academy of Sleep Medicine 2014; American Psychiatric Association 2013). OSA severity is classified by AHI as follows: mild, 5–15; moderate, 16–30; and severe, >30.

The prevalence of at least moderate OSA is 6%–17% in the general adult population and as high as 49% in older age groups (Senaratna et al. 2017). One of the top three risk factors for OSA is greater age, along with male sex and greater BMI (Senaratna et al. 2017). The association between BMI and odds of OSA significantly decreases with age (Young et al. 2002). Apneas and hypopneas are generally terminated by arousal (brief awakening), which results in sleep fragmentation. Key symptoms include loud snoring, witnessed apneas, gasping or choking during sleep, fatigue, and daytime sleepiness. The long-term sequelae from untreated severe OSA include motor vehicle accidents, hypertension, cardiovascular and cerebrovascular morbidity, cognitive dysfunction, mood dysfunction, and premature death (Peppard and Hagen 2018).

Sleep-Related Movement Disorders

Two common sleep-related movement disorders to consider in older adults are restless legs syndrome (RLS) and periodic limb movement disorder (PLMD). A diagnosis of RLS requires the following: 1) an urge to move the legs often accompanied by an unpleasant or uncomfortable sensation; 2) occurrence or worsening during periods of rest or inactivity; 3) worsening in the evening or at night, leading to significant difficulty falling asleep, and a tendency to improve or disappear in the morning; and 4) temporary relief with movement or stretching (American Academy of Sleep Medicine 2014). RLS is estimated to occur in the general population at a rate of ~7.2%, with increased prevalence with age and a greater likelihood of occurrence in females (Allen et al. 2005). Many factors can contribute to RLS, including iron deficiency, congestive heart failure, diabetes, end-stage renal disease, multiple sclerosis, neuropathy, Parkinson's disease, rheumatoid arthritis, pregnancy, and medication use (e.g., antidepressants, antihistamines with CNS effects, dopamine antagonists, lithium, nonsteroidal anti-inflammatory agents) as well as alcohol, caffeine, and nicotine use (Benca 2012).

PLMD is diagnosed when the frequency of limb movements is >15 per hour in adults with accompanying sleep disturbance or other functional impairment (American Academy of Sleep Medicine 2014). Periodic limb movements most commonly occur in the legs, with each individual movement lasting between 0.5 and 10 seconds and between-movement periods lasting 20–40 seconds. Periodic limb movements occur over minutes to several hours of the sleep period and are common in individuals with RLS and OSA (Benca 2012). They are also frequently found in asymptomatic individuals, so their identification on polysomnography is not necessarily pathological and should be considered within the broader clinical context. The same factors associated with RLS noted in the previous paragraph are also important to consider in those with periodic limb movements (Benca 2012).

Circadian Rhythm Sleep-Wake Disorders

Circadian rhythm sleep-wake disorders include all disorders in which a person's endogenous rhythm is persistently out of alignment with the schedule required by that individual's personal or professional responsibilities, resulting in excessive sleepiness or insomnia and clinically significant distress or impairment (American Academy of Sleep Medicine 2014; American Psychiatric Association 2013). Circadian rhythm sleep-wake disorders can broadly be grouped into intrinsic and extrinsic disorders. Intrinsic disorders occur when a person's circadian rhythm functions differently from that in most of the general population (e.g., advanced or delayed sleep phase). Extrinsic disorders occur when a person's normally functioning circadian rhythm is at odds with an atypical environment (e.g., shift work, jet lag). The main circadian rhythm sleep-wake disorders to consider in older adults are advanced sleep phase type and irregular sleep-wake type. Advanced sleep phase type is when the sleep-wake schedule is earlier (i.e., advanced) by several hours than what is considered conventional or desired. Symptoms include sleepiness in the early evening hours and early morning awakenings. The prevalence of advanced phase type is 0.3%–7.1% in adults ages 20–59 years and increases significantly with age (Paine et al. 2014). Irregular sleep-wake type is defined by a lack of a distinct sleep-wake pattern with at least three fragmented sleep and wake periods over the 24-hour day (American Academy of Sleep Medicine 2014; American Psychiatric Association 2013). Irregular sleep-wake type is most commonly associated with neurodegenerative disorders, including Alzheimer's disease (AD), Parkinson's disease (PD), and Huntington's disease, and can be found in adults with less exposure to outside light and a regular routine, including those hospitalized or institutionalized (American Psychiatric Association 2013).

Psychiatric and Medical Comorbidities

Psychiatric Disorders

Psychiatric disorders are common among older adults, including depression (at a rate of ~11%) and anxiety (at a rate of ~15%) (Bryant et al. 2008; Steffens et al. 2009). The relationship between depression and insomnia has been studied the most. Prospective studies support the bidirectional nature of this relationship by demonstrating that sleep disturbance more than doubles the risk of future depression in older adults (Cole and Dendukuri 2003). The relationship between bereavement and sleep disturbance in older adults is also significant, as is the role that depressive symptoms may play in this relationship (Milic et al. 2019). For anxiety, prospective epidemiological studies demonstrate that insomnia is more likely to occur simultaneously with or after the onset of anxiety in the general population (Ohayon and Roth 2003). In comparison across the adult life span, older adults with generalized anxiety disorder were significantly more likely to have sleep disturbance and higher rates of and more severe levels of depression in comparison with younger adults with generalized anxiety disorder (Altunoz et al. 2018). Finally, it is important to consider the relationship between sleep disturbance and suicidal ideation and behavior, particularly with the increased risk of death by suicide that already exists among male older adults (King et al. 2017). One longitudinal case-control cohort study of older adults that adjusted for depression severity found that baseline poor sleep quality and nonrestorative sleep were related to a 1.3- and 2.0-times greater risk, respectively, of death by suicide (Bernert et al. 2014).

Alzheimer's Disease

In a systematic review and meta-analysis of neuropsychiatric symptoms in AD, sleep disturbance was among the most common symptoms, with an estimated prevalence of 39% (Zhao et al. 2016). Common sleep disturbances related to AD mimic a more exaggerated form of normal age-related sleep changes as discussed at the beginning of this chapter, including greater sleep fragmentation, shorter sleep duration, and less SWS and REM sleep, as well as more daytime sleep and irregular circadian rhythm (Mander et al. 2017). AD is also associated with increased risk of sleep-disordered breathing (Gaeta et al. 2020). Sleep disturbance was once thought to be a consequence of AD. However, a recent systematic review and meta-analysis of longitudinal studies with an average of 9.5 years of follow-up supports more of a bidirectional effect (Shi et al. 2018). More specifically, those with insomnia at baseline were at higher risk of incident AD, and those with sleep-disordered breathing at baseline were at higher risk of incident all-cause dementia, AD, and vascular dementia (Shi et al. 2018). Finally, emerging evidence indicates a link between behavioral rest-activity rhythm irregularity and white matter microarchitecture in older adults at risk for dementia (Palmer et al. 2021).

Parkinson's Disease

Sleep disturbance is also one of the most common nonmotor symptoms for individuals with PD and can manifest in a number of ways, including insomnia, excessive daytime sleepiness, RLS, and circadian rhythm dysregulation (Chahine et al. 2017; Leng et al. 2019). More specific to PD is a greater prevalence of REM sleep behavior disorder, disorder is defined as the presence of REM sleep without typical atonia and with repeated episodes of dream enactment behavior (American Academy of Sleep Medicine 2014). Importantly, REM sleep behavior frequently manifests years before the classical motor symptoms of PD become apparent. Thus, REM sleep behavior disorder is an important risk factor for the longitudinal development of PD and other α-synucleinopathies (Iranzo et al. 2014).

Pain

In representative samples of older adults, more than half report persistent pain concerns (Blay et al. 2007; Patel et al. 2013). Also, sleep disturbance is very common in older adults with persistent pain conditions, and vice versa (Blay et al. 2007). Historically, the relationship between sleep disturbance and pain has been viewed as sleep disturbance occurring as a secondary symptom of persistent pain. However, critical reviews of prospective and experimental research indicate that sleep disturbance reliably and more strongly predicts onset and exacerbation of persistent pain than persistent pain predicts sleep disturbance (Afolalu et al. 2018; Finan et al. 2013). The findings from these larger clinical reviews have been investigated more specifically in older adult populations, with the same conclusions, supporting the imperative to assess and treat both pain and sleep disturbance as they co-occur in older adults (Dunietz et al. 2018).

Nocturia

Nocturia is common in adults, with studies showing that ~31% of individuals wake during the night two times or more to void (Coyne et al. 2003). Additionally, studies have demonstrated a relationship between increased prevalence of nocturia and age (Coyne et al. 2003). Nocturia is related to several medical concerns in older adults, including dysfunctional bladder storage, increased 24-hour or nocturnal urine production, and sleep disorders (Vaughan and Bliwise 2018). More specifically, enlargement of the prostate, overactive bladder, medication side effects, kidney stones, congestive heart failure treated with diuretic medication, chronic kidney disease, uncontrolled diabetes, lower-extremity edema, and excessive intake of fluids should be considered in the context of nocturia. Sleep disorders, including OSA, REM sleep behavior disorder, RLS, and PLMD, may also contribute to nocturia. Nocturia in older adults is often multifactorial and requires treatment with multiple components (Vaughan and Bliwise 2018).

Chronic Obstructive Pulmonary Disease

Individuals with chronic obstructive pulmonary disease often experience hypoxemia both during the day and at night, with greater hypoxemia at night (McNicholas et al.

2013; Weitzenblum and Chaouat 2004). Hypoxemia is more likely during REM sleep and can lead to poor sleep quality and issues such as pulmonary hypertension and cardiac arrhythmias. Additionally, chronic obstructive pulmonary disease and OSA are common comorbidities, and hypoxemia is more pronounced when both conditions are present (McNicholas et al. 2013; Weitzenblum and Chaouat 2004).

Delirium

Delirium is a common occurrence among elderly medical inpatients, with one study demonstrating that about 19% of elderly medical inpatients developed delirium and about 40% of those developing delirium also had dementia (Margiotta et al. 2006). Sleep and circadian functioning have been considered as both risk factors for and symptoms of delirium. A recent systematic review and meta-analysis found that interventions aimed at sleep promotion and circadian intervention during hospitalization may be efficacious in decreasing postoperative delirium (Lu et al. 2019).

Medications

Medications can affect sleep in several ways. Particularly relevant to geriatric psychiatry is the impact of psychiatric medication on sleep. Insomnia is among the top side effects for both the selective serotonin reuptake inhibitors (SSRIs) and the serotonin-norepinephrine reuptake inhibitors (SNRIs), the most commonly prescribed antidepressants (Shelton 2019). More broadly, most antidepressants, including SSRIs, SNRIs, and tricyclic antidepressants (TCAs), suppress REM sleep, and REM rebound is a common side effect with missed doses (Rumble et al. 2015). Sleep-related movement disorders can be exacerbated by or develop in the context of TCAs, SSRIs, SNRIs, and antipsychotics (Rumble et al. 2015). Serotonergic antidepressants are also a frequent iatrogenic cause of REM sleep without atonia, periodic limb movements of sleep, and RLS (Winkelman and James 2004; Yang et al. 2005). In fact, the antidepressant mirtazapine, which is frequently used in elderly patients, has been associated with particularly high rates of RLS induction in previously asymptomatic persons (Rottach et al. 2008). Many psychiatric medications increase the arousal threshold and can lead to weight gain, making individuals more prone to developing OSA. Also relevant to geriatric psychiatry are medications from other drug classes that are commonly taken by older adults and can have a negative impact on sleep, including cholinesterase inhibitors, stimulants, antihypertensives, corticosteroids, decongestants, second-generation antihistamines, lipid-lowering agents, dopamine agonists, and diuretics (Abad and Guilleminault 2018; Zdanys and Steffens 2015).

Behaviors

Substances

Persistent substance use, as well as intoxication with and withdrawal from substances, can have negative effects on sleep as measured by polysomnography (Garcia and Salloum 2015). More specifically, for stimulants such as caffeine and nicotine, persistent use has been demonstrated to lead not only to issues falling asleep but also to decreased SWS sleep and sleep efficiency. With chronic alcohol use, individuals have increased difficulty falling asleep, decreased REM sleep, and decreased total sleep time. For those who use cannabis regularly, SWS suppression is observed (Garcia and Salloum 2015). Thus, consideration of the impact of substance use on sleep disturbance is of importance, particularly because older adults are likely to be more sensitive to substances and their impact on sleep.

Routines

Irregular routines, including inconsistent timing of daily activities such as wake time, meals, contact with others, going outside, getting exercise, and bedtime, can also have a negative impact on sleep. A study of individuals ages 20–89 years demonstrated that regularity increases with age, so older adults are likely to have more regular routines than their younger counterparts (Monk et al. 1997). At the same time, several studies in older adults have demonstrated that less routine regularity predicted worse sleep outcomes (Dautovich et al. 2015; Zisberg et al. 2010). The transition out of the workforce and subsequent loss of work-related routines can have sizable impacts on sleep-wake patterns in elderly persons. For example, retirement has been associated with longer sleep duration, later bedtimes, later wake times, and increased napping (Hagen et al. 2016; Harden et al. 2019). Furthermore, a randomized controlled trial examined whether a structured physical activity intervention in comparison with a health education intervention improved sleep quality in older adults who were considered sedentary at baseline (Vaz Fragoso et al. 2015). Results revealed that those receiving the structured physical activity intervention were 30% less likely to develop poor sleep quality over the course of follow-up for 30 months.

Assessment

Given the multifactorial and complex nature of sleep disturbance in elderly persons, the geriatric psychiatrist can inquire regularly about sleep and its impact on daily functioning and determine whether psychiatric treatment could be tailored appropriately or other forms of assessment and treatment are needed for sleep disorders and related comorbidities (Table 16–2). Using an algorithm proposed by geriatric sleep specialists (Bloom et al. 2009), the geriatric psychiatrist can start with the main sleep complaint and then consider potential options. First, if the patient is primarily having difficulty either falling or staying asleep, insomnia is the likely issue. However, the timing of sleep and potential circadian rhythm issues should be considered, as well as medical and psychiatric comorbidities, medication use, substance use, and sleep-related movement issues. Second, if the patient is primarily reporting excessive daytime sleepiness, then OSA, timing of sleep and potential circadian rhythm issues, medical or psychiatric comorbidities, medication use, and substance use disorder should be considered. Finally, if the patient primarily presents with unusual sleep-related behavior or movements, then RLS, PLMD, REM sleep behavior disorder, and delirium should be considered (Bloom et al. 2009).

Clinicians should also consider whether a referral for overnight polysomnography/sleep specialty consultation is needed. Among the sleep disorders discussed more fully in this chapter, overnight polysomnography would be indicated for suspected OSA, PLMD, and REM sleep behavior disorder. In many instances, OSA can be diagnosed

TABLE 16–2.   **Overview of assessment and treatment of sleep disorders in older adults for the geriatric psychiatrist**

Assessment

Ask regularly about sleep.

Are there any changes that need to be made with psychiatric treatment to optimize sleep?

Is there a need for referral to primary care and/or other specialties to further assess and treat medical comorbidities or issues with medications or substances?

What type of sleep issue is present: difficulty initiating or maintaining sleep, excessive daytime sleepiness, and/or unusual sleep-related behavior or movement?

As needed, refer for sleep study and/or sleep specialty consultation if OSA, PLMD, or REM sleep behavior disorder is suspected.

As needed, refer for sleep specialty consultation if insomnia disorder, circadian rhythm sleep-wake disorders, or RLS is suspected. A sleep study is not indicated for these concerns. Consider also using a sleep log in the assessment and treatment process.

Treatment

Circadian rhythm sleep-wake disorders

    Light therapy in the morning (for irregular sleep-wake type)

    Light therapy at night (for advanced sleep phase type)

Insomnia

    CBT for insomnia

    Medication as adjunctive

OSA

    Avoiding medications related to weight gain

    Avoiding sedating substances

    Oral appliance (mild OSA)

    Positive airway pressure therapy

    Supine preclusion (supine-dependent OSA)

    Weight loss

REM sleep behavior disorder

    Adapting the sleep environment to prevent injury

    Melatonin

    Clonazepam (for REM sleep behavior disorder)

RLS and PLMD

    Dopaminergic agents/$\alpha_2\delta$ agents

    Iron replacement in individuals who are iron deficient

CBT=cognitive-behavioral therapy; OSA=obstructive sleep apnea; PLMD=periodic limb movement disorder; REM=rapid eye movement; RLS=restless legs syndrome.

with in-home sleep testing, designed specifically to diagnose moderate or worse sleep-disordered breathing. In contrast, an overnight sleep study is not indicated for insomnia disorder, circadian rhythm sleep-wake disorders, and RLS because diagnosis of these sleep disorders is made from clinical interview and self-report measures. Along these lines, a daily sleep log is a helpful tool not only for making the diagnosis but also for more fully understanding patterns of sleep disturbance and highlighting specific treatment targets (Carney et al. 2012).

Treatment

Insomnia

Effective treatments are available for insomnia, including both nonpharmacological and pharmacological options. Cognitive-behavioral therapy for insomnia (CBT-I) has a strong evidence base and is recommended as the initial treatment for older adults with insomnia alone and those with comorbid insomnia (Edinger et al. 2021; Schutte-Rodin et al. 2008). CBT-I is a nonpharmacological treatment that targets unhelpful behaviors and beliefs shown to often perpetuate insomnia symptoms (Edinger and Means 2005). For example, behaviors include "chasing sleep" and having an erratic sleep schedule in response; going to bed early, sleeping in late, or napping to compensate for sleep loss; and unintentionally developing an association between the bed and wakefulness, frustration about sleep, or anxiety about sleep. Unhelpful sleep-related beliefs for an older adult might include "Everyone sleeps poorly when they get older, so there is nothing that can be done to make sleep better."

The main treatment components for CBT-I are stimulus control and sleep restriction. Stimulus control aims to reassociate the bedroom with sleep while also strengthening the circadian rhythm (Bootzin 1972). Sleep restriction aims to increase the sleep drive (Spielman et al. 1987). Other components often used within CBT-I include sleep hygiene, relaxation therapy, and cognitive therapy. Behavioral sleep medicine specialists most commonly provide CBT-I in individual and group settings; however, there is a shortage of behavioral sleep medicine providers (Thomas et al. 2016). Thus, for resources more readily available for many individuals, there are also self-help books on CBT-I (Carney and Manber 2009; Edinger and Carney 2008).

Pharmacological treatment is currently recommended as a treatment option if CBT-I is not effective or for limited use in combination with CBT-I (Abad and Guilleminault 2018). FDA-approved agents for insomnia include benzodiazepines, nonbenzodiazepines, melatonin receptor agonists, histamine receptor antagonists, and orexin receptor antagonists. Non-FDA-approved agents that are often used off-label to treat insomnia in older adults include trazodone, melatonin, diphenhydramine, tryptophan, and valerian, although minimal data support their use. If appropriate, one key consideration in selecting medications is the type and timing of the insomnia complaint. That is, for difficulty initiating sleep, medications with short half-lives would be most appropriate, whereas for sleep maintenance difficulties, intermediate- to longer-acting agents may be more appropriate (Sateia et al. 2017). Other key considerations are potential side effects, costs, and contraindications. Along these lines, benzodiazepines are generally not recommended for the treatment of insomnia in older adults because of the risk of falls, development of tolerance, and exacerbation of health comorbidities. Other medications of concern are α_1-selective benzodiazepine receptor agonists (e.g., zolpidem) in terms of amnestic behavior, trazodone in terms of dizziness and orthostatic hypotension, diphenhydramine in terms of high anticholinergic effects and toxicity, and any sedating medication in individuals with untreated OSA (Abad and Guilleminault 2018).

Obstructive Sleep Apnea

The first-line treatment for OSA is positive airway pressure (PAP) therapy, which is a treatment that helps to splint the airway open through continuous, bilevel, or automatic positive airway pressure (referred to as CPAP, BPAP, and APAP, respectively) (Benca 2012). If PAP therapy is not tolerated, some individuals with mild OSA may benefit from an oral appliance that advances the mandible to support a more patent upper airway. Other individuals who have mostly supine-dependent apnea may be able to manage OSA with supine preclusion efforts. However, most individuals with moderate to severe OSA will need PAP therapy to adequately treat OSA and to decrease the potential consequences of untreated OSA. Additional conservative treatment measures for OSA include avoiding alcohol, sedating medications, and opioid medications, which can increase the likelihood of upper airway collapse during sleep; losing weight; and optimizing nasal patency (Benca 2012).

Restless Legs Syndrome and Periodic Limb Movement Disorder

Many factors can contribute to RLS and PLMD, including iron deficiency, congestive heart failure, diabetes, end-stage renal disease, multiple sclerosis, neuropathy, PD, rheumatoid arthritis, and use of medication use (e.g., antidepressants, antihistamines with CNS effects, dopamine antagonists, lithium, nonsteroidal anti-inflammatory agents), alcohol, caffeine, or nicotine (Benca 2012). Therefore, consideration of these potential issues as a first step in treatment is likely to be helpful. In terms of iron deficiency (i.e., individuals with ferritin levels <75 µg/L), iron replacement (e.g., ferrous sulfate 325 mg with 100 mg vitamin C once or twice a day) may alleviate RLS and PLMD symptoms (Allen et al. 2018). The first-line pharmacological treatment options for RLS and PLMD have varied over time, with both $\alpha_2\delta$ calcium channel ligands ($\alpha_2\delta$ agents; e.g., gabapentin, pregabalin, gabapentin enacarbil) and dopamine agonists (e.g., pramipexole, ropinirole, rotigotine) currently considered viable initial treatment options (Garcia-Borreguero et al. 2016). If $\alpha_2\delta$ agents are used, reduced starting dosages are typically recommended (e.g., gabapentin 100 mg/day, pregabalin 50 mg/day) for persons age 65 and older (Garcia-Borreguero et al. 2016). Dopamine agonists can be very effective in treating RLS; however, over time, they are associated with risk of augmentation, defined as paradoxical worsening of RLS symptoms caused by a treating agent, which can be quite difficult for inexperienced clinicians to identify and effectively manage. Additionally, these agents have been associated with impulsive/compulsive behaviors, as well as orthostatic hypotension, which can be particularly problematic in older adults. Opioids, benzodiazepines, and other anticonvulsants are considered second-line treatment options for RLS and PLMD (Bloom et al. 2009).

Circadian Rhythm Sleep-Wake Disorders

For advanced sleep phase type in adults, light therapy has the most support as an intervention, prescribed in the evening (e.g., light therapy for 12 days at ~4,000 lux for 2 hours between 8 P.M. and 11 P.M. prior to the regular bedtime) (Auger et al. 2015).

Regarding irregular sleep-wake type, treatment recommendations are specific to individuals with irregular sleep-wake type in the context of dementia. The main recommendation for these patients is also light therapy; however, the timing of light therapy differs: it is provided in the morning (e.g., light therapy for 4–10 weeks at 2,500–5,000 lux for 1–2 hours between 9 A.M. and 11 A.M.). Additionally, there is strong evidence against sleep-promoting medications and weak evidence against melatonin or melatonin receptor agonists in older adults with irregular sleep-wake type and dementia. For both advanced sleep phase type in adults and irregular sleep-wake type in older adults with dementia, there are currently no widely accepted specific recommendations for prescribed sleep-wake scheduling, timed physical activity/exercise, strategic avoidance of light, and wakefulness-promoting medications (Auger et al. 2015).

REM Sleep Behavior Disorder

The main treatment for REM sleep behavior disorder is clonazepam, with doses ranging from 0.25 mg to 2 mg 30 minutes before bed (Aurora et al. 2010). However, clinical guidelines for treatment suggest using caution in patients with dementia, gait disorders, or OSA. Another treatment option with some evidence is melatonin 3–12 mg at bedtime. Guidelines also recommend adapting the sleeping environment to prevent sleep-related injury with movement at night (Aurora et al. 2010). Notably, reduction in dream enactment does not alter the longitudinal risk of developing a symptomatic α-synucleinopathy (e.g., PD); thus, treatment recommendations for REM sleep behavior disorder should be made as part of a collaborative risk-benefit assessment that considers the safety of the patient (and bed partner) with the potential side effects of a given therapeutic strategy.

Conclusion

More than half of older adults endorse sleep disturbance, and it is associated with a number of significant and negative health outcomes in this population. Although there are age-related changes in sleep (e.g., decreased total sleep time, sleep efficiency, and percentage of SWS and increased wake time after sleep onset), many commonly and mistakenly assume that persistent sleep disturbance is a normal part of aging. Common sleep disorders in older adults to be aware of are insomnia disorder, OSA, RLS, PLMD, circadian rhythm sleep-wake disorders (advance sleep phase and irregular sleep-wake type), and REM sleep behavior disorder. Many of these sleep issues are also comorbid with other persistent conditions in older adults that have dynamic relationships with sleep, such as depression, bereavement, anxiety, suicidal ideation and behavior, AD, PD, pain, nocturia, chronic obstructive pulmonary disease, and delirium, and may also be impacted by medication, caffeine, nicotine, alcohol, cannabis, and changes in daily routines. Importantly, epidemiological data have supported a comorbid model with often bidirectional relationships between sleep disturbance and comorbidities, emphasizing the need for assessment and treatment of sleep issues. Fortunately, there are evidence-based treatments for sleep in older adults, with options for nonpharmacological treatments, particularly CBT for insomnia. Future research should continue to consider the most optimal ways to address the assessment and treatment of sleep issues in older adults to best optimize outcomes.

Key Points

- Many older adults experience sleep disturbance, which is predictive of negative health outcomes in this population.

- Some typical age-related changes in sleep do occur but do not equate to normalization of sleep disorders in older adults.

- Common sleep disorders in older adults include insomnia disorder, obstructive sleep apnea, restless legs syndrome, periodic limb movement disorder, circadian rhythm sleep-wake disorders (advance sleep phase and irregular sleep-wake types), and rapid eye movement sleep behavior disorder.

- Comorbidities commonly present with sleep issues include psychiatric disorders, Alzheimer's disease, Parkinson's disease, pain, nocturia, chronic obstructive pulmonary disease, and delirium. The impact of medication, caffeine, nicotine, alcohol, cannabis, and daily routines should also be considered.

- An evidence-based comorbid model underscores the need for assessment and treatment of sleep issues along with comorbidities.

- Geriatric psychiatrists should regularly inquire about sleep, consider the possibilities of various sleep issues, adjust psychiatric treatment as needed, and appropriately refer for further assessment and treatment as needed.

- Geriatric psychiatrists can also be informed about the various treatment pathways for sleep disorder in older adults, including cognitive-behavioral therapy for insomnia, so that they can best support their patients' overall care.

Suggested Readings

Bloom HG, Ahmed I, Alessi CA, et al: Evidence-based recommendations for the assessment and management of sleep disorders in older persons. J Am Geriatr Soc 57(5):761–789, 2009 19484833

Duffy JF, Zitting KM, Chinoy ED: Aging and circadian rhythms. Sleep Med Clin 10(4):423–434, 2015 26568120

Ohayon MM, Carskadon MA, Guilleminault C, Vitiello MV: Meta-analysis of quantitative sleep parameters from childhood to old age in healthy individuals: developing normative sleep values across the human lifespan. Sleep 27(7):1255–1273, 2004 15586779

References

Abad VC, Guilleminault C: Insomnia in elderly patients: recommendations for pharmacological management. Drugs Aging 35(9):791–817, 2018 30058034

Afolalu EF, Ramlee F, Tang NKY: Effects of sleep changes on pain-related health outcomes in the general population: a systematic review of longitudinal studies with exploratory meta-analysis. Sleep Med Rev 39:82–97, 2018 29056414

Allen RP, Walters AS, Montplaisir J, et al: Restless legs syndrome prevalence and impact: REST general population study. Arch Intern Med 165(11):1286–1292, 2005 15956009

Allen RP, Picchietti DL, Auerbach M, et al: Evidence-based and consensus clinical practice guidelines for the iron treatment of restless legs syndrome/Willis-Ekbom disease in adults and children: an IRLSSG Task Force report. Sleep Med 41:27–44, 2018 29425576

Altunoz U, Kokurcan A, Kirici S, et al: Clinical characteristics of generalized anxiety disorder: older vs. young adults. Nord J Psychiatry 72(2):97–102, 2018 29065768

American Academy of Sleep Medicine: The AASM Manual for the Scoring of Sleep and Associated Events: Rules, Terminology and Technical Specification. Westchester, IL, American Academy of Sleep Medicine, 2007

American Academy of Sleep Medicine: International Classification of Sleep Disorders, 3rd Edition. Darien, IL, Amerian Academy of Sleep Medicine, 2014

American Psychiatric Association: Diagnostic and Statistical Manual of Mental Disorders, 5th Edition. Arlington, VA, American Psychiatric Association, 2013

Auger RR, Burgess HJ, Emens JS, et al: Clinical practice guideline for the treatment of intrinsic circadian rhythm sleep-wake disorders: advanced sleep-wake phase disorder (ASWPD), delayed sleep-wake phase disorder (DSWPD), non-24-hour sleep-wake rhythm disorder (N24SWD), and irregular sleep-wake rhythm disorder (ISWRD), an update for 2015: an American Academy of Sleep Medicine clinical practice guideline. J Clin Sleep Med 11(10):1199–1236, 2015 26414986

Aurora RN, Zak RS, Maganti RK, et al: Best practice guide for the treatment of REM sleep behavior disorder (RBD). J Clin Sleep Med 6(1):85–95, 2010 20191945

Bao YP, Han Y, Ma J, et al: Cooccurrence and bidirectional prediction of sleep disturbances and depression in older adults: meta-analysis and systematic review. Neurosci Biobehav Rev 75:257–273, 2017 28179129

Benca RM: Sleep Disorders: The Clinician's Guide to Diagnosis and Management. New York, Oxford University Press, 2012

Bernert RA, Turvey CL, Conwell Y, Joiner TE Jr: Association of poor subjective sleep quality with risk for death by suicide during a 10-year period: a longitudinal, population-based study of late life. JAMA Psychiatry 71(10):1129–1137, 2014 25133759

Bixler EO, Vgontzas AN, Lin HM, et al: Excessive daytime sleepiness in a general population sample: the role of sleep apnea, age, obesity, diabetes, and depression. J Clin Endocrinol Metab 90(8):4510–4515, 2005 15941867

Blay SL, Andreoli SB, Gastal FL: Chronic painful physical conditions, disturbed sleep and psychiatric morbidity: results from an elderly survey. Ann Clin Psychiatry 19(3):169–174, 2007 17729018

Bloom HG, Ahmed I, Alessi CA, et al: Evidence-based recommendations for the assessment and management of sleep disorders in older persons. J Am Geriatr Soc 57(5):761–789, 2009 19484833

Bootzin R: Stimulus control for insomnia. Paper presented at the 80th Annual Convention of the American Psychological Association, Honolulu, HI, September 1972

Borbély AA: A two process model of sleep regulation. Hum Neurobiol 1(3):195–204, 1982 7185792

Bryant C, Jackson H, Ames D: The prevalence of anxiety in older adults: methodological issues and a review of the literature. J Affect Disord 109(3):233–250, 2008 18155775

Buysse DJ, Browman KE, Monk TH, et al: Napping and 24-hour sleep/wake patterns in healthy elderly and young adults. J Am Geriatr Soc 40(8):779–786, 1992 1634721

Carney C, Manber R: Quiet Your Mind and Get to Sleep: Solutions to Insomnia for Those with Depression, Anxiety, or Chronic Pain. Oakland, CA, New Harbinger, 2009

Carney CE, Buysse DJ, Ancoli-Israel S, et al: The consensus sleep diary: standardizing prospective sleep self-monitoring. Sleep (Basel) 35(2):287–302, 2012 22294820

Chahine LM, Amara AW, Videnovic A: A systematic review of the literature on disorders of sleep and wakefulness in Parkinson's disease from 2005 to 2015. Sleep Med Rev 35:33–50, 2017 27863901

Cole MG, Dendukuri N: Risk factors for depression among elderly community subjects: a systematic review and meta-analysis. Am J Psychiatry 160(6):1147–1156, 2003 12777274

Coyne KS, Zhou Z, Bhattacharyya SK, et al: The prevalence of nocturia and its effect on health-related quality of life and sleep in a community sample in the USA. BJU Int 92(9):948–954, 2003 14632853

Dautovich ND, Shoji KD, McCrae CS: Variety is the spice of life: a microlongitudinal study examining age differences in intraindividual variability in daily activities in relation to sleep outcomes. J Gerontol B Psychol Sci Soc Sci 70(4):581–590, 2015 24326078

Duffy JF, Zitting KM, Chinoy ED: Aging and circadian rhythms. Sleep Med Clin 10(4):423–434, 2015 26568120

Dunietz GL, Swanson LM, Jansen EC, et al: Key insomnia symptoms and incident pain in older adults: direct and mediated pathways through depression and anxiety. Sleep (Basel) 41(9) 2018 29982769

Edinger JD, Carney C: Overcoming Insomnia: A Cognitive-Behavioral Therapy Approach Workbook. New York, Oxford University Press, 2008

Edinger JD, Means MK: Cognitive-behavioral therapy for primary insomnia. Clin Psychol Rev 25(5):539–558, 2005 15951083

Edinger JD, Arnedt JT, Bertisch SM, et al: Behavioral and psychological treatments for chronic insomnia disorder in adults: an American Academy of Sleep Medicine clinical practice guideline. J Clin Sleep Med 17(2):255–262, 2021 33164742

Finan PH, Goodin BR, Smith MT: The association of sleep and pain: an update and a path forward. J Pain 14(12):1539–1552, 2013 24290442

Foley DJ, Monjan AA, Brown SL, et al: Sleep complaints among elderly persons: an epidemiologic study of three communities. Sleep 18(6):425–432, 1995 7481413

Gaeta AM, Benitez ID, Jorge C, et al: Prevalence of obstructive sleep apnea in Alzheimer's disease patients. J Neurol 267(4):1012–1022, 2020 31832828

Garcia AN, Salloum IM: Polysomnographic sleep disturbances in nicotine, caffeine, alcohol, cocaine, opioid, and cannabis use: a focused review. Am J Addict 24(7):590–598, 2015 26346395

Garcia-Borreguero D, Silber MH, Winkelman JW, et al: Guidelines for the first-line treatment of restless legs syndrome/Willis-Ekbom disease, prevention and treatment of dopaminergic augmentation: a combined task force of the IRLSSG, EURLSSG, and the RLS Foundation. Sleep Med 21:1–11, 2016 27448465

Hagen EW, Barnet JH, Hale L, Peppard PE: Changes in sleep duration and sleep timing associated with retirement transitions. Sleep (Basel) 39(3):665–673, 2016 26564125

Harden CM, Peppard PE, Palta M, et al: One-year changes in self-reported napping behaviors across the retirement transition. Sleep Health 5(6):639–646, 2019 31727591

Iranzo A, Fernández-Arcos A, Tolosa E, et al: Neurodegenerative disorder risk in idiopathic REM sleep behavior disorder: study in 174 patients. PLoS One 9(2):e89741, 2014 24587002

King CA, Horwitz A, Czyz E, Lindsay R: Suicide risk screening in healthcare settings: identifying males and females at risk. J Clin Psychol Med Settings 24(1):8–20, 2017 28251427

Leng Y, Musiek ES, Hu K, et al: Association between circadian rhythms and neurodegenerative diseases. Lancet Neurol 18(3):307–318, 2019 30784558

Li J, Vitiello MV, Gooneratne NS: Sleep in normal aging. Sleep Med Clin 13(1):1–11, 2018 29412976

Lu Y, Li Y, Wang L, et al: Promoting sleep and circadian health may prevent postoperative delirium: a systematic review and meta-analysis of randomized controlled trials. Sleep Med Rev 48:10127, 2019 31505369

Mander BA, Winer JR, Walker MP: Sleep and human aging. Neuron 94(1):19–36, 2017 28384471

Margiotta A, Bianchetti A, Ranieri P, Trabucchi M: Clinical characteristics and risk factors of delirium in demented and not demented elderly medical inpatients. J Nutr Health Aging 10(6):535–539, 2006 17183425

McNicholas WT, Verbraecken J, Marin JM: Sleep disorders in COPD: the forgotten dimension. Eur Respir Rev 22(129):365–375, 2013 23997063

Milic J, Saavedra Perez H, Zuurbier LA, et al: The longitudinal and cross-sectional associations of grief and complicated grief with sleep quality in older adults. Behav Sleep Med 17(1):31–40, 2019 28107032

Miner B, Gill TM, Yaggi HK, et al: The epidemiology of patient-reported hypersomnia in persons with advanced age. J Am Geriatr Soc 67(12):2545–2552, 2019 31390046

Monk TH, Reynolds CF III, Kupfer DJ, et al: Differences over the life span in daily life-style regularity. Chronobiol Int 14(3):295–306, 1997 9167890

Ohayon MM: Epidemiology of insomnia: what we know and what we still need to learn. Sleep Med Rev 6(2):97–111, 2002 12531146

Ohayon MM, Roth T: Place of chronic insomnia in the course of depressive and anxiety disorders. J Psychiatr Res 37(1):9–15, 2003 12482465

Ohayon MM, Carskadon MA, Guilleminault C, Vitiello MV: Meta-analysis of quantitative sleep parameters from childhood to old age in healthy individuals: developing normative sleep values across the human lifespan. Sleep 27(7):1255–1273, 2004 15586779

Paine SJ, Fink J, Gander PH, Warman GR: Identifying advanced and delayed sleep phase disorders in the general population: a national survey of New Zealand adults. Chronobiol Int 31(5):627–636, 2014 24548144

Palmer J, Duffy S, Meares S, et al: Rest-activity functioning is related to white matter microarchitecture and modifiable risk factors in older adults at-risk for dementia. Sleep 44(7):zsab007, 2021 33428761

Patel KV, Guralnik JM, Dansie EJ, Turk DC: Prevalence and impact of pain among older adults in the United States: findings from the 2011 National Health and Aging Trends Study. Pain 154(12):2649–2657, 2013 24287107

Peppard PE, Hagen EW: The last 25 years of obstructive sleep apnea epidemiology—and the next 25? Am J Respir Crit Care Med 197(3):310–312, 2018 29035088

Rechtschaffen A, Kales A: A Manual of Standardized Terminology, Techniques, and Scoring System for Sleep Stages of Human Subjects. Los Angeles, CA, Brain Information Service/Brain Research Institute, 1968

Rottach KG, Schaner BM, Kirch MH, et al: Restless legs syndrome as side effect of second generation antidepressants. J Psychiatr Res 43(1):70–75, 2008 18468624

Rumble ME, White KH, Benca RM: Sleep disturbances in mood disorders. Psychiatr Clin North Am 38(4):743–759, 2015 26600106

Sateia MJ, Buysse DJ, Krystal AD, et al: Clinical practice guideline for the pharmacologic treatment of chronic insomnia in adults: an American Academy of Sleep Medicine clinical practice guideline. J Clin Sleep Med 13(2):307–349, 2017 27998379

Schutte-Rodin S, Broch L, Buysse D, et al: Clinical guideline for the evaluation and management of chronic insomnia in adults. J Clin Sleep Med 4(5):487–504, 2008 18853708

Senaratna CV, Perret JL, Lodge CJ, et al: Prevalence of obstructive sleep apnea in the general population: a systematic review. Sleep Med Rev 34:70–81, 2017 27568340

Shelton RC: Serotonin and norepinephrine reuptake inhibitors. Handb Exp Pharmacol 250:145–180, 2019 30838456

Shi L, Chen SJ, Ma MY, et al: Sleep disturbances increase the risk of dementia: a systematic review and meta-analysis. Sleep Med Rev 40:4–16, 2018 28890168

Spielman AJ, Saskin P, Thorpy MJ: Treatment of chronic insomnia by restriction of time in bed. Sleep 10(1):45–56, 1987 3563247

Spira AP, Covinsky K, Rebok GW, et al: Objectively measured sleep quality and nursing home placement in older women. J Am Geriatr Soc 60(7):1237–1243, 2012 22702839

Steffens DC, Fisher GG, Langa KM, et al: Prevalence of depression among older Americans: the Aging, Demographics and Memory Study. Int Psychogeriatr 21(5):879–888, 2009 19519984

Stone KL, Ancoli-Israel S, Blackwell T, et al: Actigraphy-measured sleep characteristics and risk of falls in older women. Arch Intern Med 168(16):1768–1775, 2008 18779464

Thomas A, Grandner M, Nowakowski S, et al: Where are the behavioral sleep medicine providers and where are they needed? A geographic assessment. Behav Sleep Med 14(6):687–698, 2016 27159249

Tzuang M, Owusu J, Huang J, et al: Associations of insomnia symptoms with subsequent health services use among community-dwelling U.S. older adults. Sleep 44(5):zsaa251, 2021 33231264

Vaughan CP, Bliwise DL: Sleep and nocturia in older adults. Sleep Med Clin 13(1):107–116, 2018 29412977

Vaz Fragoso CA, Miller ME, King AC, et al: Effect of structured physical activity on sleep-wake behaviors in sedentary elderly adults with mobility limitations. J Am Geriatr Soc 63(7):1381–1390, 2015 26115386

Wallace ML, Buysse DJ, Redline S, et al: Multidimensional sleep and mortality in older adults: a machine-learning comparison with other risk factors. J Gerontol A Biol Sci Med Sci 74(12):1903–1909, 2019 30778527

Weitzenblum E, Chaouat A: Sleep and chronic obstructive pulmonary disease. Sleep Med Rev 8(4):281–294, 2004 15233956

Winkelman JW, James L: Serotonergic antidepressants are associated with REM sleep without atonia. Sleep 27(2):317–321, 2004 15124729

Yang C, White DP, Winkelman JW: Antidepressants and periodic leg movements of sleep. Biol Psychiatry 58(6):510–514, 2005 16005440

Young T, Shahar E, Nieto FJ, et al: Predictors of sleep-disordered breathing in community-dwelling adults: the Sleep Heart Health Study. Arch Intern Med 162(8):893–900, 2002 11966340

Zdanys KF, Steffens DC: Sleep disturbances in the elderly. Psychiatr Clin North Am 38(4):723–741, 2015 26600105

Zhao QF, Tan L, Wang HF, et al: The prevalence of neuropsychiatric symptoms in Alzheimer's disease: systematic review and meta-analysis. J Affect Disord 190:264–271, 2016 26540080

Zisberg A, Gur-Yaish N, Shochat T: Contribution of routine to sleep quality in community elderly. Sleep 33(4):509–514, 2010 20394320

CHAPTER 17

Substance-Related and Addictive Disorders

Shahrzad Mavandadi, Ph.D.

David W. Oslin, M.D.

Alcohol and drug use disorders are associated with an array of negative physical and mental health outcomes that are exacerbated with advancing age, such as functional and cognitive decline, compromised immune function, and depression. However, much remains to be learned about the correlates and consequences of substance use among older adults. Substance misuse in later life, which encompasses misuse of alcohol and illicit, prescription, and over-the-counter (OTC) drugs, has been referred to as both an "invisible" and "emerging" epidemic (Sorocco and Ferrell 2006; Yarnell et al. 2020). Epidemiological work, which has focused on younger populations, demonstrates that beginning in the middle to late 20s, overall rates of alcohol and illicit drug use begin to decline, with most older adults reporting no substance use. Nevertheless, changes in demographic and cohort trends suggest that substance misuse in later life is a pressing public health matter and that older adults represent a group in growing need of specialized substance treatment programs and services (Chhatre et al. 2017; Grant et al. 2017).

With the aging of the U.S. population and the resultant increase in the proportion of adults living to advanced ages, a concomitant increase has occurred in the number of older adults who misuse alcohol and drugs. Not only are older adults the fastest-growing segment of the U.S. population, but in the next several decades the aging population will be composed primarily of Baby Boomers, individuals born between the years 1946 and 1964. The aging of the Baby Boom cohort poses unique challenges to providers; in addition to reporting higher rates of illicit drug and alcohol use and addiction than earlier cohorts, this cohort also is significantly larger than previous cohorts (Gfroerer et al. 2003; Kuerbis 2020).

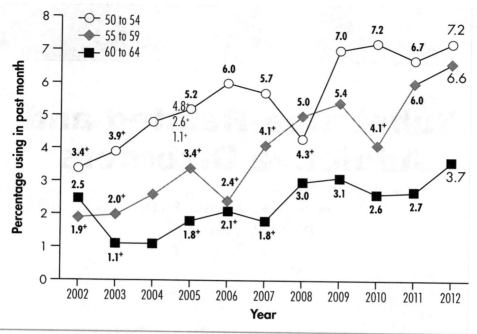

FIGURE 17–1. Past-month illicit drug use among adults ages 50–64 years: 2002–2012.
+Difference between this estimate and the 2012 estimate is statistically significant at the 0.05 level.
Source. Reprinted from Figure 2.10 (Past month illicit drug use among adults aged 50 to 64 years: 2002–2012) in Substance Abuse and Mental Health Services Administration: *Results From the 2012 National Survey on Drug Use and Health: Summary of National Findings.* NSDUH Series H-46, HHS Publication No. (SMA) 13–4795. Rockville, MD, Substance Abuse and Mental Health Services Administration, 2013. Available at: https://www.samhsa.gov/data/sites/default/files/NSDUHresults2012/NSDUHresults2012.pdf. Accessed June 1, 2020.

The potential public health impact of these demographic trends is highlighted by examining changes in rates of substance use and misuse in the past several decades. For example, it has been estimated that from the early 1990s until 2002, the prevalence of alcohol abuse or dependence (per DSM-IV criteria; American Psychiatric Association 1994) tripled to 3.1% among adults age 65 years and older (Grant et al. 2004). Subsequent analyses of alcohol use in this age group also suggest significant increases. For example, results from the National Epidemiologic Survey on Alcohol and Related Conditions (NESARC) indicate that from 2001 to 2013, rates of past-year alcohol use by older adults increased by 22.4%, high-risk drinking by 65.2%, and alcohol use disorder (AUD) by 106.7% (Grant et al. 2017). Binge drinking among adults older than 65 years also has increased, with recent reports citing rates of 10.6% (Han et al. 2019a). Reports of substance use among the Baby Boomers are notably higher; 29.3% of adults ages 50–54 years were heavy or binge drinkers in 2012, and rates of illicit drug use among those in this age group increased from 3.4% to 7.2% from 2002 to 2012 (Substance Abuse and Mental Health Services Administration 2013) (Figure 17–1). This pattern of increased binge alcohol use and AUDs among adults age 50 and older was observed in a comparison of data from the 2005 and 2014 National Survey on Drug Use and Health (NSDUH; Han et al. 2017). Recent national surveys of illicit drug use also indicate a continued increase in use among the Baby Boomers; for example, in 2020,

11.6% of adults ages 60–64 years reported the use of illicit drugs in the past month (Substance Abuse and Mental Health Services Administration 2021).

These epidemiological trends, coupled with projections that by 2030 20% of the population will be composed of adults 65 years of age or older, indicate that the number of older adults requiring treatment for substance use disorders (SUDs) will continue to significantly increase (Committee on the Mental Health Workforce for Geriatric Populations 2012; Han et al. 2009). Hence, to meet the special needs of older adults experiencing problems with alcohol and drugs, social services professionals and providers within primary and specialty care settings, particularly specialty mental health care, must learn to recognize the signs and symptoms of substance misuse and gain a firm understanding of available treatment options. Doing so will enhance efforts directed toward reducing problematic use and foster improvements in overall quality of life among older adults with SUDs.

Guidelines and Classification: A Spectrum of Use

Proper screening, diagnosis, and treatment of individuals with drug or alcohol problems require an understanding of both drinking guidelines and the full range of substance use behavior seen in older adults. Because physiological factors render older adults more sensitive not only to alcohol and illicit drugs but also to OTC and prescription medications, guidelines and recommendations for use of these substances by older adults differ from those applied to younger adults. For example, lean body mass and total water volume decrease relative to total fat volume in later life. As a result, total body volume decreases, thereby increasing the serum concentration, absorption, and distribution of alcohol and drugs in the body (Moore et al. 2007). Age-related declines in the efficiency of the metabolic enzymes that target these substances, as well as increases in CNS sensitivity, also contribute to an amplified response to drug and alcohol use among older adults. Furthermore, interactions between alcohol and OTC or prescription medications, which are commonly used by older adults for various acute and chronic medical and psychiatric conditions, may be especially harmful. Consuming alcohol in combination with taking prescription or OTC drugs may lead to exaggerated or adverse therapeutic effects or, conversely, a blunting of the effectiveness of some medications (Moore et al. 2007).

Taking these age-related factors into account, the guidelines for alcohol use stipulate lower use for older adults relative to younger adults. Recommendations set forth by the National Institute on Alcohol Abuse and Alcoholism (2007) and the Center for Substance Abuse Treatment (Blow 1998) for older adults state that adults age 65 years and older should consume no more than seven standard drinks per week (Table 17–1). Moreover, older adults should not consume more than three standard drinks on any one occasion. These drinking-limit recommendations are in accordance with data concerning the relationship between heavy consumption and alcohol-related problems and with evidence for the beneficial health effects of low-risk drinking among older adults (Klatsky 2010; Moos et al. 2009; Plunk et al. 2014).

Recommendations for the appropriate prescription and use of OTC and prescription drugs must be considered on a case-by-case basis, with special consideration

TABLE 17–1.   Alcohol conversion chart

Beverage type—one "standard" drink	Quantity
Beer or wine cooler (~5% alcohol)	12 oz
Wine (~12% alcohol)	5 oz
Fortified wine (~17% alcohol)	3–4 oz
Hard liquor (80-proof distilled spirits; ~40% alcohol)	1½ oz (i.e., 1 shot)
Malt liquor (~7% alcohol)	8½ oz
Liqueur or aperitif (~24% alcohol)	2–3 oz

Additional conversions

Beverage type/quantity	Number of standard drinks
Beer	
1 six-pack of 16-oz cans/bottles	8
1 pint	1.3
1 quart	2.7
1 liter (33.8 oz)	2.8
Wine (e.g., red, white, Chianti)	
1 bottle/1 fifth (25 oz)	5
1 bottle (40 oz)	8
1 magnum	10
½ gallon	13
Fortified wine (e.g., sherry, port; low-end wines [e.g., Night Train, Thunderbird, "bum wine"])	
1 pint	4–5
1 fifth	7
Hard liquor (e.g., bourbon, rum, gin, tequila, vodka)	
1 mixed drink	1 or more
1 fifth	17
1 pint	11
1 quart	21
½ gallon	43
1 bottle/1 fifth (25 oz)	17
1 bottle (40 oz)	27
Malt liquor (e.g., King Cobra, Olde English)	
12 oz	1½
40 oz	4½

Source.   Data modified from National Institute on Alcohol Abuse and Alcoholism: *Helping Patients Who Drink Too Much: A Clinician's Guide,* Updated 2005 Edition (NIH Publication No. 07-3769). Bethesda, MD, U.S. Department of Health and Human Services, Public Health Services, National Institutes of Health, National Institute on Alcohol Abuse and Alcoholism, reprinted September 2007. Available at: http://pubs.niaaa.nih.gov/publications/Practitioner/CliniciansGuide2005/guide.pdf. Accessed June 1, 2020.

given to the potential benefits versus the potential risks of medication use for each patient. There are no accepted safe limits for tobacco, cannabis, or illicit drug use.

Although the guidelines and recommendations for substance use address acceptable limits, there is still a great deal of variability in the degree to which older adults use alcohol and drugs. Understanding patterns of use can help inform the treatment and counseling of older adults in numerous settings. Thus, to capture this variability, or "spectrum of use," several categories have been created. The following categories and their definitions, which focus primarily on patterns of alcohol use, reflect both the clinical experience and research findings of addiction specialists (Blow 1998; National Institute on Alcohol Abuse and Alcoholism 2007).

Abstainers is the term used to describe individuals who report drinking no more than two drinks in the previous year. Past studies have indicated that ~40%–70% of older adults report abstinence and that abstinence rates increase with advancing age (Kirchner et al. 2007; Wu and Blazer 2014). These rates will likely change, however, with the aging of the population (Kuerbis 2020). Determining the reasons for abstinence has important implications for the subsequent treatment and counseling of older adults who do not drink. For example, although some individuals may have had lifelong patterns of abstinence, others may not drink because of the onset or presence of acute or chronic illness. Furthermore, some individuals may abstain from alcohol use because of a previous history of alcohol use problems or AUD. This latter group deserves special consideration and would benefit from preventive monitoring and screening. Not only could new stressors cause relapse among those with a history of problematic drinking, but past use may make older adults more vulnerable to other mental health problems such as psychiatric disorders or cognitive declines.

Low-risk, social, or *moderate drinkers* include individuals who drink within the recommended guidelines (i.e., drink no more than seven standard drinks per week and no more than three drinks on any one occasion) and do not exhibit any alcohol-related problems. Older adults in this group also observe caution when drinking; for example, they do not drink when driving a motor vehicle or boat or when using contraindicated medications.

Low-risk medication/drug use is characterized by individuals who adhere to physicians' prescriptions. Nevertheless, the number and types of medications being used by those in the low-risk category must be evaluated because harmful medication interactions may still occur among this group.

At-risk, hazardous, or *excessive substance use* is characterized by individuals who consume substances above recommended levels yet experience minimal or no substance-related health, social, or emotional problems. Although at-risk substance use in older individuals generally applies to the consumption of alcohol or prescription and OTC medications, at-risk use can also apply to any use of illicit drugs (because of the lack of quality control for these substances) (Kuerbis et al. 2014). Determining a prespecified threshold beyond which prescription drug use poses a risk is more challenging because of the high variability in appropriate pharmacological treatment regimens and recommendations that result from individuals having different medical circumstances and needs. However, identifying older adults who are taking high doses of medication and have also been taking medications for a period exceeding what would be reasonable clinical practice would help target those who may be at risk. For example, prolonged or improper use of psychoactive medications, such as benzodiazepines, presents a particularly high risk of negative health outcomes and adverse drug reactions (Lader 2014). Targeting and identifying older adults in this category is important; although they currently may not have any substance use–related problems, they may have a high risk of developing alcohol- or medication-related health problems should their substance use remain consistent or increase over time. Preventive brief interventions for at-risk users are valuable and effective, and abstinence or reductions in substance use have been shown to improve quality of life for this group.

Substance use disorder describes a pattern in which alcohol or drug consumption is at a level at which adverse medical, psychological, or social consequences have occurred or are significantly likely to occur. Thus, this category of use is not dependent on the quantity or frequency of use but rather on the extent to which substance use impairs physical or psychosocial functioning. Previously classified as two separate disorders (i.e., substance abuse and dependence) according to DSM-IV criteria, SUD spans multiple domains of functioning and falls along a continuum, with mild, moderate, and severe subclassifications (Table 17–2; American Psychiatric Association 2013). However, that criteria are based mostly on research with young to middle-aged adults and have not been sufficiently validated in older populations; therefore, the symptoms and consequences set forth in DSM-5 may not be sensitive enough to capture disorder in later life (American Psychiatric Association 2013; Kuerbis 2020; Lehmann and Fingerhood 2018). For example, some of the standard symptoms of SUD listed in DSM-5, such as employment problems or interpersonal difficulties, may not be as readily applied to older individuals given age-related factors such as retirement, widowhood, and resultant changes in occupational and social roles and network composition. As a result, the risks associated with this pattern of substance use may be underestimated. Moreover, determining whether individuals' symptoms meet diagnostic criteria relies heavily on self-reported behavioral symptoms. This is potentially problematic because self-report is susceptible to bias due to memory impairments, lack of insight or knowledge regarding the adverse effects of substance use, or unwillingness to admit symptoms. For instance, benzodiazepine misuse may go unnoticed or unreported because older adults may not link the consequences of medication use to health or social problems. Notwithstanding these limitations in diagnostic criteria, because older adults in this group are at a greater risk of negative consequences such as falls, liver disease, pancreatitis, and harmful alcohol-medication interactions, they could greatly benefit from screening, identification, and specialized treatment and services (Lehmann and Fingerhood 2018; Maust et al. 2016).

Epidemiology of Late-Life Substance Use

Alcohol

Although alcohol misuse is often underreported and thus underestimated in later life, epidemiological work suggests that alcohol problems are common and on the rise among older adults (Grant et al. 2017). For instance, the most recent NSDUH report reported that 56.5% of adults ages 60–64 years endorsed current alcohol use in the past month, 22.7% endorsed bingeing behavior, and 7.7% endorsed heavy use (Substance Abuse and Mental Health Services Administration 2021). Although rates of use were

TABLE 17–2.   **DSM-5 criteria for substance use disorder**

A. A problematic pattern of substance use leading to clinically significant impairment or distress, as manifested by at least two of the following, occurring within a 12-month period:

1. The substance is often taken in larger amounts or over a longer period than was intended.

2. There is a persistent desire or unsuccessful efforts to cut down or control the substance use.

3. A great deal of time is spent in activities necessary to obtain the substance, use the substance, or recover from its effects.

4. Craving, or a strong desire or urge to use the substance.

5. Recurrent substance use resulting in a failure to fulfill major role obligations at work, school, or home.

6. Continued substance use despite having persistent or recurrent social or interpersonal problems caused or exacerbated by the effects of the substance.

7. Important social, occupational, or recreational activities are given up or reduced because of substance use.

8. Recurrent substance use in situations in which it is physically hazardous.

9. Substance use is continued despite knowledge of having a persistent or recurrent physical or psychological problem that is likely to have been caused or exacerbated by the substance.

10. Tolerance, as defined by either of the following (note that tolerance and withdrawal alone are not sufficient for a diagnosis of a mild disorder):

    a. A need for markedly increased amounts of the substance to achieve intoxication or desired effect.

    b. A markedly diminished effect with continued use of the same amount of the substance.

11. Withdrawal, as manifested by either of the following:

    a. The characteristic withdrawal syndrome for the substance (refer to Criteria A and B of the criteria set for alcohol or other specific substance withdrawal).

    b. Substance (or closely related substance, such as benzodiazepine with alcohol) is taken to relieve or avoid withdrawal symptoms.

Specify current severity:

Mild

Moderate

Severe

Specify if (see DSM-5 text on specific disorders for definitions of course specifiers):

In early remission

In sustained remission

On maintenance therapy

In a controlled environment

Note.   Table includes only the general diagnostic criteria and specifiers for substance-related disorders; refer to DSM-5 for the full criteria sets according to substance used, including specifier descriptions and coding and reporting procedures.

Source.   American Psychiatric Association: *Diagnostic and Statistical Manual of Mental Disorders*, 5th Edition. Arlington, VA, American Psychiatric Association, 2013, pp. 485–490. Used with permission. Copyright © 2013 American Psychiatric Association.

lower for those age 65 years or older, they were nonetheless significant: 45.3% of respondents reported past-month alcohol use, 9.8% bingeing, and 3.4% heavy use.

With respect to AUD, 2.1% of adults age 65 years or older and 4.8% of adults ages 50–64 years in the 2013–2014 NSDUH reported symptoms that met DSM-IV criteria (Han et al. 2017). To estimate the rate of DSM-5 AUD in U.S. adults, Grant et al. (2015) examined data from the NESARC-III; their results indicated that 2.3% and 13.4% of adults age 65 years and older reported symptoms that met the criteria for 12-month and lifetime prevalence of AUD, respectively. These rates were higher in respondents ages 45–64; 10.0% and 28.2% reported 12-month and lifetime AUD, respectively (Grant et al. 2015). Data from the 2020 NSDUH indicate that 9.1% and 5.1% of adults ages 60–64 and 65 years and older, respectively, met criteria for past-year DSM-5 AUD (Substance Abuse and Mental Health Services Administration 2021).

Because substance misuse is more likely to be present in health care settings, rates of alcohol problems are higher among clinical than among community-based samples. For example, in their screening program of more than 12,000 primary care patients, Barry et al. (1998) found that 5% of patients screened positive for at-risk or problem drinking, as measured by alcohol consumption, binge drinking, or presence of alcohol-related problems. In another study of older adults in primary care settings, Kirchner et al. (2007) reported that of the 24,863 patients screened, 21.5% drank within recommended levels (1–7 drinks per week), whereas 4.1% were at-risk drinkers (8–14 drinks per week), and 4.5% were heavy (>14 drinks per week) or binge drinkers. The rates of AUD appear to be particularly high among patients in mental health clinics and nursing homes. In their study of 140 patients enrolled in a geriatric mental health outpatient clinic, Holroyd and Duryee (1997) reported that 8.6% of patients had symptoms that met DSM-IV criteria for alcohol dependence. Furthermore, Oslin et al. (1997b) found that 29% of male nursing home residents had a lifetime (DSM-IV) diagnosis of alcohol abuse or dependence, with 10% of residents having symptoms that met criteria for abuse or dependence within 1 year of admission to the home. Moreover, a census analysis of U.S. Department of Veterans Affairs nursing home admissions data found that 29% and 15% of residents ages 57–64 and 65–72 years, respectively, had a diagnosis of AUD (Lemke and Schaefer 2010). Evaluations of more recent clinical samples are needed to account for demographic trends and increases in alcohol use rates observed over the past decade.

Prescription and Over-the-Counter Medications

The use of pharmaceutical drugs is prevalent in older adulthood, and the risk of misusing prescription and OTC medications—which include substances such as sedatives/hypnotics, narcotic and nonnarcotic analgesics, diet aids, and decongestants—also increases with age. In one study of prescription and OTC medicine and dietary supplement use among a nationally representative sample of community-dwelling adults age 62 years and older, 87.7% of respondents reported using at least one prescription drug (Qato et al. 2016). Use of OTC drugs (37.9%) and dietary supplements (63.7%) also were quite common in the sample. Concurrent use of five or more prescription medications was reported in 35.8% of cases, with ~15.1% of these patients categorized as being at risk for a potential major drug–drug interaction (Qato et al. 2016). Indeed, polypharmacy, or the concomitant use of multiple drugs, may have negative consequences in cases in which complex medication regimens are not carefully and appropriately adhered to by patients or monitored by physicians (Maher et al. 2014).

There is evidence that the rate of prescription drug misuse, or the intentional or unintentional use of prescription drugs in a manner other than as prescribed (e.g., taking more of the medication or taking it for nonmedical purposes), has increased over time (Lehmann and Fingerhood 2018; Simoni-Wastila and Yang 2006). A large proportion of medications prescribed for older adults include psychoactive, mood-altering drugs. Psychotherapeutic medications are often subject to improper use and can lead to negative health consequences when used either alone or in combination with other drugs and alcohol. For example, ~38.5% of individuals age 50 years and older report past-year prescription opioid use, and 6.6% of past-year opioid users report misuse (Han et al. 2019b). Moreover, the use of benzodiazepines—one of the most prescribed medications in the United States—increases with age and tends to be chronic in later life. A recent analysis of the NSDUH found that adults ages 50–64 years had the highest rates of any benzodiazepine use (14.3%), with 9.7% of past-year users reporting misuse (Maust et al. 2019). In addition to their being one of the most inappropriately prescribed psychotherapeutic medications among older adults, benzodiazepine misuse is strongly associated with the misuse of prescription stimulants and opioids (Maust et al. 2014, 2019). Thus, clinicians should be cautious when prescribing or recommending a treatment, take both risks and benefits into account when determining a treatment plan, and clearly communicate guidelines for appropriate use to patients. Clinicians also should carefully consider discontinuing medications that do not prove effective. For example, medications often are continued from one care setting to another without clear justification for use as older adults are navigated through the health care system.

Illicit Drugs

Compared with rates of alcohol and prescription or OTC medication use, rates of illicit drug use among older adults have been relatively low. Based on data from the Epidemiologic Catchment Area study, analyses in the early 1990s estimated that the lifetime prevalence rate of drug abuse and dependence was 0.12% for older men and 0.06% for older women, whereas the lifetime history of illicit drug use was 2.88% for men and 0.66% for women (Anthony and Helzer 1991). More recent work, however, suggests that illicit substance use is more common in older adults than previous estimates suggested. In part because of changes in the acceptability, legality, and medicinal use of cannabis, it is the most used illicit drug among older adults. For example, data from the 2020 NSDUH showed that the prevalence of past-month cannabis use was 9.7% and 3.7% among adults ages 60–64 and age 65 and older, respectively (Substance Abuse and Mental Health Services Administration 2021). Although national estimates of the use of other illicit drugs (e.g., heroin and cocaine) are significantly lower, rates of drug use have been rising over time (Mattson et al. 2017; Wu and Blazer 2011). This is evident from trends in admissions for substance use treatment in older adults. For example, in their analysis of 12 years of Treatment Episode Data Set—Admissions data, Chhatre et al. (2017) found that the proportion of adults age 55 and older who were admitted for treatment related to cocaine/crack (4.8% in 2000 vs. 7.8% in 2012) and heroin (11.7% in 2000 vs. 14.8% in 2012) significantly increased over time. Finally, recent national surveys indicate that 2.9% and 1.5% of individuals ages 60–64 and age

65 and older, respectively, met criteria for DSM-5 illicit-drug SUD within the past year (Substance Abuse and Mental Health Services Administration 2021). Rates of illicit substance use and SUD among older adults will likely continue to rise in the next several decades because of the aging of the Baby Boom cohort.

Correlates and Consequences of Substance Use Problems

Correlates and Risk Factors of Substance Misuse

Several studies have sought to identify factors related to increased vulnerability to substance misuse and the maintenance of problematic substance use patterns in later life. Factors such as demographics (e.g., sex, ethnicity, income, employment status), medical and psychiatric comorbidity (e.g., chronic pain, cognitive impairment, other psychiatric diagnosis such as depression), history of past use, and social and family environment are all correlated with problematic substance use (Kuerbis 2020; Mejldal et al. 2020). Longitudinal work, for instance, suggests that older men tend to drink greater quantities of alcohol than older women and are more likely to have alcohol-related problems (Han et al. 2019a; Moos et al. 2009). Older men also are more likely to have had a longer history of problem drinking (Gomberg 2003). Nonetheless, there is some evidence that prevalence rates of drinking among older women are increasing faster than among older men (Breslow et al. 2017). The relationship between certain risk factors and alcohol misuse also may vary by sex; in those with AUD, women are more likely than men to have been married to a problem drinker, to report negative life events and ongoing difficulties with a spouse and other family members, and to have a history of depression (Gomberg 2003; Lemke et al. 2008). For both men and women, psychiatric comorbidity and age-related losses in social, physical, and occupational/ role domains, such as widowhood, the death of family and friends, reduced physical function, and retirement, have been associated with abusive drinking patterns in later life (Dawson et al. 2005a; Kuerbis 2020; Lemke et al. 2008). Finally, longitudinal work has shown that additional social context and life history factors, such as friends' approval of drinking and a history of heavy drinking or alcohol problems, also are related to a higher likelihood of late-life drinking problems (Moos et al. 2004). Social network factors such as loneliness and low social support are also associated with cannabis use (Kuerbis 2020).

With respect to prescription and OTC drugs, factors such as the declining physical health and physiological changes that accompany aging increase adults' exposure and reactivity to medications and thus their potential to misuse these substances in later life. Women, although they are less likely than men to use and misuse alcohol, have been shown to be more likely than men to use and misuse psychoactive medications (Simoni-Wastila and Yang 2006), particularly if they are divorced or widowed, have a lower socioeconomic status (e.g., education and income), or have been diagnosed with a mood disorder such as depression or anxiety (Closser and Blow 1993). Of note, however, more recent work suggests mixed results for the association between sex and medication misuse (Han et al. 2019b; Votaw et al. 2019). Comorbid psychiatric diagnoses, in general, increase the risk for prescription drug misuse, regardless of sex (Han et al. 2019b; Simoni-Wastila and Yang 2006). When considering the full range of factors associated with drug misuse, clinicians must recognize factors such as inappropriate prescribing practices and insufficient monitoring of drug reactions and patient adherence by health care providers (Maust et al. 2014).

Consequences of Substance Use

Although the literature presented thus far has alluded to the adverse effects of problematic substance use, some evidence suggests that low-risk or moderate alcohol consumption may have a positive impact on physical health and mental well-being. For example, low-risk or moderate alcohol consumption is associated with a reduced risk of cardiovascular disease in both men and women and also a reduced risk of cardiovascular disease–related disability (Abramson et al. 2001; Bryson et al. 2006; Kalla and Figueredo 2017). Furthermore, researchers in one study of older adults without cardiovascular disease found that alcohol consumption was related to lipoprotein subclass distribution (Mukamal et al. 2007a). Studies also have shown that moderate alcohol consumption may protect against type 2 diabetes mellitus and functional decline and may also affect additional indicators of well-being (Djoussé et al. 2007). With respect to functional decline, findings from cross-sectional work suggest that in older men, low to moderate alcohol consumption is associated with lower odds of reporting physical limitations compared with abstinence or heavy use (Cawthon et al. 2007). Finally, light to moderate alcohol use may be associated with positive subjective well-being for both men and women (Lang et al. 2007).

Although the literature cited previously does suggest that low to moderate use of alcohol can lead to various health benefits among older adults, many of these benefits may come with risks. No evidence supports the notion that recommending that nondrinkers initiate drinking will translate into reduced health risks. Moreover, there is no evidence to suggest that a person with a medical condition, such as cardiovascular disease, will benefit from continued drinking or the initiation of drinking. In fact, abstinence should still be recommended for patients taking certain medications, those who have been diagnosed with certain acute or chronic conditions (e.g., diabetes, cardiovascular disease), and those who present with a history of AUD or drug use disorder, because substance use is detrimental in these cases.

Consumption of alcohol that exceeds the levels of low-risk use should be carefully monitored and targeted for intervention, given the mounting evidence of the risks of drinking at levels above these recommendations (Lehmann and Fingerhood 2018; Oslin 2000). Even moderate alcohol use can lead to adverse health outcomes. For example, whereas moderate alcohol consumption decreases the risk of strokes caused by blocked blood vessels, it increases the risk of having a stroke caused by bleeding or hemorrhaging. Similarly, although there is a graded positive correlation between moderate alcohol use and bone mineral density at the hip, moderate use has a U-shaped relationship with risk of hip fracture (Mukamal et al. 2007b). Low to moderate consumption of alcohol also has been demonstrated to impair the ability to drive and may increase the risk of accidents and fatal injuries due to falls, motor vehicle crashes, and suicides (Sorock et al. 2006). Depression, memory problems, liver disease, cardiovascular disease, cognitive changes, and sleep problems also have been linked to moderate alcohol use, whereas alcohol dependence is associated with increased probability of morbidity and mortality from disease-specific causes such as acute pancreatitis, alcohol-induced cirrhosis, or alcohol-related cardiomyopathy (Kalla and Figueredo 2017; Rehm et al. 2009).

When assessing and treating older adults, clinicians not only need to take these factors into account but also need to consider the potential interaction between alcohol and both prescribed and OTC medications, especially psychoactive medications such as benzodiazepines, barbiturates, and antidepressants. As mentioned, alcohol use is one of the leading risk factors for the occurrence of adverse drug reactions and is known to interfere with the metabolism of medications such as digoxin and warfarin (Mallet et al. 2007; National Institute on Alcohol Abuse and Alcoholism 2014). Certain medications may themselves have a wide array of negative consequences on health if not used and prescribed carefully. For example, benzodiazepines are associated with increased risk of falls and fractures, impaired driving, disruptions in sleep cycles, and, in frail elderly adults, excessive disability (American Geriatrics Society Beers Criteria Update Expert Panel 2019). Likewise, diphenhydramine has been linked to cognitive deficits in healthy older adults, which may translate into excessive cognitive deficits in patients with dementing illnesses (Katz et al. 1998; Tannenbaum et al. 2012). Risk of death from any cause is significantly higher among older versus younger adults with opioid use disorder (Larney et al. 2015). Vulnerability to these adverse consequences is increased when the medication is used for a longer duration than intended or warranted or is improperly prescribed, such as by using an excessive dosage or prescribing the medication for the wrong indication.

Finally, mental health providers should be well versed in the impact of moderate alcohol consumption on other mental health disorders. In a study of more than 2,000 elderly patients, Oslin et al. (2000) demonstrated that reducing moderate alcohol use (one to seven drinks per week) while treating a depressive disorder enhanced treatment outcomes. Results further indicated that the greater the alcohol consumption, the larger the negative effect on the treatment of depression. Although data are sparse, there is speculation that moderate alcohol use also may have a negative impact on the prognosis and course of dementing illnesses such as Alzheimer's disease. Moreover, alcohol use may elicit the onset of or exacerbate preexisting personality changes or behavioral disturbances in patients with dementia.

Screening and Diagnosis of Substance Use Problems

Potential Barriers to Screening and Diagnosis

As outlined previously, alcohol and drug problems are common in later life. However, substance misuse remains largely underrecognized and undertreated among older adults. It has been suggested that adults age 60 years or older be screened for alcohol and prescription drug use as part of their routine mental and physical health care (Blow 1998; Wu and Blazer 2014). Routine screening would enable the identification of not only those older adults who have problematic substance use but also those who are at risk of misusing drugs and alcohol. Furthermore, proper screening helps deter-

TABLE 17–3. **Common signs and symptoms of potential substance misuse in older adults**

Anxiety	Incontinence
Blackouts, dizziness	Increased tolerance to alcohol or medications
Depression, mood swings	Legal difficulties
Disorientation, confusion	Memory loss or impairment
Falls, bruises, and burns	New difficulties in decision making
Family problems	Poor hygiene
Financial problems	Poor nutrition
Headaches	Sleep problems
Idiopathic seizures	Social isolation

Source. Adapted from Barry et al. 2002.

mine whether additional assessment is needed. Nonetheless, various factors may interfere with screening and diagnostic processes.

At the provider level, the common misconception that older substance users have a lifelong history of problem use may make it difficult for clinicians to identify individuals who either have or are at high risk of developing late-onset conditions. Although this assumption is more likely to hold for patterns of illicit drug use, up to one-third of older adults seeking treatment for alcohol problems have developed these problems in later life (Lehmann and Fingerhood 2018). Furthermore, insufficient knowledge regarding the symptoms or potential health impact of at-risk or problematic drinking may inhibit screening efforts. Diagnostic criteria and symptoms for alcohol and prescription drug misuse are not easily applied to older adults and are often confounded by symptoms of comorbid medical illnesses, further complicating the screening and diagnostic process for providers (Table 17–3). The use of multiple diagnostic terms can also lead to confusion about who should be screened, how screening should proceed, and which problems or patterns of use should be treated. A general lack of appreciation of the benefits of reduced substance use in the absence of disorder, and the belief that there are few accessible and effective treatments for substance use, can also significantly lower a clinician's motivation to screen for or to recognize at-risk or problem drinking. Assuming a clinician does assess patients for at-risk or problematic use, the self-report nature of screening instruments may interfere with accurate and appropriate decision making because of various biases related to self-report measures. Furthermore, the lack of screening instruments that assess both alcohol and drug misuse and that are validated with older adults further compounds the problems associated with recognizing substance use in later life (Dowling et al. 2008).

At the patient level, confusion as to what constitutes a substance use problem and who might benefit from an intervention also affects patients' behavior regarding seeking assessment. Like providers, older adults may perceive physical symptoms (e.g., fatigue, sleep problems, anxiety, confusion) as normative or attribute them to other medical illnesses. Also, older adults and their families may not think the substance use is problematic because of either denial or lack of knowledge regarding recommendations and guidelines for acceptable drinking and prescription/OTC drug use levels.

In addition to these factors, age- and substance-related declines in memory may contribute to the underreporting of past and current alcohol or drug use. Finally, stigma surrounding substance use may prevent some patients from providing accurate information about their use. Therefore, assessment should take a supportive, nonconfrontational approach and focus on behaviors, with potentially stigmatizing language replaced with medically accurate and neutral terminology (Kuerbis 2020).

Assessment of the Frequency and Quantity of Use

Notwithstanding the barriers just described, successful screening methods have been designed and implemented to assess the quantity and frequency of alcohol and drug use. These methods fall into three categories: prospective monitoring and recording of alcohol and drug use, retrospective accounts of daily use over some defined period (i.e., the timeline followback [TLFB] method), and questions about average consumption practices. The prospective monitoring (diary) method is considered the gold standard because it elicits the greatest number of reports of consumption and is highly associated with sales data for alcoholic beverages in younger adults (Lemmens et al. 1992; Tucker et al. 2007). However, proper completion of this type of measure is time-consuming and requires multiple visits, and therefore this method is impractical for screenings or brief assessments.

The TLFB method represents the most used technique in treatment studies for addiction. Among older adults, 7-day TLFB assessments are correlated with reports from prospective diaries. Nevertheless, certain difficulties arise with the use of this method. First, the specific week of measurement under assessment may not be representative of the person's usual drinking behavior. Second, although this method closely matches prospective diary reports for nondrinkers or daily drinkers, it underestimates consumption for less frequent users of alcohol (Lemmens et al. 1992). Given the tendency of TLFB self-reports to underestimate use, it has been suggested that to maximize accuracy, researchers and clinicians collect reports prior to the start of any procedure or effort to reduce alcohol consumption (Kaplan and Koffarnus 2019). The TLFB method also takes longer to administer than do assessments evaluating the average frequency and quantity of use, and because of the varying individual definitions of a "standard" drink, it is more effective and accurate when administered by an interviewer than when self-administered.

Finally, although general questions about the average, rather than daily, quantity and frequency of use over a specified period are least likely to match prospective diary reports and may underestimate the frequency of moderate drinking, asking questions is the method of choice among many clinicians because it is the easiest approach. Likewise, the "brown bag" approach, in which patients are asked to bring to an appointment all prescribed and OTC medications they are currently taking, is a useful and convenient aid for determining medication use and misuse. Although reports of the quantity and frequency of use can be independently used to screen and identify at-risk patients, this information must be combined with other measures when the clinician is attempting to detect problem drinking or SUD.

Standardized Screening Instruments

Brief, low-cost, convenient, standardized assessments that can be used to screen not only for frequency and quantity of alcohol use but also for drinking consequences and alcohol/medication interactions are essential to the success of efforts targeted toward prevention and early intervention for older adults at risk. As described earlier (see "Potential Barriers to Screening and Diagnosis"), screening should be a component of routine mental and physical health care and should be updated annually, before the older adult begins taking any new medications, or in response to problems that may be alcohol or medication related. Standardized screening questions can be administered by various methods, including verbal interview and paper-and-pencil or computerized questionnaire. All three methods have demonstrated equivalent reliability and validity (Berks and McCormick 2008; Conigliaro et al. 2000).

To complement questions assessing the quantity and frequency of use, the Alcohol Use Disorders Identification Test (AUDIT) and the CAGE questionnaire often are used to screen for at-risk substance use or misuse among older adults. The U.S. Preventive Task Force recommends use of the AUDIT and its abbreviated (concise) version, the AUDIT-C (Figure 17–2), for screening (Curry et al. 2018). These are simple measures that capture the frequency of drinking and bingeing in the past year (Bush et al. 1998; Dawson et al. 2005b; Rubinsky et al. 2013). The AUDIT-C is scored on a scale of 0–12, with a score of 0 indicating no alcohol use during the preceding year. For older adults, a score of 3 or more reflects a positive screen and suggests the need for further evaluation. Generally, the higher the AUDIT-C score, the more likely it is that the patient's drinking is affecting the patient's health and safety and is indicative of AUD (Bush et al. 1998; Rubinsky et al. 2013).

The CAGE questionnaire (Mayfield et al. 1974) is one of the most widely used alcohol screening tests in clinical practice. Four items regarding alcohol use are designed to assess whether patients have 1) felt that they should **C**ut down on their drinking, 2) felt **A**nnoyed that people criticized their drinking, 3) felt **G**uilty about their drinking, and 4) had a drink upon waking in the morning to get rid of a hangover—an **E**ye-opener. A modified version of the CAGE questionnaire asks only about recent problems, and the threshold is often reduced to one positive response as an indicator of problems in older adults. This modified version of the CAGE has demonstrated high specificity for detecting alcohol abuse but relatively low sensitivity for AUD (Buchsbaum et al. 1992; Moore et al. 2002). Limitations of the CAGE also include poor identification of binge drinkers and lack of distinction between lifetime and current use (Kuerbis et al. 2014).

As this last point suggests, the utility of the questionnaires may vary as a function of the category of drinking (e.g., at-risk drinking, AUD) being assessed. In one comparison of the relative sensitivity and specificity of self-administered versions of the CAGE and AUDIT, Bradley et al. (1998) showed that an augmented version of the CAGE (i.e., a measure including the CAGE items, the first two items of the AUDIT, and the question "Have you ever had a drinking problem?") performed better than the traditional versions when screening for active substance use. However, the AUDIT was superior to both versions of the CAGE in identifying heavy drinkers. Finally, although both the augmented CAGE and the AUDIT were effective in identifying both heavy drinkers and those actively dependent on alcohol, the AUDIT performed better. In sum, these results suggest that the selection of screening instruments used in clinical practice should be driven by the goals of screening. For example, when screening for both heavy drinking and AUD, clinicians might consider using the AUDIT or AUDIT-C as opposed to the CAGE (Aertgeerts et al. 2001; Rubinsky et al. 2013). Re-

1. How often did you have a drink containing alcohol in the past year?

_____ Never	(0 points)
_____ Monthly or less	(1 point)
_____ Two to four times a month	(2 points)
_____ Two to three times per week	(3 points)
_____ Four or more times a week	(4 points)

If you answered "never," score questions 2 and 3 as zero.

2. How many drinks did you have on a typical day when you were drinking in the past year?

_____ 1 or 2	(0 points)
_____ 3 or 4	(1 point)
_____ 5 or 6	(2 points)
_____ 7 to 9	(3 points)
_____ 10 or more	(4 points)

3. How often did you have six or more drinks on one occasion in the past year?

_____ Never	(0 points)
_____ Less than monthly	(1 point)
_____ Monthly	(2 points)
_____ Weekly	(3 points)
_____ Daily or almost daily	(4 points)

Possible range = 0–12. For older adults, a score of 3 or more is considered positive.

FIGURE 17–2. Alcohol use disorders Identification Test–Concise (AUDIT-C) alcohol screening.

Source. Bush K, Kivlahan DR, McDonell MB, et al.: "The AUDIT Alcohol Consumption Questions (AUDIT-C): An Effective Brief Screening Test for Problem Drinking." *Archives of Internal Medicine* 158:1789–1795, 1998. Copyright © 1998, American Medical Association. All rights reserved. Adapted with permission.

searchers and clinicians also might consider additional screening instruments, including the geriatric version of the Michigan Alcoholism Screening Test (MAST-G) and the Comorbidity Alcohol Risk Evaluation Tool (CARET) (Blow et al. 1992; Moore et al. 2002). Both of these measures are particularly effective in identifying at-risk or problematic use (Kuerbis et al. 2014).

Following administration of a screening instrument, clinicians can ask follow-up questions about the consequences, health risks, and social/family issues related to substance use. In accordance with DSM-5 criteria, to assess severity of AUD, the clinician should ask questions about alcohol-related problems, history of failed attempts to stop or cut back, and withdrawal symptoms (e.g., anxiety, tremors, sleep disturbance). The use of an assessment instrument such as the DSM criteria can assist clinicians and researchers by providing a structured approach to assessment and a checklist of items that can be evaluated across older adults. Furthermore, such assessments can inform clinicians' decision-making and help determine whether specialized alcohol treatment might be needed.

Although the screening assessments described in this section focus on alcohol use, there are also screening instruments for drug consumption, including a modified version of the CAGE questionnaire (CAGE Adapted to Include Drugs [CAGE-AID]; Hinkin et al. 2001) and the Drug and Alcohol Problem Assessment for Primary Care (DAPA-PC; Nemes et al. 2004). Although further work is needed to determine the validity of these instruments, initial findings are positive.

Use of Biological Markers for Screening

Biological markers of alcohol and drug use have proven to be less accepted in clinical practice than in research, given that they are potentially more burdensome and intrusive than other screening tools. Laboratory values that can indicate recent use or misuse include levels of blood alcohol or of acetate, which is a metabolite of alcohol (Topic and Djukic 2013). Markers of chronic alcohol use include γ-glutamyl transferase, mean corpuscular volume, high-density lipoprotein level, and carbohydrate-deficient transferrin (Hock et al. 2005; Oslin et al. 1998). Additionally, urine drug screens are useful as both screening tools and confirmation of self-report when the clinician is assessing prescription/OTC medication and illicit drug misuse. Most misused drugs will remain detectable in a urine drug screen for 4 or more days, with some still detectable after several weeks.

Treatments for Substance Use Problems

Although there are numerous potential treatment options for problematic substance use, little formal research has been conducted to compare the relative efficacy of these approaches in older adults. Moreover, past estimates indicate that only 18% of SUD treatment programs in the United States are specifically designed to address older patients' needs (Kuerbis et al. 2014). Nevertheless, the results from existing studies have been promising: older adults who engage in treatment not only have comparable or significantly better outcomes than their younger counterparts (Carew and Comiskey 2018; Lemke and Moos 2003b; Oslin et al. 2005; Satre et al. 2003, 2004a, 2012; Weiss and Petry 2013) but also are more likely to complete treatment than are younger patients (Oslin et al. 2002; Satre et al. 2004a). Brief interventions and direct-to-consumer educational interventions for alcohol and prescription medication misuse have also been shown to be effective for older adults (Jonas et al. 2012; Kuerbis and Sacco 2013; Tannenbaum et al. 2014). Therefore, despite popular belief, older adults are quite receptive and responsive to treatment, especially in programs that offer age-appropriate care and have providers who are knowledgeable about aging issues.

Brief Interventions and Therapies

Low-intensity brief interventions or brief therapies are cost-effective and practical techniques that can be used in the initial treatment of at-risk and problem drinkers in a variety of clinical settings (Jonas et al. 2012; O'Donnell et al. 2014). Brief interventions are time limited and nonconfrontational in their approach. Sessions often involve educating the patient about the substance, its impact on health, and guidelines for its use; addressing barriers and motivation to change; and offering feedback and advice. Given that these interventions are based on concepts and techniques from the behavioral self-control literature, one of the hallmarks of brief interventions is to encourage patients to change their behavior through motivational interviewing (Miller and Rollnick 1991).

Randomized clinical trials of brief interventions for alcohol problems among older populations reveal that older adults can be engaged in brief intervention protocols and find these protocols acceptable. Results also point to a greater reduction in alcohol consumption among at-risk drinkers receiving interventions than among control groups. The best evidence emerges from randomized trials of brief (10- to 15-minute) multicomponent interventions that include physician/behavioral specialist counseling visits and follow-up telephone calls from clinic staff offering advice, education, and the creation of contracts (Jonas et al. 2012). For example, in one randomized clinical study of at-risk drinkers, older primary care patients randomly assigned to a brief intervention arm were less likely to evidence at-risk and heavy drinking at 3-month follow-up and had lower rates of alcohol use at 12-month follow-up relative to those in the control group (Moore et al. 2011). Likewise, meta-analytic reviews suggest that older primary care patients randomly assigned to receive brief interventions evidence reductions in alcohol consumption at follow-up (Jonas et al. 2012). Brief interventions also have been shown to reduce prescription medication misuse among older adults (Schonfeld et al. 2010). Although most trials have been conducted in primary care settings, brief interventions for older adults are likely to be effective in mental health care settings as well. Thus, geriatric mental health providers are encouraged to gain familiarity with brief intervention therapy both as a primary treatment tool and, if needed, as a way to motivate patients toward more formal addiction treatment.

Psychosocial and Behavioral Therapies

Although the literature regarding the efficacy of psychological therapies specifically for the treatment of SUD in older adults is sparse, there is evidence that this population responds favorably to psychotherapeutic interventions (Bhatia et al. 2015; Kuerbis et al. 2014; Schonfeld and Dupree 2002). In a study of older veterans with substance abuse problems, Schonfeld et al. (2000) found that patients who completed 16 weeks of a group intervention for relapse prevention were more likely than noncompleters to still abstain at 6-month follow-up. Using cognitive-behavioral and self-management approaches, the group sessions included modules on coping with factors such as social problems, loneliness, depression, and anxiety and on dealing with high-risk situations for relapse. In another treatment study, participants age 50 years and older who completed an 18-session program that incorporated both cognitive-behavioral and self-management approaches demonstrated significant improvement in their social functioning, decreased use of nonmedical prescription drugs and alcohol, and reduced binge drinking at 6-month follow-up (Outlaw et al. 2012). Findings from a recent study that compared motivational enhancement therapy (MET) alone with MET augmented with age-adapted cognitive-behavioral therapy content in older individuals with AUD showed that at 26-week follow-up, roughly half the participants in both groups were still abstinent or had maintained low blood alcohol concentration levels (Andersen et al. 2020). Finally, behavioral therapies such as contingency management have also been linked with positive outcomes among older adults (Weiss and Petry 2013).

Self-Help Groups

A large proportion of community-based and residential treatment programs incorporate the traditional 12-step peer support model of recovery and rehabilitation. Originally developed by Alcoholics Anonymous (AA) and later adapted by groups such as Narcotics Anonymous, the 12-step model involves group support and encouragement to help members achieve and maintain sobriety. Participants share their experiences and follow the 12 steps, which include admitting one's addiction, recognizing the influence of a greater power as a source of strength, and acknowledging and atoning for past mistakes (Alcoholics Anonymous 2004).

Although self-help groups have been associated with positive outcomes for many individuals, findings regarding the rates of group engagement and outcomes among older adults remain mixed. In their matched comparison of older versus younger and middle-aged adults who participated in age-integrated residential treatment, Lemke and Moos (2003a) found that older patients engaged in 12-step programs as frequently as their younger and middle-aged counterparts when assessed at follow-up. Results also indicated that more involvement in self-help groups following treatment was associated with better outcomes across all three age groups.

Similarly, an investigation of patients who had completed an outpatient treatment program for chemical dependency yielded no age group differences in AA affiliation 5 years posttreatment (Satre et al. 2004a). Upon examination of a subset of participants in the sample who reported attending 12-step meetings in the prior year, no age group differences in the actual number of meetings attended emerged as significant. However, even though rates of attendance appeared to be comparable across age groups, the depth of involvement differed; older adults were less likely than middle-age adults to self-identify as being a 12-step group member and were less likely than younger and middle-aged adults to report calling a fellow group member for help. Comparable results were observed in examining 1-month post-discharge outcomes among alcohol-dependent patients admitted to a 12-step residential rehabilitation program (Oslin et al. 2005). Although rates of postdischarge abstinence and AA attendance did not differ across middle-aged and older adults, older adults were significantly less likely to contact a sponsor. Furthermore, older adults were less likely than middle-aged adults to engage in formal aftercare (31.2% vs. 56.4%).

Taken together, these findings highlight the importance of more careful examination of factors that may be related to 12-step program attendance, degree of engagement, and outcomes among older adults. These factors include, but are not limited to, perceived stigma, level of comfort with disclosure of personal information in group settings, degree to which age-relevant issues are addressed during group meetings, and logistical barriers, such as lack of transportation and health problems, that may preclude older adults from attending group sessions and engaging with sponsors (Oslin et al. 2005; Satre et al. 2004a).

Pharmacotherapy

Until relatively recently, the long-term treatment of older adults with alcohol dependence did not involve the use of pharmacological agents. Although disulfiram was originally the only medication approved for the treatment of alcohol dependence, its use is limited in older patients because of its potential for adverse effects and drug interactions (Lehmann and Fingerhood 2018). In 1995, the opioid antagonist naltrexone became the first pharmacological agent approved by the FDA in more than 50 years for the treatment of alcohol dependence. Approval of the drug was based on findings from clinical trials demonstrating that naltrexone was safe and effective in preventing relapse and reducing alcohol cravings (O'Malley et al. 1992; Volpicelli et al. 1992). Although these original clinical trials used samples of middle-age adults, naltrexone also has been shown to be effective in older adults. For example, results from a double-blind, placebo-controlled, randomized trial demonstrated that among older veterans ages 50–70 years, half as many patients given naltrexone relapsed to significant drinking compared with those given placebo (Oslin et al. 1997a).

Acamprosate has emerged as another potential agent in the treatment of alcohol dependence (Maisel et al. 2013). Although its exact action is still unclear, acamprosate is believed to reduce glutamate response (Kennedy et al. 2010). Clinical evidence from randomized trials suggests that it may be effective in promoting abstinence and reducing relapse to any drinking (Jonas et al. 2014; Maisel et al. 2013). Sass et al. (1996), for example, found that 43% of patients with alcohol dependence who were treated with acamprosate were abstinent at the conclusion of a 48-week randomized, placebo-controlled trial, compared with 21% of those given placebo. However, meta-analytic work has shown that while acamprosate might be more effective than naltrexone in promoting and sustaining abstinence, it has minimal effect on relapse to heavy drinking (Jonas et al. 2014; Maisel et al. 2013). Thus, naltrexone may be more effective in reducing heavy drinking and craving (Maisel et al. 2013). Unfortunately, no studies of the efficacy or safety of acamprosate, disulfiram, or buprenorphine (for the treatment of opioid use disorder) in older patients have been conducted to date (Tampi et al. 2019).

Detoxification and Withdrawal

Withdrawal symptoms are likely to occur in individuals who stop consuming substances or drastically cut down on their consumption following heavy use. During hospitalization, patients may be particularly vulnerable to alcohol or benzodiazepine withdrawal if the clinical team is unaware of the patients' problems with these substances. Considering the potential for life-threatening complications, clinicians caring for patients who misuse substances, particularly in settings in which withdrawal management or treatment is available, need to have a fundamental understanding of withdrawal symptoms and be able to provide detoxification management. Clinicians also should be aware of the anticipated time course of various symptoms.

Alcohol withdrawal symptoms can range from unnoticeable and mild to severe and life-threatening. The classic symptoms associated with alcohol withdrawal include autonomic hyperactivity (increased pulse rate, blood pressure, and temperature), restlessness, disturbed sleep, anxiety, nausea, and tremor. Severe withdrawal is marked by auditory, visual, or tactile hallucinations, delirium, seizures, and coma. Adverse functional and cognitive complications are particularly more likely to occur among older patients, with confusion often serving as the main presenting symptom (Lehmann and Fingerhood 2018). Commonly misused prescription drugs and illicit agents, such as benzodiazepines, opioids, and cocaine, cause distinct withdrawal symptoms that are also potentially life-threatening. Among older adults, the duration of withdrawal symptoms is longer, and withdrawal has the potential to complicate other medical and psychiatric illnesses. Nonetheless, no evidence suggests that older patients are more prone to alcohol withdrawal or require longer treatment for withdrawal symptoms than younger patients (Brower et al. 1994; Wojnar et al. 2001).

Moderators and Correlates of Treatment Response and Adherence

Some evidence suggests that certain factors may have an impact on the degree of treatment response and adherence in older adults receiving treatment. For example, age-specific treatment, or age matching, has been shown to improve treatment completion and to result in higher rates of attendance at group meetings compared with mixed-age treatments (Kuerbis and Sacco 2013). In one study, male veterans with alcohol problems were randomly assigned after detoxification to either age-specific treatment—which emphasized peer support, promotion of self-esteem, and time-limited goal setting—or to standard mixed-age treatment (Kashner et al. 1992). Outcomes at 6 months and 1 year showed that patients in the age-specific program were 2.9 times more likely at 6 months and 2.1 times more likely at 1 year to report abstinence compared with patients in the mixed-age group.

The type of treatment setting also may affect rates of adherence. In a study comparing engagement outcomes among older primary care patients referred to specialty mental health providers versus those referred to an integrated care model using a brief intervention, 60.4% of at-risk drinkers attended at least one visit in the integrated care model (Bartels et al. 2004). In contrast, only 33% of patients attended at least one visit to a specialty provider. These differences emerged despite efforts to address barriers to accessing specialty care, such as copayments and insurance claims, and to ensure appointments within 2 weeks of patients being identified with at-risk drinking.

Finally, certain patient-level characteristics may differentially predict treatment outcomes. For example, women may have more favorable treatment outcomes than men (Carew and Comiskey 2018; Satre et al. 2012). Satre et al. (2004b) demonstrated that 6 months after treatment at a private outpatient chemical dependency program, older women with alcohol dependency were significantly more likely than their male counterparts to report abstinence from alcohol and drugs during the prior 30 days (79.3% vs. 54.0%, $P=0.02$). Similarly, among patients who were not abstinent, men reported a mean of four heavy drinking days over the prior 30 days, whereas none of the women reported heavy drinking. Sex differences in outcomes appear to persist up to 7 years after alcohol and drug treatment; at 7-year follow-up, 76.0% of women versus 54.2% of men reported abstinence in the prior 30 days (Satre et al. 2007). In addition to sex, variables associated with older age that may be related to more favorable treatment outcomes include older adults' perceived benefit of reducing consumption (Borok et al. 2013), longer retention in treatment, and absence of individuals in the patient's close social networks (e.g., family and friends) who encourage alcohol or drug use (Satre et al. 2004b, 2007). Treatment outcomes also may be impacted by age-related changes in loss, loneliness, grief, and social network composition (Kuerbis and Sacco 2013). Thus, age-specific or age-adapted interventions and treatments that take a holistic approach and address multiple domains of functioning (e.g., emotional, cognitive, social, medical, and spiritual) and the logistic challenges that may impact treatment engagement will likely yield optimal treatment outcomes (Yarnell et al. 2020).

Medical and Psychiatric Comorbidity

The co-occurrence of problematic substance use and other medical and psychiatric conditions deserves special attention because such comorbidity may affect the course, treatment, and prognosis of both conditions. Although epidemiological studies have clearly shown that comorbidity between substance use and other psychiatric symptoms is common in younger populations, less is known about comorbidity between substance use and psychiatric illness in older adults. Nevertheless, a few studies have demonstrated that concurrent SUD is common among older adults with mental health problems (Kuerbis 2020; Wu and Blazer 2014). For example, in their study of data from the NESARC, Sacco et al. (2009) found that among high-risk alcohol users (categorized based on their pattern of alcohol use and on their symptoms meeting criteria for alcohol abuse and dependence) age 60 years and older, 24.9%, 8.8%, and 5.9% reported symptoms that met criteria for major depression, anxiety disorder, and antisocial personality disorder, respectively. In a nationally representative sample of adults ages 50 years and older, Blazer and Wu (2009) found an association between a major depressive episode and greater odds of marijuana and cocaine use in the past year. Not surprisingly, the rates of comorbidity are significantly higher among clinical samples of treatment-seeking older individuals with substance use problems (Chhatre et al. 2017; Wu and Blazer 2014).

Comorbid depressive and alcohol misuse symptoms not only are common in late life but also may have a reciprocal effect on one another. Individuals with comorbid depression and alcoholism have a more complicated clinical course of depression, marked by an increased risk of suicide and more social dysfunction, than individuals with alcoholism alone (Conwell 1991; Waern 2003). In the same vein, SUD has been associated with an increased incidence of developing a new psychiatric disorder. For example, in a longitudinal analysis of adults age 60 and older with AUD, 4% developed new-onset major depressive disorder and 2% new-onset generalized anxiety disorder over the span of 3 years, whereas 6.7% of those with a drug use disorder developed major depressive disorder (Chou et al. 2011).

Co-occurrence of substance use, mild or severe cognitive impairment, and dementing illnesses such as Alzheimer's disease is also a complex issue (Monds et al. 2017; Ridley et al. 2013). Although Wernicke-Korsakoff syndrome is well defined and is often caused by alcohol dependence, alcohol-related dementia (ARD) may be difficult to differentiate from Alzheimer's disease because of a lack of well-specified diagnostic criteria. As a result, clinical diagnostic criteria for ARD have been proposed and validated in at least one trial examining a method for distinguishing ARD, including Wernicke-Korsakoff syndrome, from other types of dementia (Oslin and Cary 2003). Despite these diagnostic issues, it is generally agreed that alcohol misuse contributes to cognitive deficits in later life. In one of the first community-based studies to include alcohol survey data, the Epidemiologic Catchment Area study found that the prevalence of a lifetime history of alcohol abuse or dependence was 1.5 times greater among individuals with mild and severe cognitive impairment than the prevalence among those with no cognitive impairment (George et al. 1991). Similarly, among older individuals seeking alcohol treatment, 23% had dementia associated with alcohol dependence (Finlayson et al. 1988), while in another study, nearly two-thirds of older adults attending an outpatient drug and alcohol treatment program screened positive for mild-to-severe cognitive impairment (Monds et al. 2017). Finally, patients with ARD who become abstinent do not show a progression in cognitive impairment comparable with that found in Alzheimer's disease (Oslin and Cary 2003).

Sleep disorders and disturbances also often co-occur with excessive drug and alcohol use. For example, in one study of patients admitted to a detoxification unit, ~70% reported sleep problems prior to admission, with 80% relating their sleep problems to their substance use (Roncero et al. 2012). Similarly, it has been estimated that between 61% and 91% of adults in early alcohol recovery report sleep disturbance (Chakravorty et al. 2016). The large body of work in this area supports the notion that the relationship between substance use and sleep problems is bidirectional; sleep disturbances increase the risk and maintenance of SUDs, while acute and chronic substance use can contribute to problems with sleep (Angarita et al. 2016; Kolla et al. 2020). Alcohol is well-known to cause changes in sleep patterns, such as decreased sleep latency, decreased stage 4 sleep, and precipitation or aggravation of sleep apnea (Angarita et al. 2016). Insomnia also has been shown to predict relapse to alcohol use, and individuals may use substances to self-medicate when experiencing insomnia and sleep disturbances (Chakravorty et al. 2016). Age-related changes in sleep patterns also occur with advancing age and include increased rapid eye movement (REM) episodes, decreased REM length and stage 3 and 4 sleep, and increased awakenings. Age-associated changes in sleep can be exacerbated by factors such as substance use. Although few studies have examined the relationship between sleep disturbance and substance misuse among older adults, there is evidence that older adults who are heavy drinkers are significantly more likely to experience poor sleep outcomes (Britton et al. 2020).

Conclusion and Future Directions

Substance misuse in older adults represents, and will represent for years to come, a pressing public health issue. In light of changes in demographic and cohort trends, recent years have seen an increase in the number of older adults who misuse alcohol and drugs. Moreover, there is a growing awareness that this group often engages in at-risk or problem substance use. Nevertheless, those in need of treatment or at risk for future problems often go unidentified and untreated. Therefore, research and clinical efforts aimed at improving screening and at identifying system-, provider-, and patient-level factors that may interfere with screening and referral processes for older adults at risk are warranted. In this vein, a better understanding among clinicians and patients of recommended drinking levels and the risks associated with moderate to heavy alcohol consumption is also needed, particularly considering the high prevalence of co-occurring medical and psychiatric problems in this age group. Clinicians also should ensure that screening is a part of routine practice when caring for older patients.

Furthermore, because both provider recommendations and patient engagement are influenced, in part, by the availability of effective treatment, better dissemination of information regarding currently available and efficacious treatments for at-risk use and SUD is needed. Treatment studies in addiction have traditionally excluded patients older than 65 years, resulting in a gap in the knowledge regarding treatment outcomes and the understanding of the neurobiology of addiction in older individuals.

Thus, research endeavors should continue to focus on developing more effective treatments for substance misuse in later life, taking into consideration and empirically assessing the various factors (e.g., patient-, treatment-, and system-related factors) that may moderate treatment engagement and outcomes. Given that these issues are particularly relevant to older adults, future work may benefit from examining nutrition, vitamin supplementation, and comorbid medical and psychiatric illnesses, both as foci for treatment and as aspects of health that may be complicated by substance use. Along these lines, more formal research that focuses on the relative efficacy of various treatment approaches, including those that employ technology and precision medicine, specifically among older adults, is needed.

Key Points

- Although demographic and cohort trends suggest that rates of substance use disorders in older adults are increasing, the misuse of alcohol and drugs in this group remains largely underrecognized and undertreated. Accordingly, substance misuse in later life has been referred to as both an invisible and emerging epidemic.

- Proper screening, diagnosis, and treatment of older adults with drug and alcohol problems require an understanding of both age-specific guidelines and the full range of substance use behavior seen among older adults.

- In light of physiological changes that accompany aging, adults age 65 years and older should consume no more than three standard drinks on any one occasion and no more than seven standard drinks in a week.

- The use of multiple pharmaceutical drugs is prevalent in older adulthood, and thus the risk of misusing prescription and over-the-counter medications increases with age. Psychotherapeutic medications, in particular, should be closely monitored because they are subject to improper use and can lead to negative health outcomes and interactions when used alone or in combination with other drugs and alcohol.

- Factors such as medical comorbidity, history of past use, sex, and social and family environment are related to increased late-life vulnerability to substance misuse and the maintenance of problematic substance use patterns.

- Diagnostic criteria and symptoms for alcohol and drug use disorders are not easily applied to older adults, because they are often confounded with symptoms of comorbid medical illnesses. Thus, when diagnosing and treating older adults, providers must be able to distinguish between symptoms of substance misuse and those stemming from comorbid conditions.

- Routine screening allows for the identification not only of older adults with substance use disorder but also of those who are at risk of misusing drugs and alcohol. Proper screening also helps determine needs for additional assessment and intervention. Standardized brief, low-cost assessments exist that can be used to assess the quantity and frequency of alcohol and drug use in clinical practice.

- A variety of treatments for substance misuse, such as brief interventions, psychotherapy, self-help groups and programs, and pharmacotherapy, have been shown to be effective among older adults.

- Special attention should be paid to co-occurrence of problematic substance use and other medical and psychiatric conditions (e.g., depression, dementia, sleep disturbance) because such comorbidity may affect the course, treatment, and prognosis of both conditions.

Suggested Readings

Blow FC (Consensus Panel Chair): Substance Abuse Among Older Adults. Treatment Improvement Protocol (TIP) Series No 26. Rockville, MD, U.S. Department of Health and Human Services, 1998

Grant BF, Goldstein RB, Saha TD, et al: Epidemiology of DSM-5 alcohol use disorder: results from the National Epidemiologic Survey on Alcohol and Related Conditions III. JAMA Psychiatry 72(8):757–766, 2015

Han BH, Moore AA, Ferris R, et al: Binge drinking among older adults in the United States, 2015 to 2017. J Am Geriatr Soc 67(10):2139–2144, 2019

Han BH, Sherman SE, Palamar JJ: Prescription opioid misuse among middle-aged and older adults in the United States, 2015–2016. Prev Med 121:94-98, 2019

Jonas DE, Amick HR, Feltner C, et al: Pharmacotherapy for adults with alcohol use disorders in outpatient settings: a systematic review and meta-analysis. JAMA 311(18):1889–1900, 2014

Kuerbis A, Sacco P: A review of existing treatments for substance abuse among the elderly and recommendations for future directions. Subst Abuse 7:13–37, 2013

Lehmann SW, Fingerhood M: Substance-use disorders in later life. N Engl J Med 379(24):2351–2360, 2018

Qato DM, Wilder J, Schumm LP, et al: Changes in prescription and over-the-counter medication and dietary supplement use among older adults in the United States, 2005 vs 2011. JAMA Intern Med 176(4):473–482, 2016

Wu L, Blazer DG: Substance use disorders and psychiatric comorbidity in mid and later life: a review. Int J Epidemiol 43(2):304–317, 2014

References

Abramson JL, Williams SA, Krumholz HM, Vaccarino V: Moderate alcohol consumption and risk of heart failure among older persons. JAMA 285(15):1971–1977, 2001 11308433

Aertgeerts B, Buntinx F, Ansoms S, Fevery J: Screening properties of questionnaires and laboratory tests for the detection of alcohol abuse or dependence in a general practice population. Br J Gen Pract 51(464):206–217, 2001 11255902

Alcoholics Anonymous: Twelve Steps and Twelve Traditions. New York, Alcoholics Anonymous, 2004

American Geriatrics Society Beers Criteria Update Expert Panel: American Geriatrics Society 2019 updated AGS Beers criteria for potentially inappropriate medication use in older adults. J Am Geriatr Soc 67(4):674–694, 2019 30693946

American Psychiatric Association: Diagnostic and Statistical Manual of Mental Disorders, 4th Edition. Washington, DC, American Psychiatric Publishing, 1994

American Psychiatric Association: Diagnostic and Statistical Manual of Mental Disorders, 5th Edition. Arlington, VA, American Psychiatric Association, 2013

Andersen K, Behrendt S, Bilberg R, et al: Evaluation of adding the community reinforcement approach to motivational enhancement therapy for adults aged 60 years and older with DSM-5 alcohol use disorder: a randomized controlled trial. Addiction 115(1):69–81, 2020 31454444

Angarita GA, Emadi N, Hodges S, Morgan PT: Sleep abnormalities associated with alcohol, cannabis, cocaine, and opiate use: a comprehensive review. Addict Sci Clin Pract 11(1):9, 2016 27117064

Anthony JC, Helzer JE: Syndromes of drug abuse and dependence, in Psychiatric Disorders in America: The Epidemiologic Catchment Area Study. Edited by Robins LN, Regier DA. New York, Free Press, 1991, pp 116–154

Barry KL, Blow FC, Walton MA, et al: Elder-specific brief alcohol intervention: 3-month outcomes. Alcohol Clin Exp Res 22:30A, 1998

Barry KL, Blow FC, Oslin DW: Substance abuse in older adults: review and recommendations for education and practice in medical settings. Subst Abus 23(3 suppl):105–131, 2002 23580990

Bartels SJ, Coakley EH, Zubritsky C, et al: Improving access to geriatric mental health services: a randomized trial comparing treatment engagement with integrated versus enhanced referral care for depression, anxiety, and at-risk alcohol use. Am J Psychiatry 161(8):1455–1462, 2004 15285973

Berks J, McCormick R: Screening for alcohol misuse in elderly primary care patients: a systematic literature review. Int Psychogeriatr 20(6):1090–1103, 2008 18538045

Bhatia U, Nadkarni A, Murthy P, et al: Recent advances in treatment for older people with substance use problems: an updated systematic and narrative review. Eur Geriatr Med 6(6):580–586, 2015

Blazer DG, Wu LT: The epidemiology of substance use and disorders among middle aged and elderly community adults: National Survey on Drug Use and Health. Am J Geriatr Psychiatry 17(3):237–245, 2009 19454850

Blow FC: Substance Abuse Among Older Adults. Treatment Improvement Protocol (TIP) Series No 26. Rockville, MD, U.S. Department of Health and Human Services, 1998

Blow FC, Brower KJ, Schulenberg JE, et al: The Michigan Alcoholism Screening Test—Geriatric version (MAST-G): a new elderly specific screening instrument. Alcohol Clin Exp Res 16(2):372, 1992

Borok J, Galier P, Dinolfo M, et al: Why do older unhealthy drinkers decide to make changes or not in their alcohol consumption? Data from the Healthy Living as You Age study. J Am Geriatr Soc 61(8):1296–1302, 2013 23889690

Bradley KA, Bush KR, McDonell MB, et al: Screening for problem drinking: comparison of CAGE and AUDIT. J Gen Intern Med 13:379–388, 1998

Breslow RA, Castle IP, Chen CM, Graubard BI: Trends in alcohol consumption among older Americans: National Health Interview Surveys, 1997 to 2014. Alcohol Clin Exp Res 41(5):976–986, 2017 28340502

Britton A, Fat LN, Neligan A: The association between alcohol consumption and sleep disorders among older people in the general population. Sci Rep 10(1):5275, 2020 32210292

Brower KJ, Mudd S, Blow FC, et al: Severity and treatment of alcohol withdrawal in elderly versus younger patients. Alcohol Clin Exp Res 18(1):196–201, 1994 8198220

Bryson CL, Mukamal KJ, Mittleman MA, et al: The association of alcohol consumption and incident heart failure: the Cardiovascular Health Study. J Am Coll Cardiol 48(2):305–311, 2006 16843180

Buchsbaum DG, Buchanan RG, Welsh J, et al: Screening for drinking disorders in the elderly using the CAGE questionnaire. J Am Geriatr Soc 40(7):662–665, 1992 1607581

Bush K, Kivlahan DR, McDonell MB, et al: The AUDIT alcohol consumption questions (AUDIT-C): an effective brief screening test for problem drinking. Ambulatory Care Quality Improvement Project (ACQUIP). Alcohol Use Disorders Identification Test. Arch Intern Med 158(16):1789–1795, 1998 9738608

Carew AM, Comiskey C: Treatment for opioid use and outcomes in older adults: a systematic literature review. Drug Alcohol Depend 182:48–57, 2018 29136566

Cawthon PM, Fink HA, Barrett-Connor E, et al: Alcohol use, physical performance, and functional limitations in older men. J Am Geriatr Soc 55(2):212–220, 2007 17302657

Chakravorty S, Chaudhary NS, Brower KJ: Alcohol dependence and its relationship with insomnia and other sleep disorders. Alcohol Clin Exp Res 40(11):2271–2282, 2016 27706838

Chhatre S, Cook R, Mallik E, Jayadevappa R: Trends in substance use admissions among older adults. BMC Health Serv Res 17(1):584, 2017 28830504

Chou KL, Mackenzie CS, Liang K, Sareen J: Three-year incidence and predictors of first-onset of DSM-IV mood, anxiety, and substance use disorders in older adults: results from Wave 2 of the National Epidemiologic Survey on Alcohol and Related Conditions. J Clin Psychiatry 72(2):144–155, 2011 21382305

Closser MH, Blow FC: Recent advances in addictive disorders. Special populations: women, ethnic minorities, and the elderly. Psychiatr Clin North Am 16(1):199–209, 1993 8456045

Committee on the Mental Health Workforce for Geriatric Populations, Board on Health Care Services, Institute of Medicine: The Mental Health and Substance Use Workforce for Older Adults: In Whose Hands? Edited by Eden J, Maslow K, Le M, Blazer D. Washington, DC, National Academies Press, 2012

Conigliaro J, Kraemer K, McNeil M: Screening and identification of older adults with alcohol problems in primary care. J Geriatr Psychiatry Neurol 13(3):106–114, 2000 11001132

Conwell Y: Suicide in elderly patients, in Diagnosis and Treatment of Depression in Late Life. Edited by Schneider LS, Reynolds CF, Lebowitz BD, et al. Washington, DC, American Psychiatric Press, 1991, pp 397–418

Curry SJ, Krist AH, Owens DK, et al: Screening and behavioral counseling interventions to reduce unhealthy alcohol use in adolescents and adults: US Preventive Services Task Force recommendation statement. JAMA 320(18):1899–1909, 2018 30422199

Dawson DA, Grant BF, Ruan WJ: The association between stress and drinking: modifying effects of gender and vulnerability. Alcohol Alcohol 40(5):453–460, 2005a 15972275

Dawson DA, Grant BF, Stinson FS, Zhou Y: Effectiveness of the derived Alcohol Use Disorders Identification Test (AUDIT-C) in screening for alcohol use disorders and risk drinking in the US general population. Alcohol Clin Exp Res 29(5):844–854, 2005b 15897730

Djoussé L, Biggs ML, Mukamal KJ, Siscovick DS: Alcohol consumption and type 2 diabetes among older adults: the Cardiovascular Health Study. Obesity (Silver Spring) 15(7):1758–1765, 2007 17636094

Dowling GJ, Weiss SR, Condon TP: Drugs of abuse and the aging brain. Neuropsychopharmacology 33(2):209–218, 2008 17406645

Finlayson RE, Hurt RD, Davis LJ Jr, Morse RM: Alcoholism in elderly persons: a study of the psychiatric and psychosocial features of 216 inpatients. Mayo Clin Proc 63(8):761–768, 1988 3398595

George LK, Landerman R, Blazer DG, et al: Cognitive impairment, in Psychiatric Disorders in America: The Epidemiologic Catchment Area Study. Edited by Robins LN, Regier DA. New York, Free Press, 1991, pp 291–327

Gfroerer J, Penne M, Pemberton M, Folsom R: Substance abuse treatment need among older adults in 2020: the impact of the aging baby-boom cohort. Drug Alcohol Depend 69(2):127–135, 2003 12609694

Gomberg ES: Treatment for alcohol-related problems: special populations: research opportunities. Recent Dev Alcohol 16:313–333, 2003 12638644

Grant BF, Goldstein RB, Saha TD, et al: Epidemiology of DSM-5 alcohol use disorder: results From the National Epidemiologic Survey on Alcohol and Related Conditions III. JAMA Psychiatry 72(8):757–766, 2015 26039070

Grant BF, Chou SP, Saha TD, et al: Prevalence of 12-month alcohol use, high-risk drinking, and DSM-IV alcohol use disorder in the United States, 2001–2002 to 2012–2013: results from the National Epidemiologic Survey on Alcohol and Related Conditions. JAMA Psychiatry 74(9):911–923, 2017 28793133

Han B, Gfroerer JC, Colliver JD, Penne MA: Substance use disorder among older adults in the United States in 2020. Addiction 104(1):88–96, 2009 19133892

Han B, Moore AA, Sherman S, et al: Demographic trends of binge alcohol use and alcohol use disorders among older adults in the United States, 2005–2014. Drug Alcohol Depend 170:198–207, 2017 27979428

Han B, Moore AA, Ferris R, Palamar JJ: Binge drinking among older adults in the United States, 2015 to 2017. J Am Geriatr Soc 67(10):2139–2144, 2019a 31364159

Han B, Sherman SE, Palamar JJ: Prescription opioid misuse among middle-aged and older adults in the United States, 2015–2016. Prev Med 121:94–98, 2019b 30763631

Hinkin CH, Castellon SA, Dickson-Fuhrman E, et al: Screening for drug and alcohol abuse among older adults using a modified version of the CAGE. Am J Addict 10(4):319–326, 2001 11783746

Hock B, Schwarz M, Domke I, et al: Validity of carbohydrate-deficient transferrin (%CDT), gamma-glutamyltransferase (gamma-GT) and mean corpuscular erythrocyte volume (MCV) as biomarkers for chronic alcohol abuse: a study in patients with alcohol dependence and liver disorders of non-alcoholic and alcoholic origin. Addiction 100(10):1477–1486, 2005 16185209

Holroyd S, Duryee JJ: Substance use disorders in a geriatric psychiatry outpatient clinic: prevalence and epidemiologic characteristics. J Nerv Ment Dis 185(10):627–632, 1997 9345253

Jonas DE, Garbutt JC, Amick HR, et al: Behavioral counseling after screening for alcohol misuse in primary care: a systematic review and meta-analysis for the U.S. Preventive Services Task Force. Ann Intern Med 157(9):645–654, 2012 23007881

Jonas DE, Amick HR, Feltner C, et al: Pharmacotherapy for adults with alcohol use disorders in outpatient settings: a systematic review and meta-analysis. JAMA 311(18):1889–1900, 2014 24825644

Kalla A, Figueredo VM: Alcohol and cardiovascular disease in the geriatric population. Clin Cardiol 40(7):444–449, 2017 28294372

Kaplan BA, Koffarnus MN: Timeline followback self-reports underestimate alcohol use prior to successful contingency management treatment. Alcohol Alcohol 54(3):258–263, 2019 31044225

Kashner TM, Rodell DE, Ogden SR, et al: Outcomes and costs of two VA inpatient treatment programs for older alcoholic patients. Hosp Community Psychiatry 43(10):985–989, 1992 1328022

Katz IR, Sands LP, Bilker W, et al: Identification of medications that cause cognitive impairment in older people: the case of oxybutynin chloride. J Am Geriatr Soc 46(1):8–13, 1998 9434659

Kennedy WK, Leloux M, Kutscher EC, et al: Acamprosate. Expert Opin Drug Metab Toxicol 6(3):363–380, 2010 20163323

Kolla BP, Mansukhani MP, Biernacka J, et al: Sleep disturbances in early alcohol recovery: prevalence and associations with clinical characteristics and severity of alcohol consumption. Drug Alcohol Depend 206:107655, 2020 31744670

Kirchner JE, Zubritsky C, Cody M, et al: Alcohol consumption among older adults in primary care. J Gen Intern Med 22(1):92–97, 2007 17351846

Klatsky AL: Alcohol and cardiovascular health. Physiol Behav 100(1):76–81, 2010 20045009

Kuerbis A: Substance use among older adults: an update on prevalence, etiology, assessment, and intervention. Gerontology 66(3):249–258, 2020 31812954

Kuerbis A, Sacco P: A review of existing treatments for substance abuse among the elderly and recommendations for future directions. Subst Abuse 7:13–37, 2013 23471422

Kuerbis A, Sacco P, Blazer DG, Moore AA: Substance abuse among older adults. Clin Geriatr Med 30(3):629–654, 2014 25037298

Lader M: Benzodiazepine harm: how can it be reduced? Br J Clin Pharmacol 77(2):295–301, 2014 22882333

Lang I, Wallace RB, Huppert FA, Melzer D: Moderate alcohol consumption in older adults is associated with better cognition and well-being than abstinence. Age Ageing 36(3):256–261, 2007 17353234

Larney S, Bohnert AS, Ganoczy D, et al: Mortality among older adults with opioid use disorders in the Veterans Health Administration, 2000–2011. Drug Alcohol Depend 147:32–37, 2015 25575652

Lehmann SW, Fingerhood M: Substance-use disorders in later life. N Engl J Med 379(24):2351–2360, 2018 30575463

Lemke S, Moos RH: Outcomes at 1 and 5 years for older patients with alcohol use disorders. J Subst Abuse Treat 24(1):43–50, 2003a 12646329

Lemke S, Moos RH: Treatment and outcomes of older patients with alcohol use disorders in community residential programs. J Stud Alcohol 64(2):219–226, 2003b 12713195

Lemke SP, Schaefer JA: Recent changes in the prevalence of psychiatric disorders among VA nursing home residents. Psychiatr Serv 61(4):356–363, 2010 20360274

Lemke S, Schutte KK, Brennan PL, Moos RH: Gender differences in social influences and stressors linked to increased drinking. J Stud Alcohol Drugs 69(5):695–702, 2008 18781244

Lemmens P, Tan ES, Knibbe RA: Measuring quantity and frequency of drinking in a general population survey: a comparison of five indices. J Stud Alcohol 53(5):476–486, 1992 1405641

Maher RL, Hanlon J, Hajjar ER: Clinical consequences of polypharmacy in elderly. Expert Opin Drug Saf 13(1):57–65, 2014 24073682

Maisel NC, Blodgett JC, Wilbourne PL, et al: Meta-analysis of naltrexone and acamprosate for treating alcohol use disorders: when are these medications most helpful? Addiction 108(2):275–293, 2013 23075288

Mallet L, Spinewine A, Huang A: The challenge of managing drug interactions in elderly people. Lancet 370(9582):185–191, 2007 17630042

Mattson M, Lipari RN, Hays C, et al: A Day In the Life of Older Adults: Substance Use Facts. The CBHSQ Report. Rockville, MD, Center for Behavioral Health Statistics and Quality, Substance Abuse and Mental Health Services Administration, 2017

Maust DT, Oslin DW, Marcus SC: Effect of age on the profile of psychotropic users: results from the 2010 National Ambulatory Medical Care Survey. J Am Geriatr Soc 62(2):358–364, 2014 24417590

Maust DT, Kales HC, Wiechers IR, et al: No end in sight: benzodiazepine use in older adults in the United States. J Am Geriatr Soc 64(12):2546–2553, 2016 27879984

Maust DT, Lin LA, Blow FC: Benzodiazepine use and misuse among adults in the United States. Psychiatr Serv 70(2):97–106, 2019 30554562

Mayfield D, McLeod G, Hall P: The CAGE questionnaire: validation of a new alcoholism screening instrument. Am J Psychiatry 131(10):1121–1123, 1974 4416585

Mejldal A, Andersen K, Behrendt S, et al: Twenty years socioeconomic trajectories in older adults with varying alcohol use: a register-based cohort study. Alcohol Alcohol 55(3):304–314, 2020 32236508

Miller W, Rollnick S: Motivational Interviewing: Preparing People to Change Addictive Behavior. New York, Guilford, 1991

Monds LA, Ridley NJ, Rivas C, et al: Cognition and adaptive functioning in older people attending drug and alcohol services. Int Psychogeriatr 29(5):815–823, 2017 28143626

Moore AA, Beck JC, Babor TF, et al: Beyond alcoholism: identifying older, at-risk drinkers in primary care. J Stud Alcohol 63(3):316–324, 2002 12086132

Moore AA, Whiteman EJ, Ward KT: Risks of combined alcohol/medication use in older adults. Am J Geriatr Pharmacother 5(1):64–74, 2007 17608249

Moore AA, Blow FC, Hoffing M, et al: Primary care-based intervention to reduce at-risk drinking in older adults: a randomized controlled trial. Addiction 106(1):111–120, 2011 21143686

Moos RH, Schutte K, Brennan P, Moos BS: Ten-year patterns of alcohol consumption and drinking problems among older women and men. Addiction 99(7):829–838, 2004 15200578

Moos RH, Schutte KK, Brennan PL, Moos BS: Older adults' alcohol consumption and late-life drinking problems: a 20-year perspective. Addiction 104(8):1293–1302, 2009 19438836

Mukamal KJ, Mackey RH, Kuller LH, et al: Alcohol consumption and lipoprotein subclasses in older adults. J Clin Endocrinol Metab 92(7):2559–2566, 2007a 17440017

Mukamal KJ, Robbins JA, Cauley JA, et al: Alcohol consumption, bone density, and hip fracture among older adults: the cardiovascular health study. Osteoporos Int 18(5):593–602, 2007b 17318666

National Institute on Alcohol Abuse and Alcoholism: Helping Patients Who Drink Too Much: A Clinician's Guide, Updated 2005 Edition (NIH Publ No. 07–3769). Bethesda, MD, U.S. Department of Health and Human Services, Public Health Services, National Institutes of Health, National Institute on Alcohol Abuse and Alcoholism, reprinted September 2007. Available at: https://pubs.niaaa.nih.gov/publications/Practitioner/Clinicians-Guide2005/guide.pdf. Accessed June 1, 2020.

National Institute on Alcohol Abuse and Alcoholism: Harmful Interactions: Mixing Alcohol With Medicines (NIH Publ No 13–5329). Bethesda, MD, U.S. Department of Health and Human Services, Public Health Services, National Institutes of Health, 2014

Nemes S, Rao PA, Zeiler C, et al: Computerized screening of substance abuse problems in a primary care setting: older vs. younger adults. Am J Drug Alcohol Abuse 30(3):627–642, 2004 15540497

O'Donnell A, Anderson P, Newbury-Birch D, et al: The impact of brief alcohol interventions in primary healthcare: a systematic review of reviews. Alcohol Alcohol 49(1):66–78, 2014 24232177

O'Malley SS, Jaffe AJ, Chang G, et al: Naltrexone and coping skills therapy for alcohol dependence: a controlled study. Arch Gen Psychiatry 49(11):881–887, 1992 1444726

Oslin DW: Alcohol use in late life: disability and comorbidity. J Geriatr Psychiatry Neurol 13(3):134–140, 2000 11001136

Oslin DW, Cary MS: Alcohol-related dementia: validation of diagnostic criteria. Am J Geriatr Psychiatry 11(4):441–447, 2003 12837673

Oslin D, Liberto JG, O'Brien J, et al: Naltrexone as an adjunctive treatment for older patients with alcohol dependence. Am J Geriatr Psychiatry 5(4):324–332, 1997a 9363289

Oslin DW, Streim JE, Parmelee P, et al: Alcohol abuse: a source of reversible functional disability among residents of a VA nursing home. Int J Geriatr Psychiatry 12(8):825–832, 1997b 9283927

Oslin DW, Pettinati HM, Luck G, et al: Clinical correlations with carbohydrate-deficient transferrin levels in women with alcoholism. Alcohol Clin Exp Res 22(9):1981–1985, 1998 9884141

Oslin DW, Katz IR, Edell WS, Ten Have TR: Effects of alcohol consumption on the treatment of depression among elderly patients. Am J Geriatr Psychiatry 8(3):215–220, 2000 10910419

Oslin DW, Pettinati H, Volpicelli JR: Alcoholism treatment adherence: older age predicts better adherence and drinking outcomes. Am J Geriatr Psychiatry 10(6):740–747, 2002 12427583

Oslin DW, Slaymaker VJ, Blow FC, et al: Treatment outcomes for alcohol dependence among middle-aged and older adults. Addict Behav 30(7):1431–1436, 2005 16022937

Outlaw FH, Marquart JM, Roy A, et al: Treatment outcomes for older adults who abuse substances. J Appl Gerontol 31:78–100, 2012

Plunk AD, Syed-Mohammed H, Cavazos-Rehg P, et al: Alcohol consumption, heavy drinking, and mortality: rethinking the j-shaped curve. Alcohol Clin Exp Res 38(2):471–478, 2014 24033586

Qato DM, Wilder J, Schumm LP, et al: Changes in prescription and over-the-counter medication and dietary supplement use among older adults in the United States, 2005 vs 2011. JAMA Intern Med 176(4):473–482, 2016 26998708

Rehm J, Mathers C, Popova S, et al: Global burden of disease and injury and economic cost attributable to alcohol use and alcohol-use disorders. Lancet 373(9682):2223–2233, 2009 19560604

Ridley NJ, Draper B, Withall A: Alcohol-related dementia: an update of the evidence. Alzheimers Res Ther 5(1):3, 2013 23347747

Roncero C, Grau-López L, Díaz-Morán S, et al: [Evaluation of sleep disorders in drug dependent inpatients]. Med Clin (Barc) 138(8):332–335, 2012 22018396

Rubinsky AD, Dawson DA, Williams EC, et al: AUDIT-C scores as a scaled marker of mean daily drinking, alcohol use disorder severity, and probability of alcohol dependence in a U.S. general population sample of drinkers. Alcohol Clin Exp Res 37(8):1380–1390, 2013 23906469

Sacco P, Bucholz KK, Spitznagel EL: Alcohol use among older adults in the National Epidemiologic Survey on Alcohol and Related Conditions: a latent class analysis. J Stud Alcohol Drugs 70(6):829–838, 2009 19895759

Sass H, Soyka M, Mann K, Zieglgänsberger W: Relapse prevention by acamprosate: results from a placebo-controlled study on alcohol dependence. Arch Gen Psychiatry 53(8):673–680, 1996 8694680

Satre DD, Mertens J, Areán PA, Weisner C: Contrasting outcomes of older versus middle-aged and younger adult chemical dependency patients in a managed care program. J Stud Alcohol 64(4):520–530, 2003 12921194

Satre DD, Mertens JR, Areán PA, Weisner C: Five-year alcohol and drug treatment outcomes of older adults versus middle-aged and younger adults in a managed care program. Addiction 99(10):1286–1297, 2004a 15369567

Satre DD, Mertens JR, Weisner C: Gender differences in treatment outcomes for alcohol dependence among older adults. J Stud Alcohol 65(5):638–642, 2004b 15536774

Satre DD, Blow FC, Chi FW, Weisner C: Gender differences in seven-year alcohol and drug treatment outcomes among older adults. Am J Addict 16(3):216–221, 2007 17612826

Satre DD, Chi FW, Mertens JR, Weisner CM: Effects of age and life transitions on alcohol and drug treatment outcome over nine years. J Stud Alcohol Drugs 73(3):459–468, 2012 22456251

Schonfeld L, Dupree LW: Age-specific cognitive behavioral and self-management treatment approaches, in Treating Alcohol and Drug Abuse in the Elderly. Edited by Gurnack AM, Atkinson RM, Osgood NJ. New York, Springer, 2002, pp 109–130

Schonfeld L, Dupree LW, Dickson-Euhrmann E, et al: Cognitive-behavioral treatment of older veterans with substance abuse problems. J Geriatr Psychiatry Neurol 13(3):124–129, 2000 11001134

Schonfeld L, King-Kallimanis BL, Duchene DM, et al: Screening and brief intervention for substance misuse among older adults: the Florida BRITE project. Am J Public Health 100(1):108–114, 2010 19443821

Simoni-Wastila L, Yang HK: Psychoactive drug abuse in older adults. Am J Geriatr Pharmacother 4(4):380–394, 2006 17296542

Sorocco KH, Ferrell SW: Alcohol use among older adults. J Gen Psychol 133(4):453–467, 2006 17128962

Sorock GS, Chen LH, Gonzalgo SR, Baker SP: Alcohol-drinking history and fatal injury in older adults. Alcohol 40(3):193–199, 2006 17418699

Substance Abuse and Mental Health Services Administration: Results From the 2012 National Survey on Drug Use and Health: Summary of National Findings, NSDUH Series H-46 (HHS Publ No SMA-13-4795). Rockville, MD, Substance Abuse and Mental Health Services Administration, 2013

Substance Abuse and Mental Health Services Administration: 2020 NSDUH detailed tables, in National Survey on Drug Use and Health (online). Rockville, MD, Center for Behavioral Health Statistics and Quality, Substance Abuse and Mental Health Services Administration, 2021. Available at: https://www.samhsa.gov/data/report/2020-nsduh-detailed-tables. Accessed November 8, 2021.

Tampi RR, Chhatlani A, Ahmad H, et al: Substance use disorders among older adults: a review of randomized controlled pharmacotherapy trials. World J Psychiatry 9(5):78–82, 2019 31559148

Tannenbaum C, Paquette A, Hilmer S, et al: A systematic review of amnestic and non-amnestic mild cognitive impairment induced by anticholinergic, antihistamine, GABAergic and opioid drugs. Drugs Aging 29(8):639–658, 2012 22812538

Tannenbaum C, Martin P, Tamblyn R, et al: Reduction of inappropriate benzodiazepine prescriptions among older adults through direct patient education: the EMPOWER cluster randomized trial. JAMA Intern Med 174(6):890–898, 2014 24733354

Topic A, Djukic M: Diagnostic characteristics and application of alcohol biomarkers. Clin Lab 59(3–4):233–245, 2013 23724610

Tucker JA, Foushee HR, Black BC, Roth DL: Agreement between prospective interactive voice response self-monitoring and structured retrospective reports of drinking and contextual variables during natural resolution attempts. J Stud Alcohol Drugs 68(4):538–542, 2007 17568958

Volpicelli JR, Alterman AI, Hayashida M, O'Brien CP: Naltrexone in the treatment of alcohol dependence. Arch Gen Psychiatry 49(11):876–880, 1992 1345133

Votaw VR, Geyer R, Rieselbach MM, McHugh RK: The epidemiology of benzodiazepine misuse: a systematic review. Drug Alcohol Depend 200:95–114, 2019 31121495

Waern M: Alcohol dependence and misuse in elderly suicides. Alcohol Alcohol 38(3):249–254, 2003 12711660

Weiss L, Petry NM: Older methadone patients achieve greater durations of cocaine abstinence with contingency management than younger patients. Am J Addict 22(2):119–126, 2013 23414496

Wojnar M, Wasilewski D, Zmigrodzka I, Grobel I: Age-related differences in the course of alcohol withdrawal in hospitalized patients. Alcohol Alcohol 36(6):577–583, 2001 11704625

Wu LT, Blazer DG: Illicit and nonmedical drug use among older adults: a review. J Aging Health 23(3):481–504, 2011 21084724

Wu LT, Blazer DG: Substance use disorders and psychiatric comorbidity in mid and later life: a review. Int J Epidemiol 43(2):304–317, 2014 24163278

Yarnell S, Li L, MacGrory B, et al: Substance use disorders in later life: a review and synthesis of the literature of an emerging public health concern. Am J Geriatr Psychiatry 28(2):226–236, 2020 31340887

CHAPTER 18

Personality Disorders

Benjamin P. Chapman, Ph.D., M.P.H.
Adam Simning, M.D., Ph.D.

Maladaptive personality tendencies, whether formally classified as a disorder or not, can wreak havoc on people's lives at any age. This chapter reviews the central aspects of personality disorder, with a focus on older adults. Although there is a large literature on personality disorders, Agronin and Maletta (2000) observed more than 20 years ago that little of it involves older adults. This appears to still be the case, with one possible reason being that few personality disorder cohorts have entered later life (Newton-Howes et al. 2015). In contrast, a great deal of work in the past two decades has focused on personality *traits* in later life. Usually, but not always, this work has involved the five-factor model of personality (FFM), which focuses on the five broad dimensions of neuroticism, extroversion, agreeableness, openness to experience, and conscientiousness. Each dimension is a combination of several more specific traits, and configurations of these traits have been proposed to match DSM-5 personality disorders (American Psychiatric Association 2013; Widiger and Mullins-Sweatt 2009). Some of this work can augment a discussion of personality disorders in older adults. Unique challenges arise in the approach and management of personality disorders in late life, particularly because neurocognitive disorders (NCDs) often present with personality changes, and psychosocial histories are often incomplete (particularly in long-term care settings). A comprehensive understanding of the personality disorders is warranted for clinicians working with older adults because these disorders are common, are associated with significant morbidity and lower quality of life, and can negatively affect the outcomes of other psychiatric disorders and medical comorbidities.

Definitions

Personality refers to an individual's "enduring patterns of perceiving, relating to, and thinking about the environment and oneself" (American Psychiatric Association 2013, p. 826). Personality consists of both temperament (i.e., genetic dispositions) and character (i.e., qualities developed through interaction with the environment) (Robinson 2005). To be diagnosed with a personality disorder, DSM-5 requires the patient have an enduring pattern of experience and behavior that is noticeably different from cultural expectations, as manifested in two or more of the following domains: cognition, affectivity, interpersonal functioning, and impulse control (American Psychiatric Association 2013). This pattern must have developed by early adulthood and must be intractable and relatively stable across the life span. A personality disorder influences a wide range of both social and personal situations and, like all DSM-5 disorders, results in significant distress or functional impairment. Finally, the enduring pattern must not be a manifestation of another mental disorder, a medical disorder, or substance use.

Several aspects of these criteria require careful consideration for older adults. First, changes in personality are often the chief complaint when an older person is brought by caregivers for a specialist evaluation (Duchek et al. 2007). It is important to clarify the timing and duration of these changes because the appearance de novo of a full-blown personality disorder in late life is untenable. Behaviors that appear symptomatic of personality disorders may reflect other medical conditions, meriting the DSM-5 diagnosis of *personality change due to another medical condition*. NCDs can produce significant behavior change. A review of personality change in Alzheimer's disease found marked consistency across studies of a pattern in which neuroticism increased and extraversion, openness, agreeableness, and conscientiousness decreased (Robins Wahlin and Byrne 2011). Changes in neuroticism and extraversion were quite large in this review, and deteriorations in conscientiousness were extreme. In terms of personality disorder symptoms, high or increasing levels of neuroticism correspond to persistent negative affect, including anxiety, depression, and anger. Low conscientiousness generally reflects a lack of impulse control and disruption of goal-directed behavior. Several personality conditions feature affective dyscontrol and impulsivity, so dementing conditions should be ruled out before assuming that these characteristics reflect a personality disorder. In fact, increasing neuroticism and decreasing conscientiousness have been noted prior to a clinical diagnosis of dementia (Balsis et al. 2005). This pattern of change also corresponds to mild behavioral impairment, a dementia prodrome (Ismail et al. 2016). Thus, clinicians must rule out existing NCDs or preceding organic changes manifesting the cognitive symptoms of NCDs when facing what appear to be personality disorder symptoms.

After making a global assessment of whether a personality disorder may be present based on the key features just listed, the next step is to identify a specific personality disorder or cluster. Since 1980, DSM has categorized three different personality disorder clusters:

- Cluster A—odd, eccentric (paranoid, schizoid, schizotypal)
- Cluster B—dramatic, emotional, erratic (antisocial, borderline, histrionic, and narcissistic)
- Cluster C—anxious, fearful (avoidant, dependent, and obsessive-compulsive)

Likewise, over the length of a life span often reaching 75–85 years, both personality and a personality disorder are likely to change somewhat; therefore, attention to identifying a cluster is particularly helpful. Some studies of self-reported personality disorder symptoms find that standard measures function differently in older compared with middle-aged or younger adults (Balsis et al. 2007; Debast et al. 2015). These studies generally show that questions about specific symptoms of various personality disorders have differing rates of endorsement in older people, suggesting that symptoms vary across the life span and that psychometric instruments sometimes do not capture personality dysfunction in later life. One framework for understanding this comes from the life span personality development concept of *heterotypic continuity* in personality characteristics, or the notion that the same underlying personality disposition can manifest in different ways at different points in the life course (Caspi and Roberts 2001). Histrionic or borderline tendencies are less likely to be manifested in sexual expressiveness or promiscuity in later life. Generally, severe impulsivity, risky behavior, and self-mutilation tend to diminish with advancing age (Zanarini et al. 2007), but self-destructive tendencies can be expressed in self-starvation, abuse of medications, and noncompliance with medical treatment (Rosowsky and Gurian 1992). Narcissistic grandiosity may focus on claims of past success rather than current achievement. Rejection sensitivity may revolve around adult children or grandchildren rather than romantic partners. In addition, considering the general impairment criteria, most older persons will be retired, so occupational impairment is not a valid indicator.

By the same token, certain normative changes occur with aging that must not be mistaken for personality pathology. Socioemotional selectivity theory, for instance, suggests that older adults naturally narrow the breadth of their social networks to focus on a smaller subset of higher-quality relationships (Carstensen et al. 2003). Loneliness and social isolation are more common experiences and may reflect transitions out of work, distance from family, or the death of friends (Hawkley and Kocherginsky 2018). Thus, small social circles do not necessarily imply schizoid tendencies. Older adults also shift from more active, externally oriented control strategies to more internally focused ones based on adjusting expectations and coping (Schulz and Heckhausen 1996). Although perceptions of control tend to be beneficial, they are naturally reduced by physical health and cognitive deterioration (Robinson and Lachman 2017). The resulting lack of motivation or initiative is not necessarily a sign of pathological dependency. Another normative aging process involves "selective optimization with compensation," or selecting certain aspects of roles or activities to maintain and emphasize while finding ways to compensate for the loss of others (Baltes 1997). This process can take many forms, including potentially odd or eccentric behaviors. For instance, a mobility-impaired person may need to crawl up stairs, and someone who is rendered cold by circulatory or other medical issues might wear winter clothes on a warm summer day. These are not evidence of Cluster C symptoms.

Many individuals may display characteristics of multiple personality disorders, in which case a "personality disorder not otherwise specified" diagnosis may be appropriate. Other options include the ability to note certain tendencies as "traits" rather than a disorder or to use the DSM-5 supplementary dimensional system for personality pathology (discussed later). Table 18–1 outlines different personality disorders and particular aging considerations. Developmental needs are noted in the table and are discussed in the section that follows.

Prevalence, Criteria, Comorbidities, and Controversies

The prevalence of personality disorders in the general population is less accurately known than that of other mental disorders, but a recent meta-analysis of adults in

TABLE 18–1.   Personality disorders and related aspects of aging

Cluster and types	Characteristics	Developmental needs	Related aspects of aging
A. Odd, eccentric			
Paranoid	Perception that people are dangerous; vigilance, suspiciousness	Trust, acceptance	Forced intimate contact from physical dependence highlights the disorder.
Schizoid	Isolation, autonomy	Reciprocity, intimacy	Disorder is relatively persistent.
Schizotypal	Bizarre behavior	Trust, social skills, abstract thinking	Individuals without the disorder who experience theft and ageism, leading to appropriate suspiciousness, may be misdiagnosed.
B. Dramatic, erratic			
Antisocial	Exploitative, taking advantage of others	Empathy	Older individuals are more law-abiding, and antisocial personality is less common in older prisoners.
Borderline	Sensitivity to rejection, feelings of abandonment	Reflection	Prevalence and/or severity of disorder declines with age.
Histrionic	Expressiveness, exhibitionism	Self-esteem beyond attractiveness, reflection	Older persons often have less energy and drive for promiscuity, shoplifting, and impulse expression.
Narcissistic	Self-aggrandizement, perceived specialness, competitiveness	Group identification, ability to share	Increased losses, such as retirement and bereavement, aggravate regulation of self-esteem.
C. Anxious, fearful			
Avoidant	Vulnerability, inhibition	Self-assertion, expressiveness	Disorder is associated with poor outcomes in major depression.
Dependent	Helplessness, attachment	Mobility, self-reliance	Individuals without the disorder who have fewer social opportunities and more medical illnesses may be subject to overdiagnosis.
Obsessive-compulsive	Perfectionism, overresponsibility, systematization	Playfulness, spontaneity	Disorder is relatively persistent.

Western countries estimated a prevalence of 8%–17% for all ages (Volkert et al. 2018). The prevalence of personality disorders in psychiatric settings is usually two to three times higher than that in the community (Schuster et al. 2013). Many general prevalence studies do not report age-stratified estimates (Quirk et al. 2016), possibly due to sample sizes that do not permit this type of subgroup analysis. In the few studies providing estimates, the prevalence of any personality disorder ranged from 5% to 10% in the general older adult population (Agronin and Maletta 2000; Schuster et al. 2013). Although personality disorders are typically thought to be less prevalent among older adults, a review of recent epidemiological studies estimated that late-life personality disorders occur in 10.6%–14.5% of community-dwelling older adults (Penders et al. 2020), similar to general adult findings. As in the general population, the prevalence of personality disorders in outpatient or inpatient samples of older persons is much higher than in community settings (Agronin and Maletta 2000; Ames and Molinari 1994). Personality disorders also appear to be more common in nursing home settings (Penders et al. 2020), although estimates in long-term care settings may be inflated due to the difficulty of diagnosing personality disorders in the presence of co-occurring or emerging NCDs.

Psychiatric comorbidities are common in patients with personality disorders. A meta-analytic review suggested that 42% and 45% of those with bipolar disorder and major depressive disorder, respectively, have a co-occurring personality disorder (Friborg et al. 2014). Similarly, co-occurring personality disorders are common across anxiety disorders (ranging from 35% in PTSD to 48% in social phobia) and are present in 52% of those with OCD (Friborg et al. 2013).

Personality disorders appear to decline in severity throughout the lifespan, especially for Cluster B disorders (Hunt 2007; Tracie Shea et al. 2009; Tyrer and Seiverwright 1988). Zanarini et al. (2007) reported the results of a 10-year follow-up study of 362 patients with personality disorders diagnosed at inpatient psychiatric admission. Twelve of 24 symptoms followed showed patterns of sharp decline, reported by <15% of the patients who reported them at baseline. Symptoms related to impulsivity (e.g., self-mutilation, suicide attempts) and entitlement resolved relatively quickly. Mood symptoms such as anger, loneliness, and emptiness were more stable. In a subsequent 16-year follow-up, Zanarini et al. (2013) found a corresponding improvement to more mature, adaptive defense mechanisms in patients with borderline personality disorder.

When evaluating the prevalence of late-life personality disorders, clinicians should also consider the possibility that the presence of a personality disorder increases mortality risk, as has been reported by some studies (Björkenstam et al. 2015; Fok et al. 2012; Tyrer et al. 2021). Among dimensional personality trait studies, lower conscientiousness and often higher neuroticism are also well-established risk factors for all-cause mortality (Graham et al. 2017). This increased mortality rate almost certainly arises from higher rates of underlying chronic disease and poorer disease management. Both higher levels of cardiovascular disease and of health service use (Lee et al. 2010; Powers et al. 2014; Quirk et al. 2016) have been reported in individuals with a personality disorder. Therefore, some evidence suggesting a decreased prevalence of personality disorders among older adults may simply reflect disproportionate early death. Reports of a lower prevalence of personality disorders in older persons have raised concerns that the assessment challenges noted earlier do not fully capture personality pathology in this group. One suggested response is to modify the criteria for personality disorders in later life (Agronin and Maletta 2000). Different explanations for the possible lower prevalence are not mutually exclusive, and other forces, such as diminished symptoms with age (Tyrer and Seiverwright 1988; Zanarini et al. 2007), also may be at work.

Prevalence estimates are challenging even in the general population at times, and this and other issues, such as the common co-occurrence of multiple disorders, have led to calls for a dimensional rather than categorical approach to personality pathology (Oldham and Skodol 2013). The FFM paradigm has proven fruitful in research in older adults examining associations between personality and depression (Hayward et al. 2013), cognitive function (Kuzma et al. 2011), dementia (Dar-Nimrod et al. 2012; Low et al. 2013), telomere length (van Ockenburg et al. 2014), health and physical functioning (Roberts et al. 2009), and mortality (Iwasa et al. 2008).

The developers of DSM-5 revisited a dimensional versus a categorical approach but ultimately remained with the DSM-IV categorical model (American Psychiatric Association 1994; Oldham and Skodol 2013). Although a dimensional approach may improve description and identification, it is less clear how the approach would be operationalized clinically, other than to revert to a categorical approach that uses cutoff scores on the dimensional scales. The dimensions represent versions of the FFM dimensions that emphasize pathological elements. This approach is called the "Alternative DSM-5 Model for Personality Disorders," and is located in Section III of DSM-5 (Widiger and Mullins-Sweatt 2009), and is proposed as a truly alternative model for clinical use, if preferred, rather than as a proposed axis for further study. The ICD-11 also recently instituted a dimensional assessment approach in which patients are first rated on severity of impairment and then on five similar pathological variants of the FFM dimensions (Bagby and Widiger 2020). These approaches were not motivated by any particular interest in aging, per se, but effectively provide a connection between the pathological personality literature and the more general personality literature based on the FFM.

Adult Development

One immediate use of the FFM literature is for understanding how traits change with age and the implications these patterns have for the course of personality pathology. People tend to decrease in neuroticism, extraversion, and openness with age while increasing in agreeableness and conscientiousness, with most changes occurring during young adulthood rather than later life (Roberts et al. 2006). This normative pattern of trait change is referred to as "maturation" and is consistent with the notion that maladaptive traits (i.e., high levels of neuroticism and low levels of conscientiousness) decrease over the life course. Perhaps most important with respect to geriatrics is that longitudinal twin studies have shown personality change in childhood to be primarily due to genetics, whereas most personality change in adulthood is environmental, including change caused by experience or disease (Roberts et al. 2006).

An interesting study of personality disorder traits in late-midlife adults (ages 55–65 years) found that, over 2.5 years, participants self-reported decreasing levels of pathological traits, whereas the informants who rated them reported stable or increasing levels (Cooper et al. 2014). Another longitudinal study of adults ages 20–60 years found marked decreases in nearly all pathological traits in an inpatient sample and similar but less pronounced changes in a community sample for whom the pathology was generally less severe (Ruiz et al. 2019). The one exception to this was for compulsive traits, which showed marked increases with age in both samples.

Studies of defense mechanisms also show a normative pattern of maturation across the life course. *Defenses* are involuntary mental mechanisms for regulating realities that persons are powerless to change. Vaillant (2012) and others (Haan 1977) classified humor, altruism, sublimation, anticipation, and suppression as mature defenses that synthesize and attenuate conflicts rather than distorting or denying them. Several studies have shown increasing reliance on mature defenses with age (Diehl et al. 1996; Glueck and Glueck 1968; Terman 1925; Vaillant 1993, 2012). Denial and other reality-distorting defenses are immature and maladaptive, and the criteria for most personality disorders suggest these defenses are used more frequently. For instance, maintaining a grandiose self-image (i.e., narcissistic personality disorder) can be thought of as a psychologically primitive defense against a fragile self-esteem. To the extent that personality disorder symptoms appear to moderate over the years, the life course of these disorders may be viewed as one that uses immature defenses and perhaps acquires slightly more mature ones with age. This may create the appearance of a developmental lag relative to an optimally functioning person, with patients with personality disorders in later life only beginning to show the level of basic coping normally seen much earlier.

To cope effectively with stress, individuals must learn to recognize the difference between situations that can and cannot be changed and then match the right coping skill with the right situation. Emotion-focused coping is used when a situation cannot be changed; problem-focused coping is used when a situation can be changed. It is only through repeated experience that these skills develop (Ryff 1999). Because personality disorders are long-standing and afflict most people for life, these patterns of coping will be delayed, never implemented, or implemented in a distorted, ineffectual fashion. Although stressful situations certainly exacerbate the symptoms of personality disorders, Neugarten (1970) pointed out how the meaning of stressful situations changes over time. People expect to experience the death of loved ones and anticipate their own declining health as they age and have time to mentally rehearse how they will respond to these "on-time" losses. When such losses occur "off-time"—at earlier stages of life—the stress is usually experienced as much greater. At any life stage, however, life stressors are likely to worsen the course of personality disorders because they present coping challenges to which people with personality disorders are not well equipped to respond. Social losses or illness later in life exacerbates personality disorder symptoms that may have been present far earlier but then diminished or remitted (Rosowsky and Gurian 1992).

Perhaps the most well-known and influential life course developmentalist is Erikson, who classified the major task of late life as resolving a crisis of "integrity vs. despair" (Erikson et al. 1986). The task that must be accomplished during later life, from this perspective, is to look back and find meaning in one's past; failure to do so leads to a state of despair, meaning that a possible mood disorder may appear superimposed on a personality pathology among older adults. Individuals with personality maladaptation lead a challenged life and may leave many failures in their wake by late life. Thus, the risk of looking back to find one's life misspent or dissatisfying is much higher for a person with a personality disorder and may serve as a target of psychotherapy if the patient is amenable to this modality.

Evaluation

Correctly identifying and diagnosing personality disorders can challenge even experienced clinicians. Contributing to this difficulty is that personality disorder and other psychiatric diagnoses often co-occur (Friborg et al. 2013, 2014), and symptoms and behaviors often span diagnostic categories. The potential role of NCDs in a patient's presentation also must be considered when evaluating older adults. Clinicians can use various methods and tools to help manage this diagnostic challenge. The Structured Clinical Interview for DSM-5 Personality Disorders (First et al. 2016) and the Personality Disorders Examination (Loranger 1988) are semistructured interviews for personality disorders that can be used to guide a diagnostic interview and increase reliability. However, these interviews follow the definitional criteria of personality disorders discussed earlier and must be conceptualized through an appropriate life-stage lens for older patients.

Historical information from medical records and from persons who have known the patient for a long period is an essential component of an accurate and valid diagnosis. Because personality disorder is not likely to appear spontaneously in later life, longitudinal inquiry about various life stages is needed to establish the historical presence of diagnostic criteria, even if not all current criteria are met. Several ancillary self-report instruments are available for initial screening purposes; however, these have a low concordance with interview methods (Perry 1992) and may overestimate the prevalence of personality disorders (Volkert et al. 2018). Additionally, a study finding that patients self-reported symptom reduction over 2.5 years, whereas their informants did not (Cooper et al. 2014), underscores the notion that people may see themselves differently than others who know them well. It is not that there will be no agreement across methods but that each method is likely to capture some unique insight into symptoms and functioning. A recent study found that self-reports, informant reports, and clinical interview ratings all contributed unique information to predicting health, marital satisfaction, and cognitive function in later life (Cruitt and Oltmanns 2018).

General personality inventories, as opposed to personality disorder instruments, may also be useful. The NEO Personality Inventory–Revised (NEO PI-R; Costa and McCrae 1992) is a comprehensive assessment of the FFM dimensions in which each dimension has six facets, or subcomponents. Considerable effort has gone into using these 30 facet scales to develop prototype profiles that correspond to various personality disorders (see Widiger and Mullins-Sweatt 2009). The NEO PI-R has also been used for personality disorders (Miller et al. 2005; Van den Broeck et al. 2013) and has been used in many studies of older adults, including inpatients with depression (e.g., Manning et al. 2017). However, this measure has 240 items, and copyright fee issues make it unwieldy for routine clinical use. Although DSM-5 did not make the recommended paradigm shift to a dimensional model of personality disorders (Oldham and Skodol 2013; Widiger and Mullins-Sweatt 2009), Section III of DSM-5 provided the alternative model described earlier that includes a five-factor personality trait model, with personality disorders understood as maladaptive variants of 5 domains and 25 facets. The Personality Inventory for DSM-5 (Krueger et al. 2012), an instrument derived from this model, is an "emerging measure" available for free at the American Psychiatric Association website (www.psychiatry.org/practice/dsm/dsm5/online-assessment-measures). For most clinicians, patients, and families, the full-length 220-item instrument is probably too cumbersome for routine use; therefore, brief forms are also available.

Perhaps the most important evaluation issue for older persons centers on distinguishing a true underlying personality disorder from NCDs. As noted, mild behavioral impairment can precede cognitive symptoms of dementia and can feature disinhibition (Ismail et al. 2016), which in turn can create the appearance of personality disorder symptoms (particularly those in Cluster B). Syndromes based on frontal lobe pathology that result in a decline in executive function present some of the most difficult diagnostic challenges, especially if the onset of symptoms is subtle, the rate of progression is slow, and the main attributes of the premorbid personality are obscure. Adults with frontal or frontotemporal lobe disease may show good preservation of memory function but are prone to trouble with mechanistic planning, verbal reasoning, or problem solving and "obeying the rules of interpersonal social behaviour, the experience of reward and punishment, and the interpretation of complex emotions" (Grafman and Litvan 1999; see also Passant et al. 2005). These difficulties are similar to some of the problems experienced by many people with borderline, narcissistic, histrionic, paranoid, and antisocial personality disorders. For many of these older adults with NCDs, diagnosing personality change due to another medical condition may be more appropriate than diagnosing a de novo personality disorder.

Treatment Issues

The broad focus of personality disorder treatment is on reducing symptoms, improving social functioning, and changing responses to the environment (Robinson 2005). Psychotherapy is typically regarded as a first-line treatment of personality disorders, with off-label use of psychotropic agents serving an adjunctive role for symptom reduction. Complicating treatment for many older adults with personality disorders, however, is that the pathology of these disorders (e.g., unstable relationships, avoidant or manipulative behaviors) can sabotage the formation of strong therapeutic alliances, adherence to treatment plans, and engagement in care.

Psychotherapy

As stated, psychotherapy is a first-line treatment of personality disorders. Review articles have suggested that cognitive-behavioral therapy (Matusiewicz et al. 2010) and long-term psychodynamic psychotherapy (Leichsenring and Rabung 2008) may be effective in treating personality disorders. A recent meta-analysis examined the effect of interventions on a wide variety of personality traits (Roberts et al. 2017). Most of the studies included (>75%) dealt with psychotherapy, and personality traits were grouped according to their FFM dimension. Most interventions were for standard presenting problems (e.g., depression, anxiety), and 12% were for personality disorders. The largest effect size was observed for neuroticism traits, which were reduced across all studies by an average of 0.5 SD. Supportive and cognitive-behavioral approaches fared best, and, in aggregate, studies indicated that ~8 weeks of treatment are needed. Studies focused on personality disorder treatment specifically showed an effect size of 0.5 SD across traits and modalities. Although these findings appear promising in general, the studies focused on patients with a mean age in their 30s and an overall age distribution, suggesting the inclusion of few, if any, older adults.

Psychotherapy focusing on older adults with personality disorders probably benefits from the general features of successful psychotherapy for geriatric patients, which include consistency, availability, empathic and respectful listening, flexibility, and open-mindedness on the part of the psychotherapist and are probably more important than a particular theoretical orientation (Clarkin et al. 2007). Some theoretical perspectives suggest that personality can change through a "bottom-up" focus on specific behaviors or patterns of daily life (Chapman et al. 2014) that views personality traits as the habitual patterns of behaviors, thoughts, and emotions occurring day in and day out. From this viewpoint, even if personality traits are assigned some higher-order, abstract existence, their manifestation in daily life is what matters for the person. For older patients, in whom behavior patterns are often quite ingrained, such an approach may be ineffective unless the patient is willing to work to alter maladaptive patterns. However, older adults experience a number of social, health, and living transitions, and such events present an opportunity to help them establish new, adaptive patterns.

Therapists who are not yet old themselves have a difficult challenge. They have no direct experience with or memory of being old (Rosowsky 1999). Some geriatric psychiatrists may be two full generations younger than their patients. Extraordinary empathy is required of these clinicians and of most practicing geriatric psychiatrists, who are usually caring for persons older than themselves.

Pharmacotherapy

Although no medications are approved by the FDA specifically for the treatment of personality disorders, patients with these disorders may be highly symptomatic, and pharmacotherapy targeted to defined symptom domains may be beneficial (Ingenhoven et al. 2010). The evidence base for these pharmacological approaches is poor, however (Bateman et al. 2015; Mazza et al. 2016). Patients with personality disorders are often on complex regimens of psychotropic medications and are at risk for polypharmacy (Starcevic and Janca 2018). Indeed, low levels of openness, extroversion, and conscientiousness have been associated with higher levels of psychotropic use (Sachs et al. 2014). Polypharmacy is particularly concerning for older adults because they are more susceptible to adverse medication reactions. Nonetheless, a personality disorder diagnosis should not preclude pharmacological treatment of concomitant psychiatric disorders, such as affective illness or psychosis, and of specific symptoms that may respond to psychotropic medications. Successful treatment of affective or psychotic symptoms may show that they were the result of these eminently treatable diseases rather than entrenched maladaptive personality traits. Personality disorder, depressive illness, and acquired brain disease share overlapping symptom constellations; symptoms such as irritability, hostility, and uncooperativeness can derive from all three.

A recent review found little evidence for the efficacy of psychotropic medication in Cluster A disorders (Mazza et al. 2016). Evidence does exist, however, for the use of selective serotonin reuptake inhibitors (SSRIs) in Cluster B disorders to improve emo-

TABLE 18–2.   **Symptom areas and pharmacotherapy classes in personality disorders**

Symptom area and types	Pharmacotherapy class
Cognition/Perception	
Loose associations, thought blocking	Antipsychotics
Overvalued ideas, delusions	
Hallucinations, depersonalization	
Affect/Mood	
Harm/avoidance	Selective serotonin reuptake inhibitors
Depression, lability	Mood stabilizers
Anger	Benzodiazepines
Anxiety	
Behavior	
Impulsivity	Mood stabilizers
Aggression	Antipsychotics
Novelty seeking	Tricyclic antidepressants, monoamine oxidase inhibitors
Reward/dependence	

tion regulation. Impulsive and aggressive symptoms may warrant consideration of mood stabilizers (Mazza et al. 2016), and second-generation antipsychotics may be useful for cognitive-perceptual symptoms (Black et al. 2014). Although Cluster C disorders lack robust evidence for medication efficacy, there is some suggestion that antidepressants may be useful, particularly SSRIs in the case of obsessive-compulsive personality disorder (Mazza et al. 2016).

Pharmacological treatment should be a systematic trial guided by three principles. First, a medication should be selected for an identified target symptom area (e.g., affect, impulsivity, aggression, anxiety) (Table 18–2). Second, trials should include a repeatable assessment strategy (e.g., global rating, self-report, or caregiver report targeted to symptom area). Third, trials should have a specified duration at the end of which a decision is made as to whether to continue the medication. SSRIs and other newer antidepressant drugs, anticonvulsants, and atypical antipsychotic drugs, used alone or in combination, may be useful in systematic trials for specified symptoms. The evidence is limited or mixed for geriatric patients, and caution is indicated, especially because of the side effects of antipsychotics (Maglione et al. 2011). Without a deliberate and thoughtful approach, patients with personality disorders are at high risk of polypharmacy (most patients with borderline personality disorder are taking three or more psychotropic medications) (Mazza et al. 2016). Exacerbating polypharmacy is that medications are unlikely to fully treat a personality disorder, and persistent residual symptoms can contribute to continual pressure on clinicians to increase and add medications.

Caregiver Education

Caregivers of patients with personality disorders are almost always aware of the patient's problems. However, they may not necessarily be aware that these patterns rise to the level of a mental disorder, albeit of a different kind than typical mood and anxiety disorders. Thus, education about a particular personality disorder or set of traits may be helpful. If dementia or a similar disorder has arisen and is superimposed on a preexisting personality disorder, clearly explain to caregivers how this may alter the patient's familiar behaviors. Patients with long-standing personality disorders can also have significant deficits in volitional capacity. Impulsivity in decision-making may render older persons more susceptible to financial scams targeting this demographic, and dependent personality features may render them more easily manipulated. At times, it may be necessary for the psychiatrist to evaluate the competence of a patient with a personality disorder and to consider proposing guardianship (Little and Little 2010). To the extent that dementia is superimposed upon a personality disorder, this decision may become more obvious.

Conclusion

Personality disorders typically begin far earlier in life, long before the patient is seen by a geriatric psychiatrist. It is important to understand the history and nature of these symptoms and how they have changed over time, if at all. Caregivers and other sources of information beyond the patient are particularly helpful in this task. Diagnostic criteria must be considered from an age-appropriate perspective, and DSM-5 offers an alternative dimensional system for characterizing personality dysfunction if an exact diagnosis is challenging. It is extremely important to distinguish between long-standing personality disorder symptoms and more recent behavior changes related to an emerging NCD. Treatment options are not well developed, and psychotherapy, pharmacotherapy, and caregiver support are the tools that must be judiciously used.

Key Points

- Personality problems may rise to the level of a formal disorder or exist in the form of subclinical maladaptive traits that impair a person's functioning to a lesser extent.

- Longitudinal history is necessary for determining whether presumed personality problems in later life are a manifestation of a personality disorder, a neurocognitive disorder, or both.

- Many issues in adult development shape the course of personality disorders over the life span, and there is some evidence that the severity of symptoms wanes. Normative age-related changes also exist and should not be mistaken for personality pathology.

- Data on the prevalence of personality disorders in older age groups are not as well developed as for younger groups. Nevertheless, some evidence suggests that personality disorders may be less prevalent among older groups. This may be due to early mortality, the inappropriateness of diagnostic criteria for older individuals, the natural remediation of symptoms with age, or some combination.

- Substantial evidence shows the negative effect of maladaptive personality traits on older adults as well as on medical and psychiatric comorbidities.

- It is possible and important to use psychotherapeutic and caregiver interventions to help older patients with personality disorders avoid behavior that significantly harms themselves or others.

- Systematic pharmacological treatment should include a target symptom area, an assessment strategy for that symptom area, and a specified duration of treatment.

Suggested Readings

Cruitt PJ, Oltmanns TF: Age-related outcomes associated with personality pathology in later life. Curr Opin Psychol 21:89–93, 2018 29073530

Oldham JM, Skodol AE: Personality and personality disorders, and the passage of time. Am J Geriatr Psychiatry 21(8):709–712, 2013 23711737

Vaillant GE: Triumphs of Experience: The Men of the Harvard Grant Study. Cambridge, MA, London, England, 2012

Tang TZ, DeRubeis RJ, Hollon SD, et al: Personality change during depression treatment: a placebo-controlled trial. Arch Gen Psychiatry 66(12):1322–1330, 2009 19996037

Winsper C, Bilgin A, Thompson A, et al: The prevalence of personality disorders in the community: a global systematic review and meta-analysis. Br J Psychiatry 216(2):69–78, 2020 31298170

References

Agronin ME, Maletta G: Personality disorders in late life: understanding and overcoming the gap in research. Am J Geriatr Psychiatry 8(1):4–18, 2000 10648290

American Psychiatric Association: Diagnostic and Statistical Manual of Mental Disorders, 4th Edition. Washington, DC, American Psychiatric Association, 1994

American Psychiatric Association: Diagnostic and Statistical Manual of Mental Disorders, 5th Edition. Arlington, VA, American Psychiatric Association, 2013

Ames A, Molinari V: Prevalence of personality disorders in community-living elderly. J Geriatr Psychiatry Neurol 7(3):189–194, 1994 7916944

Bagby RM, Widiger TA: Assessment of the ICD-11 dimensional trait model: an introduction to the special section. Psychol Assess 32(1):1–7, 2020 31750681

Balsis S, Carpenter BD, Storandt M: Personality change precedes clinical diagnosis of dementia of the Alzheimer type. J Gerontol B Psychol Sci Soc Sci 60(2):98–101, 2005 15746024

Balsis S, Gleason ME, Woods CM, Oltmanns TF: An item response theory analysis of DSM-IV personality disorder criteria across younger and older age groups. Psychol Aging 22(1):171–185, 2007 17385993

Baltes PB: On the incomplete architecture of human ontogeny: selection, optimization, and compensation as foundation of developmental theory. Am Psychol 52(4):366–380, 1997 9109347

Bateman AW, Gunderson J, Mulder R: Treatment of personality disorder. Lancet 385(9969):735–743, 2015 25706219

Björkenstam E, Björkenstam C, Holm H, et al: Excess cause-specific mortality in inpatient-treated individuals with personality disorder: 25-year nationwide population-based study. Br J Psychiatry 207(4):339–345, 2015 26159601

Black DW, Zanarini MC, Romine A, et al: Comparison of low and moderate dosages of extended-release quetiapine in borderline personality disorder: a randomized, double-blind, placebo-controlled trial. Am J Psychiatry 171(11):1174–1182, 2014 24968985

Carstensen LL, Fung HH, Charles ST: Socioemotional selectivity theory and the regulation of emotion in the second half of life. Motivation and Emotion 27(2):103–123, 2003

Caspi A, Roberts BW: Personality development across the life course: the argument for change and continuity. Psychol Inq 12(2):49–66, 2001

Chapman BP, Hampson S, Clarkin J: Personality-informed interventions for healthy aging: conclusions from a National Institute on Aging work group. Dev Psychol 50(5):1426–1441, 2014 23978300

Clarkin JF, Levy KN, Lenzenweger MF, Kernberg OF: Evaluating three treatments for borderline personality disorder: a multiwave study. Am J Psychiatry 164(6):922–928, 2007 17541052

Cooper LD, Balsis S, Oltmanns TF: Aging: empirical contribution: a longitudinal analysis of personality disorder dimensions and personality traits in a community sample of older adults: perspectives from selves and informants. J Pers Disord 28(1):151–165, 2014 24344895

Costa PT, McCrae RR: Revised NEO Personality Inventory (NEO PI-R) and NEO Five Factor Inventory (NEO-FFI) Professional Manual. Odessa, FL, Psychological Assessment Resources, 1992

Cruitt PJ, Oltmanns TF: Incremental validity of self- and informant report of personality disorders in later life. Assessment 25(3):324–335, 2018 28434236

Dar-Nimrod I, Chapman BP, Franks P, et al: Personality factors moderate the associations between apolipoprotein genotype and cognitive function as well as late onset Alzheimer disease. Am J Geriatr Psychiatry 20(12):1026–1035, 2012 23079898

Debast I, Rossi G, van Alphen SPJ, et al: Age neutrality of categorically and dimensionally measured DSM-5 Section II personality disorder symptoms. J Pers Assess 97(4):321–329, 2015 25833657

Diehl M, Coyle N, Labouvie-Vief G: Age and sex differences in strategies of coping and defense across the life span. Psychol Aging 11(1):127–139, 1996 8726378

Duchek JM, Balota DA, Storandt M, Larsen R: The power of personality in discriminating between healthy aging and early-stage Alzheimer's disease. J Gerontol B Psychol Sci Soc Sci 62(6):P353–P361, 2007 18079420

Erikson EH, Erikson JM, Kivnick HQ: Vital Involvement in Old Age. New York, WW Norton, 1986

First MB, Gibbon M, Spitzer RL, et al: Structured Clinical Interview for DSM-5 Axis II Personality Disorders. Washington, DC, American Psychiatric Publishing, 2016

Fok ML-Y, Hayes RD, Chang C-K, et al: Life expectancy at birth and all-cause mortality among people with personality disorder. J Psychosom Res 73(2):104–107, 2012 22789412

Friborg O, Martinussen M, Kaiser S, et al: Comorbidity of personality disorders in anxiety disorders: a meta-analysis of 30 years of research. J Affect Disord 145(2):143–155, 2013 22999891

Friborg O, Martinsen EW, Martinussen M, et al: Comorbidity of personality disorders in mood disorders: a meta-analytic review of 122 studies from 1988 to 2010. J Affect Disord 152–154:1–11, 2014 24120406

Glueck S, Glueck E: Delinquents and Non-Delinquents in Perspective. Cambridge, MA, Harvard University Press, 1968

Grafman J, Litvan I: Importance of deficits in executive functions. Lancet 354(9194):1921–1923, 1999 10622291

Graham EK, Rutsohn JP, Turiano NA, et al: Personality predicts mortality risk: an integrative data analysis of 15 international longitudinal studies. J Res Pers 70:174–186, 2017 29230075

Haan NA: Coping and Defending. San Francisco, CA, Jossey-Bass, 1977

Hawkley LC, Kocherginsky M: Transitions in loneliness among older adults: a 5-year follow-up in the National Social Life, Health, and Aging Project. Res Aging 40(4):365–387, 2018 29519211

Hayward RD, Taylor WD, Smoski MJ, et al: Association of five-factor model personality domains and facets with presence, onset, and treatment outcomes of major depression in older adults. Am J Geriatr Psychiatry 21(1):88–96, 2013 23290206

Hunt M: Borderline personality disorder across the lifespan. J Women Aging 19(1–2):173–191, 2007 17588886

Ingenhoven T, Lafay P, Rinne T, et al: Effectiveness of pharmacotherapy for severe personality disorders: meta-analyses of randomized controlled trials. J Clin Psychiatry 71(1):14–25, 2010 19778496

Ismail Z, Smith EE, Geda Y, et al: Neuropsychiatric symptoms as early manifestations of emergent dementia: provisional diagnostic criteria for mild behavioral impairment. Alzheimers Dement 12(2):195–202, 2016 26096665

Iwasa H, Masui Y, Gondo Y, et al: Personality and all-cause mortality among older adults dwelling in a Japanese community: a five-year population-based prospective cohort study. Am J Geriatr Psychiatry 16(5):399–405, 2008 18403571

Krueger RF, Derringer J, Markon KE, et al: Initial construction of a maladaptive personality trait model and inventory for DSM-5. Psychol Med 42(9):1879–1890, 2012 22153017

Kuzma E, Sattler C, Toro P, et al: Premorbid personality traits and their course in mild cognitive impairment: results from a prospective population-based study in Germany. Dement Geriatr Cogn Disord 32(3):171–177, 2011 22005607

Lee HB, Bienvenu OJ, Cho S-J, et al: Personality disorders and traits as predictors of incident cardiovascular disease: findings from the 23-year follow-up of the Baltimore ECA study. Psychosomatics 51(4):289–296, 2010 20587756

Leichsenring F, Rabung S: Effectiveness of long-term psychodynamic psychotherapy: a meta-analysis. JAMA 300(13):1551–1565, 2008 18827212

Little J, Little B: Borderline personality disorder: exceptions to the concept of responsible and competent. Australas Psychiatry 18(5):445–450, 2010 20863185

Loranger AW: Personality Disorders Examination (PDE) Manual. Yonkers, NY, DV Communications, 1988

Low LF, Harrison F, Lackersteen SM: Does personality affect risk for dementia? A systematic review and meta-analysis. Am J Geriatr Psychiatry 21(8):713–728, 2013 23567438

Maglione M, Maher AR, Hu J, et al: Off-Label Use of Atypical Antipsychotics: An Update. Comparative Effectiveness Reviews, No 43. Rockville, MD, Agency for Healthcare Research and Quality, 2011. Available at: http://www.ncbi.nlm.nih.gov/books/NBK66081. Accessed June 7, 2014.

Manning KJ, Chan G, Steffens DC: Neuroticism traits selectively impact long term illness course and cognitive decline in late-life depression. Am J Geriatr Psychiatry 25(3):220–229, 2017 27825555

Matusiewicz AK, Hopwood CJ, Banducci AN, Lejuez CW: The effectiveness of cognitive behavioral therapy for personality disorders. Psychiatr Clin North Am 33(3):657–685, 2010 20599139

Mazza M, Marano G, Janiri L: An update on pharmacotherapy for personality disorders. Expert Opin Pharmacother 17(15):1977–1979, 2016 27487174

Miller JD, Bagby RM, Pilkonis PA, et al: A simplified technique for scoring DSM-IV personality disorders with the five-factor model. Assessment 12(4):404–415, 2005 16244121

Neugarten BL: Dynamics of transition of middle age to old age. adaptation and the life cycle. J Geriatr Psychiatry 4(1):71–100, 1970 5527462

Newton-Howes G, Clark LA, Chanen A: Personality disorder across the life course. Lancet 385(9969):727–734, 2015 25706218

Oldham JM, Skodol AE: Personality and personality disorders, and the passage of time. Am J Geriatr Psychiatry 21(8):709–712, 2013 23711737

Passant U, Elfgren C, Englund E, Gustafson L: Psychiatric symptoms and their psychosocial consequences in frontotemporal dementia. Alzheimer Dis Assoc Disord 19(suppl 1):S15–S18, 2005 16317252

Penders KAP, Peeters IGP, Metsemakers JFM, van Alphen SPJ: Personality disorders in older
    adults: a review of epidemiology, assessment, and treatment. Curr Psychiatry Rep 22(3):14,
    2020 32025914

Perry JC: Problems and considerations in the valid assessment of personality disorders. Am J
    Psychiatry 149(12):1645–1653, 1992 1443240

Powers A, Strube MJ, Oltmanns TF: Personality pathology and increased use of medical re-
    sources in later adulthood. Am J Geriatr Psychiatry 22(12):1478–1486, 2014 24315559

Quirk SE, Berk M, Chanen AM, et al: Population prevalence of personality disorder and asso-
    ciations with physical health comorbidities and health care service utilization: a review.
    Pers Disord 7(2):136–146, 2016 26461047

Roberts BW, Walton KE, Viechtbauer W: Patterns of mean-level change in personality traits
    across the life course: a meta-analysis of longitudinal studies. Psychol Bull 132(1):1–25,
    2006 16435954

Roberts BW, Smith J, Jackson JJ, Edmonds G: Compensatory conscientiousness and health in
    older couples. Psychol Sci 20(5):553–559, 2009 19476589

Roberts BW, Luo J, Briley DA, et al: A systematic review of personality trait change through
    intervention. Psychol Bull 143(2):117–141, 2017 28054797

Robins Wahlin TB, Byrne GJ: Personality changes in Alzheimer's disease: a systematic review.
    Int J Geriatr Psychiatry 26(10):1019–1029, 2011 21905097

Robinson DJ: Field Guide to Personality Disorders, 2nd Edition. Port Huron, MI, Rapid Psy-
    chler Press, 2005

Robinson SA, Lachman ME: Perceived control and aging: a mini-review and directions for fu-
    ture research. Gerontology 63(5):435–442, 2017 28391279

Rosowsky E: Personality disorders and the difficult nursing home resident, in Personality Dis-
    orders in Older Adults: Emerging Issues in Diagnosis and Treatment. Edited by Rosowsky
    E, Abrams RC. Mahwah, NJ, Erlbaum, 1999, pp 257–274

Rosowsky E, Gurian B: Impact of borderline personality disorder in late life on systems of care.
    Hosp Community Psychiatry 43(4):386–389, 1992 1577432

Ruiz J, Gutiérrez F, Peri JM, et al: Mean-level change in pathological personality dimensions
    over 4 decades in clinical and community samples: a cross-sectional study. Personal Dis-
    ord 11(6):409–417, 2019 31855004

Ryff CD: Psychology and aging, in Principles of Geriatric Medicine and Gerontology, 4th Edi-
    tion. Edited by Hazzard WR, Blass JP, Ettinger WH, et al. New York, McGraw-Hill, 1999,
    pp 159–169

Sachs GS, Peters AT, Sylvia L, Grunze H: Polypharmacy and bipolar disorder: what's person-
    ality got to do with it? Int J Neuropsychopharmacol 17(7):1053–1061, 2014 24067291

Schulz R, Heckhausen J: A life span model of successful aging. Am Psychol 51(7):702–714, 1996
    8694390

Schuster JP, Hoertel N, Le Strat Y, et al: Personality disorders in older adults: findings from the
    National Epidemiologic Survey on Alcohol and Related Conditions. Am J Geriatr Psychi-
    atry 21(8):757–768, 2013 23567365

Starcevic V, Janca A: Pharmacotherapy of borderline personality disorder: replacing confusion
    with prudent pragmatism. Curr Opin Psychiatry 31(1):69–73, 2018 29028643

Terman LM: Genetic Studies of Genius, Vol 1: Mental and Physical Traits of a Thousand Gifted
    Children. Palo Alto, CA, Stanford University Press, 1925

Tracie Shea M, Edelen MO, Pinto A, et al: Improvement in borderline personality disorder in
    relationship to age. Acta Psychiatr Scand 119(2):143–148, 2009 18851719

Tyrer P, Seiverwright H: Studies of outcome, in Personality Disorders: Diagnosis, Management
    and Course. Edited by Tyrer P. London, Wright, 1988, pp 119–136

Tyrer P, Tyrer H, Yang M: Premature mortality of people with personality disorder in the Not-
    tingham Study of Neurotic Disorder. Pers Ment Health 15(1):32–39, 2021 31414571

Vaillant GE: The Wisdom of the Ego. Cambridge, MA, Harvard University Press, 1993

Vaillant GE: Triumphs of Experience: The Men of the Harvard Grant Study. Cambridge, MA,
    Harvard University Press, 2012

Van den Broeck J, Rossi G, De Clercq B, et al: Validation of the FFM PD count technique for screening personality pathology in later middle-aged and older adults. Aging Ment Health 17(2):180–188, 2013 22913535

van Ockenburg SL, de Jonge P, van der Harst P, et al: Does neuroticism make you old? Prospective associations between neuroticism and leukocyte telomere length. Psychol Med 44(4):723–729, 2014 23834823

Volkert J, Gablonski TC, Rabung S: Prevalence of personality disorders in the general adult population in Western countries: systematic review and meta-analysis. Br J Psychiatry 213(6):709–715, 2018 30261937

Widiger TA, Mullins-Sweatt SN: Five-factor model of personality disorder: a proposal for DSM-V. Annu Rev Clin Psychol 5:197–220, 2009 19046124

Zanarini MC, Frankenburg FR, Reich DB, et al: The subsyndromal phenomenology of borderline personality disorder: a 10-year follow-up study. Am J Psychiatry 164(6):929–935, 2007 17541053

Zanarini MC, Frankenburg FR, Fitzmaurice G: Defense mechanisms reported by patients with borderline personality disorder and Axis II comparison subjects over 16 years of prospective follow-up: description and prediction of recovery. Am J Psychiatry 170(1):111–120, 2013 23223866

CHAPTER 19

Agitation in Older Adults

Juan Joseph Young, M.D.

Rajesh R. Tampi, M.D., M.S.

Agitation has historically been one of the most difficult neuropsychiatric symptoms to treat in older adults. Unlike younger cohorts, elderly patients are more likely to present with a diverse set of both medical and psychiatric diagnoses that could contribute to the development of irritability, restlessness, anxiety, and combativeness as part of the initial presentation. Several causative factors are often associated with agitation, including new-onset delirium due to deteriorating medical conditions and worsening major neurocognitive disorders that promote aggressive verbal and physical activity, wandering, disorientation, and poor impulse control. Thus, the distress these symptoms could cause is significant and often impacts the ability of caregivers and health care providers to provide appropriate care and support to elderly adults. Consequently, agitation is one of the more common reasons for consultation with a geriatric psychiatrist (Wilson et al. 2019). This chapter focuses on the epidemiology, diagnosis, and management of agitation in elderly adults.

Epidemiology

Agitation is a part of a collective set of neuropsychiatric symptoms of dementia commonly termed "behavioral disturbances." Behavioral disturbances are common in more elderly adults and are estimated to occur in 30%–90% of patients with dementia (Müller-Spahn 2003). In addition to agitation, behavioral disturbances include depression, anxiety, psychosis, disinhibition, and sleep disturbance (Lyketsos et al. 2011). These behaviors produce elevated levels of distress in both the patient and family care-

We would like to thank Harold W. Goforth, M.D., Mugdha E. Thakur, M.D., and Lisa P. Gwyther, M.S.W., LCSW, who were coauthors of previous editions of this chapter.

givers (Gitlin et al. 2012). Agitation is one of the most common behavioral disturbances, reported to be present in ≤70% of patients with dementia (Chen et al. 2018; Ijaopo 2017), although prevalence rates of agitation vary widely depending on the geographical region (Anatchkova et al. 2019). Agitation may be described by caregivers in various ways and often includes disruptive and aggressive behaviors that create stressful situations in both long-term care facilities and the community. It is also a common component of hyperactive delirium, and patients previously diagnosed with neurocognitive disorders are more likely to exhibit both delirium and agitation (Fong et al. 2009). Agitation has been associated with lower quality of life and more severe cognitive impairment, which is consistent with postulations that neuropsychiatric symptoms, particularly agitation, are associated with worsening deficits in multiple cortical structures, including the frontal cortex, cingulate cortex, amygdala, and hippocampus (Rosenberg et al. 2015; Weissberger et al. 2017). This outcome is highly reflected in one recent study that found that residents of a large care home who were diagnosed with moderate or severe dementia were more likely to exhibit clinically significant agitation and to have a lower quality of life than residents with milder forms of dementia (Livingston et al. 2017). Other correlates with frequent agitation include advanced age, delusions, anxiety, euphoria, and irritability (Veldwijk-Rouwenhorst et al. 2017). Thus, a geriatric psychiatry clinician must be able to adequately diagnose and treat agitation due to the deleterious effects it may have on both patient and caregiver well-being (Chen et al. 2018).

Diagnosis and Evaluation

When elderly patients present with agitation, the initial step in management is a thorough and comprehensive psychiatric evaluation. The clinical course and timing of the agitation provide clues to its etiology. Agitation is also often a response to changes in the environment, routine, or the person's perspective of a caregiver. Eliciting the nature and characteristics of the reported agitation is therefore important for determining the significance of these behaviors. Expressions of discomfort and increased irritability after physical activity may suggest that the agitated behavior is a result of pain or physical issues. Disorientation and confusion could portend sensory deficits that may be alleviated with nonpharmacological interventions, such as providing corrective lenses or hearing aids after optometry and audiometry evaluation, respectively. Alternatively, agitation in the context of suspiciousness and guarded behaviors reflects a more paranoid mindset that may improve with psychotropic treatment. In this way, the clinician is more able to rule out or elevate possible etiologies of the agitated behavior and treat them appropriately. It should be noted that a suspicious and guarded demeanor may not always be explained by a psychotic thought process, and every effort should be made to investigate any potential neglect that could necessitate the involvement of adult protective services.

As mentioned, cases of sudden episodes of agitation may stem from distress due to acute medical conditions (Nordstrom et al. 2012). Developing an exhaustive differential of possible diagnoses, completing an appropriate medical workup, and providing prompt treatment of these acute medical issues often leads to the rapid resolution of agitated episodes. In these situations, a full medical evaluation and examination are necessary to rule out common medical causes of agitation and hyperactive delirium. Obtaining a detailed history of the onset and course of symptoms from the caregiver helps detect more acute processes that may cause delirium and distinguish them from the longer-term and more insidious course characteristic of dementia (Stroomer-van Wijk et al. 2016). The initial laboratory workup should include a complete blood count and a comprehensive metabolic panel because these tests could reveal an infection, anemia, or electrolyte abnormalities. In addition, obtaining a urinalysis and a urine culture would help rule out a urinary tract infection, which has been associated with irritability and aggressive behaviors in older adults (Hodgson et al. 2011). Any shortness of breath, cough, or fever should prompt clinicians to rule out a respiratory infection, and a chest X-ray should be ordered as part of the clinical workup. Focal neurological findings could be indicative of a recent stroke that could cause confusion and agitated behavior. A history of a recent fall would suggest an occult head trauma that should be evaluated utilizing neurological imaging modalities such as CT or MRI of the brain. Other reversible etiologies of agitation include adverse events from medications due to polypharmacy, poor nutrition (e.g., vitamin B_{12} or D deficiency), gastrointestinal/ genitourinary symptoms (e.g., feeling of a full bladder or constipation), and a history of alcohol or substance dependence (because withdrawal syndromes could precipitate agitated behavior).

Nonpharmacological Management

Management of agitation can be difficult and may vary depending on the setting and the resources available to caregivers and health care providers. Contemporary guidelines suggest trying both preventative and active nonpharmacological interventions before trying medications, to avoid the potential adverse effects of psychotropics—especially the atypical antipsychotics, which have been reported to have only modest short-term benefits with limited long-term therapeutic effect (Ballard et al. 2009). These strategies should focus on improving patient safety, modifying stimulation and cues, and providing a reassuring environment to ameliorate any agitated behavior that emerges, with a focus on the behaviors that are most disruptive to both the family and the patient.

It is also important to provide psychoeducation and training to caregivers regarding the nature of the dementia disease process. Families and caregivers of persons with dementia may interpret agitation in a negative light and feel personally attacked by these behaviors. Health care providers should inform caregivers that agitated behavior is neither intentional nor completely under a patient's control and that ignoring disruptive behaviors is unlikely to resolve these episodes. Caregivers should also be educated regarding common communication strategies for deescalating situations, such as maintaining an emphatic, reassuring, respectful, friendly, and calm demeanor and avoiding concrete or vague orders/responses that could project an authoritarian or potentially insulting tone and worsen the patient's agitation. Because family and caregivers are the closest to the patient, they should also be educated that it is common for people with dementia to target their frustrations on close relations while remaining civil and pleasant with strangers.

Agitated behavior typically has a triggering event or precipitating factor, but this will not always be evident. It is important to obtain a thorough history and gain insight into the patient's and family's preferences and perspectives as to the possible reasons for the disruptive behavior. Family members and caregivers should describe the type of behavior occurring because the frequency, timing, and duration are important for formulating an effective treatment plan. It should also be noted how severe the behavior is and how much the caregivers are able to tolerate it. Clinicians should also obtain information regarding caregivers' responses to the behavior that may exacerbate and worsen the patient's agitation. If the patient has been exposed to environmental changes that could cause the disorientation associated with agitated behaviors, modifying his or her daily routines or surrounding stimuli may minimize the risk of agitation. With this information, nonpharmacological interventions could be tailored to specific circumstances. If a triggering event is identified, reducing agitation would typically revolve around redirection of the agitated person's attention away from the event with calming activities that the person enjoys (e.g., going for a car ride, receiving a treat, talking about sports).

Behavioral modifications are effective tools to be implemented in the management of agitation and include approaches that are specific to individuals, such as physical and mental exercises (e.g., problem-solving tasks), enriched cues, expressive activities, and communication strategies. If agitation originates from difficulties in functioning and understanding, developing strategies to simplify tasks may help prevent the person from becoming overwhelmed because of deteriorating cognitive functioning. Slowing the pace of any activities in which a patient with dementia may partake prevents overstimulation that could then lead to frustration and anger. Optimizing cognitive and environmental factors through labeling, setting alarm clock reminders, using pictures, removing hazardous objects or risk factors (e.g., guns or fall hazards), and using lighting appropriately during the day and night may help decreasing the person's uncertainty and confusion and therefore lessen the risk of future episodes of agitation.

Regarding specific evidence-based approaches, several systematic and literature reviews have been conducted to investigate the effectiveness of nonpharmacological interventions in elderly adults (Abraha et al. 2017; Barton et al. 2016; Cammisuli et al. 2016; de Oliveira et al. 2015). Music therapy has been reported to reduce overall neuropsychiatric symptoms such as depression and anxiety in Alzheimer's disease (AD) but has not been as successful in reducing agitated behavior in the long term (Cammisuli et al. 2016; Ledger and Baker 2007). One meta-analysis suggested evidence of effectiveness (Forbes et al. 2014), although this is limited by the heterogeneity and variability of the type of music therapy intervention administered. Bright light therapy in the morning and afternoon has some evidence for alleviating agitation and aggression in patients with dementia, but the magnitude of these changes may be relatively minimal and have limited clinical effect (Burns et al. 2011; Dowling et al. 2007). In contrast, a 2014 Cochrane review of eight studies found no statistically significant effect of light therapy on cognition, sleep, or neuropsychiatric symptoms, including agitation (Forbes et al. 2014). Another systematic review reported that a limited number of studies have yielded mixed results about the effectiveness of sensory stimulation interventions, such as aromatherapy and massage therapy, in reducing agitated behaviors (Abraha et al. 2017). However, the authors found a growing body of evidence suggesting that behavioral management techniques and enhanced communication skills involving formal caregiver training in residential care were effective in reducing agitation. A similar sentiment was advocated by Caspar et al. (2018), who found that ongoing training, education, and support of caregivers, along with consideration of the physical and social environment impacting the patient, promoted the most optimal opportunities and interventions for decreasing behavioral and psychological symptoms of dementia. This supports the "person-centered care model" to alleviate agitation related to older adults' concerns that their needs are not being met (Cohen-Mansfield 2001).

Regarding postoperative delirium, the American Geriatrics Society's clinical practice guidelines recommend that an interdisciplinary team develop multicomponent nonpharmacological interventions to prevent the development of agitation after a medical procedure in at-risk older adults (American Geriatrics Society Expert Panel on Postoperative Delirium in Older Adults 2015; Oh et al. 2017). Such interventions include mobilizing and ambulating patients soon after the procedure, avoiding physical restraints, orienting to surroundings, maintaining optimal sleep hygiene, and providing adequate oxygen flow, nutritional supplementation, and fluid repletion when clinically indicated. The guidelines also recommend thorough medical evaluations to manage any other underlying or emerging organic disorders that could be contributing to the agitation and delirium. Pain management should be optimized while avoiding deliriogenic opioids. This is reflected in a study conducted by Husebo et al. (2011), who reported that implementing a pain management protocol for 8 weeks improved agitation more effectively than treatment as usual. Policies advocating the avoidance of pharmacological agents that precipitate or exacerbate delirium episodes (e.g., benzodiazepines, anticholinergic medications, and opioids) should be instituted. Optimizing the patient's vision and hearing would also decrease the risk of disorientation and subsequent agitation episodes.

Recently published National Institute for Health and Clinical Excellence guidelines and Hospital Elder Life Program protocols provide similar recommendations for decreasing the incidence of delirium in hospitalized patients. They emphasize continually reorienting the patient; optimizing cognitive functioning; treating dehydration, constipation, and hypoxia; treating infectious etiologies; providing adequate nutrition; encouraging early mobilization; adequately treating pain; discontinuing any potentially offending agents; optimizing sensory functioning; and instituting a sleep enhancement protocol (Yue et al. 2014)

Pharmacological Treatment of Agitation

Agitated behaviors can occur in the context of delirium, late-life depression, or worsening cognitive impairment in patients with dementia. It is imperative to determine the root causes of the agitation episodes so that appropriate interventions may be administered promptly. At times, psychotropics may be necessary to maintain safety and appropriate levels of care for elderly patients. However, currently no pharmacological agents have FDA approval for the treatment of agitation in dementia. Given the potential adverse effects and limited long-term efficacy associated with the psychotropic drugs commonly used to treat agitation (Ballard et al. 2009), administration of these medications must only occur under specific circumstances—that is, when agitated episodes become severe enough to put patients at acute risk of harming themselves or others or when their distress is significant enough to negatively affect their care or over-

all functioning. In these circumstances, pharmacological treatment may become necessary, but only after a thorough risk-benefit analysis has been completed and discussed
with the patient's caregivers and legal representatives. Escalating verbal and physical
aggression that is not readily redirected or alleviated by nonpharmacological interventions may warrant acute psychotropic administration, such as atypical neuroleptics, because other classes of psychotropics may either take too long to take effect, such as
antidepressants, or cause further confusion or agitation, such as benzodiazepines. (Benzodiazepine administration may worsen confusion and irritability and cause paradoxical disinhibition, although this medication class would be a suitable treatment for
managing delirium due to alcohol or benzodiazepine withdrawal.) The following sections discuss the current literature on and evidence for using different psychotropic
classes and treatment modalities for decreasing agitated behaviors.

Antipsychotics

Antipsychotics have been one of the most studied classes of psychotropics for treating
agitation in elderly adults. Presently, placebo-controlled trials demonstrating efficacy
of antipsychotics for agitation in dementia have reported improvement with risperidone, aripiprazole, haloperidol, olanzapine, and quetiapine. One systematic review
of these trials suggested a small but statistically significant effect for aripiprazole,
olanzapine, and risperidone on neuropsychiatric symptoms, including psychosis,
mood alterations, and aggression (Maglione et al. 2011). The overall effect size of these
agents is small (0.16), with haloperidol exhibiting comparable efficacy with most
atypical antipsychotics (Schneider et al. 2006). However, atypical antipsychotics have
been reported to produce a significant side effect burden and have been found to increase the risk of somnolence, urinary tract infection or incontinence, extrapyramidal
symptoms or abnormal gait, and worsening of cognition (Schneider et al. 2006; Maher
et al. 2011). The number needed to harm (NNH) for certain atypical antipsychotics
varies but is notable. The stroke NNH was 53 for risperidone, the extrapyramidal
symptoms NNH was 10 for olanzapine and 20 for risperidone, and the urinary symptoms NNH ranged from 16 to 36 (Maher et al. 2011).

Of all the adverse events associated with antipsychotic use in patients with dementia, however, clinicians must be most aware of the mortality risk and black box warning for these agents, as demonstrated by large-scale meta-analyses of clinical trials
that have reported a 1.5-fold to 1.7-fold greater risk of mortality when atypical antipsychotics were prescribed to patients with dementia (Steinberg and Lyketsos 2012).
One group was able to calculate the number needed to treat (NNT) and NNH when
using atypical antipsychotics and found that one death occurred for every 9–25 agitated patients with dementia who were treated with an atypical antipsychotic (Jeste
et al. 2008). With these data in hand, the FDA instituted a black box warning for atypical antipsychotics in 2005 and then expanded the warning in 2008 to include typical
antipsychotics (Dorsey et al. 2010). For this reason, clinicians should obtain informed
consent while educating patients or their legal representatives regarding the potential
risks and black box warnings of antipsychotics, relative to their potential benefits.

Information is limited regarding individual antipsychotic risk of increasing mortality, although Kales et al. (2012) produced a large retrospective cohort study with the
most extensive data available to answer this question. They obtained information from
the U.S. Department of Veterans Affairs (fiscal years 1999–2008) on 33,604 patients age

65 years and older who were diagnosed with dementia and began outpatient treatment with an antipsychotic (i.e., risperidone, olanzapine, quetiapine, or haloperidol) or valproic acid and its derivatives. They found that haloperidol produced the highest mortality rates (relative risk [RR] 1.54; 95% CI 1.38–1.73), followed by risperidone (used as a reference), olanzapine (RR 0.99; 95% CI 0.89–1.10), valproic acid and its derivatives (RR 0.91; 95% CI 0.78–1.06), and quetiapine (RR 0.73; 95% CI 0.67–0.80). The authors noted that the mortality risk with haloperidol was the highest in the first 30 days but decreased sharply afterward, whereas among the other agents, mortality risk was most significant in the first 120 days but declined after the first 60 days during follow-up (Kales et al. 2012). Thus, due to this significant side effect profile, antipsychotic medications should be safely tapered and withdrawn once the patient is clinically stable unless the patient would continue to benefit from them (e.g., in the presence of severe neuropsychiatric symptoms at baseline) (Declercq et al. 2013).

Mood Stabilizers

Mood stabilizers have been important alternatives to antipsychotics for agitation treatment. Unfortunately, despite their demonstrated effectiveness in treating psychiatric symptoms in younger cohorts, they are used less often in the elderly population due to the perception of relatively severe side effects and the need for strict monitoring. For example, when prescribing carbamazepine, clinicians must monitor the patient's drug levels and look for electrolyte abnormalities (e.g., hyponatremia), agranulocytosis, and drug–drug interactions due to its effect on the hepatic cytochrome P450 enzyme system. With lithium, one must monitor creatine levels, electrolytes, and kidney and thyroid function and collect regular blood levels due to its narrow therapeutic window. Valproic acid also requires regular drug level monitoring to avoid supratherapeutic levels that could lead to worsening impairment of cognition, sedation, or encephalopathy, and it is contraindicated in patients with severe hepatic dysfunction. Of the mood stabilizers used, carbamazepine and valproic acid have been the most studied for agitation in dementia, although lithium is being increasingly investigated for use in reducing the severity of agitation episodes.

Earlier studies investigating carbamazepine have found it to be associated with improvements in agitation and aggression in nursing home patients while still being well tolerated at a modal dosage of 300 mg/day (average serum level in participants 5.3 µg/mL) (Tariot et al. 1998). Another, smaller study found that a 400-mg daily dosage produced similar effects, although patients in the carbamazepine group unfortunately tended to experience worsening hallucinations (Olin et al. 2001). Alternatively, valproic acid is more widely used in clinical practice for agitation and irritability, although high rates of adverse events may prevent it from reaching therapeutic levels and, by extension, achieving its potential efficacy in older adults (Lonergan and Luxenberg 2009; Tariot et al. 2001, 2005). In a study by Tariot et al. (2001), half of the patients given valproic acid dropped out compared with only one-third of the control group; 22% of the valproic acid group was reportedly lost to attrition due to adverse effects. The recent GERI-BD study (Young et al. 2017) investigating the effectiveness of lithium and valproic acid in managing mania and hypomania in geriatric outpatients age 60 years and older suggested that study participants tolerated both mood stabilizers well, although most may have been relatively healthy and not as burdened by medical comorbidities due to the study's exclusion criteria.

Currently, data are limited regarding the use of lithium as monotherapy or as an adjunctive therapy to treat agitated behaviors in older adults, likely due to its narrow therapeutic window and relatively severe adverse effects, including worsening cognition. However, some evidence indicates that lithium may provide a therapeutic effect for agitation in patients with dementia. This is supported by a recent case series (Devanand et al. 2017) of three patients with AD and three patients with frontotemporal dementia that reported that augmenting antipsychotics and antidepressants with lithium 300–600 mg/day was associated with improvements in multiple neuropsychiatric domains, including agitation and aggression. Consequently, studies are being developed to determine if lithium could be prescribed to alleviate agitation episodes in elderly adults as an alternative to antipsychotics. The Lithium Treatment for Agitation in Alzheimer's Disease study (Devanand et al. 2018) is a randomized, double-blind, placebo-controlled trial designed to investigate the efficacy of lithium treatment for agitation or aggression in participants with AD. Patients were randomly assigned to either placebo or a low dosage of lithium (150–600 mg) with target blood levels of 0.2–0.6 mmol/L for 12 weeks. The group recently published their findings reporting improvement with lithium compared with placebo when treating delusions, irritability, lability, and overall mania symptoms ($P<0.05$), although lithium was not significantly better than placebo for agitation or aggression after conducting linear mixed effects models analyses (Devanand et al. 2021).

Antidepressants

The most prescribed antidepressants for agitation are the selective-serotonin reuptake inhibitors. Citalopram has the most data available from placebo-controlled trials. It has been demonstrated that treatment with citalopram improved agitation in patients with dementia with efficacy similar to that of antipsychotics (Pollock et al. 2002, 2007; Porsteinsson et al. 2014). A more recent study investigating the effect of citalopram augmentation with memantine to decrease neuropsychiatric symptoms in patients with AD found that although both groups (memantine + citalopram vs. memantine + placebo) had significantly improved Neuropsychiatric Inventory (NPI) total scores after a 12-week period, the group that received citalopram exhibited significantly lower scores in apathy, dysphoria, and anxiety domains (Zhou et al. 2019). However, citalopram has been associated with QT prolongation and modest worsening of cognition, which may make it intolerable in a subset of the geriatric patient population. At least a portion of its therapeutic effect on agitation may be due to its sedative effects (Newell et al. 2016), and citalopram exhibits a more significant side effect burden than its S-enantiomer, escitalopram (Ho et al. 2016). This side effect profile may be the reason why citalopram potentially provides maximal benefit only in those with milder cognitive impairment and moderate levels of agitation. One study (Schneider et al. 2016) found that citalopram administration may be potentially more harmful and less effective in those with more severe cognitive impairment and agitation compared with those with less cognitive impairment and those being treated on an outpatient basis.

As for other serotonergic agents, at least two studies have been investigated the use of escitalopram for agitation in AD. One group found that escitalopram demonstrated similar efficacy to risperidone in treating neuropsychiatric symptoms, including psychosis and agitation, while exhibiting a more favorable side effect profile, thus allowing for a higher completion rate than the antipsychotic comparator group (Barak et al. 2011). Supporting this, another group reported preliminary data indicating a decrease in agitation symptoms within 6 weeks of treatment with escitalopram (Zmuc Veranic et al. 2016). In contrast, Lyketsos et al. (2003) found sertraline to be an effective treatment of depression in patients with dementia, but it did not seem to improve neuropsychiatric symptoms except in those who responded to it for mood symptoms. One study investigating the efficacy of trazodone, haloperidol, and behavioral management techniques did not find a difference between the placebo group and any of the treatment groups (Teri et al. 2000). Another, smaller study found that trazodone was relatively effective in treating agitation in patients with frontotemporal dementia (Lebert et al. 2004).

Cholinesterase Inhibitors and NMDA Receptor Antagonists

Several studies have been conducted to determine whether improving cognition could lessen agitated behavior. The Cholinesterase Inhibitor and Atypical Neuroleptic in the Management of Agitation in Alzheimer's Disease study (Howard et al. 2007) was a placebo-controlled trial investigating the effect of donepezil 10 mg/day for the treatment of agitation in patients with dementia due to AD. The study found no significant effect with donepezil compared with placebo after 12 weeks. Rodda et al. (2009) systematically reviewed 14 randomized, placebo-controlled trials of donepezil, rivastigmine, and galantamine that studied these drugs' effect on the behavioral and psychological symptoms of dementia; nine of the studies investigated donepezil, three investigated galantamine, and two investigated rivastigmine. Only three studies reported statistically significant improvement in overall NPI scores. One of these studies (Tariot et al. 2000), investigating the effect of galantamine on agitation, found an overall decrease in NPI scores as the dosage was titrated up to 24 mg/day over the course of 5 months. The two other studies (Feldman et al. 2001; Holmes et al. 2004) found that donepezil treatment for an average duration of 24 weeks was associated with a statistically significant decrease in NPI scores compared with placebo.

Regarding treatment of agitation in patients with Lewy body dementia, McKeith et al. (2000, 2017) reported that administration of rivastigmine 12 mg/day was superior to placebo in improving behavioral and neuropsychiatric symptoms. The rivastigmine group was found to become less apathetic or anxious and to experience fewer delusions or psychosis symptoms than the placebo group. This study suggests that cholinesterase inhibitors may provide an effective alternative to the neuroleptics, which are typically avoided in patients with Lewy body pathologies.

A double-blind, placebo-controlled trial of memantine was conducted in patients with moderate to severe dementia due to AD but failed to demonstrate any efficacy in improving agitation symptoms (Fox et al. 2012). In contrast, a pooled retrospective analysis of three trials of memantine in individuals diagnosed with moderate to severe AD with agitation, aggression, or psychotic symptoms at baseline suggested efficacy and tolerability at 12 and 24 weeks (Wilcock et al. 2008). This is supported by a recent study of the effectiveness of augmenting memantine with citalopram for treating the behavioral and psychological symptoms of AD dementia (Zhou et al. 2019). That study demonstrated vastly improved NPI scores in both the placebo and the investigational groups, indicating that memantine has a significant effect in ameliorating neuropsychiatric symptoms if patients are suspected to have AD pathology (Zhou et al. 2019).

Electroconvulsive Therapy

Electroconvulsive therapy (ECT) has had several advances in recent years, including improvements in titration methods and recovery time and the minimization of cognitive side effects with the development of ultrabrief stimulation (Sackeim 2017). With ECT's undisputed effectiveness in treating multiple psychiatric disorders, several cases have emerged describing improvement of agitation symptoms in patients with dementia following ECT treatment. Several reviews have suggested that ECT is safe and effective in geriatric patients who present with agitation and aggression (Glass et al. 2017; Ujkaj et al. 2012) and has been effective for agitation related to delirium complicated by severe withdrawal symptoms (Kranaster et al. 2017; van den Berg et al. 2016). Despite these promising reports, no randomized controlled trials have yet been conducted to truly assess this efficacy due to the difficulty of obtaining a thorough informed consent in a psychiatrically and medically complex patient population (Glass et al. 2017; Acharya et al. 2015).

Other Medication Classes

α- and β-Blockers have historically been used off-label to treat agitation, anxiety, and irritability. Propranolol specifically has been investigated for treatment of agitation in patients with AD. One study (Peskind et al. 2005) found that augmentation with propranolol at an average dosage of 106 mg/day was superior to placebo for decreasing agitation when patients were maintained on stable dosages of their baseline psychotropics. However, these improvements dissipated by the 6-month follow-up. Similarly, the α-blocker prazosin was used in a small placebo-controlled trial (Wang et al. 2009) at a mean dosage of 6 mg/day for 8 weeks in patients with dementia. The authors found some efficacy in treating agitation but reported a significant dropout rate (about half of the participants), despite excluding individuals with blood pressure irregularities. Nevertheless, α- and β-blockers may be valid alternatives to other psychotropics for the acute treatment of agitation, although they should be administered in a careful and thoughtful manner due to the risks of falls and orthostasis.

One study has investigated the effect of hormone therapy with transdermal estrogen (100 μg/day) on decreasing agitated behavior in male patients with dementia (Hall et al. 2005). The authors found no significant difference in aggressive behavior after 8 weeks of treatment, although a surprising "rebound" in aggressive behavior occurred in the estrogen group following removal of the patches. A systematic review of gabapentin and pregabalin found 15 case series/case reports of patients with AD dementia being treated with these medications to alleviate agitation and aggression. These case reports provided preliminary low-grade evidence suggesting the potential benefit of these drugs in alleviating neuropsychiatric symptoms, but randomized controlled trials have not been conducted to support these anecdotal reports (Supasitthumrong et al. 2019).

Conclusion

Agitation is a complicated symptom that arises from a diverse set of potential etiologies and contributing factors, including environmental, psychological, and medical causes. Determining the root cause of agitation episodes is imperative for determining appropriate interventions that could be implemented and allowing rapid resolution of aggressive behaviors. Geriatric psychiatrists have an important role in ensuring the safety of agitated patients while also maintaining the safety of caregivers and facilitating patient care. Psychoeducation of family members and caregivers is necessary for developing the most appropriate and acceptable treatment plan for older patients in different settings. Although nonpharmacological options are always the first-line treatment in decreasing agitated behaviors, they may not always be effective or appropriate in more acute circumstances. However, it is also necessary to conduct a thorough and exhaustive risk-benefit analysis of pharmacological interventions when indicated and to offer alternatives if the potential side effect burden is too extensive for more elderly individuals. Unfortunately, there is a paucity of evidence-based studies investigating the effectiveness of safer pharmacological options in treating agitation. Future studies and randomized, placebo-controlled trials will be necessary to confirm the safety and efficacy of anecdotally effective and tolerable pharmacological agents in older adults.

Key Points

- Agitation is a frequent and distressing neuropsychiatric symptom that negatively affects patient care and quality of life.

- The potential etiologies and causes of agitation are highly varied and must be thoroughly evaluated to determine the most appropriate interventions.

- Nonpharmacological approaches are the first-line treatment for agitation in elderly adults and include music therapy and bright light therapy.

- Pharmacological interventions may become necessary when agitation episodes become too severe to be resolved by alternative management approaches.

- It is important to provide caregivers and family members a thorough summary of the risks and benefits of pharmacological agents (especially the black box warning of antipsychotics) when these drugs are used for agitation episodes.

- Medications should always be prescribed at the lowest possible dosages to minimize any potentially harmful effects.

Suggested Readings

Howard RJ, Juszszak E, Ballard CG, et al: Donepezil for the treatment of agitation in Alzheimer's disease. N Engl J Med 357:1382–1392, 2007

Schneider LS, Tariot PN, Dagerman KS, et al: Effectiveness of atypical antipsychotic drugs in patients with Alzheimer's disease. N Engl J Med 355:1528–1538, 2006

References

Abraha I, Rimland JM, Trotta FM, et al: Systematic review of systematic reviews of non-pharmacological interventions to treat behavioural disturbances in older patients with dementia: the SENATOR-OnTop series. BMJ Open 7(3):e012759, 2017 28302633

Acharya D, Harper DG, Achtyes ED, et al: Safety and utility of acute electroconvulsive therapy for agitation and aggression in dementia. Int J Geriatr Psychiatry 30(3):265–273, 2015 24838521

American Geriatrics Society Expert Panel on Postoperative Delirium in Older Adults: American Geriatrics Society abstracted clinical practice guideline for postoperative delirium in older adults. J Am Geriatr Soc 63(1):142–150, 2015 25495432

Anatchkova M, Brooks A, Swett L, et al: Agitation in patients with dementia: a systematic review of epidemiology and association with severity and course. Int Psychogeriatr 11:1–14, 2019 30855002

Ballard CG, Gauthier S, Cummings JL, et al: Management of agitation and aggression associated with Alzheimer disease. Nat Rev Neurol 5(5):245–255, 2009 19488082

Barak Y, Plopski I, Tadger S, Paleacu D: Escitalopram versus risperidone for the treatment of behavioral and psychotic symptoms associated with Alzheimer's disease: a randomized double-blind pilot study. Int Psychogeriatr 23(9):1515–1519, 2011 21492498

Barton C, Ketelle R, Merrilees J, Miller B: Non-pharmacological management of behavioral symptoms in frontotemporal and other dementias. Curr Neurol Neurosci Rep 16(2):14, 2016 26750129

Burns A, Perry E, Holmes C, et al: A double-blind placebo-controlled randomized trial of Melissa officinalis oil and donepezil for the treatment of agitation in Alzheimer's disease. Dement Geriatr Cogn Disord 31(2):158–164, 2011 21335973

Cammisuli DM, Danti S, et al: Non-pharmacological interventions for people with Alzheimer's disease: a critical review of the scientific literature from the last ten years. Eur Geriatr Med 7(1):57–64, 2016

Caspar S, Davis ED, Douziech A, Scott DR: Nonpharmacological management of behavioral and psychological symptoms of dementia: what works, in what circumstances, and why? Innov Aging 2(1):igy001, 2018 30480128

Chen P, Guarino PD, Dysken MW, et al: Neuropsychiatric symptoms and caregiver burden in individuals with Alzheimer's disease: the TEAM-AD VA cooperative study. J Geriatr Psychiatry Neurol 31(4):177–185, 2018 29966477

Cohen-Mansfield J: Nonpharmacologic interventions for inappropriate behaviors in dementia: a review, summary, and critique. Am J Geriatr Psychiatry 9(4):361–381, 2001 11739063

Declercq T, Petrovic M, Azermai M, et al: Withdrawal versus continuation of chronic antipsychotic drugs for behavioural and psychological symptoms in older people with dementia. Cochrane Database Syst Rev (3):CD007726, 2013 23543555

de Oliveira AM, Radanovic M, de Mello PC, et al: Nonpharmacological interventions to reduce behavioral and psychological symptoms of dementia: a systematic review. BioMed Res Int 2015:218980, 2015 26693477

Devanand DP, Pelton GH, D'Antonio K, et al: Low-dose lithium treatment for agitation and psychosis in Alzheimer disease and frontotemporal dementia: a case series. Alzheimer Dis Assoc Disord 31(1):73–75, 2017 27819842

Devanand DP, Strickler JG, Huey ED, et al: Lithium Treatment for Agitation in Alzheimer's Disease (Lit-AD): clinical rationale and study design. Contemp Clin Trials 71:33–39, 2018 29859917

Devanand DP, Crocco E, Forester BP, et al: Low dose lithium treatment of behavioral complications in Alzheimer's disease: Lit-AD randomized clinical. Am J Geriatr Psychiatry 2021 34059401 Epub ahead of print

Dorsey ER, Rabbani A, Gallagher SA, et al: Impact of FDA black box advisory on antipsychotic medication use. Arch Intern Med 170(1):96–103, 2010 20065205

Dowling GA, Graf CL, Hubbard EM, Luxenberg JS: Light treatment for neuropsychiatric behaviors in Alzheimer's disease. West J Nurs Res 29(8):961–975, 2007 17596638

Feldman H, Gauthier S, Hecker J, et al: A 24-week, randomized, double-blind study of done-pezil in moderate to severe Alzheimer's disease. Neurology 57(4):613–620, 2001 11524468

Fong TG, Tulebaev SR, Inouye SK: Delirium in elderly adults: diagnosis, prevention and treatment. Nat Rev Neurol 5(4):210–220, 2009 19347026

Forbes D, Blake CM, Thiessen EJ, et al: Light therapy for improving cognition, activities of daily living, sleep, challenging behaviour, and psychiatric disturbances in dementia. Cochrane Database Syst Rev (2):CD003946, 2014 24574061

Fox C, Crugel M, Maidment I, et al: Efficacy of memantine for agitation in Alzheimer's dementia: a randomised double-blind placebo controlled trial. PLoS One 7(5):e35185, 2012 22567095

Gitlin LN, Kales HC, Lyketsos CG: Nonpharmacologic management of behavioral symptoms in dementia. JAMA 308(19):2020–2029, 2012 23168825

Glass OM, Forester BP, Hermida AP: Electroconvulsive therapy (ECT) for treating agitation in dementia (major neurocognitive disorder): a promising option. Int Psychogeriatr 29(5):717–726, 2017 28095946

Hall KA, Keks NA, O'Connor DW: Transdermal estrogen patches for aggressive behavior in male patients with dementia: a randomized, controlled trial. Int Psychogeriatr 17(2):165–178, 2005 16050428

Ho T, Pollock BG, Mulsant BH, et al: R- and S-citalopram concentrations have differential effects on neuropsychiatric scores in elders with dementia and agitation. Br J Clin Pharmacol 82(3):784–792, 2016 27145364

Hodgson NA, Gitlin LN, Winter L, Czekanski K: Undiagnosed illness and neuropsychiatric behaviors in community residing older adults with dementia. Alzheimer Dis Assoc Disord 25(2):109–115, 2011 20921879

Holmes C, Wilkinson D, Dean C, et al: The efficacy of donepezil in the treatment of neuropsychiatric symptoms in Alzheimer disease. Neurology 63(2):214–219, 2004 15277611

Howard RJ, Juszczak E, Ballard CG, et al: Donepezil for the treatment of agitation in Alzheimer's disease. N Engl J Med 357(14):1382–1392, 2007 17914039

Husebo BS, Ballard C, Sandvik R, et al: Efficacy of treating pain to reduce behavioural disturbances in residents of nursing homes with dementia: cluster randomised clinical trial. BMJ 343:d4065, 2011 21765198

Ijaopo EO: Dementia-related agitation: a review of non-pharmacological interventions and analysis of risks and benefits of pharmacotherapy. Transl Psychiatry 7(10):e1250, 2017 29087372

Jeste DV, Blazer D, Casey D, et al: ACNP white paper: update on use of antipsychotic drugs in elderly persons with dementia. Neuropsychopharmacology 33(5):957–970, 2008 17637610

Kales HC, Kim HM, Zivin K, et al: Risk of mortality among individual antipsychotics in patients with dementia. Am J Psychiatry 169(1):71–79, 2012 22193526

Kranaster L, Aksay SS, Bumb JM, et al: The "forgotten" treatment of alcohol withdrawal delirium with electroconvulsive therapy: successful use in a very prolonged and severe case. Clin Neuropharmacol 40(4):183–184, 2017 28622209

Lebert F, Stekke W, Hasenbroekx C, Pasquier F: Frontotemporal dementia: a randomised, controlled trial with trazodone. Dement Geriatr Cogn Disord 17(4):355–359, 2004 15178953

Ledger AJ, Baker FA: An investigation of long-term effects of group music therapy on agitation levels of people with Alzheimer's disease. Aging Ment Health 11(3):330–338, 2007 17558584

Livingston G, Barber J, Marston L, et al: Prevalence of and associations with agitation in residents with dementia living in care homes: MARQUE cross-sectional study. BJPsych Open 3(4):171–178, 2017 28794896

Lonergan E, Luxenberg J: Valproate preparations for agitation in dementia. Cochrane Database Syst Rev (3):CD003945, 2009 19588348

Lyketsos CG, DelCampo L, Steinberg M, et al: Treating depression in Alzheimer disease: efficacy and safety of sertraline therapy, and the benefits of depression reduction: the DIADS. Arch Gen Psychiatry 60(7):737–746, 2003 12860778

Lyketsos CG, Carrillo MC, Ryan JM, et al: Neuropsychiatric symptoms in Alzheimer's disease. Alzheimers Dement 7(5):532–539, 2011 21889116

Maglione M, Maher AR, Hu J, et al: Off-Label Use of Atypical Antipsychotics: An Update. AHRQ Comparative Effectiveness Reviews. Rockville, MD, AHQR, 2011

Maher AR, Maglione M, Bagley S, et al: Efficacy and comparative effectiveness of atypical antipsychotic medications for off-label uses in adults: a systematic review and meta-analysis. JAMA 306(12):1359–1369, 2011 21954480

McKeith I, Del Ser T, Spano P, et al: Efficacy of rivastigmine in dementia with Lewy bodies: a randomised, double-blind, placebo-controlled international study. Lancet 356(9247):2031–2036, 2000 11145488

McKeith IG, Boeve BF, Dickson DW, et al: Diagnosis and management of dementia with Lewy bodies: fourth consensus report of the DLB Consortium. Neurology 89(1):88–100, 2017 28592453

Müller-Spahn F: Behavioral disturbances in dementia. Dialogues Clin Neurosci 5(1):49–59, 2003 22034255

Newell J, Yesavage JA, Taylor JL, et al: Sedation mediates part of citalopram's effect on agitation in Alzheimer's disease. J Psychiatr Res 74:17–21, 2016 26736036

Nordstrom K, Zun LS, Wilson MP, et al: Medical evaluation and triage of the agitated patient: consensus statement of the American Association for Emergency Psychiatry Project Beta Medical Evaluation Workgroup. West J Emerg Med 13(1):3–10, 2012 22461915

Oh ES, Fong TG, Hshieh TT, Inouye SK: Delirium in older persons: advances in diagnosis and treatment. JAMA 318(12):1161–1174, 2017 28973626

Olin JT, Fox LS, Pawluczyk S, et al: A pilot randomized trial of carbamazepine for behavioral symptoms in treatment-resistant outpatients with Alzheimer disease. Am J Geriatr Psychiatry 9(4):400–405, 2001 11739066

Peskind ER, Tsuang DW, Bonner LT, et al: Propranolol for disruptive behaviors in nursing home residents with probable or possible Alzheimer disease: a placebo-controlled study. Alzheimer Dis Assoc Disord 19(1):23–28, 2005 15764868

Pollock BG, Mulsant BH, Rosen J, et al: Comparison of citalopram, perphenazine, and placebo for the acute treatment of psychosis and behavioral disturbances in hospitalized, demented patients. Am J Psychiatry 159(3):460–465, 2002 11870012

Pollock BG, Mulsant BH, Rosen J, et al: A double-blind comparison of citalopram and risperidone for the treatment of behavioral and psychotic symptoms associated with dementia. Am J Geriatr Psychiatry 15(11):942–952, 2007 17846102

Porsteinsson AP, Drye LT, Pollock BG, et al: Effect of citalopram on agitation in Alzheimer disease: the CitAD randomized clinical trial. JAMA 311(7):682–691, 2014 24549548

Rodda J, Morgan S, Walker Z: Are cholinesterase inhibitors effective in the management of the behavioral and psychological symptoms of dementia in Alzheimer's disease? A systematic review of randomized, placebo-controlled trials of donepezil, rivastigmine and galantamine. Int Psychogeriatr 21(5):813–824, 2009 19538824

Rosenberg PB, Nowrangi MA, Lyketsos CG: Neuropsychiatric symptoms in Alzheimer's disease: what might be associated brain circuits? Mol Aspects Med 43–44:25–37, 2015 26049034

Sackeim HA: Modern electroconvulsive therapy: vastly improved yet greatly underused. JAMA Psychiatry 74(8):779–780, 2017 28658461

Schneider LS, Dagerman K, Insel PS: Efficacy and adverse effects of atypical antipsychotics for dementia: meta-analysis of placebo-controlled trials. Am J Geriatr Psychiatry 14(3):191–210, 2006 16505124

Schneider LS, Frangakis C, Drye LT, et al: Heterogeneity of treatment response to citalopram for patients with Alzheimer's disease with aggression or agitation: the CitAD randomized clinical trial. Am J Psychiatry 173(5):465–472, 2016 26771737

Steinberg M, Lyketsos CG: Atypical antipsychotic use in patients with dementia: managing safety concerns. Am J Psychiatry 169(9):900–906, 2012 22952071

Stroomer-van Wijk AJ, Jonker BW, Kok RM, et al: Detecting delirium in elderly outpatients with cognitive impairment. Int Psychogeriatr 28(8):1303–1311, 2016 27079735

Supasitthumrong T, Bolea-Alamanac BM, Asmer S, et al: Gabapentin and pregabalin to treat aggressivity in dementia: a systematic review and illustrative case report. Br J Clin Pharmacol 85(4):690–703, 2019 30575088

Tariot PN, Erb R, Podgorski CA, et al: Efficacy and tolerability of carbamazepine for agitation and aggression in dementia. Am J Psychiatry 155(1):54–61, 1998 9433339

Tariot PN, Solomon PR, Morris JC, et al: A 5-month, randomized, placebo-controlled trial of galantamine in AD: the Galantamine USA-10 Study Group. Neurology 54(12):2269–2276, 2000 10881251

Tariot PN, Schneider LS, Mintzer JE, et al: Safety and tolerability of divalproex sodium in the treatment of signs and symptoms of mania in elderly patients with dementia: results of a double-blind, placebo-controlled trial. Curr Ther Res Clin Exp 62(1):51–67, 2001

Tariot PN, Raman R, Jakimovich L, et al: Divalproex sodium in nursing home residents with possible or probable Alzheimer disease complicated by agitation: a randomized, controlled trial. Am J Geriatr Psychiatry 13(11):942–949, 2005 16286437

Teri L, Logsdon RG, Peskind E, et al: Treatment of agitation in AD: a randomized, placebo-controlled clinical trial. Neurology 55(9):1271–1278, 2000 11087767

Ujkaj M, Davidoff DA, Seiner SJ, et al: Safety and efficacy of electroconvulsive therapy for the treatment of agitation and aggression in patients with dementia. Am J Geriatr Psychiatry 20(1):61–72, 2012 22143072

van den Berg KS, Marijnissen RM, van Waarde JA: Electroconvulsive therapy as a powerful treatment for delirium: a case report. J ECT 32(1):65–66, 2016 25993030

Veldwijk-Rouwenhorst AE, Smalbrugge M, Wetzels R, et al: Nursing home residents with dementia and very frequent agitation: a particular group. Am J Geriatr Psychiatry 25(12):1339–1348, 2017 28886978

Wang LY, Shofer JB, Rohde K, et al: Prazosin for the treatment of behavioral symptoms in patients with Alzheimer disease with agitation and aggression. Am J Geriatr Psychiatry 17(9):744–751, 2009 19700947

Weissberger GH, Melrose RJ, Narvaez TA, et al: 18F-Fluorodeoxyglucose positron emission tomography cortical metabolic activity associated with distinct agitation behaviors in Alzheimer disease. Am J Geriatr Psychiatry 25(6):569–579, 2017 28215899

Wilcock GK, Ballard CG, Cooper JA, Loft H: Memantine for agitation/aggression and psychosis in moderately severe to severe Alzheimer's disease: a pooled analysis of 3 studies. J Clin Psychiatry 69(3):341–348, 2008 18294023

Wilson L, Power C, Owens R, Lawlor B: Psychiatric consultation in the nursing home: reasons for referral and recognition of delirium. Ir J Psychol Med 36(2):121–127, 2019 31187721

Young RC, Mulsant BH, Sajatovic M, et al: GERI-BD: a randomized double-blind controlled trial of lithium and divalproex in the treatment of mania in older patients with bipolar disorder. Am J Psychiatry 174(11):1086–1093, 2017 29088928

Yue J, Tabloski P, Dowal SL, et al: NICE to HELP: operationalizing National Institute for Health and Clinical Excellence guidelines to improve clinical practice. J Am Geriatr Soc 62(4):754–761, 2014 24697606

Zhou T, Wang J, Xin C, et al: Effect of memantine combined with citalopram on cognition of BPSD and moderate Alzheimer's disease: a clinical trial. Exp Ther Med 17(3):1625–1630, 2019 30783429

Zmuc Veranic L, Pregelj P, Jerin A: Treating agitation and aggression in patients with Alzheimer's disease with escitalopram. Psychogeriatrics 16(6):384–385, 2016

CHAPTER 20

Psychopharmacology

Benoit H. Mulsant, M.D., M.S.

Bruce G. Pollock, M.D., Ph.D.

Pharmacological intervention in late life requires special care. Older patients are more susceptible to drug-induced adverse events. Several psychotropic medications and classes have been associated with serious adverse events (Pollock et al. 2009), including increased mortality risk (Ballard and Corbett 2020; Kripke et al. 2012; Langballe et al. 2014; Lao et al. 2020; Moreno et al. 2018; Weich et al. 2014; Xu et al. 2020). Older adults are more likely to experience these events, including cardiac effects (e.g., prolonged QTc, arrhythmias, sudden death) (Beach et al. 2018), peripheral and central anticholinergic effects (e.g., constipation, urinary retention, delirium, cognitive dysfunction) (Pasina et al. 2019; Tsoutsoulas et al. 2017), antihistaminergic effects (e.g., sedation), and antiadrenergic effects (e.g., postural hypotension) that not only interfere with basic activities but also lead to falls and fractures. Other possible adverse effects in this population include hyponatremia, bleeding, and altered bone metabolism. Older patients' increased susceptibility to these adverse events may be due to the pharmacokinetic and pharmacodynamic changes associated with aging, such as diminished glomerular filtration, changes in the density and activity of target receptors, reduced liver size and hepatic blood flow, and decreased cardiac output (Pollock 2019; Reuben et al. 2019; Uchida et al. 2009) (Table 20–1).

Common illnesses that affect many older persons (e.g., diabetes, cardiac or renal failure) further diminish the processing and removal of medications from the body. In addition, polypharmacy and the associated risk of drug interactions add another level of complexity to pharmacological treatment in older patients. Poor adherence to treatment regimens—which can be a result of impaired cognition, confusing drug regimens, or lack of motivation or insight associated with the psychiatric disorder being treated—is a significant obstacle to effective and safe pharmacological treatment. Finally, psychotropic medications are not as extensively studied in older people as in younger persons or in patients without comorbid medical illness. Methods such as population pharmacokinetics can help address the lack of information about dosages

TABLE 20–1.   **Physiological changes in older persons associated with altered pharmacokinetics**

Organ system	Change	Pharmacokinetic consequence
Circulatory system	Decreased concentration of plasma albumin and increased α_1-acid glycoprotein	Increased or decreased free concentration of drugs in plasma
Gastrointestinal tract	Decreased intestinal and splanchnic blood flow	Decreased rate of drug absorption
Kidney	Decreased glomerular filtration rate	Decreased renal clearance of active metabolites
Liver	Decreased liver size; decreased hepatic blood flow; variable effects on cytochrome P450 isozyme activity	Decreased hepatic clearance
Muscle	Decreased lean body mass and increased adipose tissue	Altered volume of distribution of lipid-soluble drugs, leading to increased elimination half-life

Source.   Adapted from Pollock BG: "Psychotropic Drugs and the Aging Patient." *Geriatrics* 53(suppl 1):S20–S24, 1998. Used with permission.

and drug–drug interactions (Jin et al. 2010). Nonetheless, even with currently available knowledge, medications cause considerable morbidity in older people (Fralick et al. 2020). In a study by Laroche et al. (2007), 66% of the admissions to an acute geriatric medical unit were preceded by the prescription of at least one inappropriate medication; even among patients taking appropriate medications, the prevalence of adverse drug reactions was 16%.

Despite these challenges, psychiatric disorders can be treated successfully in late life with psychotropic drugs. In this chapter, we summarize relevant geriatric data available as of September 2021 on the efficacy, tolerability, and safety of the major psychotropic drugs used in the treatment of mental disorders.

Antidepressant Medications

Selective Serotonin Reuptake Inhibitors

Six selective serotonin reuptake inhibitors (SSRIs) are available in the United States: citalopram, escitalopram, fluoxetine, fluvoxamine, paroxetine, and sertraline. They are approved by the FDA for the treatment of major depressive disorder (MDD) (except fluvoxamine) and for several anxiety disorders (escitalopram and paroxetine for generalized anxiety disorder [GAD]; fluoxetine, fluvoxamine, paroxetine, and sertraline for OCD; fluoxetine, paroxetine, and sertraline for panic disorder; paroxetine and sertraline for PTSD; and paroxetine and sertraline for social anxiety disorder in adults). In older adults, SSRIs remain first-line antidepressants (Mulsant et al. 2014) because of their broad spectrum of action, overall efficacy (Gutsmiedl et al. 2020; Tedeschini et al. 2011), ease of use, good tolerability, and relative safety (Mulsant et al. 2014). More than 40 randomized controlled trials (RCTs) of SSRIs involving more than 6,000 geriatric patients with depression have been published and meta-analyzed (Gutsmiedl et al. 2020; Krause et al. 2019). However, as with most drugs, few clinical trials of SSRIs have been conducted under "real-life" geriatric situations (e.g., in long-term care facilities) or in very old patients. Overall, published RCTs support the efficacy and tolerability of SSRIs in older patients with MDD (Gutsmiedl et al. 2020; Krause et al. 2019; Tedeschini et al. 2011). These patients are at high risk for relapse or recurrence, and continuation or maintenance therapy with citalopram (Klysner et al. 2002), escitalopram (Gorwood et al. 2007), or paroxetine (Reynolds et al. 2006) has been shown to be effective in their prevention. SSRIs have also been shown to be helpful in older patients with melancholia (Sneed et al. 2014) or minor depression (Rocca et al. 2005) and in family caregivers with minor depression or MDD (Lavretsky et al. 2010).

Many open studies and some small controlled trials in special populations also have concluded that SSRIs are reasonably well tolerated, efficacious, and safe in patients with depression and a variety of comorbid conditions, including complicated grief (Shear et al. 2016), mild cognitive impairment (MCI) (Devanand et al. 2003; Reynolds et al. 2011), schizophrenia (Kasckow et al. 2001), cerebrovascular disease (Y. Chen et al. 2007; Murray et al. 2005; Rampello et al. 2004; Rasmussen et al. 2003; Robinson et al. 2000, 2008), Parkinson's disease (Agüera-Ortiz et al. 2021; Barone et al. 2006; Broen et al. 2016; Devos et al. 2008; Takahashi et al. 2019), traumatic brain injury (Jorge et al. 2016), cardiovascular disease (Glassman et al. 2002; Kim et al. 2015; Serebruany et al. 2003), hypertension (Fu et al. 2015), chronic obstructive pulmonary disease (He et al. 2016), end-stage renal failure and hemodialysis (Friedli et al. 2017), and terminal cancer (Sullivan et al. 2017),as well as other medical conditions (Goodnick and Hernandez 2000; Karp et al. 2005).

Two published placebo-controlled trials of citalopram (Lenze et al. 2005) and escitalopram (Lenze et al. 2009) support the efficacy of SSRIs in older patients with GAD. The use of SSRIs to treat other anxiety disorders is based on small open trials (Flint 2005; Lenze et al. 2002; Sheikh et al. 2004; Wylie et al. 2000) or extrapolation from studies in younger adults. Over the past 30 years, a series of published studies, including several RCTs, have suggested that citalopram may be efficacious in the treatment of agitation, delusions, and hallucinations associated with Alzheimer's dementia (Nyth and Gottfries 1990; Nyth et al. 1992; Pollock et al. 1997, 2002, 2007; Porsteinsson et al. 2014; Viscogliosi et al. 2017) or of response inhibition in frontotemporal dementia (Hughes et al. 2015). However, these studies used citalopram dosages above the maximum of 20 mg/day recommended by the FDA in older patients (U.S. Food and Drug Administration 2012). In a seminal randomized, placebo-controlled trial, older patients with dementia who were randomly assigned to citalopram ≤30 mg/day had longer QTc intervals and more cognitive impairment than those given placebo (Porsteinsson et al. 2014). In the same trial, the concentration of the R-citalopram enantiomer was associated with a higher proportion of adverse events (including a reduction in cognitive scores), whereas the concentration of the S-enantiomer (escitalopram) was associated with an increased probability of treatment response (Ho et al. 2016). However, the direct evidence supporting the use of escitalopram in the treatment of noncognitive symptoms associated with dementia is limited. One small ($N=40$) positive RCT supported the use of escitalopram in the treatment of behavioral and psychotic symptoms (Barak et al. 2011). In another RCT ($N=60$), no difference was found between escitalopram and placebo in patients with Alzheimer's dementia and depression (An et al. 2017). A large, multicenter RCT of escitalopram for agitation associated with Alzheimer's dementia (S-CitAD) is ongoing (Ehrhardt et al. 2019).

Several early open studies, small single-site controlled trials, or unreplicated RCTs also support the use of escitalopram or other SSRIs for the treatment of depression associated with Alzheimer's dementia (Beheydt et al. 2015; Choe et al. 2016; Katona et al. 1998; Lyketsos et al. 2003; Nyth and Gottfries 1990; Nyth et al. 1992; Olafsson et al. 1992; Petracca et al. 2001; Taragano et al. 1997). However, a larger multicenter RCT failed to confirm these results: In this study, sertraline was not more efficacious and was less well tolerated than placebo for the treatment of depression associated with Alzheimer's dementia (Rosenberg et al. 2010; Weintraub et al. 2010). Another multicenter study also demonstrated no differences in the efficacy of sertraline, mirtazapine, or placebo in treating depression in patients with Alzheimer's dementia, but the tolerability of either drug was worse than placebo (Banerjee et al. 2011; Zuidersma et al. 2019). In a double-blind, placebo-controlled discontinuation study in 128 patients with dementia and neuropsychiatric symptoms (but no depressive disorder), discontinuation of an SSRI that had been prescribed for at least 3 months was associated with a worsening of depressive symptoms compared with continuing the SSRI (Bergh et al. 2012). Taken together, these data do not support that SSRIs are superior to placebo to treat depressive symptoms in patients with Alzheimer's dementia. However, most of the participants in open studies or in randomized, placebo-controlled trials experienced significant improvement in their depressive symptoms, supporting the common practice of trialing antidepressants for severe depressive symptoms associated with dementia.

Current evidence from a very large network meta-analysis suggests some small differences in efficacy and tolerability among antidepressants in the treatment of MDD in adults (Cipriani et al. 2018). Although no such evidence exists in older adults, experts favor the use of escitalopram or sertraline over citalopram, fluvoxamine, fluoxetine, or paroxetine (Mulsant et al. 2014) because of their favorable pharmacokinetic profiles (Table 20–2) and lower potential for clinically significant drug interactions (Table 20–3) or for other adverse effects. Notably, a warning has been issued by the FDA against the use of dosages of citalopram >40 mg/day in any patient and >20 mg/day in patients older than 60 years because of a risk of prolonged QTc interval and torsades de pointes (U.S. Food and Drug Administration 2012). Some studies have confirmed this risk (Castro et al. 2013; Ho et al. 2016; Maljuric et al. 2015). However, other studies have questioned the clinical relevance of these data (Crépeau-Gendron et al. 2019; Hutton et al. 2017; McCarrell et al. 2019; Rector et al. 2016).

In older adults with depression, executive dysfunction is associated with a smaller or slower improvement from citalopram, escitalopram, or other SSRIs (Manning et al. 2015; Sneed et al. 2010). Some data suggest that SSRIs in general (and sertraline in particular) may be beneficial in terms of alleviating the cognitive impairment associated with late-life depression (Burrows et al. 2002; Doraiswamy et al. 2003; Furlan et al. 2001; Jorge et al. 2010; Newhouse et al. 2000; Savaskan et al. 2008; Victoria et al. 2017). However, other data suggest that citalopram—like other SSRIs—may have deleterious cognitive effects in some older patients (Culang et al. 2009) or in patients with dementia (Porsteinsson et al. 2014). Based on preclinical data, it has been proposed that SSRIs could be useful in preventing or even treating Alzheimer's or vascular demen-

TABLE 20–2. Pharmacokinetic properties of second-generation antidepressants

Medication	Half-life, days[a]	Proportionality of dosage to plasma concentration	Risk of uncomfortable discontinuation symptoms	Efficacious dosage range in older individuals, mg/day[b]
Selective serotonin reuptake inhibitors				
Citalopram	1–3	Linear across therapeutic range	Low	20[c]
Escitalopram	1–2	Linear across therapeutic range	Low	10–20
Fluoxetine	7–10	Nonlinear at higher dosages	Very low	20–40
Fluvoxamine	0.5–1	Nonlinear at higher dosages	Moderate	50–300
Paroxetine	1	Nonlinear at higher dosages	Moderate	20–40
Sertraline	1–3	Linear across therapeutic range	Low	50–200
Serotonin-norepinephrine reuptake inhibitors				
Desvenlafaxine	0.5	Linear up to 600 mg/day	High	50
Duloxetine	0.5	Linear across therapeutic range	Moderate	60–120
Levomilnacipran	0.5	Linear across therapeutic range	Moderate	40–120
Venlafaxine XR	0.2	Linear across therapeutic range	High	75–300
Other second-generation antidepressants				
Bupropion	1	Linear across therapeutic range	Very low	150–400 (SR);150–450 (XL)
Mirtazapine	1–2	Linear across therapeutic range	Moderate	15–45
Trazodone	5–9	Linear across therapeutic range	Low	50–600 (see text)
Vilazodone	1	Linear across therapeutic range	Moderate	20–40
Vortioxetine	2–3	Linear across therapeutic range	Low	5–20

SR=sustained release; XL=extended release; XR=extended release.

[a]Including active metabolites.

[b]Starting dosage typically half of lowest efficacious dosage; all SSRIs can be given in single daily doses except fluvoxamine, which should be given in two divided doses.

[c]The FDA has issued a drug safety communication, stating: "20 mg per day is the maximum recommended dose for patients with hepatic impairment, who are greater than 60 years of age, who are CYP 2C19 poor metabolizers, or who are taking concomitant cimetidine (Tagamet), because these factors lead to increased blood levels of citalopram, increasing the risk of QT interval prolongation and Torsade de Pointes" (U.S. Food and Drug Administration 2011).

TABLE 20–3. Second-generation antidepressants' inhibition of cytochrome P450 (CYP) and potential for causing or being involved in significant drug–drug interactions

Medication	CYP1A2	CYP2C9 and 2C19	CYP2D6	CYP3A4	Potential for causing or being involved in clinically significant drug–drug interactions	
					Causing	Being involved
Selective serotonin reuptake inhibitors						
Citalopram	+	0	+	0	Low	Moderate (2C19 inhibitors)
Escitalopram	+	0	+	0	Low	Low
Fluoxetine	+	++	+++	++	High	High
Fluvoxamine	+++	+++	+	++	High	High
Paroxetine	+	+	+++	+	Moderate	Moderate
Sertraline	+	+	+	+	Low	Low
Serotonin-norepinephrine reuptake inhibitors						
Desvenlafaxine	0	0	0	0	Minimal	Minimal
Duloxetine	0	0	+	+	Low	Low (1A2 and 2D6 inhibitors)
Levomilnacipran, milnacipran	0	0	0	0	Low	Low
Venlafaxine	0	0	0	0	Low	Low (2D6 inhibitors)
Other second-generation antidepressants						
Bupropion	0	0	++	0	Low	Moderate (2B6 inhibitors)
Nefazodone	0	+	0	+++	High	High
Trazodone	0	0	0	0	Low	Moderate (3A4 inhibitors and inducers)
Vilazodone	0	0	0	0	Low	Low (3A4 inducers and inhibitors)
Vortioxetine	0	0	0	0	Low	Low (2D6 inhibitors and 3A4 inducers)

0=minimal or no inhibition; +=mild inhibition; ++=moderate inhibition; +++=strong inhibition.

tia (Cirrito et al. 2011, 2020; Sheline et al. 2014). However, relevant human studies have had mixed results, with some studies of SSRIs in patients with dementia showing some cognitive benefits (Liu et al. 2014; Mokhber et al. 2014) and others not (Beheydt et al. 2015; Choe et al. 2016).

SSRI starting dosages for older adults (see Table 20–2) are typically half the minimal efficacious dosage in younger adults, and the dosage is usually doubled after 1 week. All of the SSRIs can be administered in a single daily dose except fluvoxamine, which should be given in two divided doses. Although frail older patients typically tolerate these drugs relatively well (Oslin et al. 2000), some experience some gastrointestinal distress (e.g., nausea) during the first few days of treatment. Significant hyponatremia resulting from the syndrome of inappropriate antidiuretic hormone secretion (SIADH) is a potentially dangerous adverse effect observed almost exclusively in older persons and typically during the first couple of weeks of treatment (Coupland et al. 2011; Fabian et al. 2004).

SSRIs and other serotonergic antidepressants (e.g., serotonin-norepinephrine reuptake inhibitors [SNRIs]) directly affect platelet activation (Pollock et al. 2000) and are associated with an increase in the risk of cerebral, gastrointestinal, or postsurgical bleeding (Auerbach et al. 2013; Hung et al. 2013; Looper 2007; Löppönen et al. 2014; Mortensen et al. 2013; Roose and Rutherford 2016; Schäfer et al. 2019; Shin et al. 2014; Wang et al. 2014). They act synergistically with other medications that increase the risk of bleeding, such as nonsteroidal anti-inflammatory drugs (NSAIDs), low-dose aspirin, or warfarin (Löppönen et al. 2014; Wang et al. 2014). Thus, SSRIs should be used cautiously in older patients taking these medications, and the prophylactic use of acid-suppressing agents could be considered in older patients at high risk for gastrointestinal bleeding (de Abajo and García-Rodríguez 2008; Yuan et al. 2006).

The antiplatelet effect of SSRIs also raises the question of whether they can be used to prevent cerebrovascular or cardiovascular events and, conversely, whether they can cause intracerebral bleeding in at-risk patients. A series of observational studies and large RCTs tried to answer these questions, and their results are mixed. Some studies have shown that SSRIs may be used to prevent ischemic strokes (Chen et al. 2019; EFFECTS Trial Collaboration 2020; He et al. 2018; Liu et al. 2020) or coronary events (J.M. Kim et al. 2018), to treat depression following a hemorrhagic stroke (Kubiszewski et al. 2020) or an ischemic stroke (Gao et al. 2017; Savadi Oskouie et al. 2017), or to treat a coronary syndrome (Kim et al. 2015). In two large retrospective studies, SSRI exposure before an ischemic stroke was not associated with adverse outcomes (including bleeding) following thrombolytic therapy (Scheitz et al. 2017; Schellen et al. 2018). In one meta-analysis, early use of SSRIs following a stroke improved functional recovery in patients undergoing rehabilitation (Gu and Wang 2018). By contrast, some studies have reported that SSRIs are not helpful in the prevention of strokes (Kim et al. 2017) or in the treatment of heart failure (Angermann et al. 2016) and contribute to intracerebral bleeding (Albrecht et al. 2018; Douros et al. 2018; Gaffey et al. 2021; Kubiszewski et al. 2020; Löppönen et al. 2014) or a number of other deleterious poststroke outcomes (AFFINITY Trial Collaboration 2020; Dennis et al. 2019; EFFECTS Trial Collaboration 2020; FOCUS Trial Collaboration 2019; Liu et al. 2020). Some data suggest that fluoxetine is significantly more likely to be associated with intracranial hemorrhage (or other types of bleeding) than other antidepressants (Kim et al. 2019). Given these data, the SSRIs or SNRIs should be avoided after a hemorrhagic stroke but can probably be utilized safely to prevent or treat depression following an ischemic stroke; it remains unclear whether they promote poststroke recovery independent of their effect on depression.

SSRIs also can be associated with bradycardia and should be started with caution in patients with low heart rates (e.g., patients taking β-blockers). In rare instances, they have been reported to cause extrapyramidal symptoms (EPS) (Mamo et al. 2000), but they are well tolerated by most patients with Parkinson's disease (Agüera-Ortiz et al. 2021; P. Chen et al. 2007; Takahashi et al. 2019) or dystonia (Zoons et al. 2018). The risk of falls and hip fracture does not differ among different classes of antidepressants (Liu et al. 1998), but there is some evidence that chronic use of SSRIs and other serotonergic drugs contributes to the risk of fractures through their direct effects on bone metabolism (Diem et al. 2007; Garfield et al. 2014; Richards et al. 2007; Shea et al. 2013).

A large pharmacoepidemiological study in patients age 66 years and older found that SSRIs, compared with non-SSRI antidepressants, are associated with a greater risk for suicide during the first month of treatment (Juurlink et al. 2006). However, the absolute risk was low, which suggests that there may be a vulnerable subgroup at risk for an idiosyncratic response. By contrast, a very large meta-analysis of controlled data available to the FDA indicated a substantial reduction in the risk for suicidal ideation in older patients taking SSRIs compared with those taking placebo (Barbui et al. 2009; Friedman and Leon 2007; Nelson et al. 2007).

Serotonin-Norepinephrine Reuptake Inhibitors

As of December 2020, the FDA had approved four SNRIs for the treatment of MDD in adults: desvenlafaxine, duloxetine, levomilnacipran, and venlafaxine. Duloxetine and venlafaxine have also been approved for the treatment of GAD, duloxetine for diabetic peripheral neuropathic pain and fibromyalgia, and venlafaxine XR (extended release) for panic disorder and social anxiety disorder. A fifth SNRI, milnacipran, is indicated solely for the treatment of fibromyalgia in the United States, although it is used to treat MDD in other countries. Because of their favorable side effect profile in younger persons and their dual mechanism of action (Chalon et al. 2003; Harvey et al. 2000), SNRIs are the preferred alternatives to SSRIs in both younger and older patients (Cooper et al. 2011; Mulsant et al. 2014). Some early meta-analyses suggested that venlafaxine may be associated with a higher rate of remission than SSRIs (e.g., Shelton et al. 2005; Thase et al. 2005a); however, a number of subsequent head-to-head trials, reviews, and meta-analyses have contradicted these early results or challenged their clinical significance in both younger patients (e.g., Bradley and Lenox-Smith 2013; Cipriani et al. 2018; Lam et al. 2010; Schueler et al. 2011; Thaler et al. 2012) and older patients (Mukai and Tampi 2009; Nelson et al. 2008; Rajji et al. 2008).

The risk-benefit ratio of SNRIs may differ between younger and older patients and may change the relative desirability of these medications in the treatment of older patients. The efficacy, tolerability, and relative safety of SNRIs in the treatment of late-life depression are supported by a series of RCTs involving nearly 2,000 older participants. Most of these RCTs used venlafaxine or duloxetine, with some additional analyses of geriatric data pooled from randomized, placebo-controlled trials of desvenlafaxine conducted in mixed-age adults (Kornstein et al. 2010a). Also, in a series of randomized comparisons of desvenlafaxine with escitalopram or placebo in perimenopausal and postmenopausal females ages 40–70 years with MDD, desvenlafaxine and escitalopram had similar efficacy and tolerability (Kornstein et al. 2010b; Soares et al. 2010), and desvenlafaxine was more efficacious than placebo (Clayton et al. 2013; Kornstein et al. 2014). Data from another randomized, placebo-controlled trial support the efficacy and tolerability of duloxetine in older patients with GAD (Alaka et al. 2014). Additional data (mostly from open-label studies or case series) support the efficacy of various SNRIs in older patients with atypical depression (Roose et al. 2004), treatment-resistant depression (Mazeh et al. 2007; Whyte et al. 2004), dysthymic disorder (Devanand et al. 2004), poststroke depression (Dahmen et al. 1999), GAD (Katz et al. 2002), stress urinary incontinence (Mariappan et al. 2005), hot flashes (Biglia et al. 2018), chronic pain syndromes (Grothe et al. 2004; Razazian et al. 2014), or pain symptoms associated with geriatric depression (Karp et al. 2010; Raskin et al. 2007; Wohlreich et al. 2009).

The only published data on the use of levomilnacipran or milnacipran in geriatric patients come from one small ($N=92$) randomized, placebo-controlled trial of milnacipran for the prevention of poststroke depression, the results of which suggest that milnacipran was well tolerated and more efficacious than placebo in preventing poststroke depression (Tsai et al. 2011). In a post hoc pooled analysis of five RCTs of levomilnacipran in patients with MDD, the 106 patients who were 60 years of age or older experienced a remission rate comparable with that of midlife patients (Montgomery et al. 2015).

The SNRIs do not significantly inhibit any major cytochrome P450 isoenzymes and therefore are unlikely to cause clinically significant drug–drug interactions (Spina et al. 2012) (see Table 20–3). However, venlafaxine and duloxetine are metabolized by CYP2D6, and their concentration can increase markedly in genetically poor metabolizers or in patients who are taking drugs that inhibit this isoenzyme (Whyte et al. 2006). The concentration of duloxetine also can be increased by medications that inhibit CYP1A2. Dosage adjustments of SNRIs are not recommended on the basis of age, but SNRIs should be used with caution in older patients with renal or liver disease (Dolder et al. 2010).

The SNRIs inhibit serotonin reuptake. Thus, they share the same side effect profile as the SSRIs, including not only nausea, diarrhea, headaches, excessive sweating, sexual dysfunction (Montejo et al. 2001), and discontinuation symptoms (Montgomery et al. 2009) but also the rarer SIADH and hyponatremia (Kirby et al. 2002), bleeding (de Abajo and García-Rodríguez 2008; Löppönen et al. 2014), serotonin syndrome (McCue and Joseph 2001; Perry 2000), and changes in bone metabolism (Garfield et al. 2014; Rauma et al. 2016; Rawson et al. 2017; Shea et al. 2013). SNRIs are also associated with adverse effects that can be linked to their action on the adrenergic system; these include dry mouth, constipation, urinary retention, increased ocular pressure, cardiovascular problems, and transient agitation (Dolder et al. 2010) and appear to be dosage dependent (Clayton et al. 2009; Liebowitz and Tourian 2010) and usually self-limiting. However, the cardiovascular effects of SNRIs are of special concern in older populations. SNRIs have been reported to cause an increase in blood pressure (Clayton et al. 2009; Thase et al. 2005c), significant orthostatic hypotension, syncope, electrocardiographic changes, arrhythmia, acute ischemia, and death in overdose (Clayton et al. 2009; Davidson et al. 2005; Johnson et al. 2006). However, in a recent observational study in 169 adults age 60 and older treated with venlafaxine ≤300 mg/day, venlafaxine did not affect electrocardiogram parameters (Behlke et al. 2020).

It is not known whether the cardiovascular risks of the various SNRIs differ; however, the bulk of the available data implicates venlafaxine. In the United Kingdom, the National Institute for Health and Clinical Excellence has recommended that venlafaxine not be prescribed to patients with preexisting heart disease, that an electrocardiogram be obtained at baseline, and that blood pressure and cardiac functions be monitored in those patients taking higher dosages (National Collaborating Centre for Mental Health 2004). A rare randomized, double-blind trial in older nursing home residents found that venlafaxine was less well tolerated than sertraline, without evidence for an increase in efficacy (Oslin et al. 2003).

In summary, it seems prudent to not use SNRIs as first-line agents in older patients and to reserve them for patients whose symptoms do not respond to one or two SSRIs (Alexopoulos et al. 2001; Mulsant et al. 2001a, 2014) or for those who present with depression and chronic pain (Karp et al. 2010; Raskin et al. 2007; Wohlreich et al. 2009). This recommendation is congruent with results from open geriatric studies (e.g., Cooper et al. 2011; Hsu et al. 2016) and results from the Sequenced Treatment Alternatives to Relieve Depression (STAR*D) study (Rush et al. 2006a, 2006b, 2008). In this seminal study, mixed-age patients who failed to respond to a first-line SSRI had similar outcomes when the next treatment step was to augment the SSRI with sustained-release bupropion or buspirone, switch to another SSRI, or switch to an agent from another class (i.e., bupropion or venlafaxine XR). The steps that followed included using a combination of venlafaxine XR and mirtazapine, with outcomes similar to those associated with switching to the monoamine oxidase inhibitor (MAOI) tranylcypromine (Rush et al. 2006a, 2006b, 2008). In a large subsequent randomized, placebo-controlled trial ($N=480$) in adults with depression who had not responded to an SSRI or an SNRI, patients randomly assigned to augmentation with mirtazapine had the same improvement but more adverse effects than those given placebo (Kessler et al. 2018). Clinicians should be cautious when combining venlafaxine and mirtazapine in older adults with cardiovascular disease, given the warning that mirtazapine can cause QTc prolongation and torsades de pointes, particularly when combined with other drugs (e.g., venlafaxine) that can also prolong the QT interval (Health Canada Advisory 2014).

Other Second-Generation Antidepressants

Only limited controlled data support the efficacy and safety of bupropion, nefazodone, mirtazapine, vilazodone, or vortioxetine in older populations. Because of their usually favorable side effect profiles and their different mechanisms of action, bupropion and mirtazapine are often used as monotherapy in older persons who cannot tolerate SSRIs or SNRIs or are used as monotherapy or in combination in older persons who do not respond to SSRIs or SNRIs (Alexopoulos et al. 2001; Mulsant et al. 2001a, 2014). There is also a growing interest in using vortioxetine as an alternative to SSRIs or SNRIs in older patients with depression due to its possible beneficial effect on cognition and function (Cumbo et al. 2019; Lenze et al. 2020; Ostuzzi et al. 2020), although most of the relevant data have been obtained in younger patients (Baune et al. 2018; Christensen et al. 2018; Mahableshwarkar et al. 2015; McIntyre et al. 2014).

Trazodone

Trazodone is indicated for the treatment of MDD, but it is now almost exclusively used off-label as a hypnotic or a sedative agent (Bossini et al. 2012; Smales et al. 2015) due to its sedative effect associated with antagonism of the serotonin 5-HT$_{2A}$ receptor and, to a lesser extent, the 5-HT$_{2B}$, 5-HT$_{1A}$, and α_1 receptors. When trazodone is used as a hypnotic agent, dosages should be kept low (e.g., 50–150 mg at bedtime) to minimize adverse effects.

Some evidence going back to the early 1990s indicates that trazodone at low to moderate dosages (50–300 mg/day) has an efficacy comparable with that of haloperidol in the treatment of agitation or aggression in patients with dementia (Henry et al. 2011; Houlihan et al. 1994; Sultzer et al. 1997; Teri et al. 2000). In a unique, small (*N*=30) RCT, trazodone (50 mg given at 10 P.M.) was more efficacious than placebo in the treatment of sleep disturbances in patients with Alzheimer's dementia; it was well tolerated and did not impair cognition (Camargos et al. 2014, 2015; McCleery and Sharpley 2020). In a related open study, trazodone was demonstrated to improve circadian rhythmicity in 30 patients with Alzheimer's dementia (Grippe et al. 2015).

With the high dosages needed to treat depression (300–600 mg/day), trazodone antagonism of α_1-adrenergic receptors may cause dry mouth, orthostatic hypotension (with syncope), QT prolongation or arrhythmias, and priapism (which is rare in older adults). Like other psychotropic medications, trazodone has been associated with hyponatremia and can be involved in serotonin syndrome, particularly when combined with SSRIs, SNRIs, or other medications that also affect the serotonergic system. In a large observational study in older primary care patients treated for depression, trazodone was associated with the highest risk of all-cause mortality among 11 commonly prescribed antidepressants (Coupland et al. 2011); however, in the absence of randomization, this association may have been due to confounding factors for which the researchers could not control. Trazodone is mostly metabolized by CYP3A4; therefore, its dosage should be reduced when it is coprescribed with medications that inhibit this liver enzyme (see Table 20–3), and drinking a large quantity of grapefruit juice should be discouraged in patients taking trazodone.

Bupropion

The antidepressant effect of bupropion has been attributed to its inhibition of norepinephrine and dopamine reuptake. It is also a nicotinic receptor antagonist approved for smoking cessation. Bupropion is a moderate inhibitor of CYP2D6 (Kotlyar et al. 2005) (see Table 20–3). It appears to be metabolized by CYP2B6 (Hesse et al. 2004), and adverse effects such as seizures or gait disturbance may be more likely in individuals who take bupropion alongside drugs that inhibit CYP2B6, such as fluoxetine or paroxetine (Joo et al. 2002).

Published data supporting the safety and efficacy of bupropion in geriatric depression are limited to small controlled trials and a small open study (Steffens et al. 2001). Expert consensus favors bupropion—alone or as an augmentation agent—in older patients with depression whose symptoms have not responded to SSRIs or who cannot tolerate them (Alexopoulos et al. 2001; Buchanan et al. 2006; Mulsant et al. 2001a, 2014). Bupropion can be helpful for patients who complain of nausea, diarrhea, unbearable fatigue, or sexual dysfunction during SSRI treatment (Nieuwstraten and Dolovich 2001; Thase et al. 2005b).

Augmentation of SSRIs or SNRIs with bupropion has been reported to be helpful in patients who were partial responders. The safety of these combinations in older patients was evaluated in a large geriatric trial (Cristancho et al. 2019). Older controlled data on the use of bupropion in adults with heart disease (Kiev et al. 1994; Roose et al. 1991) or neuropathic pain (Semenchuk et al. 2001) and in smokers (Tashkin et al. 2001) are congruent with clinical experience that bupropion is usually well tolerated by medically ill patients. Bupropion remains contraindicated in patients who have or at risk for seizure disorders (e.g., poststroke patients). However, the sustained-release preparation of bupropion has been associated with a very low incidence of seizures, comparable with that of other antidepressants (Dunner et al. 1998).

Bupropion also has been associated with onset of psychosis in case reports (Howard and Warnock 1999), and the prudent action is to avoid this medication in patients with psychosis and in agitated patients at risk for the development of psychotic symptoms. The propensity of bupropion to induce psychosis in at-risk patients has been attributed to its action on dopaminergic neurotransmission (Howard and Warnock 1999). The same mechanism has been hypothesized to underlie the association of bupropion with gait disturbance and falls in some patients (Joo et al. 2002). Because of its putative dopaminergic and noradrenergic properties, the tolerability and efficacy of bupropion (target dosage 300 mg/day) were assessed in a 12-week randomized, placebo-controlled trial in 108 patients with mild to moderate Alzheimer's disease and apathy. No group differences were found in tolerability and changes in apathy, cognition, or function; however, patients in the placebo group had more favorable outcomes in terms of neuropsychiatric symptoms and health-related quality of life (Maier et al. 2020).

Mirtazapine

The antidepressant activity of mirtazapine has been attributed to its blockade of α_2 autoreceptors, resulting in a direct enhancement of noradrenergic neurotransmission and an increase in the synaptic levels of serotonin, indirectly enhancing neurotransmission mediated by 5-HT$_{1A}$ receptors. In addition, like the antinausea drugs granisetron and ondansetron, mirtazapine inhibits 5-HT$_2$ and 5-HT$_3$ receptors. Thus, mirtazapine could be particularly helpful for individuals who do not tolerate SSRIs because of sexual dysfunction (Gelenberg et al. 2000; Montejo et al. 2001), tremor (Pact and Giduz 1999), or severe nausea (Pedersen and Klysner 1997). In one case series, mirtazapine was used successfully to treat depression in 19 mixed-age oncology patients receiving chemotherapy (Thompson 2000). It also has been combined with SSRIs (Pedersen and Klysner 1997); however, these combinations should be used with caution because they have been associated with serotonin syndrome in an older patient (Benazzi 1998). As discussed, in the STAR*D study, a combination of mirtazapine and venlafaxine XR had modest efficacy in patients with treatment-resistant depression (Rush et al. 2006a); in a subsequent large, randomized, placebo-controlled trial, participants randomly assigned to augmentation of SSRIs or SNRIs with mirtazapine experienced the same improvement but more adverse effects than those given placebo (Kessler et al. 2018). Regardless of its merits, the efficacy and safety of this combination have not been established in older patients, and it may prolong the QT interval.

No placebo-controlled trials have been published and only two comparator-controlled trials of mirtazapine in geriatric depression have been done. Consistent with this paucity of controlled data, experts favor use of mirtazapine as a third-line drug in older patients with depression who cannot tolerate or whose symptoms have not responded to SSRIs or venlafaxine (Alexopoulos et al. 2001). Mirtazapine also has been used to treat depression in frail nursing home patients (Roose et al. 2003) and in older patients with dementia (Raji and Brady 2001), but there are concerns about its effect on cognition. It has been shown to impair driving performance in two placebo- and active comparator–controlled trials in healthy volunteers (Ridout et al. 2003; Wingen et al. 2005) and cause delirium in older patients with cognitive disorders (Bailer et al. 2000). This deleterious effect on cognition may be a due to mirtazapine's antihistaminergic and sedative effects.

Other adverse effects of mirtazapine include weight gain with lipid increase (Nicholas et al. 2003), hyponatremia (Cheah et al. 2008), and, rarely, neutropenia or even agranulocytosis (Hutchison 2001). In a large observational study in older primary care patients treated for depression, mirtazapine was associated with a higher risk of stroke and mortality than other commonly prescribed antidepressants (Coupland et al. 2011); however, in the absence of randomization, one cannot rule out that this association was due to confounding factors for which the researchers could not control. In March 2014, Merck Canada issued a warning endorsed by Health Canada that mirtazapine can cause QT prolongation and torsades de pointes in association with overdose or when other risk factors for QT prolongation are present (e.g., in patients with cardiovascular disease or when combined with other medications that can cause QT prolongation) (Health Canada Advisory 2014).

Nefazodone

Nefazodone should not be used in older adults given the absence of controlled trials in this population, the mediocre outcomes of an open study (Saiz-Ruiz et al. 2002), the potentially problematic drug–drug interactions caused by its strong inhibition of CYP3A4 (see Table 20–3), and the FDA black box warning that it can cause life-threatening hepatic toxicity or even liver failure, the incidence of which has been reported to be 10- to 30-fold higher than with other antidepressants (Carvajal García-Pando et al. 2002).

Vilazodone

Vilazodone acts as both a serotonin reuptake inhibitor and a partial agonist at the serotonin 5-HT$_{1A}$ receptor, with negligible noradrenergic or dopaminergic effects. It is unlikely to cause or to be involved in drug–drug interactions (see Table 20–3). In clinical trials in adults, the most common adverse effects associated with vilazodone were diarrhea, nausea, and headache. Its efficacy in the treatment of older patients with MDD is supported by a small RCT in which 56 adults with MDD were assigned to either paroxetine or vilazodone, resulting in similar improvement in depressed mood, with vilazodone being associated with a higher reduction of proinflammatory gene expression and immune modulation than paroxetine (Eyre et al. 2017). In a post-hoc pooled analysis of four placebo-controlled RCTs of vilazodone in adults with MDD, among the 177 participants who were 60 years of age and older, those patients who were assigned to vilazodone (N=97) had greater symptomatic improvement and higher rates of response or remission than those assigned to placebo; their symptomatic improvement was also greater than that experienced by younger patients (Kornstein et al. 2018).

Vortioxetine

The antidepressant activity of vortioxetine has been attributed to its multimodal action on a variety of neurotransmitters and receptors, but it predominantly seems to be a serotonin reuptake inhibitor (Berhan and Barker 2014). It is metabolized by multiple cytochrome P450 enzymes and does not inhibit any, therefore it is unlikely to cause or to be involved in drug–drug interactions (see Table 20–3). Several RCTs of vortioxetine in older patients with MDD have been published. In the first (Katona et al. 2012), 452 patients age 65 and older (mean age 70.6 years) with a current major depressive episode and at least one previous episode prior to age 60, a Montgomery-Åsberg Depression Rating Scale score of at least 26, and a Mini-Mental State Examination (MMSE) score of <24 were assigned (1:1:1) to vortioxetine 5 mg/day, duloxetine 60 mg/day, or placebo and treated for 8 weeks under double-blind conditions. The symptomatic improvement of patients assigned to vortioxetine (−3.8±1.0) or duloxetine (−6.1±1.0) was significantly greater than that of those assigned to placebo. A similar pattern was observed in the response and remission rates (vortioxetine 53%, 29%; duloxetine 63%, 35%; placebo 35%, 19%). Both vortioxetine and duloxetine were associated with statistically significant improvement in memory (with modest effect sizes of 0.24 and 0.33, respectively); vortioxetine (but not duloxetine) was associated with significant improvement in processing speed (with effect sizes of 0.25 and 0.07). Both antidepressants were well tolerated, with nausea being the only adverse event, occurring at a significantly higher incidence with vortioxetine (21.8%) than with placebo (8.3%).

In an open-label RCT, 108 older patients (mean age 76.7±4.3 years) with mild Alzheimer's disease (MMSE score 21±3) and mild depressive symptoms (Hamilton Depression Rating Scale [Hamilton 1960] score 14±5) were randomly assigned to receive vortioxetine 15 mg/day (n=36) or other common antidepressants (i.e., escitalopram, paroxetine, bupropion, venlafaxine, or sertraline). All of the antidepressants were well tolerated, with nausea and headache the most common observed adverse effects. Over 12 months, depression and three of four cognitive measures improved significantly more in those who received vortioxetine (Cumbo et al. 2019). In another RCT, 100 patients age 65 and older with subjective cognitive impairment but without MCI or MDD received computer-based cognitive training augmented with vortioxetine or placebo for 26 weeks. Vortioxetine was associated with a higher increase in global cognitive performance than placebo only at week 12, and both groups showed similar improvement in function (Lenze et al. 2020).

Although these newer data related to the possible effect of vortioxetine on cognition or function (Jacobson et al. 2020) are encouraging, the FDA declined to grant a special indication for vortioxetine for the treatment of cognitive impairment associated with depression. However, vortioxetine appears to be a reasonable choice when treating older adults with depression and cognitive impairment. This view may change when results of the ongoing VESPA study become available (Ostuzzi et al. 2020). In other groups of older patients, as in younger patients (Koesters et al. 2017), vortioxetine does not seem to offer any advantages over more commonly used SSRIs or SNRIs; in particular, we note its apparent lack of efficacy in GAD (Mahableshwarkar et al. 2014).

Tricyclic Antidepressants and Monoamine Oxidase Inhibitors

Tricyclic antidepressants (TCAs) and MAOIs have now become fourth- and fifth-line drugs in the treatment of late-life depression because they are less well tolerated than the SSRIs or SNRIs, they have a narrow therapeutic range, and their use requires special precautions (Mulsant et al. 2001b; Rajji et al. 2008; von Wolff et al. 2013; Wilson and Mottram 2004). The tertiary-amine TCAs—amitriptyline, clomipramine, doxepin, and imipramine—can cause significant orthostatic hypotension and anticholinergic effects, including cognitive impairment, and they should be avoided in older persons (American Geriatrics Society Beers Criteria Update Expert Panel 2019). The secondary amines desipramine and nortriptyline are preferred in older patients (Mulsant et al. 2014). They have a lower propensity to cause orthostasis and falls, in addition to having linear pharmacokinetics and more modest anticholinergic effects (Chew et al. 2008). Their relatively narrow therapeutic index (i.e., the plasma level range separating efficacy and toxicity) necessitates monitoring plasma levels and electrocardiograms in older patients. A single dose is given at bedtime; 5–7 days after initiation of desipramine at 50 mg or nortriptyline at 25 mg, plasma levels should be measured and dosages adjusted linearly, with targeted plasma levels of 200–400 ng/mL for desipramine and 50–150 ng/mL for nortriptyline. These narrow ranges ensure efficacy while decreasing risks of cardiac toxicity and other side effects.

Like the tertiary-amine TCAs, desipramine and nortriptyline are type 1 antiarrhythmics: they have quinidine-like effects on cardiac conduction and should not be used in patients who have or are at risk for cardiac conduction defects (Roose et al. 1991). Most anticholinergic side effects of desipramine or nortriptyline (e.g., dry mouth, constipation) resolve with time or usually can be mitigated with symptomatic treatment (Rosen et al. 1993). TCAs have been associated with cognitive worsening compared with placebo (Reifler et al. 1989) and with less cognitive improvement than occurs with sertraline (Bondareff et al. 2000; Doraiswamy et al. 2003) or other SSRIs.

Although MAOIs have been efficacious in older patients with depression (Georgotas et al. 1986) and may have a special role in some patients with treatment-resistant depression, they are now rarely used in older patients (Shulman et al. 2009), in large part because they can cause significant hypotension or life-threatening hypertensive or serotonergic crises as a result of dietary or drug interactions. When the MAOIs are used in older patients whose symptoms have typically failed to respond to SSRIs, SNRIs, and TCAs, phenelzine is preferred to tranylcypromine because it has been more extensively studied in this population (Georgotas et al. 1986). A typical starting dosage would be 15 mg/day, with a target dosage of 45–90 mg/day in three divided doses. Patients must follow dietary restrictions (Shulman and Walker 2001) and inform their health care providers (including pharmacists) that they are taking an MAOI.

Another treatment option is the selegiline transdermal patch, which was developed to deliver selegiline blood concentrations sufficient to inhibit monoamine oxidase A and B (MAO-A and MAO-B) in the brain without inhibiting MAO-A in the gastrointestinal tract, thereby reducing the risk of hypertensive crisis (Nandagopal and DelBello 2009). No geriatric data are available. Dietary restrictions are not needed at the 6 mg/day dosage but are recommended with higher dosages (Robinson and Amsterdam 2008). The potential for lethal drug interactions or the incidence of cardiovascular or cerebrovascular events (Tadrous et al. 2021) remains a concern.

Psychostimulants, Ketamine, Esketamine, and Other Psychedelic Agents

Psychostimulants

Amphetamines. Although a handful of publications over the past 30 years have reported on the use of amphetamines in older patients with various conditions, in the absence of quality evidence supporting their safety or efficacy in these patients, they should not be used (Sassi et al. 2020).

Methylphenidate. A series of studies have assessed the use of methylphenidate in older patients with depression or cognitive impairment (Sassi et al. 2020). These studies have suggested that methylphenidate is generally well tolerated and modestly efficacious for medically burdened older individuals with depression (Satel and Nelson 1989; Wallace et al. 1995). Nevertheless, caution is advised regarding the possible exacerbation of anxiety, psychosis, anorexia, tachycardia, or hypertension (Roose and Rutherford 2016) and potential interactions with warfarin.

Several RCTs suggest that methylphenidate can be used to augment SSRIs in older patients with depression. In the largest and most recent relevant randomized, placebo-controlled trial, 143 cognitively intact older outpatients with moderate to severe MDD were assigned to methylphenidate (5–40 mg/day; mean 16 mg/day), citalopram (20–60 mg/day; mean 32 mg/day) plus placebo, or citalopram plus methylphenidate. Over 16 weeks of treatment, tolerability and improvement in cognitive performance were similar in the three groups. However, the group given citalopram plus methylphenidate experienced greater improvement and a faster change in depressive symptoms (Lavretsky et al. 2015).

Methylphenidate is also used for the treatment of apathy associated with dementia (Lanctôt et al. 2014; Rosenberg et al. 2013; van Dyck et al. 2021). A Cochrane review of three multicenter randomized, placebo-controlled trials involving 145 participants (Herrmann et al. 2008; Padala et al. 2018; Rosenberg et al. 2013) concluded that 20 mg/day of methylphenidate is well tolerated and improves apathy in patients with Alzheimer's dementia, with possible additional small benefits for cognition or functional performance. However, the evidence was deemed to be of low quality (Ruthirakuhan et al. 2018). A better-designed RCT that studied 200 patients with Alzheimer's dementia (ADMET 2) (Scherer et al. 2018) found a larger decrease over 6 months in Neuropsychiatric Inventory apathy scores in those randomized to methylphenidate than in those randomized to placebo; methylphenidate was as well tolerated as placebo, but cognitive measures and quality of life did not differ between the two groups (Mintzer et al. 2021).

Modafinil and armodafinil. The wakefulness-promoting medication modafinil and its R-enantiomer armodafinil appear to induce a calm alertness through nondopaminergic mechanisms. These agents have been used to target apathy and fatigue in adult patients taking SSRIs (Dunlop et al. 2007; Fava et al. 2007; Goss et al. 2013) or as an adjunctive treatment for the negative symptoms of schizophrenia (Lindenmayer et al. 2013). Geriatric data are limited to low-quality studies in poststroke patients (Cross et al. 2020; Poulsen et al. 2015; Visser et al. 2019), small studies of patients with Alzheimer's dementia (Frakey et al. 2012) or Lewy body dementia (Lapid et al. 2017; Varanese et al. 2013), or assessment of tolerability in older, healthy volunteer exposure (Darwish et al. 2011).

Other dopaminergic agents. Experience with other dopaminergic agents such as pergolide, piribedil, and ropinirole in older patients with psychiatric symptoms has been limited (Nagaraja and Jayashree 2001; Rektorová et al. 2003). By contrast, a series of RCTs supported the use of pramipexole in older patients with Parkinson's disease and depression (Aiken 2007; Barone et al. 2006, 2010; Rektorová et al. 2003), and experts recommend its use in these patients (Agüera-Ortiz et al. 2021; Starkstein and Brockman 2017). However, it may have a detrimental effect on cognition in some of these patients (Roy et al. 2018). Some RCTs also suggest a role for pramipexole in the treatment of adults with MDD or bipolar depression, with response rates similar to SSRIs when it is used alone (Fawcett et al. 2016; Szmulewicz et al. 2017; Tundo et al. 2019) or as an augmenting agent (Romeo et al. 2018). No such data currently exist for older adults with depression. However, the efficacy, tolerability, and safety of pramipexole in older patients with Parkinson's disease and depression suggest that it may also have a role the treatment of depression in older patients (Aiken 2007; Barone et al. 2006, 2010; Rektorová et al. 2003).

Ketamine and Esketamine

Over the past decade, the dissociative anesthetic ketamine and its S-enantiomer esketamine have been shown to have rapid antidepressant and antisuicidal properties, leading to the approval by the FDA of intranasal esketamine in conjunction with an oral antidepressant for treatment-resistant depression in adults or depressive symptoms in adults with MDD with acute suicidal ideation or behavior. The rapid antidepressant and antisuicidal effects of ketamine and esketamine have been attributed to various mechanisms, including their modulation of glutamate via the NMDA receptor (which is responsible for their anesthetic and psychotomimetic effects), downstream effect on other neurotransmitters, signaling pathways, or neurotrophic factors (Ballard and Zarate 2020; Kadriu et al. 2021; Wu et al. 2021).

Almost all evidence supporting the efficacy of ketamine or esketamine in the treatment of MDD has been obtained in physically healthy younger adults (Marcantoni et al. 2020; McIntyre et al. 2021), as is also the case for the use of ketamine in the treatment of bipolar depression or suicidality (Fornaro et al. 2020; Joseph et al. 2021; McIntyre et al. 2021). Two peer-reviewed publications reported on the treatment with ketamine of older patients with depression (George et al. 2017; Lipsitz et al. 2021), and one reported on a unique RCT in older patients with depression randomly assigned to either intranasal esketamine or placebo (Ochs-Ross et al. 2020). In a small pilot study ($N=16$), adults age 60 and older with MDD or bipolar depression whose illness did not respond to at least one antidepressant and who received weekly subcutaneous ketamine (0.2–0.5 mg/kg) experienced a significant reduction in depressive symptoms; the main adverse effects were transient dissociation, which resolved spontaneously, and increased blood pressure or heart rate (George et al. 2017). In a series of 53 patients age 60 years and older with MDD treated naturalistically with four intravenous ketamine infusions over 1–2 weeks, participants reported significant decreases in depressive symptoms, with 58% responding and 10% remitting; more than two-thirds experienced treatment-emergent hypertension, and one-fifth required an antihypertensive. A much larger and well-designed RCT ($N=138$) assessed the efficacy of flexibly dosed (28–84 mg) intranasal esketamine or placebo twice a week for 4 weeks plus a new SSRI or SNRI in adults age 65 years or older with MDD whose illness did not respond to at least two antidepressant trials (Ochs-Ross et al. 2020). The reduction in depressive scores (primary outcome) was 3.6 points greater in the esketamine/antidepressant group than in the placebo/antidepressant group but failed to reach statistical significance (P=0.059). However, esketamine was associated with significantly higher rates of response (27% vs. 13%) and remission (18% vs. 7%); also, the young-old subjects (65–74 years), but not the old-old subjects (75+ years), improved significantly. Common adverse effects were transient and included dizziness, nausea, increased blood pressure, dissociation, and headaches (Ochs-Ross et al. 2020).

Some authors have raised concerns that repeated use of ketamine may adversely affect cognition in animal models and humans (Luo et al. 2020). None of these three studies in geriatric populations (George et al. 2017; Lipsitz et al. 2021; Ochs-Ross et al. 2020) reported on cognition, but a review by Gill et al. (2021) of five studies that evaluated cognition in younger adults with treatment-resistant depression who received a subanesthetic dose of intravenous ketamine (i.e., 0.5 mg/kg subanesthetic) showed no acute worsening of cognitive function. To date, only one report has been published of the use of ketamine for treatment-resistant depression in a patient with Alzheimer's disease (Rocha et al. 2021).

Despite the lack of geriatric data, esketamine is approved by the FDA for the treatment of a major depressive episode at the same recommended dosages as in younger patients (84 mg intranasally twice per week during the induction phase and once per week during the maintenance phase), with no adjustment required for mild to moderate hepatic or renal impairment. Blood pressure needs to be measured before administration and 40 minutes later; direct observation is required for at least 2 hours after administration. Given the available data on ketamine or esketamine in older patients, these medications should not be used clinically in patients older than 75 years; in young-old patients, these medications may be used as an alternative to brain stimulation in those whose illness has not responded to other psychotropic medications (including at least one augmentation trial) (Subramanian and Lenze 2021).

Other Psychedelic Agents

The use of ketamine and esketamine in the treatment of depression or suicidality has led to a renewed interest in the use of various agents with dissociative or hallucinogenic properties, such as lysergic acid diethylamide, MDMA ("Ecstasy"), or psilocybin (De Gregorio et al. 2021; Kadriu et al. 2021). Even though some of these agents may also have rapid antidepressant properties, it would be unwise to use them in older patients until clinical trials have been conducted in this population.

Antipsychotic Medications

Atypical antipsychotics are widely prescribed to older adults, mainly for the treatment of psychotic symptoms of any etiology, various mood disorders, and psychiatric symptoms associated with dementia. In older adults, the strongest studies support the efficacy of these agents in the treatment of late-life schizophrenia and late-onset psychoses (Scott et al. 2011; Suzuki et al. 2011), MDD with psychotic features (Flint et al. 2019; Meyers et al. 2009), and agitation or psychosis associated with dementia (Maher et al. 2011) and for augmentation of antidepressants in older patients with treatment-resistant depression (Katila et al. 2013; Lenze et al. 2015). Both typical and atypical antipsychotics are also often used for the prevention or treatment of delirium, although evidence does not strongly support their use for these indications (Barbateskovic et al. 2020; Burry et al. 2019; Egberts et al. 2021; Kim et al. 2020; Marra et al. 2021; Nikooie et al. 2019; Oh et al. 2019).

The widespread use of atypical antipsychotics in patients with dementia has raised some concerns (Mulsant 2014; Salzman et al. 2008). In 2005, two highly publicized reports and an FDA warning indicated a nearly twofold increase compared with placebo in the rate of deaths among older patients with dementia treated with atypical antipsychotics (Kuehn 2005; Schneider et al. 2005). These reports have led to a reexamination of the safety of both conventional and atypical antipsychotics in older patients. A series of studies emphasized their association with mortality (Ballard et al. 2009; Langballe et al. 2014; Maust et al. 2015; Ray et al. 2009; Simoni-Wastila et al. 2016; Wang et al. 2005), stroke (Gill et al. 2005; Herrmann et al. 2004), severe hyperglycemia in patients with diabetes (Lipscombe et al. 2009), fractures (Liperoti et al. 2007), pneumonia (Boivin et al. 2019), and venous thromboembolism (Kleijer et al. 2010). However, when compared with typical antipsychotics, atypical antipsychotics appear to be associated with lower mortality (Langballe et al. 2014; Lao et al. 2020; Schneider et al. 2005), fewer falls (Hien et al. 2005; Landi et al. 2005), and fewer EPS (Lee et al. 2004; Meagher et al. 2013; Rochon et al. 2005; van Iersel et al. 2005) but more cerebrovascular events (Percudani et al. 2005), venous thromboembolism (Liperoti et al. 2005), and pancreatitis (Koller et al. 2003).

Given the increased recognition of the risks associated with the use of antipsychotics in older patients, clinicians need to consider their potential risks and benefits for each individual patient (Gauthier et al. 2010; Rajji et al. 2017; Voineskos et al. 2020). When antipsychotics are prescribed to older patients, the minimal effective dosage should be used (Tsuboi et al. 2011). Antipsychotics should be prescribed only to patients with dementia whose illness has failed to respond to nonpharmacological interventions or alternative medications (Mulsant 2014; Porsteinsson et al. 2014). Their long-term use is justified to treat schizophrenia, bipolar disorder, or MDD with psychotic features (Flint et al. 2019), and long-acting injectable (LAI) atypical antipsychotics are associated with a reduction in rehospitalization in older patients with schizophrenia (Lin et al. 2020). Discontinuation should be attempted in stable patients with disorders other than schizophrenia, bipolar disorder, or MDD with psychotic features. Although antipsychotics can be discontinued safely in most older patients with dementia, their discontinuation may be associated with recurrence of symptoms in those who present with more severe agitation or psychosis (Declercq et al. 2013).

Risperidone

Of the atypical antipsychotics, risperidone has the most published geriatric data for various conditions (Schneider et al. 2005, 2006a; Suzuki et al. 2011). Its efficacy and tolerability in the treatment of late-life schizophrenia are supported by three RCTs: one randomized comparison with olanzapine (Harvey et al. 2003; Jeste et al. 2003), one randomized open-label study of crossover from conventional antipsychotics to risperidone or olanzapine (Ritchie et al. 2003, 2006), and one RCT comparing continuing the same dosage with doubling the dosage of olanzapine or risperidone in mixed-age participants with schizophrenia whose illness had not responded to olanzapine 10 mg/day or risperidone 3 mg/day for at least 4 weeks (Sakurai et al. 2016). The randomized comparison showed similar efficacy between olanzapine and risperidone but more weight gain and less cognitive improvement with olanzapine (Harvey et al.

2003; Jeste et al. 2003). In the crossover study, patients switched to olanzapine were more likely to complete the switching process and to show an improvement in psychological quality of life (Ritchie et al. 2003, 2006). In the incremental-dosage RCT, participants randomly assigned to higher dosages did not benefit from them (Sakurai et al. 2016). The results from these three controlled trials are supported by a large body of uncontrolled data in older patients with schizophrenia and other psychotic disorders (e.g., Davidson et al. 2000; Madhusoodanan et al. 1999). In addition, an analysis of 57 patients with schizophrenia age 65 and older who participated in randomized studies of LAI ("depot") risperidone (Risperdal Consta) found that it was well tolerated and produced significant symptomatic improvements (Lasser et al. 2004).

As with other atypical antipsychotics, the efficacy and tolerability of risperidone in younger patients with bipolar disorder (and possibly other mood disorders) are well established. However, given the risks associated with antipsychotics, we continue to favor the use of mood stabilizers as first-line agents for older patients with bipolar disorder, except in the presence of severe mania or mania with psychosis, in which case the data favor combining risperidone, olanzapine, or quetiapine with a mood stabilizer (Sajatovic et al. 2005b, 2013; Young et al. 2004, 2017).

The efficacy and tolerability of risperidone in the treatment of behavioral and psychological symptoms of dementia have been reported in a series of placebo-controlled RCTs (e.g., Brodaty et al. 2003; De Deyn et al. 1999, 2005b; Katz et al. 1999; Schneider et al. 2006a, 2006b; Sink et al. 2005) and in randomized comparisons with haloperidol (Chan et al. 2001; De Deyn et al. 1999; Suh et al. 2004), promazine (Gareri et al. 2004), and olanzapine (Fontaine et al. 2003; Gareri et al. 2004; Mulsant et al. 2004). The efficacy of risperidone in the treatment of agitation or psychosis is also supported by an RCT showing that persons with Alzheimer's disease whose agitation or psychosis had responded acutely to risperidone experienced an increased risk of relapse when they were switched to placebo after 4 months (hazard ratio 1:9) or 8 months (hazard ratio 4:9) compared with those who remained on risperidone (Devanand et al. 2012). Taken together, the available data support the use of risperidone for the treatment of patients with dementia and distressing psychosis or severe agitation (Yunusa et al. 2019). However, the substantial risks associated with the use of risperidone or other atypical antipsychotics in these patients—including increased mortality (number needed to harm [NNH] 87) and stroke (NNH 53) (Maher et al. 2011; Rivière et al. 2019; Yunusa et al. 2019)—should lead to caution.

One randomized comparison with haloperidol (Han and Kim 2004) and some uncontrolled data (e.g., Mittal et al. 2004; Parellada et al. 2004) support the efficacy and tolerability of risperidone in the treatment of delirium (Boettger et al. 2015; Wang et al. 2013). In another RCT, a significantly lower incidence of delirium was observed in patients given a single 1-mg dose of risperidone just after cardiac surgery than in those given placebo (Prakanrattana and Prapaitrakool 2007; Zhang et al. 2013). However, caution is essential when using risperidone, or any antipsychotic, to treat delirium (Hale et al. 2016; D.H. Kim et al. 2018).

One small randomized comparison of risperidone and clozapine (N=10) (Ellis et al. 2000) and several open trials of low-dosage risperidone in the treatment of Parkinson's disease and drug-induced psychosis or Lewy body dementia have had inconsistent results, with a clear worsening of parkinsonian symptoms in some studies (e.g., Culo et al. 2010; Ellis et al. 2000; Iketani et al. 2019; Leopold 2000). Thus, it is prudent to avoid risperidone in these disorders (Parkinson Study Group 1999). Commonly reported adverse effects of risperidone include orthostatic hypotension (on initiation of treatment) and EPS that are dosage dependent (Katz et al. 1999). Risperidone is metabolized by CYP2D6, and poor metabolism—whether genetically determined or from CYP2D6-inhibiting medications (Mannheimer et al. 2016; Paulzen et al. 2016)—is associated with worse adverse effects. At a given dosage, concentrations of risperidone (and possibly its active metabolite paliperidone or 9-hydroxyrisperidone) seem to increase with age (Aichhorn et al. 2005). Therefore, typical dosages should be between 0.5 and 2 mg/day for older patients with dementia and <4 mg/day for older patients without dementia. Of all the atypical antipsychotics, risperidone appears to be the most likely to be associated with hyperprolactinemia (Clapham et al. 2020; Kinon et al. 2003). It is rarely associated with cognitive impairment, probably because of its low affinity for muscarinic receptors (Chew et al. 2006; Harvey et al. 2003; Mulsant et al. 2004). Like other antipsychotics, risperidone can cause weight gain, diabetes, or dyslipidemia. It is more likely to do so than aripiprazole and ziprasidone but less likely than clozapine, olanzapine, and quetiapine (American Diabetes Association et al. 2004; Feldman et al. 2004; Zheng et al. 2009).

Paliperidone

Paliperidone is the active 9-hydroxy metabolite of risperidone, and therefore some of its pharmacological action, efficacy, and side effects are similar to those of risperidone. Its once-daily extended-release formulation takes 24 hours to reach a maximum concentration, and its clearance is not affected by hepatic impairment or CYP2D6 metabolism but is affected by renal function (Mauri et al. 2018). Paliperidone carries a specific indication for the treatment of schizoaffective disorder in the United States. Its efficacy and tolerability in older patients with psychosis are supported by pooled data from 125 patients age 65 and older who participated in three 6-week registration trials that led to the medication's approval by the FDA for the treatment of schizophrenia (e.g., Davidson et al. 2007; Kane et al. 2007). Otherwise, limited available data support the efficacy and safety of paliperidone in the treatment of older patients with schizophrenia (Krause et al. 2018; Madhusoodanan and Zaveri 2010): in a 6-week randomized, placebo-controlled trial followed by a 24-week open-label extension, 114 patients age 65 and older (mean age 70 years) were given paliperidone 3–12 mg/day or placebo. Discontinuation due to adverse events and weight gain was similar in the two groups. Half of the patients who were given paliperidone experienced prolactin elevation, but this was not related to any adverse event. The efficacy was similar in both groups (Tzimos et al. 2008). Paliperidone has not yet been systematically studied in older patients with bipolar disorder or dementia, and dosages remain speculative for these populations. An LAI formulation that requires only monthly injections is an attractive option for individuals who require an LAI antipsychotic (González-Rodríguez et al. 2014; Rado and Janicak 2012), but its more widespread usage is impeded by a paucity of geriatric data.

Olanzapine

The efficacy and tolerability of olanzapine in the treatment of late-life schizophrenia have been confirmed in two randomized comparisons with haloperidol (Barak et al.

2002; Kennedy et al. 2003) and two randomized comparisons with risperidone (Harvey et al. 2003; Jeste et al. 2003; Ritchie et al. 2003, 2006). Evidence supporting the efficacy and safety of olanzapine in younger patients with bipolar disorder and other mood disorders is strong (Shelton et al. 2001; Thase 2002). Two large RCTs in which more than half of the patients were age 65 and older supported the efficacy and tolerability of olanzapine in the treatment of MDD with psychotic features (Flint et al. 2019; Meyers et al. 2009). Otherwise, there is a paucity of data relevant to older persons with mood disorders (Sajatovic et al. 2005a, 2005b; Young et al. 2017). Similarly, very few geriatric data are available on the rapidly dissolving or the intramuscular preparation of olanzapine (Belgamwar and Fenton 2005). Interestingly, although age increases olanzapine concentrations after oral administration, LAI olanzapine is unaffected by age (Tveito et al. 2018). This is probably because the injectable form bypasses age-related changes in gastrointestinal absorption or presystemic clearance.

The efficacy and tolerability of olanzapine for treating agitation or psychosis associated with dementia have been reported in several randomized, placebo-controlled trials (e.g., Clark et al. 2001; De Deyn et al. 2004; Schneider et al. 2006b; Street et al. 2000) and in randomized comparisons with haloperidol (Verhey et al. 2006), promazine or risperidone (Gareri et al. 2004), and risperidone (Fontaine et al. 2003; Mulsant et al. 2004). However, a meta-analysis of published and nonpublished randomized, placebo-controlled trials in the treatment of agitation or psychosis associated with dementia concluded that "olanzapine was not associated with efficacy overall" (Schneider et al. 2006a, p. 205). Similarly, a recent network meta-analysis concluded that olanzapine was less beneficial than aripiprazole, quetiapine, or risperidone (Yunusa et al. 2019).

In one RCT in patients with delirium, olanzapine and haloperidol were found to have comparable efficacy (Skrobik et al. 2004). In another RCT, a significantly lower incidence of delirium was observed in patients given 5 mg of olanzapine just before and just after joint replacement surgery compared with patients given placebo; however, when delirium occurred, it was longer and more severe in patients who had received olanzapine (Larsen et al. 2010; Zhang et al. 2013). Caution is needed when prescribing olanzapine for patients with delirium because some controlled trials have reported cognitive worsening in patients with dementia receiving olanzapine (Kennedy et al. 2005; Mulsant et al. 2004), and several case reports of delirium induced by olanzapine have been published. Similarly, in a systematic review and network meta-analysis, including five small RCTs of olanzapine, olanzapine worsened motor function and did not improve psychosis in patients with Parkinson's disease (Iketani et al. 2020). However, olanzapine has been demonstrated to be an effective and inexpensive antinausea treatment in patients undergoing chemotherapy (Clemmons et al. 2018; Harder et al. 2019; Slimano et al. 2018).

Based on early data, a consensus conference concluded that of the atypical antipsychotics, clozapine and olanzapine were associated with the highest risk for diabetes and caused the most weight gain and dyslipidemia (American Diabetes Association et al. 2004). Limited geriatric data show a similar risk of metabolic problems in older patients (Feldman et al. 2004; Micca et al. 2006; Zheng et al. 2009). However, some data suggest that older patients treated with olanzapine have a lower risk of weight gain or hyperlipidemia than younger patients (Flint et al. 2020; Smith et al. 2008).

TABLE 20–4. **Main receptor blockade of atypical antipsychotics**

	D_2	5-HT_2	M_1	α_1
Aripiprazole	*	++	0	+
Asenapine	+++	+++	0	+++
Brexpiprazole	*	++	0	+
Clozapine	+	++	+++	+
Iloperidone	+++	++++	0	++++
Lumateperone	*	++	0	++
Lurasidone	+++	++	0	++
Olanzapine	++	+++	++	+
Paliperidone	+++	+++	0	++
Pimavanserin	0	**	0	0
Quetiapine	+	++	+	+
Risperidone	+++	++++	0	+++
Ziprasidone	++	++	0	+

0=none; +=minimal; ++=intermediate; +++=high; ++++=very high.
Receptor types: α_1=α-adrenergic type 1; D_2=dopamine type 2; 5-HT_2=5-hydroxytryptamine (serotonin) type 2; M_1=muscarinic type 1.
*High-affinity partial agonist.
** High-affinity inverse agonist.

Other common side effects include sedation and gait disturbance. EPS appear to be dosage dependent and are rare at the lower dosages typically used in older patients (5–10 mg/day). In one RCT ($N=293$), older patients with psychosis or dementia and agitation randomly assigned to olanzapine were significantly less likely to develop EPS than those given a conventional antipsychotic; they also had a lower incidence of tardive dyskinesia (TD) over 1 year (2.5% vs. 5.5%), but the difference was not statistically significant (Kinon et al. 2015).

Olanzapine also has been associated with electroencephalographic abnormalities (Centorrino et al. 2002), and its strong blocking of the muscarinic receptor (Chew et al. 2005, 2006; Mulsant et al. 2003) (Table 20–4) may explain why it has been associated with the following effects:

- Constipation in a large series of long-term care patients (Martin et al. 2003)
- Inverted dose-response relationship, with lower efficacy in older adults with agitation or psychosis and dementia who were given 15 mg/day than in those who were given 5 mg/day, suggesting that higher dosages may be toxic in these patients (Street et al. 2000)
- Differential cognitive effect from risperidone in randomized trials involving older patients with schizophrenia (Harvey et al. 2003) or dementia (Mulsant et al. 2004)
- Worsening of cognition in a large, placebo-controlled trial in older patients with Alzheimer's disease without agitation or psychosis (Kennedy et al. 2005)
- Frank delirium in some clinical cases

Because of olanzapine's adverse effect profile, experts do not recommend it as a first-line antipsychotic in older adults at risk for anticholinergic or metabolic adverse effects (Bell et al. 2010). Individuals who are older, female, or nonsmokers or who are taking a drug that inhibits CYP1A2 (e.g., fluvoxamine or ciprofloxacin) have higher concentrations of olanzapine and may be at higher risk for adverse effects (Gex-Fabry et al. 2003). Also, in a unique randomized, placebo-controlled trial, participants given olanzapine had a significant decrease in cortical thickness over 9 months, comparable with what patients with Alzheimer's disease experience in 1 year (Voineskos et al. 2020). Although the clinical relevance of this finding is not clear, it may be another reason to avoid antipsychotics when treating psychiatric disorders for which alternative medications are available.

Quetiapine

Several uncontrolled or unblinded studies suggest that quetiapine may have a role in the treatment of older adults with primary psychotic disorders (e.g., Madhusoodanan et al. 2000; Tariot et al. 2000; Yang et al. 2005). Quetiapine also has FDA approval for treatment in adults of acute mania and depression associated with bipolar disorder and as adjunctive therapy to antidepressants for the treatment of MDD. Relevant published data from geriatric patients with bipolar disorder are limited (Carta et al. 2007; Tadger et al. 2011). By contrast, in one randomized, placebo-controlled trial of a flexible dosage (50–300 mg/day) of quetiapine in 338 older patients with MDD, remission and response rates were remarkably high (56% and 64%, respectively) and were significantly higher than with placebo (23% and 30%, respectively). Adverse events observed in >10% of the patients given quetiapine included somnolence, headache, dry mouth, and dizziness (Katila et al. 2013).

Results of several randomized, placebo-controlled trials of quetiapine in older patients with behavioral and psychological symptoms of dementia are mixed (Cheung and Stapelberg 2011; Schneider et al. 2006a). For instance, in a large trial of 333 institutionalized participants, quetiapine 200 mg/day (but not 100 mg/day) differed from placebo on global impressions and positive symptom ratings but not on the important primary outcome measures of agitation and psychosis (Zhong et al. 2007). However, in a network meta-analysis, quetiapine (like aripiprazole and risperidone) was associated with improvement (Yunusa et al. 2019).

Two small RCTs (Devlin et al. 2010, 2011; Tahir et al. 2010) and several small studies (Kim et al. 2003; Pae et al. 2004; Sasaki et al. 2003) suggest that although quetiapine may treat delirium, it may also be a causative factor in some patients (Almeida et al. 2019). Because of its low propensity to cause EPS, quetiapine is frequently used as a first-line antipsychotic in older adults with Parkinson's disease, dementia with Lewy bodies, or TD (Fernandez et al. 2002; Hershey and Coleman-Jackson 2019; Iketani et al. 2019; Poewe 2005; Yuan et al. 2017). In one systematic review and network meta-analysis that included six small RCTs, quetiapine was well tolerated and more efficacious than placebo in patients with Parkinson's disease (Iketani et al. 2020).

Due to its extensive metabolism, quetiapine has a wide dosage range. There have been several case reports of SIADH and serotonin syndrome in older patients treated with quetiapine (e.g., Atalay et al. 2007; Kohen et al. 2007). Like other antipsychotics, quetiapine can also cause somnolence or dizziness (Jaskiw et al. 2004; Katila et al. 2013; Yang et al. 2005), but the incidence of these adverse effects can be minimized by a slower dosage titration. The risk for weight gain, diabetes, or dyslipidemia associated with quetiapine appears to be similar to that associated with risperidone but lower than that associated with clozapine or olanzapine (American Diabetes Association et al. 2004; Feldman et al. 2004). As with other antipsychotics, pneumonia also remains a risk (C.S. Wu et al. 2019).

Clozapine

Clozapine is a difficult medication to use, but it is still considered the drug of choice for younger patients with treatment-resistant schizophrenia. One small case series suggested that it can be similarly helpful in older patients for the treatment of primary psychotic disorders that are refractory to other treatments (Sajatovic et al. 1997). Other data on the use of low to moderate dosages (i.e., 50–200 mg/day) in older adults with primary psychotic disorders include an RCT comparing clozapine with chlorpromazine in patients with schizophrenia (Howanitz et al. 1999) and one large case series (Barak et al. 1999; Pridan et al. 2015). Still, the strongest published studies of clozapine in geriatric populations have focused on the treatment of drug-induced psychosis in patients with Parkinson's disease (e.g., Ellis et al. 2000; Goetz et al. 2000; Parkinson Study Group 1999). The superior efficacy of clozapine over other atypical antipsychotics and pimavanserin in the treatment of psychosis in patients with Parkinson's disease was confirmed in a systematic review and network meta-analysis, including seven small RCTs of clozapine (Iketani et al. 2020). However, the use of clozapine in these patients or other older individuals is severely limited because of its significant hematological, anticholinergic (including severe constipation and ileus associated with fatalities), neurological (e.g., seizures), cognitive, metabolic, and cardiac adverse effects (Bishara and Taylor 2014; Centorrino et al. 2002; Chew et al. 2006, 2008; Das et al. 2020; Hibbard et al. 2009; Myles et al. 2018; O'Connor et al. 2010; Rajji et al. 2010). In 2020, a new FDA black box warning about potentially severe constipation was added to clozapine's label (U.S. Food and Drug Administration 2020).

Aripiprazole

Aripiprazole is FDA approved for the treatment of schizophrenia, manic or mixed episodes associated with bipolar disorder, and as an adjunctive treatment for MDD (Vasudev et al. 2018). In a large, federally funded, randomized, placebo-controlled trial, 181 older patients with MDD whose illness had not responded to 12 weeks of treatment with venlafaxine XR monotherapy (300 mg/day) were more likely to achieve remission after 12 weeks of aripiprazole augmentation (target dosage 15 mg/day) than with placebo augmentation (Lenze et al. 2015). Aripiprazole was fairly well tolerated: akathisia and parkinsonism were more frequent than with placebo, but QTc prolongation and increased adiposity, glucose, insulin, or lipids were similar in both groups (Lenze et al. 2015). The efficacy and tolerability in this relatively large RCT are congruent with the previous results of two small prospective open studies (Sajatovic et al. 2008; Sheffrin et al. 2009) and analyses of pooled geriatric data (Steffens et al. 2011; Suppes et al. 2008).

Several randomized, placebo-controlled trials of aripiprazole in older patients with agitation or psychosis associated with dementia have been published (De Deyn et al. 2005a; Mintzer et al. 2007; Streim et al. 2008). Expert opinions support the use of aripiprazole in these patients (De Deyn et al. 2013; Herrmann et al. 2013b), congruent with two meta-analyses (Maher et al. 2011; Schneider et al. 2006a) and a network meta-analysis that concluded aripiprazole "might be the most effective and safe atypical antipsychotic" for the treatment of agitation associated with dementia (Yunusa et al. 2019, p. e190828). Aripiprazole has partial dopamine type 2 (D_2) receptor agonist properties (i.e., in high dopaminergic states it acts as an antagonist and in low dopaminergic states it acts as an agonist). This may explain why it is unlikely to cause EPS, prolactin elevation, or osteoporosis even at high D_2 receptor occupancy (Mamo et al. 2007). It has only moderate affinity to the adrenergic α_1 and histamine H_1 receptors and negligible affinity to the muscarinic receptor (Chew et al. 2006, 2008). As a result, aripiprazole is less likely to cause orthostatic hypotension and antihistaminergic or anticholinergic adverse effects than other atypical agents. However, akathisia may occur in more than one-quarter of older patients; its occurrence and severity may be mitigated by slow titration or the addition of low-dosage lorazepam (Hsu et al. 2018). As is the case for paliperidone, an LAI form of aripiprazole requiring only monthly injections is available, but its safety and efficacy have not been established in patients 65 years and older.

Ziprasidone

Based on its lower effect on glucose, lipids, and weight (American Diabetes Association et al. 2004), its lack of affinity for the muscarinic receptor (Chew et al. 2006; see Table 20–4), and thus its low potential to cause cognitive impairment, ziprasidone is an attractive medication for older patients with psychosis. However, data relevant to the use of oral ziprasidone in older patients remain limited (Berkowitz 2003; Wilner et al. 2000). Three studies on the use of intramuscular ziprasidone found no adverse cardiovascular or electrocardiographic changes in a small number of older patients (Greco et al. 2005; Kohen et al. 2005; Rais et al. 2010). Moreover, after thioridazine, ziprasidone remains the antipsychotic most likely to be associated with QT prolongation (Wenzel-Seifert et al. 2011). A double-blind RCT of intravenous ziprasidone or haloperidol conducted in the intensive care unit found no benefit for either medication in patients with delirium (Girard et al. 2018). Similarly, intramuscular midazolam achieved more effective sedation than ziprasidone or olanzapine in agitated patients in the emergency department (Klein et al. 2018). In the absence of studies in geriatric populations, ziprasidone should be used with caution in older patients and should be avoided in patients with cardiac disease and those who take other drugs associated with QT prolongation.

Newer Atypical Antipsychotics and Pimavanserin

In the past decade, six other atypical antipsychotics have been approved by the FDA for use in schizophrenia or mood disorders: asenapine, brexpiprazole, cariprazine, iloperidone, lumateperone, and lurasidone (Greger et al. 2021; Mauri et al. 2018; Snyder et al. 2021). In younger adults, these newer atypical antipsychotics are thought to have better tolerability but lower efficacy than the older atypical antipsychotics (i.e., clozapine, olanzapine, or risperidone) (Antoun Reyad et al. 2020; Kantrowitz 2020). However, the geriatric literature on these newer antipsychotics is limited to two RCTs of brexpiprazole for agitation associated with dementia (Grossberg et al. 2020): a post hoc pooled analysis of older patients with bipolar disorder who participated in two placebo-controlled RCTs of lurasidone and their open-label extensions (Forester et al. 2018; Sajatovic et al. 2016), and some case series of older patients with bipolar disorder who were treated with asenapine (Baruch et al. 2013; Sajatovic et al. 2015). Otherwise, the geriatric literature consists of expert opinions based on pharmacological profiles or extrapolations from data in younger adults (Guay 2011; Rado and Janicak 2012; Vasudev et al. 2018). The limited geriatric evidence is congruent with data from younger patients, confirming the good tolerability but limited efficacy of these new antidepressants in older patients. Given the limited available evidence, principles of conservative prescribing (Schiff et al. 2011) preclude recommending the use of these newer antipsychotics in older patients at this time, despite their good tolerability.

Pimavanserin is the first medication specifically approved by the FDA for the treatment of hallucinations and psychosis associated with Parkinson's disease (Kitten et al. 2018). It has a unique mechanism of action, modulating serotonergic transmission as a selective inverse agonist of the 5-HT$_{2A}$ receptor with no appreciable effect on dopaminergic, muscarinic, histaminergic, or adrenergic receptors (Meltzer and Roth 2013). A meta-analysis of 17 RCTs confirmed its efficacy in the treatment of psychosis associated with Parkinson's disease but found it inferior to the efficacy of clozapine (Iketani et al. 2020). An analysis of data from an RCT has shown the efficacy of pimavanserin in patients with psychosis associated with Parkinson's disease who have cognitive impairment treated or untreated with cognitive enhancers; however, serious adverse events and discontinuations were more frequent in those taking cholinesterase inhibitors (Espay et al. 2018). In a retrospective cohort study, patients with Parkinson's disease or Lewy body dementia were more likely to discontinue quetiapine early than pimavanserin (Horn et al. 2019).

Pimavanserin has also been assessed for the treatment of psychosis associated with Alzheimer's disease in one small randomized, placebo-controlled trial that showed some modest efficacy (comparable with that of atypical antipsychotics) after 6 weeks but not 12 weeks; this RCT has been reported in two publications (Ballard et al. 2018, 2019) that were the subject of a systematic review (Srinivasan et al. 2020). The efficacy of pimavanserin over placebo as an augmenting agent to antidepressants in adults with MDD has also been studied in several small RCTs, with mixed results (Soogrim et al. 2021).

Common side effects of pimavanserin include peripheral edema, nausea, and confusion. Like other antipsychotics, it carries an FDA warning about its use in patients with dementia, and its use in long-term care facilities falls under federal Omnibus Budget Reconciliation Act (OBRA) regulations. Pimavanserin can cause QTc prolongation and increased mortality (Moreno et al. 2018), and caution should be exercised when co-prescribing it with cholinesterase inhibitors (Espay et al. 2018). Overall, its novel mechanism of action makes it an interesting antipsychotic agent for patients with Parkinson's disease. Its use in other groups of older patients—that is, those with treatment-resistant depression (Fava et al. 2019)—remains experimental.

Monoamine Depletors

Two vesicular monoamine transporter type 2 (VMAT2) inhibitors, deutetrabenazine and valbenazine, are approved by the FDA for the treatment of TD in adults (Touma and Scarff 2018). Like tetrabenazine, deutetrabenazine is approved for the treatment of chorea associated with Huntington's disease. Both medications decrease dopamine release and postsynaptic dopamine receptors. Their efficacy and tolerability have been evaluated in several RCTs in patients ranging in age from 18 to 85 years (Estevez-Fraga et al. 2018; Patel et al. 2019; Widschwendter and Hofer 2019). About one-third of patients with TD experience a robust response to these medications (vs. ~10% of those receiving placebo), with a number needed to treat of ~5 and NNH ~100 (Touma and Scarff 2018). Some longer-term data are available for valbenazine but not deutetrabenazine (Patel et al. 2019). Based on the available evidence, these medications can be considered in older patients with moderate to severe TD who are not candidates for a dosage reduction or change in antipsychotic. Neither medication requires a dosage adjustment based on age; however, dosages should be reduced for both medications in poor metabolizers of CYP2D6. Similarly, both may cause QT prolongation, and this risk is increased in poor metabolizers of CYP2D6, when deutetrabenazine is coadministered with a CYP2D6 inhibitor, or when valbenazine is coadministered with a CYP3A4 inhibitor or a strong CYP2D6 inhibitor.

Mood Stabilizers

As a class, mood stabilizers are high-risk options for older patients. There is a paucity of controlled studies and an abundance of concern regarding these medications' potential toxicity, problematic adverse effects, and drug–drug interactions. Beyond their approved indications, anticonvulsants have also been used in the management of agitation associated with dementia. In the GERI-BD study, the first and only RCT of the pharmacotherapy of manic or mixed episodes in older patients with bipolar disorder, participants were assigned to lithium or divalproex, and both drugs were adequately tolerated and efficacious (Young et al. 2017). No consensus exists as to which drug is preferred as a first-line mood stabilizer in older adults with bipolar disorder or secondary mania (Dunner 2017; Sajatovic et al. 2005b; Shulman 2010; Young et al. 2017). However, the neuroprotective properties of lithium (Berk et al. 2017; Damri et al. 2020; Hajek et al. 2012; Van Gestel et al. 2019) and the favorable cognitive effects of lamotrigine (Gualtieri and Johnson 2006) make them attractive agents for older patients with bipolar disorder (D'Souza et al. 2011; Sajatovic et al. 2013).

Lithium

Lithium continues to be used in older patients for the treatment of bipolar disorder (D'Souza et al. 2011; Fotso Soh et al. 2019; Shulman 2010) or, less commonly, as an augmentation agent in treatment-resistant depression (Buspavanich et al. 2019; Cooper et al. 2011; Flint and Rifat 2001; Ross 2008) or for the prevention of depressive relapse after electroconvulsive therapy (Lambrichts et al. 2021; Sackeim et al. 2001). Available data from small studies (D'Souza et al. 2011; Sajatovic et al. 2005a; Schoot et al. 2020; Shulman 2010) and one larger RCT (Young et al. 2017) suggest lithium is efficacious in the acute treatment and prophylaxis of mania in older adults. However, age-related reductions in renal clearance and decreased total body water significantly affect the pharmacokinetics of lithium in these patients, increasing the risk of toxicity (D'Souza et al. 2011). Medical comorbidities common in late life, such as impaired renal function, hyponatremia, dehydration, or heart failure, further exacerbate the risk of toxicity (D'Souza et al. 2011; Fotso Soh et al. 2019; Sajatovic et al. 2006, 2013). Thiazide diuretics, angiotensin-converting enzyme inhibitors, and NSAIDs may precipitate toxicity by further diminishing the renal clearance of lithium (Sun et al. 2018). Lithium toxicity can produce persistent CNS impairment or be fatal and is a medical emergency requiring careful correction of fluid and electrolyte imbalances and possibly the administration of mannitol (or even hemodialysis) to increase lithium excretion.

Older patients require lower lithium dosages than younger patients to reach similar serum lithium levels, and their lithium levels, electrolytes, and thyroid-stimulating hormone should be monitored regularly (D'Souza et al. 2011; Methaneethorn and Sringam 2019; Rej et al. 2014a). Also, older persons are more sensitive to the neurological side effects of lithium and experience them at lower lithium levels. This sensitivity may be a consequence of increased permeability of the blood-brain barrier and subtle changes in sodium-lithium countertransport, resulting in a higher ratio of brain-to-serum concentration in older patients than in younger patients (Forester et al. 2009). Neurotoxicity may manifest as coarse tremor, slurred speech, ataxia, hyperreflexia, and muscle fasciculations. In vitro, lithium has moderate anticholinergic activity (Chew et al. 2008). This may explain why cognitive impairment has been observed with levels well below 1 mEq/L and why frank delirium has been reported with levels as low as 1.5 mEq/L (Sproule et al. 2000). Consequently, treatment in older patients may require lithium levels to be kept as low as 0.4–0.8 mEq/L. In addition, concerns remain about the well-established association between long-term use of lithium and renal disease (Rej et al. 2014b, 2020; Schoot et al. 2020). Despite its potential toxicity, the antisuicide (Antolín-Concha et al. 2020; Kugimiya et al. 2021; Müller-Oerlinghausen and Lewitzka 2010) and neuroprotective properties (Berk et al. 2017; Damri et al. 2020; Hajek et al. 2012; Van Gestel et al. 2019) of lithium still make it an important drug in the treatment of bipolar disorder and treatment-resistant depression in late life.

Anticonvulsants

Anticonvulsants are used as alternatives to lithium in the treatment of bipolar disorder (Young et al. 2017), and there may be a subgroup of patients with bipolar disorder with dysphoria or rapid cycling who respond poorly to lithium but do well with anticonvulsants (Post et al. 1998). Some anticonvulsants (e.g., carbamazepine) are used as third-line alternatives to antipsychotics and SSRIs for the management of agitation associated with dementia (Davies et al. 2018; Herrmann et al. 2013b).

Divalproex

Divalproex, a compound of sodium valproate and valproic acid in an enteric-coated form, is a broad-spectrum anticonvulsant approved by the FDA for the treatment of acute manic or mixed episodes associated with bipolar disorder, with or without psychotic features. It also may be efficacious in the treatment of bipolar depression (Bond et al. 2010). One relatively large RCT (Young et al. 2017) and two small case series (Kando et al. 1996; Noaghiul et al. 1998) support that divalproex is relatively well tolerated by older patients with bipolar disorder; however, it should not be used in patients with dementia because several negative placebo-controlled trials have shown that divalproex is not more effective but is more toxic than placebo—including potential neurotoxicity and cognitive toxicity—in older patients with dementia and agitation (Herrmann et al. 2013b; Sink et al. 2005; Tariot et al. 2005, 2011). Sedation, nausea, weight gain, and hand tremors are common dosage-related side effects. Reversible thrombocytopenia can occur in up to half of older patients taking divalproex and may ensue at lower total drug levels than in younger patients (Fenn et al. 2006). Other dosage-related adverse effects include reversible elevations in liver enzymes and transient elevations in blood ammonia levels (which may be associated with some cognitive impairment). However, liver failure and pancreatitis are very rare. Divalproex has other metabolic effects of concern to aging patients, such as increases in bone turnover and reductions of serum folates, with concomitant elevations in plasma homocysteine concentrations (Sato et al. 2001; Schwaninger et al. 1999).

The pharmacokinetics of valproate vary according to formulation, and valproic acid, divalproex sodium, and the valproate extended-release preparation are not interchangeable. Valproate is metabolized principally by mitochondrial β-oxidation and secondarily by the cytochrome P450 system; typical half-lives are in the range of 5–16 hours and are not affected by aging alone. Concomitant administration of valproate will increase concentrations of carbamazepine, diazepam, lamotrigine, phenobarbital, and primidone. Conversely, concurrent administration of carbamazepine, lamotrigine, phenytoin, and topiramate may decrease levels of valproate. Fluoxetine and erythromycin may potentiate the effects of valproate. Changes in protein binding as a result of drug interactions are no longer considered clinically important beyond causing the misinterpretation of total (i.e., free and bound) drug levels (Benet and Hoener 2002). Because valproate binding to plasma proteins is generally reduced in older people, use of free drug levels correlates better with adverse effects (Drisaldi et al. 2019; Fenn et al. 2006).

Lamotrigine

Lamotrigine is approved by the FDA for the maintenance treatment of bipolar I disorder to prevent mood episodes (depressive, manic, or mixed episodes), and it is considered one of the first-line agents for the treatment of bipolar depression in adults (Bahji et al. 2021; Jon et al. 2020; Wang and Osser 2020). The efficacy of lamotrigine in the treatment of bipolar depression in older patients is supported by an open-label trial (Sajatovic et al. 2011) and by pooled geriatric data from two placebo-controlled maintenance RCTs (Sajatovic et al. 2005a). Open studies and case reports also suggest a possible role for lamotrigine in the treatment of bipolar mania or aggression associated with dementia (Sajatovic et al. 2007).

Clearance of lamotrigine is reduced with age (Polepally et al. 2018). However, in contrast with many other mood stabilizers and antidepressants, lamotrigine does not seem to be associated with weight gain or to cause significant drug interactions. It is also less likely than other mood stabilizers to be associated with cognitive impairment (Gualtieri and Johnson 2006). Typically, lamotrigine is well tolerated (Sajatovic et al. 2005a, 2011). Rashes are the most common reason for discontinuation, but their incidence is less frequent with lamotrigine than carbamazepine (Fenn et al. 2006; Greil et al. 2019). However, severe rashes, including Stevens-Johnson syndrome or toxic epidermal necrolysis, have been seen in ~0.3% of adult patients (Messenheimer 1998). At the first sign of rash or other evidence of hypersensitivity (e.g., fever, lymphadenopathy), lamotrigine should be discontinued, and the patient should be evaluated.

The incidence of rashes can be reduced by using a low initial dosage and a very slow titration as recommended in the FDA-approved drug summary. Because valproate increases lamotrigine concentration, the initial and target lamotrigine dosages need to be halved in patients who are taking divalproex. Conversely, carbamazepine approximately halves lamotrigine concentrations, and the initial and target lamotrigine dosages need to be doubled in patients taking carbamazepine.

In October 2020, the FDA issued a new warning that lamotrigine "exhibits Class IB antiarrhythmic activity at therapeutically relevant concentrations" and could induce sudden death. Thus, its use should be avoided in patients with second- or third-degree heart block, ischemic heart disease, or heart failure. In a follow-up communication, the FDA raised the possibility that other anticonvulsants with a similar mechanism of action (i.e., sodium channel blockers), such as carbamazepine, eslicarbazepine, oxcarbazepine, or topiramate, may have similar proarrhythmic effects (U.S. Food and Drug Administration 2021).

Carbamazepine and Oxcarbazepine

The extended-release formulation of carbamazepine is approved by the FDA for the acute treatment of manic and mixed episodes associated with bipolar disorder. In a randomized, placebo-controlled trial in 51 nursing home patients, carbamazepine was shown to be efficacious in treating agitation and aggression associated with dementia (Tariot et al. 1998). Common adverse effects in older patients include sedation, nausea, dizziness, rash, ataxia, neutropenia, and hyponatremia. Older patients are also at risk for agranulocytosis, aplastic anemia, hepatitis, falls and fractures, and problematic drug interactions (Cheng et al. 2019; Fenn et al. 2006; Perucca 2018). Carbamazepine is primarily eliminated by CYP3A4, and its clearance is reduced with aging. Its interactions with other drugs are protean: concentrations are increased to potential toxicity by CYP3A4 inhibitors such as macrolide antibiotics, antifungals, and certain antidepressants (see antidepressants that inhibit CYP3A4 in Table 20–3). CYP3A4 inducers, such as phenobarbital, phenytoin, and carbamazepine itself, lower the concentration of carbamazepine and the concentrations of many drugs metabolized by this isoenzyme, including lamotrigine, valproate, some antidepressants, and antipsychotics (Fenn et al. 2006).

Oxcarbazepine, the 10-keto analogue of carbamazepine, is a less potent CYP3A4 inducer and less likely to be involved in drug interactions. Although oxcarbazepine has been studied in a small number of younger patients with bipolar disorder, there is a paucity of data pertaining to older psychiatric patients (Sommer et al. 2007), and its use cannot be recommended in older patients.

Gabapentin and Pregabalin

Although gabapentin has been used in bipolar disorder, trials have not borne out its effectiveness, and only small case series or case reports of its use in dementia are available (Sommer et al. 2007). It has a generally favorable side effect profile and some anxiolytic and analgesic effects, particularly for neuropathic pain. Serotonin syndrome has been reported when gabapentin is combined with the analgesic tramadol (Eksi et al. 2019). Gabapentin does not bind to plasma proteins and is not metabolized but eliminated by renal excretion. In patients with renal impairment, neurological adverse effects such as ataxia, involuntary movements, disorganized thinking, excitation, and extreme sedation have been noted. Even in the absence of renal dysfunction, older individuals may be prone to excessive sedation, falls, and fractures (Cheng et al. 2019). Therefore, in older adults, initial dosages of 100 mg twice daily are more prudent than the 900 mg/day that is recommended as a starting dosage for younger patients with epilepsy.

Pregabalin is a structural congener of gabapentin. It has an improved pharmacokinetic profile and is approved by the FDA not only for the treatment of epilepsy (as adjunctive therapy for adult patients with partial-onset seizures) but also for neuropathic pain associated with diabetic peripheral neuropathy and spinal cord injury, postherpetic neuralgia, and fibromyalgia. Some published pooled geriatric data from 11 placebo-controlled RCTs show that pregabalin 150–600 mg/day is associated with clinically meaningful pain relief in older patients with painful diabetic neuropathy or postherpetic neuralgia (Semel et al. 2010). In these studies, pregabalin's main adverse effects are dizziness, somnolence, and peripheral edema, and these are dosage related. In addition, pregabalin is now frequently used off-label for the treatment of GAD (or, more rarely, other anxiety disorders) in adults. The use of 150–600 mg/day of pregabalin in older patients with GAD is supported by a randomized, placebo-controlled trial (Montgomery et al. 2008) and some open data (Karaiskos et al. 2013). Similarly, a large case series suggested it can be substituted for benzodiazepines in older patients with dementia and anxiety (Novais et al. 2019).

Uncontrolled data on the use of gabapentin or pregabalin in older patients with dementia and aggression have also been published (Supasitthumrong et al. 2019) and suggest a possible use of these medications when other evidence-based interventions have failed.

Topiramate

Early reports of the efficacy of topiramate in younger patients with bipolar disorder have not been confirmed by subsequent studies (Sommer et al. 2007). In younger patients, topiramate is one of the few psychotropic medications associated with weight loss. However, it also has been associated with cognitive impairment severe enough to interfere with functioning (Gualtieri and Johnson 2006). Additionally, because of the paucity of data pertaining to the use of topiramate in older psychiatric patients (Sommer et al. 2007), its use cannot be recommended in these patients.

Other Medications Used to Regulate Affect

Dextromethorphan 20 mg combined with quinidine 10 mg in a proprietary preparation has been specifically approved by the FDA for the treatment of pseudobulbar affect (Wahler et al. 2017). The rationale for this design is that dextromethorphan or its metabolites inhibit inappropriate crying or laughing (via an unknown mechanism); the metabolism of dextromethorphan by CYP2D6 is inhibited by quinidine (a potent CYP2D6 inhibitor). The most important concerns about this medication are the potential for QTc prolongation, falls, fatigue, dizziness, diarrhea, and precipitation of a serotonin syndrome if it is combined with SSRIs or SNRIs. It also interacts with CYP2D6 substrates (e.g., TCAs).

In a single randomized, placebo-controlled trial ($N=194$), this dextromethorphan-quinidine combination was found to be efficacious in the treatment of agitation associated with Alzheimer's dementia (Cummings et al. 2015). Serious adverse events such as falls, diarrhea, and urinary tract infection occurred about twice as frequently with this medication as with placebo. Unfortunately, the well-disseminated results of the trial led to a surge in its use in patients with dementia in long-term care homes. In

March 2018, the Centers for Medicare and Medicaid Services asked Medicare insurance providers to monitor prescriptions of this medication and to ensure that it is being appropriately prescribed (i.e., only for its indicated treatment of pseudobulbar affect) (Palmer 2018).

Anxiolytics and Sedative-Hypnotics

SSRIs and SNRIs have displaced benzodiazepines as first-line pharmacotherapy for anxiety disorders in late life. The intermediate-half-life benzodiazepine lorazepam is still being used as an adjunct medication for the short-term relief of anxiety symptoms in older patients (e.g., anxiety associated with depression). Benzodiazepine receptor agonist hypnotics (e.g., eszopiclone, zaleplon, zolpidem, zopiclone—also known as "Z-drugs") have become the preferred hypnotics in late life. Some data also support the efficacy and tolerability of suvorexant and lemborexant, two orexin receptor antagonists, for sleep maintenance in older people. Z-drugs and orexin receptor antagonists can be helpful for the treatment of primary insomnia in healthy older adults, in whom they are usually well tolerated (Abad and Guilleminault 2018). However, like benzodiazepines, these sedative-hypnotics should be used with great caution in older patients with physical or mental disorders; the lowest possible dosage should be used for the shortest possible time in all older patients.

Buspirone

The anxiolytic buspirone, a partial 5-HT_{1A} agonist, is rarely used. It may be beneficial in some patients with GAD or as an augmentation agent in treatment-resistant depression (Flint 2005; Trivedi et al. 2006). It appears to be well tolerated by older patients without the sedation or addiction liability of the benzodiazepines (Steinberg 1994). Therefore, it may be helpful for some older patients who are prone to falls, confusion, or chronic lung disease. Nonetheless, buspirone may take several weeks to exert an anxiolytic effect, has no cross-tolerance with benzodiazepines, and may cause dizziness, headache, or nervousness (Strand et al. 1990). It is of limited use for panic disorder or OCD. One large case series ($N=179$) supports the use of buspirone in patients with behavioral disturbances associated with dementia (Santa Cruz et al. 2017). The pharmacokinetics of buspirone are not affected by age or sex, but coadministration with verapamil, diltiazem, erythromycin, or itraconazole substantially increases buspirone concentrations, and its combination with serotonergic medications may result in the serotonin syndrome (Mahmood and Sahajwalla 1999).

Benzodiazepines and Benzodiazepine Receptor Agonists

Benzodiazepines

In older adults, detrimental effects of benzodiazepines have been well documented; they usually outweigh any short-term symptomatic relief that these drugs may provide and should be avoided (American Geriatrics Society Beers Criteria Update Expert Panel 2019). Single small doses of diazepam, nitrazepam, or temazepam can cause significant impairment in memory and psychomotor performance in older individuals (Breilman et al. 2019; Nikaido et al. 1990). Even benzodiazepines with shorter half-lives increase the risk of falls and hip fractures in frail older patients (Ray et al. 2000). Benzodiazepines have also been linked to adverse respiratory outcomes in older patients with chronic obstructive pulmonary disease (Vozoris et al. 2014) and possibly to an increased risk for Alzheimer's dementia (Billioti de Gage et al. 2014). They are also associated with significantly increased morbidity and mortality in older patients (Kripke et al. 2012; Weich et al. 2014).

Nevertheless, benzodiazepines are still used for prevention of alcohol withdrawal or as a temporary adjunctive treatment for anxiety symptoms or depression-related sleep disturbance when the primary pharmacotherapy is an antidepressant. Relative contraindications include heavy snoring (because it suggests sleep apnea), dementia (because patients with dementia are at increased risk for daytime confusion, impairment in activities of daily living, and daytime sleepiness), and the use of alcohol or other sedating medications (including opioids) because of pharmacodynamic interactions (discussed later). Benzodiazepines with long half-lives (i.e., chlordiazepoxide, clonazepam, clorazepate, diazepam, flurazepam, halazepam, and quazepam) are probably associated with more adverse effects and therefore should be avoided in older adults (Ballokova et al. 2014; Hemmelgarn et al. 1997). Several benzodiazepines with shorter half-lives (i.e., alprazolam, midazolam, or triazolam) undergo phase 1 hepatic metabolism by CYP3A4 that is subject to specific interactions and age-associated decline (Freudenreich and Menza 2000; Greenblatt et al. 1991). Also, sedatives with very short half-lives increase the likelihood that confused older patients will awake in the middle of the night to stagger off to the bathroom. Lorazepam and oxazepam do not undergo phase 1 hepatic metabolism, have no active metabolites, have acceptable half-lives that do not increase with age, and are not subject to drug–drug interactions. Lorazepam is available in appropriately small doses (0.5-mg divisible pills), and it is rapidly and well absorbed orally; it can also be given intravenously or intramuscularly. By contrast, oxazepam has a relatively slow and erratic absorption. Thus, lorazepam is the preferred benzodiazepine in older patients. Like other benzodiazepines, it should not be used with opioids given the twofold increase in all-cause mortality with this combination (Sharma et al. 2020; U.S. Food and Drug Administration 2016; Xu et al. 2020).

Benzodiazepine Receptor Agonists (Z-Drugs)

Although Z-drugs are efficacious in the treatment of sleep-onset insomnia (with the best evidence supporting the use of eszopiclone or zaleplon) or for sleep maintenance (with the best evidence supporting the use of eszopiclone) (Sateia et al. 2017) and are perceived to be safer than benzodiazepines, they have been associated with falls and hip fractures (Treves et al. 2018; Wang et al. 2001), cognitive impairment and traffic accidents (Glass et al. 2005; Gustavsen et al. 2008; Vermeeren et al. 2016), and overall increased morbidity and mortality in older patients (Kripke et al. 2012; Weich et al. 2014), including those with dementia (Richardson et al. 2020, 2021). Eszopiclone, zaleplon, and zolpidem undergo phase 1 hepatic metabolism by CYP3A4 that is subject to specific interactions and age-associated decline (Freudenreich and Menza 2000).

Melatonin Receptor Agonists

Ramelteon and tasimelteon are selective melatonin (MT1 and MT2) receptor agonists. Whereas tasimelteon is FDA approved for the treatment of sleep-wake disorder in patients who are blind, ramelteon is approved for up to 6 months in patients with transient or chronic sleep-onset insomnia. The efficacy of ramelteon in adults has been shown in randomized, placebo-controlled trials (Sateia et al. 2017). However, the evidence supporting its use in older persons with primary insomnia is limited (Sys et al. 2020). Like all sedative-hypnotics, its use in long-term care facilities is regulated by OBRA, and if it is used routinely for longer than 6 months, a quarterly taper should be attempted. In one small randomized, placebo-controlled trial ($N=74$), ramelteon was not helpful in alleviating the sleep disturbances associated with dementia (McCleery and Sharpley 2020). There is also some strong evidence that, like melatonin, ramelteon can help prevent the onset of delirium in hospitalized patients, particularly surgical and intensive care unit patients (Campbell et al. 2019; Khaing and Nair 2021; Kim et al. 2020; Y.C. Wu et al. 2019). However, not all relevant RCTs have been positive (Oh et al. 2021).

Ramelteon is usually well tolerated, with somnolence as its most common adverse effect. It is not associated with physical tolerance or rebound insomnia upon discontinuation. Ramelteon is primarily metabolized by CYP1A2, and it should not be administered with strong CYP1A2 inhibitors such as fluvoxamine. Conversely, smoking would be expected to decrease its concentration (through induction of CYP1A2).

Orexin (Hypocretin) Receptor Antagonists

Suvorexant

Suvorexant is the first orexin receptor antagonist approved by the FDA for treatment of insomnia characterized by difficulty with sleep onset or maintenance in adults. Orexin, also called hypocretin, is a neuropeptide that regulates wakefulness, attention, energy expenditure, and visceral function through its complex effects on the acetylcholine, dopamine, histamine, and norepinephrine systems. Loss of orexin neurons has been implicated in the pathophysiology of narcolepsy, and suvorexant can cause sleep paralysis, hypnagogic or hypnopompic hallucinations, and cataplexy-like symptoms. It can also cause nightmares or sleep terrors. Its use has also been associated with dosage-dependent worsening of depression or suicidality, and it should not be used in suicidal patients. Like all medications used for the treatment of insomnia, suvorexant can lead to physical tolerance and psychological dependence.

The half-life of suvorexant is 12 hours. It is metabolized in the liver by CYP3A4 and should be used cautiously when prescribed alongside CYP3A4 inhibitors (e.g., diltiazem, erythromycin, ketoconazole, or verapamil) (Wrishko et al. 2019). Although the package insert does not recommend different dosages in older patients, given the reduction of hepatic blood flow and increase in fat tissue associated with normal aging, these patients likely are at higher risk for all adverse effects (including drowsiness and falls). This was not demonstrated in a pre-specified pooled analysis of 839 patients age 65 and older who participated in three randomized, placebo-controlled trials for DSM-IV (American Psychiatric Association 1994) primary insomnia (Herring et al. 2017). In this analysis, suvorexant was more effective than placebo for up to 3 months. As expected, rebound insomnia was observed in some patients on discontinuation of suvorexant, but it was mild (Herring et al. 2017). Both suvorexant and placebo were well tolerated. Somnolence was the most common adverse event (occurring in 9% with 30 mg/day, 5% with 15 mg/day, 3% with placebo), and the rates of serious adverse events or falls were very low and did not differ between suvorexant and placebo. There were only five reports of sleep-related adverse events in the 521 older patients randomly assigned to suvorexant and none in the 318 assigned to placebo (Herring et al. 2017). Similarly, in another randomized, placebo- and zopiclone-controlled trial, suvorexant (unlike zopiclone) did not impair next-morning driving performance in older volunteers (Vermeeren et al. 2016). However, the older participants in these two RCTs were specifically selected to be in good physical and mental health (Herring et al. 2017; Vermeeren et al. 2016). In the largest randomized, placebo-controlled trial in patients with Alzheimer's dementia and insomnia (N=285), suvorexant improved total sleep time and was well tolerated, with somnolence again being the main adverse event (suvorexant 4.2%; placebo 1.4%) (Herring et al. 2020). This makes suvorexant one of only two medications supported by some evidence for the treatment of insomnia associated with dementia (the other is trazodone) (McCleery and Sharpley 2020). Finally, some data from two RCTs and several uncontrolled studies support the potential usefulness of suvorexant alone or in combination with ramelteon in the prevention of delirium (Adams et al. 2020; Hanazawa and Kamijo 2019).

Lemborexant

Lemborexant is an orexin receptor antagonist approved by the FDA for the treatment of insomnia characterized by difficulty with sleep onset or maintenance in adults. It shares the same pharmacological profile as suvorexant, and the same cautions apply. Evidence pooled from randomized, placebo-controlled trials (N=491) supports its efficacy and tolerability in healthy older patients (including 87 patients age 75 years and older) (Zammit and Krystal 2021); like suvorexant, it has been shown to have minimal impact on next-morning driving (Vermeeren et al. 2019). A placebo-controlled RCT compared lemborexant (5 mg and 10 mg) and zolpidem for 30 nights in 1,006 participants age 55 years and older. Lemborexant produced a larger increase in total sleep time and rapid eye movement sleep than both placebo and zolpidem (Moline et al. 2021). One network meta-analysis of four previous RCTs suggested that lemborexant is similarly tolerated (with somnolence as its more common adverse effect) and more efficacious than suvorexant or zolpidem in healthy midlife and older individuals with primary insomnia (mean age 58 years) (Kishi et al. 2020). However, given the small number of RCTs included in this meta-analysis and the absence of head-to-head comparisons of lemborexant and suvorexant, clinicians should favor use of the less expensive medication.

Cognitive Enhancers and Other Medications Used in the Treatment of Alzheimer's Dementia

Cholinesterase Inhibitors

In addition to memantine (discussed later), four cholinesterase inhibitors have received FDA approval for the symptomatic improvement of Alzheimer's dementia. Table 20–5 describes the properties of three of these drugs: donepezil, galantamine, and rivastigmine. The fourth, tacrine, is no longer recommended because of its potential hepatotoxic effects.

TABLE 20–5.   **Cholinesterase inhibitors**

Clearance	Dosing	Significant adverse effects	Pharmacodynamics
Donepezil			
Half-life 70–80 hours; CYP3A4, CYP2D6	5–10 mg/day in one dose; start at 5 mg at bedtime.	Mild nausea, diarrhea, bradycardia	Reversible ACE inhibition
Galantamine, galantamine ER			
Half-life 7 hours; CYP2D6, CYP3A4	8–24 mg/day divided into two doses; start at 8 mg/day twice daily.	Moderate nausea, vomiting, diarrhea, anorexia, tremor, insomnia	Reversible ACE inhibition; nicotinic modulation may increase acetylcholine release
Rivastigmine, rivastigmine patch			
Half-life 1.25 hours; renal	6–12 mg/day divided into two doses; start at 1.5 mg twice daily. For patch, start at 4.6 mg/day and increase after 4 weeks to 9.5 mg/day. Retitrate if drug is stopped.	Severe nausea, vomiting, anorexia, weight loss, sweating, dizziness	Pseudoirreversible ACE inhibition; also butylcholinesterase inhibition

ACE=acetylcholinesterase; CYP=cytochrome P450; ER=extended release.

Cholinesterase inhibitors produce modest improvements in cognition and function in patients with Alzheimer's dementia (Birks and Harvey 2018; Fink et al. 2020; Thancharoen et al. 2019; Tricco et al. 2018; Xu et al. 2021), including those with severe Alzheimer's dementia (Birks and Harvey 2018; Herrmann et al. 2013b; Howard et al. 2012). Thus, a trial with a cholinesterase inhibitor is recommended for most patients with this diagnosis. Some evidence favors the use of donepezil or galantamine for mild to moderate dementia (Hansen et al. 2008; Thancharoen et al. 2019) and donepezil for severe dementia (Birks and Harvey 2018; Winblad et al. 2006); however, this evidence is weak, and selection of a specific cholinesterase inhibitor should be based on its pharmacokinetic and adverse effect profile (see Table 20–5) (Herrmann et al. 2013b; Tricco et al. 2018). Cholinesterase inhibitors reduce the risk of death in patients with Alzheimer's dementia (Xu et al. 2021), but no evidence suggests that they alter the underlying neuropathology of Alzheimer's disease or its eventual progression. Thus, they should be discontinued when patients either do not respond to an adequate trial or deteriorate and require a high level of supportive care (Parsons 2016; Reeve et al. 2019; Renn et al. 2018). However, the discontinuation should be done slowly, with careful monitoring, because a rapid symptomatic deterioration may occur (Scarpini et al. 2011).

Cholinesterase inhibitors may also be beneficial for some symptoms that are common in patients with Alzheimer's dementia, such as apathy (Ruthirakuhan et al. 2018) or cognitive fatigue (Vila-Castelar et al. 2019). Current evidence does not support their use for the treatment of MCI (Freund-Levi et al. 2014; Herrmann et al. 2013b; Matsunaga et al. 2019) or the acute treatment of agitation and behavioral disturbances associated with Alzheimer's dementia (Chen et al. 2021; Fink et al. 2020; Howard et al. 2007; Rodda et al. 2009). However, several studies suggest that patients treated with cholinesterase inhibitors may be less likely to experience onset of behavioral symptoms associated with dementia, leading some experts to recommend their use for the prevention of these symptoms (Chen et al. 2021; Davies et al. 2018).

The cholinesterase inhibitors have even more modest benefit in vascular dementia (Kavirajan and Schneider 2007). In a recent network meta-analysis, donepezil 10 mg had the greatest effect on cognition, but it was associated with adverse effects (Battle et al. 2021). Some data suggest that cholinesterase inhibitors may also be efficacious in the treatment of cognitive impairment associated with other disorders, such as Lewy body dementia (Aarsland 2016; Hershey and Coleman-Jackson 2019; Li et al. 2015; Liu et al. 2019; Meng et al. 2019; Tahami Monfared et al. 2020), dementia with Parkinson's disease (Aarsland 2016; Li et al. 2015; Meng et al. 2019; Rolinski et al. 2012), frontotemporal dementia (Herrmann et al. 2013b), or late-life major depressive disorders (Reynolds et al. 2011). However, the available data are not consistent, and there is no agreement on the role of cholinesterase inhibitors in the treatment of these disorders.

In patients with diminished cognitive reserve, even small anticholinergic effects can substantially impair cognition (Mulsant et al. 2003; Nebes et al. 2005). Drugs with potent anticholinergic effects directly antagonize cholinesterase inhibitors (Chew et al. 2008; Modi et al. 2009). Thus, it is imperative that unnecessary anticholinergic medications be discontinued before initiating a cholinesterase inhibitor (Lu and Tune 2003; Modi et al. 2009; Valladales-Restrepo et al. 2019).

The main adverse effects of cholinesterase inhibitors are concentration dependent and result from their central and peripheral cholinergic actions. Nausea, diarrhea, weight loss, bradycardia, syncope, and nightmares are associated with these drugs and may lead to their discontinuation (see Table 20–5) (Gill et al. 2009; Hernandez et al. 2009; Park-Wyllie et al. 2009); gastrointestinal adverse effects may be less frequent with donepezil (Mayeux 2010). Despite theoretical concerns, the use of cholinesterase inhibitors appears to be safe in patients with chronic airway disorders (Thacker and Schneeweiss 2006). By contrast, in a placebo-controlled study in older patients with MDD receiving maintenance antidepressant pharmacotherapy, donepezil was associated with a higher rate of recurrence of depression than placebo (Reynolds et al. 2011). With these adverse effects in mind, when prescribing donepezil and galantamine, clinicians should be aware of the drugs' specific pathways of elimination and potential pharmacokinetic drug interactions with CYP2D6 or CYP3A4 inhibitors and with CYP3A4 inducers (Pilotto et al. 2009; Seritan 2008). Rivastigmine is affected by renal function, and FDA warnings have emphasized the need for careful dosage titration (and retitration if restarting) to prevent severe vomiting (Birks and Grimley Evans 2015).

NMDA Receptor Antagonist

Memantine, an NMDA receptor antagonist, has FDA approval for the treatment of moderate to severe Alzheimer's disease. As an uncompetitive antagonist with moderate affinity for NMDA receptors, memantine may attenuate neurotoxicity without interfering with glutamate's normal physiological actions. In placebo-controlled clinical trials in patients with moderate to severe Alzheimer's disease, memantine was associated with a modest delay in the deterioration of cognition and activities of daily living when administered alone (Reisberg et al. 2003) or in combination with donepezil (Fink et al. 2020; Tariot et al. 2004). Current data do not support the use of memantine for treatment of mild dementia (McShane et al. 2019; Thancharoen et al. 2019). Data on combining donepezil and memantine versus using them as monotherapy are mixed (Fink et al. 2020; Howard et al. 2012; Tariot et al. 2004), leading some guidelines to recommend against use of this combination (Herrmann et al. 2013b). In a network meta-analysis, the efficacy of the combination was ranked first, followed by donepezil, memantine, and then placebo (Guo et al. 2020), consistent with the results of an earlier meta-analysis showing that the combination of donepezil and memantine was more efficacious than donepezil alone in moderate to severe Alzheimer's dementia (Chen et al. 2017). Interestingly, memantine may increase donepezil concentrations (Yaowaluk et al. 2019).

The available data on the role of memantine in the treatment of agitation or other behavioral symptoms associated with dementia are not consistent (Cumbo and Ligori 2014; Herrmann et al. 2013a; Lockhart et al. 2011; McShane et al. 2019; Wilcock et al. 2008). Similar to the cholinesterase inhibitors, memantine may be more useful in preventing these symptoms rather than in treating them acutely (Chen et al. 2021; Fink et al. 2020), and it may also have a role in the treatment of cognitive impairment caused by Lewy body dementia or Parkinson's disease (Aarsland 2016; Aarsland et al. 2009; Emre et al. 2010; Hershey and Coleman-Jackson 2019; Matsunaga et al. 2015; Meng et al. 2019).

Memantine is usually well tolerated (Fink et al. 2020; Guo et al. 2020), although it may cause sleepiness (Fink et al. 2020) or confusion (Kavirajan 2009) in some patients. It does not appear to be implicated in drug–drug interactions, but it is excreted by the kidneys, and its dosage needs to be reduced in patients with impaired renal function.

Monoclonal Antibody to Brain Amyloid

Aducanumab is a human monoclonal antibody to brain amyloid that was assessed in two randomized placebo-controlled trials that were planned to provide 18-month outcome data in generally healthy patients who had a positive amyloid PET scan and MCI or mild dementia due to Alzheimer's disease. Aducanumab reduced amyloid beta plaques in the brain, but evidence is currently equivocal on whether it can slow cognitive decline (Alexander et al. 2021).

The FDA gave aducanumab accelerated approval in 2021; this decision was controversial (Knopman et al. 2021). The FDA is requiring an extensive Phase IV trial. Aducanumab is given by intravenous infusion every 4 weeks and requires follow-up MRI scans. Its estimated cost is $56,000 per year. The most common adverse effects with aducanumab are amyloid-related imaging abnormalities (edema and microhemorrhages), headache, falls, diarrhea, confusion, and delirium.

Conclusion

Substantial evidence now exists to support and guide the use of psychotropic medications in older adults. Most of the available data pertain to the use of SSRI or SNRI antidepressants in the treatment of MDD, atypical antipsychotics in the treatment of agitation associated with dementia, and cognitive enhancers in the treatment of cognitive impairment due to Alzheimer's dementia. Existing data also support the short- and long-term efficacy and relative safety of SSRI and SNRI antidepressants in the treatment of older adults with MDD or an anxiety disorder. In contrast, the risks associated with the use of antipsychotics outweigh their potential benefits in most older persons presenting with agitation associated with dementia. Cognitive enhancers appear to be relatively safe in older persons with dementia due to Alzheimer's disease and some other etiologies, but their efficacy is modest. Pharmacoepidemiological data show that benzodiazepines continue to be prescribed to many older people despite their potential toxicity. Empirical data to guide the use of mood stabilizers or antipsychotics in older individuals with bipolar disorder or schizophrenia are lacking. Similarly, better data are needed to inform the selection, sequencing, and combination of psychotropic medications in older persons whose symptoms do not respond to first-line pharmacological interventions.

Key Points

- Substantial evidence supports the short- and long-term efficacy and relative safety of selective serotonin reuptake inhibitor and serotonin-norepinephrine reuptake inhibitor antidepressants in the treatment of most older persons with major depressive disorder or an anxiety disorder.

- The risks associated with the use of antipsychotics outweigh their potential benefits in many older persons presenting with agitation associated with dementia.

- Cognitive enhancers appear relatively safe in older persons with dementia, but their efficacy is modest.

- Pharmacoepidemiological data show that benzodiazepines continue to be prescribed to many older persons despite their toxicity.

- Empirical data to guide the use of mood stabilizers or antipsychotics in older individuals with bipolar disorder or schizophrenia are lacking.

- Better data are needed to inform the selection, sequencing, and combination of psychotropic medications in older persons whose symptoms do not respond to first-line pharmacological interventions.

Suggested Readings

Antidepressant Medications

Gutsmiedl K, Krause M, Bighelli I, et al: How well do elderly patients with major depressive disorder respond to antidepressants? A systematic review and single-group meta-analysis. BMC Psychiatry 20(1):102, 2020 32131786

Mulsant BH, Blumberger DM, Ismail Z, et al: A systematic approach to the pharmacotherapy of geriatric major depression. Clin Geriatr Med 30(3):517–534, 2014

Antipsychotic Medications

Maher AR, Maglione M, Bagley S, et al: Efficacy and comparative effectiveness of atypical antipsychotic medications for off-label uses in adults: a systematic review and meta-analysis. JAMA 306(12):1359–1369, 2011 21954480

Nikooie R, Neufeld KJ, Oh ES, et al: Antipsychotics for treating delirium in hospitalized adults: a systematic review. Ann Intern Med 171(7):485–495, 2019 31476770

Suzuki T, Remington G, Uchida H, et al: Management of schizophrenia in late life with antipsychotic medications: a qualitative review. Drugs Aging 28(12):961–980, 2011 22117095

Vasudev A, Chaudhari S, Sethi R, et al: A review of the pharmacological and clinical profile of newer atypical antipsychotics as treatments for bipolar disorder: considerations for use in older patients. Drugs Aging 35(10):887–895, 2018 30187288

Anxiolytics and Sedative-Hypnotics

Abad VC, Guilleminault C: Insomnia in elderly patients: recommendations for pharmacological management. Drugs Aging 35(9):791–817, 2018 30058034

American Geriatrics Society Beers Criteria Update Expert Panel: American Geriatrics Society 2019 updated AGS Beers Criteria for potentially inappropriate medication use in older adults. J Am Geriatr Soc 67(4):674–694, 2019 30693946

Cognitive Enhancers

Birks JS, Harvey RJ: Donepezil for dementia due to Alzheimer's disease. Cochrane Database Syst Rev 6(6):CD001190, 2018 29923184

Fink HA, Linskens EJ, MacDonald R, et al: Benefits and harms of prescription drugs and supplements for treatment of clinical Alzheimer-type dementia. Ann Intern Med 172(10):656–668, 2020 32340037

Mood Stabilizers

Sajatovic M, Forester BP, Gildengers A, Mulsant BH: Aging changes and medical complexity in late-life bipolar disorder: emerging research findings that may help advance care. Neuropsychiatry 3(6): 621–633, 2013 24999372

Young RC, Mulsant BH, Sajatovic M, et al: GERI-BD: a randomized double-blind controlled trial of lithium and divalproex in the treatment of mania in older patients with bipolar disorder. Am J Psychiatry 174(11):1032–1033, 2017 29088928

References

Aarsland D: Cognitive impairment in Parkinson's disease and dementia with Lewy bodies. Parkinsonism Relat Disord 22(suppl 1):S144–S148, 2016 26411499

Aarsland D, Ballard C, Walker Z, et al: Memantine in patients with Parkinson's disease dementia or dementia with Lewy bodies: a double-blind, placebo-controlled, multicentre trial. Lancet Neurol 8(7):613–618, 2009 19520613

Abad VC, Guilleminault C: Insomnia in elderly patients: recommendations for pharmacological management. Drugs Aging 35(9):791–817, 2018 30058034

Adams AD, Pepin MJ, Brown JN: The role of suvorexant in the prevention of delirium during acute hospitalization: a systematic review. J Crit Care 59:1–5, 2020 32480359

AFFINITY Trial Collaboration: Safety and efficacy of fluoxetine on functional outcome after acute stroke (AFFINITY): a randomised, double-blind, placebo-controlled trial. Lancet Neurol 19(8):651–660, 2020 32702334

Agüera-Ortiz L, García-Ramos R, Grandas Pérez FJ, et al: Focus on depression in Parkinson's disease: a Delphi consensus of experts in psychiatry, neurology, and geriatrics. Parkinsons Dis 2021:6621991, 2021 33628415

Aichhorn W, Weiss U, Marksteiner J, et al: Influence of age and gender on risperidone plasma concentrations. J Psychopharmacol 19(4):395–401, 2005 15982995

Aiken CB: Pramipexole in psychiatry: a systematic review of the literature. J Clin Psychiatry 68(8):1230–1236, 2007 17854248

Alaka KJ, Noble W, Montejo A, et al: Efficacy and safety of duloxetine in the treatment of older adult patients with generalized anxiety disorder: a randomized, double-blind, placebo-controlled trial. Int J Geriatr Psychiatry 29(9):978–986, 2014 24644106

Albrecht JS, Rao V, Perfetto EM, Mullins CD: Safety of antidepressant classes used following traumatic brain injury among Medicare beneficiaries: a retrospective cohort study. Drugs Aging 35(8):763–772, 2018 30047070

Alexander GC, Knopman DS, Emerson SS, et al: Revisiting FDA approval of aducanumab. N Engl J Med 385(9):769–771, 2021 34320282

Alexopoulos GS, Katz IR, Reynolds CF III, et al: Pharmacotherapy of depression in older patients: a summary of the expert consensus guidelines. J Psychiatr Pract 7(6):361–376, 2001 15990550

Almeida F, Albuquerque E, Murta I: Delirium induced by quetiapine and the potential role of norquetiapine. Front Neurosci 13:886, 2019 31481872

American Diabetes Association, American Psychiatric Association, American Association of Clinical Endocrinologists, North American Association for the Study of Obesity: Consensus development conference on antipsychotic drugs and obesity and diabetes. Diabetes Care 27(2):596–601, 2004 14747245

American Geriatrics Society Beers Criteria Update Expert Panel: American Geriatrics Society 2019 updated AGS Beers Criteria for potentially inappropriate medication use in older adults. J Am Geriatr Soc 67(4):674–694, 2019 30693946

American Psychiatric Association: Diagnostic and Statistical Manual of Mental Disorders, 4th Edition. Washington, DC, American Psychiatric Association, 1994

An H, Choi B, Park KW, et al: The effect of escitalopram on mood and cognition in depressive Alzheimer's disease subjects. J Alzheimers Dis 55(2):727–735, 2017 27716660

Angermann CE, Gelbrich G, Störk S, et al: Effect of escitalopram on all-cause mortality and hospitalization in patients with heart failure and depression: the MOOD-HF randomized clinical trial. JAMA 315(24):2683–2693, 2016 27367876

Antolín-Concha D, Lähteenvuo M, Vattulainen P, et al: Suicide mortality and use of psychotropic drugs in patients hospitalized due to bipolar disorder: a Finnish nationwide cohort study. J Affect Disord 277:885–892, 2020 33065830

Antoun Reyad A, Girgis E, Mishriky R: Efficacy and safety of brexpiprazole in acute management of psychiatric disorders: a meta-analysis of randomized controlled trials. Int Clin Psychopharmacol 35(3):119–128, 2020 32141908

Atalay A, Turhan N, Aki OE: A challenging case of syndrome of inappropriate secretion of antidiuretic hormone in an elderly patient secondary to quetiapine. South Med J 100(8):832–833, 2007 17713312

Auerbach AD, Vittinghoff E, Maselli J, et al: Perioperative use of selective serotonin reuptake inhibitors and risks for adverse outcomes of surgery. JAMA Intern Med 173(12):1075–1081, 2013 23699725

Bahji A, Ermacora D, Stephenson C, et al: Comparative efficacy and tolerability of adjunctive pharmacotherapies for acute bipolar depression: a systematic review and network meta-analysis. Can J Psychiatry 66(3):274–288, 2021 33174452

Bailer U, Fischer P, Küfferle B, et al: Occurrence of mirtazapine-induced delirium in organic brain disorder. Int Clin Psychopharmacol 15(4):239–243, 2000 10954066

Ballard C, Corbett A: Reducing psychotropic drug use in people with dementia living in nursing homes. Int Psychogeriatr 32(3):291–294, 2020 32192559

Ballard C, Hanney ML, Theodoulou M, et al: The Dementia Antipsychotic Withdrawal Trial (DART-AD): long-term follow-up of a randomised placebo-controlled trial. Lancet Neurol 8(2):151–157, 2009 19138567

Ballard C, Banister C, Khan Z, et al: Evaluation of the safety, tolerability, and efficacy of pimavanserin versus placebo in patients with Alzheimer's disease psychosis: a Phase 2, randomised, placebo-controlled, double-blind study. Lancet Neurol 17(3):213–222, 2018 29452684

Ballard C, Youakim JM, Coate B, Stankovic S: Pimavanserin in Alzheimer's disease psychosis: efficacy in patients with more pronounced psychotic symptoms. J Prev Alzheimers Dis 6(1):27–33, 2019 30569083

Ballard ED, Zarate CA Jr: The role of dissociation in ketamine's antidepressant effects. Nat Commun 11(1):6431, 2020 33353946

Ballokova A, Peel NM, Fialova D, et al: Use of benzodiazepines and association with falls in older people admitted to hospital: a prospective cohort study. Drugs Aging 31(4):299–310, 2014 24566878

Banerjee S, Hellier J, Dewey M, et al: Sertraline or mirtazapine for depression in dementia (HTA-SADD): a randomised, multicentre, double-blind, placebo-controlled trial. Lancet 378(9789):403–411, 2011 21764118

Barak Y, Wittenberg N, Naor S, et al: Clozapine in elderly psychiatric patients: tolerability, safety, and efficacy. Compr Psychiatry 40(4):320–325, 1999 10428193

Barak Y, Shamir E, Zemishlani H, et al: Olanzapine vs. haloperidol in the treatment of elderly chronic schizophrenia patients. Prog Neuropsychopharmacol Biol Psychiatry 26(6):1199–1202, 2002 12452546

Barak Y, Plopski I, Tadger S, Paleacu D: Escitalopram versus risperidone for the treatment of behavioral and psychotic symptoms associated with Alzheimer's disease: a randomized double-blind pilot study. Int Psychogeriatr 23(9):1515–1519, 2011 21492498

Barbateskovic M, Krauss SR, Collet MO, et al: Haloperidol for the treatment of delirium in critically ill patients: a systematic review with meta-analysis and trial sequential analysis. Acta Anaesthesiol Scand 64(2):254–266, 2020 31663112

Barbui C, Esposito E, Cipriani A: Selective serotonin reuptake inhibitors and risk of suicide: a systematic review of observational studies. CMAJ 180(3):291–297, 2009 19188627

Barone P, Scarzella L, Marconi R, et al: Pramipexole versus sertraline in the treatment of depression in Parkinson's disease: a national multicenter parallel-group randomized study. J Neurol 253(5):601–607, 2006 16607468

Barone P, Poewe W, Albrecht S, et al: Pramipexole for the treatment of depressive symptoms in patients with Parkinson's disease: a randomised, double-blind, placebo-controlled trial. Lancet Neurol 9(6):573–580, 2010 20452823

Baruch Y, Tadger S, Plopski I, Barak Y: Asenapine for elderly bipolar manic patients. J Affect Disord 145(1):130–132, 2013 22877962

Battle CE, Abdul-Rahim AH, Shenkin SD, et al: Cholinesterase inhibitors for vascular dementia and other vascular cognitive impairments: a network meta-analysis. Cochrane Database Syst Rev (2):CD013306, 2021 33704781

Baune BT, Sluth LB, Olsen CK: The effects of vortioxetine on cognitive performance in working patients with major depressive disorder: a short-term, randomized, double-blind, exploratory study. J Affect Disord 229:421–428, 2018 29331703

Beach SR, Celano CM, Sugrue AM, et al: QT prolongation, torsades de pointes, and psychotropic medications: a 5-year update. Psychosomatics 59(2):105–122, 2018 29275963

Beheydt LL, Schrijvers D, Docx L, et al: Cognitive and psychomotor effects of three months of escitalopram treatment in elderly patients with major depressive disorder. J Affect Disord 188:47–52, 2015 26342888

Behlke LM, Lenze EJ, Pham V, et al: The effect of venlafaxine on electrocardiogram intervals during treatment for depression in older adults. J Clin Psychopharmacol 40(6):553–559, 2020 33044352

Belgamwar RB, Fenton M: Olanzapine IM or velotab for acutely disturbed/agitated people with suspected serious mental illnesses. Cochrane Database Syst Rev (2):CD003729, 2005 15846678

Bell JS, Taipale HT, Soini H, Pitkälä KH: Sedative load among long-term care facility residents with and without dementia: a cross-sectional study. Clin Drug Investig 30(1):63–70, 2010 19995099

Benazzi F: Serotonin syndrome with mirtazapine-fluoxetine combination. Int J Geriatr Psychiatry 13(7):495–496, 1998 9695042

Benet LZ, Hoener BA: Changes in plasma protein binding have little clinical relevance. Clin Pharmacol Ther 71(3):115–121, 2002 11907485

Bergh S, Selbæk G, Engedal K: Discontinuation of antidepressants in people with dementia and neuropsychiatric symptoms (DESEP study): double blind, randomised, parallel group, placebo controlled trial. BMJ 344:e1566, 2012 22408266

Berhan A, Barker A: Vortioxetine in the treatment of adult patients with major depressive disorder: a meta-analysis of randomized double-blind controlled trials. BMC Psychiatry 14:276, 2014 25260373

Berk M, Dandash O, Daglas R, et al: Neuroprotection after a first episode of mania: a randomized controlled maintenance trial comparing the effects of lithium and quetiapine on grey and white matter volume. Transl Psychiatry 7(1):e1011, 2017 28117843

Berkowitz A: Ziprasidone for dementia in elderly patients: case review. J Psychiatr Pract 9(6):469–473, 2003 15985971

Biglia N, Bounous VE, Susini T, et al: Duloxetine and escitalopram for hot flushes: efficacy and compliance in breast cancer survivors. Eur J Cancer Care (Engl) 27(1): 2018 26936232

Billioti de Gage S, Moride Y, Ducruet T, et al: Benzodiazepine use and risk of Alzheimer's disease: case-control study. BMJ 349:g5205, 2014 25208536

Birks JS, Grimley Evans J: Rivastigmine for Alzheimer's disease. Cochrane Database Syst Rev (4):CD001191, 2015 25858345

Birks JS, Harvey RJ: Donepezil for dementia due to Alzheimer's disease. Cochrane Database Syst Rev 6(6):CD001190, 2018 29923184

Bishara D, Taylor D: Adverse effects of clozapine in older patients: epidemiology, prevention and management. Drugs Aging 31(1):11–20, 2014 24338220

Boettger S, Jenewein J, Breitbart W: Haloperidol, risperidone, olanzapine and aripiprazole in the management of delirium: a comparison of efficacy, safety, and side effects. Palliat Support Care 13(4):1079–1085, 2015 25191793

Boivin Z, Perez MF, Atuegwu NC, et al: Association of atypical antipsychotics and mortality for patients hospitalised with pneumonia. ERJ Open Res 5(4):00223–02018, 2019 31720299

Bond DJ, Lam RW, Yatham LN: Divalproex sodium versus placebo in the treatment of acute bipolar depression: a systematic review and meta-analysis. J Affect Disord 124(3):228–234, 2010 20044142

Bondareff W, Alpert M, Friedhoff AJ, et al: Comparison of sertraline and nortriptyline in the treatment of major depressive disorder in late life. Am J Psychiatry 157(5):729–736, 2000 10784465

Bossini L, Casolaro I, Koukouna D, et al: Off-label uses of trazodone: a review. Expert Opin Pharmacother 13(12):1707–1717, 2012 22712761

Bradley AJ, Lenox-Smith AJ: Does adding noradrenaline reuptake inhibition to selective serotonin reuptake inhibition improve efficacy in patients with depression? A systematic review of meta-analyses and large randomised pragmatic trials. J Psychopharmacol 27(8):740–758, 2013 23832963

Breilmann J, Girlanda F, Guaiana G, et al: Benzodiazepines versus placebo for panic disorder in adults. Cochrane Database Syst Rev 3(3):CD010677, 2019 30921478

Brodaty H, Ames D, Snowdon J, et al: A randomized placebo-controlled trial of risperidone for the treatment of aggression, agitation, and psychosis of dementia. J Clin Psychiatry 64(2):134–143, 2003 12633121

Broen MP, Leentjens AF, Köhler S, et al: Trajectories of recovery in depressed Parkinson's disease patients treated with paroxetine or venlafaxine. Parkinsonism Relat Disord 23:80–85, 2016 26739248

Buchanan D, Tourigny-Rivard MF, Cappeliez P, et al: National guidelines for seniors' mental health: the assessment and treatment of depression. Canadian Journal of Geriatrics 9(suppl 2):S52–S58, 2006

Burrows AB, Salzman C, Satlin A, et al: A randomized, placebo-controlled trial of paroxetine in nursing home residents with non-major depression. Depress Anxiety 15(3):102–110, 2002 12001178

Burry L, Hutton B, Williamson DR, et al: Pharmacological interventions for the treatment of delirium in critically ill adults. Cochrane Database Syst Rev 9(9):CD011749, 2019 31479532

Buspavanich P, Behr J, Stamm T, et al: Treatment response of lithium augmentation in geriatric compared to non-geriatric patients with treatment-resistant depression. J Affect Disord 251:136–140, 2019 30921597

Camargos EF, Louzada LL, Quintas JL, et al: Trazodone improves sleep parameters in Alzheimer disease patients: a randomized, double-blind, and placebo-controlled study. Am J Geriatr Psychiatry 22(12):1565–1574, 2014 24495406

Camargos EF, Quintas JL, Louzada LL, et al: Trazodone and cognitive performance in Alzheimer disease. J Clin Psychopharmacol 35(1):88–89, 2015 25379952

Campbell AM, Axon DR, Martin JR, et al: Melatonin for the prevention of postoperative delirium in older adults: a systematic review and meta-analysis. BMC Geriatr 19(1):272, 2019 31619178

Carta MG, Zairo F, Mellino G, Hardoy MC: Add-on quetiapine in the treatment of major depressive disorder in elderly patients with cerebrovascular damage. Clin Pract Epidemiol Ment Health 3:28, 2007 18039392

Carvajal García-Pando A, García del Pozo J, Sánchez AS, et al: Hepatotoxicity associated with the new antidepressants. J Clin Psychiatry 63(2):135–137, 2002 11874214

Castro VM, Clements CC, Murphy SN, et al: QT interval and antidepressant use: a cross sectional study of electronic health records. BMJ 346:f288, 2013 23360890

Centorrino F, Price BH, Tuttle M, et al: EEG abnormalities during treatment with typical and atypical antipsychotics. Am J Psychiatry 159(1):109–115, 2002 11772698

Chalon SA, Granier LA, Vandenhende FR, et al: Duloxetine increases serotonin and norepinephrine availability in healthy subjects: a double-blind, controlled study. Neuropsychopharmacology 28(9):1685–1693, 2003 12784100

Chan WC, Lam LC, Choy CN, et al: A double-blind randomised comparison of risperidone and haloperidol in the treatment of behavioural and psychological symptoms in Chinese dementia patients. Int J Geriatr Psychiatry 16(12):1156–1162, 2001 11748775

Cheah CY, Ladhams B, Fegan PG: Mirtazapine associated with profound hyponatremia: two case reports. Am J Geriatr Pharmacother 6(2):91–95, 2008 18675767

Chen A, Copeli F, Metzger E, et al: The Psychopharmacology Algorithm Project at the Harvard South Shore Program: an update on management of behavioral and psychological symptoms in dementia. Psychiatry Res 295:113641, 2021 33340800

Chen H, Lin Q, Lin T, et al: A controlled study of the efficacy and safety of tandospirone citrate combined with escitalopram in the treatment of vascular depression: a pilot randomized controlled trial at a single-center in China. J Psychiatr Res 114:133–140, 2019 31075722

Chen P, Kales HC, Weintraub D, et al: Antidepressant treatment of veterans with Parkinson's disease and depression: analysis of a national sample. J Geriatr Psychiatry Neurol 20(3):161–165, 2007 17712099

Chen R, Chan PT, Chu H, et al: Treatment effects between monotherapy of donepezil versus combination with memantine for Alzheimer disease: a meta-analysis. PLoS One 12(8):e0183586, 2017 28827830

Chen Y, Patel NC, Guo JJ, Zhan S: Antidepressant prophylaxis for poststroke depression: a meta-analysis. Int Clin Psychopharmacol 22(3):159–166, 2007 17414742

Cheng HH, Huang WC, Jeng SY: Anti-epileptic drugs associated with fractures in the elderly: a preliminary population-based study. Curr Med Res Opin 35(5):903–907, 2019 30362853

Cheung G, Stapelberg J: Quetiapine for the treatment of behavioural and psychological symptoms of dementia (BPSD): a meta-analysis of randomised placebo-controlled trials. N Z Med J 124(1336):39–50, 2011 21946743

Chew ML, Mulsant BH, Pollock BG: Serum anticholinergic activity and cognition in patients with moderate-to-severe dementia. Am J Geriatr Psychiatry 13(6):535–538, 2005 15956274

Chew ML, Mulsant BH, Pollock BG, et al: A model of anticholinergic activity of atypical antipsychotic medications. Schizophr Res 88(1–3):63–72, 2006 16928430

Chew ML, Mulsant BH, Pollock BG, et al: Anticholinergic activity of 107 medications commonly used by older adults. J Am Geriatr Soc 56(7):1333–1341, 2008 18510583

Choe YM, Kim KW, Jhoo JH, et al: Multicenter, randomized, placebo-controlled, double-blind clinical trial of escitalopram on the progression-delaying effects in Alzheimer's disease. Int J Geriatr Psychiatry 31(7):731–739, 2016 26553313

Christensen MC, Loft H, McIntyre RS: Vortioxetine improves symptomatic and functional outcomes in major depressive disorder: a novel dual outcome measure in depressive disorders. J Affect Disord 227:787–794, 2018 29689693

Cipriani A, Furukawa TA, Salanti G, et al: Comparative efficacy and acceptability of 21 antidepressant drugs for the acute treatment of adults with major depressive disorder: a systematic review and network meta-analysis. Lancet 391(10128):1357–1366, 2018 29477251

Cirrito JR, Disabato BM, Restivo JL, et al: Serotonin signaling is associated with lower amyloid-β levels and plaques in transgenic mice and humans. Proc Natl Acad Sci USA 108(36):14968–14973, 2011 21873225

Cirrito JR, Wallace CE, Yan P, et al: Effect of escitalopram on Aβ levels and plaque load in an Alzheimer mouse model. Neurology 95(19):e2666–e2674, 2020 32913022

Clapham E, Bodén R, Reutfors J, et al: Exposure to risperidone versus other antipsychotics and risk of osteoporosis-related fractures: a population-based study. Acta Psychiatr Scand 141(1):74–83, 2020 31545521

Clark WS, Street JS, Feldman PD, Breier A: The effects of olanzapine in reducing the emergence of psychosis among nursing home patients with Alzheimer's disease. J Clin Psychiatry 62(1):34–40, 2001 11235926

Clayton AH, Kornstein SG, Rosas G, et al: An integrated analysis of the safety and tolerability of desvenlafaxine compared with placebo in the treatment of major depressive disorder. CNS Spectr 14(4):183–195, 2009 19407730

Clayton AH, Kornstein SG, Dunlop BW, et al: Efficacy and safety of desvenlafaxine 50 mg/d in a randomized, placebo-controlled study of perimenopausal and postmenopausal women with major depressive disorder. J Clin Psychiatry 74(10):1010–1017, 2013 24229754

Clemmons AB, Orr J, Andrick B, et al: Randomized, placebo-controlled, Phase III trial of fosaprepitant, ondansetron, dexamethasone (FOND) versus FOND plus olanzapine (FOND-O) for the prevention of chemotherapy-induced nausea and vomiting in patients with hematologic malignancies receiving highly emetogenic chemotherapy and hematopoietic cell transplantation regimens: the FOND-O trial. Biol Blood Marrow Transplant 24(10):2065–2071, 2018 29906570

Cooper C, Katona C, Lyketsos K, et al: A systematic review of treatments for refractory depression in older people. Am J Psychiatry 168(7):681–688, 2011 21454919

Coupland C, Dhiman P, Morriss R, et al: Antidepressant use and risk of adverse outcomes in older people: population based cohort study. BMJ 343:d4551, 2011 21810886

Crépeau-Gendron G, Brown HK, Shorey C, et al: Association between citalopram, escitalopram and QTc prolongation in a real-world geriatric setting. J Affect Disord 250:341–345, 2019 30877856

Cristancho P, Lenard E, Lenze EJ, et al: Optimizing Outcomes of Treatment-Resistant Depression in Older Adults (OPTIMUM): study design and treatment characteristics of the first 396 participants randomized. Am J Geriatr Psychiatry 27(10):1138–1152, 2019 31147244

Cross DB, Tiu J, Medicherla C, et al: Modafinil In Recovery After Stroke (MIRAS): a retrospective study. J Stroke Cerebrovasc Dis 29(4):104645, 2020 32147025

Culang ME, Sneed JR, Keilp JG, et al: Change in cognitive functioning following acute antidepressant treatment in late-life depression. Am J Geriatr Psychiatry 17(10):881–888, 2009 19916207

Culo S, Mulsant BH, Rosen J, et al: Treating neuropsychiatric symptoms in dementia with Lewy bodies: a randomized controlled trial. Alzheimer Dis Assoc Disord 24(4):360–364, 2010 20625270

Cumbo E, Ligori LD: Differential effects of current specific treatments on behavioral and psychological symptoms in patients with Alzheimer's disease: a 12-month, randomized, open-label trial. J Alzheimers Dis 39(3):477–485, 2014 24164733

Cumbo E, Cumbo S, Torregrossa S, Migliore D: Treatment effects of vortioxetine on cognitive functions in mild Alzheimer's disease patients with depressive symptoms: a 12 month, open-label, observational study. J Prev Alzheimers Dis 6(3):192–197, 2019 31062834

Cummings JL, Lyketsos CG, Peskind ER, et al: Effect of dextromethorphan-quinidine on agitation in patients with Alzheimer disease dementia: a randomized clinical trial. JAMA 314(12):1242–1254, 2015 26393847

Dahmen N, Marx J, Hopf HC, et al: Therapy of early poststroke depression with venlafaxine: safety, tolerability, and efficacy as determined in an open, uncontrolled clinical trial. Stroke 30(3):691–692, 1999 10066874

Damri O, Shemesh N, Agam G: Is there justification to treat neurodegenerative disorders by repurposing drugs? The case of Alzheimer's disease, lithium, and autophagy. Int J Mol Sci 22(1):189, 2020 33375448

Darwish M, Kirby M, Hellriegel ET, et al: Systemic exposure to armodafinil and its tolerability in healthy elderly versus young men: an open-label, multiple-dose, parallel-group study. Drugs Aging 28(2):139–150, 2011 21275439

Das A, Minner R, Krain L, Spollen J: Delirium on clozapine: a tale of friend turned foe: a case report. Int J Psychiatry Med :91217420972827, 2020 33148081

Davidson J, Watkins L, Owens M, et al: Effects of paroxetine and venlafaxine XR on heart rate variability in depression. J Clin Psychopharmacol 25(5):480–484, 2005 16160626

Davidson M, Harvey PD, Vervarcke J, et al: A long-term, multicenter, open-label study of risperidone in elderly patients with psychosis. On behalf of the Risperidone Working Group. Int J Geriatr Psychiatry 15(6):506–514, 2000 10861916

Davidson M, Emsley R, Kramer M, et al: Efficacy, safety and early response of paliperidone extended-release tablets (paliperidone ER): results of a 6-week, randomized, placebo-controlled study. Schizophr Res 93(1–3):117–130, 2007 17466492

Davies SJ, Burhan AM, Kim D, et al: Sequential drug treatment algorithm for agitation and aggression in Alzheimer's and mixed dementia. J Psychopharmacol 32(5):509–523, 2018 29338602

de Abajo FJ, García-Rodríguez LA: Risk of upper gastrointestinal tract bleeding associated with selective serotonin reuptake inhibitors and venlafaxine therapy: interaction with nonsteroidal anti-inflammatory drugs and effect of acid-suppressing agents. Arch Gen Psychiatry 65(7):795–803, 2008 18606952

Declercq T, Petrovic M, Azermai M, et al: Withdrawal versus continuation of chronic antipsychotic drugs for behavioural and psychological symptoms in older people with dementia. Cochrane Database Syst Rev (3):CD007726, 2013 23543555

De Deyn PP, Rabheru K, Rasmussen A, et al: A randomized trial of risperidone, placebo, and haloperidol for behavioral symptoms of dementia. Neurology 53(5):946–955, 1999 10496251

De Deyn PP, Carrasco MM, Deberdt W, et al: Olanzapine versus placebo in the treatment of psychosis with or without associated behavioral disturbances in patients with Alzheimer's disease. Int J Geriatr Psychiatry 19(2):115–126, 2004 14758577

De Deyn P, Jeste DV, Swanink R, et al: Aripiprazole for the treatment of psychosis in patients with Alzheimer's disease: a randomized, placebo-controlled study. J Clin Psychopharmacol 25(5):463–467, 2005a 16160622

De Deyn PP, Katz IR, Brodaty H, et al: Management of agitation, aggression, and psychosis associated with dementia: a pooled analysis including three randomized, placebo-controlled double-blind trials in nursing home residents treated with risperidone. Clin Neurol Neurosurg 107(6):497–508, 2005b 15922506

De Deyn PP, Drenth AF, Kremer BP, et al: Aripiprazole in the treatment of Alzheimer's disease. Expert Opin Pharmacother 14(4):459–474, 2013 23350964

De Gregorio D, Aguilar-Valles A, Preller KH, et al: Hallucinogens in mental health: preclinical and clinical studies on LSD, psilocybin, MDMA, and ketamine. J Neurosci 41(5):891–900, 2021 33257322

Dennis M, Forbes J, Graham C, et al: Fluoxetine and fractures after stroke: exploratory analyses from the focus trial. Stroke 50(11):3280–3282, 2019 31426731

Devanand DP, Pelton GH, Marston K, et al: Sertraline treatment of elderly patients with depression and cognitive impairment. Int J Geriatr Psychiatry 18(2):123–130, 2003 12571820

Devanand DP, Juszczak N, Nobler MS, et al: An open treatment trial of venlafaxine for elderly patients with dysthymic disorder. J Geriatr Psychiatry Neurol 17(4):219–224, 2004 15533993

Devanand DP, Mintzer J, Schultz SK, et al: Relapse risk after discontinuation of risperidone in Alzheimer's disease. N Engl J Med 367(16):1497–1507, 2012 23075176

Devlin JW, Roberts RJ, Fong JJ, et al: Efficacy and safety of quetiapine in critically ill patients with delirium: a prospective, multicenter, randomized, double-blind, placebo-controlled pilot study. Crit Care Med 38(2):419–427, 2010 19915454

Devlin JW, Skrobik Y, Riker RR, et al: Impact of quetiapine on resolution of individual delirium symptoms in critically ill patients with delirium: a post-hoc analysis of a double-blind, randomized, placebo-controlled study. Crit Care 15(5):R215, 2011 21923923

Devos D, Dujardin K, Poirot I, et al: Comparison of desipramine and citalopram treatments for depression in Parkinson's disease: a double-blind, randomized, placebo-controlled study. Mov Disord 23(6):850–857, 2008 18311826

Diem SJ, Blackwell TL, Stone KL, et al: Use of antidepressants and rates of hip bone loss in older women: the study of osteoporotic fractures. Arch Intern Med 167(12):1240–1245, 2007 17592096

Dolder C, Nelson M, Stump A: Pharmacological and clinical profile of newer antidepressants: implications for the treatment of elderly patients. Drugs Aging 27(8):625–640, 2010 20658791

Doraiswamy PM, Krishnan KR, Oxman T, et al: Does antidepressant therapy improve cognition in elderly depressed patients? J Gerontol A Biol Sci Med Sci 58(12):M1137–M1144, 2003 14684712

Douros A, Ades M, Renoux C: Risk of intracranial hemorrhage associated with the use of antidepressants inhibiting serotonin reuptake: a systematic review. CNS Drugs 32(4):321–334, 2018 29536379

Drisaldi A, Weeda E, Neyens R, et al: Accuracy of valproic acid concentration correction based on serum albumin. Neurocrit Care 30(2):301–306, 2019 30328046

D'Souza R, Rajji TK, Mulsant BH, Pollock BG: Use of lithium in the treatment of bipolar disorder in late-life. Curr Psychiatry Rep 13(6):488–492, 2011 21847537

Dunlop BW, Crits-Christoph P, Evans DL, et al: Coadministration of modafinil and a selective serotonin reuptake inhibitor from the initiation of treatment of major depressive disorder with fatigue and sleepiness: a double-blind, placebo-controlled study. J Clin Psychopharmacol 27(6):614–619, 2007 18004129

Dunner DL: Treatment of bipolar disorder in the elderly. Am J Psychiatry 174(11):1032–1033, 2017 29088940

Dunner DL, Zisook S, Billow AA, et al: A prospective safety surveillance study for bupropion sustained-release in the treatment of depression. J Clin Psychiatry 59(7):366–373, 1998 9714265

EFFECTS Trial Collaboration: Safety and efficacy of fluoxetine on functional recovery after acute stroke (EFFECTS): a randomised, double-blind, placebo-controlled trial. Lancet Neurol 19(8):661–669, 2020 32702335

Egberts A, Alan H, Ziere G, Mattace-Raso FUS: Antipsychotics and lorazepam during delirium: are we harming older patients? A real-life data study. Drugs Aging 38(1):53–62, 2021 33164161

Ehrhardt S, Porsteinsson AP, Munro CA, et al: Escitalopram for agitation in Alzheimer's disease (S-CitAD): methods and design of an investigator-initiated, randomized, controlled, multicenter clinical trial. Alzheimers Dement 15(11):1427–1436, 2019 31587995

Eksi MS, Turgut VU, Özcan-Eksi EE, et al: Serotonin syndrome following tramadol and gabapentin use after spine surgery. World Neurosurg 126:261–263, 2019 30898741

Ellis T, Cudkowicz ME, Sexton PM, Growdon JH: Clozapine and risperidone treatment of psychosis in Parkinson's disease. J Neuropsychiatry Clin Neurosci 12(3):364–369, 2000 10956570

Emre M, Tsolaki M, Bonuccelli U, et al: Memantine for patients with Parkinson's disease dementia or dementia with Lewy bodies: a randomised, double-blind, placebo-controlled trial. Lancet Neurol 9(10):969–977, 2010 20729148

Espay AJ, Guskey MT, Norton JC, et al: Pimavanserin for Parkinson's disease psychosis: effects stratified by baseline cognition and use of cognitive-enhancing medications. Mov Disord 33(11):1769–1776, 2018 30387904

Estevez-Fraga C, Zeun P, López-Sendón Moreno JL: Current methods for the treatment and prevention of drug-induced parkinsonism and tardive dyskinesia in the elderly. Drugs Aging 35(11):959–971, 2018 30357723

Eyre H, Siddarth P, Cyr N, et al: Comparing the immune-genomic effects of vilazodone and paroxetine in late-life depression: a pilot study. Pharmacopsychiatry 50(6):256–263, 2017 28444658

Fabian TJ, Amico JA, Kroboth PD, et al: Paroxetine-induced hyponatremia in older adults: a 12-week prospective study. Arch Intern Med 164(3):327–332, 2004 14769630

Fava M, Thase ME, DeBattista C, et al: Modafinil augmentation of selective serotonin reuptake inhibitor therapy in MDD partial responders with persistent fatigue and sleepiness. Ann Clin Psychiatry 19(3):153–159, 2007 17729016

Fava M, Dirks B, Freeman MP, et al: A phase 2, randomized, double-blind, placebo-controlled study of adjunctive pimavanserin in patients with major depressive disorder and an inadequate response to therapy (CLARITY). J Clin Psychiatry 80(6):19m12928, 2019

Fawcett J, Rush AJ, Vukelich J, et al: Clinical experience with high-dosage pramipexole in patients with treatment-resistant depressive episodes in unipolar and bipolar depression. Am J Psychiatry 173(2):107–111, 2016 26844792

Feldman PD, Hay LK, Deberdt W, et al: Retrospective cohort study of diabetes mellitus and antipsychotic treatment in a geriatric population in the United States. J Am Med Dir Assoc 5(1):38–46, 2004 14706127

Fenn HH, Sommer BR, Ketter TA, Alldredge B: Safety and tolerability of mood-stabilising anticonvulsants in the elderly. Expert Opin Drug Saf 5(3):401–416, 2006 16610969

Fernandez HH, Trieschmann ME, Burke MA, Friedman JH: Quetiapine for psychosis in Parkinson's disease versus dementia with Lewy bodies. J Clin Psychiatry 63(6):513–515, 2002 12088163

Fink HA, Linskens EJ, MacDonald R, et al: Benefits and harms of prescription drugs and supplements for treatment of clinical Alzheimer-type dementia. Ann Intern Med 172(10):656–668, 2020 32340037

Flint AJ: Generalised anxiety disorder in elderly patients: epidemiology, diagnosis and treatment options. Drugs Aging 22(2):101–114, 2005 15733018

Flint AJ, Rifat SL: Nonresponse to first-line pharmacotherapy may predict relapse and recurrence of remitted geriatric depression. Depress Anxiety 13(3):125–131, 2001 11387732

Flint AJ, Meyers BS, Rothschild AJ, et al: Effect of continuing olanzapine vs placebo on relapse among patients with psychotic depression in remission: the STOP-PD II randomized clinical trial. JAMA 322(7):622–631, 2019 31429896

Flint AJ, Rothschild AJ, Whyte EM, et al: Effect of older vs younger age on anthropometric and metabolic variables during treatment of psychotic depression with sertraline plus olanzapine: the STOP-PD II study. Am J Geriatr Psychiatry 2020 Epub ahead of print

FOCUS Trial Collaboration: Effects of fluoxetine on functional outcomes after acute stroke (FOCUS): a pragmatic, double-blind, randomised, controlled trial. Lancet 393(10168):265–274, 2019 30528472

Fontaine CS, Hynan LS, Koch K, et al: A double-blind comparison of olanzapine versus risperidone in the acute treatment of dementia-related behavioral disturbances in extended care facilities. J Clin Psychiatry 64(6):726–730, 2003 12823090

Forester BP, Streeter CC, Berlow YA, et al: Brain lithium levels and effects on cognition and mood in geriatric bipolar disorder: a lithium-7 magnetic resonance spectroscopy study. Am J Geriatr Psychiatry 17(1):13–23, 2009 18626002

Forester BP, Sajatovic M, Tsai J, et al: Safety and effectiveness of long-term treatment with lur-asidone in older adults with bipolar depression: post-hoc analysis of a 6-month, open-label study. Am J Geriatr Psychiatry 26(2):150–159, 2018 29146409

Fornaro M, Carvalho AF, Fusco A, et al: The concept and management of acute episodes of treatment-resistant bipolar disorder: a systematic review and exploratory meta-analysis of randomized controlled trials. J Affect Disord 276:970–983, 2020 32750614

Fotso Soh J, Klil-Drori S, Rej S: Using lithium in older age bipolar disorder: special consider-ations. Drugs Aging 36(2):147–154, 2019 30613911

Frakey LL, Salloway S, Buelow M, Malloy P: A randomized, double-blind, placebo-controlled trial of modafinil for the treatment of apathy in individuals with mild-to-moderate Alzhei-mer's disease. J Clin Psychiatry 73(6):796–801, 2012 22687392

Fralick M, Bartsch E, Ritchie CS, Sacks CA: Estimating the use of potentially inappropriate medications among older adults in the United States. J Am Geriatr Soc 68(12):2927–2930, 2020 32841366

Freudenreich O, Menza M: Zolpidem-related delirium: a case report. J Clin Psychiatry 61(6):449–450, 2000 10901348

Freund-Levi Y, Jedenius E, Tysen-Bäckström AC, et al: Galantamine versus risperidone treat-ment of neuropsychiatric symptoms in patients with probable dementia: an open random-ized trial. Am J Geriatr Psychiatry 22(4):341–348, 2014 24035407

Friedli K, Guirguis A, Almond M, et al: Sertraline versus placebo in patients with major depres-sive disorder undergoing hemodialysis: a randomized, controlled feasibility trial. Clin J Am Soc Nephrol 12(2):280–286, 2017 28126706

Friedman RA, Leon AC: Expanding the black box: depression, antidepressants, and the risk of suicide. N Engl J Med 356(23):2343–2346, 2007 17485726

Fu W, Ma L, Zhao X, et al: Antidepressant medication can improve hypertension in elderly pa-tients with depression. J Clin Neurosci 22(12):1911–1915, 2015 26256065

Furlan PM, Kallan MJ, Ten Have T, et al: Cognitive and psychomotor effects of paroxetine and ser-traline on healthy elderly volunteers. Am J Geriatr Psychiatry 9(4):429–438, 2001 11739070

Gaffey AE, Rosman L, Burg MM, et al: Posttraumatic stress disorder, antidepressant use, and hemorrhagic stroke in young men and women: a 13-year cohort study. Stroke 52(1):121–129, 2021 33297868

Gao J, Lin M, Zhao J, et al: Different interventions for post-ischaemic stroke depression in dif-ferent time periods: a single-blind randomized controlled trial with stratification by time after stroke. Clin Rehabil 31(1):71–81, 2017 26817808

Gareri P, Cotroneo A, Lacava R, et al: Comparison of the efficacy of new and conventional an-tipsychotic drugs in the treatment of behavioral and psychological symptoms of dementia (BPSD). Arch Gerontol Geriatr Suppl 38(suppl 9):207–215, 2004 15207416

Garfield LD, Müller DJ, Kennedy JL, et al: Genetic variation in the serotonin transporter and HTR1B receptor predicts reduced bone formation during serotonin reuptake inhibitor treatment in older adults. World J Biol Psychiatry 15(5):404–410, 2014 24074042

Gauthier S, Cummings J, Ballard C, et al: Management of behavioral problems in Alzheimer's disease. Int Psychogeriatr 22(3):346–372, 2010 20096151

Gelenberg AJ, McGahuey C, Laukes C, et al: Mirtazapine substitution in SSRI-induced sexual dysfunction. J Clin Psychiatry 61(5):356–360, 2000 10847310

George D, Gálvez V, Martin D, et al: Pilot randomized controlled trial of titrated subcutaneous ketamine in older patients with treatment-resistant depression. Am J Geriatr Psychiatry 25(11):1199–1209, 2017 28739263

Georgotas A, McCue RE, Hapworth W, et al: Comparative efficacy and safety of MAOIs versus TCAs in treating depression in the elderly. Biol Psychiatry 21(12):1155–1166, 1986 3756264

Gex-Fabry M, Balant-Gorgia AE, Balant LP: Therapeutic drug monitoring of olanzapine: the combined effect of age, gender, smoking, and comedication. Ther Drug Monit 25(1):46–53, 2003 12548144

Gill H, Gill B, Rodrigues NB, et al: The effects of ketamine on cognition in treatment-resistant depression: a systematic review and priority avenues for future research. Neurosci Biobe-hav Rev 120:78–85, 2021 33242561

Gill SS, Rochon PA, Herrmann N, et al: Atypical antipsychotic drugs and risk of ischaemic stroke: population based retrospective cohort study. BMJ 330(7489):445, 2005 15668211

Gill SS, Anderson GM, Fischer HD, et al: Syncope and its consequences in patients with dementia receiving cholinesterase inhibitors: a population-based cohort study. Arch Intern Med 169(9):867–873, 2009 19433698

Girard TD, Exline MC, Carson SS, et al: Haloperidol and ziprasidone for treatment of delirium in critical illness. N Engl J Med 379(26):2506–2516, 2018 30346242

Glass J, Lanctôt KL, Herrmann N, et al: Sedative hypnotics in older people with insomnia: meta-analysis of risks and benefits. BMJ 331(7526):1169, 2005 16284208

Glassman AH, O'Connor CM, Califf RM, et al: Sertraline treatment of major depression in patients with acute MI or unstable angina. JAMA 288(6):701–709, 2002 12169073

Goetz CG, Blasucci LM, Leurgans S, Pappert EJ: Olanzapine and clozapine: comparative effects on motor function in hallucinating PD patients. Neurology 55(6):789–794, 2000 10993997

González-Rodríguez A, Molina-Andreu O, Penadés R, et al: Effectiveness of long-acting injectable antipsychotics in delusional disorders with nonprominent hallucinations and without hallucinations. Int Clin Psychopharmacol 29(3):177–180, 2014 24681811

Goodnick PJ, Hernandez M: Treatment of depression in comorbid medical illness. Expert Opin Pharmacother 1(7):1367–1384, 2000 11249471

Gorwood P, Weiller E, Lemming O, Katona C: Escitalopram prevents relapse in older patients with major depressive disorder. Am J Geriatr Psychiatry 15(7):581–593, 2007 17586783

Goss AJ, Kaser M, Costafreda SG, et al: Modafinil augmentation therapy in unipolar and bipolar depression: a systematic review and meta-analysis of randomized controlled trials. J Clin Psychiatry 74(11):1101–1107, 2013 24330897

Greco KE, Tune LE, Brown FW, Van Horn WA: A retrospective study of the safety of intramuscular ziprasidone in agitated elderly patients. J Clin Psychiatry 66(7):928–929, 2005 16013910

Greenblatt DJ, Harmatz JS, Shapiro L, et al: Sensitivity to triazolam in the elderly. N Engl J Med 324(24):1691–1698, 1991 2034245

Greger J, Aladeen T, Lewandowski E, et al: Comparison of the metabolic characteristics of newer second generation antipsychotics: brexpiprazole, lurasidone, asenapine, cariprazine, and iloperidone with olanzapine as a comparator. J Clin Psychopharmacol 41(1):5–12, 2021 33177350

Greil W, Zhang X, Stassen H, et al: Cutaneous adverse drug reactions to psychotropic drugs and their risk factors: a case-control study. Eur Neuropsychopharmacol 29(1):111–121, 2019 30424913

Grippe TC, Gonçalves BS, Louzada LL, et al: Circadian rhythm in Alzheimer disease after trazodone use. Chronobiol Int 32(9):1311–1314, 2015 26376345

Grossberg GT, Kohegyi E, Mergel V, et al: Efficacy and safety of brexpiprazole for the treatment of agitation in Alzheimer's dementia: two 12-week, randomized, double-blind, placebo-controlled trials. Am J Geriatr Psychiatry 28(4):383–400, 2020 31708380

Grothe DR, Scheckner B, Albano D: Treatment of pain syndromes with venlafaxine. Pharmacotherapy 24(5):621–629, 2004 15162896

Gu SC, Wang CD: Early selective serotonin reuptake inhibitors for recovery after stroke: a meta-analysis and trial sequential analysis. J Stroke Cerebrovasc Dis 27(5):1178–1189, 2018 29276014

Gualtieri CT, Johnson LG: Comparative neurocognitive effects of 5 psychotropic anticonvulsants and lithium. MedGenMed 8(3):46, 2006 17406176

Guay DR: Comment on the potential utility of the new atypical antipsychotic lurasidone in the geriatric population. Consult Pharm 26(8):579–582, 2011 21840821

Guo J, Wang Z, Liu R, et al: Memantine, donepezil, or combination therapy: what is the best therapy for Alzheimer's disease? A network meta-analysis. Brain Behav 10(11):e01831, 2020 32914577

Gustavsen I, Bramness JG, Skurtveit S, et al: Road traffic accident risk related to prescriptions of the hypnotics zopiclone, zolpidem, flunitrazepam and nitrazepam. Sleep Med 9(8):818–822, 2008 18226959

Gutsmiedl K, Krause M, Bighelli I, et al: How well do elderly patients with major depressive disorder respond to antidepressants: a systematic review and single-group meta-analysis. BMC Psychiatry 20(1):102, 2020 32131786

Hajek T, Kopecek M, Höschl C, Alda M: Smaller hippocampal volumes in patients with bipolar disorder are masked by exposure to lithium: a meta-analysis. J Psychiatry Neurosci 37(5):333–343, 2012 22498078

Hale GM, Kane-Gill SL, Groetzinger L, Smithburger PL: An evaluation of adverse drug reactions associated with antipsychotic use for the treatment of delirium in the intensive care unit. J Pharm Pract 29(4):355–360, 2016 25609664

Hamilton M: A rating scale for depression. J Neurol Neurosurg Psychiatry 23:56–62, 1960

Han CS, Kim YK: A double-blind trial of risperidone and haloperidol for the treatment of delirium. Psychosomatics 45(4):297–301, 2004 15232043

Hanazawa T, Kamijo Y: Effect of suvorexant on nocturnal delirium in elderly patients with Alzheimer's disease: a case-series study. Clin Psychopharmacol Neurosci 17(4):547–550, 2019 31671494

Hansen RA, Gartlehner G, Webb AP, et al: Efficacy and safety of donepezil, galantamine, and rivastigmine for the treatment of Alzheimer's disease: a systematic review and meta-analysis. Clin Interv Aging 3(2):211–225, 2008 18686744

Harder S, Groenvold M, Isaksen J, et al: Antiemetic use of olanzapine in patients with advanced cancer: results from an open-label multicenter study. Support Care Cancer 27(8):2849–2856, 2019 30552594

Harvey AT, Rudolph RL, Preskorn SH: Evidence of the dual mechanisms of action of venlafaxine. Arch Gen Psychiatry 57(5):503–509, 2000 10807491

Harvey PD, Napolitano JA, Mao L, Gharabawi G: Comparative effects of risperidone and olanzapine on cognition in elderly patients with schizophrenia or schizoaffective disorder. Int J Geriatr Psychiatry 18(9):820–829, 2003 12949850

He Y, Zheng Y, Xu C, et al: Sertraline hydrochloride treatment for patients with stable chronic obstructive pulmonary disease complicated with depression: a randomized controlled trial. Clin Respir J 10(3):318–325, 2016 25308771

He Y, Cai Z, Zeng S, et al: Effect of fluoxetine on three-year recurrence in acute ischemic stroke: a randomized controlled clinical study. Clin Neurol Neurosurg 168:1–6, 2018 29494855

Health Canada Advisory: Remeron/Remeron RD (mirtazapine)—Abnormal Heart Rhythm. Ottawa, ON, Health Canada, March 2014. Available at: http://healthycanadians.gc.ca/recall-alert-rappel-avis/hc-sc/2014/38709a-eng.php. Accessed April 11, 2021.

Hemmelgarn B, Suissa S, Huang A, et al: Benzodiazepine use and the risk of motor vehicle crash in the elderly. JAMA 278(1):27–31, 1997 9207334

Henry G, Williamson D, Tampi RR: Efficacy and tolerability of antidepressants in the treatment of behavioral and psychological symptoms of dementia, a literature review of evidence. Am J Alzheimers Dis Other Demen 26(3):169–183, 2011 21429956

Hernandez RK, Farwell W, Cantor MD, Lawler EV: Cholinesterase inhibitors and incidence of bradycardia in patients with dementia in the Veterans Affairs New England healthcare system. J Am Geriatr Soc 57(11):1997–2003, 2009 19793162

Herring WJ, Connor KM, Snyder E, et al: Suvorexant in elderly patients with insomnia: pooled analyses of data from Phase III randomized controlled clinical trials. Am J Geriatr Psychiatry 25(7):791–802, 2017 28427826

Herring WJ, Ceesay P, Snyder E, et al: Polysomnographic assessment of suvorexant in patients with probable Alzheimer's disease dementia and insomnia: a randomized trial. Alzheimers Dement 16(3):541–551, 2020 31944580

Herrmann N, Mamdani M, Lanctôt KL: Atypical antipsychotics and risk of cerebrovascular accidents. Am J Psychiatry 161(6):1113–1115, 2004 15169702

Herrmann N, Rothenburg LS, Black SE, et al: Methylphenidate for the treatment of apathy in Alzheimer disease: prediction of response using dextroamphetamine challenge. J Clin Psychopharmacol 28(3):296–301, 2008 18480686

Herrmann N, Gauthier S, Boneva N, Lemming OM: A randomized, double-blind, placebo-controlled trial of memantine in a behaviorally enriched sample of patients with moderate-to-severe Alzheimer's disease. Int Psychogeriatr 25(6):919–927, 2013a 23472619

Herrmann N, Lanctôt KL, Hogan DB: Pharmacological recommendations for the symptomatic treatment of dementia: the Canadian Consensus Conference on the Diagnosis and Treatment of Dementia 2012. Alzheimers Res Ther 5(suppl 1):S5, 2013b 24565367

Hershey LA, Coleman-Jackson R: Pharmacological management of dementia with Lewy bodies. Drugs Aging 36(4):309–319, 2019 30680679

Hesse LM, He P, Krishnaswamy S, et al: Pharmacogenetic determinants of interindividual variability in bupropion hydroxylation by cytochrome P450 2B6 in human liver microsomes. Pharmacogenetics 14(4):225–238, 2004 15083067

Hibbard KR, Propst A, Frank DE, Wyse J: Fatalities associated with clozapine-related constipation and bowel obstruction: a literature review and two case reports. Psychosomatics 50(4):416–419, 2009 19687183

Hien TT, Cumming RG, Cameron ID, et al: Atypical antipsychotic medications and risk of falls in residents of aged care facilities. J Am Geriatr Soc 53(8):1290–1295, 2005 16078953

Ho T, Pollock BG, Mulsant BH, et al: R- and S-citalopram concentrations have differential effects on neuropsychiatric scores in elders with dementia and agitation. Br J Clin Pharmacol 82(3):784–792, 2016 27145364

Horn S, Richardson H, Xie SX, et al: Pimavanserin versus quetiapine for the treatment of psychosis in Parkinson's disease and dementia with Lewy bodies. Parkinsonism Relat Disord 69:119–124, 2019 31751863

Houlihan DJ, Mulsant BH, Sweet RA, et al: A naturalistic study of trazodone in the treatment of behavioral complications of dementia. Am J Geriatr Psychiatry 2(1):78–85, 1994 21629010

Howanitz E, Pardo M, Smelson DA, et al: The efficacy and safety of clozapine versus chlorpromazine in geriatric schizophrenia. J Clin Psychiatry 60(1):41–44, 1999 10074877

Howard R, Juszczak E, Ballard CG, et al: Donepezil for the treatment of agitation in Alzheimer's disease. N Engl J Med 357(14):1382–1392, 2007 17914039

Howard R, McShane R, Lindesay J, et al: Donepezil and memantine for moderate-to-severe Alzheimer's disease. N Engl J Med 366(10):893–903, 2012 22397651

Howard WT, Warnock JK: Bupropion-induced psychosis. Am J Psychiatry 156(12):2017–2018, 1999 10588428

Hsu JH, Mulsant BH, Lenze EJ, et al: Impact of prior treatment on remission of late-life depression with venlafaxine and subsequent aripiprazole or placebo augmentation. Am J Geriatr Psychiatry 24(10):918–922, 2016 27538352

Hsu JH, Mulsant BH, Lenze EJ, et al: Clinical predictors of extrapyramidal symptoms associated with aripiprazole augmentation for the treatment of late-life depression in a randomized controlled trial. J Clin Psychiatry 79(4):17m11764, 2018

Hughes LE, Rittman T, Regenthal R, et al: Improving response inhibition systems in frontotemporal dementia with citalopram. Brain 138(pt 7):1961–1975, 2015 26001387

Hung CC, Lin CH, Lan TH, Chan CH: The association of selective serotonin reuptake inhibitors use and stroke in geriatric population. Am J Geriatr Psychiatry 21(8):811–815, 2013 23567390

Hutchison LC: Mirtazapine and bone marrow suppression: a case report. J Am Geriatr Soc 49(8):1129–1130, 2001 11555082

Hutton LMJ, Cave AJ, St-Jean R, Banh HL: Should we be worried about QTc prolongation using citalopram? A review. J Pharm Pract 30(3):353–358, 2017 26763342

Iketani R, Imai S, Horiguchi H, et al: Comparison of the association of risperidone and quetiapine with deteriorating performance in walking and dressing in subjects with Parkinson's disease: a retrospective cohort study using administrative claims data. Int Clin Psychopharmacol 34(5):234–240, 2019 31136320

Iketani R, Furushima D, Imai S, Yamada H: Efficacy and safety of atypical antipsychotics for psychosis in Parkinson's disease: a systematic review and Bayesian network meta-analysis. Parkinsonism Relat Disord 78:82–90, 2020 32755800

Jacobson W, Zhong W, Nomikos GG, et al: Effects of vortioxetine on functional capacity across different levels of functional impairment in patients with major depressive disorder: a University of California, San Diego Performance-based Skills Assessment (UPSA) analysis. Curr Med Res Opin 36(1):117–124, 2020 31422713

Jaskiw GE, Thyrum PT, Fuller MA, et al: Pharmacokinetics of quetiapine in elderly patients with selected psychotic disorders. Clin Pharmacokinet 43(14):1025–1035, 2004 15530131

Jeste DV, Barak Y, Madhusoodanan S, et al: International multisite double-blind trial of the atypical antipsychotics risperidone and olanzapine in 175 elderly patients with chronic schizophrenia. Am J Geriatr Psychiatry 11(6):638–647, 2003 14609804

Jin Y, Pollock BG, Frank E, et al: Effect of age, weight, and CYP2C19 genotype on escitalopram exposure. J Clin Pharmacol 50(1):62–72, 2010 19841156

Johnson EM, Whyte E, Mulsant BH, et al: Cardiovascular changes associated with venlafaxine in the treatment of late-life depression. Am J Geriatr Psychiatry 14(9):796–802, 2006 16943176

Jon DI, Woo YS, Seo JS, et al: The Korean Medication Algorithm Project for Bipolar Disorder (KMAP-BP): changes in preferred treatment strategies and medications over 16 years and five editions. Bipolar Disord 22(5):461–471, 2020 32202033

Joo JH, Lenze EJ, Mulsant BH, et al: Risk factors for falls during treatment of late-life depression. J Clin Psychiatry 63(10):936–941, 2002 12416604

Jorge RE, Acion L, Moser D, et al: Escitalopram and enhancement of cognitive recovery following stroke. Arch Gen Psychiatry 67(2):187–196, 2010 20124118

Jorge RE, Acion L, Burin DI, Robinson RG: Sertraline for preventing mood disorders following traumatic brain injury: a randomized clinical trial. JAMA Psychiatry 73(10):1041–1047, 2016 27626622

Joseph B, Parsaik AK, Ahmed AT, et al: A systematic review on the efficacy of intravenous racemic ketamine for bipolar depression. J Clin Psychopharmacol 41(1):71–75, 2021 33347027

Juurlink DN, Mamdani MM, Kopp A, Redelmeier DA: The risk of suicide with selective serotonin reuptake inhibitors in the elderly. Am J Psychiatry 163(5):813–821, 2006 16648321

Kadriu B, Greenwald M, Henter ID, et al: Ketamine and serotonergic psychedelics: common mechanisms underlying the effects of rapid-acting antidepressants. Int J Neuropsychopharmacol 24(1):8–21, 2021 33252694

Kando JC, Tohen M, Castillo J, Zarate CA Jr: The use of valproate in an elderly population with affective symptoms. J Clin Psychiatry 57(6):238–240, 1996 8666559

Kane J, Canas F, Kramer M, et al: Treatment of schizophrenia with paliperidone extended-release tablets: a 6-week placebo-controlled trial. Schizophr Res 90(1–3):147–161, 2007 17092691

Kantrowitz JT: The potential role of lumateperone: something borrowed? Something new? JAMA Psychiatry 77(4):343–344, 2020 31913409

Karaiskos D, Pappa D, Tzavellas E, et al: Pregabalin augmentation of antidepressants in older patients with comorbid depression and generalized anxiety disorder: an open-label study. Int J Geriatr Psychiatry 28(1):100–105, 2013 22431439

Karp JF, Weiner D, Seligman K, et al: Body pain and treatment response in late-life depression. Am J Geriatr Psychiatry 13(3):188–194, 2005 15728749

Karp JF, Weiner DK, Dew MA, et al: Duloxetine and care management treatment of older adults with comorbid major depressive disorder and chronic low back pain: results of an open-label pilot study. Int J Geriatr Psychiatry 25(6):633–642, 2010 19750557

Kasckow JW, Mohamed S, Thallasinos A, et al: Citalopram augmentation of antipsychotic treatment in older schizophrenia patients. Int J Geriatr Psychiatry 16(12):1163–1167, 2001 11748776

Katila H, Mezhebovsky I, Mulroy A, et al: Randomized, double-blind study of the efficacy and tolerability of extended release quetiapine fumarate (quetiapine XR) monotherapy in elderly patients with major depressive disorder. Am J Geriatr Psychiatry 21(8):769–784, 2013 23567397

Katona C, Hunter BN, Bray J: A double-blind comparison of the efficacy and safely of paroxetine and imipramine in the treatment of depression with dementia. Int J Geriatr Psychiatry 13(2):100–108, 1998 9526179

Katona C, Hansen T, Olsen CK: A randomized, double-blind, placebo-controlled, duloxetine-referenced, fixed-dose study comparing the efficacy and safety of Lu AA21004 in elderly patients with major depressive disorder. Int Clin Psychopharmacol 27(4):215–223, 2012 22572889

Katz IR, Jeste DV, Mintzer JE, et al: Comparison of risperidone and placebo for psychosis and behavioral disturbances associated with dementia: a randomized, double-blind trial. J Clin Psychiatry 60(2):107–115, 1999 10084637

Katz IR, Reynolds CF III, Alexopoulos GS, Hackett D: Venlafaxine ER as a treatment for generalized anxiety disorder in older adults: pooled analysis of five randomized placebo-controlled clinical trials. J Am Geriatr Soc 50(1):18–25, 2002 12028242

Kavirajan H: Memantine: a comprehensive review of safety and efficacy. Expert Opin Drug Saf 8(1):89–109, 2009 19236221

Kavirajan H, Schneider LS: Efficacy and adverse effects of cholinesterase inhibitors and memantine in vascular dementia: a meta-analysis of randomised controlled trials. Lancet Neurol 6(9):782–792, 2007 17689146

Kennedy J, Jeste D, Kaiser CJ, et al: Olanzapine vs haloperidol in geriatric schizophrenia: analysis of data from a double-blind controlled trial. Int J Geriatr Psychiatry 18(11):1013–1020, 2003 14618553

Kennedy J, Deberdt W, Siegal A, et al: Olanzapine does not enhance cognition in non-agitated and non-psychotic patients with mild to moderate Alzheimer's dementia. Int J Geriatr Psychiatry 20(11):1020–1027, 2005 16250069

Kessler DS, MacNeill SJ, Tallon D, et al: Mirtazapine added to SSRIs or SNRIs for treatment resistant depression in primary care: Phase III randomised placebo controlled trial (MIR). BMJ 363:k4218, 2018 30381374

Khaing K, Nair BR: Melatonin for delirium prevention in hospitalized patients: a systematic review and meta-analysis. J Psychiatr Res 133:181–190, 2021 33348252

Kiev A, Masco HL, Wenger TL, et al: The cardiovascular effects of bupropion and nortriptyline in depressed outpatients. Ann Clin Psychiatry 6(2):107–115, 1994 7804386

Kim DH, Mahesri M, Bateman BT, et al: Longitudinal trends and variation in antipsychotic use in older adults after cardiac surgery. J Am Geriatr Soc 66(8):1491–1498, 2018 30125337

Kim JM, Bae KY, Stewart R, et al: Escitalopram treatment for depressive disorder following acute coronary syndrome: a 24-week double-blind, placebo-controlled trial. J Clin Psychiatry 76(1):62–68, 2015 25375836

Kim JM, Stewart R, Lee YS, et al: Effect of escitalopram vs placebo treatment for depression on long-term cardiac outcomes in patients with acute coronary syndrome: a randomized clinical trial. JAMA 320(4):350–358, 2018 30043065

Kim JS, Lee EJ, Chang DI, et al: Efficacy of early administration of escitalopram on depressive and emotional symptoms and neurological dysfunction after stroke: a multicentre, double-blind, randomised, placebo-controlled study. Lancet Psychiatry 4(1):33–41, 2017 28012485

Kim KY, Bader GM, Kotlyar V, Gropper D: Treatment of delirium in older adults with quetiapine. J Geriatr Psychiatry Neurol 16(1):29–31, 2003 12641370

Kim MS, Rhim HC, Park A, et al: Comparative efficacy and acceptability of pharmacological interventions for the treatment and prevention of delirium: a systematic review and network meta-analysis. J Psychiatr Res 125:164–176, 2020 32302794

Kim S, Ko YJ, Park K, et al: Fluoxetine and risk of bleeding in patients aged 60 years and older using the Korea adverse event reporting system database: a case/noncase study. J Clin Psychopharmacol 39(4):362–366, 2019 31206390

Kinon BJ, Stauffer VL, McGuire HC, et al: The effects of antipsychotic drug treatment on prolactin concentrations in elderly patients. J Am Med Dir Assoc 4(4):189–194, 2003 12837139

Kinon BJ, Kollack-Walker S, Jeste D, et al: Incidence of tardive dyskinesia in older adult patients treated with olanzapine or conventional antipsychotics. J Geriatr Psychiatry Neurol 28(1):67–79, 2015 25009161

Kirby D, Harrigan S, Ames D: Hyponatraemia in elderly psychiatric patients treated with selective serotonin reuptake inhibitors and venlafaxine: a retrospective controlled study in an inpatient unit. Int J Geriatr Psychiatry 17(3):231–237, 2002 11921151

Kishi T, Nomura I, Matsuda Y, et al: Lemborexant vs suvorexant for insomnia: a systematic review and network meta-analysis. J Psychiatr Res 128:68–74, 2020 32531478

Kitten AK, Hallowell SA, Saklad SR, Evoy KE: Pimavanserin: a novel drug approved to treat Parkinson's disease psychosis. Innov Clin Neurosci 15(1–2):16–22, 2018 29497575

Kleijer BC, Heerdink ER, Egberts TC, et al: Antipsychotic drug use and the risk of venous thromboembolism in elderly patients. J Clin Psychopharmacol 30(5):526–530, 2010 20814323

Klein LR, Driver BE, Miner JR, et al: Intramuscular midazolam, olanzapine, ziprasidone, or haloperidol for treating acute agitation in the emergency department. Ann Emerg Med 72(4):374–385, 2018 29885904

Klysner R, Bent-Hansen J, Hansen HL, et al: Efficacy of citalopram in the prevention of recurrent depression in elderly patients: placebo-controlled study of maintenance therapy. Br J Psychiatry 181:29–35, 2002 12091260

Knopman DS, Jones DT, Greicius MD: Failure to demonstrate efficacy of aducanumab: an analysis of the EMERGE and ENGAGE trials as reported by Biogen, December 2019. Alzheimers Dement 17(4):696–701, 2021 33135381

Koesters M, Ostuzzi G, Guaiana G, et al: Vortioxetine for depression in adults. Cochrane Database Syst Rev 7(7):CD011520, 2017 28677828

Kohen I, Preval H, Southard R, Francis A: Naturalistic study of intramuscular ziprasidone versus conventional agents in agitated elderly patients: retrospective findings from a psychiatric emergency service. Am J Geriatr Pharmacother 3(4):240–245, 2005 16503319

Kohen I, Gordon ML, Manu P: Serotonin syndrome in elderly patients treated for psychotic depression with atypical antipsychotics and antidepressants: two case reports. CNS Spectr 12(8):596–598, 2007 17667887

Koller EA, Cross JT, Doraiswamy PM, Malozowski SN: Pancreatitis associated with atypical antipsychotics: from the Food and Drug Administration's MedWatch surveillance system and published reports. Pharmacotherapy 23(9):1123–1130, 2003 14524644

Kornstein SG, Clayton AH, Soares CN, et al: Analysis by age and sex of efficacy data from placebo-controlled trials of desvenlafaxine in outpatients with major depressive disorder. J Clin Psychopharmacol 30(3):294–299, 2010a 20473066

Kornstein SG, Jiang Q, Reddy S, et al: Short-term efficacy and safety of desvenlafaxine in a randomized, placebo-controlled study of perimenopausal and postmenopausal women with major depressive disorder. J Clin Psychiatry 71(8):1088–1096, 2010b 20797382

Kornstein SG, Clayton A, Bao W, Guico-Pabia CJ: Post hoc analysis of the efficacy and safety of desvenlafaxine 50 mg/day in a randomized, placebo-controlled study of perimenopausal and postmenopausal women with major depressive disorder. Menopause 21(8):799–806, 2014 24448103

Kornstein S, Chang CT, Gommoll CP, Edwards J: Vilazodone efficacy in subgroups of patients with major depressive disorder: a post-hoc analysis of four randomized, double-blind, placebo-controlled trials. Int Clin Psychopharmacol 33(4):217–223, 2018 29608461

Kotlyar M, Brauer LH, Tracy TS, et al: Inhibition of CYP2D6 activity by bupropion. J Clin Psychopharmacol 25(3):226–229, 2005 15876900

Krause M, Huhn M, Schneider-Thoma J, et al: Antipsychotic drugs for elderly patients with schizophrenia: a systematic review and meta-analysis. Eur Neuropsychopharmacol 28(12):1360–1370, 2018 30243680

Krause M, Gutsmiedl K, Bighelli I, et al: Efficacy and tolerability of pharmacological and nonpharmacological interventions in older patients with major depressive disorder: a systematic review, pairwise and network meta-analysis. Eur Neuropsychopharmacol 29(9):1003–1022, 2019 31327506

Kripke DF, Langer RD, Kline LE: Hypnotics' association with mortality or cancer: a matched cohort study. BMJ Open 2(1):e000850, 2012 22371848

Kubiszewski P, Sugita L, Kourkoulis C, et al: Association of selective serotonin reuptake inhibitor use after intracerebral hemorrhage with hemorrhage recurrence and depression severity. JAMA Neurol 78(1):1–8, 2020 32865558

Kuehn BM: FDA warns antipsychotic drugs may be risky for elderly. JAMA 293(20):2462, 2005 15914734

Kugimiya T, Ishii N, Kohno K, et al: Lithium in drinking water and suicide prevention: the largest nationwide epidemiological study from Japan. Bipolar Disord 23(1):33–40, 2021 32780508

Lam RW, Lönn SL, Despiégel N: Escitalopram versus serotonin noradrenaline reuptake inhibitors as second step treatment for patients with major depressive disorder: a pooled analysis. Int Clin Psychopharmacol 25(4):199–203, 2010 20357664

Lambrichts S, Detraux J, Vansteelandt K, et al: Does lithium prevent relapse following successful electroconvulsive therapy for major depression? A systematic review and meta-analysis. Acta Psychiatr Scand 143(4):294–306, 2021 33506961

Lanctôt KL, Chau SA, Herrmann N, et al: Effect of methylphenidate on attention in apathetic AD patients in a randomized, placebo-controlled trial. Int Psychogeriatr 26(2):239–246, 2014 24169147

Landi F, Onder G, Cesari M, et al: Psychotropic medications and risk for falls among community-dwelling frail older people: an observational study. J Gerontol A Biol Sci Med Sci 60(5):622–626, 2005 15972615

Langballe EM, Engdahl B, Nordeng H, et al: Short- and long-term mortality risk associated with the use of antipsychotics among 26,940 dementia outpatients: a population-based study. Am J Geriatr Psychiatry 22(4):321–331, 2014 24016844

Lao KSJ, Wong AYS, Wong ICK, et al: Mortality risk associated with haloperidol use compared with other antipsychotics: an 11-year population-based propensity-score-matched cohort study. CNS Drugs 34(2):197–206, 2020 31916101

Lapid MI, Kuntz KM, Mason SS, et al: Efficacy, safety, and tolerability of armodafinil therapy for hypersomnia associated with dementia with Lewy bodies: a pilot Study. Dement Geriatr Cogn Disord 43(5–6):269–280, 2017 28448998

Laroche ML, Charmes JP, Nouaille Y, et al: Is inappropriate medication use a major cause of adverse drug reactions in the elderly? Br J Clin Pharmacol 63(2):177–186, 2007 17166186

Larsen KA, Kelly SE, Stern TA, et al: Administration of olanzapine to prevent postoperative delirium in elderly joint-replacement patients: a randomized, controlled trial. Psychosomatics 51(5):409–418, 2010 20833940

Lasser RA, Bossie CA, Zhu Y, et al: Efficacy and safety of long-acting risperidone in elderly patients with schizophrenia and schizoaffective disorder. Int J Geriatr Psychiatry 19(9):898–905, 2004 15352149

Lavretsky H, Siddarth P, Irwin MR: Improving depression and enhancing resilience in family dementia caregivers: a pilot randomized placebo-controlled trial of escitalopram. Am J Geriatr Psychiatry 18(2):154–162, 2010 20104071

Lavretsky H, Reinlieb M, St Cyr N, et al: Citalopram, methylphenidate, or their combination in geriatric depression: a randomized, double-blind, placebo-controlled trial. Am J Psychiatry 172(6):561–569, 2015 25677354

Lee PE, Gill SS, Freedman M, et al: Atypical antipsychotic drugs in the treatment of behavioural and psychological symptoms of dementia: systematic review. BMJ 329(7457):75, 2004 15194601

Lenze EJ, Mulsant BH, Shear MK, et al: Anxiety symptoms in elderly patients with depression: what is the best approach to treatment? Drugs Aging 19(10):753–760, 2002 12390052

Lenze EJ, Mulsant BH, Shear MK, et al: Efficacy and tolerability of citalopram in the treatment of late-life anxiety disorders: results from an 8-week randomized, placebo-controlled trial. Am J Psychiatry 162(1):146–150, 2005 15625213

Lenze EJ, Rollman BL, Shear MK, et al: Escitalopram for older adults with generalized anxiety disorder: a randomized controlled trial. JAMA 301(3):295–303, 2009 19155456

Lenze EJ, Mulsant BH, Blumberger DM, et al: Efficacy, safety, and tolerability of augmentation pharmacotherapy with aripiprazole for treatment-resistant depression in late life: a randomised, double-blind, placebo-controlled trial. Lancet 386(10011):2404–2412, 2015 26423182

Lenze EJ, Stevens A, Waring JD, et al: Augmenting computerized cognitive training with vortioxetine for age-related cognitive decline: a randomized controlled trial. Am J Psychiatry 177(6):548–555, 2020 32212856

Leopold NA: Risperidone treatment of drug-related psychosis in patients with parkinsonism. Mov Disord 15(2):301–304, 2000 10752580

Li Y, Hai S, Zhou Y, Dong BR: Cholinesterase inhibitors for rarer dementias associated with neurological conditions. Cochrane Database Syst Rev (3):CD009444, 2015 25734590

Liebowitz MR, Tourian KA: Efficacy, safety, and tolerability of desvenlafaxine 50 mg/d for the treatment of major depressive disorder: a systematic review of clinical trials. Prim Care Companion J Clin Psychiatry 12(3):PCC.09r00845, 2010 20944767

Lin CH, Chen FC, Chan HY, Hsu CC: A comparison of long-acting injectable antipsychotics with oral antipsychotics on time to rehospitalization within 1 year of discharge in elderly patients with schizophrenia. Am J Geriatr Psychiatry 28(1):23–30, 2020 31481273

Lindenmayer JP, Nasrallah H, Pucci M, et al: A systematic review of psychostimulant treatment of negative symptoms of schizophrenia: challenges and therapeutic opportunities. Schizophr Res 147(2–3):241–252, 2013 23619055

Liperoti R, Pedone C, Lapane KL, et al: Venous thromboembolism among elderly patients treated with atypical and conventional antipsychotic agents. Arch Intern Med 165(22):2677–2682, 2005 16344428

Liperoti R, Onder G, Lapane KL, et al: Conventional or atypical antipsychotics and the risk of femur fracture among elderly patients: results of a case-control study. J Clin Psychiatry 68(6):929–934, 2007 17592919

Lipscombe LL, Lévesque L, Gruneir A, et al: Antipsychotic drugs and hyperglycemia in older patients with diabetes. Arch Intern Med 169(14):1282–1289, 2009 19636029

Lipsitz O, Di Vincenzo JD, Rodrigues NB, et al: Safety, tolerability, and real-world effectiveness of intravenous ketamine in older adults with treatment-resistant depression: a case series. Am J Geriatr Psychiatry 2021 33478865 Epub ahead of print

Liu B, Anderson G, Mittmann N, et al: Use of selective serotonin-reuptake inhibitors or tricyclic antidepressants and risk of hip fractures in elderly people. Lancet 351(9112):1303–1307, 1998 9643791

Liu J, Cooper CA, Weintraub D, Dahodwala N: Pharmacological treatment of apathy in Lewy body disorders: a systematic review. Parkinsonism Relat Disord 60:14–24, 2019 30470658

Liu L, Fuller M, Behymer TP, et al: Selective serotonin reuptake inhibitors and intracerebral hemorrhage risk and outcome. Stroke 51(4):1135–1141, 2020 32126942

Liu X, Zhang J, Sun D, et al: Effects of fluoxetine on brain-derived neurotrophic factor serum concentration and cognition in patients with vascular dementia. Clin Interv Aging 9:411–418, 2014 24648723

Lockhart IA, Orme ME, Mitchell SA: The efficacy of licensed-indication use of donepezil and memantine monotherapies for treating behavioural and psychological symptoms of dementia in patients with Alzheimer's disease: systematic review and meta-analysis. Dement Geriatr Cogn Disord Extra 1(1):212–227, 2011 22163246

Looper KJ: Potential medical and surgical complications of serotonergic antidepressant medications. Psychosomatics 48(1):1–9, 2007 17209143

Löppönen P, Tetri S, Juvela S, et al: Association between warfarin combined with serotonin-modulating antidepressants and increased case fatality in primary intracerebral hemorrhage: a population-based study. J Neurosurg 120(6):1358–1363, 2014 24506245

Lu CJ, Tune LE: Chronic exposure to anticholinergic medications adversely affects the course of Alzheimer disease. Am J Geriatr Psychiatry 11(4):458–461, 2003 12837675

Luo Y, Yu Y, Zhang M, et al: Chronic administration of ketamine induces cognitive deterioration by restraining synaptic signaling. Mol Psychiatry 2020 32488127 Epub ahead of print

Lyketsos CG, DelCampo L, Steinberg M, et al: Treating depression in Alzheimer disease: efficacy and safety of sertraline therapy, and the benefits of depression reduction: the DIADS. Arch Gen Psychiatry 60(7):737–746, 2003 12860778

Madhusoodanan S, Zaveri D: Paliperidone use in the elderly. Curr Drug Saf 5(2):149–152, 2010 20406162

Madhusoodanan S, Suresh P, Brenner R, Pillai R: Experience with the atypical antipsychotics: risperidone and olanzapine in the elderly. Ann Clin Psychiatry 11(3):113–118, 1999 10482120

Madhusoodanan S, Brenner R, Alcantra A: Clinical experience with quetiapine in elderly patients with psychotic disorders. J Geriatr Psychiatry Neurol 13(1):28–32, 2000 10753004

Mahableshwarkar AR, Jacobsen PL, Chen Y, Simon JS: A randomised, double-blind, placebo-controlled, duloxetine-referenced study of the efficacy and tolerability of vortioxetine in the acute treatment of adults with generalised anxiety disorder. Int J Clin Pract 68(1):49–59, 2014 24341301

Mahableshwarkar AR, Zajecka J, Jacobson W, et al: A randomized, placebo-controlled, active-reference, double-blind, flexible-dose study of the efficacy of vortioxetine on cognitive function in major depressive disorder. Neuropsychopharmacology 40(8):2025–2037, 2015 25687662

Maher AR, Maglione M, Bagley S, et al: Efficacy and comparative effectiveness of atypical antipsychotic medications for off-label uses in adults: a systematic review and meta-analysis. JAMA 306(12):1359–1369, 2011 21954480

Mahmood I, Sahajwalla C: Clinical pharmacokinetics and pharmacodynamics of buspirone, an anxiolytic drug. Clin Pharmacokinet 36(4):277–287, 1999 10320950

Maier F, Spottke A, Bach JP, et al: Bupropion for the treatment of apathy in Alzheimer disease: a randomized clinical trial. JAMA Netw Open 3(5):e206027, 2020 32463470

Maljuric NM, Noordam R, Aarts N, et al: Use of selective serotonin re-uptake inhibitors and the heart rate corrected QT interval in a real-life setting: the population-based Rotterdam Study. Br J Clin Pharmacol 80(4):698–705, 2015 25966843

Mamo D, Sweet RA, Mulsant BH, et al: Effect of nortriptyline and paroxetine on extrapyramidal signs and symptoms: a prospective double-blind study in depressed elderly patients. Am J Geriatr Psychiatry 8(3):226–231, 2000 10910421

Mamo D, Graff A, Mizrahi R, et al: Differential effects of aripiprazole on D(2), 5-HT(2), and 5-HT(1A) receptor occupancy in patients with schizophrenia: a triple tracer PET study. Am J Psychiatry 164(9):1411–1417, 2007 17728427

Mannheimer B, Haslemo T, Lindh JD, et al: Risperidone and venlafaxine metabolic ratios strongly predict a CYP2D6 poor metabolizing genotype. Ther Drug Monit 38(1):127–134, 2016 26418700

Manning KJ, Alexopoulos GS, Banerjee S, et al: Executive functioning complaints and escitalopram treatment response in late-life depression. Am J Geriatr Psychiatry 23(5):440–445, 2015 24388222

Marcantoni WS, Akoumba BS, Wassef M, et al: A systematic review and meta-analysis of the efficacy of intravenous ketamine infusion for treatment resistant depression: January 2009–January 2019. J Affect Disord 277:831–841, 2020 33065824

Mariappan P, Ballantyne Z, N'Dow JM, Alhasso AA: Serotonin and noradrenaline reuptake inhibitors (SNRI) for stress urinary incontinence in adults. Cochrane Database Syst Rev (3):CD004742, 2005 16034945

Marra A, Vargas M, Buonanno P, et al: Haloperidol for preventing delirium in ICU patients: a systematic review and meta-analysis. Eur Rev Med Pharmacol Sci 25(3):1582–1591, 2021 33629327

Martin H, Slyk MP, Deymann S, Cornacchione MJ: Safety profile assessment of risperidone and olanzapine in long-term care patients with dementia. J Am Med Dir Assoc 4(4):183–188, 2003 12837138

Matsunaga S, Kishi T, Iwata N: Memantine for Lewy body disorders: systematic review and meta-analysis. Am J Geriatr Psychiatry 23(4):373–383, 2015 24406251

Matsunaga S, Fujishiro H, Takechi H: Efficacy and safety of cholinesterase inhibitors for mild cognitive impairment: a systematic review and meta-analysis. J Alzheimers Dis 71(2):513–523, 2019 31424411

Mauri MC, Paletta S, Di Pace C, et al: Clinical pharmacokinetics of atypical antipsychotics: an update. Clin Pharmacokinet 57(12):1493–1528, 2018 29915922

Maust DT, Kim HM, Seyfried LS, et al: Antipsychotics, other psychotropics, and the risk of death in patients with dementia: number needed to harm. JAMA Psychiatry 72(5):438–445, 2015 25786075

Mayeux R: Clinical practice: early Alzheimer's disease. N Engl J Med 362(23):2194–2201, 2010 20558370

Mazeh D, Shahal B, Aviv A, et al: A randomized, single-blind, comparison of venlafaxine with paroxetine in elderly patients suffering from resistant depression. Int Clin Psychopharmacol 22(6):371–375, 2007 17917556

McCarrell JL, Bailey TA, Duncan NA, et al: A review of citalopram dose restrictions in the treatment of neuropsychiatric disorders in older adults. Ment Health Clin 9(4):280–286, 2019 31293848

McCleery J, Sharpley AL: Pharmacotherapies for sleep disturbances in dementia. Cochrane Database Syst Rev (11):CD009178, 2020 33189083

McCue RE, Joseph M: Venlafaxine- and trazodone-induced serotonin syndrome. Am J Psychiatry 158(12):2088–2089, 2001 11729039

McIntyre RS, Lophaven S, Olsen CK: A randomized, double-blind, placebo-controlled study of vortioxetine on cognitive function in depressed adults. Int J Neuropsychopharmacol 17(10):1557–1567, 2014 24787143

McIntyre RS, Rosenblat JD, Nemeroff CB, et al: Synthesizing the evidence for ketamine and esketamine in treatment-resistant depression: an international expert opinion on the available evidence and implementation. Am J Psychiatry 178(5):383–399, 2021 33726522

McShane R, Westby MJ, Roberts E, et al: Memantine for dementia. Cochrane Database Syst Rev 3(3):CD003154, 2019 30891742

Meagher DJ, McLoughlin L, Leonard M, et al: What do we really know about the treatment of delirium with antipsychotics? Ten key issues for delirium pharmacotherapy. Am J Geriatr Psychiatry 21(12):1223–1238, 2013 23567421

Meltzer HY, Roth BL: Lorcaserin and pimavanserin: emerging selectivity of serotonin receptor subtype-targeted drugs. J Clin Invest 123(12):4986–4991, 2013 24292660

Meng YH, Wang PP, Song YX, Wang JH: Cholinesterase inhibitors and memantine for Parkinson's disease dementia and Lewy body dementia: a meta-analysis. Exp Ther Med 17(3):1611–1624, 2019 30783428

Messenheimer JA: Rash in adult and pediatric patients treated with lamotrigine. Can J Neurol Sci 25(4):S14–S18, 1998 9827240

Methaneethorn J, Sringam S: Factors influencing lithium pharmacokinetics in patients with acute mania: a population pharmacokinetic analysis. Hum Psychopharmacol 34(3):e2697, 2019 31025773

Meyers BS, Flint AJ, Rothschild AJ, et al: A double-blind randomized controlled trial of olanzapine plus sertraline vs olanzapine plus placebo for psychotic depression: the study of pharmacotherapy of psychotic depression (STOP-PD). Arch Gen Psychiatry 66(8):838–847, 2009 19652123

Micca JL, Hoffmann VP, Lipkovich I, et al: Retrospective analysis of diabetes risk in elderly patients with dementia in olanzapine clinical trials. Am J Geriatr Psychiatry 14(1):62–70, 2006 16407583

Mintzer JE, Tune LE, Breder CD, et al: Aripiprazole for the treatment of psychoses in institutionalized patients with Alzheimer dementia: a multicenter, randomized, double-blind, placebo-controlled assessment of three fixed doses. Am J Geriatr Psychiatry 15(11):918–931, 2007 17974864

Mintzer J, Lanctôt KL, Scherer RW, et al: Effect of methylphenidate on apathy in patients with Alzheimer disease: the ADMET 2 randomized clinical trial. JAMA Neurol e213356, 2021 34570180 Epub ahead of print

Mittal D, Jimerson NA, Neely EP, et al: Risperidone in the treatment of delirium: results from a prospective open-label trial. J Clin Psychiatry 65(5):662–667, 2004 15163252

Modi A, Weiner M, Craig BA, et al: Concomitant use of anticholinergics with acetylcholinesterase inhibitors in Medicaid recipients with dementia and residing in nursing homes. J Am Geriatr Soc 57(7):1238–1244, 2009 19467148

Mokhber N, Abdollahian E, Soltanifar A, et al: Comparison of sertraline, venlafaxine and desipramine effects on depression, cognition and the daily living activities in Alzheimer patients. Pharmacopsychiatry 47(4–5):131–140, 2014 24955552

Moline M, Zammit G, Cheng J, et al: Comparison of the effect of lemborexant with placebo and zolpidem tartrate extended release on sleep architecture in older adults with insomnia disorder. J Clin Sleep Med 17(6):11667–1174, 2021 33590823

Montejo AL, Llorca G, Izquierdo JA, Rico-Villademoros F: Incidence of sexual dysfunction associated with antidepressant agents: a prospective multicenter study of 1022 outpatients. J Clin Psychiatry 62(suppl 3):10–21, 2001 11229449

Montgomery S, Chatamra K, Pauer L, et al: Efficacy and safety of pregabalin in elderly people with generalised anxiety disorder. Br J Psychiatry 193(5):389–394, 2008 18978320

Montgomery SA, Fava M, Padmanabhan SK, et al: Discontinuation symptoms and taper/post-study-emergent adverse events with desvenlafaxine treatment for major depressive disorder. Int Clin Psychopharmacol 24(6):296–305, 2009 19779354

Montgomery SA, Gommoll CP, Chen C, Greenberg WM: Efficacy of levomilnacipran extended-release in major depressive disorder: pooled analysis of 5 double-blind, placebo-controlled trials. CNS Spectr 20(2):148–156, 2015 24902007

Moreno GM, Gandhi R, Lessig SL, et al: Mortality in patients with Parkinson disease psychosis receiving pimavanserin and quetiapine. Neurology 91(17):797–799, 2018 30258020

Mortensen JK, Larsson H, Johnsen SP, Andersen G: Post stroke use of selective serotonin reuptake inhibitors and clinical outcome among patients with ischemic stroke: a nationwide propensity score-matched follow-up study. Stroke 44(2):420–426, 2013 23306326

Mukai Y, Tampi RR: Treatment of depression in the elderly: a review of the recent literature on the efficacy of single- versus dual-action antidepressants. Clin Ther 31(5):945–961, 2009 19539096

Müller-Oerlinghausen B, Lewitzka U: Lithium reduces pathological aggression and suicidality: a mini-review. Neuropsychobiology 62(1):43–49, 2010 20453534

Mulsant BH: Challenges of the treatment of neuropsychiatric symptoms associated with dementia. Am J Geriatr Psychiatry 22(4):317–320, 2014 24635993

Mulsant BH, Alexopoulos GS, Reynolds CF III, et al: Pharmacological treatment of depression in older primary care patients: the PROSPECT algorithm. Int J Geriatr Psychiatry 16(6):585–592, 2001a 11424167

Mulsant BH, Pollock BG, Nebes R, et al: A twelve-week, double-blind, randomized comparison of nortriptyline and paroxetine in older depressed inpatients and outpatients. Am J Geriatr Psychiatry 9(4):406–414, 2001b 11739067

Mulsant BH, Pollock BG, Kirshner M, et al: Serum anticholinergic activity in a community-based sample of older adults: relationship with cognitive performance. Arch Gen Psychiatry 60(2):198–203, 2003 12578438

Mulsant BH, Gharabawi GM, Bossie CA, et al: Correlates of anticholinergic activity in patients with dementia and psychosis treated with risperidone or olanzapine. J Clin Psychiatry 65(12):1708–1714, 2004 15641877

Mulsant BH, Blumberger DM, Ismail Z, et al: A systematic approach to pharmacotherapy for geriatric major depression. Clin Geriatr Med 30(3):517–534, 2014 25037293

Murray V, von Arbin M, Bartfai A, et al: Double-blind comparison of sertraline and placebo in stroke patients with minor depression and less severe major depression. J Clin Psychiatry 66(6):708–716, 2005 15960563

Myles N, Myles H, Xia S, et al: Meta-analysis examining the epidemiology of clozapine-associated neutropenia. Acta Psychiatr Scand 138(2):101–109, 2018 29786829

Nagaraja D, Jayashree S: Randomized study of the dopamine receptor agonist piribedil in the treatment of mild cognitive impairment. Am J Psychiatry 158(9):1517–1519, 2001 11532743

Nandagopal JJ, DelBello MP: Selegiline transdermal system: a novel treatment option for major depressive disorder. Expert Opin Pharmacother 10(10):1665–1673, 2009 19527191

National Collaborating Centre for Mental Health: Management of Depression in Primary and Secondary Care (Clinical Guideline 23). London, National Institute for Clinical Excellence, 2004

Nebes RD, Pollock BG, Meltzer CC, et al: Serum anticholinergic activity, white matter hyperintensities, and cognitive performance. Neurology 65(9):1487–1489, 2005 16275844

Nelson JC, Delucchi K, Schneider L: Suicidal thinking and behavior during treatment with sertraline in late-life depression. Am J Geriatr Psychiatry 15(7):573–580, 2007 17586782

Nelson JC, Delucchi K, Schneider LS: Efficacy of second generation antidepressants in late-life depression: a meta-analysis of the evidence. Am J Geriatr Psychiatry 16(7):558–567, 2008 18591576

Newhouse PA, Krishnan KR, Doraiswamy PM, et al: A double-blind comparison of sertraline and fluoxetine in depressed elderly outpatients. J Clin Psychiatry 61(8):559–568, 2000 10982198

Nicholas LM, Ford AL, Esposito SM, et al: The effects of mirtazapine on plasma lipid profiles in healthy subjects. J Clin Psychiatry 64(8):883–889, 2003 12927002

Nieuwstraten CE, Dolovich LR: Bupropion versus selective serotonin-reuptake inhibitors for treatment of depression. Ann Pharmacother 35(12):1608–1613, 2001 11793630

Nikaido AM, Ellinwood EH Jr, Heatherly DG, Gupta SK: Age-related increase in CNS sensitivity to benzodiazepines as assessed by task difficulty. Psychopharmacology (Berl) 100(1):90–97, 1990 1967500

Nikooie R, Neufeld KJ, Oh ES, et al: Antipsychotics for treating delirium in hospitalized adults: a systematic review. Ann Intern Med 171(7):485–495, 2019 31476770

Noaghiul S, Narayan M, Nelson JC: Divalproex treatment of mania in elderly patients. Am J Geriatr Psychiatry 6(3):257–262, 1998 9659958

Novais T, Doutone A, Gombault C, et al: description of the treatment course by pregabalin for anxiety in patients with a major neurocognitive disorder. J Clin Psychopharmacol 39(3):261–263, 2019 30939590

Nyth AL, Gottfries CG: The clinical efficacy of citalopram in treatment of emotional disturbances in dementia disorders: a Nordic multicentre study. Br J Psychiatry 157:894–901, 1990 1705151

Nyth AL, Gottfries CG, Lyby K, et al: A controlled multicenter clinical study of citalopram and placebo in elderly depressed patients with and without concomitant dementia. Acta Psychiatr Scand 86(2):138–145, 1992 1529737

Ochs-Ross R, Daly EJ, Zhang Y, et al: Efficacy and safety of esketamine nasal spray plus an oral antidepressant in elderly patients with treatment-resistant depression: TRANSFORM-3. Am J Geriatr Psychiatry 28(2):121–141, 2020 31734084

O'Connor DW, Sierakowski C, Chin LF, Singh D: The safety and tolerability of clozapine in aged patients: a retrospective clinical file review. World J Biol Psychiatry 11(6):788–791, 2010 20586532

Oh ES, Needham DM, Nikooie R, et al: Antipsychotics for preventing delirium in hospitalized adults: a systematic review. Ann Intern Med 171(7):474–484, 2019 31476766

Oh ES, Leoutsakos JM, Rosenberg PB, et al: Effects of ramelteon on the prevention of postoperative delirium in older patients undergoing orthopedic surgery: the RECOVER randomized controlled trial. Am J Geriatr Psychiatry 29(1):90–100, 2021 32532654

Olafsson K, Jørgensen S, Jensen HV, et al: Fluvoxamine in the treatment of demented elderly patients: a double-blind, placebo-controlled study. Acta Psychiatr Scand 85(6):453–456, 1992 1642129

Oslin DW, Streim JE, Katz IR, et al: Heuristic comparison of sertraline with nortriptyline for the treatment of depression in frail elderly patients. Am J Geriatr Psychiatry 8(2):141–149, 2000 10804075

Oslin DW, Ten Have TR, Streim JE, et al: Probing the safety of medications in the frail elderly: evidence from a randomized clinical trial of sertraline and venlafaxine in depressed nursing home residents. J Clin Psychiatry 64(8):875–882, 2003 12927001

Ostuzzi G, Gastaldon C, Barbato A, et al: Tolerability and efficacy of vortioxetine versus SSRIs in elderly with major depression. Study protocol of the VESPA study: a pragmatic, multi-centre, open-label, parallel-group, superiority, randomized trial. Trials 21(1):695, 2020 32746941

Pact V, Giduz T: Mirtazapine treats resting tremor, essential tremor, and levodopa-induced dyskinesias. Neurology 53(5):1154, 1999 10496290

Padala PR, Padala KP, Lensing SY, et al: Methylphenidate for apathy in community-dwelling older veterans with mild Alzheimer's disease: a double-blind, randomized, placebo-controlled trial. Am J Psychiatry 175(2):159–168, 2018 28945120

Pae CU, Lee SJ, Lee CU, et al: A pilot trial of quetiapine for the treatment of patients with delirium. Hum Psychopharmacol 19(2):125–127, 2004 14994323

Palmer E: Medicare wants insurers to monitor suspicious prescribing of Nuedexta, neurological drug for outbursts of laughing. Fierce Pharma, June 4, 2018. Available at: https://www.fiercepharma.com/pharma/medicare-wants-insurers-to-monitor-suspicious-prescribing-laughing-drug-nuedexta. Accessed March 31, 2021

Parellada E, Baeza I, de Pablo J, Martínez G: Risperidone in the treatment of patients with delirium. J Clin Psychiatry 65(3):348–353, 2004 15096074

Park-Wyllie LY, Mamdani MM, Li P, et al: Cholinesterase inhibitors and hospitalization for bradycardia: a population-based study. PLoS Med 6(9):e1000157, 2009 19787032

Parkinson Study Group: Low-dose clozapine for the treatment of drug-induced psychosis in Parkinson's disease. N Engl J Med 340(10):757–763, 1999 10072410

Parsons C: Withdrawal of antidementia drugs in older people: who, when and how? Drugs Aging 33(8):545–556, 2016 27393698

Pasina L, Colzani L, Cortesi L, et al: Relation between delirium and anticholinergic drug burden in a cohort of hospitalized older patients: an observational study. Drugs Aging 36(1):85–91, 2019 30484239

Patel RS, Mansuri Z, Motiwala F, et al: A systematic review on treatment of tardive dyskinesia with valbenazine and deutetrabenazine. Ther Adv Psychopharmacol 9:2045125319847882, 2019 31205680

Paulzen M, Haen E, Gründer G, et al: Pharmacokinetic considerations in the treatment of hypertension in risperidone-medicated patients: thinking of clinically relevant CYP2D6 interactions. J Psychopharmacol 30(8):803–809, 2016 27251417

Pedersen L, Klysner R: Antagonism of selective serotonin reuptake inhibitor-induced nausea by mirtazapine. Int Clin Psychopharmacol 12(1):59–60, 1997 9179636

Percudani M, Barbui C, Fortino I, et al: Second-generation antipsychotics and risk of cerebrovascular accidents in the elderly. J Clin Psychopharmacol 25(5):468–470, 2005 16160623

Perry NK: Venlafaxine-induced serotonin syndrome with relapse following amitriptyline. Postgrad Med J 76(894):254–256, 2000 10727586

Perucca E: Drug interactions with carbamazepine: an ever expanding list? Epilepsy Res 147:119–120, 2018 30220619

Petracca GM, Chemerinski E, Starkstein SE: A double-blind, placebo-controlled study of fluoxetine in depressed patients with Alzheimer's disease. Int Psychogeriatr 13(2):233–240, 2001 11495397

Pilotto A, Franceschi M, D'Onofrio G, et al: Effect of a CYP2D6 polymorphism on the efficacy of donepezil in patients with Alzheimer disease. Neurology 73(10):761–767, 2009 19738170

Poewe W: Treatment of dementia with Lewy bodies and Parkinson's disease dementia. Mov Disord 20(suppl 12):S77–S82, 2005 16092095

Polepally AR, Brundage RC, Remmel RP, et al: Lamotrigine pharmacokinetics following oral and stable-labeled intravenous administration in young and elderly adult epilepsy patients: effect of age. Epilepsia 59(9):1718–1726, 2018 30101556

Pollock BG: Primum non nocere: prescription of potentially inappropriate psychotropic medications to older adults. Am J Geriatr Psychiatry 27(2):186–187, 2019 30396765

Pollock BG, Mulsant BH, Sweet R, et al: An open pilot study of citalopram for behavioral disturbances of dementia: plasma levels and real-time observations. Am J Geriatr Psychiatry 5(1):70–78, 1997 9169247

Pollock BG, Laghrissi-Thode F, Wagner WR: Evaluation of platelet activation in depressed patients with ischemic heart disease after paroxetine or nortriptyline treatment. J Clin Psychopharmacol 20(2):137–140, 2000 10770450

Pollock BG, Mulsant BH, Rosen J, et al: Comparison of citalopram, perphenazine, and placebo for the acute treatment of psychosis and behavioral disturbances in hospitalized, demented patients. Am J Psychiatry 159(3):460–465, 2002 11870012

Pollock BG, Mulsant BH, Rosen J, et al: A double-blind comparison of citalopram and risperidone for the treatment of behavioral and psychotic symptoms associated with dementia. Am J Geriatr Psychiatry 15(11):942–952, 2007 17846102

Pollock B, Forsyth C, Bies R: The critical role of clinical pharmacology in geriatric psychopharmacology. Clin Pharmacol Ther 85(1):89–93, 2009 19037202

Porsteinsson AP, Drye LT, Pollock BG, et al: Effect of citalopram on agitation in Alzheimer disease: the CitAD randomized clinical trial. JAMA 311(7):682–691, 2014 24549548

Post RM, Frye MA, Denicoff KD, et al: Beyond lithium in the treatment of bipolar illness. Neuropsychopharmacology 19(3):206–219, 1998 9653709

Poulsen MB, Damgaard B, Zerahn B, et al: Modafinil may alleviate poststroke fatigue: a randomized, placebo-controlled, double-blinded trial. Stroke 46(12):3470–3477, 2015 26534969

Prakanrattana U, Prapaitrakool S: Efficacy of risperidone for prevention of postoperative delirium in cardiac surgery. Anaesth Intensive Care 35(5):714–719, 2007 17933157

Pridan S, Swartz M, Baruch Y, et al: Effectiveness and safety of clozapine in elderly patients with chronic resistant schizophrenia. Int Psychogeriatr 27(1):131–134, 2015 25166892

Rado J, Janicak PG: Pharmacological and clinical profile of recently approved second-generation antipsychotics: implications for treatment of schizophrenia in older patients. Drugs Aging 29(10):783–791, 2012 23018584

Rais AR, Williams K, Rais T, et al: Use of intramuscular ziprasidone for the control of acute psychosis or agitation in an inpatient geriatric population: an open-label study. Psychiatry (Edgmont) 7(1):17–24, 2010 20386633

Raji MA, Brady SR: Mirtazapine for treatment of depression and comorbidities in Alzheimer disease. Ann Pharmacother 35(9):1024–1027, 2001 11573849

Rajji TK, Mulsant BH, Lotrich FE, et al: Use of antidepressants in late-life depression. Drugs Aging 25(10):841–853, 2008 18808208

Rajji TK, Uchida H, Ismail Z, et al: Clozapine and global cognition in schizophrenia. J Clin Psychopharmacol 30(4):431–436, 2010 20631560

Rajji TK, Mulsant BH, Nakajima S, et al: Cognition and dopamine D2 receptor availability in the striatum in older patients with schizophrenia. Am J Geriatr Psychiatry 25(1):1–10, 2017 27745822

Rampello L, Chiechio S, Nicoletti G, et al: Prediction of the response to citalopram and reboxetine in post-stroke depressed patients. Psychopharmacology (Berl) 173(1–2):73–78, 2004 14685645

Raskin J, Wiltse CG, Siegal A, et al: Efficacy of duloxetine on cognition, depression, and pain in elderly patients with major depressive disorder: an 8-week, double-blind, placebo-controlled trial. Am J Psychiatry 164(6):900–909, 2007 17541049

Rasmussen A, Lunde M, Poulsen DL, et al: A double-blind, placebo-controlled study of sertraline in the prevention of depression in stroke patients. Psychosomatics 44(3):216–221, 2003 12724503

Rauma PH, Honkanen RJ, Williams LJ, et al: Effects of antidepressants on postmenopausal bone loss: a 5-year longitudinal study from the OSTPRE cohort. Bone 89:25–31, 2016 27179631

Rawson KS, Dixon D, Civitelli R, et al: Bone turnover with venlafaxine treatment in older adults with depression. J Am Geriatr Soc 65(9):2057–2063, 2017 28555718

Ray WA, Thapa PB, Gideon P: Benzodiazepines and the risk of falls in nursing home residents. J Am Geriatr Soc 48(6):682–685, 2000 10855607

Ray WA, Chung CP, Murray KT, et al: Atypical antipsychotic drugs and the risk of sudden cardiac death. N Engl J Med 360(3):225–235, 2009 19144938

Razazian N, Baziyar M, Moradian N, et al: Evaluation of the efficacy and safety of pregabalin, venlafaxine, and carbamazepine in patients with painful diabetic peripheral neuropathy: a randomized, double-blind trial. Neurosciences (Riyadh) 19(3):192–198, 2014 24983280

Rector TS, Adabag S, Cunningham F, et al: Outcomes of citalopram dosage risk mitigation in a veteran population. Am J Psychiatry 173(9):896–902, 2016 27166093

Reeve E, Farrell B, Thompson W, et al: Deprescribing cholinesterase inhibitors and memantine in dementia: guideline summary. Med J Aust 210(4):174–179, 2019 30771226

Reifler BV, Teri L, Raskind M, et al: Double-blind trial of imipramine in Alzheimer's disease patients with and without depression. Am J Psychiatry 146(1):45–49, 1989 2643356

Reisberg B, Doody R, Stöffler A, et al: Memantine in moderate-to-severe Alzheimer's disease. N Engl J Med 348(14):1333–1341, 2003 12672860

Rej S, Beaulieu S, Segal M, et al: Lithium dosing and serum concentrations across the age spectrum: from early adulthood to the tenth decade of life. Drugs Aging 31(12):911–916, 2014a 25331906

Rej S, Shulman K, Herrmann N, et al: Prevalence and correlates of renal disease in older lithium users: a population-based study. Am J Geriatr Psychiatry 22(11):1075–1082, 2014b 24566239

Rej S, Herrmann N, Gruneir A, et al: Association of lithium use and a higher serum concentration of lithium with the risk of declining renal function in older adults: a population-based cohort study. J Clin Psychiatry 81(5):19m13045, 2020

Rektorová I, Rektor I, Bares M, et al: Pramipexole and pergolide in the treatment of depression in Parkinson's disease: a national multicentre prospective randomized study. Eur J Neurol 10(4):399–406, 2003 12823492

Renn BN, Asghar-Ali AA, Thielke S, et al: A systematic review of practice guidelines and recommendations for discontinuation of cholinesterase inhibitors in dementia. Am J Geriatr Psychiatry 26(2):134–147, 2018 29167065

Reuben DB, Herr KA, Pacala JT, et al: Geriatrics At Your Fingertips, 21st Edition. New York, The American Geriatrics Society, 2019

Reynolds CF III, Dew MA, Pollock BG, et al: Maintenance treatment of major depression in old age. N Engl J Med 354(11):1130–1138, 2006

Reynolds CF III, Butters MA, Lopez O, et al: Maintenance treatment of depression in old age: a randomized, double-blind, placebo-controlled evaluation of the efficacy and safety of donepezil combined with antidepressant pharmacotherapy. Arch Gen Psychiatry 68(1):51–60, 2011 21199965

Richards JB, Papaioannou A, Adachi JD, et al: Effect of selective serotonin reuptake inhibitors on the risk of fracture. Arch Intern Med 167(2):188–194, 2007 17242321

Richardson K, Loke YK, Fox C, et al: Adverse effects of Z-drugs for sleep disturbance in people living with dementia: a population-based cohort study. BMC Med 18(1):351, 2020 33228664

Richardson K, Savva GM, Boyd PJ, et al: Non-benzodiazepine hypnotic use for sleep disturbance in people aged over 55 years living with dementia: a series of cohort studies. Health Technol Assess 25(1):1–202, 2021

Ridout F, Meadows R, Johnsen S, Hindmarch I: A placebo controlled investigation into the effects of paroxetine and mirtazapine on measures related to car driving performance. Hum Psychopharmacol 18(4):261–269, 2003 12766930

Ritchie CW, Chiu E, Harrigan S, et al: The impact upon extra-pyramidal side effects, clinical symptoms and quality of life of a switch from conventional to atypical antipsychotics (risperidone or olanzapine) in elderly patients with schizophrenia. Int J Geriatr Psychiatry 18(5):432–440, 2003 12766921

Ritchie CW, Chiu E, Harrigan S, et al: A comparison of the efficacy and safety of olanzapine and risperidone in the treatment of elderly patients with schizophrenia: an open study of six months duration. Int J Geriatr Psychiatry 21(2):171–179, 2006 16416458

Rivière J, van der Mast RC, Vandenberghe J, Van Den Eede F: Efficacy and tolerability of atypical antipsychotics in the treatment of delirium: a systematic review of the literature. Psychosomatics 60(1):18–26, 2019 30181002

Robinson DS, Amsterdam JD: The selegiline transdermal system in major depressive disorder: a systematic review of safety and tolerability. J Affect Disord 105(1–3):15–23, 2008 17568687

Robinson RG, Schultz SK, Castillo C, et al: Nortriptyline versus fluoxetine in the treatment of depression and in short-term recovery after stroke: a placebo-controlled, double-blind study. Am J Psychiatry 157(3):351–359, 2000 10698809

Robinson RG, Jorge RE, Moser DJ, et al: Escitalopram and problem-solving therapy for prevention of poststroke depression: a randomized controlled trial. JAMA 299(20):2391–2400, 2008 18505948

Rocca P, Calvarese P, Faggiano F, et al: Citalopram versus sertraline in late-life nonmajor clinically significant depression: a 1-year follow-up clinical trial. J Clin Psychiatry 66(3):360–369, 2005 15766303

Rocha FL, de Vasconcelos Cunha UG, Paschoalin RC, et al: Use of subcutaneous ketamine to rapidly improve severe treatment-resistant depression in a patient with Alzheimer's disease. Int Clin Psychopharmacol 36(2):104–105, 2021 33230024

Rochon PA, Stukel TA, Sykora K, et al: Atypical antipsychotics and parkinsonism. Arch Intern Med 165(16):1882–1888, 2005 16157833

Rodda J, Morgan S, Walker Z: Are cholinesterase inhibitors effective in the management of the behavioral and psychological symptoms of dementia in Alzheimer's disease? A systematic review of randomized, placebo-controlled trials of donepezil, rivastigmine and galantamine. Int Psychogeriatr 21(5):813–824, 2009 19538824

Rolinski M, Fox C, Maidment I, McShane R: Cholinsesterase inhibitors for dementia with Lewy bodies, Parkinson's disease dementia and cognitive impairment in Parkinson's disease. Cochrane Database Syst Rev 3(3):CD006504, 2012 22419314

Romeo B, Blecha L, Locatelli K, et al: Meta-analysis and review of dopamine agonists in acute episodes of mood disorder: efficacy and safety. J Psychopharmacol 32(4):385–396, 2018 29543103

Roose SP, Rutherford BR: Selective serotonin reuptake inhibitors and operative bleeding risk: a review of the literature. J Clin Psychopharmacol 36(6):704–709, 2016 27684291

Roose SP, Dalack GW, Glassman AH, et al: Cardiovascular effects of bupropion in depressed patients with heart disease. Am J Psychiatry 148(4):512–516, 1991 1900980

Roose SP, Nelson JC, Salzman C, et al: Open-label study of mirtazapine orally disintegrating tablets in depressed patients in the nursing home. Curr Med Res Opin 19(8):737–746, 2003 14687445

Roose SP, Miyazaki M, Devanand D, et al: An open trial of venlafaxine for the treatment of late-life atypical depression. Int J Geriatr Psychiatry 19(10):989–994, 2004 15449363

Rosen J, Sweet R, Pollock BG, Mulsant BH: Nortriptyline in the hospitalized elderly: tolerance and side effect reduction. Psychopharmacol Bull 29(2):327–331, 1993 8290682

Rosenberg PB, Drye LT, Martin BK, et al: Sertraline for the treatment of depression in Alzheimer disease. Am J Geriatr Psychiatry 18(2):136–145, 2010 20087081

Rosenberg PB, Lanctôt KL, Drye LT, et al: Safety and efficacy of methylphenidate for apathy in Alzheimer's disease: a randomized, placebo-controlled trial. J Clin Psychiatry 74(8):810–816, 2013 24021498

Ross J: Discontinuation of lithium augmentation in geriatric patients with unipolar depression: a systematic review. Can J Psychiatry 53(2):117–120, 2008 18357930

Roy MA, Doiron M, Talon-Croteau J, et al: Effects of antiparkinson medication on cognition in Parkinson's disease: a systematic review. Can J Neurol Sci 45(4):375–404, 2018 29747716

Rush AJ, Trivedi MH, Wisniewski SR, et al: Acute and longer-term outcomes in depressed outpatients requiring one or several treatment steps: a STAR*D report. Am J Psychiatry 163(11):1905–1917, 2006a 17074942

Rush AJ, Trivedi MH, Wisniewski SR, et al: Bupropion-SR, sertraline, or venlafaxine-XR after failure of SSRIs for depression. N Engl J Med 354(12):1231–1242, 2006b 16554525

Rush AJ, Wisniewski SR, Warden D, et al: Selecting among second-step antidepressant medication monotherapies: predictive value of clinical, demographic, or first-step treatment features. Arch Gen Psychiatry 65(8):870–880, 2008 18678792

Ruthirakuhan MT, Herrmann N, Abraham EH, et al: Pharmacological interventions for apathy in Alzheimer's disease. Cochrane Database Syst Rev 5(5):CD012197, 2018 29727467

Sackeim HA, Haskett RF, Mulsant BH, et al: Continuation pharmacotherapy in the prevention of relapse following electroconvulsive therapy: a randomized controlled trial. JAMA 285(10):1299–1307, 2001 11255384

Saiz-Ruiz J, Ibañez A, Díaz-Marsá M, et al: Nefazodone in the treatment of elderly patients with depressive disorders: a prospective, observational study. CNS Drugs 16(9):635–643, 2002 12153334

Sajatovic M, Jaskiw G, Konicki PE, et al: Outcome of clozapine therapy for elderly patients with refractory primary psychosis. Int J Geriatr Psychiatry 12(5):553–558, 1997 9193964

Sajatovic M, Gyulai L, Calabrese JR, et al: Maintenance treatment outcomes in older patients with bipolar I disorder. Am J Geriatr Psychiatry 13(4):305–311, 2005a 15845756

Sajatovic M, Madhusoodanan S, Coconcea N: Managing bipolar disorder in the elderly: defining the role of the newer agents. Drugs Aging 22(1):39–54, 2005b 15663348

Sajatovic M, Blow FC, Ignacio RV: Psychiatric comorbidity in older adults with bipolar disorder. Int J Geriatr Psychiatry 21(6):582–587, 2006 16783798

Sajatovic M, Ramsay E, Nanry K, Thompson T: Lamotrigine therapy in elderly patients with epilepsy, bipolar disorder or dementia. Int J Geriatr Psychiatry 22(10):945–950, 2007 17326238

Sajatovic M, Coconcea N, Ignacio RV, et al: Aripiprazole therapy in 20 older adults with bipolar disorder: a 12-week, open-label trial. J Clin Psychiatry 69(1):41–46, 2008 18312036

Sajatovic M, Gildengers A, Al Jurdi RK, et al: Multisite, open-label, prospective trial of lamotrigine for geriatric bipolar depression: a preliminary report. Bipolar Disord 13(3):294–302, 2011 21676132

Sajatovic M, Forester BP, Gildengers A, Mulsant BH: Aging changes and medical complexity in late-life bipolar disorder: emerging research findings that may help advance care. Neuropsychiatry (London) 3(6):621–633, 2013 24999372

Sajatovic M, Dines P, Fuentes-Casiano E, et al: Asenapine in the treatment of older adults with bipolar disorder. Int J Geriatr Psychiatry 30(7):710–719, 2015 25335125

Sajatovic M, Forester BP, Tsai J, et al: Efficacy of lurasidone in adults aged 55 years and older with bipolar depression: post hoc analysis of 2 double-blind, placebo-controlled studies. J Clin Psychiatry 77(10):e1324–e1331, 2016 27529375

Sakurai H, Suzuki T, Bies RR, et al: Increasing versus maintaining the dose of olanzapine or risperidone in schizophrenia patients who did not respond to a modest dosage: a double-blind randomized controlled trial. J Clin Psychiatry 77(10):1381–1390, 2016 27788310

Salzman C, Jeste DV, Meyer RE, et al: Elderly patients with dementia-related symptoms of severe agitation and aggression: consensus statement on treatment options, clinical trials methodology, and policy. J Clin Psychiatry 69(6):889–898, 2008 18494535

Santa Cruz MR, Hidalgo PC, Lee MS, et al: Buspirone for the treatment of dementia with behavioral disturbance. Int Psychogeriatr 29(5):859–862, 2017 28124634

Sasaki Y, Matsuyama T, Inoue S, et al: A prospective, open-label, flexible-dose study of quetiapine in the treatment of delirium. J Clin Psychiatry 64(11):1316–1321, 2003 14658945

Sassi KLM, Rocha NP, Colpo GD, et al: Amphetamine use in the elderly: a systematic review of the literature. Curr Neuropharmacol 18(2):126–135, 2020 31660835

Sateia MJ, Buysse DJ, Krystal AD, et al: Clinical practice guideline for the pharmacologic treatment of chronic insomnia in adults: an American Academy of Sleep Medicine Clinical Practice Guideline. J Clin Sleep Med 13(2):307–349, 2017 27998379

Satel SL, Nelson JC: Stimulants in the treatment of depression: a critical overview. J Clin Psychiatry 50(7):241–249, 1989 2567730

Sato Y, Kondo I, Ishida S, et al: Decreased bone mass and increased bone turnover with valproate therapy in adults with epilepsy. Neurology 57(3):445–449, 2001 11502911

Savadi Oskouie D, Sharifipour E, Sadeghi Bazargani H, et al: Efficacy of citalopram on acute ischemic stroke outcome: a randomized clinical trial. Neurorehabil Neural Repair 31(7):638–647, 2017 28454498

Savaskan E, Müller SE, Böhringer A, et al: Antidepressive therapy with escitalopram improves mood, cognitive symptoms, and identity memory for angry faces in elderly depressed patients. Int J Neuropsychopharmacol 11(3):381–388, 2008 17697395

Scarpini E, Bruno G, Zappalà G, et al: Cessation versus continuation of galantamine treatment after 12 months of therapy in patients with Alzheimer's disease: a randomized, double blind, placebo controlled withdrawal trial. J Alzheimers Dis 26(2):211–220, 2011 21606568

Schäfer W, Princk C, Kollhorst B, Schink T: Antidepressants and the risk of hemorrhagic stroke in the elderly: a nested case-control study. Drug Saf 42(9):1081–1089, 2019 31165430

Scheitz JF, Turc G, Kujala L, et al: Intracerebral hemorrhage and outcome after thrombolysis in stroke patients using selective serotonin-reuptake inhibitors. Stroke 48(12):3239–3244, 2017 29127269

Schellen C, Ferrari J, Lang W, Sykora M: Effects of SSRI exposure on hemorrhagic complications and outcome following thrombolysis in ischemic stroke. Int J Stroke 13(5):511–517, 2018 29134925

Scherer RW, Drye L, Mintzer J, et al: The Apathy in Dementia Methylphenidate Trial 2 (ADMET 2): study protocol for a randomized controlled trial. Trials 19(1):46, 2018 29347996

Schiff GD, Galanter WL, Duhig J, et al: Principles of conservative prescribing. Arch Intern Med 171(16):1433–1440, 2011 21670331

Schneider LS, Dagerman KS, Insel P: Risk of death with atypical antipsychotic drug treatment for dementia: meta-analysis of randomized placebo-controlled trials. JAMA 294(15):1934–1943, 2005 16234500

Schneider LS, Dagerman K, Insel PS: Efficacy and adverse effects of atypical antipsychotics for dementia: meta-analysis of randomized, placebo-controlled trials. Am J Geriatr Psychiatry 14(3):191–210, 2006a 16505124

Schneider LS, Tariot PN, Dagerman KS, et al: Effectiveness of atypical antipsychotic drugs in patients with Alzheimer's disease. N Engl J Med 355(15):1525–1538, 2006b 17035647

Schoot TS, Molmans THJ, Grootens KP, Kerckhoffs APM: Systematic review and practical guideline for the prevention and management of the renal side effects of lithium therapy. Eur Neuropsychopharmacol 31:16–32, 2020 31837914

Schueler YB, Koesters M, Wieseler B, et al: A systematic review of duloxetine and venlafaxine in major depression, including unpublished data. Acta Psychiatr Scand 123(4):247–265, 2011

Schwaninger M, Ringleb P, Winter R, et al: Elevated plasma concentrations of homocysteine in antiepileptic drug treatment. Epilepsia 40(3):345–350, 1999 10080517

Scott J, Greenwald BS, Kramer E, Shuwall M: Atypical (second generation) antipsychotic treatment response in very late-onset schizophrenia-like psychosis. Int Psychogeriatr 23(5):742–748, 2011 21118614

Semel D, Murphy TK, Zlateva G, et al: Evaluation of the safety and efficacy of pregabalin in older patients with neuropathic pain: results from a pooled analysis of 11 clinical studies. BMC Fam Pract 11:85, 2010 21054853

Semenchuk MR, Sherman S, Davis B: Double-blind, randomized trial of bupropion SR for the treatment of neuropathic pain. Neurology 57(9):1583–1588, 2001 11706096

Serebruany VL, Glassman AH, Malinin AI, et al: Platelet/endothelial biomarkers in depressed patients treated with the selective serotonin reuptake inhibitor sertraline after acute coronary events: the Sertraline AntiDepressant Heart Attack Randomized Trial (SADHART) Platelet Substudy. Circulation 108(8):939–944, 2003 12912814

Seritan AL: Prevent drug-drug interactions with cholinesterase inhibitors: avoid adverse events when prescribing medications for patients with dementia. Curr Psychiatr 7:57–67, 2008

Sharma V, Simpson SH, Samanani S, et al: Concurrent use of opioids and benzodiazepines/Z-drugs in Alberta, Canada and the risk of hospitalisation and death: a case cross-over study. BMJ Open 10(11):e038692, 2020 33444187

Shea ML, Garfield LD, Teitelbaum S, et al: Serotonin-norepinephrine reuptake inhibitor therapy in late-life depression is associated with increased marker of bone resorption. Osteoporos Int 24(5):1741–1749, 2013 23358607

Shear MK, Reynolds CF III, Simon NM, et al: Optimizing treatment of complicated grief: a randomized clinical trial. JAMA Psychiatry 73(7):685–694, 2016 27276373

Sheffrin M, Driscoll HC, Lenze EJ, et al: Pilot study of augmentation with aripiprazole for incomplete response in late-life depression: getting to remission. J Clin Psychiatry 70(2):208–213, 2009 19210951

Sheikh JI, Lauderdale SA, Cassidy EL: Efficacy of sertraline for panic disorder in older adults: a preliminary open-label trial. Am J Geriatr Psychiatry 12(2):230, 2004 15010352

Sheline YI, West T, Yarasheski K, et al: An antidepressant decreases CSF Aβ production in healthy individuals and in transgenic AD mice. Sci Transl Med 6(236):236re4, 2014 24828079

Shelton C, Entsuah R, Padmanabhan SK, Vinall PE: Venlafaxine XR demonstrates higher rates of sustained remission compared to fluoxetine, paroxetine or placebo. Int Clin Psychopharmacol 20(4):233–238, 2005 15933485

Shelton RC, Tollefson GD, Tohen M, et al: A novel augmentation strategy for treating resistant major depression. Am J Psychiatry 158(1):131–134, 2001 11136647

Shin D, Oh YH, Eom CS, Park SM: Use of selective serotonin reuptake inhibitors and risk of stroke: a systematic review and meta-analysis. J Neurol 261(4):686–695, 2014 24477492

Shulman KI: Lithium for older adults with bipolar disorder: should it still be considered a first-line agent? Drugs Aging 27(8):607–615, 2010 20658789

Shulman KI, Walker SE: A reevaluation of dietary restrictions for irreversible monoamine oxidase inhibitors. Psychiatr Ann 31:378–384, 2001

Shulman KI, Fischer HD, Herrmann N, et al: Current prescription patterns and safety profile of irreversible monoamine oxidase inhibitors: a population-based cohort study of older adults. J Clin Psychiatry 70(12):1681–1686, 2009 19852903

Simoni-Wastila L, Wei YJ, Lucas JA, et al: Mortality risk of antipsychotic dose and duration in nursing home residents with chronic or acute indications. J Am Geriatr Soc 64(5):973–980, 2016 27166586

Sink KM, Holden KF, Yaffe K: Pharmacological treatment of neuropsychiatric symptoms of dementia: a review of the evidence. JAMA 293(5):596–608, 2005 15687315

Skrobik YK, Bergeron N, Dumont M, Gottfried SB: Olanzapine vs haloperidol: treating delirium in a critical care setting. Intensive Care Med 30(3):444–449, 2004 14685663

Slimano F, Netzer F, Borget I, et al: Olanzapine as antiemetic drug in oncology: a retrospective study in non-responders to standard antiemetic therapy. Int J Clin Pharm 40(5):1265–1271, 2018 29744791

Smales ET, Edwards BA, Deyoung PN, et al: Trazodone effects on obstructive sleep apnea and non-REM arousal threshold. Ann Am Thorac Soc 12(5):758–764, 2015 25719754

Smith E, Rothschild AJ, Heo M, et al: Weight gain during olanzapine treatment for psychotic depression: effects of dose and age. Int Clin Psychopharmacol 23(3):130–137, 2008 18408527

Sneed JR, Culang ME, Keilp JG, et al: Antidepressant medication and executive dysfunction: a deleterious interaction in late-life depression. Am J Geriatr Psychiatry 18(2):128–135, 2010 20104069

Sneed JR, Reinlieb ME, Rutherford BR, et al: Antidepressant treatment of melancholia in older adults. Am J Geriatr Psychiatry 22(1):46–52, 2014 24119858

Snyder GL, Vanover KE, Davis RE, et al: A review of the pharmacology and clinical profile of lumateperone for the treatment of schizophrenia. Adv Pharmacol 90:253–276, 2021 33706936

Soares CN, Thase ME, Clayton A, et al: Desvenlafaxine and escitalopram for the treatment of postmenopausal women with major depressive disorder. Menopause 17(4):700–711, 2010 20539246

Sommer BR, Fenn HH, Ketter TA: Safety and efficacy of anticonvulsants in elderly patients with psychiatric disorders: oxcarbazepine, topiramate and gabapentin. Expert Opin Drug Saf 6(2):133–145, 2007 17367259

Soogrim V, Ruberto VL, Murrough J, Jha MK: Spotlight on pimavanserin tartrate and its therapeutic potential in the treatment of major depressive disorder: the evidence to date. Drug Des Devel Ther 15:151–157, 2021 33469267

Spina E, Trifirò G, Caraci F: Clinically significant drug interactions with newer antidepressants. CNS Drugs 26(1):39–67, 2012 22171584

Sproule BA, Hardy BG, Shulman KI: Differential pharmacokinetics of lithium in elderly patients. Drugs Aging 16(3):165–177, 2000 10803857

Srinivasan S, Tampi RR, Balaram K, Kapoor A: Pimavanserin for the treatment of psychosis in Alzheimer's disease: a literature review. World J Psychiatry 10(7):162–174, 2020 32844093

Starkstein SE, Brockman S: Management of depression in parkinson's disease: a systematic review. Mov Disord Clin Pract (Hoboken) 4(4):470–477, 2017 30363415

Steffens DC, Doraiswamy PM, McQuoid DR: Bupropion SR in the naturalistic treatment of elderly patients with major depression. Int J Geriatr Psychiatry 16(9):862–865, 2001 11571765

Steffens DC, Nelson JC, Eudicone JM, et al: Efficacy and safety of adjunctive aripiprazole in major depressive disorder in older patients: a pooled subpopulation analysis. Int J Geriatr Psychiatry 26(6):564–572, 2011 20827794

Steinberg JR: Anxiety in elderly patients: a comparison of azapirones and benzodiazepines. Drugs Aging 5(5):335–345, 1994 7833587

Strand M, Hetta J, Rosen A, et al: A double-blind, controlled trial in primary care patients with generalized anxiety: a comparison between buspirone and oxazepam. J Clin Psychiatry 51(suppl):40–45, 1990 2211567

Street JS, Clark WS, Gannon KS, et al: Olanzapine treatment of psychotic and behavioral symptoms in patients with Alzheimer disease in nursing care facilities: a double-blind, randomized, placebo-controlled trial. Arch Gen Psychiatry 57(10):968–976, 2000 11015815

Streim JE, Porsteinsson AP, Breder CD, et al: A randomized, double-blind, placebo-controlled study of aripiprazole for the treatment of psychosis in nursing home patients with Alzheimer disease. Am J Geriatr Psychiatry 16(7):537–550, 2008 18591574

Subramanian S, Lenze EJ: Ketamine for depression in older adults. Am J Geriatr Psychiatry 29(9):914–916, 2021 33509675

Suh GH, Son HG, Ju YS, et al: A randomized, double-blind, crossover comparison of risperidone and haloperidol in Korean dementia patients with behavioral disturbances. Am J Geriatr Psychiatry 12(5):509–516, 2004 15353389

Sullivan DR, Mongoue-Tchokote S, Mori M, et al: Randomized, double-blind, placebo-controlled study of methylphenidate for the treatment of depression in SSRI-treated cancer patients receiving palliative care. Psychooncology 26(11):1763–1769, 2017 27429350

Sultzer DL, Gray KF, Gunay I, et al: A double-blind comparison of trazodone and haloperidol for treatment of agitation in patients with dementia. Am J Geriatr Psychiatry 5(1):60–69, 1997 9169246

Sun M, Herrmann N, Shulman KI: Lithium toxicity in older adults: a systematic review of case reports. Clin Drug Investig 38(3):201–209, 2018 29189921

Supasitthumrong T, Bolea-Alamanac BM, Asmer S, et al: Gabapentin and pregabalin to treat aggressivity in dementia: a systematic review and illustrative case report. Br J Clin Pharmacol 85(4):690–703, 2019 30575088

Suppes T, Eudicone J, McQuade R, et al: Efficacy and safety of aripiprazole in subpopulations with acute manic or mixed episodes of bipolar I disorder. J Affect Disord 107(1–3):145–154, 2008 17904226

Suzuki T, Remington G, Uchida H, et al: Management of schizophrenia in late life with antipsychotic medications: a qualitative review. Drugs Aging 28(12):961–980, 2011 22117095

Sys J, Van Cleynenbreugel S, Deschodt M, et al: Efficacy and safety of non-benzodiazepine and non-Z-drug hypnotic medication for insomnia in older people: a systematic literature review. Eur J Clin Pharmacol 76(3):363–381, 2020 31838549

Szmulewicz AG, Angriman F, Samamé C, et al: Dopaminergic agents in the treatment of bipolar depression: a systematic review and meta-analysis. Acta Psychiatr Scand 135(6):527–538, 2017 28256707

Tadger S, Paleacu D, Barak Y: Quetiapine augmentation of antidepressant treatment in elderly patients suffering from depressive symptoms: a retrospective chart review. Arch Gerontol Geriatr 53(1):104–105, 2011 20678815

Tadrous M, Shakeri A, Chu C, et al: Assessment of stimulant use and cardiovascular event risks among older adults. JAMA Netw Open 4(10):e2130795, 2021 34694389

Tahami Monfared AA, Desai M, Hughes R, et al: Treatment options for dementia with Lewy bodies: a network meta-analysis of randomised control trials. Neurol Ther 9(2):521–534, 2020 32495063

Tahir TA, Eeles E, Karapareddy V, et al: A randomized controlled trial of quetiapine versus placebo in the treatment of delirium. J Psychosom Res 69(5):485–490, 2010 20955868

Takahashi M, Tabu H, Ozaki A, et al: Antidepressants for depression, apathy, and gait instability in Parkinson's disease: a multicenter randomized study. Intern Med 58(3):361–368, 2019 30146591

Taragano FE, Lyketsos CG, Mangone CA, et al: A double-blind, randomized, fixed-dose trial of fluoxetine vs. amitriptyline in the treatment of major depression complicating Alzheimer's disease. Psychosomatics 38(3):246–252, 1997 9136253

Tariot PN, Erb R, Podgorski CA, et al: Efficacy and tolerability of carbamazepine for agitation and aggression in dementia. Am J Psychiatry 155(1):54–61, 1998 9433339

Tariot PN, Salzman C, Yeung PP, et al: Long-Term use of quetiapine in elderly patients with psychotic disorders. Clin Ther 22(9):1068–1084, 2000 11048905

Tariot PN, Farlow MR, Grossberg GT, et al: Memantine treatment in patients with moderate to severe Alzheimer disease already receiving donepezil: a randomized controlled trial. JAMA 291(3):317–324, 2004 14734594

Tariot PN, Raman R, Jakimovich L, et al: Divalproex sodium in nursing home residents with possible or probable Alzheimer disease complicated by agitation: a randomized, controlled trial. Am J Geriatr Psychiatry 13(11):942–949, 2005 16286437

Tariot PN, Schneider LS, Cummings J, et al: Chronic divalproex sodium to attenuate agitation and clinical progression of Alzheimer disease. Arch Gen Psychiatry 68(8):853–861, 2011 21810649

Tashkin D, Kanner R, Bailey W, et al: Smoking cessation in patients with chronic obstructive pulmonary disease: a double-blind, placebo-controlled, randomised trial. Lancet 357(9268):1571–1575, 2001 11377644

Tedeschini E, Levkovitz Y, Iovieno N, et al: Efficacy of antidepressants for late-life depression: a meta-analysis and meta-regression of placebo-controlled randomized trials. J Clin Psychiatry 72(12):1660–1668, 2011 22244025

Teri L, Logsdon RG, Peskind E, et al: Treatment of agitation in AD: a randomized, placebo-controlled clinical trial. Neurology 55(9):1271–1278, 2000 11087767

Thacker EL, Schneeweiss S: Initiation of acetylcholinesterase inhibitors and complications of chronic airways disorders in elderly patients. Drug Saf 29(11):1077–1085, 2006 17061913

Thaler KJ, Morgan LC, Van Noord M, et al: Comparative effectiveness of second-generation antidepressants for accompanying anxiety, insomnia, and pain in depressed patients: a systematic review. Depress Anxiety 29(6):495–505, 2012 22553134

Thancharoen O, Limwattananon C, Waleekhachonloet O, et al: Ginkgo biloba extract (EGb761), cholinesterase inhibitors, and memantine for the treatment of mild-to-moderate Alzheimer's disease: a network meta-analysis. Drugs Aging 36(5):435–452, 2019 30937879

Thase ME: What role do atypical antipsychotic drugs have in treatment-resistant depression? J Clin Psychiatry 63(2):95–103, 2002 11874227

Thase ME, Entsuah R, Cantillon M, Kornstein SG: Relative antidepressant efficacy of venlafaxine and SSRIs: sex-age interactions. J Womens Health (Larchmt) 14(7):609–616, 2005a 16181017

Thase ME, Haight BR, Richard N, et al: Remission rates following antidepressant therapy with bupropion or selective serotonin reuptake inhibitors: a meta-analysis of original data from 7 randomized controlled trials. J Clin Psychiatry 66(8):974–981, 2005b 16086611

Thase ME, Tran PV, Wiltse C, et al: Cardiovascular profile of duloxetine, a dual reuptake inhibitor of serotonin and norepinephrine. J Clin Psychopharmacol 25(2):132–140, 2005c 15738744

Thompson DS: Mirtazapine for the treatment of depression and nausea in breast and gynecological oncology. Psychosomatics 41(4):356–359, 2000 10906359

Touma KTB, Scarff JR: Valbenazine and deutetrabenazine for tardive dyskinesia. Innov Clin Neurosci 15(5–6):13–16, 2018 30013814

Treves N, Perlman A, Kolenberg Geron L, et al: Z-drugs and risk for falls and fractures in older adults-a systematic review and meta-analysis. Age Ageing 47(2):201–208, 2018 29077902

Tricco AC, Ashoor HM, Soobiah C, et al: Comparative effectiveness and safety of cognitive enhancers for treating Alzheimer's disease: systematic review and network metaanalysis. J Am Geriatr Soc 66(1):170–178, 2018 29131306

Trivedi MH, Fava M, Wisniewski SR, et al: Medication augmentation after the failure of SSRIs for depression. N Engl J Med 354(12):1243–1252, 2006 16554526

Tsai CS, Wu CL, Chou SY, et al: Prevention of poststroke depression with milnacipran in patients with acute ischemic stroke: a double-blind randomized placebo-controlled trial. Int Clin Psychopharmacol 26(5):263–267, 2011 21811172

Tsoutsoulas C, Mulsant BH, Kumar S, et al: Anticholinergic burden and cognition in older patients with schizophrenia. J Clin Psychiatry 78(9):e1284–e1290, 2017 29188908

Tsuboi T, Suzuki T, Uchida H: A tipping point in drug dosing in late-life schizophrenia. Curr Psychiatry Rep 13(3):225–233, 2011 21327902

Tundo A, de Filippis R, De Crescenzo F: Pramipexole in the treatment of unipolar and bipolar depression: a systematic review and meta-analysis. Acta Psychiatr Scand 140(2):116–125, 2019 31111467

Tveito M, Smith RL, Molden E, et al: Age impacts olanzapine exposure differently during use of oral versus long-acting injectable formulations: an observational study including 8,288 patients. J Clin Psychopharmacol 38(6):570–576, 2018 30300295

Tzimos A, Samokhvalov V, Kramer M, et al: Safety and tolerability of oral paliperidone extended-release tablets in elderly patients with schizophrenia: a double-blind, placebo-controlled study with six-month open-label extension. Am J Geriatr Psychiatry 16(1):31–43, 2008 18165460

Uchida H, Mamo DC, Mulsant BH, et al: Increased antipsychotic sensitivity in elderly patients: evidence and mechanisms. J Clin Psychiatry 70(3):397–405, 2009 19192476

U.S. Food and Drug Administration: FDA Drug Safety Communication: Abnormal heart rhythms associated with high doses of Celexa (citalopram hydrobromide). Silver Spring, MD, U.S. Food and Drug Administration, August 2011. Available at: https://www.fda.gov/drugs/drug-safety-and-availability/fda-drug-safety-communication-abnormal-heart-rhythms-associated-high-doses-celexa-citalopram. Accessed March 3, 2021.

U.S. Food and Drug Administration: FDA Drug Safety Communication: Revised recommendations for Celexa (citalopram hydrobromide) related to a potential risk of abnormal heart rhythms with high doses. Silver Spring, MD, U.S. Food and Drug Administration, March 2012. Available at: http://www.fda.gov/Drugs/DrugSafety/ucm297391.htm. Accessed April 11, 2021.

U.S. Food and Drug Administration: FDA Drug Safety Communication: FDA warns about serious risks and death when combining opioid pain or cough medicines with benzodiazepines; requires its strongest warning. Silver Spring, MD, U.S. Food and Drug Administration, August 2016. Available at: https://www.fda.gov/drugs/drug-safety-and-availability/fda-drug-safety-communication-fda-warns-about-serious-risks-and-death-when-combining-opioid-pain-or. Accessed October 21, 2021.

U.S. Food and Drug Administration: U.S. FDA Drug Safety Communication: FDA strengthens warning that untreated constipation caused by schizophrenia medicine clozapine (Clozaril) can lead to serious bowel problems. Silver Spring, MD, U.S. Food and Drug Administration, January 2020. Available at: https://www.fda.gov/drugs/drug-safety-and-availability/fda-strengthens-warning-untreated-constipation-caused-schizophrenia-medicine-clozapine-clozaril-can. Accessed April 12, 2021

U.S. Food and Drug Administration: Lamictal (lamotrigine): Drug Safety Communication—Studies show increased risk of heart rhythm problems in patients with heart disease. Silver Spring, MD, U.S. Food and Drug Administration, March 2021. Available at: https://www.fda.gov/safety/medical-product-safety-information/lamictal-lamotrigine-drug-safety-communication-studies-show-increased-risk-heart-rhythm-problems. Accessed April 3, 2021.

Valladales-Restrepo LF, Duran-Lengua M, Machado-Alba JE: Potentially inappropriate prescriptions of anticholinergics drugs in Alzheimer's disease patients. Geriatr Gerontol Int 19(9):913–917, 2019 31342625

van Dyck CH, Arnsten AFT, Padala PR, et al: Neurobiologic rationale for treatment of apathy in Alzheimer's disease with methylphenidate. Am J Geriatr Psychiatry 29(1):51–62, 2021 32461027

Van Gestel H, Franke K, Petite J, et al: Brain age in bipolar disorders: effects of lithium treatment. Aust N Z J Psychiatry 53(12):1179–1188, 2019 31244332

van Iersel MB, Zuidema SU, Koopmans RT, et al: Antipsychotics for behavioural and psychological problems in elderly people with dementia: a systematic review of adverse events. Drugs Aging 22(10):845–858, 2005 16245958

Varanese S, Perfetti B, Gilbert-Wolf R, et al: Modafinil and armodafinil improve attention and global mental status in Lewy bodies disorders: preliminary evidence. Int J Geriatr Psychiatry 28(10):1095–1097, 2013 24038163

Vasudev A, Chaudhari S, Sethi R, et al: A review of the pharmacological and clinical profile of newer atypical antipsychotics as treatments for bipolar disorder: considerations for use in older patients. Drugs Aging 35(10):887–895, 2018 30187288

Verhey FR, Verkaaik M, Lousberg R, et al: Olanzapine versus haloperidol in the treatment of agitation in elderly patients with dementia: results of a randomized controlled double-blind trial. Dement Geriatr Cogn Disord 21(1):1–8, 2006 16244481

Vermeeren A, Vets E, Vuurman EF, et al: On-the-road driving performance the morning after bedtime use of suvorexant 15 and 30 mg in healthy elderly. Psychopharmacology (Berl) 233(18):3341–3351, 2016 27424295

Vermeeren A, Jongen S, Murphy P, et al: On-the-road driving performance the morning after bedtime administration of lemborexant in healthy adult and elderly volunteers. Sleep (Basel) 42(4):zsy260, 2019 30597112

Victoria LW, Whyte EM, Butters MA, et al: Improvement in depression is associated with improvement in cognition in late-life psychotic depression. Am J Geriatr Psychiatry 25(6):672–679, 2017 28285771

Vila-Castelar C, Ly JJ, Kaplan L, et al: Attention measures of accuracy, variability, and fatigue detect early response to donepezil in Alzheimer's disease: a randomized, double-blind, placebo-controlled pilot trial. Arch Clin Neuropsychol 34(3):277–289, 2019 29635383

Viscogliosi G, Chiriac IM, Ettorre E: Efficacy and safety of citalopram compared to atypical antipsychotics on agitation in nursing home residents with Alzheimer dementia. J Am Med Dir Assoc 18(9):799–802, 2017 28739492

Visser MM, Maréchal B, Goodin P, et al: Predicting modafinil-treatment response in poststroke fatigue using brain morphometry and functional connectivity. Stroke 50(3):602–609, 2019 30777001

Voineskos AN, Mulsant BH, Dickie EW, et al: Effects of antipsychotic medication on brain structure in patients with major depressive disorder and psychotic features: neuroimaging findings in the context of a randomized placebo-controlled clinical trial. JAMA Psychiatry 77(7):674–683, 2020 32101271

von Wolff A, Hölzel LP, Westphal A, et al: Selective serotonin reuptake inhibitors and tricyclic antidepressants in the acute treatment of chronic depression and dysthymia: a systematic review and meta-analysis. J Affect Disord 144(1–2):7–15, 2013 22963896

Vozoris NT, Fischer HD, Wang X, et al: Benzodiazepine drug use and adverse respiratory outcomes among older adults with COPD. Eur Respir J 44(2):332–340, 2014 24743966

Wahler RG Jr, Reiman AT, Schrader JV: Use of compounded dextromethorphan-quinidine suspension for pseudobulbar affect in hospice patients. J Palliat Med 20(3):294–297, 2017 27997281

Wallace AE, Kofoed LL, West AN: Double-blind, placebo-controlled trial of methylphenidate in older, depressed, medically ill patients. Am J Psychiatry 152(6):929–931, 1995 7755127

Wang D, Osser DN: The Psychopharmacology Algorithm Project at the Harvard South Shore Program: an update on bipolar depression. Bipolar Disord 22(5):472–489, 2020 31650675

Wang HR, Woo YS, Bahk WM: Atypical antipsychotics in the treatment of delirium. Psychiatry Clin Neurosci 67(5):323–331, 2013 23859663

Wang PS, Bohn RL, Glynn RJ, et al: Zolpidem use and hip fractures in older people. J Am Geriatr Soc 49(12):1685–1690, 2001 11844004

Wang PS, Schneeweiss S, Avorn J, et al: Risk of death in elderly users of conventional vs. atypical antipsychotic medications. N Engl J Med 353(22):2335–2341, 2005 16319382

Wang YP, Chen YT, Tsai CF, et al: Short-term use of serotonin reuptake inhibitors and risk of upper gastrointestinal bleeding. Am J Psychiatry 171(1):54–61, 2014 24030313

Weich S, Pearce HL, Croft P, et al: Effect of anxiolytic and hypnotic drug prescriptions on mortality hazards: retrospective cohort study. BMJ 348:g1996, 2014 24647164

Weintraub D, Rosenberg PB, Drye LT, et al: Sertraline for the treatment of depression in Alzheimer disease: week-24 outcomes. Am J Geriatr Psychiatry 18(4):332–340, 2010 20220589

Wenzel-Seifert K, Wittmann M, Haen E: QTc prolongation by psychotropic drugs and the risk of torsade de pointes. Dtsch Arztebl Int 108(41):687–693, 2011 22114630

Whyte EM, Basinski J, Farhi P, et al: Geriatric depression treatment in nonresponders to selective serotonin reuptake inhibitors. J Clin Psychiatry 65(12):1634–1641, 2004 15641868

Whyte EM, Romkes M, Mulsant BH, et al: CYP2D6 genotype and venlafaxine-XR concentrations in depressed elderly. Int J Geriatr Psychiatry 21(6):542–549, 2006 16642541

Widschwendter CG, Hofer A: Antipsychotic-induced tardive dyskinesia: update on epidemiology and management. Curr Opin Psychiatry 32(3):179–184, 2019 30720484

Wilcock GK, Ballard CG, Cooper JA, Loft H: Memantine for agitation/aggression and psychosis in moderately severe to severe Alzheimer's disease: a pooled analysis of 3 studies. J Clin Psychiatry 69(3):341–348, 2008 18294023

Wilner KD, Tensfeldt TG, Baris B, et al: Single- and multiple-dose pharmacokinetics of ziprasidone in healthy young and elderly volunteers. Br J Clin Pharmacol 49(suppl 1):15S–20S, 2000 10771449

Wilson K, Mottram P: A comparison of side effects of selective serotonin reuptake inhibitors and tricyclic antidepressants in older depressed patients: a meta-analysis. Int J Geriatr Psychiatry 19(8):754–762, 2004 15290699

Winblad B, Kilander L, Eriksson S, et al: Donepezil in patients with severe Alzheimer's disease: double-blind, parallel-group, placebo-controlled study. Lancet 367(9516):1057–1065, 2006 16581404

Wingen M, Bothmer J, Langer S, Ramaekers JG: Actual driving performance and psychomotor function in healthy subjects after acute and subchronic treatment with escitalopram, mirtazapine, and placebo: a crossover trial. J Clin Psychiatry 66(4):436–443, 2005 15816785

Wohlreich MM, Sullivan MD, Mallinckrodt CH, et al: Duloxetine for the treatment of recurrent major depressive disorder in elderly patients: treatment outcomes in patients with comorbid arthritis. Psychosomatics 50(4):402–412, 2009 19687181

Wrishko RE, McCrea JB, Yee KL, et al: Effect of CYP3A inhibition and induction on the pharmacokinetics of suvorexant: two Phase I, open-label, fixed-sequence trials in healthy subjects. Clin Drug Investig 39(5):441–451, 2019 30810914

Wu CS, Chen TY, Tsai SY, et al: Estimating the risk of pneumonia in patients with schizophrenia newly receiving clozapine: a nationwide cohort study. J Clin Psychopharmacol 39(4):297–304, 2019 31188233

Wu M, Minkowicz S, Dumrongprechachan V, et al: Ketamine rapidly enhances glutamate-evoked dendritic spinogenesis in medial prefrontal cortex through dopaminergic mechanisms. Biol Psychiatry 89(11):1096–1105, 2021 33637303

Wu YC, Tseng PT, Tu YK, et al: Association of delirium response and safety of pharmacological interventions for the management and prevention of delirium: a network meta-analysis. JAMA Psychiatry 76(5):526–535, 2019 30810723

Wylie ME, Miller MD, Shear MK, et al: Fluvoxamine pharmacotherapy of anxiety disorders in later life: preliminary open-trial data. J Geriatr Psychiatry Neurol 13(1):43–48, 2000 10753007

Xu H, Garcia-Ptacek S, Jönsson L, et al: Long-term effects of cholinesterase inhibitors on cognitive decline and mortality. Neurology 96(17):e2220–e2230, 2021 33741639 Epub ahead of print

Xu KY, Hartz SM, Borodovsky JT, et al: Association between benzodiazepine use with or without opioid use and all-cause mortality in the United States, 1999–2015. JAMA Netw Open 3(12):e2028557, 2020 33295972

Yang CH, Tsai SJ, Hwang JP: The efficacy and safety of quetiapine for treatment of geriatric psychosis. J Psychopharmacol 19(6):661–666, 2005 16272189

Yaowaluk T, Senanarong V, Limwongse C, et al: Influence of CYP2D6, CYP3A5, ABCB1, APOE polymorphisms and nongenetic factors on donepezil treatment in patients with Alzheimer's disease and vascular dementia. Pharm Genomics Pers Med 12:209–224, 2019 31564952

Young RC, Gyulai L, Mulsant BH, et al: Pharmacotherapy of bipolar disorder in old age: review and recommendations. Am J Geriatr Psychiatry 12(4):342–357, 2004 15249272

Young RC, Mulsant BH, Sajatovic M, et al: GERI-BD: a randomized double-blind controlled trial of lithium and divalproex in the treatment of mania in older patients with bipolar disorder. Am J Psychiatry 174(11):1086–1093, 2017 29088928

Yuan M, Sperry L, Malhado-Chang N, et al: Atypical antipsychotic therapy in Parkinson's disease psychosis: a retrospective study. Brain Behav 7(6):e00639, 2017 28638698

Yuan Y, Tsoi K, Hunt RH: Selective serotonin reuptake inhibitors and risk of upper GI bleeding: confusion or confounding? Am J Med 119(9):719–727, 2006 16945603

Yunusa I, Alsumali A, Garba AE, et al: Assessment of reported comparative effectiveness and safety of atypical antipsychotics in the treatment of behavioral and psychological symptoms of dementia: a network meta-analysis. JAMA Netw Open 2(3):e190828, 2019 30901041

Zammit G, Krystal A: Evaluating lemborexant for the treatment of insomnia. Expert Opin Pharmacother 22(10)L1235–1243, 2021 33711243

Zhang H, Lu Y, Liu M, et al: Strategies for prevention of postoperative delirium: a systematic review and meta-analysis of randomized trials. Crit Care 17(2):R47, 2013 23506796

Zheng L, Mack WJ, Dagerman KS, et al: Metabolic changes associated with second-generation antipsychotic use in Alzheimer's disease patients: the CATIE-AD study. Am J Psychiatry 166(5):583–590, 2009 19369318

Zhong KX, Tariot PN, Mintzer J, et al: Quetiapine to treat agitation in dementia: a randomized, double-blind, placebo-controlled study. Curr Alzheimer Res 4(1):81–93, 2007 17316169

Zoons E, Booij J, Delnooz CCS, et al: Randomised controlled trial of escitalopram for cervical dystonia with dystonic jerks/tremor. J Neurol Neurosurg Psychiatry 89(6):579–585, 2018 29326295

Zuidersma M, Chua KC, Hellier J, et al: Sertraline and mirtazapine versus placebo in subgroups of depression in dementia: findings from the HTA-SADD randomized controlled trial. Am J Geriatr Psychiatry 27(9):920–931, 2019 31084994

CHAPTER 21

Electroconvulsive Therapy and Other Forms of Brain Stimulation

Richard D. Weiner, M.D., Ph.D.

Mustafa M. Husain, M.B.B.S.

Jonathan R. Young, M.D.

Elisa Kallioniemi, Ph.D.

Brain stimulation techniques, in particular electroconvulsive therapy (ECT) and transcranial magnetic stimulation (TMS), have become a rapidly evolving area in geropsychiatric practice. This chapter begins with a discussion of ECT, which involves the electrical induction of a series of seizures as a treatment for mental disorders, most notably major depressive disorder (MDD). Coverage of this topic includes the history of ECT, its indications and risks, the evaluation of patients, ECT technique (including a recently proposed experimental modification called focal electrically administered seizure therapy [FEAST]), and the management of patients following completion of an acute (i.e., index) ECT course, including the use of ECT to prevent relapse (maintenance ECT). Later sections cover other types of brain stimulation techniques, including magnetic seizure therapy (MST), TMS, transcranial direct current stimulation (tDCS), vagus nerve stimulation (VNS), and deep brain stimulation (DBS), particularly in the treatment of elderly patients. Finally, the chapter ends with a brief discussion of what can be expected in the future of brain stimulation therapies.

History

In 1935, Hungarian neuropsychiatrist Ladislas Meduna chemically induced seizures in a small series of patients with schizophrenia (Shorter and Healy 2007). His rationale for doing so was based on the hypothesis (later shown to be incorrect) that individuals with epilepsy had a reduced incidence of schizophrenia. Having achieved some partial success in therapeutic outcome, Meduna's new pharmacoconvulsive therapy was greeted with great acclaim as a way of managing what had been an otherwise untreatable illness. When this treatment modality spread to Italy shortly thereafter, another neuropsychiatrist, Ugo Cerletti, was impressed its efficacy but frustrated by its technical complexity (Shorter and Healy 2007). Through his work as an experimental epileptologist, Cerletti was aware of an electrical model of seizure induction that had been used in animal research and offered the opportunity for a more efficient and less complex treatment than pharmacoconvulsive therapy. After further experimentation, Cerletti and his assistant, Lucio Bini, were successful in using electrical seizure induction to treat some of their patients with schizophrenia, and ECT rapidly replaced pharmacoconvulsive therapy.

Although ECT was first used in the treatment of schizophrenia, clinicians soon discovered that its highest therapeutic potency was in treating mood disorders. The peak in ECT utilization was from the early 1940s through the mid-1950s, at which point the first effective antipsychotic and antidepressant medications were introduced into clinical use, followed by antimanic agents in the 1960s (Braslow and Marder 2019). Although these new psychopharmacological agents obviated the need for ECT in many patients with these disorders, ECT remains the most rapid and effective means to induce remission in MDD (Hermida et al. 2018; U.K. ECT Review Group 2003) and continues to be of substantial therapeutic benefit for individuals with treatment-resistant mania (Medda et al. 2014) and schizophrenia spectrum disorders (Sanghani et al. 2018), as well as those with catatonia associated with either psychiatric or medical etiologies (Luchini et al. 2015).

In the early days of ECT, considerable fear surrounded its use in older adults, largely because of the medical comorbidity common in this population. The cardiovascular physiology of ECT was not yet well understood, and more recent procedural innovations—such as oxygenation, muscular relaxation, general anesthesia, and physiological monitoring—had not yet been instituted. Furthermore, ECT procedures during that early period were performed in a distinctly nonmedical setting, often in psychiatrists' offices, without the presence of other medical staff or medical support resources. As ECT methodology became more refined, practitioners became more willing to use it with older patients and others with significant medical comorbidity. In Texas, which mandates reporting of ECT use, 18.5% of ECT treatment courses were administered to individuals age 65 years and older between September 1, 2018, and August 31, 2019 (Texas Department of State Health Services 2020). At present, ECT is considered to be a mainstay of psychiatric treatment in elderly patients, particularly those with MDD (Kerner and Prudic 2014; McDonald 2016; Meyer et al. 2020), although racial disparities persist in the use of this important treatment modality (Jones et al. 2019).

Acute ECT Use

Diagnostic Indications

Mood Disorders

The most common diagnostic indication for ECT is MDD (American Psychiatric Association 2001). A significant body of literature not only supports the efficacy of ECT for MDD (American Psychiatric Association 2010) but also suggests that it is the most rapidly effective treatment for this condition (Agarkar et al. 2018; Husain et al. 2004). This literature includes a series of randomized, double-blind, placebo-controlled studies in which the control was "sham ECT" whereby the subjects received all aspects of a usual clinical ECT treatment except the electrical stimulus (Brandon 1986). The evidence from meta-analytical studies also suggests greater efficacy with ECT than with antidepressant medication (Janicak et al. 1985; U.K. ECT Review Group 2003). Regarding subtypes of depression, ECT appears to be effective in treating both melancholic and severe nonmelancholic depression (Fink et al. 2007; Sackeim and Rush 1995), including in elderly populations (Birkenhäger et al. 2010; Sackeim 1998; Veltman et al. 2019). Patients with bipolar depression do at least as well as those with unipolar depression (Bahji et al. 2019). However, ECT is particularly effective in treating MDD with psychotic features (Petrides et al. 2001; Sobin et al. 1996; van Diermen et al. 2018).

Although ECT is used more frequently for MDD than for other illnesses, and the vast majority of ECT research studies have focused on this condition, evidence suggests that ECT has efficacy in treating several other mental disorders as well. Multiple reviews of ECT in the treatment of bipolar disorder, including mania, mixed states, and depressive episodes, have reported substantial efficacy (Dierckx et al. 2012; Elias et al. 2021; Perugi et al. 2017; Versiani et al. 2011). In this regard, ECT has been reported to achieve a response rate as high as 80%, to have efficacy equal to that of lithium, and to have a significant advantage over lithium in patients who have not responded to lithium or antipsychotic medication. The relative efficacy of ECT compared with anticonvulsant antimanic agents has not yet been studied, and no systematic studies exist to indicate the utility of ECT in individuals with rapid-cycling bipolar disorder. However, there are some case-series data regarding a potential role for maintenance ECT in the management of rapid-cycling bipolar disorder (Minnai et al. 2011).

Schizophrenia Spectrum Disorders

As noted, ECT was first employed as a treatment for individuals with schizophrenia. However, the superior response to ECT of patients with mood disorders was soon evident. Following the development of antipsychotic medications in the late 1950s, the use of ECT as a treatment for schizophrenia gradually declined. Regardless, studies have suggested that antipsychotic medications and ECT have comparable efficacy for management of psychotic, or "positive," symptoms (Chanpattana and Sackeim 2010; Pompili et al. 2013; Sanghani et al. 2018), particularly as supplementation to antipsychotic medications (Klapheke 1993). However, no evidence indicates that ECT has efficacy for the treatment of deficit, or "negative," symptoms of schizophrenia.

The acute benefits of ECT added to clozapine in patients whose illness does not respond to clozapine alone were studied by Petrides et al. (2015) in a controlled crossover investigation, with 50% of subjects receiving the combined treatment showing a clinically significant response in positive symptoms, versus 0% for those continued on clozapine alone. When the clozapine-alone group (none of whose illness responded during the initial study phase) was switched to ECT plus clozapine, 47% showed response, indicating that the benefit of combination treatment was a real effect. The presence of affective symptoms appears to increase the likelihood of response to ECT in patients with schizophrenia (Pompili et al. 2013). In this regard, case reports and case series suggest that individuals with schizoaffective disorder may respond better to ECT than do those with schizophrenia (American Psychiatric Association 2001; Sanghani et al. 2018).

Catatonia

Catatonia, a syndrome characterized by abnormal motor activity associated with severe mood, schizophrenia spectrum, and some medical disorders, has been found to be more common in elderly persons (Luchini et al. 2015). ECT is highly effective in the treatment of catatonia (Fink 2019; Krystal and Coffey 1997), including geriatric populations (Suzuki et al. 2002), although it seems to produce greater response in the context of a mood disorder than a schizophrenia spectrum disorder (Luchini et al. 2015). ECT has even been found to be effective when the patient's catatonia is associated with medical conditions, such as systemic lupus erythematosus, uremia, hepatic encephalopathy, porphyria, hyperparathyroidism, and autoimmune encephalitis (Fricchione et al. 1990; Rummans and Bassingthwaighte 1991; Warren et al. 2019). Although it is typically used after attempting treatment with benzodiazepines, ECT should be considered a first-line intervention in severe cases in which catatonic features occur in the context of etiologies such as malignant catatonia, neuroleptic malignant syndrome, delirious mania, or severe catatonic excitement (Medda et al. 2015; Morcos et al. 2019; Wittenauer Welsh et al. 2016). When treating such cases, it is important that appropriate, standardized outcome measures be used (Bush et al. 1996).

Neurological Disorders

ECT can be a useful treatment for Parkinson's disease when medication management fails or is poorly tolerated (Williams et al. 2017). However, it should also be noted that patients with Parkinson's disease may be at increased risk for developing cognitive side effects and delirium with ECT (Figiel et al. 1991). In addition, the benefits gained with ECT in Parkinson's symptoms and signs are transient, necessitating the use of maintenance ECT in such cases (Wengel et al. 1998). ECT has successfully been used to manage extreme agitation, aggression, or other severe behavioral disturbances related to psychotic thought processes in individuals with dementia (Acharya et al. 2015; Hermida et al. 2020b). In such cases, ECT is used for its antipsychotic effect rather than for behavioral control.

Another neurological condition for which there is evidence of a potential benefit for ECT—albeit based on multiple case reports and case series rather than controlled trials—is treatment-resistant status epilepticus (Pinchotti et al. 2018; San-Juan et al. 2019). Any success in the electrically induced seizure aborting the ongoing episode of status epilepticus is believed to be related to its powerful postictal inhibitory response, which lasts considerably longer than the induced seizure itself. In this regard, a series of ECT treatments may be necessary, possibly at least daily, in order to produce a lasting anticonvulsant effect. It should also be recognized that these are extremely challenging cases given the typical presence of high dosages of concurrent anticonvulsant medications.

Response in Older Adults

Several prospective studies suggest that ECT is a highly effective treatment for MDD in elderly individuals (Kamat et al. 2003; Kerner and Prudic 2014; O'Connor et al. 2001; Riva-Posse et al. 2013; Tew et al. 1999; van der Wurff et al. 2003; Wesson et al. 1997). In this regard, a large study by the Consortium for Research in ECT involving 253 patients split into three age groups (≥65 years, 46–64 years, and ≤45 years) found that whereas remission rates for the older two groups were equivalent (90% for both), a lower proportion of younger patients (70%) remitted (O'Connor et al. 2001). A more recent European study reported similar findings (van Diermen et al. 2018), as did a large multicenter trial in the United States, which showed conservative acute response and remission rates of 70% and 62%, respectively, after an acute treatment course (Kellner et al. 2016b). Furthermore, there is also evidence that elderly patients receiving ECT for treatment of MDD experienced greater improvement in quality-of-life indicators than younger patients (Güney et al. 2020). Finally, when acutely effective, ECT has a significant longitudinal positive impact on older adults not only in terms of efficacy but also in regard to long-term morbidity and mortality rates (Philibert et al. 1995).

ECT as a Maintenance Treatment

Although ECT is a highly effective acute treatment for several neuropsychiatric conditions, it is not a cure in the sense that it does not ensure that future episodes will not occur (American Psychiatric Association 2001). Also, evidence indicates that the relapse rates of MDD following an acute ECT course are high, ranging from 35% to 80% over 1 year (Bourgon and Kellner 2000; Huuhka et al. 2004). Therefore, it is important to institute some form of therapy to minimize relapse risk. Such therapy could consist of pharmacotherapy, psychotherapy, or intermittent single ECT treatments (or some combination thereof).

This substantial risk of relapse is underscored by findings from a study by Sackeim et al. (2001a) in which roughly 80% of patients successfully treated with ECT for MDD relapsed within 6 months. Nevertheless, prophylactic pharmacotherapy on its own is not universally effective; roughly 50%–60% of patients with depression relapse within 1 year of completing an acute ECT course when treated with typical single-agent pharmacotherapy (Sackeim et al. 1990, 2001a). The relapse rate after ECT appears to be even higher among individuals whose depression was resistant to medication before the acute ECT course (Sackeim et al. 1990). One study suggested that, rather than single-agent monotherapy, more aggressive pharmacotherapy—specifically the combination of nortriptyline and lithium—is associated with a decrease in the relapse rate to ~40% within 6 months after ECT (Sackeim et al. 2001a).

An alternative to continuation or maintenance pharmacotherapy is continuation or maintenance ECT. "Continuation" ECT is historically applied in the first 6 months following an acute ECT series (based on the unproven assumption that subliminal aspects of the acute episode are still present over that period), whereas "maintenance" ECT is the long-term prophylactic use of ECT for relapse prevention. In this chapter, we use *maintenance ECT* to refer to both such uses. Although this section discusses the general indications and efficacy for maintenance ECT, a later section covers more technical aspects of maintenance ECT delivery.

Several case series and retrospective reports have suggested the efficacy of continuation or maintenance ECT (Petrides et al. 2011; van Schaik et al. 2012). However, a randomized controlled trial of maintenance ECT versus maintenance pharmacotherapy was not carried out until the mid-2000s, when Kellner et al. (2006) reported similar 6-month outcomes for patients treated with maintenance bilateral ECT or a combination of lithium and nortriptyline maintenance pharmacotherapy. Since that trial, two multicenter controlled clinical trials in responders to acute ECT treatment for MDD have been published that compared maintenance ECT plus aggressive pharmacotherapy with aggressive pharmacotherapy alone (Kellner et al. 2016a; Nordenskjöld et al. 2013). Both trials showed a decrease in relapse risk over the applicable study interval (1 year and 6 months, respectively). The trial by Kellner et al. (2016a) is particularly notable because it required subjects to have been full remitters to a highly structured acute ECT course and required that the aggressive pharmacotherapy regimen (venlafaxine plus lithium) be the same for all subjects.

The indications and efficacy for maintenance ECT for patients with bipolar disorder who received an acute series of ECT for treatment of a depressive episode is believed to be the same as for patients with unipolar depression (Vaidya et al. 2003), as well as for patients who received an acute ECT series for a manic episode (Elias et al. 2021). An interesting subgroup consists of patients with rapid-cycling bipolar disorder, a condition that is notoriously difficult to treat. In severe, medication-resistant cases, there is limited evidence that a symptom-titrated maintenance ECT regimen can sometimes serve to increase the interval between episodes (Minnai et al. 2011).

The risk of relapse for patients who received their acute ECT course for a schizophrenic or schizoaffective episode is extremely high, even with antipsychotic medication prophylaxis, and long-term maintenance ECT in association with antipsychotic medication is almost always indicated (Isserles et al. 2020; Youn et al. 2019). In such cases, there is often a "critical interval" beyond which positive symptoms recur (Ward et al. 2018). Although there is not a clear evidence base in the psychiatric literature, a similar critical interval situation is believed to be present for many patients with ECT-responsive Parkinson's disease. For patients who received an acute ECT course for treatment of catatonia, the mortality and morbidity associated with recurrence is sufficiently high that at least short-term maintenance ECT should be considered.

Risks of ECT and Use in Patients With Neurological and Medical Disorders

Because the decision about whether to pursue a course of ECT should involve an evaluation of both the expected risks and benefits of ECT, clinicians should carry out and document an assessment of the likelihood of potential adverse sequelae for each patient. Furthermore, they should communicate the presence and implications of high-risk medical conditions as part of the informed consent process. It is important to understand and to convey that the risk of any medical procedure is "relative"—that is, the "true" risk basically relates to the risk of having the procedure versus the risk of viable treatment alternatives, including the risks associated with the underlying illness itself—and can be substantial for individuals referred for ECT, particularly those who have prominent suicidal ideation or behavior and those with severe catatonia or medical debilitation related to the psychiatric episode.

Mortality

In terms of acute mortality, the overall mortality rate for ECT has been estimated as ~2 deaths per 100,000 treatments (Shiwach et al. 2001). A more recent meta-analysis of 15 studies involving more than 750,000 ECT treatments in 32 countries estimated the mortality rate at 2.1 per 100,000 treatments (Tørring et al. 2017). This relatively low mortality rate appears to be comparable with the rate associated with minor surgery (Mullen et al. 2017). This low general mortality rate covers the entire ECT population as a whole and cannot be expected to apply to patients who are in the high-risk category, as discussed later, most of whom are elderly. Age-stratified mortality risk for all patients receiving ECT in Ontario from 2003 to 2011 was reported by Blumberger et al. (2017), with those ages 65–85 years having a 3.85 times greater ECT-related mortality rate within 7 days of ECT than those younger than 65 years. The 7-day mortality was 8.87 times greater for those older than 85 years than for those younger than 65 years.

Regardless of age, a patient-specific level of risk, particularly from a relative risk standpoint, must be determined for those perceived to be at high risk, and this information must be conveyed as part of the informed consent process and be documented in the medical record.

General Acute Adverse Effects

ECT is usually well tolerated. However, several common minor acute physical side effects are important to monitor and address when present, including headache, muscle ache, nausea, and fatigue (Bryson et al 2017; Meyer et al. 2020). Headache is observed in as much as 45% of patients during and shortly after the postictal period, and ECT may exacerbate a preexisting headache syndrome (Haghighi et al. 2016). Generalized muscle soreness is typically due to fasciculations induced by the depolarizing muscle relaxant succinylcholine but will not occur with a nondepolarizing agent (American Psychiatric Association 2001). Treatment for headaches and muscle soreness is symptomatic, and aspirin, acetaminophen, and nonsteroidal anti-inflammatory drugs are typically effective. For patients who experience frequent post-ECT headaches or soreness, prophylactic treatment with these agents may be beneficial (American Psychiatric Association 2001). Nausea on awakening is usually transient and may be treated with serotonin 5-HT$_3$ receptor antagonists, such as ondansetron, or dopamine antagonists, such as metoclopramide (American Psychiatric Association 2001).

More serious, but typically rare, medical complications of ECT and its associated anesthesia are pneumonia, prolonged apnea, malignant cardiac arrhythmias, myocardial infarction, stroke, and status epilepticus (Blumberger et al. 2017). Except for status epilepticus, these events are more likely with elderly patients, particularly those with significant medical comorbidity, and are discussed in a later section. *Status epilepticus* is defined as a seizure lasting longer than 5 minutes or multiple seizures occurring within a <5-minute interval (Horváth et al. 2019) and requires immediate neurological intervention. It is important to differentiate status epilepticus from prolonged seizures with ECT, which are infrequent but not rare and are typically easy to manage; these are discussed later in the "Technique" section. Although there is a rare risk of spontaneous seizures during or following an ECT course, there does not appear to be an increased risk of developing epilepsy, especially in elderly patients (Bøg et al. 2018).

Another, and often overlooked, medical risk of ECT is falls. Frail elderly adults, who are often debilitated or dehydrated, are at particular risk for falls, which can lead to broken bones and other traumatic outcomes (Blumberger et al. 2017). Acute psychiatric side effects include treatment-emergent mania. Although uncommon, mania or hypomania may be induced in patients with depression or those in mixed affective states during the ECT course (Devanand et al. 1992). This may be most common in patients with bipolar disorder. For patients who have increasing severity of manic symptoms with further ECT, treatment-emergent mania must be distinguished from delirium with euphoria, which can be identified by continuous confusion, disorientation, and more pronounced memory impairment (Devanand et al. 1988). Delirium may resolve by increasing the interval between treatments, decreasing stimulus intensity, or modifying electrode placement from bilateral to unilateral (American Psychiatric Association 2001). Postictal delirium or excitement occurs in a minority of patients and is characterized by motor agitation, disorientation, and inability to follow commands (Devanand et al. 1989). See the "Anesthetic Considerations" section later in the chapter for management recommendations.

Cognitive Side Effects

The most important side effect with ECT is cognitive dysfunction, which remains a key factor limiting the use of this treatment modality (American Psychiatric Association 2001). The most common objectively accessible cognitive side effects are anterograde amnesia (difficulty retaining new information) and retrograde amnesia (difficulty recalling information learned in the past) (Semkovska and McLoughlin 2010). Both anterograde and retrograde memory effects tend to most strongly impact information encountered during the period closest to the ECT treatment course. Anterograde amnesia typically resolves within a few weeks after the treatment course, whereas retrograde amnesia tends to resolve more slowly (Weiner et al. 1986).

Although most evidence indicates that objective cognitive deficits with ECT are transient, patient reports of persistent and even permanent memory impairment, particularly but not exclusively autobiographical in nature, sometimes occur (Sigström et al. 2020). The causes of such persistent subjective deficits are unclear and are likely multifactorial and not always directly related to the ECT itself. Despite objective evidence that memory performance transiently decreases after ECT, some patients indicate that their memory function improves, likely a result of the lifting of depressive symptoms (American Psychiatric Association 2001; Weiner et al. 1986). This finding appears to be present in older adults as well as in younger individuals, particularly those in whom the severity of depression-related cognitive deficits presents as a pseudodementia (Bosboom and Deijen 2006). Reviews of ECT's effects on cognitive functioning in elderly adults indicate that such deficits are not substantially greater than those experienced by younger individuals (Kumar et al. 2016; Tielkes et al. 2008).

Both the degree and the duration of objective and subjective memory side effects of ECT vary substantially in patients who receive ECT. Research studies have identified factors that can affect objective memory side effects of ECT (McClintock et al. 2014). Compared with unilateral placement of stimulus electrodes, bilateral placement has repeatedly been shown to increase the risk of amnesia, including in elderly populations (O'Connor et al. 2010; Stoppe et al. 2006). In addition, greater risk is associated with higher stimulus intensity (compared with the seizure threshold), larger numbers of ECT treatments, higher doses of barbiturate anesthetic, and less time between treatments. Furthermore, some patients—including those taking lithium and medications with anticholinergic properties, as well as those with preexisting cerebral disease—appear to be at increased risk of cognitive side effects (Patel et al. 2020). Individuals with diseases affecting the basal ganglia and subcortical white matter may be at particular risk (Figiel et al. 1990).

Given their importance, the nature, likelihood, and persistence of both objective and subjective cognitive adverse effects of ECT should be covered in the informed consent process, and monitoring of these effects should take place during and at least immediately following an acute ECT course (Porter et al. 2020; U.S. Food and Drug Administration 2018). There is presently no clear consensus on which instrument to use for such monitoring. Given the operational challenges involved, such as the setting, time constraints, and difficulty in productively engaging very psychiatrically ill individuals, any such measure needs to be sensitive, brief, and easy to reliably administer. Given the FDA's preference for a broader assessment tool than one focusing on memory (U.S. Food and Drug Administration 2018), many practitioners have implemented use of instruments such as the Mini-Mental State Examination or the Montreal Cognitive Assessment for this purpose, even though their overall sensitivity to ECT effects is low, including in the elderly population (Hebbrecht et al. 2020; Obbels et al. 2019). A new instrument, the ElectroConvulsive Therapy Cognitive Assessment, was recently developed and shows early evidence of increased ECT sensitivity compared with the Montreal Cognitive Assessment (Hermida et al. 2020a). Although use of instruments such as these is optimal, at a minimum, some form of memory assessment should be used, such as a simple delayed verbal recall task combined with a brief global subjective memory rating tool.

Tolerability and Risks Associated With Medical Comorbidities

It is important to identify individuals at risk for medical complications with ECT and to be aware of modifications in ECT technique that may minimize risks. Elderly patients referred for ECT frequently have preexisting medical illnesses that need to be considered in the clinical assessment (Christopher 2003; Weiner and Krystal 2001). Although some illnesses appear to increase the risk of adverse effects with ECT (Zielinski et al. 1993), no illness should be considered an absolute contraindication for the use of ECT, given that risk is relative rather than absolute. The decision about whether to pursue a course of ECT should always involve a careful weighing of the individual patient's risks and benefits both for carrying out ECT and for selecting a different and likely less effective treatment modality. Conditions for which evidence has suggested an increased risk with ECT are discussed in the following subsections.

Central Nervous System Disorders

In addition to the neurological indications for ECT, many individuals referred for ECT for treatment of psychiatric indications have comorbid neurological disorders, particularly elderly patients. A major risk for CNS adverse outcomes with ECT originates from an increase in intracranial and intravascular pressure (Krystal and Coffey 1997); however, despite this, the CNS complication rate is generally quite low. Several CNS disorders leave patients more susceptible to complications related to increases in intracranial and intravascular pressure. For example, those with a space-occupying CNS lesion, such as a tumor, subdural hematoma, or intracranial arachnoid cyst, have historically been thought to be at increased risk for noncardiogenic pulmonary edema, cerebral edema, brain hemorrhage, and cerebral herniation (Krystal and Coffey 1997). Although space-occupying cerebral lesions were once considered an absolute contraindication to ECT, patients with small lesions without edema or elevated intracranial pressure can usually be safely treated with ECT (Dauleac et al. 2019). For the remainder of patients with space-occupying CNS lesions, risks may be diminished (although not removed) by pretreating with an antihypertensive agent, osmotic diuretics, and steroids and by employing hyperventilation during treatment (Buday et al. 2020).

The increase in intravascular pressure that occurs with ECT theoretically could also lead to an increased risk of intracranial hemorrhage; however, such events are very rare (Hsieh et al. 2019). Nonetheless, individuals with recent strokes, arteriovenous malformations, and aneurysms are considered at increased risk (Krystal and Coffey 1997). Anecdotally, ECT has been safely administered in patients with intracranial aneurysms who have been treated by clipping the aneurysm or by placement of intravascular coils or stents (Pickett and Hazelton 2019). Nevertheless, decisions regarding any delay in ECT treatment should consider the severity of the stroke and extent of recovery, as well as the urgency of ECT (American Psychiatric Association 2001). Antihypertensive agents given at the time of ECT should be considered to diminish the rise in intravascular pressure in patients with a history of hemorrhagic stroke. However, such prophylaxis may be counterproductive in individuals who have had cerebral ischemic events, and care should also be taken to avoid hypotension during the acute postictal period.

As noted earlier, patients with preexisting cerebral disease, including dementia, may be particularly likely to experience problems with ECT-related amnesia. At times, even frank delirium may occur. These risks, which appear to be most prominent in individuals with dementia or basal ganglia disease, can be minimized by decreasing the frequency of treatments and using unilateral electrode placement. However, the coexistence of ECT-responsive disorders with a known or possible neurocognitive disorder should not be a deterrent to the use of ECT, particularly because at least a portion of cognitive dysfunction in such individuals may represent pseudodementia that might resolve with treatment (Isserles et al. 2017).

Cardiovascular Disorders

The physiology of ECT prominently involves the cardiovascular system (Bryson et al. 2013). Fluctuations in heart rate and blood pressure that occur during ECT treatments place strain on the cardiac system and in high-risk patients may be associated with cardiovascular complications. Immediately following the stimulus, parasympathetic tone increases, which can lead to a sudden but transient decrease in heart rate and not uncommonly presents as a brief period of asystole. The subsequent induced seizure, however, is associated with a sympathetic surge that markedly increases both blood pressure and heart rate and is then followed by a relative increase in parasympathetic tone as the induced seizure ends (Suzuki et al. 2019).

Despite these autonomic fluctuations, cardiovascular complications rarely occur with ECT in patients without preexisting cardiovascular risk factors (Nordenskjöld et al. 2021; Weiner et al. 2000). Cardiac conditions that increase this risk include recent myocardial infarction, uncompensated congestive heart failure, severe valvular disease, unstable aneurysm, unstable angina or active cardiac ischemia, uncontrolled hypertension, and severe aortic stenosis (Applegate 1997; Singla and Grover 2018). A finding of good functional status indicates that the risk is low; otherwise, further cardiac evaluation is indicated.

Patients with coronary artery disease are at risk for ischemia during both periods of relative parasympathetic tone and periods of increased sympathetic system tone (Christopher 2003). When parasympathetic tone is increased, there is a risk of ischemia due to hypoperfusion, whereas when sympathetic activity rises, the increased cardiac workload can lead to complications whose risks can be decreased pharmacologically. Anticholinergic medications such as atropine or glycopyrrolate can be used to decrease the occurrence and severity of bradycardia; β-adrenergic blockers can be used to decrease cardiac workload; and calcium channel blockers may be used to decrease the risks of ischemia (Kellner and Bryson 2013). Typically, patients who are receiving medications for the treatment of coronary artery disease at the time of referral for ECT are maintained on those medications throughout the ECT course, including administration before ECT on treatment days (American Psychiatric Association 2001). Changes to the medication regimen or the addition of other medications to decrease the risks of cardiac complications should generally be considered in consideration with a cardiology consultant.

Individuals with pathologies associated with low cardiac output, such as heart failure, or those with severe valvular disease are at particular risk during the sympathetic surge because of the increase in afterload and decreased diastolic filling time (Stern et al. 1997). Such patients should not be administered large volumes of fluid (Rayburn 1997). Several medications have been suggested as means to decrease risks in these situations, including β-adrenergic blockers, α-adrenergic blockers, nitrites, digitalis, and anticholinergic agents; however, the use of such agents is controversial (Weiner et al. 2000). No single regimen appears to be optimal for all patients with these diseases, and the treatment plan should be individualized based on risk-benefit considerations.

Arrhythmias may increase the risks of ECT (Takada et al. 2005). Bradyarrhythmias are typically best managed acutely with atropine to prevent exacerbation during increases in parasympathetic tone. Because of the anticonvulsant effects of lidocaine, ventricular ectopy should be treated with other agents before the ECT treatment (Hood and Mecca 1983). Patients with atrial fibrillation may experience spontaneous cardioversion with ECT that can lead to an embolic event (Petrides and Fink 1996). Thus, consideration should be given to echocardiography (to rule out a mural thrombus) and the use of anticoagulants (Weiner et al. 2000). ECT appears to be safe in patients with implanted cardiac pacemakers and defibrillators, although no controlled trials have been done (Dolenc et al. 2004).

Endocrinological Disorders

Several endocrinological disorders require special consideration before ECT. The most common is diabetes mellitus. Patients with diabetes are more likely than other ECT patients to have problems stemming from the need to fast from midnight until the time of the ECT treatment. Blood glucose levels should be measured prior to each treatment, which should be performed relatively early in the day. Insulin doses may need to be adjusted, particularly with increased food intake due to clinical improvement (Netzel et al. 2002).

In patients with hyperthyroidism or pheochromocytoma, β-adrenergic blockers are typically administered to prevent the development of a thyroid storm or hypertensive crisis, respectively, which can be elicited by the sympathetic surge (Weiner et al. 2000). In cases of pheochromocytoma, α-adrenergic and tyrosine hydroxylase blockers may also be needed.

Metabolic Disorders

The primary metabolic problems in the context of ECT are hyperkalemia and hypokalemia, both of which may lead to cardiac arrhythmias. Hyperkalemia is of particular concern because of the transient rise in serum potassium caused by succinylcholine and the muscle activity that may occur during the induced seizures (Christopher 2003; Weiner et al. 2000). In patients with hyperkalemia, prolonged paralysis and associated apnea induced by succinylcholine may be seen. Although it is best to correct these conditions before administering ECT, the use of paralytic agents other than succinylcholine should be considered for cases in which correction of hyperkalemia is not possible.

Hematological Disorders

Thrombophlebitis carries a risk of embolism with ECT, although this can generally be mitigated with the use of anticoagulant medications. Patients with prolonged immobility, such as in catatonia, are at particular risk for deep vein thrombosis, which, if untreated, may develop a pulmonary embolism during ECT (Mamah et al. 2005). This risk is considered higher when a thrombus is located more proximally (above the knee) as opposed to distally (Kearon 2003). The use of warfarin has been recommended, with a goal of achieving an international normalized ratio between 1.5 and 2.5 (Petrides and Fink 1996), although heparin and low-molecular-weight heparin have also been successfully used (Inagawa et al. 2018).

Pulmonary Disorders

Patients with asthma or chronic obstructive pulmonary disease are at increased risk of posttreatment bronchospasm, which may be mitigated by their use of an inhaler medication before each treatment (Weiner et al. 2000). Theophylline should be avoided if possible or used at a minimal dose because of an increased risk of prolonged seizures and status epilepticus (American Psychiatric Association 2001). In addition, although pre-ECT oxygenation is important (see "Anesthetic Considerations" section), it should be used with care in patients with chronic obstructive pulmonary disease because excessive oxygen could further blunt their respiratory response, which is often dependent on relative hypoxia (Schak et al. 2008).

Gastrointestinal Disorders

Patients with gastroesophageal reflux disease are often encountered in the practice of ECT. The risk of aspiration may be reduced with the use of a pretreatment histamine type 2 antagonist or a proton pump inhibitor the morning of treatment (Weiner et al. 2000). To increase gastric emptying, pretreatment metoclopramide may be considered, and sodium citrate may be used to neutralize the acidity of stomach contents. Such precautions may be particularly useful in high-risk patients, such as those with a history of bariatric surgery (Lubit et al. 2016). Although only a single case of gastric rupture has been reported (van Schaik et al. 2006), fecal impaction may be a risk factor for intestinal rupture with ECT (Weiner et al. 2000). Consequently, it is important to address constipation in patients referred for ECT, which is particularly common in the elderly population.

Genitourinary Disorders

Urinary retention carries a potential risk of bladder rupture with ECT. This complication is rare, reported in one patient with a full bladder receiving unmodified ECT and psychotropic medications with anticholinergic effects (O'Brien and Morgan 1991) and in another with a history of prostate disease. As a result, it has been recommended that patients void before ECT, and urinary catheterization should be considered for those with significant obstruction or difficulty urinating. In addition, anticholinergic premedication at the time of ECT may last for up to several hours and increase the risk of urinary retention in susceptible patients.

Musculoskeletal Disorders

Musculoskeletal conditions, such as osteoporosis, unstable fractures, and loose or damaged teeth, are common in older adults and carry an increased risk of complications with ECT. Patients with osteoporosis or recent or unstable fractures are at risk for bone damage during the induced convulsion and should be considered at high risk for falls. Care must be taken to ensure complete muscle relaxation in such patients (Bryson et al. 2015). The contraction of the jaw muscles that leads to teeth clenching cannot be diminished with the use of paralytic agents, however, because it occurs by direct electrical stimulation of the muscle tissue and not via neuromuscular transmission. Therefore, the use of a mouth guard is always necessary. Patients with loose or damaged teeth may require customized devices, dental treatment, or tooth extraction before ECT. These efforts result in a minimal risk of dental fracture during ECT, with an estimated incidence at 0.2% per series in a large Swedish register-based study (Göterfelt et al. 2020).

Other Medical Conditions

Because ECT is associated with an acute increase in intraocular pressure (lasting minutes rather than hours), this may be a risk for patients with glaucoma (Song et al. 2004), although no evidence of any lasting sequelae has been found. Still, patients receiving ongoing medication for glaucoma should receive this prior to ECT on treatment days.

Despite a lack of evidence, ECT was listed as a contraindication on package inserts for cochlear implant devices, presumably on the basis of a theoretical concern regarding potential electrical damage to the device from the ECT stimulus. However, multiple reports have since indicated that ECT can be safely performed without device damage (Jiam et al. 2020).

Adverse Effects Specific to Older Adults

Advanced age itself does not appear to increase the medical risks of ECT. As a group, however, older individuals have a higher incidence of comorbid medical conditions that increase the risks of treatment, as outlined in the preceding subsections (Blumberger et al. 2017; Kujala et al. 2002; Nuttall et al. 2004; Sutor and Rasmussen 2016; Takada et al. 2005). Although early studies reported that older adults in general tend to have greater and more prolonged cognitive impairment with ECT (American Psychiatric Association 2001; Sackeim et al. 2007), such increased risk has more recently been questioned (Tielkes et al. 2008; Verwijk et al. 2014). Nonetheless, particularly for those with preexisting cognitive impairment, modifications of treatment technique should be considered to minimize cognitive side effects.

The greater frequency of comorbid medical disease in elderly persons also increases the risks associated with pharmacological management of their neuropsychiatric conditions. In some cases, these risks can make pharmacological management extremely difficult and may lead to a referral for ECT. Manly et al. (2000) compared the frequency of side effects associated with ECT and with pharmacotherapy in a group of patients older than 75 years with depression who were matched for age, sex, and diagnosis. They reported that ECT resulted in fewer side effects (particularly cardiovascular and gastrointestinal) and greater efficacy than pharmacological management. This study underscores that ECT is a relatively safe treatment for older adults and that, in many cases, it may be both the safest and most effective option.

Pre-ECT Evaluation

Basic Components of the Evaluation

The pre-ECT evaluation should include assessments completed by a clinician privileged to administer ECT and by an anesthesia provider. This evaluation should include 1) a thorough psychiatric history and examination, including any history of response to ECT and other treatments; 2) a medical history and examination, with special attention paid to cardiovascular, respiratory, neurological, and musculoskeletal systems; 3) presence of skull defects; 4) a history of dental problems, including dentures and examination for loose or missing teeth; and 5) a history of personal and familial adverse effects with general anesthesia (American Psychiatric Association 2001; Sundsted et al. 2014; Tess and Smetana 2009). Although there is no consensus regarding routine laboratory tests to carry out prior to initiating ECT, a complete blood count, serum chemistry (including sodium and potassium), and electrocardiogram are generally ordered (American Psychiatric Association 2001). A chest x-ray is indicated in patients with cardiovascular or pulmonary disease or a history of smoking (American Psychiatric Association 2001).

The decision regarding whether to pursue testing of cerebral function and structure (e.g., electroencephalographic, neuroradiological, or neuropsychological assessment) should be made on an individual basis, guided by the patient's history and examination. Further testing or medical/surgical consultation should be considered when the potential risks of ECT are unclear or when there is uncertainty about whether and how to modify ECT technique to decrease these risks. In every case, the pre-ECT assessment should include an evaluation of the risks of cognitive impairment based on the considerations described in the earlier section "Cognitive Side Effects" and the information obtained in the history, examination, and testing. This evaluation should play a key role in recommendations about treatment technique in terms of stimulus electrode placement, treatment frequency, stimulus dosing, and medication adjustments.

Decision About Whether to Administer ECT

The decision about whether to recommend ECT should be based on a history of treatment resistance, careful assessment of risks and benefits of ECT versus alternative treatments, other data obtained in the pre-ECT evaluation, urgency of need for a rapid response, and patient preference. ECT should be seriously considered only when the patient has a disorder for which there is evidence of ECT efficacy (American Psychiatric Association 2001).

In severe MDD, for which ECT is the most effective treatment known, it has been demonstrated that the greater the severity of illness, the stronger the indication for ECT (Weiner and Krystal 2001). Although generally used on a secondary basis for patients with treatment-resistant MDD, ECT is often the treatment of choice and has been recommended as first-line (primary) treatment when psychosis is present; when there is a high risk of mortality due to suicidality, dehydration, or malnutrition; or when the patient is unable to cooperate with necessary medical treatment (Kellner et al. 2020). No consensus guidelines exist categorizing the extent of treatment refractoriness necessary for secondary intervention with ECT in terms of medication dosage, duration, or number of failed trials (American Psychiatric Association 2010). Acute illness severity, risks associated with the underlying psychiatric episode, and patient preference all play a role in the decision to recommend ECT. Multiple studies support the use of ECT following medication failure, indicating that a significant number of patients respond to ECT after one or more failed medication trials (Avery and Lubrano 1979; Paul et al. 1981; Prudic et al. 1996).

Informed Consent

The collaborative aspect of decision-making has been formalized as the legal doctrine of informed consent (American Psychiatric Association 2001). No patient with the capacity to give voluntary consent should be treated with ECT without giving written informed consent. Although there is no clear consensus regarding how to determine capacity to give consent, this capacity has generally been interpreted as evidence that the patient can understand information about the procedure and can act responsibly based on this information (American Psychiatric Association 2001). The process of determining competency, the process for giving ECT involuntarily in emergent cases, and the specific procedures for obtaining informed consent should be carried out as specified by applicable state statutes (Livingston et al. 2018). Because of the increased likelihood of cognitive dysfunction in older adults, capacity to consent is of particular concern (Rabheru 2001).

At a minimum, written consent should be obtained before the initial course of ECT, if an acute treatment course involves an unusually large number of treatments, and before initiating continuation or maintenance ECT (American Psychiatric Association 2001). To adequately convey the risks and benefits, the consent form should include the following information (American Psychiatric Association 2001):

1. Description of treatment alternatives
2. Detailed description of how, when, and where ECT will be carried out
3. Discussion of options regarding electrode placement
4. Typical range of number of treatments
5. Statement that there is no guarantee the treatment will be successful
6. Statement that some continuation or maintenance treatment will be necessary
7. Discussion of the possible risks, including death, cardiac dysfunction, confusion, and memory impairment
8. Statement that the consent also applies to emergency treatment that may be clinically necessary at times when the patient is unconscious
9. List of patient requirements during the ECT course, such as taking nothing by mouth after midnight before treatment
10. Statement that there has been an opportunity to ask questions and an indication of who can be contacted with further questions
11. Statement that consent is voluntary and can be withdrawn at any time

Informed consent involves more than just signing a consent form; it requires a consent discussion with the patient or surrogate (and, if possible, a significant other). The consent discussion should include any significant differences in likelihood of benefit or extent of risk from that depicted in the consent form, and mention of such discussion should be briefly documented in the patient's medical record.

Management of Medications

The pre-ECT assessment should include a review of all medications to optimize the patient's medical status and avoid potential adverse effects from drug–drug and drug–treatment interactions (American Psychiatric Association 2001). This review should be followed by recommendations for any applicable medication changes before the start of the ECT course, as well as how medications should be taken during the ECT series.

Medications that have a protective effect against potential ECT medical adverse effects should be continued (American Psychiatric Association 2001). However, some medications make it more difficult to induce a therapeutic seizure with ECT or increase the risk of adverse effects. In such cases, unless there is a compelling reason to continue the agent, the dosage should be decreased or discontinued, taking into account the possibility of withdrawal effects. Whenever appropriate, the patient's medical provider should be contacted about any potential nonpsychiatric medication changes. The following medications are among those best avoided or maintained at the lowest possible levels during an ECT course: 1) lithium, which may increase the risks for delirium or prolonged seizures (Patel et al. 2020); 2) benzodiazepines, whose anticonvulsant properties may decrease efficacy (but can be reversed with flumazenil at the time of ECT) (Krystal et al. 1998); and 3) antiepileptic drugs, whose anticonvulsant properties may decrease efficacy (however, if used to control epilepsy or brittle bipolar disorder, the medication should be withheld the night before and the morning of treatment). Antiepileptic medications have been found to increase the seizure threshold and to decrease seizure duration, although the clinical significance is unclear (Ak and Yalçin 2018).

There are considerable differences of opinion and in practice regarding the use of other psychotropic medications during the acute ECT course. Compelling evidence exists for a potentiating effect of psychotropic medication on ECT with the use of antipsychotic agents in individuals with schizophrenia (and inferentially in those with psychotic depression) (Haskett and Loo 2010). The literature regarding the benefits of antidepressant medication to augment ECT response is unclear, although it does not appear that such a combination is associated with significantly increased risk, and there is some evidence that newer antidepressant agents may be of benefit (Sackeim et al. 2009). In addition to the possibility of potentiating efficacy, antidepressant medication augmentation may also be necessary because it may be difficult to accomplish complete drug withdrawal before instituting ECT or because there is a desire to decrease the risk of early relapse after ECT.

On the days of ECT, medications that should be administered before each treatment are those that optimize medical status or are thought to exert a protective effect in the context of ECT-induced physiological changes. Medications that are taken the morning of treatment should be taken with a sip of water. These include antihypertensive and antianginal medications, antiarrhythmic agents (except lidocaine and analogues, due to negative effects on seizure elicitation) (Devanand and Sackeim 1988), antireflux medications, bronchodilators (except theophylline, given the risk of prolonged seizures), glaucoma medication (except long-acting cholinesterase inhibitors), and corticosteroids (although extra "stress doses" are unnecessary in ECT practice) (Rasmussen et al. 2008).

Medications that should be withheld on ECT days until after the treatment include all psychotropic medications, which is particularly important for lithium, benzodiazepines, and anticonvulsant medications. Medications that can interfere with seizure induction should also be withheld the night before treatment. Other medications that should be withheld until after treatment include diuretics, because these may increase the risk of incontinence and bladder rupture. For diabetic patients, some practitioners split the morning dose of long-acting insulin into before- and after-treatment doses; however, it is important to monitor blood glucose levels and to adjust insulin dosing as necessary, involving medical consultation as needed (Netzel et al. 2002).

Technique

Inpatient Versus Outpatient Administration

Although ECT has traditionally been used primarily in the inpatient setting, a shift has occurred over time—much like the one that has occurred for surgical procedures—to offer it on an outpatient basis (American Psychiatric Association 2001). At present, inpatient ECT is reserved for situations in which either the patient's psychiatric illness itself requires an inpatient level of care or in which it is necessary to ensure that ECT can be safely administered (e.g., for patients with high medical risk factors and no social support system). These situations are particularly likely to occur with older adults. Even when inpatient treatments are initially required, consideration should be given to switching to outpatient treatment when it is clinically feasible, particularly for those who have improved cognitive and functional status, a medically uncomplicated course, and a responsible adult at home (Lapid et al. 2018).

Anesthetic Considerations

ECT is a procedure involving general anesthesia and muscle paralysis. Airway management, the administration of medications necessary for anesthesia, and the handling of medical emergencies during and immediately following the ECT procedure are the responsibility of the anesthesia provider (American Psychiatric Association 2001). Appropriate medical backup should be readily available, particularly for high-risk cases. With older adults, it is important to recognize that lower doses of anesthetic medications may be indicated because of altered metabolism or tolerance. In addition, time to effect may be longer in elderly patients. On the other hand, under some circumstances, higher doses may be necessary (e.g., more relaxant agent may be needed for a patient with osteoporosis).

The patient is ventilated by mask with 100% oxygen throughout the procedure, beginning at least a few minutes before anesthesia induction and lasting until a satisfactory level of spontaneous respiration and blood oxygenation is maintained. General anesthesia is usually induced with intravenous methohexital, typically 1 mg/kg (Ding and White 2002; Saito 2005). It is best to avoid using propofol as the general anesthetic due to its negative effects on both seizure duration and seizure quality (Vaidya et al. 2012). Because seizure threshold (the amount of electricity necessary to induce a seizure) appears to increase with age and the stimulus output of ECT devices is limited by the FDA (U.S. Food and Drug Administration 2018), difficulties in seizure induction can be experienced with older adults, particularly late in an index ECT course. In such situations, the anesthetic can be switched to one with fewer anticonvulsant properties (e.g., etomidate [Singh et al. 2015] or ketamine [McGirr et al. 2015]).

After the patient loses consciousness, the muscle relaxant succinylcholine is administered intravenously, typically 1 mg/kg, to minimize the ictal motor response (American Psychiatric Association 2001). Succinylcholine has long been used during ECT because of its rapid onset and short duration of action. However, it is contraindicated in patients with hyperkalemia, extensive motor rigidity, inherited or acquired pseudocholinesterase deficiency (e.g., severe liver disease or prolonged malnutrition), and some neuromuscular diseases (e.g., muscular dystrophy). In such cases, rocuronium, with reversal via sugammadex, is typically used (Hoshi et al. 2011). When succinylcholine is used, optimal muscular relaxation can be ascertained by the disappearance of relaxant-induced fasciculations and the loss of muscle tone, deep tendon reflexes, or twitch response to a peripheral nerve stimulator. Prior to application of the electrical stimulus, a mouth guard should be placed and the patient's chin held manually, closing the mouth during stimulus delivery to prevent oral trauma due to direct stimulation of masseter muscles.

The anticholinergic medication glycopyrrolate (which is less likely to be associated with postictal delirium than atropine) may be administered before general anesthesia to minimize the risk of stimulus-related asystole and postictal oral secretions. However, such agents should be used selectively because they may potentiate tachycardia throughout the procedure. When hypertension and tachycardia are severe or when prophylaxis is indicated based on preexisting cardiovascular disease, β-blocking medications (e.g., labetalol) and other antihypertensive agents (e.g., nicardipine or hydralazine) can be used to minimize these effects. However, these agents should also be used selectively given the risk of bradycardia and hypotension postictally.

Anesthetic considerations for postictal agitation or delirium, which is more common in elderly patients, include providing reassurance and maintaining a quiet, low-light environment during the postictal recovery process. However, when necessary, pharmacological management can include intravenous agents, such as midazolam (1 mg IV), the α_2 agonist dexmedetomidine (10–40 μg IV), haloperidol (2–5 mg IV), or propofol (0.5 mg/kg IV). Dexmedetomidine is interesting because if it is administered preictally, it will also blunt the sympathetically mediated rise in heart rate and blood pressure during the induced seizure (Aydogan et al. 2013).

During 2020, the severe worldwide COVID-19 viral pandemic impacted the delivery of medical care, particularly treatments that involved direct airway management, including ECT. The provision of nonurgent procedures and surgery became heavily curtailed, and those that did take place required major revision in technique, particularly with respect to anesthesia administration. Although these practice revisions varied in scope, expert consensus recommendations for overall ECT patient populations during the pandemic surge were provided by Lapid et al. (2020), and recommendations for ECT administration to COVID-19 patients were provided by Braithwaite et al. (2020).

Physiological Monitoring

During ECT, as with any procedure using general anesthesia, vital signs and pulse oximetry are monitored throughout the procedure and during the immediate postictal period until stabilized. After spontaneous respiration resumes and vital signs and oxygen saturation begin trending toward baseline, the patient is moved to a postanesthesia care unit or area (previously referred to as a recovery room), where monitoring of vital signs and oxygenation continues.

Both the motor and electroencephalographic representations of seizure activity are monitored during ECT. To allow monitoring of the motor response in a patient whose muscles are relaxed, a blood pressure cuff is placed around the ankle and inflated to ~200 mm Hg just before administration of the muscle relaxant. This action prevents muscle activity distal to the cuff from being suppressed during the seizure. Ictal electroencephalographic recordings are made using recording leads placed on the head in conjunction with amplification and display capabilities built into the ECT device. Two electroencephalographic channels should be recorded so that seizure activity from both the left and the right cerebral hemispheres can be monitored. Such recording can be accomplished by placing one pair of recording electrodes over the left prefrontal and left mastoid areas and the other pair over the homologous areas on the right.

Stimulus Electrode Placement

There are presently three major types of ECT stimulus electrode placement: bitemporal, bifrontal, and unilateral nondominant (the right side for most individuals). Bitemporal

ECT involves placing both stimulus electrodes over the frontotemporal regions, with the center of each electrode ~1 inch above the midpoint of a line transecting the external canthus of the eye and the tragus of the ear. Bifrontal electrode placement involves locating the center of the stimulus electrodes ~5 cm superior to each external canthus. The preferred type of unilateral nondominant placement involves putting one electrode over the right frontotemporal area (as described for bitemporal ECT) and the other over the right centroparietal area, just to the right of the vertex of the scalp, a point defined by the intersection of lines between the inion and nasion and between the tragi of both ears.

There is significant controversy over the choice of stimulus electrode placement (American Psychiatric Association 2001). Although unilateral ECT appears to be effective in many patients as long as stimulus intensity is sufficient (see "Stimulus Dosing" section and a recent meta-analysis by Kolshus et al. 2017), some patients may preferentially respond to brief-pulse bitemporal ECT. On the other hand, ECT-associated amnesia is greater with bitemporal ECT. A reasonable trade-off is to use unilateral ECT initially unless an urgent response is necessary or the patient has indicated a preference for or has shown a past preferential response to bitemporal ECT. Data are mixed regarding bifrontal electrode placement, the newest of the three techniques (Bailine et al. 2000), with some studies suggesting that both the efficacy and the cognitive effects of bifrontal ECT may be less than with bitemporal ECT and perhaps slightly greater than with unilateral ECT. However, a large multicenter trial did not show an advantage for bifrontal ECT (Kellner et al. 2010).

The choice of stimulus electrode placement is particularly challenging in older patients. An urgent need for a rapid response is often present in these individuals, yet adverse cognitive effects are of concern, especially in patients with preexisting cerebral impairment. One study reported that high-dose brief-pulse unilateral ECT was as effective as bitemporal ECT in older adults (Stoppe et al. 2006), although the placement controversy is still not resolved.

Recently, there has been renewed interest in optimizing stimulus electrode placement, based in part on a belief that minimizing stimulus current flow in areas vital to memory recall (e.g., left hippocampus) would be associated with a substantial decrease in ECT-induced amnesia (Bai et al. 2017). One investigational approach, FEAST, involves the use of a novel stimulus electrode placement with a relatively small right prefrontal electrode and a large rectangular electrode placed over the right precentral region (Nahas et al. 2013). An additional innovative feature of the FEAST technique is the use of a unidirectional electrical stimulus that acts to provide a more efficient activation of prefrontal structures. A recent small controlled clinical trial comparing FEAST with ultrabrief-pulse right unilateral ECT reported some promising but not statistically significant cognitive advantage for FEAST over ECT (Sahlem et al. 2020), and a larger multicenter trial is presently under way.

An additional innovative focal seizure therapy approach is MST, which, because it involves a magnetic stimulus device, is discussed later in the section "Other Brain Stimulation Modalities."

Stimulus Waveform

All contemporary ECT devices used in the United States use a bidirectional, constant-current, brief-pulse stimulus waveform. This is more efficient than the older sine-wave stimulus for inducing seizures and allows ECT to be administered with fewer adverse cognitive effects (Weiner et al. 1986). More recently, these devices have incorporated the use of the ultrabrief-pulse stimulus, defined as a pulse width duration of <0.5 ms. The ultrabrief-pulse stimulus is a more efficient way to induce seizures (Loo et al. 2007) and is associated with less memory impairment. Although ultrabrief-pulse unilateral ECT may also be associated with a slightly more delayed antidepressant effect than unilateral ECT with brief-pulse stimuli (Luccarelli et al. 2020; Sackeim et al. 2008), most patients do just as well.

Stimulus Dosing

Regardless of stimulus waveform type, the paradigm for the choice of stimulus dose intensity remains as controversial as the choice of electrode placement. The disagreement centers on whether to dose with respect to an empirically determined seizure threshold estimate obtained at the first treatment (dose-titration technique) or to use a formula based on factors such as age, sex, and electrode placement (formula-based technique) (American Psychiatric Association 2001). Coffey et al. (1995) found that the dose-titration technique is better because it offers a more precise means to determine the patient's seizure threshold (which can vary manyfold) and thereby allows the practitioner to more effectively individualize and control stimulus intensity. In practice, seizure threshold is estimated at the first treatment by incrementally increasing the dosage from a low level until a seizure is induced.

Compelling evidence now indicates that stimulus intensity for unilateral brief-pulse ECT should be somewhere between 2.5 and 8 times the seizure threshold (in terms of electrical charge), with the range reflecting uncertainty as to the minimum dosage necessary to optimize therapeutic outcome (McCall et al. 2000). Notably, increasing stimulus intensity also increases the severity of ECT-associated memory impairment, although to a lesser degree than a switch to bitemporal ECT. Stimulus intensity is less of an issue with bitemporal brief-pulse ECT, in which a stimulus 1.5 times the seizure threshold appears to be sufficient. However, stimulus intensity is of most concern with ultrabrief-pulse ECT, certainly for unilateral electrode placement but likely also for bitemporal and bifrontal placement (Sackeim et al. 2008). Although evidence-based guidance in this regard is presently limited, it is recommended for ultrabrief-pulse stimuli that a stimulus intensity six to eight times the seizure threshold be used for unilateral ECT and four to six times the seizure threshold for bitemporal treatments.

As alluded to earlier (see "Anesthetic Considerations"), seizure threshold is a function of age, with substantially higher thresholds present in older adults. This higher threshold leaves these patients at greater risk for being unable to receive a stimulus of sufficient intensity because the maximum output of the ECT devices used in the United States is limited by FDA regulations (Krystal et al. 2000a). The risk that the threshold will exceed the maximum available stimulus intensity is highest late in the treatment course because the seizure threshold rises to a varying extent with the number of treatments. However, recent evidence has shown that a trial of high-intensity, brief-pulse bitemporal ECT might be effective for patients with MDD who have failed to respond to trials with alternative ECT modalities (Sackeim et al. 2020), although it is understood that this exposes these individuals to an increased risk of adverse cognitive effects.

Determination of Seizure Adequacy

ECT-induced seizures are identical to spontaneous grand mal seizures except that with ECT the motor response is attenuated by a muscle relaxant agent. The electroencephalographic recording during ECT (ictal electroencephalogram) exhibits the typical features of a grand mal seizure, with irregular polyspike activity marking the tonic portion of the seizure and repetitive polyspike and slow-wave discharges during the clonic component. During the immediate postictal period, a relative suppression (i.e., flattening) of electroencephalographic activity can typically be seen (Weiner et al. 1991).

Compelling evidence indicates that not all seizures are equally potent from a therapeutic perspective. With unilateral ECT, barely suprathreshold seizures—despite having identical durations to seizures from more moderately suprathreshold stimuli—are only minimally therapeutic (Sackeim et al. 1993), and newer data support a similar finding for ultrabrief-pulse bitemporal stimulus electrode placement. Based on findings that seizures with higher stimulus intensity exhibit attributes such as higher amplitude, greater regularity in shape, and greater postictal electroencephalographic suppression (Krystal et al. 1995) and that such features appear to be associated with therapeutic response to ECT, a growing interest has developed in the possibility that electroencephalographically based stimulus dosing may one day be feasible. This type of innovation is attractive because it would allow practitioners a means to tailor the stimulus intensity to the minimum therapeutic dosage for each patient and control for the variable rise in seizure threshold that occurs over the ECT course (Krystal et al. 2000b). ECT device manufacturers in the United States have incorporated "seizure quality" features into their devices, although the utility of these features in routine clinical use remains to be established (American Psychiatric Association 2001; Francis-Taylor et al. 2020; Rasmussen et al. 2007). This utility is particularly questionable for ultrabrief-pulse ECT, in which the seizures appear less intense than with brief-pulse ECT and the postictal electroencephalographic suppression is less apparent (qualities that also may make determination of seizure endpoint more challenging). Regardless of stimulus waveform, seizure quality determinations can be more difficult with elderly patients, possibly due to the effects of age-related neuronal loss on the extent of ictal hypersynchrony.

Frequency and Number of Acute Treatments

In the United States, ECT is typically administered three times a week, with an acute or index course usually lasting between 6 and 12 treatments, although more or fewer are sometimes necessary. The frequency of acute ECT may be reduced to twice a week or even once a week if amnesia or confusion becomes a major problem (American Psychiatric Association 2001), which is not infrequent with elderly patients. In many other countries, acute ECT is administered twice a week throughout the course, with a controlled comparison study showing equal overall efficacy and slower response, fewer treatments, and fewer cognitive deficits with twice-weekly versus thrice-weekly treatments (Charlson et al. 2012).

The decision about when to end the index ECT course depends on treatment outcome. In general, the index course is considered complete when a therapeutic plateau has occurred—that is, when the patient has reached a maximum level of response. If no substantial improvement occurs by the sixth treatment, consideration should be given to making changes in the ECT technique, such as increasing stimulus intensity, changing stimulus pulse duration, switching stimulus electrode placement, or discontinuing any medications with anticonvulsant properties. If no response occurs after 12 ECT treatments, alternative treatment modalities should be considered, such as combination pharmacotherapy using multiple agents of different classes.

Maintenance Therapy

As discussed earlier, the diagnoses for which ECT is utilized are typically recurrent in nature. The risk of relapse is extremely high, particularly in the first 6 months (Tew et al. 2007), especially for patients with psychotic depression and those whose illness was resistant to medications prior to ECT (Flint and Rifat 1998; Sackeim et al. 1990), necessitating an aggressive program of maintenance treatment to minimize the likelihood of relapse. Maintenance treatment may be pharmacological or in the form of maintenance ECT (given at much greater intervals).

Pharmacological Maintenance Therapy

Pharmacological maintenance treatment is usually attempted after the initial acute ECT course unless the patient has a strong preference for maintenance ECT. There does not appear to be a benefit to starting an antidepressant during the acute course (Prudic et al. 2013). With MDD, evidence suggests that a combination of antidepressant and mood stabilizer may be more effective in maintaining remission than an antidepressant medication alone (Sackeim et al. 2001a). Unfortunately, medication resistance during the index episode may diminish the likelihood of a sustained prophylactic effect (Prudic et al. 2013; Sackeim et al. 1990). Maintenance pharmacotherapy following ECT treatment of mania or schizophrenia has not been well studied, although it has been recommended that patients with mania receive a mood stabilizer and possibly an antipsychotic medication and that patients with schizophrenia receive antipsychotic agents (Sackeim 1994). In the absence of applicable data, an aggressive regimen of different drug classes should be considered.

Maintenance ECT

The efficacy of maintenance ECT for patients with various diagnoses has already been discussed. The high relapse rate after an ECT series, even with pharmacological maintenance therapy, continues to generate ongoing interest in the technique and optimization of maintenance ECT, often combined with pharmacotherapy, psychotherapy, or both. Although there are no established guidelines for a maintenance ECT regimen, practitioners traditionally begin with weekly treatments for 2–4 weeks, followed by 1–2 months of biweekly treatments, and then by 3-week and then 4-week intervals. After 6–12 months, treatments is either stopped or continued at an even lower frequency. Although many patients receiving maintenance ECT do well with such a regimen, others seem to require more frequent treatments or further augmentation with psychotropic medications or psychotherapy. Some patients eventually relapse, leading to another acute ECT course or a switch to alternative treatment modalities.

In recent decades, many providers have shifted toward a more symptom-titrated dosing frequency for maintenance ECT treatments, which represents a trade-off between minimizing the number of treatments and minimizing the likelihood of relapse. Such a regimen works best when there is good ongoing communication between the ECT provider, other mental health practitioners, and the patient and family. Based on data from a multicenter trial of maintenance ECT versus maintenance pharmacotherapy, Lisanby et al. (2008) suggested a highly structured symptom-based approach to maintenance ECT for patients with MDD whose illness responded well to an acute course of ECT. With this approach, the patient is administered four weekly treatments followed by close monitoring for at least 6 months; recurrence of depressive symptoms is followed by one or two ECT treatments during the following week. That approach, combined with maintenance pharmacotherapy and lithium, was tested in a large, multicenter, controlled 6-month trial of patients whose illness remitted with ECT. Patients who received ECT plus pharmacotherapy were compared with a group of patients who received only the dual-agent pharmacotherapy (Kellner et al. 2016a). The combination treatment group showed significantly less relapse than the pharmacotherapy-only group, even though most of the ECT plus pharmacotherapy group's subjects did not require any maintenance treatments after the initial four weekly ECTs.

In terms of cognitive effects, maintenance ECT is significantly better tolerated than acute ECT, particularly if the interval between treatments is kept large. A review of the cognitive effects of maintenance ECT in elderly patients suggests that this group is not at particularly increased risk in this regard (Tielkes et al. 2008). However, some patients requiring frequent maintenance ECT do experience cumulative difficulties with amnesia, and this possibility should be considered in treatment planning. Given the general good tolerance of maintenance ECT, there is no maximum lifetime number of ECT treatments.

Other Brain Stimulation Modalities

In recent years, major research initiatives have been undertaken to study and further develop alternative brain stimulation approaches for the treatment of depression. Most of these trials have been conducted in the general adult population, and thus these approaches have not been tested exhaustively in elderly patients despite their potential of these approaches for successfully treating late-life depression. Nevertheless, results from TMS, MST, tDCS, VNS, and DBS use in adult populations are promising. For the purposes of the present chapter, these treatments can be divided into noninvasive (i.e., not requiring surgery), which includes TMS, MST, and tDCS, and invasive (i.e., surgical), which includes VNS and DBS.

Noninvasive Approaches

Transcranial Magnetic Stimulation

TMS is presently the most common alternative brain stimulation approach to ECT. It involves the noninvasive and nonconvulsive use of time-varying electromagnetic fields to stimulate the surface of the brain (Barker et al. 1985; Ilmoniemi et al. 1999). The basic principle is that a rapidly alternating electric current is run through a stimulation coil placed above the target brain area. This changing electric current produces a magnetic field that passes through the scalp and skull unimpeded. When the magnetic field pulse reaches the surface of the brain, it induces an electric field that depolarizes the affected neurons. Most of this activation occurs directly under the stimulation coil, but TMS has also been shown to modulate remote brain regions by stimulating structurally connected networks (Bestmann et al. 2004).

When a train involving multiple TMS pulses is delivered, known as repetitive TMS (rTMS), the stimulation can produce long-lasting plastic changes in the brain. Depending on the stimulation frequency applied, these changes may either be inhibitory or excitatory. Repeating TMS pulses with a low frequency (≤ 1 Hz) inhibit brain function, whereas high frequencies (≥ 5 Hz) excite function. In the treatment of MDD, excitatory rTMS (commonly 10–20 Hz) is applied to the left dorsolateral prefrontal cortex (DLPFC) or inhibitory rTMS (typically 1 Hz) is delivered to the right DLPFC. The rationale for these stimulation protocols is based on the characteristic hypoactivity of the left DLPFC and the hyperactivity of the right DLPFC in the context of depression, as identified by early PET and functional MRI studies (Grimm et al. 2008). However, in depression protocols, it is common only to provide excitatory rTMS to the left DLPFC.

High-frequency rTMS applied to the left DLPFC has been approved by the FDA to treat mild to moderate depression in patients with a maximum age of 69 years whose illness has failed to respond to at least one antidepressant medication (Gellersen and Kedzior 2019). Typically, rTMS is given 5 days a week for 4–6 weeks. Recently, accelerated protocols—that is, several sessions per day—have also emerged (Baeken 2018). The antidepressant efficacy associated with currently available protocols is comparable with that of pharmacotherapeutic interventions (Lefaucheur et al. 2020). In previous studies, the degree of prior treatment resistance, shorter current episode of depression, and absence of comorbid anxiety disorder have been linked with a higher antidepressant efficacy (Demitrack and Thase 2009).

A few variations of rTMS configuration have arisen with similar antidepressant efficacies. One coil design modification has established deep TMS (dTMS), which was approved by the FDA for depression in 2013 (Kaster et al. 2018) and for OCD in 2018 (Carmi et al. 2018). dTMS uses an H-shaped coil that allows stimulation of slightly deeper structures than the figure-of-eight coil, but with a trade-off of losing the focality of the stimulation. A second rTMS variation relating to the temporal characteristics of the stimulation pattern is theta-burst stimulation (TBS), which received FDA approval in 2018 (Blumberger et al. 2018). In TBS, stimulation is applied with a figure-of-eight coil using bursts of three TMS pulses given at 50 Hz frequency and repeated every 200 ms (i.e., at theta frequency). TBS includes two protocols: continuous TBS, in which the repeated stimulation bursts are provided without any pauses, resulting in inhibition of underlying brain activity, and intermittent TBS, in which the repeated bursts are given in trains of 2 seconds followed by an 8-second pause. Intermittent TBS results in enhanced brain activity. Due to increased stimulation frequency compared with standard rTMS and dTMS, more pulses can be given in a shorter time. Thus, TBS treatment can be delivered in a few minutes, compared with 30–40 minutes in conventional rTMS and dTMS treatments. There is preliminary evidence that a further innovation with intermittent TBS, in which it is given multiple times a day, may allow very rapid improvement in patients with MDD (Cole et al. 2020).

For rTMS to be an optimally efficient treatment, the TMS pulses should be targeted to a specific cortical region (Lefaucheur et al. 2007). Targeting can be done using a standardized 10–20 electroencephalography electrode location (e.g., F3 for left DLPFC) or by using other scalp-based measures or stereotactic systems. The most accurate localization method is MRI-guided neuronavigation, which continuously visualizes the TMS coil location with respect to the surface of the brain. This also allows the targeting of TMS to a functionally determined area that can be based on, for example, functional MRI findings (Cash et al. 2020).

Overall, rTMS has had a strong safety record accompanied by minimal side effects, which is important in the treatment of elderly adults (Loo et al. 2008; O'Reardon et al. 2007; Rossi et al. 2009). Studies have consistently shown that rTMS is relatively well tolerated and accepted by patients. The procedure has resulted in only mild adverse effects, the most common of which are transient headaches and muscle twitches and pain at the stimulation site (George et al. 2010; O'Reardon et al. 2007). These effects may be minimized by adjusting the stimulation parameters or coil location. Also important for elderly patients is that no significant adverse cognitive effects have been noted; in fact, rTMS may even improve cognition (Martin et al. 2017). A more serious risk posed by the potential for inadvertent seizure induction is rare, and many instances of reported seizures have involved neurologically compromised patients or rTMS parameters that did not follow the recommended guidelines (Lerner et al. 2019; Rossi et al. 2021; Wani et al. 2013).

The recent COVID-19 pandemic has temporarily impacted rTMS utilization and safety, as it has for many other medical treatments requiring direct in-person management, with pertinent clinical guidelines for its use recently made available (Bikson et al. 2020). The common contraindications for rTMS are nonremovable implanted ferromagnetic devices or other magnetic-sensitive metal implants in or near the head. However, the presence of metal may not be an absolute contraindication if it is located far from the stimulated area (Rossi et al. 2009). Other common contraindications are epilepsy and a history of seizures (Downar et al. 2016; Lerner et al. 2019).

In summary, small sample sizes and varying rTMS parameters in previous studies limit drawing extensive conclusions on the efficacy of rTMS in geriatric populations. Geriatric patients also have unique neurobiological features that must be considered in rTMS applications, notably prefrontal atrophy. Cortical atrophy increases the distance that the magnetic field needs to travel, which attenuates the field; thus, the stimulation intensity needs to be increased accordingly (Nahas et al. 2004). Due to these anatomical changes, some of the older studies in which rTMS was provided to geriatric populations with the same parameters as in younger adult populations found rTMS to be ineffective in the elderly subjects. However, results from recent studies, in which the stimulation intensity was increased to overcome mild atrophy, have instead supported efficacy in geriatric patients (Blumberger et al. 2015). Another rTMS parameter that is an age-dependent moderator of efficacy is the number of TMS pulses. Most studies showing effectiveness in elderly patients have used a higher number of pulses than those reporting an age-related reduction in efficacy (Sabesan et al. 2015).

In terms of future developments, existing rTMS technology continues to evolve, allowing greater precision in targeting the optimal area and the fine-tuning of stimulus parameters. Many recent studies on adult populations have concentrated on using new pulse frequencies and delivery patterns, optimizing dosage and duration of treatment, finding optimal target locations and biomarkers, and developing efficient maintenance protocols. Future studies are also needed to optimize treatment parameters in geriatric populations.

Magnetic Seizure Therapy

MST is a noninvasive brain stimulation method that is being investigated for the treatment of depression (Lisanby et al. 2001). MST methodology is based on both rTMS and ECT, with the aim of inducing a similar therapeutic seizure to that in ECT but using time-varying electromagnetic fields. To induce a seizure, the applied stimulation frequencies, pulse-train durations, and intensities need to be much higher than in conventional rTMS. The rationale behind MST is that the magnetic field–induced electric fields are more focal and can be better controlled in comparison with electric fields applied directly on the scalp, as in ECT and FEAST. Also, MST-induced electric fields only affect directly underlying cortical regions and not deeper brain structures like those in ECT. This may explain the diminished cognitive side effects with MST.

The first MST treatments were given with stimulation frequencies varying between 40 Hz and 50 Hz, but recent studies have increased the frequency up to 100 Hz because this can induce seizures more reliably (Spellman et al. 2008). Currently, a twin coil consisting of two cone-shaped coils placed bilaterally is used, but round, double-cone, and cap-cone stimulation coils have also been used (Kallioniemi et al. 2019).

The current treatment protocol in MST is very similar to that in ECT (Kallioniemi et al. 2019). The treatments are always administered under low-level general anesthesia and a paralytic agent. The dosage of stimulation is individualized for each patient by measuring the seizure threshold, determined by increasing the MST stimulation duration until motor activity in a cuffed limb and ictal electroencephalogram can be clearly seen. Treatments are provided with a suprathreshold duration, two or three times per week, until the patient's illness has remitted. Available evidence shows that MST-induced seizures differ from those of ECT because they have lower electroencephalographic amplitude during the ictal phase, have less postictal suppression, and may be briefer than with ECT (Backhouse et al. 2018; Hoy and Fitzgerald 2011).

Present research suggests that MST may induce a comparable antidepressant outcome as with ECT but with fewer associated cognitive side effects (Daskalakis et al. 2020; McClintock et al. 2011). Also, MST is efficient in reducing suicidality (Sun et al. 2016). The recovery and reorientation times associated with MST are much shorter than for ECT, and most patients can recover and reorient within a few minutes after the seizure (McClintock et al. 2011). MST may also be associated with less headache and nausea than ECT but otherwise involves similar anesthesia-related side effects as ECT (Kallioniemi et al. 2019).

Preliminary evidence for the efficacy of MST still awaits confirmation in large-scale controlled clinical trials, and it has not yet been explicitly applied in the geriatric population. Furthermore, knowledge on optimal MST parameters remains scarce. However, if proven effective, MST may provide a cognitively safer antidepressant option for geriatric populations. MST has not yet been approved by the FDA (as of October 2021).

Transcranial Direct Current Stimulation

tDCS is a noninvasive brain stimulation method that uses a weak subconvulsive level of constant direct current (commonly 1–2.5 mA) that is subthreshold for inducing action potentials but can alter neuronal excitability (Arul-Anandam and Loo 2009). The method remains under development and has not received FDA approval for the treatment of depression (as of October 2021). Administration involves placing two stimulus electrodes at targeted areas on the patient's head, such that the electric current passing between them flows through the underlying cortical tissue. The anode (i.e., the positively charged electrode) increases cortical excitability, whereas the cathode— the negatively charged electrode—induces an inhibitory effect in the underlying brain tissue. To treat depression, the anode is commonly placed over the left DLPFC and the cathode on the right hemisphere (Arul-Anandam and Loo 2009). Stimulation is given for 20–30 minutes and repeated daily for 4–6 weeks.

Because it is in the early phases of development, tDCS has not yet been extensively tested in the geriatric population, but in the general adult population it has demonstrated small to moderate antidepressant effects (Kalu et al. 2012). As in rTMS, mood effects usually occur after several weeks of treatment; thus, tDCS cannot induce a rapid response like ECT. Several factors, such as the length and frequency of treatment, lead placement, and patient characteristics, influence treatment outcomes (Brunoni et al. 2012). tDCS is attractive as a brain stimulation treatment due to its demonstrated minimal risk of severe adverse effects. Minor adverse effects commonly reported by patients include burning, tingling, and itching sensations at the stimulation site during treatment (Bikson et al. 2016). Thus, should tDCS prove efficacious in the treatment of MDD, it could serve as a promising simpler, lower-risk, and potentially at-home noninvasive treatment that provides a viable alternative with minimal side effects in the treatment of late-life depression.

Invasive Approaches

Vagus Nerve Stimulation

VNS is an invasive neuromodulatory treatment initially approved by the FDA for the treatment of refractory epilepsy in 1997. After mood improvements were seen in patients, its efficacy in depression was investigated (Manepalli and Sapkota 2014). The vagus nerve is thought to affect depression via its relationship with areas of the brain associated with mood regulation, which is supported by some neuroimaging studies (Daban et al. 2008). In 2005, VNS was approved by the FDA for treatment-resistant depression. Indications include severe and recurrent major depressive episodes lasting ≥2 years and failure of four other treatments.

VNS involves the implantation of a small, battery-operated electrical pulse generator the size of a cardiac pacemaker in the patient's chest to provide intermittent electrical stimulation to the left vagus nerve. An external programming device is used to activate the device and to adjust stimulus dosing. The most reported side effects of VNS are voice alteration and increased cough (Sackeim et al. 2001b), but these effects often resolve as the patient develops tolerance to the stimulation. Physicians can also alter the stimulation levels to reduce side effects and potentiate efficacy. Due to the surgical procedures involved, VNS may lead to acute complications and serious adverse events, although these are rare.

So far, the efficacy of VNS in treating depression has been limited, with low effect sizes and evidence of effectiveness only after several months of stimulation (Manepalli and Sapkota 2014). However, ongoing research indicates that any beneficial effects may be long-lasting (McAllister-Williams et al. 2020). The safety and efficacy data in geriatric patients are currently insufficient, but a few case studies suggest that VNS is safe and reasonably well tolerated in this patient population (Merrill et al. 2006; Sirven et al. 2000).

Deep Brain Stimulation

DBS is an investigational invasive neuromodulation modality that continues to be evaluated for severe treatment-resistant depression. It was approved by the FDA for the treatment of Parkinson's disease in 2002 and has since been approved for a Humanitarian Device Exemption for the treatment of highly refractory OCD. It has not yet been approved by the FDA for treatment of depression (as of October 2021). Many patients being treated for Parkinson's disease with DBS implants report concomitant improvement in mood symptoms (Kuehn 2007), and this finding generated interest in DBS as an approach to treat severe depression.

DBS involves stereotactic surgical implantation of electrodes in a targeted area deep within the brain, such as the subgenual cingulate (i.e., Brodmann area 25) in depression. Other brain regions have also been tested, including the ventral striatum and nucleus accumbens (Schlaepfer et al. 2008, 2014). The implanted electrodes are attached to an electrical pulse generator implanted in the patient's chest wall, and constant electrical stimulation is delivered. As with VNS, the frequency and intensity of this current can be controlled with a small handheld programming device. Despite the invasive nature of DBS, an important strength is that it has not been shown to affect cognitive functioning (Mayberg et al. 2005). Still, there are risks associated with the surgical procedure, including infection, bleeding, and seizures. In addition, irritability, headaches, and pain at the generator site have been reported (Lozano et al. 2008). Further research is attempting to identify other subcortical regions for targeting stimulation and to establish techniques and procedures that minimize such side effects (Crowell et al. 2019; Schlaepfer et al. 2014).

Future of ECT and Other Brain Stimulation Therapies

The clinical importance of ECT has persisted for more than 80 years despite the development of many alternative treatment options. Its continued viability in the future, however, depends not only on the extent and value of further innovations in alternative treatments but also on the success of ongoing and future ECT optimization efforts to maximize efficacy and minimize adverse cognitive effects. As noted, research is under way to improve on the available options for both stimulus electrode placement and electrical stimulus parameters. Other work is being done to enable practitioners to better predict which patients might be ECT responders.

Future alternatives to ECT include not only new psychopharmacological agents but also new types of brain stimulation therapies, such as TMS, MST, tDCS, VNS, and DBS. Although these innovative alternative brain stimulation techniques are still in their early phases of development and only limited data are available to support their present use in the geriatric population, they are conceptually appealing due to the absence of the neurocognitive and systemic side effects typically associated with both ECT and pharmacological treatments. Table 21–1 delineates the respective advantages and disadvantages of the different types of brain stimulation modalities that have been discussed in this chapter.

TABLE 21–1. Advantages and disadvantages of different types of brain stimulation in the treatment of psychiatric disorders

Treatment	Invasive vs. noninvasive	Advantages	Disadvantages
Deep brain stimulation (DBS)	Invasive	Automatic continuous stimulation	Surgical implantation with associated complications; replacement of device every few years
Electroconvulsive therapy (ECT)	Noninvasive	Efficacious and rapid response	Neurocognitive adverse effects; involves general anesthesia
Focal electrically administered seizure therapy (FEAST)	Noninvasive	Fewer neurocognitive effects than ECT (efficacy and speed of response uncertain)	Involves general anesthesia
Magnetic seizure therapy (MST)	Noninvasive	Fewer neurocognitive effects than ECT (efficacy and speed of response uncertain)	Involves general anesthesia
Transcranial magnetic stimulation (TMS) and transcranial direct current stimulation (tDCS)	Noninvasive	Minimal risk; no significant neurocognitive adverse events	Daily treatments; compliance issues; depth of stimulation needed for elderly patients
Vagus nerve stimulation (VNS)	Invasive	Automatic continuous stimulation	Surgical implantation with associated complications; replacement of device stimulator every few years

Additional studies are needed to explore the efficacy of these interventions in the treatment of severe treatment-resistant depression and other psychiatric disorders in elderly patients. In the meantime, a clear role remains for ECT in the treatment of various disorders, most notably MDD, for which older adults are at particularly high risk.

Key Points

- Electroconvulsive therapy (ECT) is the most rapid and effective treatment for major depressive episodes in older adults but is associated with varying degrees of cognitive dysfunction, particularly acutely.

- Major medical risks of ECT are largely a function of medical comorbidity.

- An acute ECT treatment course can be ended once a therapeutic plateau has been reached.

- The risk for relapse after an acute course of ECT is high, and aggressive maintenance treatment is needed.

- Other brain stimulation therapies for the treatment of depression include transcranial magnetic stimulation, magnetic seizure therapy, focal electrically administered seizure therapy, transcranial direct current stimulation, vagus nerve stimulation, and deep brain stimulation.

- Most non-ECT brain stimulation therapies have been studied primarily in the general adult population, and data supporting their efficacy in older adults are limited.

- Future clinical trials are needed to test the benefit of these and future brain stimulation therapies in the geriatric population.

Suggested Readings

Dukakis K, Tye L: Shock: The Healing Power of Electroconvulsive Therapy. New York, Avery, 2006

Endler NS: Holiday of Darkness, Revised. Toronto, ON, Wall and Davis, 1990

Fink M: Electroconvulsive Therapy: A Guide for Professionals and Their Patients, 2nd Edition. New York, Oxford University Press, 2010

Higgins ES, George MS: Brain Stimulation Therapies for Clinicians, 2nd Edition. Washington, DC, American Psychiatric Association Publishing, 2020

Kellner CH: Handbook of ECT: A Guide to Electroconvulsive Therapy for Practitioners. New York, Cambridge University Press, 2019

Mankad MV, Beyer JL, Weiner RD, et al: Clinical Manual of Electroconvulsive Therapy. Washington, DC, American Psychiatric Publishing, 2010

Manning M: Undercurrents: A Life Beneath the Surface. San Francisco, CA, HarperCollins, 1995

Rasmussen KG: Principles and Practice of Electroconvulsive Therapy. Washington, DC, American Psychiatric Association Publishing, 2019

Reti IM: Brain Stimulation: Methodologies and Interventions. New York, Wiley, 2015

Shorter E, Healy D: Shock Therapy: A History of Electroconvulsive Treatment in Mental Illness. New Brunswick, NJ, Rutgers University Press, 2007

Weiner RD (ed): The Practice of ECT: Recommendations for Treatment, Training, and Privileging, 2nd Edition. Washington, DC, American Psychiatric Publishing, 2001

References

Acharya D, Harper DG, Achtyes ED, et al: Safety and utility of acute electroconvulsive therapy for agitation and aggression in dementia. Int J Geriatr Psychiatry 30(3):265–273, 2015 24838521

Agarkar S, Hurt SW, Young RC: Speed of antidepressant response to electroconvulsive therapy in bipolar disorder vs. major depressive disorder. Psychiatry Res 265:355–359, 2018 29803951

Ak S, Yalçin N: Do antiepileptic drugs used during electroconvulsive therapy impact treatment process? J Clin Psychopharmacol 38(4):344–348, 2018 29912793

American Psychiatric Association: The Practice of Electroconvulsive Therapy: Recommendations for Treatment, Training, and Privileging, 2nd Edition. Washington, DC, American Psychiatric Publishing, 2001

American Psychiatric Association: Practice Guideline for the Treatment of Patients With Major Depressive Disorder, 3rd Edition. Washington, DC, American Psychiatric Association, 2010

Applegate RJ: Diagnosis and management of ischemic heart disease in the patient scheduled to undergo electroconvulsive therapy. Convuls Ther 13(3):128–144, 1997 9342129

Arul-Anandam AP, Loo C: Transcranial direct current stimulation: a new tool for the treatment of depression? J Affect Disord 117(3):137–145, 2009 19201483

Avery D, Lubrano A: Depression treated with imipramine and ECT: the DeCarolis study reconsidered. Am J Psychiatry 136(4B):559–562, 1979 426143

Aydogan MS, Yücel A, Begec Z, et al: The hemodynamic effects of dexmedetomidine and esmolol in electroconvulsive therapy: a retrospective comparison. J ECT 29(4):308–311, 2013 23774056

Backhouse FA, Noda Y, Knyahnytska Y, et al: Characteristics of ictal EEG in magnetic seizure therapy at various stimulation frequencies. Clin Neurophysiol 129(8):1770–1779, 2018 29735419

Baeken C: Accelerated rTMS: a potential treatment to alleviate refractory depression. Front Psychol 9:2017, 2018 30429807

Bahji A, Hawken ER, Sepehry AA, et al: ECT beyond unipolar major depression: systematic review and meta-analysis of electroconvulsive therapy in bipolar depression. Acta Psychiatr Scand 139(3):214–226, 2019 30506992

Bai S, Gálvez V, Dokos S, et al: Computational models of bitemporal, bifrontal and right unilateral ECT predict differential stimulation of brain regions associated with efficacy and cognitive side effects. Eur Psychiatry 41:21–29, 2017 28049077

Bailine SH, Rifkin A, Kayne E, et al: Comparison of bifrontal and bitemporal ECT for major depression. Am J Psychiatry 157(1):121–123, 2000 10618025

Barker AT, Jalinous R, Freeston IL: Non-invasive magnetic stimulation of human motor cortex. Lancet 325(8437):1106–1107, 1985 2860322

Bestmann S, Baudewig J, Siebner HR, et al: Functional MRI of the immediate impact of transcranial magnetic stimulation on cortical and subcortical motor circuits. Eur J Neurosci 19(7):1950–1962, 2004 15078569

Bikson M, Grossman P, Thomas C, et al: Safety of transcranial direct current stimulation: evidence based update. Brain Stimul 9(5):641–661, 2016 27372845

Bikson M, Hanlon CA, Woods AJ, et al: Guidelines for TMS/tES clinical services and research through the COVID-19 pandemic. Brain Stimul 13(4):1124–1149, 2020 32413554

Birkenhäger TK, Pluijms EM, Ju MR, et al: Influence of age on the efficacy of electroconvulsive therapy in major depression: a retrospective study. J Affect Disord 126(1–2):257–261, 2010 20303601

Blumberger DM, Hsu JH, Daskalakis ZJ: A review of brain stimulation treatments for late-life depression. Curr Treat Options Psychiatry 2(4):413–421, 2015 27398288

Blumberger DM, Seitz DP, Herrmann N, et al: Low medical morbidity and mortality after acute courses of electroconvulsive therapy in a population-based sample. Acta Psychiatr Scand 136(6):583–593, 2017 28922451

Blumberger DM, Vila-Rodriguez F, Thorpe KE, et al: Effectiveness of theta burst versus high-frequency repetitive transcranial magnetic stimulation in patients with depression (THREE-D): a randomised non-inferiority trial. Lancet 391(10131):1683–1692, 2018 29726344

Bøg FK, Jørgensen MB, Andersen ZJ, Osler M: Electroconvulsive therapy and subsequent epilepsy in patients with affective disorders: a register-based Danish cohort study. Brain Stimul 11(2):411–415, 2018 29203131

Bosboom PR, Deijen JB: Age-related cognitive effects of ECT and ECT-induced mood improvement in depressive patients. Depress Anxiety 23(2):93–101, 2006 16400627

Bourgon LN, Kellner CH: Relapse of depression after ECT: a review. J ECT 16(1):19–31, 2000 10735328

Braithwaite R, McKeown HL, Lawrence VJ, Cramer O: Successful electroconvulsive therapy in a patient with confirmed, symptomatic COVID-19. J ECT 36(3):222–223, 2020 32453191

Brandon S: Efficacy of ECT in depression: controlled trials. Psychopharmacol Bull 22:465–468, 1986

Braslow JT, Marder SR: History of psychopharmacology. Annu Rev Clin Psychol 15(15):25–50, 2019 30786241

Brunoni AR, Ferrucci R, Fregni F, et al: Transcranial direct current stimulation for the treatment of major depressive disorder: a summary of preclinical, clinical and translational findings. Prog Neuropsychopharmacol Biol Psychiatry 39(1):9–16, 2012 22651961

Bryson EO, Popeo D, Briggs M, et al: Electroconvulsive therapy (ECT) in patients with cardiac disease: hemodynamic changes. J ECT 29(1):76–77, 2013 23422523

Bryson EO, Liebman L, Nazarian R, Kellner CH: Safe resumption of maintenance electroconvulsive therapy 12 days after surgical repair of hip fracture. J ECT 31(2):81–82, 2015 25313642

Bryson EO, Aloysi AS, Farber KG, Kellner CH: Individualized anesthetic management for patients undergoing electroconvulsive therapy: a review of current practice. Anesth Analg 124(6):1943–1956, 2017 28277323

Buday J, Albrecht J, Mareš T, et al: Brain tumors and electroconvulsive therapy: a literature overview of the last 80 years. Front Neurol 11:723, 2020 32849199

Bush G, Fink M, Petrides G, et al: Catatonia, I: rating scale and standardized examination. Acta Psychiatr Scand 93(2):129–136, 1996 8686483

Carmi L, Alyagon U, Barnea-Ygael N, et al: Clinical and electrophysiological outcomes of deep TMS over the medial prefrontal and anterior cingulate cortices in OCD patients. Brain Stimul 11(1):158–165, 2018 28927961

Cash RFH, Weigand A, Zalesky A, et al: Using brain imaging to improve spatial targeting of TMS for depression. Biol Psychiatry 7, 2020 Epub ahead of print

Chanpattana W, Sackeim HA: Electroconvulsive therapy in treatment-resistant schizophrenia: prediction of response and the nature of symptomatic improvement. J ECT 26(4):289–298, 2010 20375701

Charlson F, Siskind D, Doi SA, et al: ECT efficacy and treatment course: a systematic review and meta-analysis of twice vs thrice weekly schedules. J Affect Disord 138(1–2):1–8, 2012 21501875

Christopher EJ: Electroconvulsive therapy in the medically ill. Curr Psychiatry Rep 5(3):225–230, 2003 12773277

Coffey CE, Lucke J, Weiner RD, et al: Seizure threshold in electroconvulsive therapy, I: initial seizure threshold. Biol Psychiatry 37(10):713–720, 1995 7640326

Cole EJ, Stimpson KH, Bentzley BS, et al: Stanford accelerated intelligent neuromodulation therapy for treatment-resistant depression. Am J Psychiatry 177(8):716–726, 2020 32252538

Crowell AL, Riva-Posse P, Holtzheimer PE, et al: Long-term outcomes of subcallosal cingulate deep brain stimulation for treatment-resistant depression. Am J Psychiatry 176(11):949–956, 2019 31581800

Daban C, Martinez-Aran A, Cruz N, Vieta E: Safety and efficacy of vagus nerve stimulation in treatment-resistant depression: a systematic review. J Affect Disord 110(1–2):1–15, 2008 18374988

Daskalakis ZJ, Dimitrova J, McClintock SM, et al: Magnetic seizure therapy (MST) for major depressive disorder. Neuropsychopharmacology 45(2):276–282, 2020 31486777

Dauleac C, Vinckier F, Bourdillon P: Subdural hematoma and electroconvulsive therapy: a case report and review of the literature. Neurochirurgie 65(1):40–42, 2019 30554774

Demitrack MA, Thase ME: Clinical significance of transcranial magnetic stimulation (TMS) in the treatment of pharmacoresistant depression: synthesis of recent data. Psychopharmacol Bull 42(2):5–38, 2009 19629020

Devanand DP, Sackeim HA: Seizure elicitation blocked by pretreatment with lidocaine. Convuls Ther 4(3):225–229, 1988 11940969

Devanand DP, Sackeim HA, Decina P, Prudic J: The development of mania and organic euphoria during ECT. J Clin Psychiatry 49(2):69–71, 1988 3338979

Devanand DP, Briscoe KM, Sackeim HA: Clinical features and predictors of postictal excitement. Convuls Ther 5(2):140–146, 1989 11941004

Devanand DP, Prudic J, Sackeim HA: Electroconvulsive therapy-induced hypomania is uncommon. Convuls Ther 8(4):296–298, 1992 11941183

Dierckx B, Heijnen WT, van den Broek WW, Birkenhäger TK: Efficacy of electroconvulsive therapy in bipolar versus unipolar major depression: a meta-analysis. Bipolar Disord 14(2):146–150, 2012 22420590

Ding Z, White PF: Anesthesia for electroconvulsive therapy. Anesth Analg 94(5):1351–1364, 2002 11973219

Dolenc TJ, Barnes RD, Hayes DL, Rasmussen KG: Electroconvulsive therapy in patients with cardiac pacemakers and implantable cardioverter defibrillators. Pacing Clin Electrophysiol 27(9):1257–1263, 2004 15461716

Downar J, Blumberger DM, Daskalakis ZJ: Repetitive transcranial magnetic stimulation: an emerging treatment for medication-resistant depression. CMAJ 188(16):1175–1177, 2016 27551033

Elias A, Thomas N, Sackeim HA: Electroconvulsive therapy in mania: a review of 80 years of clinical experience. Am J Psychiatry 178(3):229–239, 2021

Figiel GS, Coffey CE, Djang WT, et al: Brain magnetic resonance imaging findings in ECT-induced delirium. J Neuropsychiatry Clin Neurosci 2(1):53–58, 1990 2136061

Figiel GS, Hassen MA, Zorumski C, et al: ECT-induced delirium in depressed patients with Parkinson's disease. J Neuropsychiatry Clin Neurosci 3(4):405–411, 1991 1821261

Fink M: Electroshock therapy and catatonia: a productive synergism. J ECT 35(4):219–221, 2019 31764441

Fink M, Rush AJ, Knapp R, et al: DSM melancholic features are unreliable predictors of ECT response: a CORE publication. J ECT 23(3):139–146, 2007 17804986

Flint AJ, Rifat SL: Two-year outcome of psychotic depression in late life. Am J Psychiatry 155(2):178–183, 1998 9464195

Francis-Taylor R, Ophel G, Martin D, Loo C: The ictal EEG in ECT: a systematic review of the relationships between ictal features, ECT technique, seizure threshold and outcomes. Brain Stimul 13(6):1644–1654, 2020 32998055

Fricchione GL, Kaufman LD, Gruber BL, Fink M: Electroconvulsive therapy and cyclophosphamide in combination for severe neuropsychiatric lupus with catatonia. Am J Med 88(4):442–443, 1990 2327432

Gellersen HM, Kedzior KK: Antidepressant outcomes of high-frequency repetitive transcranial magnetic stimulation (rTMS) with F8-coil and deep transcranial magnetic stimulation (DTMS) with H1-coil in major depression: a systematic review and meta-analysis. BMC Psychiatry 19(1):139, 2019 31064328

George MS, Lisanby SH, Avery D, et al: Daily left prefrontal transcranial magnetic stimulation therapy for major depressive disorder: a sham-controlled randomized trial. Arch Gen Psychiatry 67(5):507–516, 2010 20439832

Göterfelt L, Ekman CJ, Hammar Å, et al: The incidence of dental fracturing in electroconvulsive therapy in Sweden. J ECT 36(3):168–171, 2020 31972668

Grimm S, Beck J, Schuepbach D, et al: Imbalance between left and right dorsolateral prefrontal cortex in major depression is linked to negative emotional judgment: an fMRI study in severe major depressive disorder. Biol Psychiatry 63(4):369–376, 2008 17888408

Güney P, Ekman CJ, Hammar Å, et al: Electroconvulsive therapy in depression: improvement in quality of life depending on age and sex. J ECT 36(4):242–246, 2020 32108666

Haghighi M, Sedighinejad A, Naderi Nabi B, et al: The incidence and predictors of headache and myalgia in patients after electroconvulsive therapy (ECT). Anesth Pain Med 6(3):e33724, 2016 27761416

Haskett RF, Loo C: Adjunctive psychotropic medications during electroconvulsive therapy in the treatment of depression, mania, and schizophrenia. J ECT 26(3):196–201, 2010 20805728

Hebbrecht K, Giltay EJ, Birkenhäger TK, et al: Cognitive change after electroconvulsive therapy in mood disorders measured with the Montreal Cognitive Assessment. Acta Psychiatr Scand 142(5):413–422, 2020 32895922

Hermida AP, Glass OM, Shafi H, McDonald WM: Electroconvulsive therapy in depression: current practice and future direction. Psychiatr Clin North Am 41(3):341–353, 2018 30098649

Hermida AP, Goldstein FC, Loring DW, et al: ElectroConvulsive therapy Cognitive Assessment (ECCA) tool: a new instrument to monitor cognitive function in patients undergoing ECT. J Affect Disord 269:36–42, 2020a 32217341

Hermida AP, Tang YL, Glass O, et al: Efficacy and safety of ECT for behavioral and psychological symptoms of dementia (BPSD): a retrospective chart review. Am J Geriatr Psychiatry 28(2):157–163, 2020b 31668364

Hood DD, Mecca RS: Failure to initiate electroconvulsive seizures in a patient pretreated with lidocaine. Anesthesiology 58(4):379–381, 1983 6837980

Horváth L, Fekete I, Molnár M, et al: The outcome of status epilepticus and long-term follow-up. Front Neurol 10:427, 2019 31105639

Hoshi H, Kadoi Y, Kamiyama J, et al: Use of rocuronium-sugammadex, an alternative to succinylcholine, as a muscle relaxant during electroconvulsive therapy. J Anesth 25(2):286–290, 2011 21293886

Hoy KE, Fitzgerald PB: Magnetic seizure therapy for treatment-resistant depression. Expert Rev Med Devices 8(6):723–732, 2011 22029469

Hsieh KY, Tsai KY, Chou FH, Chou YM: Reduced risk of stroke among psychiatric patients receiving ECT: a population-based cohort study in Taiwan. Psychiatry Res 276:107–111, 2019 31048180

Husain MM, Rush AJ, Fink M, et al: Speed of response and remission in major depressive disorder with acute electroconvulsive therapy (ECT): a Consortium for Research in ECT (CORE) report. J Clin Psychiatry 65(4):485–491, 2004 15119910

Huuhka M, Korpisammal L, Haataja R, Leinonen E: One-year outcome of elderly inpatients with major depressive disorder treated with ECT and antidepressants. J ECT 20(3):179–185, 2004 15343003

Ilmoniemi RJ, Ruohonen J, Karhu J: Transcranial magnetic stimulation: a new tool for functional imaging of the brain. Crit Rev Biomed Eng 27(3–5):241–284, 1999 10864281

Inagawa Y, Saito S, Okada T, et al: Electroconvulsive therapy for catatonia with deep venous thrombosis: a case series. Prim Care Companion CNS Disord 20(4):18, 2018 29995361

Isserles M, Daskalakis ZJ, Kumar S, et al: Clinical effectiveness and tolerability of electroconvulsive therapy in patients with neuropsychiatric symptoms of dementia. J Alzheimers Dis 57(1):45–51, 2017 28222513

Isserles M, Remington J, Kaster TS, et al: Clinical effectiveness of maintenance electroconvulsive therapy in patient with schizophrenia: a retrospective cohort study. J ECT 36(1):42–46, 2020 31192873

Janicak PG, Davis JM, Gibbons RD, et al: Efficacy of ECT: a meta-analysis. Am J Psychiatry 142(3):297–302, 1985 3882006

Jiam NT, Li D, Kramer K, Limb CJ: Preserved cochlear implant function after multiple electroconvulsive therapy treatments. Laryngoscope 131(5):E1695–E1698, 2020 33252138

Jones KC, Salemi JL, Dongarwar D, et al: Racial/Ethnic disparities in receipt of electroconvulsive therapy for elderly patients with a principal diagnosis of depression in inpatient settings. Am J Geriatr Psychiatry 27(3):266–278, 2019 30587412

Kallioniemi E, McClintock SM, Deng Z-D, et al: Magnetic seizure therapy: towards personalized seizure therapy for major depression. Pers Med Psychiatry 17–18:37–42, 2019 32832741

Kalu UG, Sexton CE, Loo CK, Ebmeier KP: Transcranial direct current stimulation in the treatment of major depression: a meta-analysis. Psychol Med 42(9):1791–1800, 2012 22236735

Kamat SM, Lefevre PJ, Grossberg GT: Electroconvulsive therapy in the elderly. Clin Geriatr Med 19(4):825–839, 2003 15024814

Kaster TS, Daskalakis ZJ, Noda Y, et al: Efficacy, tolerability, and cognitive effects of deep transcranial magnetic stimulation for late-life depression: a prospective randomized controlled trial. Neuropsychopharmacology 43(11):2231–2238, 2018 29946106

Kearon C: Natural history of venous thromboembolism. Circulation 107(suppl 1):I22–I30, 2003

Kellner CH, Bryson EO: Electroconvulsive therapy anesthesia technique: minimalist versus maximally managed. J ECT 29(3):153–155, 2013 23965604

Kellner CH, Knapp RG, Petrides G, et al: Continuation electroconvulsive therapy vs pharmacotherapy for relapse prevention in major depression: a multisite study from the Consortium for Research in Electroconvulsive Therapy (CORE). Arch Gen Psychiatry 63(12):1337–1344, 2006 17146008

Kellner CH, Knapp R, Husain MM, et al: Bifrontal, bitemporal and right unilateral electrode placement in ECT: randomised trial. Br J Psychiatry 196(3):226–234, 2010 20194546

Kellner CH, Husain MM, Knapp RG, et al: A novel strategy for continuation ECT in geriatric depression: phase 2 of the PRIDE study. Am J Psychiatry 173(11):1110–1118, 2016a 27418381

Kellner CH, Husain MM, Knapp RG, et al: Right unilateral ultrabrief pulse ECT in geriatric depression: phase 1 of the PRIDE study. Am J Psychiatry 173(11):1101–1109, 2016b 27418379

Kellner CH, Obbels J, Sienaert P: When to consider electroconvulsive therapy (ECT). Acta Psychiatr Scand 141(4):304–315, 2020 31774547

Kerner N, Prudic J: Current electroconvulsive therapy practice and research in the geriatric population. Neuropsychiatry (London) 4(1):33–54, 2014 24778709

Klapheke MM: Combining ECT and antipsychotic agents: benefits and risks. Convuls Ther 9(4):241–255, 1993 11941220

Kolshus E, Jelovac A, McLoughlin DM: Bitemporal v. high-dose right unilateral electroconvulsive therapy for depression: a systematic review and meta-analysis of randomized controlled trials. Psychol Med 47(3):518–530, 2017 27780482

Krystal AD, Coffey CE: Neuropsychiatric considerations in the use of electroconvulsive therapy. J Neuropsychiatry Clin Neurosci 9(2):283–292, 1997 9144111

Krystal AD, Weiner RD, Coffey CE: The ictal EEG as a marker of adequate stimulus intensity with unilateral ECT. J Neuropsychiatry Clin Neurosci 7(3):295–303, 1995 7580187

Krystal AD, Watts BV, Weiner RD, et al: The use of flumazenil in the anxious and benzodiazepine-dependent ECT patient. J ECT 14(1):5–14, 1998 9661088

Krystal AD, Dean MD, Weiner RD, et al: ECT stimulus intensity: are present ECT devices too limited? Am J Psychiatry 157(6):963–967, 2000a 10831477

Krystal AD, Weiner RD, Lindahl V, Massie R: The development and retrospective testing of an electroencephalographic seizure quality-based stimulus dosing paradigm with ECT. J ECT 16(4):338–349, 2000b 11314871

Kuehn BM: Scientists probe deep brain stimulation: some promise for brain injury, psychiatric illness. JAMA 298(19):2249–2251, 2007 18029821

Kujala I, Rosenvinge B, Bekkelund SI: Clinical outcome and adverse effects of electroconvulsive therapy in elderly psychiatric patients. J Geriatr Psychiatry Neurol 15(2):73–76, 2002 12083596

Kumar S, Mulsant BH, Liu AY, et al: Systematic review of cognitive effects of electroconvulsive therapy in late-life depression. Am J Geriatr Psychiatry 24(7):547–565, 2016 27067067

Lapid MI, McNally Forsyth D, Hegard TL, et al: Characteristics of successful transitions from inpatient to outpatient electroconvulsive therapy. J Psychiatr Pract 24(3):140–145, 2018 30015784

Lapid MI, Seiner S, Heintz H, et al: Electroconvulsive therapy practice changes in older individuals due to COVID-19: expert consensus statement. Am J Geriatr Psychiatry 28(11):1133–1145, 2020 32863137

Lefaucheur J-P, Brugières P, Ménard-Lefaucheur I, et al: The value of navigation-guided rTMS for the treatment of depression: an illustrative case. Neurophysiol Clin 37(4):265–271, 2007 17996815

Lefaucheur J-P, Aleman A, Baeken C, et al: Evidence-based guidelines on the therapeutic use of repetitive transcranial magnetic stimulation (rTMS): an update (2014–2018). Clin Neurophysiol 131(2):474–528, 2020 31901449

Lerner AJ, Wassermann EM, Tamir DI: Seizures from transcranial magnetic stimulation 2012–2016: results of a survey of active laboratories and clinics. Clin Neurophysiol 130(8):1409–1416, 2019 31104898

Lisanby SH, Schlaepfer TE, Fisch HU, Sackeim HA: Magnetic seizure therapy of major depression. Arch Gen Psychiatry 58(3):303–305, 2001 11231838

Lisanby SH, Sampson S, Husain MM, et al: Toward individualized post-electroconvulsive therapy care: piloting the Symptom-Titrated, Algorithm-Based Longitudinal ECT (STABLE) intervention. J ECT 24(3):179–182, 2008 18708943

Livingston R, Wu C, Mu K, Coffey MJ: Regulation of electroconvulsive therapy: a systematic review of US state laws. J ECT 34(1):60–68, 2018 28991068

Loo C, Sheehan P, Pigot M, Lyndon W: A report on mood and cognitive outcomes with right unilateral ultrabrief pulsewidth (0.3 ms) ECT and retrospective comparison with standard pulsewidth right unilateral ECT. J Affect Disord 103(1–3):277–281, 2007 17706790

Loo C, McFarquhar TF, Mitchell PB: A review of the safety of repetitive transcranial magnetic stimulation as a clinical treatment for depression. Int J Neuropsychopharmacol 11(1):131–147, 2008 17880752

Lozano AM, Mayberg HS, Giacobbe P, et al: Subcallosal cingulate gyrus deep brain stimulation for treatment-resistant depression. Biol Psychiatry 64(6):461–467, 2008 18639234

Lubit EB, Fetterman TC, Ying P: Recurrent aspiration in a patient with gastric band undergoing electroconvulsive therapy. J ECT 32(2):134–135, 2016 26075693

Luccarelli J, McCoy TH Jr, Shannon AP, et al: Rate of continuing acute course treatment using right unilateral ultrabrief pulse electroconvulsive therapy at a large academic medical center. Eur Arch Psychiatry Clin Neurosci 271(1):191–197, 2020 33196856

Luchini F, Medda P, Mariani MG, et al: Electroconvulsive therapy in catatonic patients: efficacy and predictors of response. World J Psychiatry 5(2):182–192, 2015 26110120

Mamah D, Lammle M, Isenberg KE: Pulmonary embolism after ECT. J ECT 21(1):39–40, 2005

Manepalli J, Sapkota N: Neuromodulation therapies in the elderly depressed patient. Curr Geriatr Rep 3(4):229–236, 2014

Manly DT, Oakley SP Jr, Bloch RM: Electroconvulsive therapy in old-old patients. Am J Geriatr Psychiatry 8(3):232–236, 2000 10910422

Martin DM, McClintock SM, Forster JJ, et al: Cognitive enhancing effects of rTMS administered to the prefrontal cortex in patients with depression: a systematic review and meta-analysis of individual task effects. Depress Anxiety 34(11):1029–1039, 2017 28543994

Mayberg HS, Lozano AM, Voon V, et al: Deep brain stimulation for treatment-resistant depression. Neuron 45(5):651–660, 2005 15748841

McAllister-Williams RH, Sousa S, Kumar A, et al: The effects of vagus nerve stimulation on the course and outcomes of patients with bipolar disorder in a treatment-resistant depressive episode: a 5-year prospective registry. Int J Bipolar Disord 8(1):13, 2020 32358769

McCall WV, Reboussin DM, Weiner RD, Sackeim HA: Titrated moderately suprathreshold vs fixed high-dose right unilateral electroconvulsive therapy: acute antidepressant and cognitive effects. Arch Gen Psychiatry 57(5):438–444, 2000 10807483

McClintock SM, Tirmizi O, Chansard M, Husain MM: A systematic review of the neurocognitive effects of magnetic seizure therapy. Int Rev Psychiatry 23(5):413–423, 2011 22200131

McClintock SM, Choi J, Deng ZD, et al: Multifactorial determinants of the neurocognitive effects of electroconvulsive therapy. J ECT 30(2):165–176, 2014 24820942

McDonald WM: Neuromodulation treatments for geriatric mood and cognitive disorders. Am J Geriatr Psychiatry 24(12):1130–1141, 2016 27889282

McGirr A, Berlim MT, Bond DJ, et al: A systematic review and meta-analysis of randomized controlled trials of adjunctive ketamine in electroconvulsive therapy: efficacy and tolerability. J Psychiatr Res 62:23–30, 2015 25684151

Medda P, Toni C, Perugi G: The mood-stabilizing effects of electroconvulsive therapy. J ECT 30(4):275–282, 2014 25010031

Medda P, Toni C, Luchini F, et al: Catatonia in 26 patients with bipolar diorder: clinical features and risponse to electroconvulsive therapy. Bipolar Disord 17(8):892–901, 2015 26643014

Merrill CA, Jonsson MA, Minthon L, et al: Vagus nerve stimulation in patients with Alzheimer's disease: additional follow-up results of a pilot study through 1 year. J Clin Psychiatry 67(8):1171–1178, 2006 16965193

Meyer JP, Swetter SK, Kellner CH: Electroconvulsive therapy in geriatric psychiatry: a selective review. Clin Geriatr Med 36(2):265–279, 2020 32222301

Minnai GP, Salis PG, Oppo R, et al: Effectiveness of maintenance electroconvulsive therapy in rapid-cycling bipolar disorder. J ECT 27(2):123–126, 2011 20559148

Morcos N, Rosinski A, Maixner DF: Electroconvulsive therapy for neuroleptic malignant syndrome: a case series. J ECT 35(4):225–230, 2019 31764444

Mullen MG, Michaels AD, Mehaffey JH, et al: Risk associated with complications and mortality after urgent surgery vs elective and emergency surgery: implications for defining "quality" and reporting outcomes for urgent surgery. JAMA Surg 152(8):768–774, 2017 28492821

Nahas Z, Li X, Kozel FA, et al: Safety and benefits of distance-adjusted prefrontal transcranial magnetic stimulation in depressed patients 55–75 years of age: a pilot study. Depress Anxiety 19(4):249–256, 2004 15274174

Nahas Z, Short B, Burns C, et al: A feasibility study of a new method for electrically producing seizures in man: focal electrically administered seizure therapy [FEAST]. Brain Stimul 6(3):403–408, 2013 23518262

Netzel PJ, Mueller PS, Rummans TA, et al: Safety, efficacy, and effects on glycemic control of electroconvulsive therapy in insulin-requiring type 2 diabetic patients. J ECT 18(1):16–21, 2002 11925516

Nordenskjöld A, von Knorring L, Ljung T, et al: Continuation electroconvulsive therapy with pharmacotherapy versus pharmacotherapy alone for prevention of relapse of depression: a randomized controlled trial. J ECT 29(2):86–92, 2013 23303421

Nordenskjöld A, Güney P, Nordenskjöld AM: Major adverse cardiovascular events following electroconvulsive therapy in depression: a register-based nationwide Swedish cohort study with 1-year follow-up. J Affect Disord 296:298–304, 2021 34606801

Nuttall GA, Bowersox MR, Douglass SB, et al: Morbidity and mortality in the use of electroconvulsive therapy. J ECT 20(4):237–241, 2004 15591857

Obbels J, Vansteelandt K, Verwijk E, et al: MMSE changes during and after ECT in late-life depression: a prospective study. Am J Geriatr Psychiatry 27(9):934–944, 2019 31104967

O'Brien PD, Morgan DH: Bladder rupture during ECT. Convuls Ther 7(1):56–59, 1991 11941099

O'Connor DW, Gardner B, Eppingstall B, Tofler D: Cognition in elderly patients receiving unilateral and bilateral electroconvulsive therapy: a prospective, naturalistic comparison. J Affect Disord 124(3):235–240, 2010 20053457

O'Connor MK, Knapp R, Husain M, et al: The influence of age on the response of major depression to electroconvulsive therapy: a C.O.R.E. Report. Am J Geriatr Psychiatry 9(4):382–390, 2001 11739064

O'Reardon JP, Solvason HB, Janicak PG, et al: Efficacy and safety of transcranial magnetic stimulation in the acute treatment of major depression: a multisite randomized controlled trial. Biol Psychiatry 62(11):1208–1216, 2007 17573044

Patel RS, Bachu A, Youssef NA: Combination of lithium and electroconvulsive therapy (ECT) is associated with higher odds of delirium and cognitive problems in a large national sample across the United States. Brain Stimul 13(1):15–19, 2020 31492631

Paul SM, Extein I, Calil HM, et al: Use of ECT with treatment-resistant depressed patients at the National Institute of Mental Health. Am J Psychiatry 138(4):486–489, 1981 6111228

Perugi G, Medda P, Toni C, et al: The role of electroconvulsive therapy (ECT) in bipolar disorder: effectiveness in 522 patients with bipolar depression, mixed-state, mania and catatonic features. Curr Neuropharmacol 15(3):359–371, 2017 28503107

Petrides G, Fink M: Atrial fibrillation, anticoagulation, and electroconvulsive therapy. Convuls Ther 12(2):91–98, 1996 8744168

Petrides G, Fink M, Husain MM, et al: ECT remission rates in psychotic versus nonpsychotic depressed patients: a report from CORE. J ECT 17(4):244–253, 2001 11731725

Petrides G, Tobias KT, Kellner CH, Rudorfer MV: Continuation and maintenance electroconvulsive therapy for mood disorders: review of the literature. Neuropsychobiology 64(3):129–140, 2011 21811083

Petrides G, Malur C, Braga RJ, et al: Electroconvulsive therapy augmentation in clozapine-resistant schizophrenia: a prospective, randomized study. Am J Psychiatry 172(1):52–58, 2015

Philibert RA, Richards L, Lynch CF, Winokur G: Effect of ECT on mortality and clinical outcome in geriatric unipolar depression. J Clin Psychiatry 56(9):390–394, 1995 7665536

Pickett GE, Hazelton L: Electroconvulsive therapy after flow diversion stenting of intracranial aneurysm. J ECT 35(2):e17–e19, 2019 30720553

Pinchotti DM, Abbott C, Quinn DK: Targeted electroconvulsive therapy for super refractory status epilepticus: a case report and literature review. Psychosomatics 59(3):302–305, 2018 29150213

Pompili M, Lester D, Dominici G, et al: Indications for electroconvulsive treatment in schizophrenia: a systematic review. Schizophr Res 146(1–3):1–9, 2013 23499244

Porter RJ, Baune BT, Morris G, et al: Cognitive side-effects of electroconvulsive therapy: what are they, how to monitor them and what to tell patients. BJPsych Open 6(3):e40, 2020 32301408

Prudic J, Haskett RF, Mulsant B, et al: Resistance to antidepressant medications and short-term clinical response to ECT. Am J Psychiatry 153(8):985–992, 1996 8678194

Prudic J, Haskett RF, McCall WV, et al: Pharmacological strategies in the prevention of relapse after electroconvulsive therapy. J ECT 29(1):3–12, 2013 23303417

Rabheru K: The use of electroconvulsive therapy in special patient populations. Can J Psychiatry 46(8):710–719, 2001 11692973

Rasmussen KG, Varghese R, Stevens SR, Ryan DA: Electrode placement and ictal EEG indices in electroconvulsive therapy. J Neuropsychiatry Clin Neurosci 19(4):453–457, 2007 18070850

Rasmussen KG, Albin SM, Mueller PS, Abel MD: Electroconvulsive therapy in patients taking steroid medication: should supplemental doses be given on the days of treatment? J ECT 24(2):128–130, 2008 18580555

Rayburn BK: Electroconvulsive therapy in patients with heart failure or valvular heart disease. Convuls Ther 13(3):145–156, 1997 9342130

Riva-Posse P, Hermida AP, McDonald WM: The role of electroconvulsive and neuromodulation therapies in the treatment of geriatric depression. Psychiatr Clin North Am 36(4):607–630, 2013 24229660

Rossi S, Hallett M, Rossini PM, et al: Safety, ethical consideration, and application guidelines for the use of transcranial magnetic stimulation in clinical practice and research. Clin Neurophysiol 120(12):2008–2039, 2009 19833552

Rossi S, Antal A, Bestmann S, et al: Safety and recommendations for TMS use in healthy subjects and patient populations, with updates on training, ethical and regulatory issues: expert guidelines. Clin Neurophysiol 132(1):269–306, 2021

Rummans TA, Bassingthwaighte ME: Severe medical and neurologic complications associated with near-lethal catatonia treated with electroconvulsive therapy. Convuls Ther 7(2):121–124, 1991 11941111

Sabesan P, Lankappa S, Khalifa N, et al: Transcranial magnetic stimulation for geriatric depression: promises and pitfalls. World J Psychiatry 5(2):170–181, 2015 26110119

Sackeim HA: Continuation therapy following ECT: directions for future research. Psychopharmacol Bull 30(3):501–521, 1994 7878189

Sackeim HA: The use of electroconvulsive therapy in late-life depression, in Clinical Geriatric Psychopharmacology, 3rd Edition. Edited by Salzman C. Baltimore, MD, Williams and Wilkins, 1998, pp 262–309

Sackeim HA, Rush AJ: Melancholia and response to ECT. Am J Psychiatry 152(8):1242–1243, 1995

Sackeim HA, Prudic J, Devanand DP, et al: The impact of medication resistance and continuation pharmacotherapy on relapse following response to electroconvulsive therapy in major depression. J Clin Psychopharmacol 10(2):96–104, 1990 2341598

Sackeim HA, Prudic J, Devanand DP, et al: Effects of stimulus intensity and electrode placement on the efficacy and cognitive effects of electroconvulsive therapy. N Engl J Med 328(12):839–846, 1993 8441428

Sackeim HA, Haskett RF, Mulsant BH, et al: Continuation pharmacotherapy in the prevention of relapse following electroconvulsive therapy: a randomized controlled trial. JAMA 285(10):1299–1307, 2001a 11255384

Sackeim HA, Rush AJ, George MS, et al: Vagus nerve stimulation (VNS) for treatment-resistant depression: efficacy, side effects, and predictors of outcome. Neuropsychopharmacology 25(5):713–728, 2001b 11682255

Sackeim HA, Prudic J, Fuller R, et al: The cognitive effects of electroconvulsive therapy in community settings. Neuropsychopharmacology 32(1):244–254, 2007 16936712

Sackeim HA, Prudic J, Nobler MS, et al: Effects of pulse width and electrode placement on the efficacy and cognitive effects of electroconvulsive therapy. Brain Stimul 1(2):71–83, 2008 19756236

Sackeim HA, Dillingham EM, Prudic J, et al: Effect of concomitant pharmacotherapy on electroconvulsive therapy outcomes: short-term efficacy and adverse effects. Arch Gen Psychiatry 66(7):729–737, 2009 19581564

Sackeim HA, Prudic J, Devanand DP, et al: The benefits and costs of changing treatment technique in electroconvulsive therapy due to insufficient improvement of a major depressive episode. Brain Stimul 13(5):1284–1295, 2020 32585354

Sahlem GL, McCall WV, Short EB, et al: A two-site, open-label, non-randomized trial comparing focal electrically administered seizure therapy (FEAST) and right unilateral ultrabrief pulse electroconvulsive therapy (RUL-UBP ECT). Brain Stimul 13(5):1416–1425, 2020

Saito S: Anesthesia management for electroconvulsive therapy: hemodynamic and respiratory management. J Anesth 19(2):142–149, 2005 15875132

Sanghani SN, Petrides G, Kellner CH: Electroconvulsive therapy (ECT) in schizophrenia: a review of recent literature. Curr Opin Psychiatry 31(3):213–222, 2018 29528902

San-Juan D, Dávila-Rodríguez DO, Jiménez CR, et al: Neuromodulation techniques for status epilepticus: A review. Brain Stimul 12(4):835–844, 2019 31053521

Schak KM, Mueller PS, Barnes RD, Rasmussen KG: The safety of ECT in patients with chronic obstructive pulmonary disease. Psychosomatics 49(3):208–211, 2008 18448774

Schlaepfer TE, Cohen MX, Frick C, et al: Deep brain stimulation to reward circuitry alleviates anhedonia in refractory major depression. Neuropsychopharmacology 33(2):368–377, 2008 17429407

Schlaepfer TE, Bewernick BH, Kayser S, et al: Deep brain stimulation of the human reward system for major depression—rationale, outcomes and outlook. Neuropsychopharmacology 39(6):1303–1314, 2014 24513970

Semkovska M, McLoughlin DM: Objective cognitive performance associated with electroconvulsive therapy for depression: a systematic review and meta-analysis. Biol Psychiatry 68(6):568–577, 2010 20673880

Shiwach RS, Reid WH, Carmody TJ: An analysis of reported deaths following electroconvulsive therapy in Texas, 1993–1998. Psychiatr Serv 52(8):1095–1097, 2001 11474057

Shorter E, Healy D: Shock Therapy: A History of Electroconvulsive Treatment in Mental Illness. New Brunswick, NJ, Rutgers University Press, 2007

Sigström R, Nordenskjöld A, Juréus A, et al: Long-term subjective memory after electroconvulsive therapy. BJPsych Open 6(2):e26, 2020 32148217

Singh PM, Arora S, Borle A, et al: Evaluation of etomidate for seizure duration in electroconvulsive therapy: a systematic review and meta-analysis. J ECT 31(4):213–225, 2015 25634566

Singla H, Grover S: Electroconvulsive therapy in an elderly patient with severe aortic stenosis: a case report and review of literature. Indian J Psychol Med 40(3):288–291, 2018 29875541

Sirven JI, Sperling M, Naritoku D, et al: Vagus nerve stimulation therapy for epilepsy in older adults. Neurology 54(5):1179–1182, 2000 10720294

Sobin C, Prudic J, Devanand DP, et al: Who responds to electroconvulsive therapy? A comparison of effective and ineffective forms of treatment. Br J Psychiatry 169(3):322–328, 1996 8879718

Song J, Lee PP, Weiner R, Challa P: The effect of surgery on intraocular pressure fluctuations with electroconvulsive therapy in a patient with severe glaucoma. J ECT 20(4):264–266, 2004 15591863

Spellman T, McClintock SM, Terrace H, et al: Differential effects of high-dose magnetic seizure therapy and electroconvulsive shock on cognitive function. Biol Psychiatry 63(12):1163–1170, 2008 18262171

Stern L, Hirschmann S, Grunhaus L: ECT in patients with major depressive disorder and low cardiac output. Convuls Ther 13(2):68–73, 1997 9253526

Stoppe A, Louzã M, Rosa M, et al: Fixed high-dose electroconvulsive therapy in the elderly with depression: a double-blind, randomized comparison of efficacy and tolerability between unilateral and bilateral electrode placement. J ECT 22(2):92–99, 2006 16801822

Sun Y, Farzan F, Mulsant BH, et al: Indicators for remission of suicidal ideation following magnetic seizure therapy in patients with treatment-resistant depression. JAMA Psychiatry 73(4):337–345, 2016 26981889

Sundsted KK, Burton MC, Shah R, Lapid MI: Preanesthesia medical evaluation for electroconvulsive therapy: a review of the literature. J ECT 30(1):35–42, 2014 24091900

Sutor B, Rasmussen KG: Clinical challenges in maintenance electroconvulsive therapy for older patients with medical comorbidity. J ECT 32(1):67–69, 2016 25993032

Suzuki K, Awata S, Matsuoka H: Short-term effect of ECT in middle-aged and elderly patients with intractable catatonic schizophrenia. J ECT 19(2):73–80, 2002 12792454

Suzuki Y, Miyajima M, Ohta K, et al: Changes in cardiac autonomic nervous system activity during a course of electroconvulsive therapy. Neuropsychopharmacol Rep 39(1):2–9, 2019 30411870

Takada JY, Solimene MC, da Luz PL, et al: Assessment of the cardiovascular effects of electroconvulsive therapy in individuals older than 50 years. Braz J Med Biol Res 38(9):1349–1357, 2005 16138218

Tess AV, Smetana GW: Medical evaluation of patients undergoing electroconvulsive therapy. N Engl J Med 360(14):1437–1444, 2009 19339723

Tew JD Jr, Mulsant BH, Haskett RF, et al: Acute efficacy of ECT in the treatment of major depression in the old-old. Am J Psychiatry 156(12):1865–1870, 1999 10588398

Tew JD Jr, Mulsant BH, Haskett RF, et al: Relapse during continuation pharmacotherapy after acute response to ECT: a comparison of usual care versus protocolized treatment. Ann Clin Psychiatry 19(1):1–4, 2007 17453654

Texas Department of State Health Services: Report on Electroconvulsive Therapy For Fiscal Year 2019. Austin, TX, Texas Department of State Health Services, April 2020. Available at: https://www.hhs.texas.gov/file/131446/download?token=XKFtMAci. Accessed October 17, 2021.

Tielkes CE, Comijs HC, Verwijk E, Stek ML: The effects of ECT on cognitive functioning in the elderly: a review. Int J Geriatr Psychiatry 23(8):789–795, 2008 18311845

Tørring N, Sanghani SN, Petrides G, et al: The mortality rate of electroconvulsive therapy: a systematic review and pooled analysis. Acta Psychiatr Scand 135(5):388–397, 2017 28332236

U.K. ECT Review Group: Efficacy and safety of electroconvulsive therapy in depressive disorders: a systematic review and meta-analysis. Lancet 361(9360):799–808, 2003 12642045

U.S. Food and Drug Administration: Neurological devices; reclassification of electroconvulsive therapy devices; effective date of requirement for premarket approval for electroconvulsive therapy devices for certain specified intended uses. Final order. Fed Regist 83(246):66103–66124, 2018 30596410

Vaidya NA, Mahableshwarkar AR, Shahid R: Continuation and maintenance ECT in treatment-resistant bipolar disorder. J ECT 19(1):10–16, 2003 12621271

Vaidya PV, Anderson EL, Bobb A, et al: A within-subject comparison of propofol and methohexital anesthesia for electroconvulsive therapy. J ECT 28(1):14–19, 2012 22330701

van der Wurff FB, Stek ML, Hoogendijk WJ, Beekman AT: The efficacy and safety of ECT in depressed older adults: a literature review. Int J Geriatr Psychiatry 18(10):894–904, 2003 14533122

van Diermen L, van den Ameele S, Kamperman AM, et al: Prediction of electroconvulsive therapy response and remission in major depression: meta-analysis. Br J Psychiatry 212(2):71–80, 2018 29436330

van Schaik AM, Klumpers UM, de Gast HM, et al: Gastric rupture after electroconvulsive therapy. J ECT 22(2):153–154, 2006 16801835

van Schaik AM, Comijs HC, Sonnenberg CM, et al: Efficacy and safety of continuation and maintenance electroconvulsive therapy in depressed elderly patients: a systematic review. Am J Geriatr Psychiatry 20(1):5–17, 2012 22183009

Veltman EM, de Boer A, Dols A, et al: Melancholia as predictor of electroconvulsive therapy outcome in later life. J ECT 35(4):231–237, 2019 31764445

Versiani M, Cheniaux E, Landeira-Fernandez J: Efficacy and safety of electroconvulsive therapy in the treatment of bipolar disorder: a systematic review. J ECT 27(2):153–164, 2011 20562714

Verwijk E, Comijs HC, Kok RM, et al: Short- and long-term neurocognitive functioning after electroconvulsive therapy in depressed elderly: a prospective naturalistic study. Int Psychogeriatr 26(2):315–324, 2014 24280446

Wani A, Trevino K, Marnell P, Husain MM: Advances in brain stimulation for depression. Ann Clin Psychiatry 25(3):217–224, 2013 23926577

Ward HB, Szabo ST, Rakesh G: Maintenance ECT in schizophrenia: a systematic review. Psychiatry Res 264:131–142, 2018 29631245

Warren N, Grote V, O'Gorman C, Siskind D: Electroconvulsive therapy for anti-N-methyl-d-aspartate (NMDA) receptor encephalitis: a systematic review of cases. Brain Stimul 12(2):329–334, 2019 30528383

Weiner RD, Krystal AD: Electroconvulsive therapy, in Treatments of Psychiatric Disorders, 3rd Edition. Edited by Gabbard GO, Rush AJ. Washington, DC, American Psychiatric Publishing, 2001, pp 1267–1293

Weiner RD, Rogers HJ, Davidson JR, Squire LR: Effects of stimulus parameters on cognitive side effects. Ann N Y Acad Sci 462:315–325, 1986 3458412

Weiner RD, Coffey CE, Krystal AD: The monitoring and management of electrically induced seizures. Psychiatr Clin North Am 14(4):845–869, 1991 1771151

Weiner RD, Coffey CE, Krystal AD: Electroconvulsive therapy in the medical and neurologic patient, in Psychiatric Care of the Medical Patient, 2nd Edition. Edited by Stoudemire A, Fogel BS, Greenberg D. New York, Oxford University Press, 2000, pp 419–428

Wengel SP, Burke WJ, Pfeiffer RF, et al: Maintenance electroconvulsive therapy for intractable Parkinson's disease. Am J Geriatr Psychiatry 6(3):263–269, 1998 9659959

Wesson ML, Wilkinson AM, Anderson DN, Cracken CM: Does age predict the long-term outcome of depression treated with ECT? (A prospective study of the long-term outcome of ECT-treated depression with respect to age.) Int J Geriatr Psychiatry 12(1):45–51, 1997 9050423

Williams NR, Bentzley BS, Sahlem GL, et al: Unilateral ultra-brief pulse electroconvulsive therapy for depression in Parkinson's disease. Acta Neurol Scand 135(4):407–411, 2017 27241213

Wittenauer Welsh J, Janjua AU, Garlow SJ, et al: Use of expert consultation in a complex case of neuroleptic malignant syndrome requiring electroconvulsive therapy. J Psychiatr Pract 22(6):484–489, 2016 27824784

Youn T, Jeong SH, Kim YS, Chung IW: Long-term clinical efficacy of maintenance electroconvulsive therapy in patients with treatment-resistant schizophrenia on clozapine. Psychiatry Res 273:759–766, 2019 31207863

Zielinski RJ, Roose SP, Devanand DP, et al: Cardiovascular complications of ECT in depressed patients with cardiac disease. Am J Psychiatry 150(6):904–909, 1993 8494067

CHAPTER 22

Individual and Group Psychotherapy

Moria J. Smoski, Ph.D.

Dimitris N. Kiosses, Ph.D.

Psychotherapy has been shown to be an effective treatment for a number of mental disorders seen in older adults. As a treatment modality it can be particularly useful for older adult psychiatric patients who cannot tolerate or will not take medication or who are dealing with stressful conditions, interpersonal difficulties, limited levels of social support, or recurrent episodes of a disorder. However, it has been estimated that only 30% of older adults in need of psychiatric services receive professional care (Byers et al. 2012), and older adults are half as likely as middle-aged adults to receive specialty care (e.g., psychologists or psychiatrists), with the bulk of mental health services provided in primary care (Crabb and Hunsley 2006). Older Black adults seek out professional mental health care about one-half as often as their white counterparts, instead turning to informal support networks as a means of coping (Conner et al. 2010). Older adults report a longer delay in initiating mental health treatment than do younger cohort groups (Wang et al. 2005).

Although many practitioners assume that older adults have negative attitudes toward psychotherapy, research in elderly samples is not conclusive. Contrary to clinical lore, growing descriptive research suggests that older adults may prefer counseling over medication treatment (Conner et al. 2010; Gum et al. 2006). Older adults have also been shown to report more positive attitudes toward mental health professionals and to be less concerned about stigma attached to seeking treatment for depression than younger adults (Rokke and Scogin 1995). However, older adults prefer that mental

---

We gratefully acknowledge the contributions of Thomas R. Lynch, Ph.D., Dawn E. Epstein, Ph.D., and Patricia A. Areán, Ph.D., to this chapter in previous editions of this textbook.

health treatment be provided in a primary care context rather than through specialty clinics; favor therapists who understand their existential and spiritual concerns and values; and, as result of their unique sociohistorical context, often feel more comfortable receiving care from practitioners who are of the same race, ethnicity, or religion as themselves (Bartels et al. 2004; Chen et al. 2006; Gum et al. 2010; Hinrichsen 2006; Snodgrass 2009). Whenever possible, patient preferences or biases regarding treatment should be considered before referral for psychotherapy.

As discussed in more detail later in the chapter, older adults will respond to many of the therapeutic interventions that are used in younger populations with little treatment modification. Although highly effective treatments that were originally developed through utilization in younger adult populations, such as cognitive-behavioral therapy (CBT) for mood and anxiety disorders and dialectical behavior therapy (DBT) for personality disorders, have been successfully modified for use in older adult populations, the adaptations are related more to issues regarding cognitive, functional, and sensory impairments than to actual patient age. For older individuals with cognitive impairments, the pace of therapy should be slower, and inclusion of significant others in therapy is advisable. For patients with vision impairments, any written materials should be in larger font sizes, and the use of audio recordings of sessions can facilitate treatment. Accounting for unique cohort-based differences (e.g., sociohistorical environment, norms and commonly held beliefs, role expectations, illness beliefs, culture) and age-specific stressors (e.g., chronic illness and disability, the loss of loved ones and therefore of sources of support, caregiving responsibilities) is also advisable. In-home mental health services may be a valuable option for patients who lack reliable transportation or who have a medical or physical disability. Alternatively, telephone- and internet-based interventions may help older adults overcome common treatment barriers (Alexander et al. 2010). A thorough pretreatment assessment and modifications that are specific to the patient's strengths and deficits can help circumvent age-related pitfalls in psychological treatment (Knight and Poon 2008; Snodgrass 2009; Yang et al. 2009). Many older individuals, particularly those between the ages of 65 and 80 years, are high functioning and may not need these age-specific modifications; therapists should get to know each patient first before making assumptions about what the patient can or cannot do.

In this chapter, we review the empirical evidence for psychosocial interventions for mental health conditions in older adults, considering both individual and group-based psychotherapies. The material is organized by type of disorder and, for each disorder, by type of therapy. Whenever possible, we evaluate the evidence with respect to quality of data, generalizability, and long-term effects of treatment.

Depressive Disorders

Individual Cognitive-Behavioral Therapies

Traditional CBT, particularly CBT for older adults, focuses on three main problematic behaviors: negativity bias, affect regulation, and behavioral activation/motivation. Therapy sessions are constructed first to ascertain the prominent areas of focus and then to teach patients a series of remedial skills to address those areas. In the first week or two of therapy, patients are asked to keep track of their activities, moods, perceptions of daily events, and work and social interactions and to note when they are feeling any kind of negative emotion. After this assessment phase, the patient and therapist work toward behavioral goals depending on the results of the assessment. If the patient has a strong negativity bias (i.e., attends only to negative or threatening social and environmental cues or overly interprets situations as negative and threatening), the work will focus on helping the patient reorient his attention toward a balanced appraisal of life events. If the assessment reveals that the patient has low motivation and limited social and physical activities, then the focus of CBT is on behavioral activation activities and on strategies to increase motivation (Serfaty et al. 2009). In the literature on depression in older adults, CBT has been the most frequently studied psychotherapy (Gould et al. 2012; Karlin et al. 2015). There is some indication that CBT may be more effective than other approaches in older adults (Cuijpers et al. 2016), and older people tend to have better outcomes with CBT than younger cohorts, potentially due to better attendance at therapy sessions (Walker and Clarke 2001).

Group-Based Cognitive-Behavioral Psychotherapies

Although group-based CBT does exist, limited research has been done on the effectiveness of this mode of delivery. Group-based CBT has been effective for older adults with cognitive disabilities (McLaughlin and McFarland 2011) and is effective as an augmentation therapy for people taking antidepressant medications (Wilkinson et al. 2009). In the general adult population, group CBT was found to be as effective as individual CBT but much less expensive to deliver (Bland 2010; Brown et al. 2011).

Individual Problem-Solving Therapy

Problem-solving therapy (PST) is a learning-based behavioral intervention that helps patients focus on solving problems that they feel are contributing to their depression (Areán et al. 1993). According to PST theory, depression is a function of patients' inability to solve important problems in their lives, either because the problems are particularly challenging or because the patients have never had the opportunity to learn effective coping skills (Nezu and Perri 1989). In PST, patients are taught a method of seven-step problem-solving skills for problems in everyday life. Common problems involve social engagement, relationships, motivation, coping with loss, and disease management. PST takes between 4 and 10 sessions and can be administered in a variety of settings, including outpatient, home care, and primary care (Kirkham et al. 2016). The main goal of treatment is to teach patients to become better problem solvers by choosing problems to work on and finding the most appropriate solution.

PST is effective in older adult populations, including low-income elderly persons (Areán et al. 2010a) and those with vision impairment (Rovner et al. 2007). This therapy is effective in telephone and video conference (Choi et al. 2014) and across service settings (Rovner et al. 2007) and can be learned and implemented by a variety of community providers (e.g., social workers, case managers) (Kiosses et al. 2010; Tasman and Rovner 2004; Unützer et al. 2001). In a meta-analysis, PST was found to be as effective as other interventions for treating depression in adults; however, there were far fewer dropouts from PST than from interventions such as CBT and interpersonal therapy (IPT) (Cuijpers et al. 2007).

Although psychotherapies for late-life depression are efficacious, they may not be easily utilized in the community. Engage therapy was developed to address this need and to streamline psychotherapy to be accessible by community therapists (Alexopoulos and Areán 2014). Engage is based on a neurobiological model of depression and uses reward exposure as its central intervention by guiding patients to participate in meaningful, rewarding activities (behavioral activation) (Alexopoulos et al. 2016). Preliminary data suggest that Engage therapy has comparable efficacy with PST in reducing depression and disability in older adults with major depression (Alexopoulos et al. 2015).

Group Problem-Solving Therapy

Very few data exist on the effectiveness of group-based PST, although manuals are available. In a study comparing group-based PST with group-based life review therapy in older adults with major depression, both treatments were effective in reducing symptoms; however, PST resulted in a far greater number of people who recovered from depression (Areán et al. 1993). In a study comparing collaborative care with usual care for depression in older adults in primary care, patients who had responded favorably to PST were offered PST maintenance groups, but very few people elected to participate in the group treatment, preferring to be seen individually for follow-up (Areán et al. 2008).

Interpersonal Psychotherapy

IPT focuses on four common psychosocial problems related to depression: loss and grief, interpersonal disputes and conflicts, role transitions, and interpersonal skill deficits. IPT consists of an assessment phase, treatment phase, maintenance phase, and relapse prevention phase (Miller 2008). IPT for older adults is very similar to that for younger adult populations. The initial assessment phase of IPT involves collecting an interpersonal inventory that helps the therapist and patient identify the primary focus of treatment. Once that focus is identified, two important techniques are used to help the patient move past the problem: communication analysis and differentiating content affect and process affect (Stuart and Noyes 2006). Communication analysis involves asking patients to describe the last time that they encountered the interpersonal problem and discussing the specific details of that problem (e.g., what was said in the encounter and how the patient felt). After the causes of the interpersonal problem are identified, patients develop new communication skills to express their needs and affect. These skills are strengthened through in-session roleplay and between-session practice of these new communication skills. During this process, the therapist works with the patient to identify the feelings that arise while discussing the incident in therapy (process affect) and the feelings that arise outside of the therapy session (content affect).

IPT in the general adult population is a very effective treatment; however, the research on IPT in older adults is mixed, owing to a relatively small database and the fact that larger trials addressed preventing recurrence of depression in those at high risk for recurrence (Areán and Cook 2002). IPT has been found to be very promising as an acute treatment in older adults with depression (Miller et al. 2001, 2003; Reynolds et al. 1999) or with suicidal ideation (Heisel et al. 2015). However, as a prevention approach, the results are not as positive (Carreira et al. 2008; Reynolds et al. 2010).

Other Psychotherapeutic Techniques

A number of other psychotherapeutic techniques for older adults have less empirical support but warrant mentioning: self-guided therapies (e.g., internet-based therapies or bibliotherapy) and life review. Self-guided treatments are those in which patients have access to the therapy in the form of a book or website and are told to follow the instructions. Self-guided therapy has been proven effective in treating depression (Cuijpers et al. 2008). A study by Naylor et al. (2010) compared a physician-delivered behavioral prescription to read *Feeling Good* (Burns 1999) versus usual care for depression in a primary care setting. Dysfunctional attitudes and depressive symptoms were similarly reduced in both treatment groups, and perceived life satisfaction and enjoyment increased. Bibliotherapy might be a viable alternative for patients who cannot afford the cost of medication, who respond partially or not at all to medication, who are reluctant to engage in tertiary psychiatric or psychological care, or who experience adverse side effects (Bowman et al. 1995; Scogin et al. 1989; van't Hof et al. 2011).

Life review and reminiscence psychotherapies are based on the patient's reexperiencing of personal memories and significant life experiences. These interventions have been empirically supported as effective therapies in the treatment of late-life depression, with reminiscence therapy showing reductions in depressive symptoms comparable with CBT in a meta-analysis performed by Pinquart et al. (2007). In a systematic review and meta-analysis of randomized or controlled clinical trials of life review therapy, this therapy was found effective in reducing depressive symptoms, but its effectiveness appears to have been be related to the duration of the intervention (Lan et al. 2017). Specifically, 8 weeks was the most effective duration of treatment. Practicing life review therapy for less than 8 weeks did not have a significant effect on depressive symptoms, and conducting the therapy beyond 8 weeks did not provide any additional benefit (Lan et al. 2017). Reminiscence therapy is often administered in a group setting, with the goal of improving one's self-esteem and sense of social cohesiveness. Recent research suggests that this is an acceptable and viable intervention for late-life depression (Preschl et al. 2012; Serrano Selva et al. 2012).

Psychosocial Interventions for Late-Life Suicide Prevention

Suicide rates in older adults are elevated, and men older than 80 years have the highest rate of suicide for any age-by-sex group (Centers for Disease Control and Prevention 2020). Despite the need for interventions, psychosocial approaches for this population are sparse. In a systematic review of interventions to prevent suicidal behaviors in elderly persons (Okolie et al. 2017), a variety of interventions were identified, including collaborative primary care programs, psychotherapies, and community-based telephone counseling and multilevel programs. Two primary care–based collaborative management programs (Prevention of Suicide in Primary Care Elderly: Collaborative Trial [PROSPECT; Alexopoulos et al. 2009; Bruce et al. 2004] and Improving Mood–Promoting Access to Collaborative Treatment [IMPACT; Unützer et al. 2002, 2006]) and two psychosocial interventions (PST and problem adaptation therapy [PATH]) were evaluated in randomized controlled trials with suicide-related outcomes (Okolie et al. 2017). Even though PROSPECT and IMPACT are collaborative programs and not considered psychosocial interventions, they offered psychosocial interventions (IPT or PST) as a treatment option.

The results from these studies are encouraging. PROSPECT participants had a faster reduction in suicidal ideation than usual-care participants over 24 months (Alexopoulos et al. 2009; Bruce et al. 2004). IMPACT participants had significantly lower rates of suicidal ideation than control subjects over 24 months (Unützer et al. 2002, 2006). PST participants had a significantly greater reduction in suicidal ideation than supportive-therapy participants among older adults with major depression and executive dysfunction (Gustavson et al. 2016). Finally, in a subanalysis of a randomized controlled trial, PATH participants and supportive-therapy participants had comparable reductions in suicidal ideation among older adults with major depression and dementia (Kiosses et al. 2015b).

Despite these encouraging results, further research is urgently needed in psychotherapies for late-life suicide prevention. Most psychotherapies for suicide prevention have been developed to reduce depression rather than suicidal ideation or suicidal behavior per se. However, the mechanism of action for reducing depression may be different from the one for reducing suicidal ideation or behavior. Furthermore, psychosocial interventions for late-life suicide prevention have been tested in older adults with depression and not in older adults who are suicidal or are at high risk for suicide. For example, PST and PATH were developed to reduce depression and disability and were tested in older adults with depression and cognitive impairment who had mild forms of suicidality or no suicidal ideation. Therefore, there is a great need for new psychosocial interventions that will identify and target potential mechanisms of action to reduce suicidal ideation and behavior and evaluate suicide-related outcomes in randomized controlled trials with older adults at risk for suicide.

Anxiety Disorders

Individual Cognitive-Behavioral Therapies

Anxiety disorders are among the most prominent mental disorders of late life, with generalized anxiety disorder (GAD) and agoraphobia (Canuto et al. 2018) being the most diagnosed (Blazer et al. 1991). Wolitzky-Taylor et al. (2010) have written a comprehensive review of anxiety disorders in older adults. Anxiety disorders in late life have been associated with significant distress, increased morbidity and health-related activity limitations, memory deficits, and significant reductions in health-related quality of life. The cumulative burden of anxiety symptoms predicts incidence of functional impairment and exacerbation of existing impairment in older adults (Simning and Seplaki 2020). Although pharmacotherapy for late-life anxiety is quite effective, unwanted side effects can limit the utility of pharmacotherapy (Stanley et al. 2009; Wetherell et al. 2013).

Research on evidence-based treatments for late-life anxiety has been growing over the past two decades, with cognitive and behavioral interventions receiving the strongest support (Ayers et al. 2007). CBT for anxiety disorders focuses on modifying anxious responses to inappropriately feared stimuli. Therapy includes repeated exposure to feared stimuli to facilitate habituation and to provide corrective learning about the actual level of danger or threat from feared stimuli (Foa and Kozak 1986; Moscovitch et al. 2009). These approaches include behavioral techniques such as imaginal and in vivo exposures and cognitive approaches that focus on modifying beliefs about potential threats. Cognitive modifications may include reducing the perceived danger of physical symptoms of anxiety in panic disorder (e.g., recognizing that heart rate increases do not indicate a threat of heart attack) or decreasing the overestimation of negative evaluation by others in social phobia (Deacon and Abramowitz 2004). CBT has been found to be effective for a range of anxiety symptoms (Barrowclough et al. 2001), with comparable effectiveness to medication management (Gorenstein et al. 2005).

In one example of a randomized trial of GAD treatment in older adults, Stanley et al. (2003) compared the efficacy of CBT with that of a minimal-contact condition. The treatment protocol included education training, relaxation training, cognitive restructuring, and exposure to anxiety-provoking stimuli. CBT participants reported significant within-group improvement in the severity of GAD symptoms at the end of the intervention and at 12-month follow-up. These findings suggest that CBT may not only provide effective immediate therapy but also promote long-term gains in the management of GAD. One meta-analysis supported the efficacy of CBT in treating GAD over wait-list or treatment-as-usual conditions, with a slight advantage over active control conditions such as supportive therapy (Hall et al. 2016). Using CBT to augment medication management of anxiety disorders in older adults may be especially effective in managing reactivity to stress (Rosnick et al. 2016), and CBT is associated with reduced relapse following discontinuation compared with discontinuation of a selective serotonin reuptake inhibitor (SSRI) (Wetherell et al. 2013). Adapting CBT for use in primary care facilities is effective (Stanley et al. 2009) and provides treatment where older individuals are most likely to look for it. Implementation of CBT in primary care also facilitates collaboration between CBT therapists and prescription providers. This integration may also be a cost-effective treatment option, as has been the case in primary care psychotherapy for depression.

Although CBT has strong promise for treating GAD in older adults, further empirical research must be conducted to verify its efficacy in this population and to determine mediators and moderators of treatment response. For example, it appears that CBT is not effective in older adults who have consistently low executive function abilities but is effective in individuals whose executive functioning improves along with their psychological symptoms (Mohlman and Gorman 2005). In addition, and in contrast to younger adult populations, older individuals with more severe anxiety at baseline as well as psychiatric comorbidities showed the greatest benefit from treatment (Wetherell et al. 2005). Although older adults do benefit from CBT, they may not benefit to the same extent as younger adults (Kishita and Laidlaw 2017; Wolitzky-Taylor et al. 2010). A greater understanding of the mechanisms and predictors of treatment response will help further refine CBT as an effective approach for late-life anxiety disorders.

Acceptance and commitment therapy (ACT) is among the newer interventions with roots in CBT that show promise for treatment of late-life anxiety. ACT focuses on increasing cognitive flexibility, decreasing experiential avoidance, and increasing engagement with values-based actions. Rather than targeting the frequency or intensity of anxious symptoms, ACT aims to increase patients' acceptance of those experiences through learning to mindfully observe them rather than attempting to push them away or inadvertently fueling them through perseverative thinking (Luoma et al. 2007). A preliminary trial that demonstrated the feasibility of utilizing ACT in older adults with anxiety disorders resulted in a lower dropout rate than that seen with conventional CBT (Wetherell et al. 2011). Preliminary evidence supports using ACT-based interventions for anxiety and depression in long-term care populations (Davison et al. 2017). Further investigation is necessary to determine whether ACT may represent an improvement over CBT in the treatment of late-life anxiety.

Relaxation Training

Relaxation training may be one of the most frequently used treatments for anxiety in older adults. Relaxation training may include techniques such as progressive muscle relaxation, relaxation breathing techniques, and guided imagery. Such techniques are associated with reduced anxiety symptoms (DeBerry 1981–1982, 1982; DeBerry et al. 1989), with maintenance of gains for a year or more (Rickard et al. 1994). Effect sizes for relaxation training across anxiety disorders are comparable with effect sizes for CBT (Thorp et al. 2009).

Relaxation training has some advantages for treating mild anxiety in older adults. The strategies can be taught in brief individual or group sessions. Theoretically, they can be delivered during a regular visit to a primary care physician. As with many behavioral strategies, relaxation training has the advantage of masquerading as skills training for patients who might avoid traditional psychotherapy. Also, patients with cognitive deficits who may have difficulty with more cognitive-based strategies may benefit from purely behavioral strategies. One caveat is that relaxation training may be counterproductive when used in combination with exposure-based treatments because intentional relaxation during exposures may provide temporary relief but interfere with learning long-term tolerance of anxiety (Abramowitz 2013).

Substance-Related Disorders

Substance use has increased worldwide in the past 25 years. Substance use is a growing health problem for older adults in the United States, with alcohol, prescription drug (e.g., opioids and benzodiazepines), and illicit drug abuse as the main substance use problems (Seim et al. 2020). With the Baby Boom generation entering late life, a cohort with higher rates of earlier life substance use than previous geriatric cohorts, a rise is expected in the number of older adults who use alcohol and illicit substances (Gfroerer et al. 2003; Yarnell et al. 2020). Despite the demand for development of age-specific treatments that are acceptable for older adults, psychosocial interventions for this population are underdeveloped (Satre et al. 2003, 2004; Schonfeld et al. 2000; Yarnell et al. 2020).

Cognitive-Behavioral Treatment and Motivational Enhancement Therapy

Although some comprehensive cognitive-behavioral interventions have shown promise for treating substance abuse in older adults, they are also plagued by high dropout rates (Schonfeld et al. 2000). Schonfeld et al. (2010) assessed the effectiveness of the Florida Brief Intervention and Treatment for Elders (BRITE) Project—a low-cost approach for older adults at risk for illicit and nonillicit substance abuse and misuse, which was based on the Screening, Brief Intervention, and Referral to Treatment (SBIRT) initiative (Schonfeld et al. 2000, 2015). Prescription medication misuse and alcohol abuse were most prevalent in the sample. The treatment protocol involved a brief, home-based intervention lasting one to five sessions that included motivational interviewing, education about relevant substances and consequences of substance use and misuse, reasons to quit substance use, and medication management. The BRITE approach resulted in a significant reduction of depression as well as alcohol and prescription medication misuse (Schonfeld et al. 2010).

In a recently published study conducted in Denmark, Germany, and the United States (Andersen et al. 2020), 693 patients ages 60 and older with alcohol use disorder (based on DSM-5 [American Psychiatric Association 2013]) were randomly assigned to receive either motivational enhancement therapy (MET) or MET plus Community Reinforcement Approach for Seniors (CRA-S) (MET+CRA-S) over 26 weeks. MET, which includes four manualized sessions, focuses on increasing motivation to change and establishing a change plan; CRA-S, which includes up to eight additional manualized sessions, focuses on helping patients implement their change plan. The primary outcome was a self-report of either total alcohol abstinence or an expected blood alcohol concentration of ≤0.05% (based on the self-reported consumption) (success) or a blood alcohol concentration of >0.05% during the follow-up period (failure) during the 30 days preceding the 26-week follow-up. MET and MET+CRA-S had comparable success rates (49% vs. 52%, respectively) over 26 weeks, and no significant differences were found between the two conditions. These results are encouraging, but further studies are recommended to establish the efficacy of MET in older adults (Andersen et al. 2020).

Screening, Brief Intervention, and Referral to Treatment

Brief interventions in primary care have received increasing attention for the treatment of alcohol use in older adults. Because primary care physicians are the most likely individuals to identify overuse of alcohol in their patients, this setting is a natural area for which to develop treatment protocols. Brief counseling by the treating physician has been found to be significantly more effective in reducing alcohol misuse in older adults than providing a general health booklet (Fleming et al. 1999). The SBIRT model was developed primarily to assist primary care clinicians in detecting and managing this illness (Babor et al. 2007) and is also used in other health care settings such as emergency departments and trauma centers (Schonfeld et al. 2015). This model provides patients with an initial brief screening to determine extent of substance use, and patients who screen positive are treated in one of two settings. Some are treated in primary care with a brief motivational intervention focusing on increasing patient awareness about substance use and the pros and cons of that use to help motivate the patients to make changes in their substance use. Those requiring a higher level of care are referred to specialty substance abuse treatment outside of the primary care setting (Young et al. 2012). In an SBIRT study in 29 agencies in 15 Florida counties, 85,001 screenings were recorded, and about 10% of the clients were at moderate or high risk of substance use (Schonfeld et al. 2015). In a random sample of clients who received brief intervention, brief treatment, or referral to treatment (N=516) in 6-month follow-up, 130 clients provided data at both baseline and 6-month follow up and revealed a significant decrease in past-30-day substance use in any alcohol and illegal drug use (Schonfeld et al. 2015). Another study found that primary care–based brief treatment for alcohol misuse in older adults was as effective as referral to specialty treatment (Oslin et al. 2006).

Previous editions of this book have indicated that there is insufficient research on the management of substance abuse in older populations. Despite the alarming need for psychosocial interventions in this area, research continues to be scarce.

Personality Disorders

Cognitive-Behavioral Therapies

Personality disorders are enduring patterns of inner experience (e.g., cognition, affect, impulse control) and behavior (e.g., interpersonal difficulties) that have an onset in adolescence or early adulthood, are stable over time, deviate considerably from normal cultural expectations, and cause distress or impairment in functioning. National survey studies have concluded that the prevalence rate for personality disorders in older adults is between 8% and 15% (Reynolds et al. 2015; Schuster et al. 2013), which is essentially analogous to the 13% prevalence rate for younger age groups (Torgersen et al. 2001). Overall, the emotionally constricted/risk-averse disorders in Cluster A (i.e., paranoid and schizoid personality disorders) and Cluster C (i.e., obsessive-compulsive, avoidant, and dependent personality disorders) are the most common disorders in late life (Kenan et al. 2000; Morse and Lynch 2004; Schuster et al. 2013; but see Reynolds et al. 2015 for commensurate rates of Cluster B disorders). In addition, personality disorder rates are even higher (~30%) among older adults with depression (Abrams 1996; Thompson et al. 1988).

Personality psychopathology has generally been associated with poorer response to treatment among older adults, whether treated with antidepressants or psychotherapy (Abrams et al. 1994; Lynch et al. 2007; Thompson et al. 1988; Zweig 2008; but see also Gradman et al. 1999; Gum et al. 2007). Older adult patients with depression and comorbid personality disorder are four times more likely to experience maintenance or reemergence of depressive symptoms than are those without personality disorder diagnoses (Morse and Lynch 2004). Despite this, and despite calls for greater attention to the development and improvement of interventions for personality disorders in late life (e.g., Videler et al. 2012), few controlled studies of the treatment of personality disorders in older adults have been published.

The only published randomized clinical trial specifically targeting personality disorders in older adults was conducted by Lynch et al. (2007). The study focused on providing standard DBT using both group and individual sessions following Linehan's (1993) manual. Participants were older adults with depression who presented with at least one comorbid personality disorder and who did not have an adequate response to an 8-week SSRI trial. Compared with patients in a medication-only condition, participants who received DBT plus medication management reached the level of remission more quickly and showed improvements in interpersonal sensitivity and aggression, although they did not show greater reductions in depressive symptoms (Lynch et al. 2007). Adaptations of standard DBT focusing on the most common older adult personality disorders (e.g., paranoid personality disorder, obsessive-compulsive personality disorder) are needed to target reducing rigidity, cognitive inflexibility, emotional constriction, and risk aversion (Lynch and Cheavens 2008). Two open/multiple-baseline trials have demonstrated promising effects for schema therapy in older adults with significant personality symptoms (Videler et al. 2014) and Cluster C disorders (Videler et al. 2018), with additional trials under way (van Donzel et al. 2021; van Dijk et al. 2019). Further randomized clinical trials are needed to demonstrate the benefits of schema therapy over existing standard treatments.

Despite the promising nature of these findings, the bulk of empirical evidence suggests that the presence of a personality disorder in an older adult seriously compromises treatment. In addition, rates of personality disorders among older adults may be only slightly lower than those in younger age groups, and subsyndromal personality disorders may be more prevalent in older populations relative to younger ones (Abrams and Bromberg 2006). It appears that psychotherapy interventions likely will be enhanced when they target the unique behavioral, cognitive, and interpersonal dynamics associated with personality disorders in older adults.

Psychotherapy With Cognitively Impaired Patients

One frequent consideration for providers and referring physicians is the degree to which an older adult with impairments in memory or executive function can engage with and benefit from individual or group psychotherapy. Cognitive difficulties in late life occur on a spectrum, ranging from a lack of any impairment to age-related cognitive decline to specific deficits or mild cognitive impairment to more frank dementia. At some point along this spectrum, patients become less able to perform and to capitalize on cognitive and behavioral changes without significant support from caregivers and environmental modifications. The challenge for providers is to assess the appropriateness of a given intervention and to make modifications as necessary to maximize benefits.

Psychotherapies, especially CBT, are thought to rely on executive functioning and memory skills (Hariri et al. 2000; Mohlman 2008; Mohlman and Gorman 2005). Cognitive reappraisal requires patients to attend to their thoughts, hold them in working memory, generate alternative thoughts, and implement those alternative thoughts. Implementing behavioral changes requires remembering the new behavior in order to implement it, planning, and sustained attention to new behaviors. Because psychotherapy requires executive and memory skills, it is hypothesized to be less effective for those with cognitive impairments. Empirical studies are mixed, with some finding reduced effectiveness in cognitively impaired patients (Mohlman and Gorman 2005) and others finding no correlation between cognitive screening measures (e.g., the Mini-Mental State Examination [Folstein et al. 1975]) and treatment outcome in older adults (Marquett et al. 2013; Wetherell et al. 2005), especially if cognitive performance improves with treatment.

Given that individuals with cognitive impairments also have a reduced response to pharmacotherapy (Manning et al. 2015; Pimontel et al. 2012), the presence of cognitive impairments does not necessarily disqualify a patient from consideration for psychotherapy. Although psychosocial interventions have been developed for older adults with depression and anxiety with comorbid cognitive impairment, most of them have been tested in small samples (<30 per group), and few have been evaluated in adequately powered randomized controlled trials (Areán et al. 2010b; Kiosses et al. 2015a; Miller and Reynolds 2007; Mohlman 2008; Orgeta et al. 2015; Raue et al. 2017;

Rodakowski et al. 2015; Simon et al. 2015; Spector et al. 2015). PST was adapted for older adults with major depression and executive dysfunction and demonstrated efficacy in reducing depression and disability versus supportive therapy in 221 older adults with depression and executive dysfunction (Alexopoulos et al. 2011; Areán et al. 2010b). Similarly, in 74 patients with major depression and advanced cognitive impairment (from mild cognitive deficits to moderate dementia), PATH resulted in a significantly greater reduction in depression and disability compared with supportive therapy (Kiosses et al. 2015a). Finally, CBT and problem-solving interventions have shown promise for reducing depression and anxiety in neurological conditions, including Parkinson's disease (Armento et al. 2012; Calleo et al. 2015), stroke (Alexopoulos et al. 2012), and multiple sclerosis (Moss-Morris et al. 2013).

Several modifications to therapy may be used to better accommodate and target cognitive impairments. One common modification is the incorporation of a caregiver in the therapy process. Caregivers can assist with the generation of treatment targets, help implement changes outside of therapy (e.g., assisting with behavioral experiments as part of cognitive therapy or helping to work past barriers to behavioral activation goals), and provide reminders and reinforcement for therapy content for patients with memory impairments. In addition to helping patients maximize insight and change from therapy, therapy can help the caregivers themselves learn to recognize their own changing roles as caregivers, learn realistic expectations for their loved ones' abilities, and maximize their effectiveness in assisting their loved one.

In cognitive-behavioral approaches, a modification strategy for individuals with milder impairment is to target cognitive change (e.g., challenge beliefs about being a "burden," generate realistic assessments about fall risks in those with fear of falling). For individuals with more moderate to severe impairment, the focus shifts to behavioral changes and environmental adaptations (e.g., reinforcing positive reminiscence over expressions of dysphoria; facilitating engagement with valued or pleasant activities; utilizing notes, calendars, step-by-step written plans) (Kiosses et al. 2015a; Teri and Gallagher-Thompson 1991). Finally, training programs that target remediation of executive dysfunction have been administered along with standard CBT, with benefits to cognitive function and reduction in worry in patients with GAD (Mohlman 2008). These programs include audiotape-and-workbook or computer-based trainings that target speed of processing, attention, and cognitive flexibility processes within in-session and at-home exercises (Anguera et al. 2013; Mohlman 2008). With these modifications, psychotherapy can lead to significant improvements in mood and behavioral symptoms.

Even within the context of mild to moderate dementia, psychosocial interventions can benefit patients' mood and behavior. Because the dementia is not expected to abate, treatment targets global quality of life, affective states, disruptive behavioral symptoms, functional impairment, and prevention of self-harm. Most psychosocial interventions for dementia are based on behavioral strategies and may target caregivers and, or in lieu of, the patients themselves (Livingston et al. 2005; Teri et al. 2005).

Transdiagnostic and Third-Wave Treatments

The past two decades have seen the rise of "third-wave" CBTs that emphasize patients' relationship with their thoughts, feelings, and behaviors, rather than the content of their thoughts per se (Hayes and Hofmann 2017). These interventions include therapies that emphasize acceptance and metacognitive awareness, such as ACT, DBT, the Unified Protocol, and mindfulness-based interventions. Third-wave CBTs emphasize the identification and treatment of psychological processes, such as rumination or avoidance, over syndrome- or diagnosis-based protocols. In this way, they are aligned with principles of the National Institute of Mental Health's Research Domain Criteria, which emphasize understanding and addressing biologically mediated processes that contribute to psychopathology (Hayes and Hofmann 2017). Given the transdiagnostic emphasis of the approaches, studies of their efficacy do not neatly fall into categories such as treatment for mood disorders or anxiety disorders. However, they may be especially promising interventions for many patients whose presentations cross diagnostic lines.

Preliminary evidence is promising for the use of third-wave interventions with older adults (Kishita et al. 2017). Mindfulness-based interventions have been shown to reduce depression and anxiety symptoms and improve quality of life and may help maintain cognitive function in older adults with memory complaints (Smoski et al. 2016). Mindfulness-based stress reduction (MBSR) may not require modification in order to be appropriate for patients with mild memory problems (Lenze et al. 2014) because standard MBSR classes are becoming available in more communities across the United States and other countries. There is growing evidence that other third-wave interventions, including ACT (Davison et al. 2017; Karlin et al. 2013; Scott et al. 2017), are acceptable and have preliminary evidence of efficacy in reducing depression, anxiety, and chronic pain symptoms, although comparison trials with other gold-standard interventions are largely lacking in older adult populations.

Conclusion

Psychotherapy offers significant promise for the treatment of psychopathology in elderly persons and at times may be the treatment of choice in terms of both efficacy and patient preference. We encourage practitioners to select treatments that have been tested in randomized clinical trials rather than basing their choices on theoretical preference or ease of application. The use of treatments without this type of empirical support can slow or reduce recovery.

Future research should continue to examine the beneficial effects of strategies combining medication and psychotherapy. In addition, research examining the mechanisms of change and issues associated with treatment response by disorder and type of therapy remains to be more fully developed. Finally, continued research is needed to focus on populations with treatment-resistant illnesses, such as personality disorders, substance use disorders, and comorbid disorders.

Key Points

- Psychotherapy is a good option for treating mental disorders in older adults who have trouble tolerating medications, who prefer psychotherapy over medication treatment, or who have conditions for which psychotherapy is the most effective treatment.

- Modifications of traditional therapies may be necessary to compensate for age-related problems with vision, hearing, mobility, and cognition.

- Effective treatments for depression include several different individual and group cognitive-behavioral therapies, interpersonal psychotherapy, and short-term psychodynamic therapy.

- The most common anxiety disorder among older adults is generalized anxiety disorder. Behavioral treatments such as relaxation training and cognitive-behavioral therapy are the most effective treatments for this disorder.

- Patients with personality pathology have poorer response to treatment of other comorbid conditions, such as depression and anxiety. Few treatments targeting personality disorder in older adults have been tested. One promising and empirically validated treatment is a modification of dialectical behavior therapy for older adults.

- Although cognitive impairments may limit the effectiveness of psychotherapy, modifications such as the inclusion of a caregiver in the therapy process or adjunctive cognitive remediation techniques can improve outcomes.

- There is a great need for psychotherapies addressing late-life suicide prevention that are based on mechanisms of action for reducing suicidal ideation and behavior in this population.

- Psychotherapies for late-life suicide prevention need to also focus on older adults at high risk for suicide.

- Development of interventions designed to meet the unique needs of underrepresented minority groups is needed, as well as greater training in culturally competent care to address the needs of all older adults with mental health concerns.

Suggested Readings

Alexopoulos GS, Arean P: A model for streamlining psychotherapy in the RDoC era: the example of "Engage." Mol Psychiatry 19(1):14–19, 2014

Barrowclough C, King P, Colville J, et al: A randomized trial of the effectiveness of cognitive-behavioral therapy and supportive counseling for anxiety symptoms in older adults. J Consult Clin Psychol 69:756–762, 2001

Bartels SJ, Coakley EH, Zubritsky C, et al: Improving access to geriatric mental health services: a randomized trial comparing treatment engagement with integrated versus enhanced referral care for depression, anxiety, and at-risk alcohol use. Am J Psychiatry 161:1455–1462, 2004

Bruce ML, Ten Have TR, Reynolds CF, et al: Reducing suicidal ideation and depressive symptoms in depressed older primary care patients. JAMA 291:1081–1091, 2004

Livingston G, Johnston K, Katona C, et al: Systematic review of psychological approaches to the management of neuropsychiatric symptoms of dementia. Am J Psychiatry 162:1996–2021, 2005

Lynch TR, Cheavens JS, Cukrowicz KC, et al: Treatment of older adults with co-morbid personality disorder and depression: a dialectical behavior therapy approach. Int J Geriatr Psychiatry 22:131–143, 2007

Mohlman J, Gorman JM: The role of executive functioning in CBT: a pilot study with anxious older adults. Behav Res Ther 43:447–465, 2004

Oslin DW, Grantham S, Coakley E, et al: PRISM-E: comparison of integrated care and enhanced specialty referral in managing at-risk alcohol use. Psychiatr Serv 57:954–958, 2006

Thompson LW, Coon DW, Gallagher-Thompson D, et al: Comparison of desipramine and cognitive/behavioral therapy in the treatment of elderly outpatients with mild-to-moderate depression. Am J Geriatr Psychiatry 9:225–240, 2001

Unützer JM, Katon WM, Williams JWJ, et al: Improving primary care for depression in late life: the design of a multicenter randomized trial. Med Care 39:785–799, 2001

Unützer J, Tang L, Oishi S, et al: Reducing suicidal ideation in depressed older primary care patients. J Am Geriatr Soc 54(10):1550–1556, 2006

References

Abramowitz JS: The practice of exposure therapy: relevance of cognitive-behavioral theory and extinction theory. Behav Ther 44(4):548–558, 2013 24094780

Abrams RC: Personality disorders in the elderly. Int J Geriatr Psychiatry 11:759–763, 1996

Abrams RC, Bromberg CE: Personality disorders in the elderly: a flagging field of inquiry. Int J Geriatr Psychiatry 21(11):1013–1017, 2006 17061248

Abrams RC, Rosendahl E, Card C, Alexopoulos GS: Personality disorder correlates of late and early onset depression. J Am Geriatr Soc 42(7):727–731, 1994 8014347

Alexander CL, Arnkoff DB, Glass CR: Bringing psychotherapy to primary care: innovations and challenges. Clin Psychol Sci Pract 17(3):191–214, 2010

Alexopoulos GS, Areán P: A model for streamlining psychotherapy in the RDoC era: the example of "Engage." Mol Psychiatry 19(1):14–19, 2014 24280983

Alexopoulos GS, Reynolds CF III, Bruce ML, et al: Reducing suicidal ideation and depression in older primary care patients: 24-month outcomes of the PROSPECT study. Am J Psychiatry 166(8):882–890, 2009 19528195

Alexopoulos GS, Raue PJ, Kiosses DN, et al: Problem-solving therapy and supportive therapy in older adults with major depression and executive dysfunction: effect on disability. Arch Gen Psychiatry 68(1):33–41, 2011 21199963

Alexopoulos GS, Wilkins VM, Marino P, et al: Ecosystem focused therapy in poststroke depression: a preliminary study. Int J Geriatr Psychiatry 27(10):1053–1060, 2012 22249997

Alexopoulos GS, Raue PJ, Kiosses DN, et al: Comparing engage with PST in late-life major depression: a preliminary report. Am J Geriatr Psychiatry 23(5):506–513, 2015 25081818

Alexopoulos GS, Raue PJ, Gunning F, et al: "Engage" therapy: behavioral activation and improvement of late-life major depression. Am J Geriatr Psychiatry 24(4):320–326, 2016 26905044

American Psychiatric Association: Diagnostic and Statistical Manual of Mental Disorders, 5th Edition. Arlington, VA, American Psychiatric Association, 2013

Andersen K, Behrendt S, Bilberg R, et al: Evaluation of adding the community reinforcement approach to motivational enhancement therapy for adults aged 60 years and older with DSM-5 alcohol use disorder: a randomized controlled trial. Addiction 115(1):69–81, 2020 31454444

Anguera JA, Boccanfuso J, Rintoul JL, et al: Video game training enhances cognitive control in older adults. Nature 501(7465):97–101, 2013 24005416

Areán PA, Cook BL: Psychotherapy and combined psychotherapy/pharmacotherapy for late life depression. Biol Psychiatry 52(3):293–303, 2002 12182934

Areán PA, Perri MG, Nezu AM, et al: Comparative effectiveness of social problem-solving therapy and reminiscence therapy as treatments for depression in older adults. J Consult Clin Psychol 61(6):1003–1010, 1993 8113478

Areán P, Hegel M, Vannoy S, et al: Effectiveness of problem-solving therapy for older, primary care patients with depression: results from the IMPACT project. Gerontologist 48(3):311–323, 2008 18591356

Areán PA, Mackin S, Vargas-Dwyer E, et al: Treating depression in disabled, low-income elderly: a conceptual model and recommendations for care. Int J Geriatr Psychiatry 25(8):765–769, 2010a 20602424

Areán PA, Raue P, Mackin RS, et al: Problem-solving therapy and supportive therapy in older adults with major depression and executive dysfunction. Am J Psychiatry 167(11):1391–1398, 2010b 20516155

Armento ME, Stanley MA, Marsh L, et al: Cognitive behavioral therapy for depression and anxiety in Parkinson's disease: a clinical review. J Parkinsons Dis 2(2):135–151, 2012 23939438

Ayers CR, Sorrell JT, Thorp SR, Wetherell JL: Evidence-based psychological treatments for late-life anxiety. Psychol Aging 22(1):8–17, 2007 17385978

Babor TF, McRee BG, Kassebaum PA, et al: Screening, brief intervention, and referral to treatment (SBIRT): toward a public health approach to the management of substance abuse. Subst Abus 28(3):7–30, 2007 18077300

Barrowclough C, King P, Colville J, et al: A randomized trial of the effectiveness of cognitive-behavioral therapy and supportive counseling for anxiety symptoms in older adults. J Consult Clin Psychol 69(5):756–762, 2001 11680552

Bartels SJ, Coakley EH, Zubritsky C, et al: Improving access to geriatric mental health services: a randomized trial comparing treatment engagement with integrated versus enhanced referral care for depression, anxiety, and at-risk alcohol use. Am J Psychiatry 161(8):1455–1462, 2004 15285973

Bland P: Group CBT is a cost-effective option for persistent back pain. Practitioner 254(1728):7, 2010

Blazer D, George LK, Hughes D: The epidemiology of anxiety disorders: an age comparison, in Anxiety in the Elderly: Treatment and Research. Edited by Salzman C, Lebowitz BD. New York, Springer, 1991, pp 17–30

Bowman D, Scogin F, Lyrene B: The efficacy of self-examination therapy and cognitive bibliotherapy in the treatment of mild to moderate depression. Psychother Res 5:131–140, 1995

Brown JS, Sellwood K, Beecham JK, et al: Outcome, costs and patient engagement for group and individual CBT for depression: a naturalistic clinical study. Behav Cogn Psychother 39(3):355–358, 2011 21406135

Bruce ML, Ten Have TR, Reynolds CF III, et al: Reducing suicidal ideation and depressive symptoms in depressed older primary care patients: a randomized controlled trial. JAMA 291(9):1081–1091, 2004 14996777

Burns DD: Feeling Good: The New Mood Therapy. New York, William Morrow, 1999

Byers AL, Arean PA, Yaffe K: Low use of mental health services among older Americans with mood and anxiety disorders. Psychiatr Serv 63(1):66–72, 2012 22227762

Calleo JS, Amspoker AB, Sarwar AI, et al: A pilot study of a cognitive-behavioral treatment for anxiety and depression in patients with Parkinson disease. J Geriatr Psychiatry Neurol 28(3):210–217, 2015 26047635

Canuto A, Weber K, Baertschi M, et al: Anxiety disorders in old age: psychiatric comorbidities, quality of life, and prevalence according to age, gender, and country. Am J Geriatr Psychiatry 26(2):174–185, 2018 29031568

Carreira K, Miller MD, Frank E, et al: A controlled evaluation of monthly maintenance interpersonal psychotherapy in late-life depression with varying levels of cognitive function. Int J Geriatr Psychiatry 23(11):1110–1113, 2008 18457338

Centers for Disease Control and Prevention: WISQARS: Fatal Injury Reports, National, Regional and State, 1981–2019. Atlanta, GA, Centers for Disease Control and Prevention, 2020. Available at: https://wisqars.cdc.gov/fatal-reports. Accessed March 2020.

Chen H, Coakley EH, Cheal K, et al: Satisfaction with mental health services in older primary care patients. Am J Geriatr Psychiatry 14(4):371–379, 2006 16582046

Choi NG, Hegel MT, Marti N, et al: Telehealth problem-solving therapy for depressed low-income homebound older adults. Am J Geriatr Psychiatry 22(3):263–271, 2014 23567376

Conner KO, Copeland VC, Grote NK, et al: Barriers to treatment and culturally endorsed coping strategies among depressed African-American older adults. Aging Ment Health 14(8):971–983, 2010 21069603

Crabb R, Hunsley J: Utilization of mental health care services among older adults with depression. J Clin Psychol 62(3):299–312, 2006 16400646

Cuijpers P, van Straten A, Warmerdam L: Problem solving therapies for depression: a meta-analysis. Eur Psychiatry 22(1):9–15, 2007 17194572

Cuijpers P, van Straten A, Warmerdam L, Andersson G: Psychological treatment of depression: a meta-analytic database of randomized studies. BMC Psychiatry 8:36, 2008 18485191

Cuijpers P, Ebert DD, Acarturk C, et al: Personalized psychotherapy for adult depression: a meta-analytic review. Behav Ther 47(6):966–980, 2016 27993344

Davison TE, Eppingstall B, Runci S, O'Connor DW: A pilot trial of acceptance and commitment therapy for symptoms of depression and anxiety in older adults residing in long-term care facilities. Aging Ment Health 21(7):766–773, 2017 26942691

Deacon BJ, Abramowitz JS: Cognitive and behavioral treatments for anxiety disorders: a review of meta-analytic findings. J Clin Psychol 60(4):429–441, 2004 15022272

DeBerry S: An evaluation of progressive muscle relaxation on stress related symptoms in a geriatric population. Int J Aging Hum Dev 14(4):255–269, 1981–1982 7345035

DeBerry S: The effects of meditation-relaxation on anxiety and depression in a geriatric population. Psychotherapy (Chic) 19:512–521, 1982

DeBerry S, Davis S, Reinhard KE: A comparison of meditation-relaxation and cognitive/behavioral techniques for reducing anxiety and depression in a geriatric population. J Geriatr Psychiatry 22(2):231–247, 1989 2701175

Fleming MF, Manwell LB, Barry KL, et al: Brief physician advice for alcohol problems in older adults: a randomized community-based trial. J Fam Pract 48(5):378–384, 1999 10334615

Foa EB, Kozak MJ: Emotional processing of fear: exposure to corrective information. Psychol Bull 99(1):20–35, 1986 2871574

Folstein MF, Folstein SE, McHugh PR: "Mini-mental state": a practical method for grading the cognitive state of patients for the clinician. J Psychiatr Res 12(3):189–198, 1975 1202204

Gfroerer J, Penne M, Pemberton M, Folsom R: Substance abuse treatment need among older adults in 2020: the impact of the aging baby-boom cohort. Drug Alcohol Depend 69(2):127–135, 2003 12609694

Gorenstein EE, Kleber MS, Mohlman J, et al: Cognitive-behavioral therapy for management of anxiety and medication taper in older adults. Am J Geriatr Psychiatry 13(10):901–909, 2005 16223969

Gould RL, Coulson MC, Howard RJ: Cognitive behavioral therapy for depression in older people: a meta-analysis and meta-regression of randomized controlled trials. J Am Geriatr Soc 60(10):1817–1830, 2012 23003115

Gradman TJ, Thompson LW, Gallagher-Thompson D: Personality disorders and treatment outcome, in Personality Disorders in Older Adults: Emerging Issues in Diagnosis and Treatment. Edited by Rosowsky E, Abrams RC. Mahwah, NJ, Erlbaum, 1999, pp 69–94

Gum AM, Areán PA, Hunkeler E, et al: Depression treatment preferences in older primary care patients. Gerontologist 46(1):14–22, 2006 16452280

Gum AM, Areán PA, Bostrom A: Low-income depressed older adults with psychiatric comorbidity: secondary analyses of response to psychotherapy and case management. Int J Geriatr Psychiatry 22(2):124–130, 2007 17096464

Gum AM, Iser L, Petkus A: Behavioral health service utilization and preferences of older adults receiving home-based aging services. Am J Geriatr Psychiatry 18(6):491–501, 2010 21217560

Gustavson KA, Alexopoulos GS, Niu GC, et al: Problem-solving therapy reduces suicidal ideation in depressed older adults with executive dysfunction. Am J Geriatr Psychiatry 24(1):11–17, 2016 26743100

Hall J, Kellett S, Berrios R, et al: Efficacy of cognitive behavioral therapy for generalized anxiety disorder in older adults: systematic review, meta-analysis, and meta-regression. Am J Geriatr Psychiatry 24(11):1063–1073, 2016 27687212

Hariri AR, Bookheimer SY, Mazziotta JC: Modulating emotional responses: effects of a neocortical network on the limbic system. Neuroreport 11(1):43–48, 2000 10683827

Hayes SC, Hofmann SG: The third wave of cognitive behavioral therapy and the rise of process-based care. World Psychiatry 16(3):245–246, 2017 28941087

Heisel MJ, Talbot NL, King DA, et al: Adapting interpersonal psychotherapy for older adults at risk for suicide. Am J Geriatr Psychiatry 23(1):87–98, 2015 24840611

Hinrichsen GA: Why multicultural issues matter for practitioners working with older adults. Prof Psychol Res Pr 37(1):29–35, 2006

Karlin BE, Walser RD, Yesavage J, et al: Effectiveness of acceptance and commitment therapy for depression: comparison among older and younger veterans. Aging Ment Health 17(5):555–563, 2013 23607328

Karlin BE, Trockel M, Brown GK, et al: Comparison of the effectiveness of cognitive behavioral therapy for depression among older versus younger veterans: results of a national evaluation. J Gerontol B Psychol Sci Soc Sci 70(1):3–12, 2015 24218096

Kenan MM, Kendjelic EM, Molinari VA, et al: Age-related differences in the frequency of personality disorders among inpatient veterans. Int J Geriatr Psychiatry 15(9):831–837, 2000 10984730

Kiosses DN, Areán PA, Teri L, Alexopoulos GS: Home-delivered problem adaptation therapy (PATH) for depressed, cognitively impaired, disabled elders: a preliminary study. Am J Geriatr Psychiatry 18(11):988–998, 2010 20808092

Kiosses DN, Ravdin LD, Gross JJ, et al: Problem adaptation therapy for older adults with major depression and cognitive impairment: a randomized clinical trial. JAMA Psychiatry 72(1):22–30, 2015a 25372657

Kiosses DN, Rosenberg PB, McGovern A, et al: Depression and suicidal ideation during two psychosocial treatments in older adults with major depression and dementia. J Alzheimers Dis 48(2):453–462, 2015b 26402009

Kirkham JG, Choi N, Seitz DP: Meta-analysis of problem solving therapy for the treatment of major depressive disorder in older adults. Int J Geriatr Psychiatry 31(5):526–535, 2016 26437368

Kishita N, Laidlaw K: Cognitive behaviour therapy for generalized anxiety disorder: is CBT equally efficacious in adults of working age and older adults? Clin Psychol Rev 52:124–136, 2017 28119196

Kishita N, Takei Y, Stewart I: A meta-analysis of third wave mindfulness-based cognitive behavioral therapies for older people. Int J Geriatr Psychiatry 32(12):1352–1361, 2017 27862293

Knight BG, Poon CY: Contextual adult life span theory for adapting psychotherapy with older adults. J Ration-Emot Cogn-Behav Ther 26(4):232–249, 2008

Lan X, Xiao H, Chen Y: Effects of life review interventions on psychosocial outcomes among older adults: a systematic review and meta-analysis. Geriatr Gerontol Int 17(10):1344–1357, 2017 28124828

Lenze EJ, Hickman S, Hershey T, et al: Mindfulness-based stress reduction for older adults with worry symptoms and co-occurring cognitive dysfunction. Int J Geriatr Psychiatry 29(10):991–1000, 2014 24677282

Linehan MM: Cognitive-Behavioral Treatment of Borderline Personality Disorder. New York, Guilford, 1993

Livingston G, Johnston K, Katona C, et al: Systematic review of psychological approaches to the management of neuropsychiatric symptoms of dementia. Am J Psychiatry 162(11):1996–2021, 2005 16263837

Luoma JB, Hayes SC, Walser RD: Learning ACT: An Acceptance and Commitment Therapy Skills-Training Manual for Therapists. Oakland, CA, New Harbinger, 2007

Lynch TR, Cheavens JS: Dialectical behavior therapy for comorbid personality disorders. J Clin Psychol 64(2):154–167, 2008 18186120

Lynch TR, Cheavens JS, Cukrowicz KC, et al: Treatment of older adults with co-morbid personality disorder and depression: a dialectical behavior therapy approach. Int J Geriatr Psychiatry 22(2):131–143, 2007 17096462

Manning KJ, Alexopoulos GS, Banerjee S, et al: Executive functioning complaints and escitalopram treatment response in late-life depression. Am J Geriatr Psychiatry 23(5):440–445, 2015 24388222

Marquett RM, Thompson LW, Reiser RP, et al: Psychosocial predictors of treatment response to cognitive-behavior therapy for late-life depression: an exploratory study. Aging Ment Health 17(7):830–838, 2013 23631698

McLaughlin DP, McFarland K: A randomized trial of a group based cognitive behavior therapy program for older adults with epilepsy: the impact on seizure frequency, depression and psychosocial well-being. J Behav Med 34(3):201–207, 2011 20927577

Miller MD: Using interpersonal therapy (IPT) with older adults today and tomorrow: a review of the literature and new developments. Curr Psychiatry Rep 10(1):16–22, 2008 18269890

Miller MD, Reynolds CF III: Expanding the usefulness of interpersonal psychotherapy (IPT) for depressed elders with co-morbid cognitive impairment. Int J Geriatr Psychiatry 22(2):101–105, 2007 17096459

Miller MD, Cornes C, Frank E, et al: Interpersonal psychotherapy for late-life depression: past, present, and future. J Psychother Pract Res 10(4):231–238, 2001 11696649

Miller MD, Frank E, Cornes C, et al: The value of maintenance interpersonal psychotherapy (IPT) in older adults with different IPT foci. Am J Geriatr Psychiatry 11(1):97–102, 2003 12527545

Mohlman J: More power to the executive? A preliminary test of CBT plus executive skills training for treatment of late-life GAD. Cognit Behav Pract 15:306–316, 2008

Mohlman J, Gorman JM: The role of executive functioning in CBT: a pilot study with anxious older adults. Behav Res Ther 43(4):447–465, 2005 15701356

Morse JQ, Lynch TR: A preliminary investigation of self-reported personality disorders in late life: prevalence, predictors of depressive severity, and clinical correlates. Aging Ment Health 8(4):307–315, 2004 15370047

Moscovitch DA, Antony MM, Swinson RP: Exposure-based treatments for anxiety disorders, in Oxford Handbook of Anxiety and Related Disorders. Edited by Antony MM, Stein MB. New York, Oxford University Press, 2009, pp 461–475

Moss-Morris R, Dennison L, Landau S, et al: A randomized controlled trial of cognitive behavioral therapy (CBT) for adjusting to multiple sclerosis (the saMS trial): does CBT work and for whom does it work? J Consult Clin Psychol 81(2):251–262, 2013 22730954

Naylor EV, Antonuccio DO, Litt M, et al: Bibliotherapy as a treatment for depression in primary care. J Clin Psychol Med Settings 17(3):258–271, 2010 20803165

Nezu AM, Perri MG: Social problem-solving therapy for unipolar depression: an initial dismantling investigation. J Consult Clin Psychol 57(3):408–413, 1989 2738213

Okolie C, Dennis M, Simon Thomas E, John A: A systematic review of interventions to prevent suicidal behaviors and reduce suicidal ideation in older people. Int Psychogeriatr 29(11):1801–1824, 2017 28766474

Orgeta V, Qazi A, Spector A, Orrell M: Psychological treatments for depression and anxiety in dementia and mild cognitive impairment: systematic review and meta-analysis. Br J Psychiatry 207(4):293–298, 2015 26429684

Oslin DW, Grantham S, Coakley E, et al: PRISM-E: comparison of integrated care and enhanced specialty referral in managing at-risk alcohol use. Psychiatr Serv 57(7):954–958, 2006 16816279

Pimontel MA, Culang-Reinlieb ME, Morimoto SS, Sneed JR: Executive dysfunction and treatment response in late-life depression. Int J Geriatr Psychiatry 27(9):893–899, 2012 22009869

Pinquart M, Duberstein PR, Lyness JM: Effects of psychotherapy and other behavioral interventions on clinically depressed older adults: a meta-analysis. Aging Ment Health 11(6):645–657, 2007 18074252

Preschl B, Maercker A, Wagner B, et al: Life-review therapy with computer supplements for depression in the elderly: a randomized controlled trial. Aging Ment Health 16(8):964–974, 2012 22788983

Raue PJ, McGovern AR, Kiosses DN, Sirey JA: Advances in psychotherapy for depressed older adults. Curr Psychiatry Rep 19(9):57, 2017 28726061

Reynolds CF III, Frank E, Perel JM, et al: Nortriptyline and interpersonal psychotherapy as maintenance therapies for recurrent major depression: a randomized controlled trial in patients older than 59 years. JAMA 281(1):39–45, 1999

Reynolds CF III, Dew MA, Martire LM, et al: Treating depression to remission in older adults: a controlled evaluation of combined escitalopram with interpersonal psychotherapy versus escitalopram with depression care management. Int J Geriatr Psychiatry 25(11):1134–1141, 2010

Reynolds K, Pietrzak RH, El-Gabalawy R, et al: Prevalence of psychiatric disorders in U.S. older adults: findings from a nationally representative survey. World Psychiatry 14(1):74–81, 2015

Rickard HC, Scogin F, Keith S: A one-year follow-up of relaxation training for elders with subjective anxiety. Gerontologist 34(1):121–122, 1994 8150300

Rodakowski J, Saghafi E, Butters MA, Skidmore ER: Non-pharmacological interventions for adults with mild cognitive impairment and early stage dementia: an updated scoping review. Mol Aspects Med 43–44:38–53, 2015 26070444

Rokke PD, Scogin F: Depression treatment preferences in younger and older adults. J Clin Geropsychol 1:243–257, 1995

Rosnick CB, Wetherell JL, White KS, et al: Cognitive-behavioral therapy augmentation of SSRI reduces cortisol levels in older adults with generalized anxiety disorder: a randomized clinical trial. J Consult Clin Psychol 84(4):345–352, 2016 26881447

Rovner BW, Casten RJ, Hegel MT, et al: Preventing depression in age-related macular degeneration. Arch Gen Psychiatry 64(8):886–892, 2007 17679633

Satre DD, Mertens J, Areán PA, Weisner C: Contrasting outcomes of older versus middle-aged and younger adult chemical dependency patients in a managed care program. J Stud Alcohol 64(4):520–530, 2003 12921194

Satre DD, Mertens JR, Areán PA, Weisner C: Five-year alcohol and drug treatment outcomes of older adults versus middle-aged and younger adults in a managed care program. Addiction 99(10):1286–1297, 2004 15369567

Schonfeld L, Dupree LW, Dickson-Euhrmann E, et al: Cognitive-behavioral treatment of older veterans with substance abuse problems. J Geriatr Psychiatry Neurol 13(3):124–129, 2000 11001134

Schonfeld L, King-Kallimanis BL, Duchene DM, et al: Screening and brief intervention for substance misuse among older adults: the Florida BRITE project. Am J Public Health 100(1):108–114, 2010 19443821

Schonfeld L, Hazlett RW, Hedgecock DK, et al: Screening, Brief Intervention, and Referral to Treatment for older adults with substance misuse. Am J Public Health 105(1):205–211, 2015 24832147

Schuster J-P, Hoertel N, Le Strat Y, et al: Personality disorders in older adults: findings from the National Epidemiologic Survey on Alcohol and Related Conditions. Am J Geriatr Psychiatry 21(8):757–768, 2013 23567365

Scogin F, Jamison C, Gochneaur K: Comparative efficacy of cognitive and behavioral bibliotherapy for mildly and moderately depressed older adults. J Consult Clin Psychol 57(3):403–407, 1989 2738212

Scott W, Daly A, Yu L, McCracken LM: Treatment of chronic pain for adults 65 and over: analyses of outcomes and changes in psychological flexibility following interdisciplinary acceptance and commitment therapy (ACT). Pain Med 18(2):252–264, 2017 28204691

Seim L, Vijapura P, Pagali S, Burton MC: Common substance use disorders in older adults. Hosp Pract 48(suppl 1):48–55, 2020

Serfaty MA, Haworth D, Blanchard M, et al: Clinical effectiveness of individual cognitive behavioral therapy for depressed older people in primary care: a randomized controlled trial. Arch Gen Psychiatry 66(12):1332–1340, 2009 19996038

Serrano Selva JP, Latorre Postigo JM, Ros Segura L, et al: Life review therapy using autobiographical retrieval practice for older adults with clinical depression. Psicothema 24(2):224–229, 2012 22420349

Simning A, Seplaki CL: Association of the cumulative burden of late-life anxiety and depressive symptoms with functional impairment. Int J Geriatr Psychiatry 35(1):80–90, 2020 31650615

Simon SS, Cordás TA, Bottino CM: Cognitive behavioral therapies in older adults with depression and cognitive deficits: a systematic review. Int J Geriatr Psychiatry 30(3):223–233, 2015 25521935

Smoski MJ, McClintock A, Keeling L: Mindfulness training for emotional and cognitive health in late life. Curr Behav Neurosci Rep 3(4):301–307, 2016

Snodgrass J: Toward holistic care: integrating spirituality and cognitive behavioral therapy for older adults. J Relig Spirit Aging 21(3):219–236, 2009

Spector A, Charlesworth G, King M, et al: Cognitive-behavioural therapy for anxiety in dementia: pilot randomised controlled trial. Br J Psychiatry 206(6):509–516, 2015 25698766

Stanley MA, Beck JG, Novy DM, et al: Cognitive-behavioral treatment of late-life generalized anxiety disorder. J Consult Clin Psychol 71(2):309–319, 2003 12699025

Stanley MA, Wilson NL, Novy DM, et al: Cognitive behavior therapy for generalized anxiety disorder among older adults in primary care: a randomized clinical trial. JAMA 301(14):1460–1467, 2009 19351943

Stuart S, Noyes R Jr: Interpersonal psychotherapy for somatizing patients. Psychother Psychosom 75(4):209–219, 2006 16785770

Tasman W, Rovner B: Age-related macular degeneration: treating the whole patient. Arch Ophthalmol 122(4):648–649, 2004 15078685

Teri L, Gallagher-Thompson D: Cognitive-behavioral interventions for treatment of depression in Alzheimer's patients. Gerontologist 31(3):413–416, 1991 1879719

Teri L, McKenzie G, LaFazia D: Psychosocial treatment of depression in older adults with dementia. Clin Psychol Sci Pract 12:303–316, 2005

Thompson LW, Gallagher D, Czirr R: Personality disorder and outcome in the treatment of late-life depression. J Geriatr Psychiatry 21(2):133–153, 1988 3216093

Thorp SR, Ayers CR, Nuevo R, et al: Meta-analysis comparing different behavioral treatments for late-life anxiety. Am J Geriatr Psychiatry 17(2):105–115, 2009 19155744

Torgersen S, Kringlen E, Cramer V: The prevalence of personality disorders in a community sample. Arch Gen Psychiatry 58(6):590–596, 2001 11386989

Unützer J, Katon W, Williams JW Jr, et al: Improving primary care for depression in late life: the design of a multicenter randomized trial. Med Care 39(8):785–799, 2001 11468498

Unützer J, Katon W, Callahan CM, et al: Collaborative care management of late-life depression in the primary care setting: a randomized controlled trial. JAMA 288(22):2836–2845, 2002 12472325

Unützer J, Tang L, Oishi S, et al: Reducing suicidal ideation in depressed older primary care patients. J Am Geriatr Soc 54(10):1550–1556, 2006 17038073

van Dijk SDM, Veenstra MS, Bouman R, et al: Group schema-focused therapy enriched with psychomotor therapy versus treatment as usual for older adults with Cluster B and/or C personality disorders: a randomized trial. BMC Psychiatry 19(1):26, 2019 30646879

van Donzel L, Ouwens MA, van Alphen SPJ, et al: The effectiveness of adapted schema therapy for cluster C personality disorders in older adults: integrating positive schemas. Contemp Clin Trials Commun 21:100715, 2021 33604483

van't Hof E, Stein DJ, Marks I, et al: The effectiveness of problem solving therapy in deprived South African communities: results from a pilot study. BMC Psychiatry 11:156, 2011 21961801

Videler AC, van Royen RJJ, van Alphen SPJ: Schema therapy with older adults: call for evidence. Int Psychogeriatr 24(7):1186–1187, 2012 22340711

Videler AC, Rossi G, Schoevaars M, et al: Effects of schema group therapy in older outpatients: a proof of concept study. Int Psychogeriatr 26(10):1709–1717, 2014 24990412

Videler AC, van Alphen SPJ, van Royen RJJ, et al: Schema therapy for personality disorders in older adults: a multiple-baseline study. Aging Ment Health 22(6):738–747, 2018 28429623

Walker DA, Clarke M: Cognitive behavioural psychotherapy: a comparison between younger and older adults in two inner city mental health teams. Aging Ment Health 5(2):197–199, 2001 11511068

Wang PS, Berglund P, Olfson M, et al: Failure and delay in initial treatment contact after first onset of mental disorders in the National Comorbidity Survey Replication. Arch Gen Psychiatry 62(6):603–613, 2005 15939838

Wetherell JL, Hopko DR, Diefenbach GJ, et al: Cognitive-behavioral therapy for late-life generalized anxiety disorder: who gets better? Behav Ther 36:147–156, 2005

Wetherell JL, Afari N, Ayers CR, et al: Acceptance and commitment therapy for generalized anxiety disorder in older adults: a preliminary report. Behav Ther 42(1):127–134, 2011 21292059

Wetherell JL, Petkus AJ, White KS, et al: Antidepressant medication augmented with cognitive-behavioral therapy for generalized anxiety disorder in older adults. Am J Psychiatry 170(7):782–789, 2013 23680817

Wilkinson P, Alder N, Juszczak E, et al: A pilot randomised controlled trial of a brief cognitive behavioural group intervention to reduce recurrence rates in late life depression. Int J Geriatr Psychiatry 24(1):68–75, 2009 18615497

Wolitzky-Taylor KB, Castriotta N, Lenze EJ, et al: Anxiety disorders in older adults: a comprehensive review. Depress Anxiety 27(2):190–211, 2010 20099273

Yang JA, Garis J, Jackson C, et al: Providing psychotherapy to older adults in home: benefits, challenges, and decision-making guidelines. Clin Gerontol 32(4):333–346, 2009

Yarnell S, Li L, MacGrory B, et al: Substance use disorders in later life: a review and synthesis of the literature of an emerging public health concern. Am J Geriatr Psychiatry 28(2):226–236, 2020 31340887

Young MM, Stevens A, Porath-Waller A, et al: Effectiveness of brief interventions as part of the Screening, Brief Intervention and Referral to Treatment (SBIRT) model for reducing the non-medical use of psychoactive substances: a systematic review protocol. Syst Rev 1:22, 2012 22587894

Zweig RA: Personality disorder in older adults: assessment challenges and strategies. Prof Psychol Res Pr 39(3):298–305, 2008

CHAPTER 23

Working With Families of Older Adults

Richard H. Fortinsky, Ph.D.

Lisa P. Gwyther, M.S.W., L.C.S.W.

Families in the United States are the foundational care providers for older adults with chronic illnesses and disabilities who are living in the community. According to a landmark study sponsored by the National Academies of Sciences, Engineering, and Medicine (2016), at least 17.7 million individuals in the United States are family caregivers of older adults (age ≥65 years) who need help because of a limitation in their physical, mental, or cognitive functioning. The number of family caregivers is expected to grow in a corresponding fashion with the projected steady growth of the older population over the next several decades. Additionally, the racial and ethnic diversity of the older population, and hence of the family caregiving population, will also continue to grow in the decades ahead (National Academies of Sciences, Engineering, and Medicine 2016). These trends present tremendous challenges as well as opportunities for psychiatrists and other health professionals who work with families caring for older adults.

In this chapter, we first provide a profile of family caregivers for older adults living at home, in terms of caregivers' relationship to those they care for, their racial and ethnic diversity, the types of health-related needs they address, and the psychological and physical health consequences they face due to their care responsibilities. We then compare the caregiving circumstances of family caregivers of older adults with cognitive impairment due to Alzheimer's disease and related dementia (ADRD) with those of family caregivers of older adults without ADRD. Next, we provide an update on the numerous types of psychoeducational, skill-building, and multicomponent interventions—known collectively as *nonpharmacological interventions*—that have been tested for efficacy with family caregivers of older adults with ADRD. Following this review, we focus on caring for older adults amid the COVID-19 pandemic, about which little is yet known but which is now receiving a tremendous amount of recent attention in the geriatric and psychiatric scientific literature. Finally, we discuss important, clinically relevant topics pertinent to family caregiving for older adults along with recommendations for psychiatrists and other health professionals working with families of older adults.

Care of Older Adults by Families in the United States

When we think about caregiving by family members and other informal helpers, the most common feature is that the caregiver's involvement is spurred primarily by a personal relationship, not by the reward of financial compensation. Beyond that generalization, the circumstances of individual caregivers and the caregiver context vary greatly. For example, family caregivers may live with, near to, or far from the older relative for whom they care. Family caregivers may help with transportation, money management, or household tasks; self-care activities such as bathing, dressing, eating, or toileting; or medically complex tasks such as managing medications and administering injections. The frequency of care they provide may be daily or more occasional and of shorter or longer duration. The older individual may have dementia, which usually requires constant supervision (National Academies of Sciences, Engineering, and Medicine 2016). Finally, if older adults cannot manage their own affairs, caregivers become the navigator linking their relative with the array of health, social, and legal services that might be required to sustain independent living. Therefore, when working with families, clinicians must first gain a portrait of the caregiving situation along all of these dimensions to most effectively support the family.

Over the period from 1999 through 2015, there were several important trends in national profiles of older adults who received help with self-care activities of daily living or indoor mobility from family members or other unpaid caregivers. Older adults receiving such help in 2015, compared with in 1999, were less likely to be non-Hispanic white (80% vs 87%, respectively), more likely to be married (62% vs 50%, respectively), and less likely to be widowed (29% vs 43%, respectively). About one-third of these older adults had ADRD, and a similar proportion needed help with three or more self-care activities or indoor mobility; these proportions did not change over time (Wolff et al. 2018). Growing racial and ethnic diversity, as well as consistently sizable proportions of older adults with cognitive impairment and substantial physical disability, is an important trend and one that likely will affect the types of support that families of older adults will need in the years ahead.

Among caregivers of these older adults, in 2015, most were spouses (49%) or adult children (36%), and 95% of all caregivers lived within a 30-minute drive of the older individual needing help; these proportions did not change over time. However, older adults with adult child caregivers were more functionally impaired in 2015 than in 1999. Caregiving arrangements were long-standing and quite intense over time, especially for adult child caregivers, and the proportion of these caregivers who lived in a household with a child younger than 18 years doubled during this time, from 13% in 1999 to 26% in 2015. Although nearly 25% of adult child caregivers reported substantial emotional difficulty due to caregiving across this period, among spouses the proportion reporting such emotional difficulty actually declined considerably, from 23% in 1999 to 11% in 2015 (Wolff et al. 2018). Taken together, these trends indicate that adult child caregivers are especially susceptible to stress and to other psychological problems related to their caregiving responsibilities, including facing caregiving for parents with substantial disabilities in addition to caring for their own children.

No single model exists for working with families of older adults. Clinicians need to provide both patients and families with person- and family-centered assessment and treatment, considering issues of context, diversity, and heterogeneity. Despite the need for family-specific treatment, patterns of family issues consistently emerge based on trajectories of psychiatric illness. Perhaps the most specific guidance in the literature comes from meta-analyses and reviews of clinical research on families of older adults with progressive degenerative dementias (Adelman et al. 2014; Gallagher-Thompson and Coon 2007; Gillick 2013; Pinquart and Sörensen 2006; Reinhard et al. 2012; Weimer and Sager 2009).

Family Care for Older Adults With Alzheimer's Disease and Related Dementia

ADRD presents unique challenges to families providing care for older adults, especially as the disease process progresses and older adults lose the cognitive capacity to conduct their self-care and other daily activities independently. Compared with family caregivers of older adults with normal cognition, family caregivers of older adults with Alzheimer's disease (AD) spend more hours per week providing care, with measurable negative impacts on caregivers' mental health, personal and family time (Alzheimer's Association 2020; Langa et al. 2001), and family relationships (Gwyther 2005). Based on data from national caregiver surveys, Figure 23–1 illustrates the proportion of caregivers who provide help with daily activities to older adults with versus without ADRD. Caregivers of older adults with ADRD provide the most disproportionate amounts of help with self-care activities that are very personal, including bathing or showering, feeding, getting to and from the toilet, and dealing with incontinence (Alzheimer's Association 2020).

Psychiatrists working with families of persons with dementia should expect to treat both vulnerable primary family caregivers and families in conflict (Rabins et al. 2006). AD has forced long-term care services, policy, and treatment to move from a narrow focus on aging to a more dynamic family focus that is more inclusive of the person with dementia (Batsch and Mittelman 2012). Over the course of an older person's degenerative dementia, families will confront depression, delusions, agitation, behavioral changes, and other psychiatric symptoms in their cognitively impaired relative (Gitlin et al. 2012; Lyketsos et al. 2000; Olin et al. 2002; Tractenberg et al. 2002). The burden on the family can be great, available information can be insufficient, and doubt can be overwhelming (Gwyther 2000). Families that are caring for older members with dementia need reminders from psychiatrists to focus on maintaining family quality of life and quality of care within the constraints imposed by psychiatric, functional, and behavioral changes (Hughes et al. 1999).

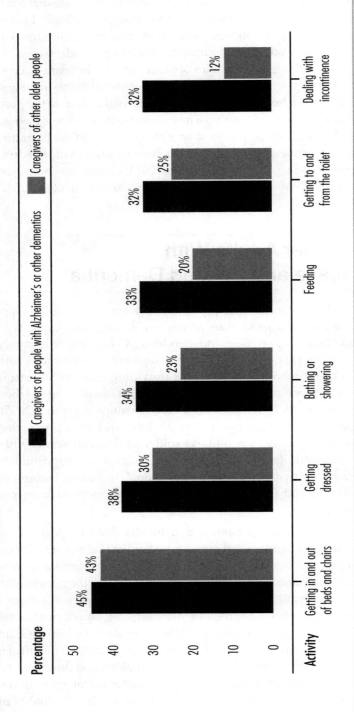

FIGURE 23–1. Proportion of caregivers of people with Alzheimer's or other dementias versus caregivers of other older people who provide help with specific activities of daily living, United States, 2015.

Source. Alzheimer's Association: 2020 Alzheimer's Disease Facts and Figures. *Alzheimer's and Dementia* 16(3):391–460, 2020. Used with permission.

Half of family caregivers live with the impaired older adult over a disease course lasting 3–20 years. Despite the high rates of shared residence, evidence suggests that 30% of older adults with moderate to severe dementia live alone, often with extensive supervision and assistance from local and long-distance family caregivers (Tierney et al. 2004). Certain trends have emerged from studies of family care in dementia. A shift is occurring away from the direct provision of care by families and toward more long-distance care or family care coordination. Dementia care may necessitate that people move to be closer to one another, and moves and daily proximity may increase stress as well. An increasing number of adult children have become primary caregivers, and many are still working part- or full-time. Although employment might lead to burdensome role overload, some caregivers experience unanticipated benefits from continuing to work. Dementia care frequently precipitates the family's first experience with seeking help from agencies and from other family members. Increasing evidence shows that the lack of an available and affordable long-term care system is pushing the limits of family capacity and solidarity (Hurd et al. 2013).

Despite the apparent investment of families in care for older adults, some families never comprehend the minimal safety risks associated with dementia care. Elder mistreatment—whether abuse or passive or active neglect—may be associated with exceeding these family members' limits (Fulmer et al. 2005). Families may feel powerless and overwhelmed when they cannot predictably control the symptoms and course of dementia. The psychiatrist working with the family has several tasks: assessment of tolerance limits, education, treatment of psychiatric consequences of caregiver burden, and management of family expectations of the disease course and of themselves. Additionally, psychiatrists working with families must realize that despite assumptions about a single primary family caregiver, changes in primary caregivers often occur when a spouse or partner dies or cognitively declines or when siblings pass a cognitively impaired parent among themselves in a futile attempt to equalize responsibility.

Increasing dependency, loss, and grief are realities for families caring for a loved one with AD, but not all family outcomes are negative or burdensome (Tschanz et al. 2013). Although depression and anxiety are the most frequently reported psychiatric symptoms among caregivers of patients with AD, some families express pride in their care as a legacy of their commitment to family values. Recent studies report both health benefits and decrements from assuming family care (Roth et al. 2013). The following reminders about family care may prove useful to clinicians and families:

1. Family care is an adaptive challenge: the family is not necessarily the problem, nor is the family necessarily the obstacle to effective care. Few incentives (financial, religious, or counseling) will make an unwilling family assume care. The reverse is equally true: few disincentives will keep a determined spouse, partner, or child from honoring his or her commitment.
2. The family rarely has one voice. Different perceptions and expectations of close and distant family members frequently precipitate family conflict. There is no perfectly fair and equal division of family care responsibility. Families can expect a permanent imbalance in the normal give-and-take of family relationships while working toward a more equitable sharing of responsibility.
3. Few families have the luxury of only one person needing care at a time.

4. Manipulation by dependent elders is much less common than are real unmet dependency needs. More underuse of services and underreporting of burden occur than overuse and overreporting.

5. There is no one right way or ideal place to offer family care. Many families are forced to choose between equally unacceptable options. Successful family caregivers gather information, take direct action when possible, and often reframe things that they cannot change into more positive terms (e.g., "It could be worse—at least she is still with me").

6. Successful family caregivers are flexible in adjusting expectations of themselves, the older adult, other family members, and professionals as they work to fit the needs and capacities of all. Coping with family care is facilitated by a sense of humor, a strong faith or value system, creativity, practical problem-solving skills, and emotional support from other family members or friends.

7. Families caring for older adults with dementia must define and negotiate complex situations, perform physically intimate tasks, manage emotions and communication, modify expectations, and capitalize on the older adult's preserved capacities.

8. A family caregiver's awareness of an available service, need for the service, or knowledge of how to access the service does not necessarily lead to the appropriate or timely use of that service.

9. There is no perfect control in a family care situation. Families are better off if they work on their reactions to stress or lack of control.

10. Denial is a common defense of family caregivers. Some people need to deny the inevitable outcome (e.g., loss of a beloved spouse or partner, eventual placement of a parent in a nursing home) to provide hopeful, consistent daily care.

11. A primary caregiver at home is efficient and preferred. However, these caregivers need breaks, respite, backup people, and services to supplement their personalized care. Even in ideal situations, contingency plans are necessary (Derence 2005; Lund et al. 2009).

Evidence-Based Interventions to Support Families

Psychiatrists working with families of older adults living with ADRD also should be aware that numerous nonpharmacological interventions designed to help persons living with ADRD and their caregivers have been implemented and evaluated over the past 15 years in the United States. Although there is not a single classification system for these types of interventions, Table 23–1 summarizes the various types of interventions found to be successful with caregivers (Alzheimer's Association 2020). Meta-analyses and scoping reviews of these interventions have found evidence of efficacious programs, particularly those that improve skill building and psychological outcomes of caregivers of persons living with ADRD (Butler et al. 2020; Cheng and Zhang 2020; Gaugler et al. 2020; Gitlin et al. 2020). Investigators are increasingly turning their attention to replicating or adapting efficacious interventions for older adults living with ADRD and their caregivers in "real world" health care and social service systems and settings. Such efforts have involved translational studies that identify the adaptations to evidence-based programs in dementia care required to embed them in

TABLE 23–1.   **Type and focus of caregiver interventions**

Type	Focus
Case management	Provides assessment, information, planning, referral, care coordination, and/or advocacy for family caregivers.
Psychoeducational approaches	Include structured programs that provide information about the disease, resources, and services and about how to expand skills to effectively respond to symptoms of the disease (e.g., cognitive impairment, behavioral symptoms, care-related needs). Include lectures, discussions, and written materials and are led by professionals with specialized training.
Counseling	Aims to resolve preexisting personal problems that complicate caregiving to reduce conflicts between caregivers and care recipients and/or improve family functioning.
Psychotherapeutic approaches	Involve the establishment of a therapeutic relationship between the caregiver and a professional therapist (e.g., cognitive-behavioral therapy for caregivers to focus on identifying and modifying beliefs related to emotional distress, developing new behaviors to deal with caregiving demands, and fostering activities that can promote caregiver well-being).
Respite	Provides planned, temporary relief for the caregiver through the provision of substitute care (e.g., adult day services and in-home or institutional respite care for a certain number of weekly hours).
Support groups	Are less structured than psychoeducational or psychotherapeutic interventions. Provide caregivers the opportunity to share personal feelings and concerns to overcome feelings of isolation.
Multicomponent approaches	Are characterized by intensive support strategies that combine multiple forms of intervention, such as education, support, and respite, into a single long-term service (often provided for 12 months or more).

Source.   Alzheimer's Association: 2020 Alzheimer's Disease Facts and Figures. *Alzheimer's and Dementia* 16(3):391, 2020, Figure 8, p 35. Used with permission.

health care systems in a more pragmatic fashion (Fortinsky et al. 2016, 2020; Gitlin and Czaja 2016; Gitlin et al. 2015). Most recently, published translational studies using single-group pre- and posttest designs found that beneficial outcomes for persons living with ADRD and caregivers could be achieved when efficacious interventions were incorporated into community service settings (Bass et al. 2019; Cho et al. 2019; Hodgson and Gitlin 2020). Psychiatrists and their health care colleagues interested in learning more about what interventions have been tested can refer to a free online database of these evidence-based programs (Best Practice Caregiving, https://bpc.caregiver.org).

Caregiving in the COVID-19 Pandemic

The rapid evolution of the COVID-19 pandemic across the world in 2020 changed life everywhere and presented a new and completely unexpected twist to the challenges of caring for an older family member at home. At this time, there is limited published empirical research on the consequences of quarantine and social distancing, the fear of transmitting and contracting the coronavirus within families and households in the highly vulnerable older population, and the disproportionate impact of COVID-19 on families of Black, Latinx, Asian American, and Native American heritage in the United States who are caring for older adults. The caregivers of older adults with chronic illnesses and associated disabilities who are living at home face serious challenges related to COVID-19 restrictions, such as how to keep older adults and themselves occupied and socially engaged at home to avoid loneliness and social isolation, and how to manage older adults' and their own health care needs by navigating the health care system to wisely use telehealth medical care with physicians and minimize the need for emergency department visits or hospital admissions.

Most published work in this area is based on clinically guided recommendations from authors in several countries to help families navigate health and social services during the pandemic. Within the United States, Duong and Karlawish (2020) recommended that the family and other informal caregivers practice behaviors that reduce virus exposure, such as wearing personal protective equipment when helping frail older adults with daily activities and using technology creatively to reach caregivers at home, to train them about how to avoid unnecessary hospital visits. Similar recommendations regarding need for greater use of technology to reach caregivers and services to support caregivers have been made by the Veterans Health Affairs network (Dang et al. 2020). Greenberg et al. (2020) focused on the caregivers of older adults with dementia, emphasizing that they are at risk for increased physical and mental health problems due to loneliness and social isolation, especially if they experience unavailability of community-based services such as respite care and if they assume greater care responsibilities because of a shortage of in-home workers. Similar themes have been struck by other recent articles (Kent et al. 2020; Lightfoot and Moone 2020; Stokes and Patterson 2020), while Makaroun et al. (2020) pointed out the increased risk for elder abuse under conditions of home confinement among vulnerable older adults and their caregivers. Depending on the trajectory of coronavirus (COVID-19) infection in different geographical areas and on the relative success of vaccines, families might have to face caring for their older relatives at home amid restrictions of the COVID-19 era for some time to come. Psychiatrists working with these families should be prepared to refine the use of remote technologies and to help ensure these technologies are equitably available to families across the racial, ethnic, and socioeconomic spectrum to optimize the success of treatment and support.

As of November 20, 2021, a total of 47.66 million COVID-19 cases had been reported in the United States. Trends indicated increasing case counts in northern-region states and decreasing case counts in southern-region states, consistent with greater indoor activity in late autumn in northern regions. A total of 769,643 deaths due to COVID-19 had been reported, with a daily average of 1,115 reported deaths. Although the percentage of the population of all ages who were fully vaccinated stood at 59%, corresponding percentages for the populations age 12 years and older and 65 years and older stood at 69% and 86%, respectively (The New York Times 2021). Additionally, on November 19, 2021, federal regulators recommended that all American adults who were at least 6 months removed from their second doses receive COVID-19 booster shots (Putterman 2021).

Goals in Working With Families of Older Adults

Clinical goals with families of older adults will vary depending on the presenting problems and family resources. Common goals, however, are to normalize variability; address safety, autonomy, and capacity issues; mobilize secondary family social support; facilitate appropriate decision-making at care transitions (particularly with requests for medications to treat agitation, aggression, or sleep disturbance); and help family members accept help or let go of direct care as necessary. In essence, the family is forced to constantly adapt family life over a prolonged period and often with conflicting perceptions of needs by different family members and the person with dementia. Well-timed psychiatric help can assist primary family members and elders in accepting new realities, promote appropriate decision-making, and facilitate tough care transitions.

Other goals of working with family caregivers include treating their own mood, substance-related, or anxiety disorders (particularly during the COVID-19 pandemic) and providing individual and family treatment around issues of grief, loss, or conflict in family relationships that limit the effectiveness of care. In general, family treatment should enhance the effectiveness of family care and coping, the self-efficacy of caregivers (Semiatin and O'Connor 2012), and the family's satisfaction with their preferred levels of involvement.

Psychiatrists working with family caregivers over time will monitor the quality of family care; mental health, capacity, and vulnerability of caregivers; and impact of the demands of care on family relationships (Sun et al. 2013). Psychiatrists should be alert to anxiety, self-neglect, suicidal ideation, depression, or anger in caregivers, as well as abuse, exploitation, or neglect of patients. These indications should prompt immediate recommendations for treatment, respite, or relinquishment of caregiving responsibilities. Exigent negative caregiver outcomes on which to focus therapy include decrements in mental health, social participation, and personal or family time, as well as loss of privacy.

Interdisciplinary Partnerships

Focused treatment with families of older adults holds great potential for positive outcomes, particularly in the context of an interprofessional partnership or team (Bass et al. 2013; Fortinsky et al. 2014; Possin et al. 2019). Research suggests that social workers' individual and family counseling with spouse caregivers can mobilize and sustain community and secondary family support, reduce and prevent further primary caregiver depression, preserve caregiver self-reported health, change negative appraisals of behavioral symptoms, and even delay nursing home placement by more than 1 year compared with a control group (Mittelman et al. 1996, 2004, 2007).

Psychiatrists may work collaboratively with social workers or nurses who can help provide timely or sustained assistance during particularly vulnerable times of care transitions (Boustani et al. 2011; Jennings et al. 2020). The psychiatrist's role is to assess and treat a family caregiver's psychiatric illness and to treat the cognitively impaired patient's psychiatric symptoms. Over time, the social worker or nurse may provide care management and monitor family capacity and tolerance while educating the family about common symptoms and care transitions (Callahan et al. 2012).

Some families will initially resist referrals to a social worker but may become more amenable if the social worker is described as an expert consumer guide or family consultant. At care transition times, a family consultant can provide assessment, intervention, and resource information. The family consultant can help families become more effective care managers and increase their level of independence in handling the requisite tasks. The consultant may serve as a teacher, coach, advocate, counselor, cheerleader, or support person who can provide continuity, energy, and a fresh perspective to promote family resilience.

Referrals to well-developed and validated psychoeducational group treatment programs have demonstrated equally positive results (Hepburn et al. 2007; Livingston et al. 2013). One helpful resource is the Rosalynn Carter Institute for Caregivers (www.rosalynncarter.org), which offers an evidence-based caregiver intervention resource center and detailed information on interventions and training that have been found to positively affect caregiver outcomes. Another is Maslow's (2012) review of more than 40 evidence-based family interventions.

Another way to monitor goals in the psychiatric treatment of families of older adults is to base treatment on the known precipitants of the breakdown in family care. Major precipitants of nursing home placement include both patient and caregiver factors (Yaffe et al. 2002). Patient factors that strongly predict placement are disruptive psychiatric and behavioral symptoms, incontinence, and disrupted sleep. Changes in behavior and personality are also major causes of caregiver burden and depression. To the extent that psychiatric consultation is available to the older adult for treatment of psychiatric symptoms, and to the extent that the family can be taught nonpharmacological approaches (see Chapter 19, "Agitation in Older Adults"), the health of the family and caregivers and effective home care for the older adult can be preserved.

Other predictors of family care breakdown include unresolved family conflicts or mood disorders, substance use disorders, or anxiety disorders in the primary caregiver. Treating depression in a family caregiver generally has a positive impact on the mood, functioning, and behavior of the older person with cognitive impairment (Teri et al. 1997), and vice versa.

Family As Information Seeker

Families are more likely than older adults with dementia to initiate and seek psychiatric care throughout the course of the illness. The stigma of psychiatric illness often delays psychiatric diagnosis (Werner et al. 2012), and ethnic and cultural beliefs that equate cognitive decline with normal aging or laziness can produce the same result. Psychiatrists must remind families that a specific diagnosis suggests treatment options. Stigma is best addressed by correcting misconceptions or lack of information. An unconvinced family can be told that AD is a brain disorder that can and does happen to anyone. The brain becomes the vulnerable organ in dementia, and psychiatric symptoms are brain symptoms just as angina is a symptom of a heart disorder. When damaged, both organs require special diagnosis and care.

Many family caregivers do not seek a diagnosis until psychiatric symptoms (e.g., suspiciousness) emerge or personality changes (e.g., uncharacteristic irritability) disrupt family life. Unfortunately, the patient is most likely to resist an evaluation once these symptoms emerge. Psychiatrists typically are reluctant to speak with a patient's family members without that patient's consent. An evaluation can be facilitated if the psychiatrist agrees to see the patient about a less threatening symptom, such as headaches, loss of interest, or low energy.

Diagnostic Office Visits

Although the patient is entitled to time alone with the psychiatrist initially, time alone with family informants later can be invaluable as the psychiatrist assesses the effects of functional loss and other family stressors. Most family caregivers prefer to talk privately with the psychiatrist to avoid confronting older relatives about their symptoms and declining condition. It may be helpful to have two family members accompany the patient to an evaluation. One family member can be with the older adult while the other speaks privately with the psychiatrist.

Initial Communication With Older Adults and Their Families

Initially, communication with patients and their family members will likely be in response to the common emotional reactions to hearing a diagnosis of degenerative dementia. One husband described the physician's diagnostic disclosure of his wife's early-stage AD as emotionally more devastating than being shot down during the Vietnam conflict. Elder persons and family members may also express doubt about the diagnosis. Rather than confront their doubt or denial, the clinician might suggest that they behave as though the diagnosis of AD has been confirmed while awaiting confirmation based on symptoms or progression of the disease. Asking directly about common early changes, such as difficulty handling money, problems managing medications, or increased irritability, may highlight expectable mental status changes while offering a preview of psychiatric expertise. Sometimes, explaining the symptoms of apathy and loss of executive function can help families understand why their efforts to get the elder person to try harder at tasks are likely to prove frustrating and futile.

Initial family sessions often elicit fear from family caregivers about their interdependent future or risks of heritability. Frustration is another common theme that emerges in early family treatment. Family caregivers frequently express frustration with the elder adult's obsessive need for repetition and reassurance. Clinicians can help families cope by offering information to clear up misconceptions about the presumed intentionality of the elder person's resistance. Additionally, confabulations are typical and predictable attempts by older adults with dementia to fill in gaps in their failing memory. Encouraging the family to get angry at the disease rather than at professionals, the services, or each other can be extremely helpful. Families should be reminded that conflict among their members will only limit needed help (Coon et al. 2003).

The family must understand that the elder person's realistic dependency does not imply weakness of character or lack of will. Families of patients with early or mild dementia should be encouraged to take advantage of education and support programs offered by the Alzheimer's Disease Research Centers and the Alzheimer's Association (Logsdon et al. 2010). These groups provide vital information and a community for both the patient and the family at times when they may be most reluctant to share the diagnosis with family and friends. These programs, along with online and written materials, help both the patient and the caregivers reduce the risks associated with early isolation, reduced social engagement, and lack of meaningful or purposeful activity. Many programs designed for individuals living with dementia that provide educational webinars for families and support groups for both have pivoted rapidly and successfully to online or virtual platforms, increasing access and participation.

Fatigue and exhaustion, often expressed as feeling "overwhelmed," emerge frequently among primary family caregivers. Encouraging restorative sleep hygiene, respite, exercise, and energy economies can be helpful for family members. Another common theme in family work is the guilt that members feel about losing patience or missing early opportunities to recognize distress in a relative. They appreciate reminders from clinicians that everyone experiences regret based on unique but certain limits. Most well-intentioned families seeking psychiatric treatment have done what seemed best given limited understanding at the time. They can be reminded that it would have been worse if they had done nothing. Families overwhelmed by guilt benefit from specific reminders to expect and accept negative feelings and resentment, to forgive themselves when efforts go awry, to establish time and energy priorities based on current quality-of-life preferences, to set limits, to say "no" and mean it, and to act from love or a values commitment. It helps to remind them that regret is inevitable but that unexpected resilience can often help family members pick themselves up and learn from their experience and that of others in a support group.

Following the psychiatric evaluation, key themes should be highlighted and noted in writing for absent family members. Older spouses in first marriages are generally more comfortable facing threatening health information together, and a healthy spouse may be put off by attempts to separate him or her from the impaired spouse. Providing the same information to both spouses at the same time helps older couples preserve their couple identity and accept the psychiatric recommendations as a mutual and shared adaptive challenge.

Family Expectations of Psychiatrists

Vulnerable family caregivers may seek a private place and time, undivided professional attention, and the comfort of initial familiar, polite small talk. Families want psychiatrists to listen without rushing to implied understanding or suggestions. Families of older adults expect to be asked what they have tried in coping with their relative's impairment. Even more, these families appreciate the psychiatrist's asking about what else is going on in their lives.

Wandering and getting lost are common in dementia. Caregivers may expect expert advice and immediate cures for these disruptive symptoms, and they often seek explanations for why medications do not "treat" wandering as well as environmental, communication, and activity strategies do. They should be given specific referrals to the Medic Alert + Alzheimer's Association 24/7 Wandering Support for a Safe Return program (www.alz.org/care/dementia-medic-alert-safe-return.asp) or newer technologies if affordable, such as global positioning systems or monitoring devices. They also need help in accepting respite to cope with the toll of the prolonged hypervigilance required to protect their family member from safety risks to themselves, such as getting lost, exploited, or hurt or from posing risks to others.

Families of older adults want psychiatrists to tailor information and education relevant to their immediate, pressing concerns. For example, a family concerned about the combative behavior of an older adult may be helped by a psychiatrist who responds, "First, let's talk about guns in the house" (Lynch et al. 2008). When depleted primary caregivers are confronting the range of behavioral symptoms of an older adult with AD, they may look to the psychiatrist to lend positivity, optimism, a proactive attitude, perspective, and objectivity. They may want acknowledgment of their contributions to the older adult's quality of life and forgiveness for what they were unable to accomplish despite their best intentions. The psychiatrist must be careful with well-intentioned attempts to commend families for doing "a great job." A family caregiver might be quick to point out, "I am not performing a job—I am her husband, and I promised to take care of her in sickness and in health."

Families also appreciate preventive self-care reminders from psychiatrists, but vague suggestions that caregivers take care of themselves often frustrate overwhelmed families with few resources. Family members need help translating principles of respite and meaningful use of respite time in ways congruent with their personal values and cultural expectations. Specific examples may help. For instance, some family members respond to statements such as "Family care without respite is like expecting your car to run on empty—it doesn't." Respite options can be presented as opportunities to "recharge your battery" (Gitlin et al. 2006). Enduring evidence also shows that encouraging physical activity (King and Brassington 1997; Teri et al. 2003) and actively assessing and treating sleep disorders in older adults and family caregivers are associated with positive care and family outcomes (McCurry et al. 2005, 2011).

Families look to psychiatrists for support in making certain decisions and may ask for help in mobilizing other family members. Expertise in family communication and family systems theory is particularly helpful and relevant at these junctures (Eisdorfer et al. 2003). Family caregivers expect psychiatrists to let them express their feelings, even when these feelings are judged to be unacceptable (e.g., "Sometimes I almost wish she would just die—I never expected her to live this long"). They may want help managing their anger toward the older adult, other family members, service providers, or God. These families appreciate psychiatrists who create new choices by reframing the problem or situation. For example, a family caregiver may seek permission from the psychiatrist to be less than perfect or "good enough for now." At such times, a psychiatrist's use of humor and compassion can produce dramatic relief.

Assessing the Family of the Older Adult

A targeted assessment of the family of an older adult may result in referrals to Alzheimer's Association services, private or public geriatric care management, family counseling, home help, day programs, assisted living, or nursing home care. Cultural values, expectations, and health beliefs will influence how and when families decide to pursue referrals, as well as their receptivity to family treatment by psychiatrists. Pinquart and Sörensen (2005) investigated ethnic differences in stressors, resources, and psychological outcomes of family caregiving. They suggested that more specific theories are needed to explain some of the differential effects of minority groups of caregivers. In addition to ethnic minorities, other groups that deserve clinical and research attention are older adults, partners, and families with issues of sexual and gender diversity. In many regions of the country, LGBTQ communities still do not have legal protections or fully sanctioned empowerment to make care decisions for their partners or families. Some helpful resources are the National Resource Center on LGBT Aging (www.lgbtagingcenter.org), the Family Caregiver Alliance's LGBT Community Online Support Group (www.caregiver.org/connecting-caregivers/support-groups), and SAGE: Advocacy and Services for LGBT Elders (www.sageusa.org).

One of the most useful ways to elicit a picture of family functioning is to ask the family to describe a typical day. Clues about how long the patient is left alone and about potential safety risks come from such open-ended questions. The psychiatrist should probe further if the caregiver hints about increased use of alcohol or psychoactive medications in response to stress. Asking questions about a typical day may elicit family anger at the patient's apathy and social withdrawal or reveal a family's lack of awareness of safety issues. The family may complain that the older adult with cognitive impairment is becoming more irritable or jealous of grandchildren. Probing further may reveal that this grandparent is still providing childcare despite significant declines in judgment or capabilities.

It is important to assess the home and neighborhood environment. People with dementia are easy targets for exploitation by telephone, email, and mail fraud and from people who come to the door. High-crime neighborhoods pose additional risks. An older adult who spends time at the corner store buying alcohol and cigarettes or at the bank withdrawing money may be especially vulnerable.

The psychiatrist should ask specifically about the primary caregiver's health, being alert to offhand comments such as "I'm fine as long as he can drive me to chemotherapy." Caregivers should be asked about their own sleep and how it is affected by the sleep pattern of the adult receiving care. Many family caregivers report being frustrated, overwhelmed, edgy, or exhausted but will deny having depression, anxiety, or psychiatric symptoms. Although psychiatrists are well advised to respond promptly to poorly controlled rage or suicidal or violent threats, skillful probing may be required to elicit other symptoms.

A review of family relationships may elicit new or historical family conflicts that can complicate care. For example, a distant, estranged sibling might insist that the family caregiver is exaggerating symptoms in an attempt to take control. A written explanation from the psychiatrist about objective functional loss and level-of-care needs can help clarify the situation, corroborate the caregiver's experiences, and give credence to what is truly needed. Another key to effective family assessment is to ask about other family commitments. For example, a daughter backing up her mother's care of her father may be distracted by anxiety about her husband's failing business or a child's drug addiction. Cultural expectations must be carefully assessed along with each family member's subjective perceptions of financial resources. When paid or formal services are needed, family decision-making is often related to subjective perceptions of future financial adequacy rather than the objective cost or affordability of services. Some family members may be saving for a rainy day, whereas others may value preserving their inheritance above meeting the elder person's current care needs. It is also wise to assess family strengths, skills, and goals. For example, some families may cope well with providing care for incontinence or end-of-life care but be unable to tolerate the disruptive behaviors or sleep patterns of moderate dementia. Families that have coped with chronic mental illness or substance abuse in other family members may have well-developed coping strategies or support systems (e.g., Alcoholics Anonymous) that can help them adapt to care for their impaired relative.

Finally, assessment should include some review of the family's experience with previous and current help from family members or paid services. Some key issues include the adequacy, quality, cost, and dependability of the help. For example, if a previous home care worker stole from them or failed to show up, the family would be less likely to accept another home care referral. Previous conflict over elder care is likely to limit the family's willingness to ask for help. If a family believes that the help they give each other is adequate, dependable, or sufficient, they often are unwilling to consider formal services because they do not perceive a need.

Selecting Interventions for Families of Older Adults

Families of persons with dementia need a continuing source of reliable information. Referrals to the Alzheimer's Association (www.alz.org) and the Alzheimer's Disease Education and Referral Center of the National Institute on Aging (www.nia.nih.gov/health/about-adear-center) help meet this need. Multicomponent interventions have been demonstrated to enhance positive caregiver outcomes (Belle et al. 2006). The most effective of these interventions for family caregivers emphasize problem solving and active participatory skill-building strategies for behavior change over purely didactic educational approaches. Effective multicomponent approaches are flexible and tailored to individual risk factors. They are timed to key transition points or to stressors in care trajectories and are offered at sufficient dosages or with sufficient amounts of assistance over time to ensure sustained outcomes. Combining individual and family counseling, family education, support group participation, and care management is associated with decreased caregiver burden and depression. This also results in decreases in the elder person's disruptive symptoms and increases in caregiver satisfaction, subjective well-being, and self-efficacy.

Psychoeducational and skill-building approaches tested over time in diverse settings and even virtual platforms may be especially useful (Griffiths et al. 2018). For example, a multimodal approach for treating an older adult's agitation could include treatment of depression in the elder person or in the family caregiver with pharmacological and nonpharmacological strategies; participation by the family caregiver in psychoeducational, skills training, or caregiver support groups; and participation by the elder person and the family caregiver in structured exercise programs.

Nonpharmacological approaches to the treatment of depression in elder-care family dyads could be based on increasing the frequency of individually selected pleasant events (Teri et al. 1997). Once the older adult and caregiver have identified which activities are the most enjoyable, the goal becomes increasing the frequency and duration of these activities. In a dyadic intervention study, Whitlatch et al. (2006) found that patients with early-stage dementia and their family caregivers were able to participate in and benefit from a structured intervention focused on care planning for future needs.

Referrals to support groups should be balanced, and benefits should not be oversold. The benefits of participation in support groups are derived from experiential similarity, consumer information, coping and survivor models, expressive or advocacy outlets, and, for some, the creation of substitute family or social outlets. Participants may feel less isolated and misunderstood than nonparticipants. Clinical experience in working with families over time and during the pandemic suggests that, for some families, support groups offer a low-cost, readily available venue to share difficult feelings such as anger, regret, and frustration. Support groups can be a safe place to express disappointment in services, professionals, or other family members. Well-facilitated support groups help families recognize that they are not failures and receive immediate practical help unavailable elsewhere. Increasingly, online groups enhance access to a broader range of working participants. Most support group participants are in and out of groups over a prolonged illness course. There are few opportunities to measure ideal dose or exposure for specific benefits of participation, and few evidence-based studies have documented the benefits of caregiver support group participation.

One support group does not fit all. Black individuals frequently do not feel the need to talk about family business among strangers but may respond to a church-based group on family care. In an open mutual help group with revolving membership, not all participants will be dealing with the same care issues. The exclusive focus on dementia as just one aspect of family life may not meet certain families' needs. Some families cannot get to meetings regularly or use online platforms, and some groups are not consistently available. These factors limit the benefits of such a minimalist intervention. The benefits of participation can be enhanced by encouraging families to shop around for a group that best meets their needs and reminding them that they may be able to obtain comparable social support from groups to which they already belong, such as a church, synagogue, or employee or retiree organization.

Information available online is increasingly useful for finding resources at care transition points. For example, if a move to residential care becomes an issue, information about quality care and finding nursing homes and assisted living facilities is available online from Centers for Medicare and Medicaid Services (www.medicare.gov) and the National Consumer Voice for Quality Long-Term Care (www.theconsumervoice.org). State ombudsman offices also offer online information about local facilities. Online discussion boards and disease-specific residential care considerations can be helpful from groups such as the Association for Frontotemporal Degeneration (theaftd.org).

Educational Strategies With Families of Older Adults

Many families are too overwhelmed at a first psychiatric consultation or diagnostic evaluation to absorb information or instructions. Teachable moments with family members come at crisis points with specific psychiatric symptoms, such as when an older individual with dementia makes accusations of family theft or spousal infidelity or when the patient insists that his or her spouse or partner is an imposter. A medicine metaphor is appropriate: the timing and "dosing" of information may enhance effective use of that information in adapting care over time. Some families may have read or heard inaccurate or partially correct information about symptoms that can be easily corrected. Some may have heard myths that all elderly persons with dementia are aggressive. Some families have been overwhelmed by too much questionably credible information online. Just like medication management in geriatrics, the maxim "start low

---

TABLE 23–2.   **Key messages for family caregivers**

1. Be willing to listen to and validate the feelings of the older adult but understand that you cannot fix or do everything he or she may want or need. Know that it will not necessarily get easier, but things will change, and the experience will change you forever.
2. You are living with a situation you did not create, and your choices are limited by circumstances beyond your control. Seek options that are good enough for now.
3. You can only do what seems best at the time. Identify what you can and will tolerate, then set limits and call in reinforcements. Doubts or regrets are inevitable.
4. Find someone with whom you can be brutally honest, express those doubts and negative feelings, and move on.
5. Solving problems is much easier than living with the solutions. It is tempting for distant relatives to second-guess or criticize. Hope for the best but plan for the worst.
6. It is not always possible to compare how one person handles things with how another relative would handle them if the positions were reversed.
7. The older adult is not unhappy or upset because of what you have done. He or she is living with unwanted dependency. Sick people often take out their frustration on close family members.
8. Considering what is best for your family involves compromise among competing needs, loyalties, and commitments. Everyone may get some of what he or she needs. Think twice before giving up that job, club, or church group. Make realistic commitments and avoid making promises that include the words *always, never,* or *forever.*
9. Find ways to let your older relative give to or help you. He or she needs to feel purposeful, appreciated, and loved.
10. Take time to celebrate small victories when things go well.

---

and go slow" applies equally well to family education about dementia. Overwhelming families with too many treatment suggestions or referrals is just as likely to lead to poor compliance as is changing multiple medication regimens all at once. Finally, information should be presented in hopeful terms, such as "Treating your depression should have positive effects on your partner's mood as well" or "Many families surprise themselves with their resilience." Presenting information in a timed and dosed manner also offers opportunities for repetition of key themes. The key messages for family caregivers listed in Table 23–2 can be presented at intervals and in "doses" that are based on the frequency of contact with the family, the family's need to know, and the family's capacity to understand.

Responding to Families During the Course of Progressive Impairment

Over the course of a patient's dementia, family caregivers become not only information seekers but also care managers, consumer advocates, surrogate decision-makers, and health care providers. Negotiating these complex roles can be difficult, and even more so if the family caregiver is burdened by role overload. Evaluate caregiver vulnerability by asking family members to self-assess their pressure points or signs of overwhelming caregiver overload (U.S. Department of Veterans Affairs 2014). Clinical red flags may signal imminent danger due to the caregiver's own precarious health. Unsubtle hints may be a caregiver's comments such as "after my last stroke," "before he totaled the car," or "sometimes I feel like just letting him wander away." Pursuing such threads with standard clinical protocols is certainly warranted.

Other issues surface when working with the families of moderately impaired older adults. Isolation of the caregiver and patient is common as friends drop off in response to disruptive behavioral symptoms or the need for constant supervision of the older adult. This has become critical during the pandemic when the person with dementia cannot understand or will not follow precautions, day and home services are less available or safe, and the family is providing more care in isolation. Families need to be reminded that being vulnerable does not make older people grateful or lovable and that cabin fever among cohabiting elder persons and family caregivers can be a real threat to mental health and safety. Families are especially sensitive to relatives who confuse or mistake family identities or suggest that family members are impostors. Making suggestions that family caregivers say something like "I'll try to do it like your mother would" may help them understand and respond to accusations of this type.

Family members must be warned not to give up their cherished activities—social engagement has positive mental health effects at any age. Maintenance of a strong religious faith or community has also been shown to have positive effects on elder persons and family caregivers. Expressive outlets such as sports, the arts, or advocacy can help families cope with frustration and anger. Prayer, meditation, exercise, massage, and yoga, in combination with active treatment of depression or anxiety, are all worthy treatment recommendations. An older person's participation at an adult day center can be presented to the family as a vital source of social stimulation for the elder person and a stress-reduction strategy for the family caregiver (Zarit et al. 2014).

Helping Families Assess Capacity of Older Adults

Many families turn to psychiatrists to assess the judgment and decision-making capacity of older members, whether the concerns are related to handling money, making health decisions, living alone, or driving. Money-handling and health care decisions should be addressed soon after diagnosis to ensure time for patients to select a surrogate. Often families seek psychiatric consultation when conflict surfaces over the patient's selection of a surrogate or the surrogate's handling of the older adult's funds. Questions about whether the patient had sufficient capacity at the time he or she wrote a will or assigned power of attorney can become adversarial and unrelated to family treatment. Effective work with families regarding capacity should be done early, with a preventive focus. It is wise for one family member to make sure bills are paid. This can be done with different levels of the patient's involvement, from making decisions about which bills to pay to signing checks or establishing online autopay or representative payeeship.

Assessment of and Limitations on Driving

The clinician can encourage the family to assess driving capacity based on observations of the patient's current driving and provide the family with reminders that dementia affects judgment, reaction time, and problem solving. Psychiatric assessment

TABLE 23–3.   Signs of decline in driving skills

Trouble navigating turns
Moving into the wrong lane
Stopping in advance of or after exits
Leaving the car in inappropriate places
Driving uncharacteristically slow or fast
Delayed responses to unexpected situations
Failure to anticipate dangerous situations
Scrapes or dents on car, garage, or mailbox
Becoming lost in familiar places
Arriving unusually late from a short-distance drive
Receiving moving violations or warnings
Confusing the brake and the accelerator
Stopping in traffic for no apparent reason

of the patient or a more intensive driving evaluation from a trained occupational therapist, along with current observations from the family, will provide direction on when the patient's driving should be limited. Unfortunately, by the time there is evidence of a decline in driving ability, many patients cannot adequately report or judge their safety on the road. Anonymous reports to the Department of Motor Vehicles may or may not lead to required testing or removal of the patient's license, but the absence of a license, taking of the keys, or even dismantling the car rarely stops a determined older adult with dementia.

Driving is one area in which the family must be encouraged and prepared to assess the patient's capacity over time. The signs of decline in driving skills listed in Table 23–3 may help guide family observations and reports to the psychiatrist. Psychiatrists may suggest a range of successful ways to limit driving, such as the following:

- A prescriptive reminder to stop driving can be tempered with a qualifier such as "until we determine your diagnosis or treatment." Families appreciate a physician's willingness to be the source of such unwelcome news. However, patients have been known to keep driving, making comments such as "That doctor doesn't know anything." Families also report that patients are unlikely to "forget" those responsible for taking their keys, and patients may continue to blame family members for their loss of driving independence.
- Shaving the patient's keys, substituting an incorrect key, removing a distributor cap, or otherwise disabling a car can sometimes reduce the need to confront the patient with lost skills. However, patients have been known to fix the car, replace the keys, or even buy a new car while the old one was "in the shop." Some families believe these strategies are not ethical and will not consider anything short of direct "truthful" confrontation.
- The car could be sold, given to a family member who needs it for school or work, moved to an undisclosed location, or put up on blocks. One family of a taxi driver put the taxi on blocks in the backyard to help the patient remember that it was "broken."

- The family can also arrange for solutions that limit the need for driving—delivery services, senior vans, or offers of regular rides to church or for visits. Some families find that having a taxi charge account, privately hired driver, or helpful younger family member drive and escort the patient works best.

Addressing Questions of Capacity to Live Alone

Families may go to extremes to keep an older adult with dementia in a familiar environment, allowing values of autonomy and choice to temporarily trump safety. The psychiatrist, in addition to performing a psychiatric assessment of the patient's cognition, judgment, functional impairment, and decision-making capacity, can suggest that the family consider the following questions:

- Can the family member with dementia use the telephone to call for help from a family member or from 911? Will the person respond inappropriately to telemarketers or to mail or email scams? Have mysterious packages or bills for unusual items begun appearing? Does the person make repetitive calls every few minutes to the police or to the same family member at work or at home? Are any suspicious new friends accompanying the patient to the bank?
- Can the family member with dementia get to the store or to regular activities? Does the patient over- or under-buy certain items?
- Can the individual handle money and pay bills or, if not, is he or she willing to let others do this or to have bills forwarded or paid online?
- Can the patient take medicine appropriately, on time, and in correct doses? Does he or she self-medicate or risk overdoses of unnecessary medications?
- Is the family member bathing, changing clothes, and dressing appropriately for the weather?
- Is the person leaving the house after dark or traveling in dangerous areas alone? Does the patient let strangers in or buy from or contribute to questionable causes?
- Is the person having problems positioning his or her body to use a toilet, or is he or she urinating in wastebaskets or outdoors?
- Is the patient falling or getting lost by wandering outside a safe area?
- Are there significant changes in the family member's appetite, weight, sleep, appearance, or eating habits?
- Is discreet surveillance by neighbors, friends, or family readily available?

The last question regarding discreet surveillance is paramount. Individuals with moderate dementia may live alone successfully if they have regular contact with, surveillance by, or checking from neighbors or family members. Environmental demand varies considerably and must be assessed along with patient variables.

Families and Institutionalization of the Older Adult

Family stress does not stop at the door of the nursing home. Indeed, ample evidence shows that families experience great burden, disruption, and conflict in the time immediately before and after placing their family member in assisted living or a nursing home (Gaugler et al. 2009). Visiting limitations during the pandemic brought issues of the effects of social isolation, loneliness, and limits on family access to supplement or monitor care to the national forefront. Family members may seek psychiatric services to deal with guilt and grief and often with their anger toward the nursing facility, the lack of affordable care options, and each other. Many families are disappointed by the lack of medical or psychiatric treatment available to the residents of assisted living or nursing homes. Families should be encouraged to work with the facility and nursing home ombudsman while dealing with their affective, anxiety, and grief symptoms.

Conclusion

Clinical work with families of older adults is about helping them adapt to change, uncertainty, variability, and loss. Much of the psychiatric care of families helps them to modify their expectations for new dependency while celebrating retained capacities and learning to forgive themselves and others for inevitable doubts and mistakes. Interprofessional partnerships and teamwork with the Alzheimer's Association, health or primary care coordination or care transition initiatives, or nurses or social workers offer the most effective and efficient models of psychiatric services for families of older adults. There is often as much need for "timed and dosed" patient and family education as for treatment of psychotic, depressive, anxious, or other psychiatric symptoms or syndromes of the elder person or family members. Families expect psychiatrists to provide active treatment and monitoring of psychiatric symptoms, reassurance, interpretation of information, and referrals. In addition, it is always helpful to acknowledge the losses and contributions to care by individual family members, to encourage caregiver self-care, to offer authoritative absolution for inevitable mistakes, and to offer decisional support, especially with regard to transitions in care and earlier moves to palliative or hospice care.

Key Points

- Psychiatric treatment of families helps them modify expectations for their family member's progressive cognitive decline and learn to forgive themselves and others for inevitable doubts and mistakes.

- Interprofessional consultation, partnerships, and teamwork with the Alzheimer's Association and with health, aging, and social services offer the most effective and efficient models for psychiatric services to families of older adults.

- Psychiatrists should provide active treatment and monitoring of family caregivers' psychiatric symptoms, outline reasonable expectations, and offer families information about outcomes of treatment.

- It is helpful to acknowledge family caregivers' losses and their contributions to care. It is also important to encourage their own self-care and to offer them expert decisional support during transitions in care.

Suggested Readings

AARP, National Alliance for Caregiving: Caregiving in the United States 2020. Washington, DC, AARP, May 2020

Adelman RD, Tmanova LL, Delgado D, et al: Caregiver burden: a clinical review. JAMA 311(10):1052–1060, 2014

Gallagher-Thompson D, Coon DW: Evidence-based psychological treatments for distress in family caregivers of older adults. Psychol Aging 22(1): 37–51, 2007

Gaugler JE, Jutkowitz E, Gitlin LN: Non-Pharmacological Interventions for Persons Living with Alzheimer's Disease: Decadal Review and Recommendations. Washington, DC, National Academies of Sciences, Engineering, and Medicine, 2020. Available at: https://sites.nationalacademies.org/cs/groups/dbassesite/documents/webpage/dbasse_198207.pdf.

Gitlin LN, Marx K, Stanley IH, Hodgson N: Translating evidence-based dementia caregiving interventions into practice: state-of-the-science and next steps. Gerontologist 55(2):210–226, 2015

Gitlin LN, Jutkowitz E, Gaugler JE: Dementia Caregiver Intervention Research Now and into the Future: Review and Recommendations. Washington, DC, National Academies of Sciences, Engineering and Medicine, 2020. Available at: https://sites.nationalacademies.org/cs/groups/dbassesite/documents/webpage/dbasse_198208.pdf

Mittelman MS, Roth DL, Clay OJ, Haley WE: Preserving health of Alzheimer caregivers: impact of a spouse caregiver intervention. Am J Geriatr Psychiatry 15(9):780–789, 2007

Rabins PV, Lyketsos C, Steele C: Practical Dementia Care. New York, Oxford University Press, 2006

References

Adelman RD, Tmanova LL, Delgado D, et al: Caregiver burden: a clinical review. JAMA 311(10):1052–1060, 2014 24618967

Alzheimer's Association: 2020 Alzheimer's disease facts and figures. Alzheimers Dement 16(3):391–460, 2020

Bass DM, Judge KS, Snow AL, et al: Caregiver outcomes of partners in dementia care: effect of a care coordination program for veterans with dementia and their family members and friends. J Am Geriatr Soc 61(8):1377–1386, 2013 23869899

Bass DM, Hornick T, Kunik M, et al: Findings from a real-world translation study of the evidence-based "Partners in Dementia Care." Innov Aging 3(3):igz031, 2019 31660442

Batsch NL, Mittelman MS: World Alzheimer Report 2012: Overcoming the Stigma of Dementia. London, Alzheimer's Disease International, 2012. Available at: https://www.alzint.org/resource/world-alzheimer-report-2012. Accessed June 11, 2014.

Belle SH, Burgio L, Burns R, et al: Enhancing the quality of life of dementia caregivers from different ethnic or racial groups: a randomized, controlled trial. Ann Intern Med 145(10):727–738, 2006 17116917

Boustani MA, Sachs GA, Alder CA, et al: Implementing innovative models of dementia care: the Healthy Aging Brain Center. Aging Ment Health 15(1):13–22, 2011 21271387

Butler M, Gaugler JE, Talley KMC, et al: Care Interventions for People Living With Dementia and Their Caregivers. Comparative Effectiveness Review No 231. AHRQ Publ No 20-EHC023. Rockville, MD, Agency for Healthcare Research and Quality, July 2020

Callahan CM, Arling G, Tu W, et al: Transitions in care for older adults with and without dementia. J Am Geriatr Soc 60(5):813–820, 2012 22587849

Cheng ST, Zhang F: A comprehensive meta-review of systematic reviews and meta-analyses on nonpharmacological interventions for informal dementia caregivers. BMC Geriatr 20(1):137, 2020 32293325

Cho J, Luk-Jones S, Smith DR, Stevens AB: Evaluation of REACH-TX: a community-based approach to the REACH II intervention. Innov Aging 3(3):igz022, 2019

Coon DW, Thompson L, Steffen A, et al: Anger and depression management: psychoeducational skill training interventions for women caregivers of a relative with dementia. Gerontologist 43(5):678–689, 2003 14570964

Dang S, Penney LS, Trivedi R, et al: Caring for caregivers during COVID-19. J Am Geriatr Soc 68(10):2197–2201, 2020 32638348

Derence K: Dementia-specific respite: the key to effective caregiver support. N C Med J 66(1):48–51, 2005 15786679

Duong MT, Karlawish J: Caregiving at a physical distance: initial thoughts for COVID-19 and beyond. J Am Geriatr Soc 68(6):1170–1172, 2020 32311070

Eisdorfer C, Czaja SJ, Loewenstein DA, et al: The effect of a family therapy and technology-based intervention on caregiver depression. Gerontologist 43(4):521–531, 2003 12937331

Fortinsky RH, Delaney C, Harel O, et al: Results and lessons learned from a nurse practitioner-guided dementia care intervention for primary care patients and their family caregivers. Res Gerontol Nurs 7(3):126–137, 2014 24444453

Fortinsky RH, Gitlin LN, Pizzi LT, et al: Translation of the Care of Persons with Dementia in their Environments (COPE) intervention in a publicly funded home care context: rationale and research design. Contemp Clin Trials 49:155–165, 2016 27394383

Fortinsky RH, Gitlin LN, Pizzi LT, et al: Effectiveness of the Care of Persons with Dementia in their Environments intervention when embedded in a publicly funded home and community-based service program. Innov Aging 4(6):a053, 2020 33367114

Fulmer T, Paveza G, VandeWeerd C, et al: Dyadic vulnerability and risk profiling for elder neglect. Gerontologist 45(4):525–534, 2005 16051915

Gallagher-Thompson D, Coon DW: Evidence-based psychological treatments for distress in family caregivers of older adults. Psychol Aging 22(1):37–51, 2007 17385981

Gaugler JE, Mittelman MS, Hepburn K, Newcomer R: Predictors of change in caregiver burden and depressive symptoms following nursing home admission. Psychol Aging 24(2):385–396, 2009 19485656

Gaugler JE, Jutkowitz E, Gitlin LN: Non-Pharmacological Interventions for Persons Living with Alzheimer's Disease: Decadal Review and Recommendations. Washington, DC, National Academies of Sciences, Engineering, and Medicine, 2020. Available at: https://sites.nationalacademies.org/cs/groups/dbassesite/documents/webpage/dbasse_198207.pdf. Accessed September 5, 2020.

Gillick MR: The critical role of caregivers in achieving patient-centered care. JAMA 310(6):575–576, 2013 23867885

Gitlin LN, Czaja S: Lessons learned from implementing proven interventions into real world contexts, in Behavioral Intervention Research: Designing, Evaluating, and Implementing. Edited by Sussman S. Berlin, Springer, 2016, pp 379–398

Gitlin LN, Reever K, Dennis MP, et al: Enhancing quality of life of families who use adult day services: short- and long-term effects of the adult day services plus program. Gerontologist 46(5):630–639, 2006 17050754

Gitlin LN, Kales HC, Lyketsos CG: Nonpharmacologic management of behavioral symptoms in dementia. JAMA 308(19):2020–2029, 2012 23168825

Gitlin LN, Marx K, Stanley IH, Hodgson N: Translating evidence-based dementia caregiving interventions into practice: state-of-the-science and next steps. Gerontologist 55(2):210–226, 2015 26035597

Gitlin LN, Jutkowitz E, Gaugler JE: Dementia Caregiver Intervention Research Now and into the Future: Review and Recommendations. Washington, DC, National Academies of Sciences, Engineering, and Medicine, 2020. Available at: https://sites.nationalacademies.org/cs/groups/dbassesite/documents/webpage/dbasse_198208.pdf. Accessed September 5, 2020.

Greenberg NE, Wallick A, Brown LM: Impact of COVID-19 pandemic restrictions on community-dwelling caregivers and persons with dementia. Psychol Trauma 12(S1):S220–S221, 2020 32584105

Griffiths PC, Kovaleva M, Higgins M, et al: Tele-Savvy: an online program for dementia care-givers. Am J Alzheimers Dis Other Demen 33(5):269–276, 2018 29544342

Gwyther LP: Family issues in dementia: finding a new normal. Neurol Clin 18(4):993–1010, 2000 11072271

Gwyther LP: Family care and Alzheimer's disease: what do we know? What can we do? NC Med J 66(1):37–40, 42, 2005

Hepburn K, Lewis M, Tornatore J, et al: The Savvy Caregiver program: the demonstrated effectiveness of a transportable dementia caregiver psychoeducation program. J Gerontol Nurs 33(3):30–36, 2007 17378189

Hodgson N, Gitlin LN: Implementing and sustaining family care programs in real world settings: barriers and facilitators, in Bridging the Family Care Gap. Edited by Gaugler JE. Amsterdam, Elsevier, 2020

Hughes SL, Giobbie-Hurder A, Weaver FM, et al: Relationship between caregiver burden and health-related quality of life. Gerontologist 39(5):534–545, 1999 10568078

Hurd MD, Martorell P, Delavande A, et al: Monetary costs of dementia in the United States. N Engl J Med 368(14):1326–1334, 2013 23550670

Jennings LA, Hollands S, Keeler E, et al: The effects of dementia care co-management on acute care, hospice and long-term care utilization. J Am Geriatr Soc 68(11):2500–2507, 2020

Kent EE, Ornstein KA, Dionne-Odom JN: The family caregiving crisis meets an actual pandemic. J Pain Symptom Manage 60(1):e66–e69, 2020 32283220

King AC, Brassington G: Enhancing physical and psychological functioning in older family caregivers: the role of regular physical activity. Ann Behav Med 19(2):91–100, 1997 9603683

Langa KM, Chernew ME, Kabeto MU, et al: National estimates of the quantity and cost of informal caregiving for the elderly with dementia. J Gen Intern Med 16(11):770–778, 2001 11722692

Lightfoot E, Moone RP: Caregiving in times of uncertainty: helping adult children of aging parents find support during the COVID-19 outbreak. J Gerontol Soc Work 63(6–7):542–552, 2020 32449648

Livingston G, Barber J, Rapaport P, et al: Clinical effectiveness of a manual based coping strategy programme (START, STrAtegies for RelaTives) in promoting the mental health of carers of family members with dementia: pragmatic randomised controlled trial. BMJ 347:f6276, 2013 24162942

Logsdon RG, Pike KC, McCurry SM, et al: Early stage memory loss support groups: outcomes from a randomized controlled clinical trial. J Gerontol B Psychol Sci Soc Sci 65(6):691–697, 2010 20693265

Lund D, Utz R, Casarta M, et al: Examining what caregivers do during respite time to make respite more effective. J Appl Gerontol 28(1):109–131, 2009

Lyketsos CG, Steinberg M, Tschanz JT, et al: Mental and behavioral disturbances in dementia: findings from the Cache County Study on Memory in Aging. Am J Psychiatry 157(5):708–714, 2000 10784462

Lynch CA, Moran M, Lawlor BA: Firearms and dementia: a smoking gun? Int J Geriatr Psychiatry 23(1):1–6, 2008 18081001

Makaroun LK, Bachrach RL, Rosland A-M: Elder abuse in the time of COVID-19: increased risks for older adults and their caregivers. Am J Geriatr Psychiatry 28(8):876–880, 2020

Maslow K: Translating Innovation to Impact: Evidence-Based Interventions to Support People With Alzheimer's Disease and Their Caregivers at Home and in the Community. A White Paper. Washington, DC, Alliance for Aging Research, Administration on Aging, MetLife Foundation, September 2012. Available at: http://www.aoa.gov/AoA_Programs/HPW/Alz_Grants/docs/TranslatingInnovationtoImpactAlzheimersDisease.pdf. Accessed October 31, 2014.

McCurry SM, Gibbons LE, Logsdon RG, et al: Nighttime insomnia treatment and education for Alzheimer's disease: a randomized, controlled trial. J Am Geriatr Soc 53(5):793–802, 2005 15877554

McCurry SM, Pike KC, Vitiello MV, et al: Increasing walking and bright light exposure to improve sleep in community-dwelling persons with Alzheimer's disease: results of a randomized, controlled trial. J Am Geriatr Soc 59(8):1393–1402, 2011 21797835

Mittelman MS, Ferris SH, Shulman E, et al: A family intervention to delay nursing home placement of patients with Alzheimer disease: a randomized controlled trial. JAMA 276(21):1725–1731, 1996 8940320

Mittelman MS, Roth DL, Haley WE, Zarit SH: Effects of a caregiver intervention on negative caregiver appraisals of behavior problems in patients with Alzheimer's disease: results of a randomized trial. J Gerontol B Psychol Sci Soc Sci 59(1):27–34, 2004 14722336

Mittelman MS, Roth DL, Clay OJ, Haley WE: Preserving health of Alzheimer caregivers: impact of a spouse caregiver intervention. Am J Geriatr Psychiatry 15(9):780–789, 2007 17804831

National Academies of Sciences, Engineering, and Medicine: Families Caring for an Aging America. Washington, DC, National Academies of Medicine, Engineering, and Medicine, 2016

The New York Times: Coronavirus in the U.S.: latest map and case count. The New York Times, November 21, 2021. Available at: https://www.nytimes.com/interactive/2021/us/covid-cases.html. Accessed November 21, 2021.

Olin JT, Schneider LS, Katz IR, et al: Provisional diagnostic criteria for depression of Alzheimer disease. Am J Geriatr Psychiatry 10(2):125–128, 2002 11925273

Pinquart M, Sörensen S: Ethnic differences in stressors, resources, and psychological outcomes of family caregiving: a meta-analysis. Gerontologist 45(1):90–106, 2005 15695420

Pinquart M, Sörensen S: Helping caregivers of persons with dementia: which interventions work and how large are the effects? Int Psychogeriatr 18:577–595, 2006 16686964

Possin KL, Merrilees JJ, Dulaney S, et al: Effect of collaborative dementia care via telephone and internet on quality of life, caregiver well-being, and health care use: the care ecosystem randomized clinical trial. JAMA Intern Med 179(12):1658–1667, 2019 31566651

Putterman A: If you're 18 or older and six months past your second COVID-19 vaccine dose, you're now eligible for a booster. Here's what you need to know. Hartford Courant, November 20, 2021. Available at: https://www.courant.com/coronavirus/hc-news-coronavirus-connecticut-booster-shots-what-to-know-20211120-sspz3odd3rfy3npxhyw2capequ-story.html. Accessed November 20, 2021.

Rabins PV, Lyketsos C, Steele C: Practical Dementia Care. New York, Oxford University Press, 2006

Reinhard SC, Levine C, Samis S: Home Alone: Family Caregivers Providing Complex Chronic Care. Washington, DC, AARP Public Policy Institute, 2012. Available at: http://www.aarp.org/home-family/caregiving/info-10–2012/home-alone-family caregivers-providing-complex-chronic-care.html. Accessed June 13, 2014.

Roth DL, Haley WE, Hovater M, et al: Family caregiving and all-cause mortality: findings from a population-based propensity-matched analysis. Am J Epidemiol 178(10):1571–1578, 2013 24091890

Semiatin AM, O'Connor MK: The relationship between self-efficacy and positive aspects of caregiving in Alzheimer's disease caregivers. Aging Ment Health 16(6):683–688, 2012 22360626

Stokes JE, Patterson SE: Intergenerational relationships, family caregiving policy, and COVID-19 in the United States. J Aging Soc Policy 32(4–5):416–424, 2020 32489144

Sun F, Durkin DW, Hilgeman MM, et al: Predicting desire for institutional placement among racially diverse dementia family caregivers: the role of quality of care. Gerontologist 53(3):418–429, 2013 22961466

Teri L, Logsdon RG, Uomoto J, McCurry SM: Behavioral treatment of depression in dementia patients: a controlled clinical trial. J Gerontol B Psychol Sci Soc Sci 52(4):159–166, 1997 9224439

Teri L, Gibbons LE, McCurry SM, et al: Exercise plus behavioral management in patients with Alzheimer disease: a randomized controlled trial. JAMA 290(15):2015–2022, 2003 14559955

Tierney MC, Charles J, Naglie G, et al: Risk factors for harm in cognitively impaired seniors who live alone: a prospective study. J Am Geriatr Soc 52(9):1435–1441, 2004 15341543

Tractenberg RE, Weiner MF, Thal LJ: Estimating the prevalence of agitation in community-dwelling persons with Alzheimer's disease. J Neuropsychiatry Clin Neurosci 14(1):11–18, 2002 11884649

Tschanz JT, Piercy K, Corcoran CD, et al: Caregiver coping strategies predict cognitive and functional decline in dementia: the Cache County Dementia Progression Study. Am J Geriatr Psychiatry 21(1):57–66, 2013 23290203

U.S. Department of Veterans Affairs: Caregiver Self-Assessment Worksheet. Washington, DC, U.S. Department of Veterans Affairs, 2014. Available at: http://va.gov/GERIATRICS/Guide/LongTermCare/Caregiver_Self_Assessment.pdf#zoom=100. Accessed June 11, 2014.

Weimer DL, Sager MA: Early identification and treatment of Alzheimer's disease: social and fiscal outcomes. Alzheimers Dement 5(3):215–226, 2009 19362885

Werner P, Mittelman MS, Goldstein D, Heinik J: Family stigma and caregiver burden in Alzheimer's disease. Gerontologist 52(1):89–97, 2012 22048807

Whitlatch CJ, Judge K, Zarit SH, Femia E: Dyadic intervention for family caregivers and care receivers in early stage dementia. Gerontologist 46(5):688–694, 2006 17050761

Wolff JL, Mulcahy J, Huang J, et al: Family caregivers of older adults, 1999–2015: trends in characteristics, circumstances, and role-related appraisal. Gerontologist 58(6):1021–1032, 2018 28637266

Yaffe K, Fox P, Newcomer R, et al: Patient and caregiver characteristics and nursing home placement in patients with dementia. JAMA 287(16):2090–2097, 2002 11966383

Zarit SH, Whetzel CA, Kim K, et al: Daily stressors and adult day service use by family caregivers: effects on depressive symptoms, positive mood, and dehydroepiandrosterone-sulfate. Am J Geriatr Psychiatry 22(12):1592–1602, 2014 24566240

CHAPTER 24

Clinical Psychiatry in the Nursing Home

Melinda Lantz, M.D.

Kecia-Ann Blissett, D.O.

Joel Streim, M.D.

Nursing homes provide long-term care for elderly patients with chronic illness and disability as well as rehabilitation and convalescent care for individuals recovering from acute illness. As documented in previous reviews (Streim and Katz 2009), clinical studies have consistently provided evidence that the diagnosis, management, and treatment of mental disorders are important components of nursing home care. The delivery of mental health services in nursing homes continues to be shaped by several factors, including growing scientific knowledge, availability of new treatments, evolving federal regulations, measurement-based care, the public dissemination of quality measures, and changes in the medical marketplace. In this chapter, we review historical trends and current information on the psychiatric problems common in the nursing home, discuss current trends affecting clinical care, and present a conceptual model for the organization of mental health services in the nursing home setting.

Nursing Home Populations

The Centers for Medicare and Medicaid Services (CMS) *Nursing Home Data Compendium 2015 Edition* indicates that 1.4 million people are living in 15,600 nursing homes across the United States (Centers for Medicare and Medicaid Services 2016). Of these, 15% are younger than 65 years, 43% are between 65 and 84 years, and 42% are age 85 years and older. There has been a small decline of 0.1% in the nursing home population over the past 30 years, which also reflects a reduction in long-term care facilities by roughly 3% nationwide. The greatest increase in nursing home type is reflected in the for-profit sector, which operates 70% of nursing facilities and includes 72% of all nursing home beds in the United States. Historically, the National Nursing Home Survey (NNHS) was first conducted in 1973–1974 and was repeated in 1977, 1985, 1995, 1997, 1999, and 2004 (National Center for Health Statistics 2004). According to the most recent NNHS, 4% of Americans age 65 years and older—1.5 million people—were residing in 16,100 long-term care facilities (Jones et al. 2009). Compared with 1995 survey data from the National Center for Health Statistics (Dey 1997), this represents a 0.11% decline, although the proportion of residents in the oldest age groups has been continuously increasing.

Although the number of Americans older than 65 years residing in nursing homes for extended periods of time has been decreasing steadily over the past decade, the use of nursing home beds for short-term stays has increased significantly. These beds are usually for skilled nursing services and have a rehabilitation aspect to their treatment. The payers for this type of stay are Medicare and commercial insurers. In 2014, 1.7 million fee-for-service Medicare beneficiaries received skilled nursing care treatment in 15,000 nursing facilities at the cost of $28.6 billion in Medicare funds. Approximately 20% of all fee-for-service Medicare beneficiaries are discharged from their acute care hospital admission to a nursing home that provides skilled nursing or rehabilitative care. These post–acute care referrals to nursing homes are associated with shorter hospital stays, lower hospital costs, and reported improved patient health and quality of life. Many of these same nursing facilities that provide short-term skilled nursing or rehabilitative care also provide residential long-term care.

The population in nursing homes, whether for short- or long-term care, consists primarily of older female patients (66% of residents; Centers for Medicare and Medicaid Services 2016) with multiple impairments in activities of daily living (ADLs). Cognitive impairments of varying degrees may also be present in this population. Although most persons admitted will be 65 years or older, a small cohort younger than 65 years also receive care in nursing facilities. However, their presentation and needs will be different, usually consisting of traumatic brain injuries, substance use disorders, or psychiatric illness.

Considering the increasing aging population in the United States, the need for nursing home care may be expected to increase. However, recent data have indicated that nursing home utilization has declined over time. From 2000 to 2010, use of nursing homes by individuals 65 years or older decreased. In that same period, the number of nursing homes also declined but then stabilized in 2014. This decline in utilization may be the result of many factors, including increasing use of in-home care and assisted care facility services and reimbursement policy changes by Medicare and Medicaid. For example, the availability of Medicare reimbursement for the first 100 days of nursing home care following discharge after a stay of at least 72 hours in an acute care facility led to nursing home admissions for subacute rehabilitation of hospitalized patients who were too disabled to return home immediately following hospital discharge. A Rand Corporation study of post-hospital care for Medicare beneficiaries found that post-acute use of formal care in skilled nursing facilities increased with age (Steiner and Neu 1993).

Persons living in nursing homes since the year 2000 have tended to be very disabled: 96% required help with bathing, 86% with dressing, 57% with toileting, and 45% with feeding. Thirty percent had ambulatory dysfunction, and 24% needed help getting in and out of bed. Among residents age 65 years and older, 27% had visual impairment and 23% had hearing impairment (Krauss and Altman 1998; Rhoades and Krauss 1999). The most disabled—those with five ADL impairments and severe cognitive loss—represent 15% of the nursing home population. Although cognitive and functional impairment are common among nursing home residents, recent data show that ≤20% have no ADL limitations. Approximately 34% of nursing home residents had severe incontinence of both bladder and bowel. Physical restraint use has become uncommon, with only 1% of residents having been restrained in the past 7 days. Antipsychotic medications use is common, with 22% of residents receiving these drugs in the past 7 days (Centers for Medicare and Medicaid Services 2016).

Prevalence of Psychiatric Disorders

The prevalence of all types psychiatric disorders among residents of nursing homes is high overall, with Alzheimer's disease (AD) and related dementias by far the most common disorders identified in the 2004 National Nursing Home Survey and validated in additional studies using the Minimum Data Set 3.0 (MDS 3.0) (Seitz et al. 2010; Ulbricht et al. 2017). The MDS 3.0 is a standardized clinical assessment that is federally mandated for all nursing home admissions to Medicare- and Medicaid-certified facilities. Data are collected upon patient admission and quarterly regarding any cognitive impairment, mood, behavior, and health conditions, including delirium (Centers for Medicare and Medicaid Services 2016). Older studies that were conducted between 1986 and 1993 and were based on psychiatric interviews using DSM-III (American Psychiatric Association 1980) or DSM-III-R (American Psychiatric Association 1987) diagnostic criteria, reported prevalences of psychiatric disorders between 80% and 94% (Chandler and Chandler 1988; Parmelee et al. 1989; Rovner et al. 1986, 1990a; Tariot et al. 1993). Although no interview-based epidemiological studies in nursing homes have been published since 1993, MDS 3.0 data indicate that ≤26% of nursing home residents have depression and 62% have experienced cognitive loss (Ulbricht et al. 2017).

Current prevalence estimates rely on MDS 3.0 data and limited literature reviews regarding shifts in diagnostic trends. Version 3.0, implemented in October 2010, is the most recent version of the standardized resident assessment system required by CMS, with the mandate to describe and report domains of nursing home resident health and quality of life. The MDS 3.0 includes structured resident interviews to assess mood, cognition, and delirium (Centers for Medicare and Medicaid Services 2016; Saliba et al. 2012). Definitions of *hallucinations, delusions,* and *clarity of behavioral disturbances* were enhanced in the MDS 3.0 to allow for the frequency and severity of symptoms to be identified. Impact on nursing home resident life is noted. Rejection and resistance to care is identified as a separate MDS 3.0 item, and wandering is assessed separately as a behavior to be addressed and accommodated by facilities but not grouped with all behavioral disturbances (Seitz et al. 2010; Ulbricht et al. 2017). Historical reviews of MDS data from 2005 indicate that the number of nursing home residents who had mental illnesses such as schizophrenia, bipolar disorder, depression, or anxiety comprised 27% of admissions (Grabowski et al. 2009). More recent findings from the *Nursing Home Data Compendium 2015 Edition* (Centers for Medicare and Medicaid Services 2016) indicate that 62% of residents have moderate to severe cognitive loss. Together, these prevalence data, whether based on clinical interviews, chart review, or MDS data, strongly suggest that nursing homes serve as de facto neuropsychiatric institutions, although they were not originally intended for this purpose. The challenge of providing short- and long-term care services in nursing homes is therefore complicated by the extensive psychiatric comorbidity found in this setting (Reichman and Conn 2010). Fullerton et al. (2009) ascertained that more than a half-million people with mental illnesses (excluding dementia) resided in U.S. nursing homes on any given day, exceeding the number in all other health care institutions combined. Using MDS 2.0 data from 2005, Grabowski et al. (2009) determined that 27.4% of the 1.2 million new U.S. nursing home patients admitted that year had schizophrenia, bipolar disorder, depression, or anxiety ("broad mental illness definition"). These investigators found that by 2005, the number of patients admitted with mental illness exceeded by 50% the number admitted with dementia only. Most of this shift was explained by a sharp increase in the proportion of patients admitted with depression and expanding options for those with dementia to receive care at home or in assisted-living facilities. However, dementia (with or without comorbid mental illness) remains a common condition among nursing home residents, accounting for 36.5% of new admissions in 2004. A review of epidemiological studies and the 2004 NNHS in this population found that the median prevalence of dementia was 58%; behavioral and psychological symptoms of dementia, 78%; major depression, 10%; and depressive symptoms, 29% (National Center for Health Statistics 2004; Seitz et al. 2010).

Disturbing trends in nursing home care among racial and ethnic minority groups have been identified (Bowblis et al. 2021; Fashaw-Walters et al. 2021; Li et al. 2015, 2019). Black nursing home residents are more likely than white residents to receive antipsychotic medications, be physically restrained, have a urinary catheter, and receive a feeding tube. Concerns have been identified regarding the appropriate treatment of pain among Black nursing home residents and the provision of recommended vaccinations and preventative care (Luo et al. 2014; Rahman and Foster 2015). In a large-scale study analyzing 4 million sets of MDS 3.0 assessments from 2011 to 2015, Black nursing home residents with AD or other dementias had a 1.7% increase in diagnoses of schizophrenia compared with non-Black residents, who displayed a 1.7% decrease in schizophrenia (Fashaw-Walters et al. 2021). Mortality related to the COVID-19 pandemic was overly represented in nursing homes serving persons of color and their communities compared with nursing homes with a low representation of minorities (Cai et al. 2021).

Cognitive Disorders and Behavioral Disturbances

The most common psychiatric disorder in nursing homes is dementia, with prevalence rates ranging from 50% to 75% found over the past 50 years (Chandler and Chandler 1988; Katz et al. 1989; Parmelee et al. 1989; Rovner et al. 1986, 1990a; Seitz et al. 2010; Tariot et al. 1993; Teeter et al. 1976). Most recent data from the *Nursing Home Data Compendium 2015 Edition* show a slight decline in the rate of admissions of residents with moderate or greater cognitive loss from 65% in 2011 to 62% in 2014 using MDS 3.0 assessments (Centers for Medicare and Medicaid Services 2016). Historical data indicate that AD (DSM-III-R primary degenerative dementia) accounted for ~50%–60% of dementia cases and that vascular dementia accounted for ~25%–30% (Barnes and Raskind 1981; Rovner et al. 1986, 1990a). Other causes of dementia were also reported, with lower prevalence rates and greater variability between sites. More recently, a study of 714 residents in three private nursing facilities found a 7.7% prevalence rate of Parkinson's disease and a 3.7% rate of Parkinson's disease dementia (Hoegh et al. 2013). The prevalence rates of dementia with Lewy bodies and frontotemporal dementia have not been specifically ascertained in nursing home populations.

Delirium is common in nursing homes and occurs primarily in patients made more vulnerable by a dementing illness. Available studies indicate that ~6%–7% of residents are delirious at the time of evaluation (Barnes and Raskind 1981; Rovner et al. 1986, 1990a). However, this figure probably underestimates the number of patients who have cognitive impairment associated with reversible toxic or metabolic factors. In one study, investigators found that nearly 25% of impaired residents had potentially reversible conditions (Sabin et al. 1982); another study found that 6%–12% of residential care patients with dementia improved in cognitive performance over the course of 1 year (Katz et al. 1991). A large study of residents with severe cognitive impairment found improvement at 6-month follow-up in 14% of the sample, associated with the following baseline findings: higher function, antidepressant medication use, and falls (Buttar et al. 2003). In nursing homes, as in other settings, a common reversible cause of cognitive impairment may be cognitive toxicity from drugs used to treat medical or psychiatric disorders. However, evidence indicates that long-acting opioids, previously thought to have adverse effects on cognitive function, may lead to improvements in functional status and social engagement without decrements in cognitive status or increases in the rate of delirium among nursing home residents treated for nonmalignant chronic pain (Won et al. 2006). For residents admitted to the nursing home for post–acute care rehabilitation, unresolved delirium is associated with poor functional recovery (Kiely et al. 2006). Severity of cognitive impairment and depressive symptoms at the time of initial assessment has been found to predict the trajectory and course of delirium in nursing home residents (von Gunten et al. 2013).

The clinical features of dementing disorders that can contribute to disability include treatable behavioral and psychological symptoms of dementia, such as hallucinations, delusions, depression, anxiety, and agitation. The combined 1-year prevalence of psychosis, agitation, and depression has been estimated to be between 76% and 82% (Ballard et al. 2001), and the 2-year prevalence of neuropsychiatric symptoms was found to be 96.6% among residents with dementia (Wetzels et al. 2010). In nursing home populations, psychotic symptoms have been reported in ~25%–50% of residents with a primary dementing illness (Berrios and Brook 1985; Chandler and Chandler 1988; Rovner et al. 1986, 1990a; Teeter et al. 1976). Clinically significant depression is seen in ~25% of patients with dementia. Dementia complicated by mixed agitation and depression accounts for more than one-third of complicated dementia in nursing home populations and is associated with multiple psychiatric and medical needs, psychotropic drug use, and hospital admissions (Bartels et al. 2003).

Medical Expenditure Panel Survey data revealed that 30% of residents exhibit behavioral problems, including verbal abuse (11.8%), physical abuse (9.1%), socially inappropriate behavior (14.5%), resistance to care (12.5%), and wandering (9.4%) (Krauss and Altman 1998). In nursing homes operated by the U.S. Department of Veterans Affairs (VA) health care system, ~70% of residents with dementia exhibited some type of challenging behavior (McCarthy et al. 2004). A prospective cohort study of nursing home residents with dementia found a point prevalence of agitation or aggression ranging from 20.5% to 29.1%, with a 2-year cumulative prevalence of 53.8%; a point prevalence of irritability ranging from 21.4% to 28.2%, with a 2-year cumulative prevalence of 58.1%; and a point prevalence of aberrant motor behavior fluctuating between 18.8% and 26.5%, with a cumulative prevalence of 50.4% (Wetzels et al. 2010). Disturbances of behavior, in addition to impaired ability to perform ADLs, have been identified as the most common reasons that patients with dementia are admitted to nursing homes (Steele et al. 1990), and disruptive behaviors often complicate care after admission (Cohen-Mansfield et al. 1989; Teeter et al. 1976; Zimmer et al. 1984).

Most psychiatric consultations in long-term care settings are for the evaluation and treatment of behavioral disturbances such as pacing and wandering, verbal abusiveness, disruptive shouting, physical aggression, destructive acts, and resistance to necessary care (Fenton et al. 2004; Loebel et al. 1991). Behavioral disturbances occur most often in patients with dementia and patients with psychotic symptoms—an association that remains even after controlling for level of cognitive impairment (Rovner et al. 1990b). Agitation and hyperactivity are also commonly associated with depression (Heeren et al. 2003; Volicer et al. 2012), as are delirium, sensory deprivation or overload, occult physical illness, pain, constipation, urinary retention, and adverse drug effects (including akathisia due to neuroleptics) (Cohen-Mansfield and Billig 1986). Depressive symptoms are associated with disruptive vocalizations in nursing home residents, even after adjustment for sex, age, and cognitive status (Dwyer and Byrne 2000). In a study comparing verbal and physical nonaggressive agitation, verbal agitation was correlated with female sex, depressed affect, poor performance of ADLs, and impaired social functioning (Cohen-Mansfield and Libin 2005). In addition to agitation, symptoms such as apathy, inactivity, and withdrawal occur in nursing home residents with and without depression. Apathy has been found to increase over time, with a 2-year cumulative incidence of 42.1% (Wetzels et al. 2010). Although these symptoms are less disturbing to staff and less frequently lead to psychiatric consultation (Fenton et al. 2004), they can be disabling and may be associated with decreases in socialization and self-care.

Depression

Depression increases the risk of nursing home admission among elder community-dwelling persons in the United States and Europe (Ahmed et al. 2007; Harris and Cooper 2006; Onder et al. 2007); this association remains even after controlling for age, physical illness, and functional status (Harris 2007). Among nursing home residents, depressive disorders represent the second most common psychiatric diagnosis after dementia. This prevalence is highly variable based on method of evaluation. Physician diagnosis of depression ranges from 17% to 60%, with significant variability among populations with dementia and those of varied ethnic and cultural backgrounds (Li et al. 2019; Ulbricht et al. 2017). Depressive symptoms are highly prevalent, affecting nearly 50% of nursing home residents (Harris-Kojetin et al. 2016). Cultural, ethnic, and language barriers appear to impact the assessment and reporting of depressive symptoms among nursing home residents. Li et al. (2019) found a reduced likelihood of reporting depression based on Patient Health Questionnaire–9 (PHQ-9) scores in racial and ethnic minority residents compared with non-Hispanic white persons, using the 2014 MDS. This difference could not be attributed to variations in functional status, medical diagnoses, facility type, or location, which suggests that cultural competency needs should be addressed in long term care facilities (Li et al. 2019). Most studies in U.S. nursing homes have historically identified depression prevalence rates of 15%–50% depending on the population studied, the instrument used, and whether major depressive disorder (MDD) or depressive symptoms are being reported (Baker and Miller 1991; Chandler and Chandler 1988; Hyer and Blazer 1982; Katz et al. 1989; Kaup et al. 2007; Lesher 1986; Levin et al. 2007; McCusker et al. 2014; Parmelee et al. 1989; Rovner et al. 1986, 1990a, 1991; Tariot et al. 1993; Teeter et al. 1976). Studies from other countries have shown similar rates (Ames 1990, 1991; Ames et al. 1988; Barca et al. 2010; Chahine et al. 2007; Harrison et al. 1990; Horiguchi and Inami 1991; Jongenelis et al. 2004; Mann et al. 1984; Rozzini et al. 1996; Snowdon 1986; Snowdon and Donnelly 1986; Spagnoli et al. 1986; Trichard et al. 1982). Approximately 6%–10% of all nursing home residents, and 20%–25% of those who are cognitively intact, have symptoms that meet criteria for MDD; this figure is an order of magnitude greater than the rates in community-dwelling elderly persons (Blazer and Williams 1980; Kramer et al. 1985).

The prevalence of less severe but clinically significant (e.g., minor or subsyndromal) depression among residents in long-term care settings is even higher. In one study, Parmelee et al. (1992) reported that the 1-year incidence of MDD was 9.4% and that patients with preexisting minor depression were at increased risk; the incidence of minor depression among individuals who were euthymic at baseline was 7.4%. Similarly, McCusker et al. (2014) found that baseline depression score was an independent risk factor for incident depression. These data demonstrate that minor or subsyndromal depression in nursing home residents appears to be a risk factor for MDD and might represent an opportunity for preventive treatment in this population. Other risk factors include age, pain, visual impairment, stroke, functional limitations, negative life events, loneliness, lack of social support, and perceived inadequacy of care (Jongenelis et al. 2004).

Depression in nursing home residents tends to be persistent. Although self-rated depression may decrease moderately in the initial 2 weeks to 6 months following nursing home admission (Engle and Graney 1993; Smalbrugge et al. 2006), Ames et al. (1988) found that only 17% of patients with diagnosable depressive disorders had recovered after an average of 3.6 years of follow-up. Smalbrugge et al. (2006) found persistence of symptoms in two-thirds of residents at 6-month follow-up, although rates were significantly higher among those with more severe symptoms at baseline.

Evidence of morbidity associated with depression comes from studies that showed an increase in pain complaints among residents with depression (McCusker et al. 2014; Parmelee et al. 1991), an association between depression and biochemical markers of subnutrition (Katz et al. 1993), and independent associations of delirium and diabetes with depression (McCusker et al. 2014). Depression in nursing home residents, both those with and those without dementia, is associated with disability (Kaup et al. 2007). Among patients admitted to nursing homes for post–acute care rehabilitation, those with depression have poorer functional outcomes (Webber et al. 2005). In addition to its association with morbidity and disability, depression in nursing home populations has been found to be associated with an increase in mortality rate, with effect sizes ranging from 1.6 to 3.0 (Ashby et al. 1991; Katz et al. 1989; Parmelee et al. 1992; Rovner et al. 1991; Sutcliffe et al. 2007). Whereas Rovner et al. (1991) reported that the increased mortality rate remained apparent after controlling for the patients' medical diagnoses and level of disability, Parmelee et al. (1992) found that the effect could be attributed to the interrelationships among depression, disability, and physical illness.

In addition to the medical comorbidity, disability, and mortality that characterize MDD among nursing home residents, evidence has shown that heterogeneity in these patients may reflect the existence of clinically relevant subtypes of depression. A treatment study by Katz et al. (1990) demonstrated that measures of self-care deficits and serum levels of albumin were highly intercorrelated and that both predicted a lack of response to treatment with nortriptyline. Although this study demonstrated that MDD is a specific, treatable disorder—even for patients with medical comorbidity residing in long-term care—there is also evidence in this setting for a treatment-relevant subtype of depression characterized by high levels of disability and low levels of serum albumin. This latter condition may be related to the syndrome of frailty that has been well described in the geriatric medical literature (Malmstrom et al. 2014).

As described later in this chapter (see "Pharmacotherapy"), evidence also indicates that depression among nursing home residents with dementia may differ from that among residents who are depressed and cognitively intact. Several studies of nursing home residents have shown poorer response to treatment with noradrenergic and serotonergic antidepressant drugs among very old residents with comorbid cognitive impairment or dementia (Magai et al. 2000; Oslin et al. 2000; Rosen et al. 2000; Streim et al. 2000; Trappler and Cohen 1996, 1998). These findings provide evidence of another treatment-relevant depression subtype, although this condition may not be specific to nursing homes. Similarly poor antidepressant treatment responses have been amply demonstrated in very old outpatients whose depressive symptoms are associated with vascular risk factors and executive dysfunction (Sneed et al. 2007, 2008).

Progress in the Treatment of Psychiatric Disorders in the Nursing Home

An appreciation of the unique characteristics of nursing home populations—particularly the extremes of old age and the high prevalence rates of cognitive impairment, psychiatric and medical comorbidity, and disability—has led to increased recognition that the results of efficacy studies conducted in general adult outpatient populations may not be readily generalizable to nursing home residents. This recognition points to the need for treatment studies conducted specifically in nursing home patients. Although the number of randomized controlled trials (RCTs) is limited, there is a growing body of literature on treatment outcomes in the nursing home.

Nonpharmacological Management of Behavioral Disturbances

Since 1990, numerous studies have been published describing nonpharmacological interventions for behavioral disturbances associated with dementia in the nursing home setting. Few of these have been RCTs. Comprehensive reviews of these studies have been written by Cohen-Mansfield (2001), Olazarán et al. (2010), Teri et al. (2002), Snowden et al. (2003), and Livingston et al. (2005).

Several nonpharmacological interventions have proven effective, although only behavior management therapies (Cohen-Mansfield et al. 2012; Karlin et al. 2014), specific types of caregiver and residential care staff education (Deudon et al. 2009), and possibly sensory and cognitive stimulation appear to have lasting effectiveness (Livingston et al. 2005). Although effective interventions have been developed, their implementation has been limited by many barriers, including a lack of specialized staff training and inadequate reimbursement for this type of care (Cody et al. 2002; Lawrence et al. 2012). One promising approach combined enhanced activities, guidelines for the use of psychotropic medication, and educational rounds for nursing home staff (Rovner et al. 1996). In a randomized clinical trial, this approach was shown to reduce the prevalence of problem behaviors and the use of antipsychotic drugs and physical restraints. Individualized consultation for staff nurses about the management of patients with dementia was also shown to diminish the use of physical restraints (Evans et al. 1997). Reductions in agitation were observed in a study of a daytime physical activity intervention combined with a nighttime program to decrease noise and sleep-disruptive nursing care practices (Alessi et al. 1999).

A few multisensory stimulation methods have shown promising results, although RCTs are still needed. Namaste Care, a program developed for nursing home residents with advanced dementia, emphasizes the calming effects of touch, sound, smell, and taste (Fullarton and Volicer 2013; Simard and Volicer 2010). Snoezelen rooms provide stimulation to meet patients' multisensory needs (Berg et al. 2010; van Weert et al. 2005). Bright light therapy has been shown to increase observed nocturnal sleep time but not to improve agitated behavior in nursing home residents with dementia (Lyketsos et al. 1999). Although some studies have claimed that aromatherapy with lavender oil is effective in reducing agitated behaviors, results have not been consistently replicated when controlling for nonolfactory aspects of treatment in residents with severe dementia (Snow et al. 2004). Music therapy has been shown to reduce agitation, but a comparison with general recreational activities demonstrated no additional beneficial effects of music (Vink et al. 2013). Humor therapy was found to significantly reduce agitation but not depression (Low et al. 2013). Individualized activities matched to the skills and interests of residents with dementia have also been shown to reduce agitation and negative affect (Kolanowski et al. 2005). A randomized, placebo-controlled trial of nonpharmacological individualized interventions for unmet patient needs demonstrated significant declines in total, physical nonaggressive, and verbal agitation (Cohen-Mansfield et al. 2012).

The largest trial of nonpharmacological interventions to date was conducted in the VA Community Living Centers, which are residential nursing facilities that offer dementia care for veterans (Karlin et al. 2014). In this trial, a psychologist served as the primary interventionist and behavioral coordinator and worked closely with facility staff to develop and implement a behavioral intervention plan to address challenging behaviors associated with dementia. The multicomponent psychosocial approach was based on a model developed by Teri et al. (2005) for training direct care workers in assisted-living residences. This program, when adapted to the VA Community Living Center setting, achieved a 35% reduction in the frequency and 46% reduction in the severity of challenging dementia-related behaviors. Although not specific to nursing homes, recommendations from a multidisciplinary expert panel on the nonpharmacological management of neuropsychiatric dementia symptoms were provided by Kales et al. (2014).

Psychotherapy

Evidence for the efficacy of psychotherapy in other settings suggests that it may be of value for treating mental disorders of aging in patients whose cognitive abilities allow them to participate. However, a search of the PsycINFO, PubMed, and Cochrane databases for the terms *psychotherapy* and *nursing homes* from 1987 to 2021 identified only a limited number of controlled studies of the effectiveness of specific individual or group psychotherapeutic modalities for nursing home residents (Table 24–1). Bharucha et al. (2006) identified and reviewed 18 controlled studies of "talk" psychotherapy for depression and psychological well-being in nursing home populations and found that most demonstrated at least short-term benefits on measures of mood, hopelessness, perceived control, self-esteem, and other psychological variables. However, the interpretation of many of these studies' findings was limited by their small sample sizes, variable study entry criteria, short trial durations, heterogeneous outcome assessment methods, and lack of detail on intervention methods. Controlled research on psychotherapeutic interventions has included studies of task-oriented versus insight-oriented therapy (Moran and Gatz 1987); reality orientation (Baines et al. 1987); reminiscence groups (Baines et al. 1987; Chao et al. 2006; Goldwasser et al. 1987; Haslam et al. 2010; McMurdo and Rennie 1993; Orten et al. 1989; Politis et al. 2004; Rattenbury and Stones 1989; Youssef 1990); exercise, activity, and progressive relaxation groups (Bensink et al. 1992; McMurdo and Rennie 1993); supportive group psychotherapy (Goldwasser et al. 1987; Szczepanska-Gieracha et al. 2014; Williams-Barnard and Lindell 1992); validation therapy (Tondi et al. 2007; Toseland et al. 1997); cognitive or cognitive-behavioral group therapies (Abraham et al. 1992; Zerhusen et al. 1991); focused visual imagery therapy (Abraham et al. 1997); and a psychosocial activity intervention (Beck et al. 2002). Except in the investigations by Abraham et al. (1992, 1997), patients were selected based not on specific psychiatric symptoms or syndromes but rather on age, cognitive status, or mobility.

Some of these studies reported improvements on measures of communication, behavior, cognitive performance, mood, social withdrawal, physical function, somatic preoccupation, self-esteem, perceived locus of control, quality of life, and life satisfaction. Case reports and demonstration projects by experienced clinicians have also documented the value of psychotherapy for treating depression in nursing home residents (Leszcz et al. 1985; Ollech 2006; Sadavoy 1991). Overall, there is a paucity of research on the outcomes of well-described psychotherapies among nursing home residents who have well-characterized psychiatric disorders. Nevertheless, the available evidence from nursing home research, considered together with outcomes of psychotherapy for older adults in other clinical settings, suggests that psychotherapy should be regarded as an important component of mental health treatment for the more cognitively intact nursing home residents with depression.

Pharmacotherapy

Pharmacological treatments are commonly used in nursing homes for dementia and its associated psychological and behavioral symptoms and for depression. More comprehensive reviews of the evidence for pharmacological treatment of neuropsychiat-

TABLE 24–1. Randomized controlled studies of the outcomes of psychotherapeutic interventions in elderly nursing home residents

Study	Type of intervention	Sample	Outcome measures	Results and comments
Baines et al. 1987	Reality orientation *vs.* reminiscence therapy *vs.* no-therapy control group (crossover design)	*N*=15; mean age 81.5 years; moderate to severe cognitive impairment	Cognitive function, life satisfaction, communication, behavior, staff knowledge of residents	Only the group that received reality orientation first and then reminiscence therapy showed sustained improvement in communication and behavior and nonsustained improvement in function (information/orientation). No improvement in other groups. Intervention associated with improved staff knowledge of residents.
Goldwasser et al. 1987	Reminiscence group therapy *vs.* supportive group therapy *vs.* no-treatment control group	*N*=27; dementia (MMSE score range 1–22; mean 10.4)	Depression; cognitive function; behavioral/ADL function	Reminiscence group showed nonsustained improvement in self-reported depression on BDI. Neither intervention showed significant effects on cognitive or behavioral function.
Moran and Gatz 1987	Task-oriented group *vs.* insight-oriented group *vs.* waiting-room control group	*N*=59; mean age 76.3 years; mobile, conversant	Self-reported psychosocial competence in 1) sense of control, 2) trust, 3) active coping, and 4) striving for social approval; life satisfaction	Task group improved on all measures except trust. Task group had significant increase in life satisfaction compared with insight and control groups. Insight group improved on sense of control and trust.
Orten et al. 1989	Reminiscence group *vs.* control group	*N*=56; mean age 82.6 years; moderate confusion	Social behavior, ADL function, agitation, somatic complaining, attitude	Significant improvement for one of three experimental groups; no improvement when all groups analyzed together. Investigators suggest therapist skills are an important variable.

TABLE 24–1. Randomized controlled studies of the outcomes of psychotherapeutic interventions in elderly nursing home residents *(continued)*

Study	Type of intervention	Sample	Outcome measures	Results and comments
Rattenbury and Stones 1989	Reminiscence group vs. current topics discussion group vs. no group	*N*=24; mean age 83–87 years; no cognitive impairment as judged by nursing home staff	Psychological well-being (happiness-depression scale), activity level, functional level, mood	Both intervention groups improved on the happiness-depression scale. No improvement on other measures, including mood scale. Positive correlation between happiness scores and increased verbal activity level between week 1 and week 4.
Ames 1990	Psychogeriatric team recommendations vs. routine clinical care	*N*=93; mean age 82.3 years	Depression, ADL performance	No difference between intervention and control groups. Only 27 of 81 recommended interventions were implemented (e.g., medication changes, referral for mental health services). Role of psychogeriatric services in management of facilities and medical care of residents not clearly defined.
Youssef 1990	Group reminiscence counseling for young-old subjects vs. old-old subjects vs. control group	*N*=60, all female; young-old ages 65–74 years; old-old age ≥75 years	Depression	Young-old group had significant improvement in depression scores on BDI. Old-old group showed improvement only on social withdrawal and somatic preoccupation items but not on total BDI scores. Control condition not described.
Zerhusen et al. 1991	Group cognitive therapy vs. music group (control) vs. routine clinical care (control)	*N*=60; mean age 77 years	Depression, performance ratings of group leaders	Cognitive therapy group had 30% improvement in self-rated depression scores on BDI; no significant improvement in control subjects. Group gains did not vary with group leader ratings.

TABLE 24–1. Randomized controlled studies of the outcomes of psychotherapeutic interventions in elderly nursing home residents *(continued)*

Study	Type of intervention	Sample	Outcome measures	Results and comments
Abraham et al. 1992	Group CBT vs. group focused visual imagery therapy vs. education-discussion control groups (16 meetings for experimental groups vs. 3 for control)	$N=76$; mean age 84 years; depressed and with mild to moderate cognitive impairment	Cognitive function, depression, hopelessness, life satisfaction	No effects of group therapy on geriatric depression, hopelessness, or life satisfaction. Both intervention groups showed improved cognitive function on modified MMSE, with greater gains in focused visual imagery participants. No significant cognitive change in control groups.
Bensink et al. 1992	Progressive relaxation group vs. activity group (control)	$N=28$; age ≥ 65 years; mean age 77 years; MMSE score ≥ 20	Locus of control, self-esteem	Only progressive relaxation group showed increase in perceived internal locus of control. Both groups showed improvement in self-esteem, with greater effect in progressive relaxation group.
Williams-Barnard and Lindell 1992	Group therapy with high nurse prizing vs. low nurse prizing vs. control group (16 meetings for experimental groups vs. 3 for control)	$N=73$; age ≥ 65 years	Self-concept	Self-concept improved in 68.4% of residents in high-prizing group, 29.4% in low-prizing groups, and 10.8% in control group. Declined in 40% of low-prizing group and 5.3% of high-prizing group.
McMurdo and Rennie 1993	Exercise sessions vs. reminiscence groups	$N=49$; mean age 81 years	Physical function, ADL performance, depression, life satisfaction, cognitive function	Physical function improved in exercise group and declined in reminiscence group. Self-reported depression (BDI scores) declined in both. Exercise group had significantly greater improvement than reminiscence group.

TABLE 24–1. Randomized controlled studies of the outcomes of psychotherapeutic interventions in elderly nursing home residents (*continued*)

Study	Type of intervention	Sample	Outcome measures	Results and comments
Abraham et al. 1997	Group CBT *vs.* group focused visual imagery therapy *vs.* control groups	*N*=76; mean age 84 years; depressed and with mild to moderate cognitive impairment	Depression factors, cognitive factors	Secondary analyses. Both interventions reduced depressive symptoms over 24 weeks.
Toseland et al. 1997	Validation therapy group *vs.* social contact group (control) *vs.* usual-care group (control)	*N*=88; mean age 87 years; dementia	Behavioral disturbances, depression, use of physical restraints and psychotropic medication	Less physical and verbal aggression and less depression in validation therapy group than in other groups. Validation therapy not effective in reducing use of physical restraints or psychotropic drugs. Social contact and usual-care groups had greater reductions in nonaggressive behavioral problems.
Beck et al. 2002	ADL group *vs.* psychosocial activity intervention *vs.* both *vs.* placebo *vs.* no intervention	*N*=127; mean age 83 years; MMSE mean score 10; disruptive behaviors	Positive and negative affect, frequency of disruptive behaviors	Significantly more positive affect in treatment groups; no decrease in negative affect and no change in disruptive behaviors.
Politis et al. 2004	Reminiscence-based activity intervention *vs.* "time and attention" one-on-one meetings with activities therapist (control)	*N*=37; dementia	Apathy, quality of life, activity level	Significant reduction in NPI apathy scores in both groups. No difference between groups; greater within-group improvement on quality-of-life measure for control group only.
Chao et al. 2006	Reminiscence group therapy *vs.* usual care (matched control subjects)	*N*=24	Depression, self-esteem, life satisfaction	Significant improvement on self-esteem measure; no significant effects on depression or life satisfaction.

TABLE 24–1. Randomized controlled studies of the outcomes of psychotherapeutic interventions in elderly nursing home residents *(continued)*

Study	Type of intervention	Sample	Outcome measures	Results and comments
Haslam et al. 2010	Individual vs. group reminiscence vs. social activity (control); weekly for 6 weeks	N=73; age range 58–93 years; living in standard-care or specialized-care nursing home units; MMSE mean score 16.6	Memory performance, well-being	Group reminiscence enhanced memory; social activity control condition enhanced well-being.
Graessel et al. 2011	Cognitive (and motor) stimulation group vs. usual-care group (control)	N=98; mean age 85.1 years; dementia	Cognitive function, ADL performance, mean MMSE score 14.6	Cognitive function and ADL performance stable in treatment group at 12-month follow-up; control group declined on both measures.
Olsen et al. 2016	Animal-assisted interventions for depression, agitation, and quality of life	N=51; mean age 82.9 years (intervention), 84.1 years (control)	Depression, agitation, quality of life, CSDD, BARS, QUALID	Significant effect on depression and quality of life for participants with severe dementia at follow-up. Significant effect on quality of life with animal-assisted activities immediately after intervention. No effects on agitation.
Van der Ploeg et al. 2016	Internet video chat on agitation	N=9; mean age 86.7 years; dementia	Agitation	Internet video chat (Skype) with family led to decrease in agitation count by 24.1 from baseline compared with standard landline phone calls.
Wahnschaffe et al. 2017	Dynamic lighting on agitation	N=12; mean age 79.1 years; dementia	Agitation; CMAI mean score 27.92	Dynamic lighting in living room significantly reduced agitated behavior in patients with dementia, indicating short-term benefits from higher daily light exposures.

ADL=activity of daily living; BARS=Brief Agitation Rating Scale (Finkel et al. 1993); BDI=Beck Depression Inventory (Beck et al. 1961); CBT=cognitive-behavioral therapy; CMAI=Cohen-Mansfield Agitation Inventory (Cohen-Mansfield et al. 1989); CSDD=Cornell Scale for Depression in Dementia (Alexopoulos et al. 1988); MMSE=Mini-Mental State Examination (Folstein et al. 1975); NPI=Neuropsychiatric Inventory (Wood et al. 2000); QUALID=Quality of Life in Late-stage Dementia (Weiner et al. 2000).

ric symptoms of dementia specifically in the nursing home setting are provided by Bharani and Snowden (2005) and Seitz et al. (2013).

Randomized, placebo-controlled clinical trials of psychotropic drugs conducted specifically in nursing home populations are summarized in Table 24–2. Some of the earlier studies provided evidence for the efficacy of antipsychotic drugs in managing agitation and related symptoms in residents with dementia, but the effect sizes were frequently modest, and high placebo response rates were common (Barnes et al. 1982; Schneider et al. 1990; Sunderland and Silver 1988). Subsequently, several multicenter, randomized, double-blind, placebo-controlled clinical trials demonstrated the efficacy of some of the atypical antipsychotic agents for the treatment of psychotic symptoms and agitated behavior in nursing home residents with dementia. These include published studies of risperidone (Brodaty et al. 2003; Katz et al. 1999), olanzapine (Meehan et al. 2002; Street et al. 2000), quetiapine (Zhong et al. 2007), and aripiprazole (Mintzer et al. 2007; Rappaport et al. 2009). Secondary analyses of data from the nursing home trials of risperidone showed that the medication had antipsychotic effects and had independent effects on aggression or agitation. Other studies of atypical antipsychotic drugs in nursing home residents with dementia failed to show statistically significant benefits on the a priori designated primary outcome measures related to psychosis or behavioral disturbances (De Deyn et al. 1999, 2005; Mintzer et al. 2006; Streim et al. 2008), although some of these studies found possible benefits on secondary behavioral measures. Widespread interest in studying the atypical antipsychotics for treatment of elderly nursing home residents was partly attributable to the expectation that atypical antipsychotics would be better tolerated than conventional antipsychotics in this population. Studies have evaluated data from RCTs in nursing home residents with dementia and found an increase in all-cause mortality among patients treated with antipsychotic medications, with first-generation antipsychotics having a slightly higher risk than second-generation agents. The higher risk of hip fracture and thromboembolic events is noted and of obvious clinical concern (Chiu et al. 2015).

Use of antipsychotic medications for patients with dementia has been a complex and controversial issue for decades. The additional FDA black box warnings regarding increased mortality among patients with dementia who are treated with antipsychotic agents should give any clinician pause prior to the use of these agents and has led to many facilities creating policies around informed consent from patients or surrogates prior to initiating antipsychotic medication, although this is not required by the CMS (Lester et al. 2011). Medications are needed that help alleviate the suffering associated with overt paranoia and hallucinations while balancing the adverse effects and overt risks. Dextromethorphan-quinidine, dextromethorphan-bupropion, and pimavanserin are some drugs that show promise, but clinical data are limited (Ahmed et al. 2019). There is some evidence that using low-dosage, fixed-schedule administration of antipsychotic medications for limited periods of time may reduce symptoms if careful monitoring is provided (Chiu et al. 2015).

These controlled clinical trials have examined only the acute effects of treatment, typically for 6–12 weeks of treatment, and little is known about the effectiveness of treatment for longer periods. However, evidence suggests that the need for and benefits from antipsychotic drug treatment change over the course of months in nursing home patients with dementia. Several double-blind, placebo-controlled discontinuation studies have demonstrated that most patients receiving long-term treatment with

TABLE 24–2. Randomized, placebo-controlled studies of the efficacy of psychotropic medications in elderly nursing home residents

Study	Medication and dosage (mg/day)	Sample	Efficacy measures	Results and comments
Beber 1965	Oxazepam (10–80) vs. PBO	N=100; mean age 79 years; nonpsychotic with chronic brain syndrome (n=28), mixed anxiety/depression (n=26), anxiety (n=43), or depression (n=3)	Anxiety and tension; depression, lethargy, autonomic reactions; irritability, insomnia, agitation, phobic reactions	Improvement in all parameters significantly greater in oxazepam group than in PBO group; 44 subjects received concomitant treatment with other drugs, including neuroleptics, antidepressants, hypnotics, antiparkinsonian agents, and analgesics.
Barnes et al. 1982	Thioridazine (mean 62.5) vs. loxapine (mean 10.5) vs. PBO	N=53; mean age 83 years; dementia and ≥3 behavioral symptoms	BPRS, SCAG, NOSIE, CGI	Total scores and global ratings showed modest efficacy with thioridazine and loxapine but not statistically better vs. PBO. High PBO response rate. Significant improvement in anxiety, excitement, emotional lability, and uncooperativeness in active treatment groups; no significant differences in overall efficacy between thioridazine and loxapine. Significant improvement on BPRS and SCAG only in subjects with high-severity baseline scores.
Stotsky 1984	Thioridazine (10–200) vs. diazepam (20–40) vs. PBO	N=237 nursing home patients; mean age 80 years; all nonpsychotic with cognitive impairment, emotional lability, ADL dysfunction, and agitation, anxiety, depressed mood, or sleep disturbance[a]	Modified Ham-A; modified NOSIE; global evaluations	Thioridazine well tolerated, with few side effects. Thioridazine group improved significantly more vs. PBO group on all Ham-A items (74% vs. 42%) and global evaluations and improved significantly more vs. diazepam group on NOSIE and global ratings. Insomnia responded better to diazepam, but more overall improvement on Ham-A rating with thioridazine.

TABLE 24–2. Randomized, placebo-controlled studies of the efficacy of psychotropic medications in elderly nursing home residents *(continued)*

Study	Medication and dosage *(mg/day)*	Sample	Efficacy measures	Results and comments
Dehlin et al. 1985	Alaproclate (SRI; 400) vs. PBO	N=40; mean age 82 years; primary degenerative, multi-infarct, or mixed dementia; not selected on basis of affective or behavioral symptoms	Intellectual function, motor function (ADLs), emotional function (including depressive symptoms), clinical global evaluation	No difference in efficacy found between alaproclate and PBO. Severity of dementia ranged from mild to severe. Behavioral problems not described.
Katz et al. 1990	Nortriptyline (mean 65.25) vs. PBO	N=30 residents of nursing home or congregate housing; mean age 84 years; MDD (Ham-D score ≥18)	Ham-D[b], GDS, CGI	Significant improvement in patients treated with nortriptyline vs. PBO on Ham-D and CGI but not on GDS. Location (nursing home vs. congregate housing) not significantly related to response. Trend toward decreased nortriptyline response related to higher levels of disability and lower serum albumin in nursing home patients.
Nyth and Gottfries 1990	Citalopram (10–30; mean 25) vs. PBO	N=98; mean age 77.6 years; primary degenerative (AD) or multi-infarct dementia (VaD)	GBS, CGI, MADRS	Patients with AD in citalopram group had significant reduction in irritability and depressed mood on GBS vs. control group; from baseline to week 4, they improved significantly on MADRS and on GBS emotional blunting, confusion, irritability, anxiety, fear-panic, depressed mood, and restlessness. No treatment benefits in patients with VaD. Placebo group worsened on CGI. Few adverse effects occurred; no drug–PBO differences.

TABLE 24–2.	Randomized, placebo-controlled studies of the efficacy of psychotropic medications in elderly nursing home residents *(continued)*			
Study	**Medication and dosage *(mg/day)***	**Sample**	**Efficacy measures**	**Results and comments**
Finkel et al. 1995	Thiothixene (0.25–18; mean 4.6) vs. PBO	*N*=33; mean age 85 years; dementia with agitated or aggressive behavior	CMAI, MMSE, Global Deterioration Scale (Reisberg et al. 1988), ADLs	Thiothixene group had significantly greater reduction in agitation vs. PBO group after 11 weeks of treatment and 6 weeks after crossover from PBO; no between-group differences on MMSE, Global Deterioration Scale, or ADLs.
Tariot et al. 1998	Carbamazepine (modal dose 300; mean serum level 5.3 µg/mL) vs. PBO	*N*=51; dementia with agitation	BPRS, CGI, agitation, aggression, cognition, functional status, staff time	Carbamazepine group had significantly greater improvement on BPRS vs. PBO group at 6 weeks; global improvement occurred in 77% and 22%, respectively. Secondary analyses showed improvement attributable to decreased agitation and aggression. Nurses reported perception of decreased time required to manage agitation in carbamazepine group. Significantly more adverse events seen with carbamazepine (59%) vs. PBO (29%).
De Deyn et al. 1999	Risperidone (0.5–4; mean 1.1) vs. haloperidol (0.5–4; mean 1.2) vs. PBO; 12 weeks	*N*=344; AD dementia, VaD, and mixed dementia (MMSE mean score 8.7)	BEHAVE-AD[b], CMAI, CGI, MMSE	No significant difference in response rates on the BEHAVE-AD for risperidone vs. PBO; total and aggression subscale and CMAI aggression item scores lower and CGI significantly greater with risperidone than PBO. Post hoc analysis showed significantly greater reduction in BEHAVE-AD aggression scores with risperidone vs. haloperidol. Somnolence greater with risperidone (12.2%) vs. PBO (4.4%). EPS significantly greater with haloperidol (22%) vs. risperidone (15%) or PBO (11%). Slight but significant decline in MMSE scores in haloperidol group. Response defined as ≥30% reduction on BEHAVE-AD.

TABLE 24–2. Randomized, placebo-controlled studies of the efficacy of psychotropic medications in elderly nursing home residents *(continued)*

Study	Medication and dosage *(mg/day)*	Sample	Efficacy measures	Results and comments
Katz et al. 1999	Risperidone (0.5–2) vs. PBO; 12 weeks	N=625; mean age 82.7 years; psychotic and behavioral symptoms and AD, VaD, or mixed AD and VaD (MMSE mean score 6.6)	BEHAVE-AD[b], CMAI, CGI, MMSE, FAST, PSMS	Significantly greater reductions in BEHAVE-AD total and aggression and psychosis subscale scores with risperidone 1 mg and 2 mg vs. with PBO. Response rates significantly greater with 1 mg (45%) and 2 mg (50%) vs. with PBO (33%). More EPS and somnolence with 2 mg vs. 1 mg. Optimal dosage for nursing home patients with severe dementia appears to be 1 mg. Response defined as ≥50% reduction on BEHAVE-AD.
Magai et al. 2000	Sertraline vs. PBO	N=31; all females with late-stage AD and depression	Depression, facial affect	Both groups improved at 8 weeks; sertraline had no significant benefits over PBO. "Knit-brow" facial response approached significance for treatment × time effect.
Street et al. 2000	Olanzapine (5, 10, 15) vs. PBO; 6 weeks	N=206; mean age 83.8 years; AD with psychotic and/or behavioral symptoms (MMSE mean score 6.9)	NPI-NH core[b] and total (including occupational disruptiveness scores), BPRS, MMSE	Significant improvement with olanzapine 5 mg and 10 mg in summary measures of agitation, aggression, and psychosis and significantly reduced disruptive effects on caregivers vs. PBO. Olanzapine associated with somnolence and gait disturbance but not increased EPS, central anticholinergic effects, or cognitive impairment vs. PBO; 18% of PBO and 44% of olanzapine group dropouts were due to adverse events.
Olin et al. 2001	Carbamazepine (mean 388) vs. PBO; 6 weeks	N=21; AD dementia (MMSE mean score 6.0)	BPRS[b], CGI-C, Ham-D	Both groups improved on CGI-C (56% on carbamazepine, 58% on PBO); no significant differences seen on BPRS, CGI, or Ham-D. Adverse events mild and similar for drug and PBO.

TABLE 24–2. Randomized, placebo-controlled studies of the efficacy of psychotropic medications in elderly nursing home residents *(continued)*

Study	Medication and dosage *(mg/day)*	Sample	Efficacy measures	Results and comments
Porsteinsson et al. 2001	Divalproex (mean 826; mean serum level 45.4 μg/mL) vs. PBO; 6 weeks	N=56; mean age 85 years; probable or possible AD, VaD, or mixed dementia with agitation (MMSE mean score 6.8)	BPRS[b], OAS, BRSD, CMAI, CGI-C	Divalproex group showed significant improvement on BPRS at 6 weeks vs. PBO only in a secondary analysis after adjustment for several covariates; 68% of divalproex group and 52% of PBO group had reduced agitation on CGI (NS). Significantly more side effects (generally mild) reported in divalproex vs. PBO group (68% vs. 33%), but sedation was 39% with divalproex vs. 11% with PBO.
Tariot et al. 2001a	Donepezil (5–10) vs. PBO	N=208; mean age 85.7 years; probable or possible AD or AD with cerebrovascular disease (MMSE mean score 14.4)	NPI-NH, CDR-SB, MMSE, PSMS	Both groups improved on NPI-NH; no significant difference between donepezil and PBO. Significantly greater improvement seen with donepezil than PBO on CDR-SB at week 24 and on MMSE at weeks 8, 16, and 20, but not on PSMS. Improvement not influenced by advanced age. No difference in adverse events found for drug vs. PBO.
Tariot et al. 2001b	Divalproex (mean 1,000) vs. PBO; 6 weeks	N=172; AD, VaD, or mixed dementia with symptoms of mania (MMSE mean score 7.4)	BRMS[b], BPRS, CMAI, CGI-C	Study discontinued early due to significantly greater rate of adverse events with divalproex, especially somnolence.
Burrows et al. 2002	Paroxetine (10–30) vs. PBO	N=24; age ≥80 years; nonmajor depression	CSD, Ham-D	No significant benefit found with paroxetine for treatment of nonmajor depression.
Meehan et al. 2002	Olanzapine (2.5–5 IM single dose) vs. lorazepam vs. PBO; 24 hours	N=204 from nursing home *and* hospital sites; AD dementia, VaD, and mixed AD dementia-VaD (MMSE mean score 11.8)	PANSS-EC[b], ACES	Significantly greater mean reduction in PANSS-EC scores seen 2 hours post dose for olanzapine 2.5 and 5 mg vs. PBO. No difference between olanzapine and lorazepam. Adverse events not significantly different across groups.

TABLE 24–2. Randomized, placebo-controlled studies of the efficacy of psychotropic medications in elderly nursing home residents *(continued)*

Study	Medication and dosage *(mg/day)*	Sample	Efficacy measures	Results and comments
Brodaty et al. 2003	Risperidone (0.5–2; mean 0.95) vs. PBO; 12 weeks	N=345; mean age 83 years; AD dementia, VaD, or mixed dementia, with aggressive behavior (MMSE mean score 5.5)	CMAI aggression[b], CMAI nonaggression subscales, BEHAVE-AD, CGI-S, CGI-C	Significant improvement on CMAI total aggression and nonaggressive agitation scores, BEHAVE-AD total scores and psychosis subscale, and CGI severity and change scores for risperidone vs. PBO group. Risperidone group had more somnolence, falls, UTIs, and CVAE, but no drug–PBO difference found in EPS.
De Deyn et al. 2005	Olanzapine (1, 2.5, 5, or 7.5) vs. PBO; 10 weeks	N=652; AD dementia with psychosis (MMSE mean score 13.7)	NPI-NH psychosis subscale[b]; CGI-C[b], NPI total, individual item, and occupational disruptiveness scores	No significant difference seen between any dosage of olanzapine and PBO on primary outcomes. More weight gain with olanzapine, but no difference found in anticholinergic effects or EPS or in dropout rates due to adverse effects.
Tariot et al. 2005	Divalproex (800) vs. PBO; 6 weeks	N=153; probable or possible AD with agitation	BPRS agitation factor[b] and total, CGI-C, CMAI	Trial completed by 72% of enrolled subjects. No significant drug–PBO differences found on primary or secondary outcome measures.
Mintzer et al. 2006	Risperidone (1 or 1.5; mean 1.03) vs. PBO; 8 weeks	N=473; AD dementia with psychosis (MMSE mean score 12.4)	BEHAVE-AD psychosis subscale[b], CGI-C[b]	Both groups improved; no significant differences on primary outcome measures. Subgroup analysis showed patients with MMSE score <10 had significantly greater improvement on CGI-C with risperidone. No difference in discontinuation rates between groups, but risperidone group had higher rates of somnolence (16.2% vs. 4.6%) and death (3.8% vs. 2.5%).

TABLE 24–2. Randomized, placebo-controlled studies of the efficacy of psychotropic medications in elderly nursing home residents *(continued)*

Study	Medication and dosage *(mg/day)*	Sample	Efficacy measures	Results and comments
Winblad et al. 2006	Donepezil (10) *vs.* PBO; 26 weeks	N=248; severe AD (MMSE score range 1–10)	SIB[b], ADCS-ADL severe[b], MMSE, NPI, CGI-I	Significant improvement in SIB scores and less decline in ADL function seen in donepezil group at 6 months. CGI-I significant for donepezil in completer analysis only. No significant behavioral benefits seen. Adverse events comparable between groups, but more patients in donepezil group discontinued treatment due to adverse events.
Mintzer et al. 2007	Aripiprazole (2, 5, or 10 fixed dosage) *vs.* PBO; 10 weeks	N=487; mean age 82.5 years; AD dementia with psychosis (MMSE mean score 12.4)	NPI-NH psychosis subscale[b] and total, CGI-S, CGI-I, BPRS psychosis core and total score, CMAI; response defined as ≥50% decrease in NPI score	Aripiprazole 10 mg group had significantly greater improvement vs. PBO group on NPI-NH psychosis scores and response rates, BPRS core and total scores, and CMAI scores. Aripiprazole 5 mg group had significantly greater improvement only on BPRS and CMAI. Aripiprazole 2 mg not efficacious. Dosage-dependent occurrence of CVAE in active groups. Death rates in PBO and 2-, 5-, and 10-mg groups 3%, 3%, 2%, and 7%, respectively; differences not statistically significant.
Zhong et al. 2007	Quetiapine (100 or 200) *vs.* PBO; 10 weeks	N=333; Alzheimer's and mixed dementia	PANSS-EC[b], CGI-C, NPI-NH, CMAI	No significant differences between quetiapine and PBO by LOCF analysis of PANSS-EC, NPI-NH, or CMAI scores at endpoint. Quetiapine 200 mg (but not 100 mg) significantly better than PBO on CGI-C scores and response rates using both LOCF and OC analyses and on PANSS-EC using OC analysis. No differences in incidence of postural hypotension, falls, and CVAE. More deaths with quetiapine; rates not statistically different from PBO. Response defined as ≥40% reduction in PANSS-EC or much/very much improved on CGI-C.

TABLE 24–2. Randomized, placebo-controlled studies of the efficacy of psychotropic medications in elderly nursing home residents *(continued)*

Study	Medication and dosage *(mg/day)*	Sample	Efficacy measures	Results and comments
Streim et al. 2008	Aripiprazole (2, 5, 10, or 15 flexible dosage titration) *vs.* PBO; 10 weeks	*N*=256; mean age 83 years; AD dementia with psychosis (MMSE mean score 13.6)	NPI-NH psychosis subscale[b], CGI-S[b], NPI-NH total; BPRS psychosis, core, and total scores; CMAI; CSDD; NPI caregiver distress; ADCS ADL scores; CGI-I	No significant difference between aripiprazole and PBO on NPI-NH psychosis or CGI-S at endpoint. Significantly greater improvement in aripiprazole group on secondary outcomes: NPI and BPRS total scores, CMAI, CGI-I, CSDD. More somnolence seen with aripiprazole (14%) vs. PBO (4%); other adverse effects similar for both, with low rate of EPS. Response defined as ≥50% decrease in NPI scores.
Rappaport et al. 2009	Aripiprazole (5–15 IM) *vs.* PBO (IM); 24 hours	*N*=129; mean age 80 years; AD dementia, VaD, mixed dementia with agitation (MMSE mean score 13.3)	PANSS-EC, ACES	Greater improvements seen on PANSS-EC scores with aripiprazole 10 and 15 mg vs. PBO; double the incidence of adverse events seen with aripiprazole (50%–60%) vs. PBO (32%).
Ballard et al. 2019	Pimavanserin 34 mg vs PBO; 12 weeks	*N*=181; mean age 82 years; AD with psychosis	NPI-NH psychosis subscores	Greater improvement in NPI-NH psychosis scores found in subset of patients with severe symptoms, NPI-NH psychosis ≥12 at baseline. Subset included *n*=27 in pimavanserin group and *n*=30 in PBO group. Improvement defined as 50% reduction from baseline. Fewer dropouts in pimavanserin group vs. PBO group.
Sommer et al. 2009	Oxcarbazepine (300–900) *vs.* PBO; 8 weeks	*N*=103; mean age 83.5 years; AD dementia, VaD, or mixed dementia with agitation and aggression	NPI-NH agitation and aggression subscores; NPI caregiver burden scale; BARS	After 8 weeks, no statistically significant differences between groups on any outcome measures. Trend observed in favor of the oxcarbazepine group in reduction in scores on the BARS.

TABLE 24–2. Randomized, placebo-controlled studies of the efficacy of psychotropic medications in elderly nursing home residents (*continued*)

Study	Medication and dosage (*mg/day*)	Sample	Efficacy measures	Results and comments

ACES=Agitation-Calmness Evaluation Scale; AD=Alzheimer's disease; ADCS-ADL=Alzheimer's Disease Cooperative Study–Activities of Daily Living Inventory (Galasko et al. 1997); ADL=activity of daily living; BARS=Brief Agitation Rating Scale (Finkel et al. 1993); BEHAVE-AD=Behavioral Pathology in Alzheimer's Disease (Reisberg et al. 1996); BPRS=Brief Psychiatric Rating Scale (Overall and Gorham 1962); BRMS=Bech-Rafaelsen Mania Scale (Bech et al. 1979); BRSD=Behavior Rating Scale for Dementia (Mack et al. 1999); CDR-SB=Clinical Dementia Rating (Nursing Home Version)—Sum of the Boxes (Hughes et al. 2000); CGI=Clinical Global Impression Scale (Guy 1976); CGI-C=CGI Change (Guy 1976; Schneider et al. 1997); CGI-I=CGI Improvement (Guy 1976); CGI-S=CGI of Severity (Guy 1976); CMAI=Cohen-Mansfield Agitation Inventory (Cohen-Mansfield et al. 1989); CSD=Cornell Scale for Depression; CSDD=Cornell Scale for Depression in Dementia (Alexopoulos et al. 1988); CVAE=cerebrovascular adverse events; EPS=extrapyramidal symptoms; FAST=Functional Assessment Staging (Reisberg 1988); GBS=Gottfries-Bråne-Steen Geriatric Rating Scale (Gottfries et al. 1982); GDS=Geriatric Depression Scale (Yesavage et al. 1982–1983); Ham-A=Hamilton Anxiety Scale (Hamilton 1959); Ham-D=Hamilton Rating Scale for Depression (Hamilton 1960); IM=intramuscular; LOCF=last observation carried forward; MADRS=Montgomery-Åsberg Depression Rating Scale (Montgomery and Åsberg 1979); MDD=major depressive disorder; MMSE=Mini-Mental State Examination (Folstein et al. 1975); NOSIE=Nurses' Observation Scale for Inpatient Evaluation (Honigfeld et al. 1966); NPI-NH=Neuropsychiatric Inventory–Nursing Home Version (Wood et al. 2000); NS=nonsignificant; OAS=Overt Aggression Scale (Yudofsky et al. 1986); OC=observed case; PANSS-EC=Positive and Negative Symptom Scale–Excited Component (Kay et al. 1987); PBO=placebo; PSMS=Physical Self-Maintenance Scale (Lawton and Brody 1969); SCAG=Sandoz Clinical Assessment—Geriatric (Shader et al. 1974); SIB=self-injurious behavior; SRI=serotonin reuptake inhibitor; UTI=urinary tract infection; VaD=vascular dementia.

[a]Also studied were 273 patients on geriatric wards of state hospitals.

[b]Primary outcome measure.

antipsychotics could be withdrawn from these agents without experiencing a reemergence of psychosis or agitated behaviors (Bridges-Parlet et al. 1997; Cohen-Mansfield et al. 1999; Ruths et al. 2004). These data are consistent with findings from older discontinuation studies (Barton and Hurst 1966; Risse et al. 1987). Therefore, it is important to periodically reevaluate the need for continuing antipsychotic drug treatment.

Since 2003, analyses of safety data from RCTs of atypical antipsychotic drugs in elderly adults with dementia, including the aforementioned nursing home studies, have revealed significantly increased risks of cerebrovascular adverse events and mortality in this population. Although elevated risks were not found in every study, pooled analyses showed that the rate of cerebrovascular adverse events (including stroke and transient ischemic attacks) was greater than that with placebo (Dorsey et al. 2010; U.S. Food and Drug Administration 2003). Most of the affected patients had known cerebrovascular risk factors prior to starting drug treatment. These findings led to regulatory warnings in the United States, Canada, and the United Kingdom regarding the safety of these drugs in elderly patients with dementia.

The FDA also warns that elderly patients with dementia-related psychosis treated with atypical antipsychotics have a risk of death ~1.7 times greater than that for those given placebo (4.5% vs. 2.6%) and provides a reminder that atypical antipsychotics do not have FDA approval for the treatment of patients with dementia-related psychosis (Dorsey et al. 2010; U.S. Food and Drug Administration 2005). Consistent with this FDA warning, a meta-analysis by Schneider et al. (2005) examining results of 15 RCTs, many of which were conducted in nursing home patients, found that the risk of mortality was 3.5% for elderly patients treated with atypical antipsychotics versus 2.3% for patients treated with placebo. Although no placebo-controlled trials of ziprasidone or clozapine are known to have been conducted in elderly patients with dementia, it is reasonable to view the increased mortality as a class effect. Wang et al. (2005) found a significantly higher adjusted risk of death for elderly patients taking conventional antipsychotics compared with those taking atypical antipsychotics, regardless of whether they had dementia or resided in a nursing home. The authors suggested that conventional antipsychotic medications are at least as likely as atypical agents to increase the risk of death in older adults. Subsequent comparisons in community-dwelling populations revealed higher mortality rates among nursing home residents with dementia who were newly started on antipsychotic drugs (Gill et al. 2007; Rochon et al. 2008).

Regarding concerns about risks of antipsychotic drugs in elderly nursing home residents with dementia, experts in the field have suggested that nonpharmacological approaches be considered first for the treatment of noncognitive behavioral symptoms (Blazer 2013). For those nursing home patients whose behavioral symptoms do not respond to nonpharmacological interventions, the decision to use an atypical antipsychotic should be based on a careful assessment of each patient's risk-benefit profile.

Six randomized clinical trials evaluated the efficacy of mood-stabilizing anticonvulsant drugs for the treatment of agitation and aggression in nursing home residents. The first was a study of carbamazepine that demonstrated it to be effective for agitation and aggression but not for psychotic symptoms such as delusions and hallucinations (Tariot et al. 1998). In this study, nursing reports indicated that less staff time was needed for patient care in the carbamazepine group. Another trial of carbamazepine reported high rates of improvement in both drug- and placebo-treated patients, with nonsignificant between-group differences (Olin et al. 2001). A subsequent study of oxcarbazepine failed to show efficacy for treatment of agitation and aggression (Sommer et al. 2009). A number of placebo-controlled studies evaluated divalproex, with few encouraging results; one trial was discontinued before completion because of adverse effects in the drug treatment group. Overall, these studies failed to provide evidence for efficacy in reducing agitated behavior (Porsteinsson et al. 2001; Tariot et al. 2001b, 2005). The tolerability of divalproex was limited by somnolence, weakness, and diminished oral intake in this population.

Acetylcholinesterase inhibitors have been shown to delay the decline in cognitive function in individuals with mild to severe AD. Although few studies have been conducted specifically in nursing home samples, the 2004 NNHS found that of the 49.1% of survey participants with dementia, 30% were receiving cholinesterase inhibitors (Seitz et al. 2009). A randomized clinical trial of donepezil in nursing home residents showed effects on cognitive performance that were comparable with those observed in less impaired outpatients (Tariot et al. 2001a). A subsequent study demonstrated that donepezil improves cognition and preserves function in patients with AD and severe dementia who are residing in nursing homes (Winblad et al. 2006). These studies also examined the effects of donepezil on behavioral disturbances as a secondary outcome measure and did not find significant benefits. Ballard et al. (2005) compared the effects of quetiapine, rivastigmine, and placebo on agitation and cognition in nursing home patients with dementia and found that neither drug was effective for the treatment of agitation and that quetiapine was associated with significantly greater cognitive decline. Recent research (Ballard et al. 2019, 2020) has reported promising data of likely efficacy in decreasing AD psychosis and related agitation and aggression. A study by Tariot et al. (2004) reported significant improvement in Neuropsychiatric Inventory scores in patients for whom memantine rather than placebo was added to stable doses of donepezil, but memantine has not yet been studied prospectively in the nursing home setting. Survival analyses in an observational study suggest that adding memantine to a cholinesterase inhibitor may delay the time to nursing home placement (Lopez et al. 2009).

Only five RCTs have evaluated the effects of antidepressants in nursing home residents. The first study found no differences in intellectual, emotional, or functional status in residents with dementia who were treated with alaproclate (Dehlin et al. 1985). The second study, which was also placebo controlled, showed a positive response to nortriptyline for treatment of MDD in a long-term care population with high levels of medical comorbidity (Katz et al. 1990). In the third study, patients were randomly assigned to receive regular or low-dosage nortriptyline, and significant plasma level–response relationships were demonstrated in cognitively intact patients (Streim et al. 2000). These findings confirmed the validity of the diagnosis of depression in nursing home residents in the context of significant medical comorbidity and disability. However, in patients with dementia, the plasma level–response relationship was significantly different, suggesting that the depression occurring in dementia might be a treatment-relevant subtype of MDD or a distinct disorder. The fourth, a controlled antidepressant trial in nursing home residents with late-stage AD, showed no significant benefits of sertraline over placebo (Magai et al. 2000). In the fifth study, a randomized placebo-controlled trial of paroxetine in very old residents with non-major depression, no significant benefit was found for drug over placebo (Burrows et al. 2002).

Available open-label studies of the efficacy of selective serotonin reuptake inhibitors (SSRIs) in nursing home residents with depression have had mixed results, some consistent with the findings of Magai et al. (2000) suggesting that SSRIs may be less effective for depression in patients with dementia than in those who are cognitively intact (Oslin et al. 2000; Rosen et al. 2000; Trappler and Cohen 1996, 1998). Findings from nonrandomized open-label antidepressant trials in nursing home residents with depression are summarized in a review by Boyce et al. (2012).

Although the SSRIs might be expected to be well tolerated by frail elderly nursing home patients because of their side effect profiles, there is evidence that these drugs can cause serious adverse events in this population. Thapa et al. (1998) demonstrated that the use of SSRIs was associated with a nearly twofold increase in the risk of falls in nursing home residents, comparable with the risk found with tricyclic antidepressants. Investigators in the United Kingdom reported that antidepressant use was associated with better physical functioning but a greater frequency of falls in residential care patients (Arthur et al. 2002). A randomized, double-blind comparison trial found that venlafaxine was less well tolerated than sertraline in frail nursing home patients without conferring more treatment benefits, as might be expected from an agent with mixed serotonergic and noradrenergic effects (Oslin et al. 2003).

More recent studies have again focused on the use of serotonin reuptake inhibitors for the treatment of agitation, noting the safety of citalopram and escitalopram among patients with dementia (Ahmed et al. 2019; Viscogliosi et al. 2017). As prior studies have suggested, these agents may have a more favorable side effect profile overall, but concerns of efficacy and risk of falls with injury still require investigation. Concerns about QTc prolongation with dosages of citalopram >20 mg have led to an FDA warning regarding dosing and need for more cautious electroencephalographic monitoring (Kales et al. 2015).

History of Deficient Mental Health Care as an Impetus for Nursing Home Reform

Although psychiatric disorders are extraordinarily common in nursing home residents and efficacious treatments do exist, psychiatric services are often not adequate in these settings. Historically, nursing home design, staffing, programs, services, and funding have not evolved to meet the needs of patients with mental disorders (Reichman and Conn 2010; Streim and Katz 1994). In the 1980s, it was estimated that as many as two-thirds of nursing home residents with psychiatric disorders had been misdiagnosed (German et al. 1986; Sabin et al. 1982) and that as little as 5% of nursing home residents' needs for mental health services were being met (Burns and Taube 1990). This mismatch of psychiatric needs and available treatment led not only to neglect but also to inappropriate treatment; psychiatric problems were often mismanaged with the use of physical or chemical restraints.

Physical Restraints

The 1977 NNHS showed that 25% of 1.3 million U.S. nursing home residents had been restrained by geriatric chairs, cuffs, belts, or similar devices, primarily to control behavioral symptoms (National Center for Health Statistics 1979). Other early surveys found rates of restraint use as high as 85%. In addition to agitation and behavior problems, patient factors predicting the use of restraints include age, cognitive impairment, risk of injuries to self (e.g., from falls) or others (e.g., from combative behavior), physical frailty, the presence of monitoring or treatment devices, and the need to promote body alignment. Institutional and systemic factors associated with restraint use include pressure to avoid litigation, staff attitudes, insufficient staffing, and availability of restraint devices. Potential adverse effects include increased risk of falls and other injuries (Capezuti et al. 1996), functional decline, skin breakdown, physiological effects of immobilization stress, disorganized behavior, and demoralization. Although mechanical restraints have often been used in attempts to control agitation, they do not in fact decrease behavioral disturbances (Werner et al. 1989), and cross-national studies indicate that nursing home residents can be managed without such measures (Cape 1983; Evans and Strumpf 1989; Innes and Turman 1983).

Misuse of Psychotropic Drugs

Concerns about inadequate and inappropriate care have also focused on the overuse of psychotropic drugs in nursing home residents, especially the misuse of these drugs as chemical restraints to control behaviors. Studies in the 1970s and 1980s reported that ~50% of residents had orders for psychotropic medications, with 20%–40% given antipsychotic drugs, 10%–40% given anxiolytics or hypnotics, and 5%–10% given antidepressants (Avorn et al. 1989; Beers et al. 1988; Buck 1988; Burns et al. 1988; Cohen-Mansfield 1986; Custer et al. 1984; DeLeo et al. 1989; Ray et al. 1980; Teeter et al. 1976; Zimmer et al. 1984). Psychotropic drugs were frequently prescribed without adequate regard for the residents' psychiatric diagnosis or medical status. Zimmer et al. (1984) reported that only 15% of residents given psychotropic drugs had received a psychiatric consultation. Other studies reported that 21% of patients without a psychiatric diagnosis were given psychotropic medication (Burns et al. 1988), that physicians'— as opposed to the patients'—characteristics predicted drug dosages (Ray et al. 1980), and that psychotropic drugs were often prescribed in the absence of any documentation of the patient's mental status in the clinical record (Avorn et al. 1989).

In light of concerns about balancing the safety and efficacy of antipsychotics with managing psychosis and agitation in nursing home residents with dementia, patients with nonpsychotic behavioral problems should be managed with other medications, behavioral treatments, interpersonal approaches, or environmental interventions when possible. Moreover, although all evidence for the efficacy of antipsychotic medications comes from short-term studies, they are often prescribed for long-term treatment. Concerns regarding the overuse of antipsychotic medications were supported by findings from drug discontinuation studies (see "Pharmacotherapy"). One classic double-blind study of antipsychotic withdrawal showed that only 16% of patients who had been receiving medications on a chronic basis exhibited significant deterioration when the drugs were withdrawn (Barton and Hurst 1966). A subsequent small-scale withdrawal study in patients who had been receiving antipsychotic drugs for several months showed that 22% experienced increased agitation on withdrawal, indicating benefit from continued treatment, but that 22% were unchanged and 55% showed improvement (Risse et al. 1987).

The need to identify target symptoms that may respond to antipsychotic medications to reduce distress and limit unsafe aggression has been the focus of multiple best-practice pathways devised to help caregivers and professionals identify target symptoms; find behavioral, environmental, and interpersonal interventions; and decide whether psychotropic medications are warranted. These interventions, such as DICE (describe, investigate, create, evaluate), are person centered and help clinicians with documentation, interventions, and follow-up monitoring (Kales et al. 2015).

Inadequate Treatment of Depression

Although the focus of public concern and regulatory scrutiny in the 1970s and 1980s was on the overprescription of antipsychotic medications in patients with dementia, undertreatment of other psychiatric conditions in the nursing home has also been a serious problem. In a report that did much to stimulate nursing home reform, the Institute of Medicine Committee on Nursing Home Regulation (1986) highlighted problems both in the overuse of antipsychotics and in the underuse of antidepressants for treatment of affective disorders. Similarly, in a review of epidemiological studies on the use of psychotropic medications in nursing homes, Murphy (1989) noted that antidepressants were the one class of drugs that appeared to be underused and that, as a result, MDD in this setting often remained untreated during the 1970s and 1980s. Before 1990, less than 15% of residents with a known diagnosis of depression were receiving antidepressant medication (Heston et al. 1992).

Interventions designed to recognize and treat conditions such as unrecognized pain along with mood symptoms are associated with high-quality care. MDS 3.0 assessments indicate that 14.1% of residents have a new diagnosis of depression 90 days after admission (Yuan et al. 2019).

Federal Regulations and Psychiatric Care in the Nursing Home

The misuse of physical and chemical restraints was a rallying point for advocacy groups that urged the federal government to institute nursing home reform. In addition, the U.S. General Accounting Office was concerned that states were admitting patients with chronic and severe psychiatric problems to Medicaid-certified nursing homes not because the patients needed this type of care but because their admission would shift a substantial portion of the costs of their care from the state to the federal government. Apparently in response to both sets of concerns, Congress enacted the Nursing Home Reform Act as part of the Omnibus Budget Reconciliation Act of 1987 (OBRA-87). This legislation provided for government regulation of nursing facilities and of the care that they provide (Elon and Pawlson 1992), and it directed the Health Care Financing Administration (reorganized and renamed in 2001 as the CMS) to issue regulations that operationalize the laws (Health Care Financing Administration 1991) and to develop guidelines that help federal and state surveyors interpret regulations and determine whether facilities are complying(Centers for Medicare and Medicaid Services 2014).

These regulations and survey processes were implemented in 1990. Mental health screening, assessment, care planning, and treatment are addressed under sections of the regulations that pertain to resident assessment, resident rights and facility practices, and quality of care (Health Care Financing Administration 1991, 1992a, 1992b). Regulations include provisions for preadmission screening and annual resident review that require the assessment of each resident prior to admission to any federally funded nursing facility (Health Care Financing Administration 1992a). When an initial first-stage screening reveals that a serious mental disorder (other than dementia) might be present, a second-stage assessment including a psychiatric evaluation must be made to ascertain whether the patient has a mental disorder, to make a specific psychiatric diagnosis, and to determine whether acute psychiatric care is needed that precludes adequate or appropriate treatment in a nursing home. Patients who are found to have dementia on the initial screening are exempt from the preadmission psychiatric evaluation. Thus, the preadmission screening is intended 1) to prevent inappropriate admission to nursing homes of patients who do not have dementia but who have severe psychiatric disorders and 2) to help ensure that patients with disabilities due to treatable psychiatric disorders are not placed in long-term care facilities before they receive the benefits of adequate psychiatric treatment.

For eligible patients admitted to a nursing home, an annual reassessment must be made to determine whether nursing home care remains appropriate. Regulations requiring comprehensive assessment of all residents (Health Care Financing Administration 1991) led to the development of a uniform Resident Assessment Instrument, which includes the MDS (Centers for Medicare and Medicaid Services 2013; Morris et al. 1990). MDS 3.0 was implemented in 2010 (Centers for Medicare and Medicaid Services 2006; Saliba et al. 2012). Members of an interdisciplinary health care team must administer this instrument on at least a quarterly basis and report the results to CMS (Health Care Financing Administration 1992c). Areas of assessment that are relevant to mental health include hearing, speech, and vision; cognitive patterns; mood; behavior; functional status; health conditions; swallowing and nutritional status; medications; special treatments and procedures (including rehabilitative, respite, and hospice care); and restraints. Responses on the MDS may indicate changes in a patient's clinical status that warrant further evaluation and possible need for changes in the care plan. Changes in a resident's status may trigger requests for psychiatric consultation.

Nursing facilities are highly regulated by both federal and state guidelines. Most nursing homes participate in federal programs and are subject to the evolving regulations that began in 1986 when the Institute of Medicine issued a comprehensive report detailing significant quality issues in long-term care facilities (Institute of Medicine Committee on Nursing Home Regulation 1986). This report inspired a series of regulatory changes that included specific language related to psychotropic medications and unnecessary drugs. Regulations related to resident rights and facility practices restrict the use of physical restraints and antipsychotic drugs when "administered for purposes of discipline or convenience and not required to treat the resident's medical symptoms" (Health Care Financing Administration 1991, p. 48,875). Regulations related to quality of care further require that residents not receive "unnecessary drugs" and that antipsychotic medications not be given unless "necessary to treat a specific condition as diagnosed and documented in the clinical record" (p. 48,910). An *unnec-*

essary drug is defined as any drug used 1) in excessive dosages (including duplicate therapy), 2) for excessive duration, 3) without adequate monitoring, 4) without adequate indications for its use, 5) in the presence of adverse consequences that indicate that it should be reduced or discontinued, or 6) for any combination of the first five reasons (Health Care Financing Administration 1991). The surveyor guidelines based on these regulations further limit the use of antipsychotic medications, antianxiety agents, sedative-hypnotics, and related medications (Centers for Medicare and Medicaid Services 2014). For each of these classes, the guidelines specify a list of acceptable indications, upper limits for daily dosages, requirements for monitoring treatment and adverse effects, and time frames for attempting dosage reductions and discontinuation. These guidelines are periodically updated to reflect new clinical knowledge and the availability of new drugs approved by the FDA, with a recent revision posted to the CMS website in 2014 (Centers for Medicare and Medicaid Services 2014).

To minimize concerns about federal interference with medical practice, the current guidelines include qualifying statements that recognize cases in which strict adherence to prescribing limits or gradual dosage reduction or discontinuation is "clinically contraindicated." Although the focus is on limiting the use of psychotropic drugs, the guidelines acknowledge that appropriate medical treatment can involve continuing treatment with psychotropic medications. Thus, physicians' options for treating nursing home residents need not be unduly restricted by regulations if the clinical rationale—explaining that the benefits of treatment (in terms of symptom relief, improved health status, or improved function) outweigh the risks—is clearly documented in the medical record. Although the facility, not the physician, is accountable for compliance with regulations, the physician's clinical reasoning and judgment play a critical role in the process of ensuring quality care.

In 2012, the CMS, in collaboration with state agencies, advocacy groups, and concerned stakeholders, launched the National Partnership to Improve Dementia Care, which included a major impetus on reducing the use of antipsychotic medications in nursing facilities. Outcomes of the program included a decline in the rate of antipsychotic drug prescriptions from 25.5% in 2011 to 21.7% in 2014 (Crystal et al. 2020). Concern has been expressed about an increase in prescriptions for mood stabilizers for patients with dementia that may represent a shift in prescribing patterns (Maust et al. 2018; Zhao et al. 2020).

In 2016, the CMS finalized an update to nursing home regulations following a comprehensive review and public comment (Unroe et al. 2018). These included specific increases in the monitoring of patients receiving any type of psychotropic medications, including antipsychotic, antidepressant, antianxiety, and hypnotic drugs. Although evaluation specifically by a psychiatrist is not required, facilities are mandated to have monthly reviews by a clinical pharmacist for those patients who receive psychotropic medications. There is increased emphasis on clinical justification of the diagnosis and the rationale for the use of psychiatric medication (Centers for Medicare and Medicaid Services HHS 2016; Unroe et al. 2018). These regulations were accompanied by provisions for interdisciplinary care planning and trainings for staff in dementia care, abuse, and neglect. Facilities are tasked even more than before to justify the need for psychotropic medications and to provide treatment of psychological and psychosocial problems. Although the role of a psychiatrist is not mandated, mental health care of nursing facility residents will clearly be an increasing subject of regulation and oversight (Fashaw et al. 2020; Unroe et al. 2018).

Concerns have been raised that reporting of schizophrenia diagnoses has increased at a disproportionate rate since these regulations were implemented. From 1985 to 2015, the percentage of nursing home residents with a diagnosis of schizophrenia increased from 6% to 11% (Fashaw et al. 2020). Although this confirms the use of nursing homes as mental health care facilities, it raises the issues of the appropriateness of diagnoses, the need for increasing care, and the role of the psychiatrist in guiding resident treatment.

In addition to addressing the use of psychotropic drugs, the interpretive guidelines also outline conditions for the use of physical restraints. According to the guidelines, restraints are not permitted unless there is documentation that their use is necessary to enable the resident to achieve or maintain the highest practicable level of function. Physical or occupational therapists should be consulted and should provide documentation if restraints are deemed necessary to enhance body positioning or improve mobility.

Although the federal regulations emphasize eliminating inappropriate treatment, their requirements also call for the provision of necessary and appropriate care for residents with mental health problems. Under the provisions designed to ensure quality of care, federal regulations define a need for geriatric psychiatry services in nursing homes, requiring that "the facility must ensure that a resident who displays mental or psychosocial adjustment difficulties receives appropriate services to correct the assessed problem" (Health Care Financing Administration 1991, p. 48,896).

In 1999, 12 years after the nursing home reform amendments were passed into law by Congress, the Health Care Financing Administration developed quality indicators that were derived from resident assessment data (Center for Health Systems Research and Analysis 1999) in order to provide surveyors with benchmarks for measuring and comparing the quality of care provided by individual nursing homes. In 2002, CMS expanded these efforts by introducing the Nursing Home Quality Initiative, which derives quality measures from regularly reported MDS data and posts these on the Medicare.gov website in a program called Nursing Home Compare (Medicare.gov 2014a). This publicly accessible website enables health care consumers to compare the quality of care delivered by individual facilities in the same region or across the nation. At the time this chapter was written, 5 short-stay quality measures and 13 long-stay quality measures had been posted. Quality measures that are directly or may be indirectly relevant to the mental health of nursing home residents are listed in Table 24–3. These measures include the percentage of residents experiencing moderate to severe pain, falls with injuries, depressive symptoms, weight loss, increased need for help with ADLs, physical restraint, and receipt of antipsychotic medication.

In 2007, CMS also began a national rollout of the Quality Indicator Survey, which was designed to make the nursing home survey process more resident centered, comprehensive, and consistent (Lin and Kramer 2013). Whenever a state survey finds that a percentile threshold has been exceeded in any of these areas, a citation of deficiency can be issued to the nursing home. The facility is then required to develop and submit a plan of correction for approval by the state licensing agency. This system represents an advance in monitoring quality of care and promoting cultural change in U.S. nurs-

TABLE 24–3.   **Centers for Medicare and Medicaid Services nursing home quality measures with relevance to the mental health of residents**

Short-stay quality measures

  Percentage of residents who self-report moderate to severe pain

  Percentage of short-stay residents who newly received an antipsychotic medication

Long-stay quality measures

  Percentage of residents experiencing one or more falls with a major injury

  Percentage of residents who self-report moderate to severe pain

  Percentage of residents who were physically restrained

  Percentage of residents whose need for help with activities of daily living has increased

  Percentage of residents who have lost too much weight

  Percentage of residents who have depressive symptoms

  Percentage of long-stay residents who received an antipsychotic medication

Source.   Medicare.gov 2014a.

ing homes, although the limits of risk adjustment for some of the quality indicators have been questioned, and the results of quality surveys may be difficult to interpret. Nevertheless, the Nursing Home Quality Initiative is widely considered to represent a major step forward in measurement-based care and public access to quality data. In 2012 CMS responded to issues in the survey process by founding the National Partnership to Improve Dementia Care in Nursing Homes. The goal of this multifaceted program included a reduction in the use of inappropriate antipsychotic use within nursing facilities over several years. This initiative showed some early success in that most facilities met the target reduction of 15% in the first year, but significant variability by state remains in citations and the survey process (Urick et al. 2016).

In June 2008 CMS launched an initiative to provide public access to nursing home ratings on the Nursing Home Compare website, posting a five-star rating system along with facility characteristics. Facilities must be prepared for intense public scrutiny of not only five-star ratings but also online reviews through commonly used sites such as Yelp (Johari et al. 2018).

Changing Patterns of Psychiatric Care

Since the passage of the Nursing Home Reform Act in 1987 and implementation of the resultant regulations in 1990, significant changes have been made in nursing home care, including mental health care. Some of these changes may be attributed to the process of conducting surveys and enforcing federal regulations. However, several other factors appear to have contributed, including the dissemination of information about regulatory requirements, availability and marketing of new medications, advances in scientific knowledge from nursing home research, and cumulative effects of professional education regarding patient safety and good clinical practice. Public reporting of quality measures and increasing consumer awareness are also likely to be playing a role.

Shifts in Antipsychotic Medication Use

Studies of the effect of federal regulations in the early years after their implementation showed a substantial decline in the use of antipsychotic drugs (Shorr et al. 1994) and physical restraints (Hawes et al. 1997) and an increase in the use of antidepressants (Lantz et al. 1996). Between 1991 and 1997, a 52.2% decrease (from 33.7% to 16.1%) in the use of antipsychotic medications was reported (Hughes et al. 2000). One study reported that greater reductions in antipsychotic use during this period were found in nursing facilities that emphasized psychosocial care, had a a less severe case mix, and had a higher nurse-to-resident ratio (Svarstad et al. 2001). Soon after the regulations were introduced, several investigators developed educational programs for physicians, nurses, and aides to teach practice principles consistent with federal guidelines. Studies evaluating these educational interventions demonstrated reductions of 23%–72% in the use of antipsychotics (Avorn et al. 1992; Meador et al. 1997; Ray et al. 1993; Rovner et al. 1992; Schnelle et al. 1992). In the study showing the most substantial reductions, the frequency of behavior problems was not found to increase (Ray et al. 1993). Studies of the appropriateness of antipsychotic use that examined documentation of CMS-approved diagnostic indications, appropriate target symptoms, and dosing within recommended limits in the surveyor guidelines suggested relatively high rates of compliance with federal regulations (Llorente et al. 1998; Siegler et al. 1997).

Although the changes found by these studies were generally interpreted as an indication of improvement in care, the studies did not examine health care outcomes or effects on residents' quality of life (Snowden and Roy-Byrne 1998) and did not address concerns that reductions in medication use might have an adverse effect on patients who required antipsychotic treatment, such as those with a diagnosis of chronic schizophrenia or mood disorder with psychosis. A retrospective study in a single nursing facility, which described attempts to discontinue or lower the dosage of antipsychotic drugs in 75% of subjects studied, found that residents with appropriate indications for antipsychotic use according to the federal regulations were significantly less likely to have their antipsychotic agents stopped (Semla et al. 1994). Nevertheless, for 20% of residents whose antipsychotic was discontinued or reduced in dosage, either the agent was subsequently resumed or its dosage was increased. This result, which is consistent with reports from earlier discontinuation studies, suggests that the finding of a reduction in overall rates of antipsychotic use may reflect a beneficial trend for most patients but cannot be interpreted as an indication of across-the-board improvement in the quality of residents' care (Lantz et al. 1996).

In contrast to declining rates of antipsychotic use in the early 1990s, Online Survey Certification and Reporting (OSCAR) data showed a reversal in this trend from 1995 to 1999, with the national rate of antipsychotic drug use in nursing homes increasing from 16% to 19.4% during that period (American Society of Consultant Pharmacists 2000). Despite this increase, a survey conducted by the Office of the Inspector General of the Department of Health and Human Services, using data from the year 2000, found that psychotropic drugs had been appropriately prescribed in 85% of the 485 cases reviewed (Office of Inspector General 2001c). However, these findings were contradicted by a large retrospective analysis of Medicare databases merged to MDS assessments from the same period (Briesacher et al. 2005). In this analysis, 27.6% of all

Medicare beneficiaries in nursing homes received antipsychotic medications between 2000 and 2001; of the treated patients, only 41.8% received antipsychotic therapy that was within federal prescribing guidelines. A cross-sectional analysis of the 2004 NNHS similarly identified that 26% of nursing home residents in the survey received antipsychotic medication, and 40% of these cases were without appropriate indications for antipsychotic use (Stevenson et al. 2010).

The increased rates of antipsychotic medication use, coupled with the safety concerns about the risk of cerebrovascular adverse events and mortality, have prompted a closer look at alternatives to antipsychotic drug treatment for behavioral disturbances in nursing home residents with dementia. A study by Fossey et al. (2006), conducted in the wake of the safety findings described earlier in this chapter (see "Pharmacotherapy"), examined 12-month outcomes of an intervention that provided training and support to nursing home staff in psychosocial approaches for managing agitated behavior associated with dementia. The rate of antipsychotic medication use was 19.1% lower in the intervention homes, with no significant differences in the level of agitated or disruptive behavior between intervention and control facilities. Thus, it appears that a significant proportion of residents may be managed with less risk and without a concomitant increase in behavioral problems.

Over the past decade, CMS has also contracted with quality improvement organizations (QIOs, which are private, nonprofit entities formerly called peer review organizations) in all 50 states, the District of Columbia, Puerto Rico, and the U.S. Virgin Islands to promote population-based quality improvement in nursing home care (Rollow et al. 2006; Stevenson and Mor 2009). In 2012, CMS launched a National Partnership to Improve Dementia Care, which uses a multidimensional approach to reduce the inappropriate use of antipsychotic drugs in these settings (Medicare.gov 2014b). As a component of this partnership, the scope of work for QIOs currently involves extensive dementia care training for nursing home staff, supported by training materials that focus on nonpharmacological management of dementia-related behaviors. Data from this period reported on the Nursing Home Compare website reveal a 9% decline in the national rate of antipsychotic use from 23.9% at the end of 2011 to 21.7% at the beginning of 2013. State-level data for this period show reductions ranging from 2.3% to 23.3%.

Increase in Antidepressant Drug Use

Despite the decline in use of antipsychotics in the early 1990s, overall use of psychotherapeutic medications in U.S. nursing homes increased, from 21.7% in 1991 to 46.1% in 1997 (Health Care Financing Administration 1998). This increase was partly attributable to a rise in antidepressant use from 12.6% to 24.9% (97.6% increase) during that period. In the United Kingdom, rates of antidepressant use also increased by 72%, from 11% in 1990 to 18.9% in 1997 (Arthur et al. 2002). From the mid-1990s to the mid-2000s, the prevalence of antidepressant medication use in the United States more than doubled again. A study of 12 Pennsylvania nursing homes found that 47.6% of residents were taking antidepressants (Datto et al. 2002). OSCAR data showed that this was part of a national trend, with more than 12,000 U.S. nursing homes reporting an increase in antidepressant prescribing: from 21.9% in 1996 to 35.5% in 2001 to 47.5% in 2006 (American Society of Consultant Pharmacists 2000; Hanlon et al. 2010). The 2004 NNHS found the overall prevalence of antidepressant use among elderly nursing home residents to be 46.2%, with half of those prescribed these drugs being age 85 years and older (Karkare et al.

2011). The most-prescribed class of antidepressants was SSRIs (31.1%), followed by se-rotonin modulators (4.7%), serotonin-norepinephrine reuptake inhibitors (2.8%), tricy-clic antidepressants (2.3%), and monoamine oxidase inhibitors (0.01%).

Considered together, these data represent an extraordinary change in the pattern of drug use in a population that traditionally received inadequate pharmacotherapy for depression. The dramatic increase in antidepressant prescriptions is probably due in part to the wide availability of newer antidepressants that are perceived to be safer and better tolerated among elderly nursing home residents with medical and psychi-atric comorbidity. Education of primary care physicians about the morbidity, disabil-ity, mortality, and costs associated with untreated depression may also have played a role, as well as aggressive marketing by pharmaceutical companies. With current an-tidepressant drug use rates that appear comparable with or greater than the estimated prevalence of depression among nursing home residents, it is possible that a signifi-cant proportion of antidepressant prescriptions are intended for indications other than depression, such as sleep, pain, anxiety, or agitation. Research is needed to de-termine whether the reported changes in prescribing have had a positive effect on the mental health of nursing home residents with depression.

Decline in Physical Restraint Use

Although the early effects of federal nursing home regulations on trends in psychotropic drug use during the 1990s were difficult to discern (Lantz et al. 1996), the effect of the fed-eral regulations on restraints appeared to be uniformly positive, with several studies showing significant reductions in use (Castle et al. 1997). One study found restraint use rates of 37.4% in 1990 (before OBRA-87 implementation in October 1990) and 28.1% in 1993 (following introduction of the standardized Resident Assessment Instrument re-quired by OBRA-87) (Hawes et al. 1997). Siegler et al. (1997) found that restraint use could be significantly reduced without a resultant increase in antipsychotic or benzodiaz-epine use. No evidence has been published of an increase in fall-related injuries associated with lower rates of physical restraint use. Despite this overall decline in use, deaths asso-ciated with physical restraints, although rare, continue to occur and are largely due to neck compression and asphyxia (Bellenger et al. 2018). Physical restraint combined with antipsychotic medication use is found among the most vulnerable nursing home residents with severe cognitive loss and functional decline (Foebel et al. 2016).

Special Care Units

Encouraged by consumer demand to better meet the needs of nursing home residents with dementia, by 1991 10% of U.S. nursing homes had established special care units (SCUs). A decade later, it was estimated that 22% of nursing homes had designated SCUs for patients with dementia. In the 2004 NNHS, 23.8% of facilities reported hav-ing special programs for the management of behavior problems, although not all of these were provided exclusively on a dedicated SCU (National Center for Health Sta-tistics 2004). To characterize the population served by these units, Holmes et al. (1990) reported that SCU patients had more severe cognitive, behavioral, and functional deficits than non-SCU patients with dementia who lived in the same nursing home. More than 90% of residents in SCUs had behavior problems (Wagner et al. 1995).

Research on the effectiveness of SCUs is difficult to interpret and generalize be-cause of the heterogeneity of these facilities (Office of Technology Assessment 1992;

Ohta and Ohta 1988), lack of adjustment for differences between comparator groups, and absence of any RCTs (Lai et al. 2009). Some studies indicate that the facilities, services, and programs offered by SCUs may not be significantly better than those available on conventional nursing home units. A study of Minnesota nursing homes described unit and facility characteristics, noting that the designation of SCU was not associated with more services or more individualized dementia care than was provided in units without the designation; however, the study found that some dementia-specific features were less likely to be found in the regular units of nursing homes that also had designated SCUs (Grant et al. 1995).

A case-control study of 625 patients on 31 SCUs and 32 traditional units found that residence on an SCU was associated with reduced use of physical restraints but not with less use of so-called pharmacological restraints (Sloane et al. 1991). A subsequent study that included data on more than 1,100 residents on 48 SCUs reported that the use of physical restraints was not different and that the likelihood of psychotropic medication use was actually greater for patients on SCUs than for their counterparts on traditional units (Phillips et al. 2000). A study of 430 patients with dementia residing in SCUs for patients with AD and traditional nursing facilities in Italy found lower odds of physical restraint use and higher rates of withdrawal from antipsychotics in the SCU group, with no differences in falls, hospitalization rates, or mortality (Nobili et al. 2008). Although Saxton et al. (1998) reported evidence suggesting that mobility may be maintained for longer periods of time among SCU residents, Phillips et al. (1997) found that the rate of decline in ADL function is not significantly slower for SCU residents. Studies showing benefits of SCUs for behavioral disturbances are limited, although one randomized clinical trial reported a reduced frequency of catastrophic reactions (Swanson et al. 1993)—sudden agitated behavior in response to overwhelming external stimuli—as a positive outcome for residence on a dementia SCU. Some studies have demonstrated psychological benefits not only for SCU patients (Lawton et al. 1998) but also for caregivers (Kutner et al. 1999; Wells and Jorm 1987), with evidence of increased family involvement (Hansen et al. 1988; Sloane et al. 1998).

Studies have also examined the extent to which agitation is associated with aspects of the treatment environment in SCUs. Independent correlates of low agitation levels in these units included low rates of physical restraint use, high proportion of residents in bed during the day, small unit size, fewer comorbid conditions, low levels of functional dependency, and favorable scores on measures of physical environment and unit activities. More recent studies have shown an association between residence on dementia SCUs and reduction in inappropriate antipsychotic use (–9.75%), physical restraints (–9.6%), pressure ulcers (–3.3%), feeding tubes (–8.3%), and overall hospitalizations (–14.7%) from data collected using the MDS. This study included an impressively large sample of more than 7,000,000 subjects who resided in nursing homes between 2005 and 2010 (Joyce et al. 2018). Social interactions of patients residing on dementia SCUs are higher than for those on traditional nursing home units, although nursing home residents are highly dependent on staff to initiate such interactions (Adlbrecht et al. 2021).

Subacute Care in Nursing Homes

Since 1983, when the Medicare Prospective Payment System established reimbursement for acute care hospitals on the basis of diagnosis-related groups rather than number of inpatient days, hospitals have had a strong incentive to limit lengths of stay by discharging patients earlier. In the 1990s, Medicare reimbursement rates for the first 100 days of nursing home care, computed according to the Resource Utilization Groups system, were substantially higher for short-stay patients who received rehabilitation services than for long-term care patients. Thus, nursing homes had an incentive to admit a higher proportion of short-stay patients with subacute rehabilitation needs. These financial incentives for early hospital discharge to nursing homes serving as step-down facilities for subacute medical treatment, convalescent care, and rehabilitation services resulted in significant increases in Medicare costs for subacute-care patients in the nursing home setting. Alarm about the increase in spending occurring in the late 1990s prompted changes in Medicare reimbursement that resulted in dramatic reductions in payments to nursing homes from the late 1990s onward.

In general, short-stay nursing home residents—patients who, after relatively brief stays in nursing homes, are discharged to the community or die—differ from long-term care patients in that they are younger; more likely to be admitted directly from an acute care hospital; less likely to have irreversible cognitive impairment, incontinence, or ambulatory dysfunction; and more likely to have a primary diagnosis of hip fracture, stroke, or cancer. The objectives of mental health care for short-stay patients are related not so much to managing behavior problems associated with dementia as to helping patients cope with disease and disability, screening for delirium and reversible causes of cognitive impairment, and treating disorders such as depression and anxiety that can impede rehabilitation and recovery. A high prevalence of potentially treatable neuropsychiatric symptoms—including depression in 33%, nighttime disturbances in 19%, anxiety in 15%, and irritability and disinhibition in 12%—was found in post-stroke patients who could not be successfully discharged from the nursing home where they received subacute rehabilitative care (Buijck et al. 2012). In short, the objectives of mental health care for these patients are similar to goals of traditional consultation-liaison psychiatry in the general hospital. As the opportunities for psychiatric intervention follow these patients from the acute care hospital into the nursing homes, the services required may need to be more frequent or intensive than those usually available to long-term care residents. A study by Lenze et al. (2012) demonstrated the benefits of applying motivational and behavioral skills in physical and occupational therapy to improve patient engagement, therapy intensity, and functional outcomes for older adults in post-acute rehabilitation. For subacute care patients in nursing homes, an investment in psychiatric care can lead to improved participation in rehabilitation efforts, with a more efficient recovery and return to independent functioning and a higher likelihood of successful discharge to the community.

Adequacy of Mental Health Care

The high prevalence of psychiatric problems and the federal mandate to ensure quality of care define a need for geriatric mental health services in nursing homes (Smith et al. 1990). Although the OBRA-87 regulations had the intended impact (Snowden and Roy-Byrne 1998) and have resulted in measurable improvements in several aspects of patient care, concurrent improvements in access to mental health care, receipt of appropriate care, or improved mental health outcomes have not been seen. Medicare claims data from 1992—2 years after implementation of the Nursing Home Reform Act of 1987—indicated that only 26% of all nursing home residents and 36% of those with a mental illness received psychiatric services (Smyer et al. 1994). Although Medicare payments for psychiatric services in nursing facilities increased in the mid-1990s, expenditures declined from $221 million in 1996 to $194 million in 1999 (Office of Inspector General 2001a). Evidence since then shows continued low levels of mental health treatment in nursing homes (Reichman and Conn 2010; Shea et al. 2000).

Historically, part of the problem has been attributable to poor case identification. Borson et al. (1997) found the required preadmission assessment to be inadequate for identifying nursing home applicants who require mental health services, in part because patients with dementia are exempt from initial psychiatric evaluation, and thus, many patients with the behavioral and psychological symptoms of dementia are not identified. Although 88% of patients in this sample had been appropriately placed on the basis of their personal and nursing care needs, 55% had unmet mental health needs. As described earlier in this chapter (see "Prevalence of Psychiatric Disorders"), individuals with serious mental illness constitute an increasing proportion of admissions to nursing homes for subacute care (Fullerton et al. 2009), and despite a relatively low level of skilled nursing care needs, they are more likely to become long-stay residents (Aschbrenner et al. 2011b). Aschbrenner et al. (2011a) suggested that a substantial number of adults with serious mental illness residing in nursing homes may have the functional capacity to live in less restrictive environments.

Also, for nearly two decades there were concerns that the required periodic assessments using MDS 2.0 *after* admission did not provide adequate detection of depression (Brown et al. 2002; McCurren 2002; Office of Inspector General 2001b; Schnelle et al. 2001; Snowden 2004). McCurren (2002) found poor correlation between MDS 2.0 mood disturbance items and the Geriatric Depression Scale, a well-validated screening instrument for depression in older individuals. In examining the data from 1,492 nursing homes across five states, Brown et al. (2002) found that 11% of residents were identified on the MDS 2.0 as depressed, half the rate expected on the basis of epidemiological studies that used direct clinical assessments. Ruckdeschel et al. (2004) subsequently showed evidence supporting the use of a self-report approach to detection of depression by the MDS. This led to the eventual testing, validation, and adoption of the PHQ-9 as the standardized measure of mood that is currently embedded in MDS 3.0 (Saliba et al. 2012). This newer version of the MDS was shown to perform better than MDS 2.0 and better than the Geriatric Depression Scale for detecting clinical depression among nursing home residents. It is hoped that improved measurement of depression will lead to improved rates of treatment and remission. However, in the study by Brown et al. (2002), of the 11% of residents identified by MDS as having depression, only 55% received antidepressant therapy. Thus, expected improvements in detection of mental disorders will not, by themselves, necessarily lead to improved rates of treatment.

Limited access to care appears to be a significant part of the problem. In a survey of nursing homes across six states conducted by Reichman et al. (1998), 47.6% of 899 respondents indicated that the frequency of on-site psychiatric consultation was inadequate. The 2004 NNHS similarly reported that only 40.4% of nursing homes had mental health services available at the facility, and only 48.5% had formal contracts for psychology or psychiatry services (National Center for Health Statistics 2004). Directors of nursing judged 38% of nursing home residents as needing a psychiatric evaluation, but more than one-fourth of rural facilities and more than one-fifth of small facilities reported that no psychiatric consultant was available to them. Meeting the demand for mental health treatment may also be more difficult for nursing facilities that are part of a chain or that contain Medicaid beds (Castle and Shea 1997). Thus, evidence indicates that the federal requirement that patients receive services to "attain or maintain the highest practicable physical, mental, and psychosocial well-being" (Health Care Financing Administration 1991, p. 48910) has not remedied the problem of access to mental health services in U.S. nursing homes (Colenda et al. 1999; Grabowski et al. 2010). Despite evidence for the continuing lack of available services, the Office of the Inspector General reported in 2001 that 27% of mental health services provided in nursing homes and paid for by Medicare were "medically unnecessary" (Office of Inspector General 2001a). However, many of the services identified as resulting in "inappropriate" payments were specifically for excessive psychological testing and group psychotherapy for patients with severe cognitive impairment who were determined by reviewers to be incapable of benefiting from these specific procedures. This survey by the Office of the Inspector General did not examine the adequacy of appropriate, medically necessary psychiatric care.

Evidence shows that even among patients whose mental disorders are recognized and for whom treatment is initiated, that treatment is often inadequate. The report by Brown et al. (2002) indicated that of nursing home residents with depression who were receiving antidepressants, 32% were prescribed dosages lower than the manufacturers' recommended minimum effective dosage for treating depression. In a survey of 12 nursing homes, Datto et al. (2002) found that 47% of patients were taking antidepressants but that nearly half of these patients were still depressed. Although a small proportion of these residents may have been in the early stages of treatment, before a response could reasonably be expected, it appears likely that many of those not responsive to initial treatment did not receive proper follow-up care with required dosage adjustments or changes in therapy. This finding points to a need for improved adherence to practice guidelines for follow-up care to achieve remission of depression symptoms. A more comprehensive treatment of this subject is available in the consensus recommendations for improving the quality of mental health care in nursing homes (American Geriatrics Society and American Association for Geriatric Psychiatry 2003).

Expansion of telehealth and telepsychiatry programs shows significant promise in expanding access to mental health assessment and services for nursing home residents. On March 6, 2020, CMS granted a waiver for telehealth services provided to Medicare beneficiaries in all settings, including nursing homes (Centers for Medicare and Medicaid Services 2020). This was granted for the duration of the COVID-19 public health emergency. Although limited data are available to track the increase in services provided specifically to nursing homes, by late March 2020, all telehealth visits to Medicare beneficiaries had increased from 10,000 per week to 300,000 per week. The program is considered successful, and there is strong sentiment that the waiver should be extended indefinitely, even by CMS administration.

Mental Health Care in Nursing Homes: A Model for Service Delivery

The high prevalence of psychiatric disorders in nursing homes argues for the importance of establishing systems that incorporate mental health into the basic services provided (Borson et al. 1987). In addition, the following factors attest to the importance of the professional components of care: 1) the complex nature of the psychiatric disorders exhibited by nursing home residents, 2) the need to evaluate medical as well as social and environmental factors as causes of mental health problems, 3) the potential benefits of specific treatments, and 4) the need for careful monitoring to assess treatment responses and prevent serious adverse effects of medications. Thus, clinical needs demand that mental health services in nursing homes have two distinct but interacting systems: one that is intrinsic to the facility and contextual and another that is professional and concerned primarily with the delivery of specific treatments. To conduct valid assessments and make diagnoses, mental health professionals must rely on nursing home staff to report their shift-by-shift observations of residents' behavior and other clinical signs and to implement and monitor the treatments they prescribe. Conversely, to succeed in providing appropriate mental health care to nursing home residents, staff members in the intrinsic system must have access to ongoing consultation with anddirect support from mental health professionals knowledgeable in geriatrics.

It has been suggested that facility staff should receive mental health training in basic assessment and clinical management skills to help them handle problems that occur when specific professional services are lacking. However, the intrinsic and professional systems cannot readily replace each other, and adequate care requires both. Although staff training is needed, a realistic goal is to develop staff skills that complement rather than replace the activities of mental health professionals. This two-system model has obvious implications with respect to the financing of mental health services in nursing homes: it demonstrates the need to fund mental health care as both a necessary part of the per diem costs of nursing home care and a reimbursable professional service.

Although the intrinsic and professional systems for mental health services are distinct, they are inherently interdependent: geriatric psychiatrists and psychologists and geropsychiatric nurse practitioners also play important intrinsic roles as administrative and staff consultants, in-service educators, case conference moderators, interdisciplinary team meeting participants, and contributors in other activities familiar to consultation-liaison psychiatrists. Facility staff must be effective in recognizing problems, facilitating referral, supporting treatment, and monitoring outcome to enable the professional system to function optimally. The increased availability of telepsychiatry services offers the opportunity for virtual and remote staff training and involvement of mental health professionals at team meetings, in family conferences, and in behavioral care planning. Billing and coding for involvement in these services remain problematic, however, even with current CMS telehealth waivers. Facility infrastructure will need to be mindful of services that will likely require financial support (Centers for Medicare and Medicaid Services 2020).

Intrinsic System

The intrinsic system of mental health care in nursing homes can be conceptualized as including a wide range of components: design of the environment; implementation of psychosocial programs; formulation of institutional policies and procedures for assessment, care delivery, monitoring, and quality improvement; and optimization of the ways in which staff and residents interact. The importance of the intrinsic system is recognized in nursing home regulations that require training of nursing aides; in the nursing staff assessments required for completion of the MDS; and in OBRA-87 requirements that nursing homes provide assessments, treatment planning, and services to attain or maintain the highest practicable level of mental and physical well-being for each resident. Because psychiatric disorders are common in nursing home patients, nurses and aides should be knowledgeable about the nature of the cognitive and functional deficits associated with dementia and the manifestations of delirium and depression. Staff members should understand how to modify their approach to working with residents when cognitive impairment or communication deficits interfere with care. Staff should also know how to apply basic principles of behavioral psychology to identify the causes of agitation and related behavioral symptoms in patients with dementia, as well as how to plan environmental and behavioral interventions.

Several approaches to providing such training have been developed. Evaluation studies have demonstrated that improved mental health care through staff training is an attainable goal and have identified barriers to overcome (Smyer et al. 1992). As mental health care is incorporated into the basic fabric of the nursing home, it must include provisions for patients with variable degrees of cognitive impairment and depression in the extent of residents' autonomy, the availability of staff supervision and assistance, and the design of activities. The idea that key components of mental health services should be intrinsic to the nursing home is perhaps most evident in the design of SCUs for patients with dementia. Nonetheless, the need for these services applies to all patients, not only to those with cognitive impairment. Moreover, the potential benefits of such services are not limited to their effects on residents with diagnosed disorders; there is also the potential for prevention. For example, opportunities for pleasurable events and activities can have positive effects on mood and behavior for residents with and without a diagnosis of depression. In addition, evidence indicates that contextual interventions designed to encourage a sense of empowerment in residents can have positive effects on both mental and physical health.

Knowledge about the benefits of encouraging autonomy is derived from the classic study by Langer and Rodin (1976), who evaluated a controlled intervention designed to increase nursing home residents' sense of control over day-to-day events. Residents were randomly assigned to one of two groups: a treatment group, in which staff gave the message that residents were responsible for making decisions for themselves, or a control condition group, in which the message conveyed was that staff were responsible for residents' care. Both immediately after the intervention and at 18-month follow-up, the treatment groups exhibited benefits in mood, alertness, and active participation. The effects of control-enhancing interventions have been confirmed in several other studies (e.g., Banziger and Roush 1983; Schulz 1976; Thomasma et al. 1990) and have been discussed in terms of "learned helplessness" models (Avorn and Langer 1982). The benefits of interventions designed to enhance the predictability of the environment have also been confirmed (Krantz and Schulz 1980). In summary, these studies show that the social environment in which care is provided can have a significant effect on nursing home residents and that environmental design should be viewed as a component of mental health care.

Professional System

The intrinsic system for mental health services as just described is necessary but not sufficient to meet the needs of nursing home residents. The services of mental health professionals are also important for evaluating the interactions between medical and mental health problems, establishing psychiatric diagnoses, and planning and administering specific treatments for mental disorders. This component of the professional system must encompass medically oriented psychiatric care, including psychopharmacological treatment. A position statement by the major provider groups in this field (Board of Directors of the American Association for Geriatric Psychiatry et al. 1992) acknowledged the history of psychotropic drug misuse in nursing homes but emphasized that psychopharmacological treatment of diagnosed mental disorders is an important part of the medical and mental health care of nursing home residents. The complexity of psychopharmacological treatment in frail nursing home residents with medical comorbidities requires that psychiatrists knowledgeable in geriatrics be an integral part of the professional system.

The professional system should include care with both a psychosocial and a biomedical focus. For example, psychiatrists, psychologists, and psychiatric nurse practitioners and advanced practice nurses with specific expertise in behavioral treatment may be successful in evaluating the antecedents and causes of behavioral and psychological symptoms of dementia and in developing environmental and behavioral interventions, even when efforts by the facility's nursing staff have proven ineffective (Teri et al. 2002). As described earlier, psychotherapy may be of value for residents whose cognitive abilities allow them to participate. Further research is needed to determine how existing treatments should be modified and how they can be administered to optimize their effectiveness in the nursing home. Despite the need for more research, psychotherapy for more cognitively intact nursing home residents with depression should be considered an important treatment among the professional mental health services available to nursing home residents.

COVID-19 Impact on Nursing Homes

COVID-19 has highlighted many deficiencies in nursing homes related to reimbursement and organizational structure. Although the nursing home population accounts for ~0.5% of U.S. population, the mortality from this pandemic for nursing home residents at this time is ~25% (Chidambaram 2020; Grabowski and Mor 2020). Because of this impact on the system, regulatory agencies have established emergency response action plans that provide guidance for keeping their residents safe during the pandemic. The guidelines include considerations on resident cohorting, new admissions (or readmissions) to the facility, and requirements for reporting suspected or confirmed

COVID-19 cases among residents and staff alike. Waves of change have washed ashore upon many facilities to slow the spread of infection, one of which has been the restriction of visitors, which has left many residents without physical interaction with family and friends. The psychological impact on residents faced with social isolation has become a real concern.

As staff assess and address the physical symptoms related to COVID-19, they must be made aware of the mental health impact, remain vigilant in their mental health assessment, and address issues appropriately. However, once at-risk residents are identified, treatment implementation may be met with barriers. Access to mental health care has become an even greater concern during the pandemic. Virtual engagement, once less thought of and rarely used, is now the subject of new and revived interest. Many nursing homes are using virtual applications, such as Facetime or Zoom, to have residents speak with and see family members. In addition, mental health providers who are not able to come to facilities can now conduct telepsychiatry appointments with residents and recommend treatments for staff to implement.

Conclusion

The high prevalence of mental health problems among nursing home residents underscores the importance of psychiatric care in nursing homes. Psychiatry in U.S. nursing homes has evolved substantially over several decades, with changes driven by a combination of factors, including scientific knowledge, availability of new treatments, evolving federal regulations, measurement-based care, public dissemination of quality measures, and recognition of the need for integrated approaches to the delivery of mental health services.

Key Points

- According to the 2004 National Nursing Home Survey, 4% of Americans age 65 years and older—1.5 million people—resided in 16,100 long-term care facilities.

- Epidemiological studies have consistently shown that 80%–94% of nursing home residents have diagnosable psychiatric disorders, which suggests that nursing homes are serving as de facto neuropsychiatric institutions, although they were not originally intended for this purpose.

- Since the implementation of federal nursing home regulations in the early 1990s, the rate of antipsychotic medication use has declined and antidepressant use has increased. However, approximately half of nursing home residents who are receiving antidepressant medications continue to have symptoms of depression.

- Since 2003, analyses of safety data from randomized controlled studies of atypical antipsychotic drugs in elderly patients with dementia, including nursing home studies, have revealed significantly increased risks of cerebrovascular adverse events and mortality in this population. This led to initiatives by the

Centers for Medicare and Medicaid Services to improve the quality of dementia care in nursing homes, including the goal of reducing antipsychotic drug use.

- Although mechanical restraints have often been used in attempts to control agitation, they do not decrease behavioral disturbances, and cross-national studies have indicated that it is possible to manage nursing home residents more safely without such measures.

- The social environment within which care is provided can have a significant effect on nursing home residents; environmental design should be viewed as a component of mental health care.

Suggested Readings

American Geriatrics Society, American Association for Geriatric Psychiatry: The American Geriatrics Society and American Association for Geriatric Psychiatry recommendations for policies in support of quality mental health care in U.S. nursing homes. J Am Geriatr Soc 51(9):1299–1304, 2003

Bharucha AJ, Dew MA, Miller MD, et al: Psychotherapy in long-term care: a review. J Am Med Dir Assoc 7(9):568–580, 2006

Boyce RD, Hanlon JT, Karp JF, et al: A review of the effectiveness of antidepressant medications for depressed nursing home residents. J Am Med Dir Assoc 13(4):326–331, 2012

Centers for Medicare and Medicaid: State Operations Manual, Appendix PP: Guidance to Surveyors for Long Term Care Facilities. Rev 107, 04-04-14. Baltimore, MD, Centers for Medicare and Medicaid, 2014. Available at: https://www.cms.gov/Regulations-and-Guidance/Guidance/Manuals/downloads/som107ap_pp_guidelines_ltcf.pdf. Accessed June 12, 2014.

Karlin BE, Visnic S, Shealy McGee J, et al: Results from the multisite implementation of STAR-VA: a multicomponent psychosocial intervention for managing challenging dementia-related behaviors of veterans. Psychol Serv 11(2):200–208, 2014

Saliba D, Jones M, Streim J, et al: Overview of significant changes in the Minimum Data Set for nursing homes version 3.0. J Am Med Dir Assoc 13(7):595–601, 2012

References

Abraham IL, Neundorfer MM, Currie LJ: Effects of group interventions on cognition and depression in nursing home residents. Nurs Res 41(4):196–202, 1992 1383947

Abraham IL, Onega LL, Reel SJ, et al: Effects of cognitive group interventions on depressed frail nursing home residents, in Depression in Long Term and Residential Care: Advances in Research and Treatment. Edited by Rubinstein RL, Lawton MP. New York, Springer, 1997, pp 154–168

Adlbrecht L, Bartholomeyczik S, Hildebrandt C, et al: Social interactions of persons with dementia living in special care units in long-term care: a mixed-methods systematic review. Dementia 20(3):967–984, 2021

Ahmed A, Lefante CM, Alam N: Depression and nursing home admission among hospitalized older adults with coronary artery disease: a propensity score analysis. Am J Geriatr Cardiol 16(2):76–83, 2007 17380615

Ahmed M, Malik M, Teselink J, et al: Current agents in development for treating behavioral and psychological symptoms associated with dementia. Drugs Aging 36(7):589–605, 2019 30957198

Alessi CA, Yoon EJ, Schnelle JF, et al: A randomized trial of a combined physical activity and environmental intervention in nursing home residents: do sleep and agitation improve? J Am Geriatr Soc 47(7):784–791, 1999 10404920

Alexopoulos GS, Abrams RC, Young RC, Shamoian CA: Cornell Scale for Depression in Dementia. Biol Psychiatry 23(3):271–284, 1988 3337862

American Geriatrics Society, American Association for Geriatric Psychiatry: The American Geriatrics Society and American Association for Geriatric Psychiatry recommendations for policies in support of quality mental health care in U.S. nursing homes. J Am Geriatr Soc 51(9):1299–1304, 2003 12919244

American Psychiatric Association: Diagnostic and Statistical Manual of Mental Disorders, 3rd Edition. Washington, DC, American Psychiatric Association, 1980

American Psychiatric Association: Diagnostic and Statistical Manual of Mental Disorders, 3rd Edition, Revised. Washington, DC, American Psychiatric Association, 1987

American Society of Consultant Pharmacists: Fact Sheet. Alexandria, VA, American Society of Consultant Pharmacists, September 2000

Ames D: Depression among elderly residents of local-authority residential homes: its nature and the efficacy of intervention. Br J Psychiatry 156:667–675, 1990 2095943

Ames D: Epidemiological studies of depression among the elderly in residential and nursing homes. Int J Geriatr Psychiatry 6(6):347–354, 1991

Ames D, Ashby D, Mann AH, Graham N: Psychiatric illness in elderly residents of Part III homes in one London borough: prognosis and review. Age Ageing 17(4):249–256, 1988 3262986

Arthur A, Matthews R, Jagger C, Lindesay J: Factors associated with antidepressant treatment in residential care: changes between 1990 and 1997. Int J Geriatr Psychiatry 17(1):54–60, 2002 11802231

Aschbrenner KA, Cai S, Grabowski DC, et al: Medical comorbidity and functional status among adults with major mental illness newly admitted to nursing homes. Psychiatr Serv 62(9):1098–1100, 2011a 21885592

Aschbrenner K, Grabowski DC, Cai S, et al: Nursing home admissions and long-stay conversions among persons with and without serious mental illness. J Aging Soc Policy 23(3):286–304, 2011b 21740203

Ashby D, Ames D, West CR, et al: Psychiatric morbidity as predictor of mortality for residents of local authority homes for the elderly. Int J Geriatr Psychiatry 6(8):567–575, 1991

Avorn J, Langer E: Induced disability in nursing home patients: a controlled trial. J Am Geriatr Soc 30(6):397–400, 1982 7077022

Avorn J, Dreyer P, Connelly K, Soumerai SB: Use of psychoactive medication and the quality of care in rest homes: findings and policy implications of a statewide study. N Engl J Med 320(4):227–232, 1989 2911307

Avorn J, Soumerai SB, Everitt DE, et al: A randomized trial of a program to reduce the use of psychoactive drugs in nursing homes. N Engl J Med 327(3):168–173, 1992 1608408

Baines S, Saxby P, Ehlert K: Reality orientation and reminiscence therapy: a controlled crossover study of elderly confused people. Br J Psychiatry 151:222–231, 1987 3318991

Baker FM, Miller CL: Screening a skilled nursing home population for depression. J Geriatr Psychiatry Neurol 4(4):218–221, 1991 1789910

Ballard CG, Margallo-Lana M, Fossey J, et al: A 1-year follow-up study of behavioral and psychological symptoms in dementia among people in care environments. J Clin Psychiatry 62(8):631–636, 2001 11561936

Ballard CG, Margallo-Lana M, Juszczak E, et al: Quetiapine and rivastigmine and cognitive decline in Alzheimer's disease: randomised double blind placebo controlled trial. BMJ 330(7496):874–877, 2005 15722369

Ballard CG, Youakim JM, Coate B, Stankovic S: Pimavanserin in Alzheimer's disease psychosis: efficacy in patients with more pronounced psychotic symptoms. J Prev Alzheimers Dis 6(1):27–33, 2019 30569083

Ballard CG, Coate B, Abler V, et al: Evaluation of the efficacy of pimavanserin in the treatment of agitation and aggression in patients with Alzheimer's disease psychosis: a post hoc analysis. Int J Geriatr Psychiatry 35(11):1402–1408, 2020 32729631

Banziger G, Roush S: Nursing homes for the birds: a control-relevant intervention with bird feeders. Gerontologist 23:527–531, 1983

Barca ML, Engedal K, Laks J, Selbaek G: A 12 months follow-up study of depression among nursing-home patients in Norway. J Affect Disord 120(1–3):141–148, 2010 19467560

Barnes R, Raskind MA: DSM-III criteria and the clinical diagnosis of dementia: a nursing home study. J Gerontol 36(1):20–27, 1981 7451830

Barnes R, Veith R, Okimoto J, et al: Efficacy of antipsychotic medications in behaviorally disturbed dementia patients. Am J Psychiatry 139(9):1170–1174, 1982 7114310

Bartels SJ, Horn SD, Smout RJ, et al: Agitation and depression in frail nursing home elderly patients with dementia: treatment characteristics and service use. Am J Geriatr Psychiatry 11(2):231–238, 2003 12611753

Barton R, Hurst L: Unnecessary use of tranquilizers in elderly patients. Br J Psychiatry 112(491):989–990, 1966 5339369

Beber CR: Management of behavior in the institutionalized aged. Dis Nerv Syst 26(9):591–595, 1965 5319033

Bech P, Bolwig TG, Kramp P, Rafaelsen OJ: The Bech-Rafaelsen Mania Scale and the Hamilton Depression Scale. Acta Psychiatr Scand 59(4):420–430, 1979 433633

Beck AT, Ward CH, Mendelson M, et al: An inventory for measuring depression. Arch Gen Psychiatry 4:561–571, 1961 13688369

Beck CK, Vogelpohl TS, Rasin JH, et al: Effects of behavioral interventions on disruptive behavior and affect in demented nursing home residents. Nurs Res 51(4):219–228, 2002 12131234

Beers M, Avorn J, Soumerai SB, et al: Psychoactive medication use in intermediate-care facility residents. JAMA 260(20):3016–3020, 1988 2903260

Bellenger EN, Ibrahim JE, Lovell JJ, Bugeja L: The nature and extent of physical restraint-related deaths in nursing homes: a systematic review. J Aging Health 30(7):1042–1061, 2018 28553823

Bensink GW, Godbey KL, Marshall MJ, Yarandi HN: Institutionalized elderly: relaxation, locus of control, self-esteem. J Gerontol Nurs 18(4):30–38, 1992 1569298

Berg A, Sadowski K, Beyrodt M, et al: Snoezelen, structured reminiscence therapy and 10-minutes activation in long term care residents with dementia (WISDE): study protocol of a cluster randomized controlled trial. BMC Geriatr 10:5, 2010 20113526

Berrios GE, Brook P: Delusions and the psychopathology of the elderly with dementia. Acta Psychiatr Scand 72(3):296–301, 1985 4072730

Bharani N, Snowden M: Evidence-based interventions for nursing home residents with dementia-related behavioral symptoms. Psychiatr Clin North Am 28(4):985–1005, 2005

Bharucha AJ, Dew MA, Miller MD, et al: Psychotherapy in long-term care: a review. J Am Med Dir Assoc 7(9):568–580, 2006 17095422

Blazer D: Antipsychotics and dementia: where do we go from here? J Am Med Dir Assoc 14(4):307–308, 2013 23415842

Blazer D, Williams CD: Epidemiology of dysphoria and depression in an elderly population. Am J Psychiatry 137(4):439–444, 1980 7361929

Board of Directors of the American Association for Geriatric Psychiatry, Clinical Practice Committee of the American Geriatrics Society, Committee on Long-Term Care and Treatment for the Elderly, American Psychiatric Association: Psychotherapeutic medications in the nursing home. J Am Geriatr Soc 40:946–949, 1992 1512392

Borson S, Liptzin B, Nininger J, Rabins P: Psychiatry and the nursing home. Am J Psychiatry 144(11):1412–1418, 1987 3314537

Borson S, Loebel JP, Kitchell M, et al: Psychiatric assessments of nursing home residents under OBRA-87: should PASARR be reformed? Pre-Admission Screening and Annual Review. J Am Geriatr Soc 45(10):1173–1181, 1997 9329477

Bowblis JR, Ng W, Akosionu O, Shippee TP: Decomposing racial and ethnic disparities in nursing home quality of life. J Appl Gerontol 40(9):1051–1061, 2021 32772869

Boyce RD, Hanlon JT, Karp JF, et al: A review of the effectiveness of antidepressant medications for depressed nursing home residents. J Am Med Dir Assoc 13(4):326–331, 2012 22019084

Bridges-Parlet S, Knopman D, Steffes S: Withdrawal of neuroleptic medications from institutionalized dementia patients: results of a double-blind, baseline-treatment-controlled pilot study. J Geriatr Psychiatry Neurol 10(3):119–126, 1997 9322135

Briesacher BA, Limcangco MR, Simoni-Wastila L, et al: The quality of antipsychotic drug prescribing in nursing homes. Arch Intern Med 165(11):1280–1285, 2005 15956008

Brodaty H, Ames D, Snowdon J, et al: A randomized placebo-controlled trial of risperidone for the treatment of aggression, agitation, and psychosis of dementia. J Clin Psychiatry 64(2):134–143, 2003 12633121

Brown MN, Lapane KL, Luisi AF: The management of depression in older nursing home residents. J Am Geriatr Soc 50(1):69–76, 2002 12028249

Buck JA: Psychotropic drug practice in nursing homes. J Am Geriatr Soc 36(5):409–418, 1988 3283198

Buijck BI, Zuidema SU, Spruit-van Eijk M, et al: Neuropsychiatric symptoms in geriatric patients admitted to skilled nursing facilities in nursing homes for rehabilitation after stroke: a longitudinal multicenter study. Int J Geriatr Psychiatry 27(7):734–741, 2012 21932248

Burns BJ, Taube CA: Mental health services in general medical care and in nursing homes, in Mental Health Policy for Older Americans: Protecting Minds at Risk. Edited by Fogel BS, Furino A, Gottlieb GL. Washington, DC, American Psychiatric Press, 1990, pp 63–84

Burns BJ, Larson DB, Goldstrom ID, et al: Mental disorder among nursing home patients: preliminary findings from the National Nursing Home Survey Pretest. Int J Geriatr Psychiatry 3(1):27–35, 1988

Burrows AB, Salzman C, Satlin A, et al: A randomized, placebo-controlled trial of paroxetine in nursing home residents with non-major depression. Depress Anxiety 15(3):102–110, 2002 12001178

Buttar AB, Mhyre J, Fries BE, Blaum CS: Six-month cognitive improvement in nursing home residents with severe cognitive impairment. J Geriatr Psychiatry Neurol 16(2):100–108, 2003 12801160

Cai S, Yan D, Intrator O: COVID-19 cases and death in nursing homes: the role of racial and ethnic composition of facilities and their communities. J Am Med Dir Assoc 22(7):1345–1351, 2021 34062147

Cape RD: Freedom from restraint. Gerontologist 23:217, 1983

Capezuti E, Evans L, Strumpf N, Maislin G: Physical restraint use and falls in nursing home residents. J Am Geriatr Soc 44(6):627–633, 1996 8642150

Castle NG, Shea D: Institutional factors of nursing homes that predict the provision of mental health services. J Ment Health Adm 24(1):44–54, 1997 9033155

Castle NG, Fogel B, Mor V: Risk factors for physical restraint use in nursing homes: pre- and post-implementation of the Nursing Home Reform Act. Gerontologist 37(6):737–747, 1997 9432990

Center for Health Systems Research and Analysis: Facility Guide for the Nursing Home Quality Indicators. Madison, WI, University of Wisconsin-Madison, 1999

Centers for Medicare and Medicaid Services: Minimum Data Set, Version 3.0. Baltimore, MD, Centers for Medicare and Medicaid Services, 2006. Available at: http://www.cms.gov/Medicare/Quality-Initiatives-Patient-Assessment-Instruments/NursingHomeQualityInits/downloads/MDS30Draft.pdf. Accessed June 12, 2014.

Centers for Medicare and Medicaid Services: Minimum Data Set 3.0 Resident Assessment Instrument Manual. Baltimore, MD, Centers for Medicare and Medicaid Services, 2013. Available at: http://www.cms.gov/Medicare/Quality-Initiatives-Patient-Assessment-Instruments/NursingHomeQualityInits/MDS30RAIManual.html. Accessed June 12, 2014.

Centers for Medicare and Medicaid Services: Appendix PP: guidance to surveyors for long term care facilities, in State Operations Manual, Rev 107, 04-04-14. Baltimore, MD, Centers for Medicare and Medicaid Services, 2014. Available at: https://www.cms.gov/Regulations-and-Guidance/Guidance/Manuals/downloads/som107ap_pp_guidelines_ltcf.pdf. Accessed June, 12, 2014.

Centers for Medicare and Medicaid Services: Nursing Home Data Compendium 2015 Edition. Independence, MO, Centers for Medicare and Medicaid Services, 2016. Available at: http://cms.gov/Medicare/Provider-Enrollment-and-Certification/ CertificationandComplianc/Downloads/nursinghomedatacompendium_508-2015.pdf. Accessed November 10, 2021.

Centers for Medicare and Medicaid Services: Medicare Telemedicine Health Care Provider Fact Sheet. Baltimore, MD, Centers for Medicare and Medicaid Services, March 17, 2020. Available at https://www.cms.gov/Medicare/Telemedicine. Accessed July 26, 2020.

Centers for Medicare and Medicaid Services HHS: Medicare and Medicaid Programs; reform of requirements for long-term care facilities. Final rule. Fed Regist 81(192):68688–68872, 2016 27731960

Chahine LM, Bijlsma A, Hospers AP, Chemali Z: Dementia and depression among nursing home residents in Lebanon: a pilot study. Int J Geriatr Psychiatry 22(4):283–285, 2007 16977675

Chandler JD, Chandler JE: The prevalence of neuropsychiatric disorders in a nursing home population. J Geriatr Psychiatry Neurol 1(2):71–76, 1988 3266998

Chao SY, Liu HY, Wu CY, et al: The effects of group reminiscence therapy on depression, self esteem, and life satisfaction of elderly nursing home residents. J Nurs Res 14(1):36–45, 2006 16547904

Chidambaram P: State reporting of cases and deaths due to COVID-19 in long-term care facilities. Kaiser Family Foundation Issue Brief, April 23, 2020. https://www.kff.org/medicaid/issue-brief/state-reporting-of-cases-and-deaths-due-to-covid-19-in-long-term-care-facilities. Accessed April 26, 2020.

Chiu Y, Bero L, Hessol NA, et al: A literature review of clinical outcomes associated with antipsychotic medication use in North American nursing home residents. Health Policy 119(6):802–813, 2015 25791166

Cody M, Beck C, Svarstad BL: Challenges to the use of nonpharmacologic interventions in nursing homes. Psychiatr Serv 53(11):1402–1406, 2002 12407267

Cohen-Mansfield J: Agitated behaviors in the elderly, II: preliminary results in the cognitively deteriorated. J Am Geriatr Soc 34(10):722–727, 1986 3760436

Cohen-Mansfield J: Nonpharmacologic interventions for inappropriate behaviors in dementia: a review, summary, and critique. Am J Geriatr Psychiatry 9(4):361–381, 2001 11739063

Cohen-Mansfield J, Billig N: Agitated behaviors in the elderly, I: a conceptual review. J Am Geriatr Soc 34(10):711–721, 1986 3531296

Cohen-Mansfield J, Libin A: Verbal and physical non-aggressive agitated behaviors in elderly persons with dementia: robustness of syndromes. J Psychiatr Res 39(3):325–332, 2005 15725431

Cohen-Mansfield J, Marx MS, Rosenthal AS: A description of agitation in a nursing home. J Gerontol 44(3):M77–M84, 1989 2715584

Cohen-Mansfield J, Lipson S, Werner P, et al: Withdrawal of haloperidol, thioridazine, and lorazepam in the nursing home: a controlled, double-blind study. Arch Intern Med 159(15):1733–1740, 1999 10448776

Cohen-Mansfield J, Thein K, Marx MS, et al: Efficacy of nonpharmacologic interventions for agitation in advanced dementia: a randomized, placebo-controlled trial. J Clin Psychiatry 73(9):1255–1261, 2012 23059151

Colenda CC, Streim J, Greene JA, et al: The impact of OBRA '87 on psychiatric services in nursing homes: joint testimony of the American Psychiatric Association and the American Association for Geriatric Psychiatry. Am J Geriatr Psychiatry 7(1):12–17, 1999 9919316

Crystal S, Jarrín OF, Rosenthal M, et al: National Partnership to Improve Dementia Care in Nursing Homes Campaign: state and facility strategies, impact, and antipsychotic reduction outcomes. Innov Aging 4(3):igaa018, 2020 32699827

Custer RL, Davis JE, Gee SC: Psychiatric drug usage in VA nursing home care units. Psychiatr Ann 14(4):285–292, 1984

Datto CJ, Oslin DW, Streim JE, et al: Pharmacologic treatment of depression in nursing home residents: a mental health services perspective. J Geriatr Psychiatry Neurol 15(3):141–146, 2002 12230084

De Deyn PP, Rabheru K, Rasmussen A, et al: A randomized trial of risperidone, placebo, and haloperidol for behavioral symptoms of dementia. Neurology 53(5):946–955, 1999 10496251

De Deyn PP, Katz IR, Brodaty H, et al: Management of agitation, aggression, and psychosis associated with dementia: a pooled analysis including three randomized, placebo-controlled double-blind trials in nursing home residents treated with risperidone. Clin Neurol Neurosurg 107(6):497–508, 2005 15922506

Dehlin O, Hedenrud B, Jansson P, Nörgård J: A double-blind comparison of alaproclate and placebo in the treatment of patients with senile dementia. Acta Psychiatr Scand 71(2):190–196, 1985 3883697

DeLeo D, Stella AG, Spagnoli A: Prescription of psychotropic drugs in geriatric institutions. Int J Geriatr Psychiatry 4:11–16, 1989

Deudon A, Maubourguet N, Gervais X, et al: Non-pharmacological management of behavioural symptoms in nursing homes. Int J Geriatr Psychiatry 24(12):1386–1395, 2009 19370714

Dey AN: Characteristics of elderly nursing home residents: data from the 1995 National Nursing Home Survey. Adv Data (289):1–8, 1997 10182808

Dorsey ER, Rabbani A, Gallagher SA, et al: Impact of FDA black box advisory on antipsychotic medication use. Arch Intern Med 170(1):96–103, 2010 20065205

Dwyer M, Byrne GJ: Disruptive vocalization and depression in older nursing home residents. Int Psychogeriatr 12(4):463–471, 2000 11263713

Elon R, Pawlson LG: The impact of OBRA on medical practice within nursing facilities. J Am Geriatr Soc 40(9):958–963, 1992 1512394

Engle VF, Graney MJ: Stability and improvement of health after nursing home admission. J Gerontol 48(1):S17–S23, 1993 8418151

Evans LK, Strumpf NE: Tying down the elderly: a review of the literature on physical restraint. J Am Geriatr Soc 37(1):65–74, 198, 1989

Evans LK, Strumpf NE, Allen-Taylor SL, et al: A clinical trial to reduce restraints in nursing homes. J Am Geriatr Soc 45(6):675–681, 1997 9180659

Fashaw SA, Thomas KS, McCreedy E, Mor V: Thirty-year trends in nursing home composition and quality since the passage of the Omnibus Reconciliation Act. J Am Med Dir Assoc 21(2):233–239, 2020 31451383

Fashaw-Walters SA, McCreedy E, Bynum JPW, et al: Disproportionate increases in schizophrenia diagnoses among Black nursing home residents with ADRD. J Am Geriatr Soc 2021 34590709 Epub ahead of print

Fenton J, Raskin A, Gruber-Baldini AL, et al: Some predictors of psychiatric consultation in nursing home residents. Am J Geriatr Psychiatry 12(3):297–304, 2004 15126231

Finkel SI, Lyons JS, Anderson RL: A brief agitation rating scale (BARS) for nursing home elderly. J Am Geriatr Soc 41(1):50–52, 1993 8418123

Finkel SI, Lyons JS, Anderson RL, et al: A randomized, placebo-controlled trial of thiothixene in agitated, demented nursing home patients. Int J Geriatr Psychiatry 10:129–136, 1995

Foebel AD, Onder G, Finne-Soveri H, et al: Physical restraint and antipsychotic medication use among nursing home residents with dementia. J Am Med Dir Assoc 17(2):184.e9–184.e14, 2016 26778491

Folstein MF, Folstein SE, McHugh PR: "Mini-mental state": a practical method for grading the cognitive state of patients for the clinician. J Psychiatr Res 12(3):189–198, 1975 1202204

Fossey J, Ballard C, Juszczak E, et al: Effect of enhanced psychosocial care on antipsychotic use in nursing home residents with severe dementia: cluster randomised trial. BMJ 332(7544):756–761, 2006 16543297

Fullarton J, Volicer L: Reductions of antipsychotic and hypnotic medications in Namaste Care. J Am Med Dir Assoc 14(9):708–709, 2013 23890761

Fullerton CA, McGuire TG, Feng Z, et al: Trends in mental health admissions to nursing homes, 1999–2005. Psychiatr Serv 60(7):965–971, 2009 19564228

Galasko D, Bennett D, Sano M, et al: An inventory to assess activities of daily living for clinical trials in Alzheimer's disease: the Alzheimer's Disease Cooperative Study. Alzheimer Dis Assoc Disord 11(suppl 2):S33–S39, 1997 9236950

German PS, Shapiro S, Kramer M: Nursing home study of eastern Baltimore Epidemiologic Catchment Area, in Mental Illness in Nursing Homes: Agenda for Research. Edited by Harper MS, Lebowitz BD. Rockville, MD, National Institute of Mental Health, 1986, pp 21–40

Gill SS, Bronskill SE, Normand SL, et al: Antipsychotic drug use and mortality in older adults with dementia. Ann Intern Med 146(11):775–786, 2007 17548409

Goldwasser AN, Auerbach SM, Harkins SW: Cognitive, affective, and behavioral effects of reminiscence group therapy on demented elderly. Int J Aging Hum Dev 25(3):209–222, 1987 3429043

Gottfries CG, Bråne G, Gullberg B, Steen G: A new rating scale for dementia syndromes. Arch Gerontol Geriatr 1(4):311–330, 1982 7186327

Grabowski DC, Mor V: Nursing home care in crisis in the wake of COVID-19. JAMA 324(1):23–24, 2020 32442303

Grabowski DC, Aschbrenner KA, Feng Z, Mor V: Mental illness in nursing homes: variations across states. Health Aff 28(3):689–700, 2009 19414877

Grabowski DC, Aschbrenner KA, Rome VF, Bartels SJ: Quality of mental health care for nursing home residents: a literature review. Med Care Res Rev 67(6):627–656, 2010 20223943

Graessel E, Stemmer R, Eichenseer B, et al: Non-pharmacological, multicomponent group therapy in patients with degenerative dementia: a 12-month randomized, controlled trial. BMC Med 9:129, 2011 22133165

Grant LA, Kane RA, Stark AJ: Beyond labels: nursing home care for Alzheimer's disease in and out of special care units. J Am Geriatr Soc 43(5):569–576, 1995 7730542

Guy W (ed): ECDEU Assessment Manual for Psychopharmacology, Revised (DHEW Publ No ADM-76-388). Rockville, MD, U.S. Department of Health, Education and Welfare, 1976

Hamilton M: The assessment of anxiety states by rating. Br J Med Psychol 32(1):50–55, 1959 13638508

Hamilton M: A rating scale for depression. J Neurol Neurosurg Psychiatry 23:56–62, 1960 14399272

Hanlon JT, Handler SM, Castle NG: Antidepressant prescribing in US nursing homes between 1996 and 2006 and its relationship to staffing patterns and use of other psychotropic medications. J Am Med Dir Assoc 11(5):320–324, 2010 20511098

Hansen SS, Patterson MA, Wilson RW: Family involvement on a dementia unit: the Resident Enrichment and Activity Program. Gerontologist 28(4):508–510, 1988 3224863

Harris Y: Depression as a risk factor for nursing home admission among older individuals. J Am Med Dir Assoc 8(1):14–20, 2007 17210498

Harris Y, Cooper JK: Depressive symptoms in older people predict nursing home admission. J Am Geriatr Soc 54(4):593–597, 2006 16686868

Harris-Kojetin L, Sengupta M, Park-Lee E, et al: Long-term care providers and services users in the United States: data from the National Study of Long-Term Care Providers, 2013–2014. Vital Health Stat 3 (38):x–xii, 1–105, 2016 27023287

Harrison R, Savla N, Kafetz K: Dementia, depression and physical disability in a London borough: a survey of elderly people in and out of residential care and implications for future developments. Age Ageing 19(2):97–103, 1990 2140005

Haslam C, Haslam SA, Jetten J, et al: The social treatment: the benefits of group interventions in residential care settings. Psychol Aging 25(1):157–167, 2010 20230136

Hawes C, Mor V, Phillips CD, et al: The OBRA-87 nursing home regulations and implementation of the Resident Assessment Instrument: effects on process quality. J Am Geriatr Soc 45(8):977–985, 1997 9256852

Health Care Financing Administration: Medicare and Medicaid: requirements for long-term care facilities—HCFA. Final rule. Fed Regist 56:48865–48921, 1991

Health Care Financing Administration: Medicare and Medicaid programs; preadmission screening and annual resident review—HCFA. Final rule with comment period. Fed Regist 57(230):56450–56514, 1992a 10122884

Health Care Financing Administration: Medicare and Medicaid: resident assessment in long-term care facilities—HCFA. Final rule. Fed Regist 57:61614–61733, 1992b

Health Care Financing Administration: State Operations Manual: Provider Certification (Transmittal No 250). Washington, DC, Health Care Financing Administration, 1992c

Health Care Financing Administration: Report to Congress: Study of Private Accreditation (Deeming) of Nursing Homes, Regulatory Incentives and Non-Regulatory Incentives, and Effectiveness of the Survey and Certification System. Washington, DC, Health Care Financing Administration, 1998

Heeren O, Borin L, Raskin A, et al: Association of depression with agitation in elderly nursing home residents. J Geriatr Psychiatry Neurol 16(1):4–7, 2003 12641365

Heston LL, Garrard J, Makris L, et al: Inadequate treatment of depressed nursing home elderly. J Am Geriatr Soc 40(11):1117–1122, 1992 1401696

Hoegh M, Ibrahim AK, Chibnall J, et al: Prevalence of Parkinson disease and Parkinson disease dementia in community nursing homes. Am J Geriatr Psychiatry 21(6):529–535, 2013 23567411

Holmes D, Teresi J, Weiner A, et al: Impacts associated with special care units in long-term care facilities. Gerontologist 30(2):178–183, 1990 2189792

Honigfeld G, Gillis RD, Klett CJ: NOSIE-30: a treatment-sensitive ward behavior scale. Psychol Rep 19(1):180–182, 1966 5942082

Horiguchi J, Inami Y: A survey of the living conditions and psychological states of elderly people admitted to nursing homes in Japan. Acta Psychiatr Scand 83(5):338–341, 1991 1853725

Hughes CM, Lapane KL, Mor V: Influence of facility characteristics on use of antipsychotic medications in nursing homes. Med Care 38(12):1164–1173, 2000 11186295

Hyer L, Blazer DG: Depressive symptoms: impact and problems in long term care facilities. International Journal of Behavioral Gerontology 1:33–44, 1982

Innes EM, Turman WG: Evaluation of patient falls. QRB Qual Rev Bull 9(2):30–35, 1983 6403903

Institute of Medicine Committee on Nursing Home Regulation: Improving the Quality of Care in Nursing Homes. Washington, DC, National Academy Press, 1986

Johari K, Kellogg C, Vazquez K, et al: Ratings game: an analysis of Nursing Home Compare and Yelp ratings. BMJ Qual Saf 27(8):619–624, 2018 29133461

Jones AL, Dwyer LL, Bercovitz AR, Strahan GW: The National Nursing Home Survey: 2004 overview. Vital Health Stat 13(167):1–155, 2009 19655659

Jongenelis K, Pot AM, Eisses AM, et al: Prevalence and risk indicators of depression in elderly nursing home patients: the AGED study. J Affect Disord 83(2–3):135–142, 2004 15555706

Joyce NR, McGuire TG, Bartels SJ, et al: The impact of dementia special care units on quality of care: an instrumental variables analysis. Health Serv Res 53(5):3657–3679, 2018 29736944

Kales HC, Gitlin LN, Lyketsos CG: Management of neuropsychiatric symptoms of dementia in clinic settings: recommendations from a multidisciplinary expert panel. J Am Geriatr Soc 62(4):762–769, 2014 24635665

Kales HC, Gitlin LN, Lyketsos CG: Assessment and management of behavioral and psychological symptoms of dementia. BMJ 350:h369, 2015 25731881

Karkare SU, Bhattacharjee S, Kamble P, Aparasu R: Prevalence and predictors of antidepressant prescribing in nursing home residents in the United States. Am J Geriatr Pharmacother 9(2):109–119, 2011 21565710

Karlin BE, Visnic S, McGee JS, Teri L: Results from the multisite implementation of STAR-VA: a multicomponent psychosocial intervention for managing challenging dementia-related behaviors of veterans. Psychol Serv 11(2):200–208, 2014 23937081

Katz IR, Lesher E, Kleban M, et al: Clinical features of depression in the nursing home. Int Psychogeriatr 1(1):5–15, 1989 2518789

Katz IR, Simpson GM, Curlik SM, et al: Pharmacologic treatment of major depression for elderly patients in residential care settings. J Clin Psychiatry 51(suppl):41–47, discussion 48, 1990 2195013

Katz IR, Parmelee P, Brubaker K: Toxic and metabolic encephalopathies in long-term care patients. Int Psychogeriatr 3(2):337–347, 1991 1811786

Katz IR, Beaston-Wimmer P, Parmelee P, et al: Failure to thrive in the elderly: exploration of the concept and delineation of psychiatric components. J Geriatr Psychiatry Neurol 6(3):161–169, 1993 8397760

Katz IR, Jeste DV, Mintzer JE, et al: Comparison of risperidone and placebo for psychosis and behavioral disturbances associated with dementia: a randomized, double-blind trial. J Clin Psychiatry 60(2):107–115, 1999 10084637

Kaup BA, Loreck D, Gruber-Baldini AL, et al: Depression and its relationship to function and medical status, by dementia status, in nursing home admissions. Am J Geriatr Psychiatry 15(5):438–442, 2007 17463194

Kay SR, Fiszbein A, Opler LA: The Positive and Negative Syndrome Scale (PANSS) for schizophrenia. Schizophr Bull 13(2):261–276, 1987 3616518

Kiely DK, Jones RN, Bergmann MA, et al: Association between delirium resolution and functional recovery among newly admitted postacute facility patients. J Gerontol A Biol Sci Med Sci 61(2):204–208, 2006 16510867

Kolanowski AM, Litaker M, Buettner L: Efficacy of theory-based activities for behavioral symptoms of dementia. Nurs Res 54(4):219–228, 2005 16027564

Kramer M, German PS, Anthony JC, et al: Patterns of mental disorders among the elderly residents of eastern Baltimore. J Am Geriatr Soc 33(4):236–245, 1985 3989184

Krantz DS, Schulz PR: Personal control and health: some applications to crises of middle and old age. Advances in Environmental Psychology 2:23–57, 1980

Krauss NA, Altman BM: Characteristics of Nursing Home Residents, 1996. MEPS Research Findings No 5 (AHCPR Publ No 99–0006). Rockville, MD, Agency for Health Care Policy and Research, 1998

Kutner N, Mistretta E, Barnhart H, et al: Family members' perceptions of quality of life change in dementia SCU residents. J Appl Gerontol 18:423–439, 1999

Lai CK, Yeung JH, Mok V, Chi I: Special care units for dementia individuals with behavioural problems. Cochrane Database Syst Rev (4):CD006470, 2009 19821370

Langer EJ, Rodin J: The effects of choice and enhanced personal responsibility for the aged: a field experiment in an institutional setting. J Pers Soc Psychol 34(2):191–198, 1976 1011073

Lantz MS, Giambanco V, Buchalter EN: A ten-year review of the effect of OBRA-87 on psychotropic prescribing practices in an academic nursing home. Psychiatr Serv 47(9):951–955, 1996 8875659

Lawrence V, Fossey J, Ballard C, et al: Improving quality of life for people with dementia in care homes: making psychosocial interventions work. Br J Psychiatry 201(5):344–351, 2012 23118034

Lawton MP, Brody EM: Assessment of older people: self-maintaining and instrumental activities of daily living. Gerontologist 9(3):179–186, 1969 5349366

Lawton MP, Van Haitsma K, Klapper J, et al: A stimulation-retreat special care unit for elders with dementing illness. Int Psychogeriatr 10(4):379–395, 1998 9924833

Lenze EJ, Host HH, Hildebrand MW, et al: Enhanced medical rehabilitation increases therapy intensity and engagement and improves functional outcomes in postacute rehabilitation of older adults: a randomized-controlled trial. J Am Med Dir Assoc 13(8):708–712, 2012 22863663

Lesher E: Validation of the Geriatric Depression Scale among nursing home residents. Clin Gerontol 4:21–28, 1986

Lester P, Kohen I, Stefanacci RG, Feuerman M: Antipsychotic drug use since the FDA black box warning: survey of nursing home policies. J Am Med Dir Assoc 12(8):573–577, 2011 21450177

Leszcz M, Feigenbaum E, Sadavoy J, Robinson A: A men's group: psychotherapy of elderly men. Int J Group Psychother 35(2):177–196, 1985 4008130

Levin CA, Wei W, Akincigil A, et al: Prevalence and treatment of diagnosed depression among elderly nursing home residents in Ohio. J Am Med Dir Assoc 8(9):585–594, 2007 17998115

Li Y, Harrington C, Temkin-Greener H, et al: Deficiencies in care at nursing homes and racial/ethnic disparities across homes fell, 2006–11. Health Aff (Millwood) 34(7):1139–1146, 2015 26153308

Li Y, Cai X, Harrington C, et al: Racial and ethnic differences in the prevalence of depressive symptoms among U.S. nursing home residents. J Aging Soc Policy 31(1):30–48, 2019 29883281

Lin MK, Kramer AM: The Quality Indicator Survey: background, implementation, and wide-spread change. J Aging Soc Policy 25(1):10–29, 2013 23256556

Linkins KW, Lucca AM, Housman M, Smith SA: Use of PASRR programs to assess serious mental illness and service access in nursing homes. Psychiatr Serv 57(3):325–332, 2006 16524989

Livingston G, Johnston K, Katona C, et al: Systematic review of psychological approaches to the management of neuropsychiatric symptoms of dementia. Am J Psychiatry 162(11):1996–2021, 2005 16263837

Llorente MD, Olsen EJ, Leyva O, et al: Use of antipsychotic drugs in nursing homes: current compliance with OBRA regulations. J Am Geriatr Soc 46(2):198–201, 1998 9475449

Loebel JP, Borson S, Hyde T, et al: Relationships between requests for psychiatric consultations and psychiatric diagnoses in long-term-care facilities. Am J Psychiatry 148(7):898–903, 1991 2053630

Lopez OL, Becker JT, Wahed AS, et al: Long-term effects of the concomitant use of memantine with cholinesterase inhibition in Alzheimer disease. J Neurol Neurosurg Psychiatry 80(6):600–607, 2009 19204022

Low LF, Brodaty H, Goodenough B, et al: The Sydney Multisite Intervention of LaughterBosses and ElderClowns (SMILE) study: cluster randomised trial of humour therapy in nursing homes. BMJ Open 3(1):e002072, 2013 23315520

Luo H, Zhang X, Cook B, et al: Racial/Ethnic disparities in preventive care practice among U.S. nursing home residents. J Aging Health 26(4):519–539, 2014 24626378

Lyketsos CG, Lindell Veiel L, Baker A, Steele C: A randomized, controlled trial of bright light therapy for agitated behaviors in dementia patients residing in long-term care. Int J Geriatr Psychiatry 14(7):520–525, 1999 10440971

Mack JL, Patterson MB, Tariot PN: Behavior Rating Scale for Dementia: development of test scales and presentation of data for 555 individuals with Alzheimer's disease. J Geriatr Psychiatry Neurol 12(4):211–223, 1999 10616870

Magai C, Kennedy G, Cohen CI, Gomberg D: A controlled clinical trial of sertraline in the treatment of depression in nursing home patients with late-stage Alzheimer's disease. Am J Geriatr Psychiatry 8(1):66–74, 2000 10648297

Malmstrom TK, Miller DK, Morley JE: A comparison of four frailty models. J Am Geriatr Soc 62(4):721–726, 2014 24635726

Mann AH, Graham N, Ashby D: Psychiatric illness in residential homes for the elderly: a survey in one London borough. Age Ageing 13(5):257–265, 1984 6496236

Maust DT, Kim HM, Chiang C, Kales HC: Association of the Centers for Medicare & Medicaid Services' national partnership to improve dementia care with the use of antipsychotics and other psychotropics in long-term care in the United States from 2009 to 2014. JAMA Intern Med 178(5):640–647, 2018 29550856

McCarthy JF, Blow FC, Kales HC: Disruptive behaviors in Veterans Affairs nursing home residents: how different are residents with serious mental illness? J Am Geriatr Soc 52(12):2031–2038, 2004 15571538

McCurren C: Assessment for depression among nursing home elders: evaluation of the MDS mood assessment. Geriatr Nurs 23(2):103–108, 2002 11956523

McCusker J, Cole MG, Voyer P, et al: Observer-rated depression in long-term care: frequency and risk factors. Arch Gerontol Geriatr 58(3):332–338, 2014 24345307

McMurdo MET, Rennie L: A controlled trial of exercise by residents of old people's homes. Age Ageing 22(1):11–15, 1993 8438659

Meador KG, Taylor JA, Thapa PB, et al: Predictors of antipsychotic withdrawal or dose reduction in a randomized controlled trial of provider education. J Am Geriatr Soc 45(2):207–210, 1997 9033521

Medicare.gov: Find and Compare Nursing Homes, Hospitals and Other Providers Near You. Baltimore, MD, Centers for Medicare and Medicaid Services, 2014a. Available at: http://www.medicare.gov/nursinghomecompare/search.html?AspxAutoDetectCookie-Support=1. Accessed January 5, 2015.

Medicare.gov: Quality Improvement Organizations. Baltimore, MD, Centers for Medicare and Medicaid Services, 2014b. Available at: https://www.cms.gov/Medicare/Quality-Initiatives-Patient-Assessment-Instruments/QualityImprovementOrgs/index.html?redirect=/qualityimprovementorgs. Accessed June 11, 2014.

Meehan KM, Wang H, David SR, et al: Comparison of rapidly acting intramuscular olanzapine, lorazepam, and placebo: a double-blind, randomized study in acutely agitated patients with dementia. Neuropsychopharmacology 26(4):494–504, 2002 11927174

Mintzer J, Greenspan A, Caers I, et al: Risperidone in the treatment of psychosis of Alzheimer disease: results from a prospective clinical trial. Am J Geriatr Psychiatry 14(3):280–291, 2006 16505133

Mintzer JE, Tune LE, Breder CD, et al: Aripiprazole for the treatment of psychoses in institutionalized patients with Alzheimer dementia: a multicenter, randomized, double-blind, placebo-controlled assessment of three fixed doses. Am J Geriatr Psychiatry 15(11):918–931, 2007 17974864

Montgomery SA, Åsberg M: A new depression scale designed to be sensitive to change. Br J Psychiatry 134:382–389, 1979 444788

Moran JA, Gatz M: Group therapies for nursing home adults: an evaluation of two treatment approaches. Gerontologist 27(5):588–591, 1987 3678897

Morris JN, Hawes C, Fries BE, et al: Designing the national resident assessment instrument for nursing homes. Gerontologist 30(3):293–307, 1990 2354790

Murphy E: The use of psychotropic drugs in long-term care (editorial). Int J Geriatr Psychiatry 4:1–2, 1989

National Center for Health Statistics: The National Nursing Home Survey (DHEW Publ No PHS-79-1794). Hyattsville, MD, National Center for Health Statistics, 1979

National Center for Health Statistics: The National Nursing Home Survey. Hyattsville, MD, National Center for Health Statistics, 2004. Available at: https://www.cdc.gov/nchs/nnhs/about_nnhs.htm. Accessed June 11, 2014.

Nobili A, Piana I, Balossi L, et al: Alzheimer special care units compared with traditional nursing home for dementia care: are there differences at admission and in clinical outcomes? Alzheimer Dis Assoc Disord 22(4):352–361, 2008 18978601

Nyth AL, Gottfries CG: The clinical efficacy of citalopram in treatment of emotional disturbances in dementia disorders: a Nordic multicentre study. Br J Psychiatry 157:894–901, 1990 1705151

Office of Inspector General: Medicare Payments for Psychiatric Services in Nursing Homes: A Follow-Up (Publ No OEI-02-99-00140). Washington, DC, U.S. Department of Health and Human Services. 2001a. Available at: https://oig.hhs.gov/oei/reports/oei-02-99-00140.pdf. Accessed June 11, 2014.

Office of Inspector General: Nursing Home Resident Assessment: Quality of Care (Publ No OEI-02-99-00040). Washington, DC, U.S. Department of Health and Human Services, 2001b. Available at: https://oig.hhs.gov/oei/reports/oei-02-99-00040.pdf. Accessed June 11, 2014.

Office of Inspector General: Psychotropic Drug Use in Nursing Homes (Publ No OEI-02-00-00490). Washington, DC, U.S. Department of Health and Human Services, 2001c. Available at: https://oig.hhs.gov/oei/reports/oei-02-00-00490.pdf. Accessed June 11, 2014.

Office of Technology Assessment: Special Care Units for People With Alzheimer's and Other Dementias: Consumer Education, Research, Regulatory, and Reimbursement Issues (OTA-H-543). Washington, DC, U.S. Government Printing Office, August 1992

Ohta RJ, Ohta BM: Special units for Alzheimer's disease patients: a critical look. Gerontologist 28(6):803–808, 1988 3150963

Olazarán J, Reisberg B, Clare L, et al: Nonpharmacological therapies in Alzheimer's disease: a systematic review of efficacy. Dement Geriatr Cogn Disord 30(2):161–178, 2010 20838046

Olin JT, Fox LS, Pawluczyk S, et al: A pilot randomized trial of carbamazepine for behavioral symptoms in treatment-resistant outpatients with Alzheimer disease. Am J Geriatr Psychiatry 9(4):400–405, 2001 11739066

Ollech D: An analyst's experience working in a skilled nursing facility: a case study. Am J Psychoanal 66(4):381–390, 2006 17115282

Olsen C, Pedersen I, Bergland A, et al: Effect of animal-assisted interventions on depression, agitation and quality of life in nursing home residents suffering from cognitive impairment or dementia: a cluster randomized controlled trial. Int J Geriatr Psychiatry 31(12):1312–1321, 2016 26807956

Omnibus Budget Reconciliation Act of 1987, Pub L No 100-203. Subtitle C: Nursing home reform.

Onder G, Liperoti R, Soldato M, et al: Depression and risk of nursing home admission among older adults in home care in Europe: results from the Aged in Home Care (AdHOC) study. J Clin Psychiatry 68(9):1392–1398, 2007 17915978

Orten JD, Allen M, Cook J: Reminiscence groups with confused nursing center residents: an experimental study. Soc Work Health Care 14(1):73–86, 1989 2781444

Oslin DW, Streim JE, Katz IR, et al: Heuristic comparison of sertraline with nortriptyline for the treatment of depression in frail elderly patients. Am J Geriatr Psychiatry 8(2):141–149, 2000 10804075

Oslin DW, Ten Have TR, Streim JE, et al: Probing the safety of medications in the frail elderly: evidence from a randomized clinical trial of sertraline and venlafaxine in depressed nursing home residents. J Clin Psychiatry 64(8):875–882, 2003 12927001

Overall JE, Gorham DR: The Brief Psychiatric Rating Scale. Psychol Rep 10:799–812, 1962

Parmelee PA, Katz IR, Lawton MP: Depression among institutionalized aged: assessment and prevalence estimation. J Gerontol 44(1):M22–M29, 1989 2783434

Parmelee PA, Katz IR, Lawton MP: The relation of pain to depression among institutionalized aged. J Gerontol 46(1):p15–p21, 1991 1986040

Parmelee PA, Katz IR, Lawton MP: Incidence of depression in long-term care settings. J Gerontol 47(6):M189–M196, 1992 1430853

Phillips CD, Sloane PD, Hawes C, et al: Effects of residence in Alzheimer disease special care units on functional outcomes. JAMA 278(16):1340–1344, 1997 9343465

Phillips CD, Spry KM, Sloane PD, Hawes C: Use of physical restraints and psychotropic medications in Alzheimer special care units in nursing homes. Am J Public Health 90(1):92–96, 2000 10630143

Politis AM, Vozzella S, Mayer LS, et al: A randomized, controlled, clinical trial of activity therapy for apathy in patients with dementia residing in long-term care. Int J Geriatr Psychiatry 19(11):1087–1094, 2004 15481065

Porsteinsson AP, Tariot PN, Erb R, et al: Placebo-controlled study of divalproex sodium for agitation in dementia. Am J Geriatr Psychiatry 9(1):58–66, 2001 11156753

Rahman M, Foster AD: Racial segregation and quality of care disparity in US nursing homes. J Health Econ 39:1–16, 2015 25461895

Rappaport SA, Marcus RN, Manos G, et al: A randomized, double-blind, placebo-controlled tolerability study of intramuscular aripiprazole in acutely agitated patients with Alzheimer's, vascular, or mixed dementia. J Am Med Dir Assoc 10(1):21–27, 2009 19111849

Rattenbury C, Stones MJ: A controlled evaluation of reminiscence and current topics discussion groups in a nursing home context. Gerontologist 29(6):768–771, 1989 2620839

Ray WA, Federspiel CF, Schaffner W: A study of antipsychotic drug use in nursing homes: epidemiologic evidence suggesting misuse. Am J Public Health 70(5):485–491, 1980 6103676

Ray WA, Taylor JA, Meador KG, et al: Reducing antipsychotic drug use in nursing homes: a controlled trial of provider education. Arch Intern Med 153(6):713–721, 1993 8447709

Reichman WE, Conn DK: Nursing home psychiatry: is it time for a reappraisal? Am J Geriatr Psychiatry 18(12):1049–1053, 2010 21155142

Reichman WE, Coyne AC, Borson S, et al: Psychiatric consultation in the nursing home: a survey of six states. Am J Geriatr Psychiatry 6(4):320–327, 1998 9793580

Reisberg B: Functional assessment staging (FAST). Psychopharmacol Bull 24(4):653–659, 1988 3249767

Reisberg B, Ferris SH, de Leon MJ, Crook T: Global Deterioration Scale (GDS). Psychopharmacol Bull 24(4):661–663, 1988 3249768

Reisberg B, Auer SR, Monteiro IM: Behavioral pathology in Alzheimer's disease (BEHAVE-AD) rating scale. Int Psychogeriatr 8(suppl 3):301–308, discussion 351–354, 1996 9154579

Rhoades J, Krauss N: Nursing Home Trends, 1987 and 1996. MEPS Chartbook No 3 (AHCPR Publ No 99–0032). Rockville, MD, Agency for Health Care Policy and Research, 1999

Risse SC, Cubberley L, Lampe TH, et al: Acute effects of neuroleptic withdrawal in elderly dementia patients. J Geriatr Drug Ther 2:65–77, 1987

Rochon PA, Normand SL, Gomes T, et al: Antipsychotic therapy and short-term serious events in older adults with dementia. Arch Intern Med 168(10):1090–1096, 2008 18504337

Rollow W, Lied TR, McGann P, et al: Assessment of the Medicare quality improvement organization program. Ann Intern Med 145(5):342–353, 2006 16908911

Rosen J, Mulsant BH, Pollock BG: Sertraline in the treatment of minor depression in nursing home residents: a pilot study. Int J Geriatr Psychiatry 15(2):177–180, 2000 10679849

Rovner BW, Kafonek S, Filipp L, et al: Prevalence of mental illness in a community nursing home. Am J Psychiatry 143(11):1446–1449, 1986 3777239

Rovner BW, German PS, Broadhead J, et al: The prevalence and management of dementia and other psychiatric disorders in nursing homes. Int Psychogeriatr 2(1):13–24, 1990a 2101294

Rovner BW, Lucas-Blaustein J, Folstein MF, et al: Stability over one year in patients admitted to a nursing home dementia unit. Int J Geriatr Psychiatry 5:77–82, 1990b

Rovner BW, German PS, Brant LJ, et al: Depression and mortality in nursing homes. JAMA 265(8):993–996, 1991 1992213

Rovner BW, Edelman BA, Cox MP, Shmuely Y: The impact of antipsychotic drug regulations on psychotropic prescribing practices in nursing homes. Am J Psychiatry 149(10):1390–1392, 1992 1530076

Rovner BW, Steele CD, Shmuely Y, Folstein MF: A randomized trial of dementia care in nursing homes. J Am Geriatr Soc 44(1):7–13, 1996 8537594

Rozzini R, Boffelli S, Franzoni S: Prevalence and predictors of depressive symptoms in a nursing home. J Geriatr Psychiatry 11:629–634, 1996

Ruckdeschel K, Thompson R, Datto CJ, et al: Using the minimum data set 2.0 mood disturbance items as a self-report screening instrument for depression in nursing home residents. Am J Geriatr Psychiatry 12(1):43–49, 2004 14729558

Ruths S, Straand J, Nygaard HA, et al: Effect of antipsychotic withdrawal on behavior and sleep/wake activity in nursing home residents with dementia: a randomized, placebo-controlled, double-blinded study: the Bergen District Nursing Home Study. J Am Geriatr Soc 52(10):1737–1743, 2004 15450054

Sabin TD, Vitug AJ, Mark VH: Are nursing home diagnosis and treatment inadequate? JAMA 248(3):321–322, 1982 7087125

Sadavoy J: Psychotherapy for the institutionalized elderly, in Practical Psychiatry in the Nursing Home: A Handbook for Staff. Edited by Conn DK, Herrman N, Kaye A, et al. Toronto, ON, Canada, Hogrefe and Huber, 1991, pp 217–236

Saliba D, Jones M, Streim J, et al: Overview of significant changes in the Minimum Data Set for nursing homes version 3.0. J Am Med Dir Assoc 13(7):595–601, 2012 22784698

Saxton J, Silverman M, Ricci E, et al: Maintenance of mobility in residents of an Alzheimer special care facility. Int Psychogeriatr 10(2):213–224, 1998 9677508

Schneider LS, Pollock VE, Lyness SA: A metaanalysis of controlled trials of neuroleptic treatment in dementia. J Am Geriatr Soc 38(5):553–563, 1990 1970586

Schneider LS, Olin JT, Doody RS, et al: Validity and reliability of the Alzheimer's Disease Cooperative Study–Clinical Global Impression of Change. Alzheimer Dis Assoc Disord 11(suppl 2):S22–S32, 1997 9236949

Schneider LS, Dagerman KS, Insel P: Risk of death with atypical antipsychotic drug treatment for dementia: meta-analysis of randomized placebo-controlled trials. JAMA 294(15):1934–1943, 2005 16234500

Schnelle JF, Newman DR, White M, et al: Reducing and managing restraints in long-term-care facilities. J Am Geriatr Soc 40(4):381–385, 1992 1556366

Schnelle JF, Wood S, Schnelle ER, Simmons SF: Measurement sensitivity and the Minimum Data Set depression quality indicator. Gerontologist 41(3):401–405, 2001 11405438

Schulz R: Effects of control and predictability on the physical and psychological well-being of the institutionalized aged. J Pers Soc Psychol 33(5):563–573, 1976 1271225

Seitz DP, Gruneir A, Conn DK, Rochon PA: Cholinesterase inhibitor use in U.S. nursing homes: results from the National Nursing Home Survey. J Am Geriatr Soc 57(12):2269–2274, 2009 19874411

Seitz D, Purandare N, Conn D: Prevalence of psychiatric disorders among older adults in long-term care homes: a systematic review. Int Psychogeriatr 22(7):1025–1039, 2010 20522279

Seitz DP, Gill SS, Herrmann N, et al: Pharmacological treatments for neuropsychiatric symptoms of dementia in long-term care: a systematic review. Int Psychogeriatr 25(2):185–203, 2013 23083438

Semla TP, Palla K, Poddig B, Brauner DJ: Effect of the Omnibus Reconciliation Act 1987 on antipsychotic prescribing in nursing home residents. J Am Geriatr Soc 42(6):648–652, 1994 7911134

Shader RI, Harmatz JS, Salzman C: A new scale for clinical assessment in geriatric populations: Sandoz Clinical Assessment—Geriatric (SCAG). J Am Geriatr Soc 22(3):107–113, 1974 4464879

Shea DG, Russo PA, Smyer MA: Use of mental health services by persons with a mental illness in nursing facilities: initial impacts of OBRA87. J Aging Health 12(4):560–578, 2000 11503732

Shorr RI, Fought RL, Ray WA: Changes in antipsychotic drug use in nursing homes during implementation of the OBRA-87 regulations. JAMA 271(5):358–362, 1994 8283585

Siegler EL, Capezuti E, Maislin G, et al: Effects of a restraint reduction intervention and OBRA '87 regulations on psychoactive drug use in nursing homes. J Am Geriatr Soc 45(7):791–796, 1997 9215327

Simard J, Volicer L: Effects of Namaste Care on residents who do not benefit from usual activities. Am J Alzheimers Dis Other Demen 25(1):46–50, 2010 19332652

Sloane PD, Mathew LJ, Scarborough M, et al: Physical and pharmacologic restraint of nursing home patients with dementia. Impact of specialized units. JAMA 265(10):1278–1282, 1991 1995975

Sloane PD, Mitchell CM, Preisser JS, et al: Environmental correlates of resident agitation in Alzheimer's disease special care units. J Am Geriatr Soc 46(7):862–869, 1998 9670873

Smalbrugge M, Jongenelis L, Pot AM, et al: Incidence and outcome of depressive symptoms in nursing home patients in the Netherlands. Am J Geriatr Psychiatry 14(12):1069–1076, 2006 17138812

Smith M, Buckwalter KC, Albanese M: Geropsychiatric education programs: providing skills and understanding. J Psychosoc Nurs Ment Health Serv 28(12):8–12, 1990 2126559

Smyer M, Brannon D, Cohn M: Improving nursing home care through training and job redesign. Gerontologist 32(3):327–333, 1992 1499997

Smyer MA, Shea DG, Streit A: The provision and use of mental health services in nursing homes: results from the National Medical Expenditure Survey. Am J Public Health 84(2):284–287, 1994 8296955

Sneed JR, Roose SP, Keilp JG, et al: Response inhibition predicts poor antidepressant treatment response in very old depressed patients. Am J Geriatr Psychiatry 15(7):553–563, 2007 17586780

Sneed JR, Keilp JG, Brickman AM, Roose SP: The specificity of neuropsychological impairment in predicting antidepressant non-response in the very old depressed. Int J Geriatr Psychiatry 23(3):319–323, 2008 17726720

Snow LA, Hovanec L, Brandt J: A controlled trial of aromatherapy for agitation in nursing home patients with dementia. J Altern Complement Med 10(3):431–437, 2004 15253846

Snowden MB: The Minimum Data Set Depression Rating Scale (MDSDRS) lacks reliability for identifying depression among older adults living in nursing homes. Evid Based Ment Health 7(1):7, 2004 14769651

Snowden M, Roy-Byrne P: Mental illness and nursing home reform: OBRA-87 ten years later. Psychiatr Serv 49(2):229–233, 1998 9575011

Snowden M, Sato K, Roy-Byrne P: Assessment and treatment of nursing home residents with depression or behavioral symptoms associated with dementia: a review of the literature. J Am Geriatr Soc 51(9):1305–1317, 2003 12919245

Snowdon J: Dementia, depression, and life satisfaction in nursing homes. Int J Geriatr Psychiatry 1:85–91, 1986

Snowdon J, Donnelly N: A study of depression in nursing homes. J Psychiatr Res 20(4):327–333, 1986 3806427

Sommer OH, Aga O, Cvancarova M, et al: Effect of oxcarbazepine in the treatment of agitation and aggression in severe dementia. Dement Geriatr Cogn Disord 27(2):155–163, 2009 19182483

Spagnoli A, Foresti G, Macdonald A, et al: Dementia and depression in Italian geriatric institutions. Int J Geriatr Psychiatry 1:15–23, 1986

Steele C, Rovner B, Chase GA, Folstein M: Psychiatric symptoms and nursing home placement of patients with Alzheimer's disease. Am J Psychiatry 147(8):1049–1051, 1990 2375439

Steiner A, Neu CR: Monitoring the Changes in Use of Medicare Posthospital Services. Washington, DC, RAND/UCLA/Harvard Center for Health Care Financing Policy Research, 1993

Stevenson DG, Mor V: Targeting nursing homes under the Quality Improvement Organization program's 9th statement of work. J Am Geriatr Soc 57(9):1678–1684, 2009 19682119

Stevenson DG, Decker SL, Dwyer LL, et al: Antipsychotic and benzodiazepine use among nursing home residents: findings from the 2004 National Nursing Home Survey. Am J Geriatr Psychiatry 18(12):1078–1092, 2010 20808119

Stotsky B: Multicenter study comparing thioridazine with diazepam and placebo in elderly, nonpsychotic patients with emotional and behavioral disorders. Clin Ther 6(4):546–559, 1984 6380725

Street JS, Clark WS, Gannon KS, et al: Olanzapine treatment of psychotic and behavioral symptoms in patients with Alzheimer disease in nursing care facilities: a double-blind, randomized, placebo-controlled trial. Arch Gen Psychiatry 57(10):968–976, 2000 11015815

Streim JE, Katz IR: Federal regulations and the care of patients with dementia in the nursing home. Med Clin North Am 78(4):895–909, 1994 8022236

Streim JE, Katz IR: Psychiatric aspects of long-term care, in Comprehensive Textbook of Psychiatry, 9th Edition, Vol II. Edited by Sadock BJ, Sadock VA, Ruiz P. Philadelphia, PA, Lippincott Williams and Wilkins, 2009, pp 4195–4200

Streim JE, Oslin DW, Katz IR, et al: Drug treatment of depression in frail elderly nursing home residents. Am J Geriatr Psychiatry 8(2):150–159, 2000 10804076

Streim JE, Porsteinsson AP, Breder CD, et al: A randomized, double-blind, placebo-controlled study of aripiprazole for the treatment of psychosis in nursing home patients with Alzheimer disease. Am J Geriatr Psychiatry 16(7):537–550, 2008 18591574

Sunderland T, Silver MA: Neuroleptics in the treatment of dementia. Int J Geriatr Psychiatry 3:79–88, 1988

Sutcliffe C, Burns A, Challis D, et al: Depressed mood, cognitive impairment, and survival in older people admitted to care homes in England. Am J Geriatr Psychiatry 15(8):708–715, 2007 17504909

Svarstad BL, Mount JK, Bigelow W: Variations in the treatment culture of nursing homes and responses to regulations to reduce drug use. Psychiatr Serv 52(5):666–672, 2001 11331803

Swanson EA, Maas ML, Buckwalter KC: Catastrophic reactions and other behaviors of Alzheimer's residents: special unit compared with traditional units. Arch Psychiatr Nurs 7(5):292–299, 1993 8257198

Szczepanska-Gieracha J, Kowalska J, Pawik M, Rymaszewska J: Evaluation of a short-term group psychotherapy used as part of the rehabilitation process in nursing home patients. Disabil Rehabil 36(12):1027–1032, 2014 23962232

Tariot PN, Podgorski CA, Blazina L, Leibovici A: Mental disorders in the nursing home: another perspective. Am J Psychiatry 150(7):1063–1069, 1993 8317577

Tariot PN, Erb R, Podgorski CA, et al: Efficacy and tolerability of carbamazepine for agitation and aggression in dementia. Am J Psychiatry 155(1):54–61, 1998 9433339

Tariot PN, Cummings JL, Katz IR, et al: A randomized, double-blind, placebo-controlled study of the efficacy and safety of donepezil in patients with Alzheimer's disease in the nursing home setting. J Am Geriatr Soc 49(12):1590–1599, 2001a 11843990

Tariot PN, Schneider LS, Mintzer J, et al: Safety and tolerability of divalproex sodium in the treatment of signs and symptoms of mania in elderly patients with dementia: results of a double-blind, placebo-controlled trial. Curr Ther Res Clin Exp 62:51–67, 2001b

Tariot PN, Farlow MR, Grossberg GT, et al: Memantine treatment in patients with moderate to severe Alzheimer disease already receiving donepezil: a randomized controlled trial. JAMA 291(3):317–324, 2004 14734594

Tariot PN, Raman R, Jakimovich L, et al: Divalproex sodium in nursing home residents with possible or probable Alzheimer disease complicated by agitation: a randomized, controlled trial. Am J Geriatr Psychiatry 13(11):942–949, 2005 16286437

Teeter RB, Garetz FK, Miller WR, Heiland WF: Psychiatric disturbances of aged patients in skilled nursing homes. Am J Psychiatry 133(12):1430–1434, 1976 985657

Teri L, Logsdon RG, McCurry SM: Nonpharmacologic treatment of behavioral disturbance in dementia. Med Clin North Am 86(3):641–656, 2002 12168563

Teri L, Huda P, Gibbons L, et al: STAR: a dementia-specific training program for staff in assisted living residences. Gerontologist 45(5):686–693, 2005 16199404

Thapa PB, Gideon P, Cost TW, et al: Antidepressants and the risk of falls among nursing home residents. N Engl J Med 339(13):875–882, 1998 9744971

Thomasma M, Yeaworth RC, McCabe BW: Moving day: relocation and anxiety in institutionalized elderly. J Gerontol Nurs 16(7):18–25, 1990 2370428

Thomeer MB, Mudrazija S, Angel J: How and why does nursing home use differ by race and ethnicity? J Gerontol B Psychol Sci Soc Sci 73(4):e11–e12, 2018 29669093

Tondi L, Ribani L, Bottazzi M, et al: Validation therapy (VT) in nursing home: a case-control study. Arch Gerontol Geriatr 44(suppl 1):407–411, 2007 17317483

Toseland RW, Diehl M, Freeman K, et al: The impact of validation group therapy on nursing home residents with dementia. J Appl Gerontol 61:31–50, 1997

Trappler B, Cohen CI: Using fluoxetine in "very old" depressed nursing home residents. Am J Geriatr Psychiatry 4(3):258–262, 1996 28531085

Trappler B, Cohen CI: Use of SSRIs in "very old" depressed nursing home residents. Am J Geriatr Psychiatry 6(1):83–89, 1998 9469218

Trichard L, Zabow A, Gillis LS: Elderly persons in old-age homes: a medical, psychiatric and social investigation. S Afr Med J 61(17):624–627, 1982 7079853

Ulbricht CM, Rothschild AJ, Hunnicutt JN, Lapane KL: Depression and cognitive impairment among newly admitted nursing home residents in the USA. Int J Geriatr Psychiatry 32(11):1172–1181, 2017 28544134

Unroe KT, Ouslander JG, Saliba D: Nursing home regulations redefined: implications for providers. J Am Geriatr Soc 66(1):191–194, 2018 29155452

Urick BY, Kaskie BP, Carnahan RM: Improving antipsychotic prescribing practices in nursing facilities: the role of surveyor methods and surveying agencies in upholding the Nursing Home Reform Act. Res Social Adm Pharm 12(1):91–103, 2016 25990258

U.S. Food and Drug Administration: Risperdal (Risperidone) Dear Healthcare Professional Letter, Silver Spring, MD, U.S. Food and Drug Administration, April 2003

U.S. Food and Drug Administration: Public Health Advisory: Deaths with Antipsychotics in Elderly Patients With Behavioral Disturbances. Silver Spring, MD, U.S. Food and Drug Administration, April 11, 2005.

Van der Ploeg ES, Eppingstall B, O'Connor DW: Internet video chat (Skype) family conversations as a treatment of agitation in nursing home residents with dementia. Int Psychogeriatr 28(4):697–698, 2016 26560943

van Weert JC, van Dulmen AM, Spreeuwenberg PM, et al: Behavioral and mood effects of snoezelen integrated into 24-hour dementia care. J Am Geriatr Soc 53(1):24–33, 2005 15667372

Vink AC, Zuidersma M, Boersma F, et al: The effect of music therapy compared with general recreational activities in reducing agitation in people with dementia: a randomized controlled trial. J Geriatr Psychiatry 10:1031–1038, 2013

Viscogliosi G, Chiriac IM, Ettorre E: Efficacy and safety of citalopram compared to atypical antipsychotics on agitation in nursing home residents with Alzheimer dementia. J Am Med Dir Assoc 18(9):799–802, 2017 28739492

Volicer L, Frijters DH, Van der Steen JT: Relationship between symptoms of depression and agitation in nursing home residents with dementia. Int J Geriatr Psychiatry 27(7):749–754, 2012 21956820

von Gunten A, Mosimann UP, Antonietti JP: A longitudinal study on delirium in nursing homes. Am J Geriatr Psychiatry 21(10):963–972, 2013 23567403

Wagner AW, Teri L, Orr-Rainey N: Behavior problems of residents with dementia in special care units. Alzheimer Dis Assoc Disord 9(3):121–127, 1995 8534409

Wang PS, Schneeweiss S, Avorn J, et al: Risk of death in elderly users of conventional vs. atypical antipsychotic medications. N Engl J Med 353(22):2335–2341, 2005 16319382

Wahnschaffe A, Nowozin C, Haedel S, et al: Implementation of dynamic lighting in a nursing home: impact on agitation but not on rest-activity patterns. Curr Alzheimer Res 14(10):1076–1083, 2017 28595522

Webber AP, Martin JL, Harker JO, et al: Depression in older patients admitted for postacute nursing home rehabilitation. J Am Geriatr Soc 53(6):1017–1022, 2005 15935027

Weiner MF, Martin-Cook K, Svetlik DA, et al: The Quality of Life in Late-Stage Dementia (QUALID) scale. J Am Med Dir Assoc 1(3):114–116, 2000 12818023

Wells Y, Jorm AF: Evaluation of a special nursing home unit for dementia sufferers: a randomised controlled comparison with community care. Aust N Z J Psychiatry 21(4):524–531, 1987 3449047

Werner P, Cohen-Mansfield J, Braun J, Marx MS: Physical restraints and agitation in nursing home residents. J Am Geriatr Soc 37(12):1122–1126, 1989 2592719

Wetzels RB, Zuidema SU, de Jonghe JFM, et al: Course of neuropsychiatric symptoms in residents with dementia in nursing homes over 2-year period. Am J Geriatr Psychiatry 18(12):1054–1065, 2010 21155143

Williams-Barnard CL, Lindell AR: Therapeutic use of "prizing" and its effect on self-concept of elderly clients in nursing homes and group homes. Issues Ment Health Nurs 13(1):1–17, 1992 1737699

Winblad B, Kilander L, Eriksson S, et al: Donepezil in patients with severe Alzheimer's disease: double-blind, parallel-group, placebo-controlled study. Lancet 367(9516):1057–1065, 2006 16581404

Won A, Lapane KL, Vallow S, et al: Long-term effects of analgesics in a population of elderly nursing home residents with persistent nonmalignant pain. J Gerontol A Biol Sci Med Sci 61(2):165–169, 2006 16510860

Wood S, Cummings JL, Hsu MA, et al: The use of the neuropsychiatric inventory in nursing home residents. Characterization and measurement. Am J Geriatr Psychiatry 8(1):75–83, 2000 10648298

Yesavage JA, Brink TL, Rose TL, et al: Development and validation of a geriatric depression screening scale: a preliminary report. J Psychiatr Res 17(1):37–49, 1982–1983 7183759

Youssef FA: The impact of group reminiscence counseling on a depressed elderly population. Nurse Pract 15(4):32–42, 1990

Yuan Y, Lapane KL, Baek J, et al: Nursing home star ratings and new onset of depression in long-stay nursing home residents. J Am Med Dir Assoc 20(10):1335–1339, 2019 31281113

Yuan Y, Min HS, Lapane KL, et al: Depression symptoms and cognitive impairment in older nursing home residents in the USA: a latent class analysis. Int J Geriatr Psychiatry 35(7):769–778, 2020 32250496

Yudofsky SC, Silver JM, Jackson W, et al: The Overt Aggression Scale for the objective rating of verbal and physical aggression. Am J Psychiatry 143(1):35–39, 1986 3942284

Zerhusen JD, Boyle K, Wilson W: Out of the darkness: group cognitive therapy for depressed elderly. J Psychosoc Nurs Ment Health Serv 29(9):16–21, 1991 1941727

Zhao D, Shridharmurthy D, Alcusky MJ, et al: The prevalence and factors associated with antiepileptic drug use in US nursing home residents. Drugs Aging 37(2):137–145, 2020 31845208

Zhong KX, Tariot PN, Mintzer J, et al: Quetiapine to treat agitation in dementia: a randomized, double-blind, placebo-controlled study. Curr Alzheimer Res 4(1):81–93, 2007 17316169

Zimmer JG, Watson N, Treat A: Behavioral problems among patients in skilled nursing facilities. Am J Public Health 74(10):1118–1121, 1984 6476166

CHAPTER 25

Use of Technology in Geriatric Psychiatry

Heejung J. Kim, B.A.

Miranda D. Skurla, B.S.

Aniqa T. Rahman, B.A.

Ipsit V. Vahia, M.D.

Geriatric psychiatry is changing. Although the field has largely focused on providing primary psychiatric care to older adults, over the past decade there is a clear trend indicating the current geriatric mental health workforce is not adequately equipped to provide appropriate care to an ever-increasing population of older adults. This discrepancy is only likely to grow. A report by the National Academy of Medicine clearly identified the shortage of a geriatric workforce as a major issue of public health relevance and approaching crisis. The future of the field will depend on creating models of care that allow maximal dissemination of geriatric psychiatric expertise. Development of these models of care will need to be combined with a rethinking of the current trends and diagnostics and treatment for older adults. It has been well recognized that the presentation of most psychiatric symptoms with aging differs from that in younger populations. As the concepts of precision medicine and personalized care are effectively translated from research into clinical practice, it is becoming possible to quantify the ways in which psychiatric symptomatology in late life differs from that earlier in life. Thus, the availability of new tools to quantify presentation at the level of the individual is now beginning to create intriguing possibilities for the ways in which we measure, monitor, and provide care.

The field may also need to pay attention to the pressing issue of how to reach the largest possible number of people in need with the highest possible efficiency worldwide. Given that a lack of access to care for older adults is often driven by pragmatic issues, such as a lack of transportation, disparities in available care in rural versus urban environments, and insufficient expertise in dealing with the complexities of geriatric care, creative solutions will need to be developed that enable communication and quantified care over long distances. Although this is a significant issue in the developed world, it is even more critical in the developing world. For example, in India, there are only two fellowship programs in geriatric psychiatry to serve a total population of more than 1.3 billion individuals. Thus, in addition to maximizing the reach of geriatric psychiatry expertise, the field will also need to consider how to train a global workforce. Although the use of technological tools is not necessarily considered a core part of the training curriculum in geriatric psychiatry at present, it is crucial that such skills be systematically developed and taught for the field to evolve into a prominent role around these issues.

At the time we are writing this chapter, the world is more than 18 months into the COVID-19 pandemic. Although this pandemic has caused significant disruption in health care, it has also been a major impetus for the adoption of technologies, primarily telemedicine. In this chapter, we first discuss COVID-19, technology, and mental health, because the field of technology and mental health must adapt to the changes in health care that COVID-19 has triggered. Next, we review how older adults tend to use technologies. Following this, we present an overview of the current state of technology in mental health, including the use of technology both in diagnostics and assessment and in providing care and treatment. In these sections, we also discuss the use of electronic health records (EHRs) and telemedicine. We present special sections on technology that can aid clinicians caring for persons with limiting issues, such as living in a rural environment or facing challenges with mobility and transportation. We also present a detailed section on the issues of ethics and privacy around the use of technology and discuss policy implications for more digitized geriatric mental health care, which will be especially important in the context of a broad-scale adaptation of technology in response to COVID-19. Finally, we present a road map for how technology may be incorporated across clinical settings into geriatric mental health care so that technology-enhanced models of practice become the standard of care.

COVID-19, Technology, and Geriatric Mental Health

When we began writing this chapter, it had been only 6 months since the first recorded case of COVID-19 in the United States. At publication, the pandemic remained an acute and evolving global issue. There continue to be several unknowns regarding whether and how the pandemic may reshape geriatric mental health. However, a significant initial impact of COVID-19 was the population-wide transition from in-person care to telecare. In the span of a few months, interventions and approaches that would previously have been considered novel and cutting edge (e.g., virtual visits, text messaging, integration of health care records) became the standard of care across all clinical settings. The pandemic also accelerated the adoption of mental health applications for psychotherapy, chatbot-based psychotherapy, and support and regular use of mobile applications and platforms that support activities such as mindfulness and meditation, physical activity, or even social engagement with friends and colleagues.

It is premature at present to comment definitively on how the pandemic will impact technology use in geriatric mental health care. However, Gould and Hantke (2020) proposed a meaningful framework and clinical guidelines for deploying technologies most appropriately with older adults. They proposed the following four goals: 1) to ensure better access to technology for older adults, 2) to promote familiarity with technology and proficiency at using it, 3) to encourage patient buy-in around technology, and 4) to improve clinician familiarity with these tools. They also recommend that achieving these goals would require a concerted effort by clinicians and patients and changes at the system and policy levels. It would also involve action on the part of multiple stakeholders, including health care systems and technology companies. Suggested points of action at the policy level include the creation of low-cost data packages for older adults who are on fixed incomes and the identification and funding of programs that may provide technological support. The authors also recommended that clinicians adopt a pro-technology stance, including working with patients to establish their technological capacity (including device ownership); explaining benefits of using various technologies, including telemedicine, to patients; and becoming familiar with the technologies themselves so that they can have more informed conversations with patients.

Thus, the changes in practice triggered by the COVID-19 pandemic represent a large-scale adoption of approaches developed several years prior to the pandemic and shown in research studies to be efficacious. These new approaches provide geriatric psychiatry a stable platform on which to develop innovative, technology-based models of care that would improve access, care delivery, and ongoing support.

Use of Technology Among Older Adults

Older adults have not traditionally been considered heavy consumers of technology, but recent surveys indicate that patterns of technology use among this population are changing rapidly. Moreover, there may be generational differences among adults age 65 years and older in how they use various devices such as mobile phones, tablets, and computers. According to a Pew Research Center survey conducted in 2017 (Anderson and Perrin 2017), the overall rate of mobile phone use among older adults is >80%. This percentage includes all mobile devices, but smartphones constitute a rapidly growing share. The use of tablet devices also continues to grow rapidly: nearly one-third of older adults now own a tablet device. Expectedly, ownership and usage rates of these technologies are higher among adults between ages 65 and 75 and decrease with user age; persons age 80 and older use technologies at a substantially lower rate. The Pew survey also sheds light on barriers to effective technology use. The researchers determined that more education and higher household incomes are associated with greater use of technology. In addition, older adults report lower initial confidence, or lower "tech readiness," defined as the self-perceived ability to navigate technological devices (McClain et al. 2021). However, once older adults adopt technology, they may engage at a high level with both the technology and the digital content.

Parallel to increases in the use and ownership of technology is a steady increase in the use of social media among older adults. Although more than 35% of older adults use social networking sites, more than 60% still do not use social media. We have already noted an increase in social networking throughout the COVID-19 pandemic. Video conferencing applications, more than other forms of technological communication methods, such as email, text messaging, and social media, were identified as drivers in lowering rates of depression at follow-up (Teo et al. 2019).

Although this topic has a relatively small base of evidence thus far, the future of digital mental health in geriatric psychiatry will be contingent on clinicians' ability to assess technology ownership and proficiency and to recommend the right technology for the right application for the right patient. As rates of technology use among older adults rise worldwide, including among those with serious mental illness, clinicians are likely to find that patients already have basic access to technology by which meaningful data may be collected and interventions administered. This initial engagement with technology has laid the foundation for the development of technologies targeting both diagnostics and therapeutics, both of which we review in the following section.

Technologies for Diagnostics and Assessments

Digital Phenotyping

Recent technological developments have made mobile devices sensitive enough to capture subtle aspects of behavior, cognition, and mood. Data collected using this technology help deepen the clinician's insight into a patient's clinical profile. This process of collecting digital information from various sensors implemented in a patient's natural setting is called *digital phenotyping* (Onnela and Rauch 2016; Torous et al. 2016). Digital phenotyping methods complement the traditional evaluating methods usually based on self-reported or clinician-reported measurements and offset the disadvantages of these methods. Traditional methods have limitations in capturing an accurate clinical profile because they have the potential to introduce recall inaccuracies or reporting biases and ecological inaccuracies and can miss early signs of manifestations (Ben-Zeev and Young 2010; Komatsu et al. 2013; Trull and Ebner-Priemer 2013). These limitations necessitate the development of more objective and precise instruments to detect markers of various psychiatric and neurological disorders.

Mobile Technologies

One of the most accessible methods for digital phenotyping is through smartphone sensors. The ease of implementing monitoring features in a patient's smartphone can be attributed to its ubiquity. Within the geriatric population, smartphone use has quadrupled (Anderson and Perrin 2017). This widespread use allows smartphones to be used for various purposes, such as tracking mood changes. Although self-reported scales tracking changes in mood traditionally have been used for diagnostic purposes, the burden of adherence hinders continuous data collection, particularly in individuals with mood disorders (Palmius et al. 2017). Using unobtrusive methods to collect data passively could circumvent this issue. In patients with mood disorders, in whom early detection of relapse and prompt intervention are significant for making a good prognosis (Perry et al. 1999), data collected continuously through a smartphone could have useful applications. In one study (Palmius et al. 2017), investigators used geolocation data collected from smartphones to estimate depressive episodes. Global positioning system (GPS) data alone could detect depressive episodes with 95% accuracy, as verified by scores on the Quick Inventory of Depressive Symptomatology. The types of data collected include the amount of movement between different locations, variability in the time spent in the different locations recorded, time spent at home, transition time, and total distance. Episodes unable to be predicted by GPS data could be accounted for by individual differences in how mood relates to physical motion.

Variables besides GPS data can be collected from smartphones to track changes in psychiatric status. Ben-Zeev et al. (2015) utilized microphones, GPS, multiaxial accelerometers, and light sensors to measure changes in speech duration, geospatial activity, kinesthetic activity, and sleep duration, respectively. Compared with self-reported assessments, these measurements viably reflected patients' daily stress levels, changes in depression, and changes in loneliness. As outlined in the studies mentioned earlier, smartphone sensors offer ample possibilities in digital phenotyping and can provide opportunities for physicians to assess psychiatric states without much active involvement of the patient, increasing accessibility.

Another variable that could provide significant insights for a patient's psychiatric assessment is the patient's use of electronic and social media. A study investigating the language used in social media showed that individuals with ADHD were more likely to exhibit certain language characteristics than those who did not have ADHD (Guntuku et al. 2019). In another study, individuals who posted more frequently on social media were more likely to have a history of depression compared with those who did not post frequently (Smith et al. 2017). Findings such as these highlight the benefit of incorporating social media use into psychiatric assessments and clinical decisions. In one psychiatric teaching hospital, this practice was found to be common, and many clinicians performing psychotherapy reported that reviewing social media information improved the quality of their care (Hobbs et al. 2019).

Wearables

Another category of devices that improve clinicians' insight into patients' naturalistic environment is wearables. These devices are worn by the patient and passively collect data on the wearer's movements. One type of wearable developed was able to successfully measure gait and balance in those with Alzheimer's disease and mild cognitive impairment (Hsu et al. 2014). Individuals with Alzheimer's disease are known to experience impairments in their motor function (Alexander et al. 1995; Pettersson et al. 2005); traditionally, cameras, foot switches, electronic mats, and manual stopwatch tests are used to measure gait and balance functioning. However, these methods cannot be easily implemented in the naturalistic environment and can introduce human error. One device investigated by Hsu et al. (2014) overcame these limitations to allow evaluation of gait and balance beyond the clinic. In this study, an inertial sensor–based wearable instrument effectively measured different parameters of gait and balance. The ability of this wearable device to measure aspects of motor function could allow early detection and screen for risk factors, ultimately reducing complications such as falls. Studies have shown that the most optimal placement of the wearable device is on the user's hip (Chen and Bassett 2005; Matthews et al. 2012; Troiano et al. 2008). However, because of low compliance at this location, another viable option is the nondominant wrist (Troiano et al. 2014).

Noncontact Prototype Devices

Noncontact prototype devices expand the scope and density of symptoms measured. One such device, the Emerald, uses radio waves and signal processing algorithms to detect positioning (Vahia et al. 2020). Superimposed positional data can be utilized to measure significant motions and compare this with nurse and visitor logs for older adults with paranoia and agitation. For example, increased motion detected on family visit days versus non-visit days would suggest increased agitation. Such indications provide insight in the patient's clinical profile and help providers establish a more sensitive treatment plan. More recently, the Emerald device used similar noncontact methods to provide objective measurements of persons with dementia; for example, the number of transitions between spaces identified episodes of agitation (Au-Yeung et al. 2021).

Noncontact devices are also feasible for use in acute care settings. In one study, such devices were used to monitor vital signs, movement, and sound emissions within the geriatric-gerontopsychiatric emergency department (Kroll et al. 2020). Visual sensors, acoustic sensors, and sensory mats placed on patients' beds collected data passively throughout their stay. Closely monitoring older adults with dementia is of particular importance because they have a higher likelihood of in-hospital complications (Watkin et al. 2012). Given that changes in heart rate and blood pressure measurements suggest an increase in agitation, monitoring these indicators closely and detecting markers early on could prevent further complications (Chase et al. 2004). Other methods of monitoring vital signs with adhesives or wearables could cause discomfort and decrease patient compliance (Kroll et al. 2020). Hence, noncontact devices can counteract the disadvantages of alternative methods for monitoring patients at risk.

Digital and Web-Based Neurocognitive Testing

Traditionally, pen-and-paper neurocognitive tests have been used to evaluate cognitive function. Although shorter pen-and-paper tests were developed to decrease testing time and optimize staff time, some limitations remain, including the inability to obtain a comprehensive profile of deficit, the extensive training required to administer these tests, and the need for manual scoring (Guimond et al. 2019; Velligan et al. 2004). In recent years, researchers have developed web-based and digital-based neurocognitive tests that circumvent some limitations of the conventional batteries. In this subsection, we outline some of these new mediums and their clinical applications.

One of the most widely used Web-based instruments for evaluating schizophrenia is Cogstate. With its eight scales, Cogstate successfully evaluates the cognitive domains of processing speed, verbal learning, visual learning, reasoning, problem solving, and social cognition (Makdissi et al. 2001). This battery requires 35 minutes to complete and can be administered to patients from a wide range of ages. Compared with conventional tests, Cogstate demonstrated viability in evaluating cognitive decline in patients with mild traumatic brain injury, schizophrenia, and AIDS dementia complex, three conditions that involve more subtle impairments in cognition than those seen in conditions such as Alzheimer's disease (Maruff et al. 2009). The battery itself includes tasks that require subjects to respond as quickly and accurately as possible using the laptop keyboard when prompted on the screen. Their responses and response times are recorded in milliseconds. The investigators found that Cogstate is sensitive to even mild cognitive impairments. In addition to its ability to detect cognitive function, testing through Web-based mediums entails an added benefit of practicality and accessibility.

Mobile-based neurocognitive testing through a smartphone is another alternative to traditional pen-and-paper testing. Advantages of mobile-based tests include their ability to record the total time of testing precisely and to present prompts in a standardized manner. Jongstra et al. (2017) used a smartphone application to assess cognitive function in healthy adults older than 50 years with a family history of dementia.

Some of the scales used included Memory-Word, Trail Making, Stroop test, Reaction Time, and Letter-N-Back. Although not all patients complied with repeatedly completing the assessments over the course of the entire study, the authors noted that one of the most significant benefits of application-based neurocognitive testing is the ease with which data can be collected repeatedly over time to detect changes in cognitive function. As smartphone and computer use become more prevalent in the geriatric population, the advantages of mobile-based and Web-based neurocognitive testing, including its ease of administration, accessibility, and automatic scoring, render technology highly beneficial in diagnostics and assessment (Guimond et al. 2019).

Other Web-Based Surveys

Ecological momentary assessment (EMA) is defined as "a collection of methods for obtaining repeated real-time assessments of subjects' behavior and experience in their natural environments, to minimize recall bias, maximize ecological validity, and document variation over time" (Shiffman et al. 2008, p. 25). Patients can be prompted to complete assessments in three different ways: once daily (i.e., diaries), randomly, or every time a variable of interest occurs (Asselbergs et al. 2016; Cain et al. 2009). In one study, EMA data were used to predict depression in a geriatric population (Kim et al. 2019). Older adults were given a wearable device (Actiwatch) and were prompted four times daily to complete a mood scale on their device. The investigators found that data collection through EMA in conjunction with information on physical activities, sleep, and exposure to light was effective for predicting depression. In addition, the researchers confirmed findings from previous studies that had not used EMA, noticing a pattern of increased depressed mood preceding an increase in time at home. Incorporating EMAs into assessing changes in mood could significantly impact treatment effectiveness.

Sleep Sensors

Sleep sensors can improve psychiatric assessment through measurement of sleep duration and stages. Traditional self-report measures of sleep duration are limited and error prone (Silva et al. 2007). More accurate methods such as polysomnography may disrupt normal sleep patterns due to intrusiveness. Wrist-worn actigraphs can be useful in measuring the duration and quality of sleep with minimal disruptiveness but are limited because interpretation of their data is dependent solely on motion detection (Lauderdale et al. 2014). Bed sensors are other portable options for sleep sensing that can detect motion and physiological variables such as CNS measurements (Kortelainen et al. 2010). One case study illustrates the potential applications of unobtrusive sleep sensing in psychiatric care (Vahia and Sewell 2016):

> A patient with a complex medical and psychiatric history who initially complained of recent onset of confusion and poor decision making reported disruption of functioning, especially related to his work. He discussed hypersomnia and insomnia but denied depressed mood, anhedonia, thoughts of death, or psychomotor retardation. Obtaining sleep study was not feasible. Wrist-worn actigraph measurements of his step counts and sleep duration identified a severe psychomotor retardation, which guided development of an altered treatment plan.

Further investigation of sleep-sensing devices would refine the benefits of their unobtrusiveness and their accuracy in measuring sleep quality and duration.

Portable Electroencephalogram

The electroencephalogram (EEG) has been a useful neuroimaging tool that is widely used to evaluate various dysfunctions in cognition. Recently, wireless EEGs, synonymous with portable, mobile, or wearable EEGs, have been developed as a more convenient alternative to the traditional EEGs used primarily in clinical settings. Wireless EEGs differ from conventional EEGs by using a wireless connection through Bluetooth or Wi-Fi. Their portability allows measurements to be taken in a naturalistic environment in which movement is less restricted rather than in a constrained laboratory setting (McDowell et al. 2013), and they can have various levels of mobility depending on how the equipment is mounted. Examples include off-body, waist, or head-mounted or carried in a backpack. These EEGs allow for a range of motion from static positions such as lying, sitting, or standing to highly active positions such as climbing stairs, constrained running, and carrying (Bateson et al. 2017).

Besides their advantages in portability, the convenience and ease of use of portable EEGs can be attributed to how quickly they can be prepared. One type of portable device includes EEGs that use dry electrodes as opposed to electrodes prepared with gel or saline patches as typically used in conventional EEGs. Circumventing the laborious process of using wet preparations shortens preparation time for dry EEGs and thereby increases ease of use (Hinrichs et al. 2020; Kam et al. 2019; Lin et al. 2011). Recently, noncontact EEGs have also demonstrated promising feasibility and applicability for clinical needs (Chi and Cauwenberghs 2010; Ng et al. 2020; Sun and Yu 2016).

Digital Therapeutics

Potentially the greatest opportunity for technology to revolutionize psychiatric care is through its incorporation into direct therapeutic interventions. Technology can be used to enhance existing interventions or broaden their reach, but new tools also allow for the invention of entirely novel therapies. Often used as the foremost example of digital therapeutics is *telemedicine*, a term used to describe the use of telecommunication and videoconferencing technologies to deliver care remotely. Telemedicine brings traditional in-person psychological assessment or individual psychotherapy sessions into the patient's home without much change to the content and integrity of the intervention. In addition to telemedicine, mobile applications and sensor-based pills give clinicians greater reach into patients' lives outside of the clinic, providing ecologically valid information about patients' mood states, behavior, and medication adherence. Finally, technological advances in the realms of robotics and virtual reality can mold and manipulate existing therapies to accommodate deficits specific to the geriatric community. This section addresses the aforementioned technologies, their potential benefits, and how they are being incorporated into clinical care.

Telemedicine

The American Psychiatric Association's "Position Statement on Telemedicine in Psychiatry" states that telemedicine "is a validated and effective practice of medicine...a legitimate component of a mental health delivery system" (American Psychiatric Association 2018). Especially in the field of geriatrics, telemedicine is poised to greatly expand access to specialty care because of its ability to reach rural and underserved populations. The geriatric population experiences mobility challenges due to physical disability or transportation burden, which, alone or in combination with other barriers, can make it difficult for patients to travel to a clinic. Additionally, the overall shortage of geriatricians decreases the chances of an older adult or a caregiver finding a specialist within a reasonable traveling distance (Morley 2016).

Nursing homes and long-term care facilities may benefit most from the adoption of telemedicine services when residents have complicated medical and psychiatric conditions that require a higher level of care than the facility can provide. An important use of telemedicine is bridging the gap between an inpatient hospital stay and the long-term care setting (Ramos-Ríos et al. 2012). Creating a continuum of care between the acute hospital setting and the patient's residence may reduce or prevent future readmissions and emergency department visits (Morley 2016). In addition, the role of nonphysician clinicians is enhanced in telemedicine because nurses may be responsible for appointment preparation and the efficient communication of relevant clinical information to the specialist. Finally, the participation of a caregiver in the remote appointment is especially important because it provides an additional layer of familiarity and comfort for the patient (Ramos-Ríos et al. 2012).

A primary use for telemedicine is cognitive assessment and dementia diagnosis, as well as management of behavioral and psychological symptoms. A thorough cognitive and functional assessment is necessary for diagnosing dementia and its subtypes; however, it can be difficult to find a specialist with the credentials to perform this assessment. Telemedicine may allow us to stretch our limited pool of geriatricians to serve the greatest number of patients. The first hurdle that telemedicine faces is establishing interrater reliability and agreement between assessments conducted via videoconference and in-person assessments. Although some studies have found high rates of agreement between virtual and in-person assessment, other work has suggested that a physical and neurological examination must be performed in person to reliably diagnose the dementia subtype. Additionally, standard paper-based cognitive tests, such as the Mini-Mental State Examination (MMSE; Folstein et al. 1975), must be adapted for use via videoconferencing platforms. Previous research has suggested that patients may perform worse on the MMSE when the examination is administered through videoconferencing, something that will require innovation within the field of neuropsychology (Ramos-Ríos et al. 2012). However, clinical assessments of behavioral and psychological symptoms, such as agitation, depression and anxiety, or disturbances in sleep and appetite, may be able to be completed remotely with input from caregivers.

Telemedicine has also been proven useful in geriatric mood disorder populations and has been well tolerated and accepted by patients and their families (Harerimana et al. 2019). Videoconferencing has been used to deliver cognitive-behavioral therapy remotely, which demonstrates the ability to adapt existing therapies to the virtual form. Telemedicine can also be used as a supplement to self-guided Web-based interventions in which patients receive support from a "TeleCoach." Finally, other studies have used electronic devices to deliver educational content to patients and to facilitate an information exchange between patients and providers using questionnaires (Harerimana et al. 2019).

An overarching theme in the literature on telemedicine and other digital therapeutics is the importance of the patient's degree of comfort with and receptiveness to the technology. To make such a structural change to our existing models of care delivery, there must be support from all parties involved, including providers, caregivers, families, and, most importantly, patients themselves (Harerimana et al. 2019). Telemedicine is more than another tool at the disposal of providers; as the COVID-19 pandemic has shown, it can facilitate a complete shift in paradigm around how we conceptualize the care delivery ecosystem. It allows us to fundamentally reimagine how to most efficiently allocate scarce resources of geriatric specialty care. Given the unique challenges of the geriatric population and their perceived confidence in technology use, further investigation of improving infrastructure for telemedicine in geriatric psychiatry is urgently needed (Narasimha et al. 2017). Recently published work has demonstrated the utility of training older adults on using telemedicine, but more efficient and sustainable methods are urgently needed for the longer term (Adrien et al. 2021).

Mobile Applications

As discussed earlier, smartphones are becoming ubiquitous among the geriatric population, with ~50% of seniors now owning a smartphone (Anderson and Perrin 2017). Mobile applications are highly customizable and can be made incredibly user-friendly through the use of focus groups and small-scale feasibility studies. Because of these factors, they are a promising medium through which to connect with patients outside of the clinic in ways that feel more natural and meet patients in their environments. However, the use of applications in psychiatry faces problems with adherence and efficacy: they must be used over long periods of time to determine whether they lead to improved clinical outcomes. Applications have been tested in the dementia population to monitor a loved one for wandering or to facilitate reminiscence activities. In other psychopathology, they can be used to deliver evidence-based psychosocial interventions and psychotherapy and to support the work done in person in the clinic.

One of the significant sources of danger for the patient and worry for the caregiver in dementia is the occurrence of wandering. This behavior requires constant monitoring by caregivers, which can be especially difficult for the 15% of caregivers who live far from their loved one (Sposaro et al. 2010). One solution piloted in an assisted living facility is an application that continuously gathers data about a person's behavior to determine the probability of that person wandering. The application can then take appropriate action, such as directing the person to a safe location or calling the caregiver or 911, based on the results of its predictive modeling (Sposaro et al. 2010). As more research is done to establish factors that contribute to or increase the risk of wandering, algorithms and models within applications can be refined to be more precise and to intervene in tailored and personalized ways.

In addition to monitoring patients' behavioral symptoms, applications can be used for mindfulness-based interventions (Hawkes et al. 2020). Mindfulness in conjunction with art therapy has been used with effectiveness in various populations, but its application is less established in older adults. The feasibility of this combination has been more recently studied in conjunction with the use of digital tools such as tablets and smartphones. Its benefit in delivering mindfulness techniques and its acceptance by older adults demonstrate promising applications that can diversify the ways through which interventions can be delivered.

Other applications can be used to facilitate cognitive interventions in the home setting. For example, reminiscence therapy, and more generally reminiscence activities, are important for maintaining a sense of self in dementia. Mobile applications allow easy management and display of media, such as photos, videos, and audio recordings, that can be used as stimuli for reminiscence activities. Caregivers can upload media into the application, allowing individuals with dementia to view photos and videos and to listen to music on their own. Personal media, such as photos of the person's grandchildren or wedding, tend to be preferable to generic content, a finding consistent with other literature (Mulvenna et al. 2017).

Similar to the adaptation of reminiscence activities, evidence-based psychosocial interventions for psychiatric illnesses can also be transformed into mobile form. Applications provide tangible benefits for these types of interventions, specifically ensuring that the intervention is delivered in a standardized manner, something that is difficult to maintain across providers. Although evidence has shown that these applications are feasible, the next step is to establish their efficacy for influencing clinical outcomes. However, many intangible benefits suggest that their use would result in improved symptoms by supporting the work done in the clinic in a personalized and engaging manner. Finally, applications integrate smoothly into our health care system's shift toward preventive medicine and self-management of symptoms before they reach crisis level (Fortuna et al. 2017). By tracking depression symptoms, for example, applications can determine usual patterns of movement, communication, and activity levels. Predictive modeling then allows them to detect deviation from the norm and to alert either the patient or the caregiver (Sposaro et al. 2010). Mobile applications also give patients the proper tool and structure to better participate in their care, and this, it is hoped, will lead to lasting and significant improvement.

Finally, applications have the potential to deliver evidence-based psychotherapy if they meet basic usability standards and demonstrate empirical efficacy. There is no shortage of mental health applications available for various diagnostic categories, including mood disorders, anxiety, PTSD, and schizophrenia and schizoaffective disorders, but few of these have been rigorously evaluated. Although many studies report symptom reduction with application use, these results have not been replicated, and studies frequently lack a control group. Thus, there is a need for further research to develop empirical evidence for these applications, and it is especially important that this research be independent from the developers themselves. Across all diagnoses, however, many applications share common features, such as use of cognitive-behavioral therapy principles, capabilities for symptom monitoring, collection of information regarding skill implementation, and psychoeducation (Lui et al. 2017). Programs that incorporate these features and are generally user-friendly should be rigorously tested across various diagnostic and demographic populations, taking care to ensure that the research includes control groups and is independent from any conflicts of interest (Huguet et al. 2016). Future research will also have to investigate the efficacy of using application-based treatments in conjunction with versus in place of in-person treatment (Lui et al. 2017). Usability testing in the geriatric population specifically is important for ensuring that this population can successfully navigate and engage with the application.

Digital Tools for Medication Adherence

Older adults commonly have multiple chronic health conditions in addition to mental health diagnoses, and this greatly increases the number of medications in their daily routine. Poor medication adherence can be caused by a multitude of factors and contributes to adverse health outcomes and decreased quality of life (Tan et al. 2018). Therefore, using technology to promote medication adherence outside of the clinic is of great interest to those working with older adults. Two prominent approaches are "smart" pill boxes equipped with sensors and digital health feedback systems.

Simply adding a sensor to a typical pill box allows a wealth of data to be collected about older adults' medication adherence behavior. Temporal and frequency information about pill box access can be corroborated with intended dosing schedules, with discrepancies triggering a notification to the patient or caregiver. By identifying moments when medication regimens are not being followed, the smart pill box allows caregivers to intervene early to inform and educate patients and family members about proper adherence. However, the smart pill box is not a blanket solution to the problem of nonadherence. It must integrate seamlessly into the patient's routine and deliver personalized and real-time alerts that will ensure interventions occur in a timely manner to prevent future nonadherence (Tan et al. 2018).

Another potential solution is the "smart pill," which is an example of a digital health feedback system (DHFS). As the pill is digested, a signal is sent to a patch worn by the patient, which transmits it to a mobile application (Rosenbaum 2018). This intervention may be helpful for forgetful patients, who can check the mobile application for their medication history. The FDA has approved a DHFS system for aripiprazole, although this product is not yet widely available on the market. Like the smart pill box, however, a DHFS addresses nonadherence that may be primarily driven by cognitive challenges such as executive dysfunction or forgetfulness. Other factors such as volitional resistance or side effects can also be contributors. Hence, DHFS technology also requires clinician involvement to be effective, because clinicians can gather data from the DHFS while maintaining clinical context and addressing other factors that may be contributors (Rosenbaum 2018).

Robotics and Virtual Reality

The ability of technology to imitate and reproduce real-life experiences is meaningful in geriatric psychiatry, where patients may have deficits in mobility and be unable to participate in many activities because of physical limitations. Animal-like robots have become a potential alternative to animal-assisted therapies for older residents, particularly those in long-term care facilities, and virtual reality has emerged as a technology with endless capabilities for diagnostic assessments, interventions, and therapy.

Animal-like robots may improve mood, encourage physical activity, reduce stress, and promote social contact and communication (Jung et al. 2017). A robotic seal called PARO has been investigated as a companion for patients with dementia residing in long-term care and assisted living facilities. A handful of studies have investigated the effects of brief, nonfacilitated sessions with PARO compared with usual care on measures of agitation and sleep in patients with dementia but have found only small reductions in daytime and nighttime motor activity with the PARO intervention (Moyle et al. 2018). Unstructured interventions, however, may be less effective than facilitated interventions such as those used in animal-assisted therapy. Although free interaction with PARO may distract patients from negative moods, facilitated interaction may be more effective at promoting social contact between patients and between patients and the care team. Finally, there is an emphasis on avoiding a toylike appearance for these robots, because that may result in feelings of infantilization (Jung et al. 2017).

Service robots have also been emerging as a platform for care, although attitudes about their use vary. Although they were employed in the care of older adults prior to the COVID-19 pandemic, their use has since diversified and expanded (Ozturkcan and Merdin-Uygur 2021). Examples include disinfecting public spaces, dispensing prescriptions, and allowing health care worker telepresence and nursing home socializing. In mental health care, some barriers exist, including the perception of robots in relation to their human-likeness, especially in the case of social robots, which can have applications for emotional targets, such as loneliness (Ozturkcan and Merdin-Uygur 2021; Sekhon et al. 2021). To understand the full potential and applications of humanoid robots, a deeper understanding of needs for and attitudes toward robots is indicated.

Virtual reality (VR) provides another opportunity for older adults to interact with a world or environment not usually accessible to them. VR systems have been most heavily studied in dementia populations, although there is some evidence for their use in PTSD. Navigation and memorization tasks embedded in a virtual environment may be able to detect cognitive deficits in spatial cognition and memory earlier than standard assessments because of VR's enhanced ecological validity. It can be used as a training intervention to improve cognitive skills or ability to perform activities of daily living, such as cooking, driving, or shopping (García-Betances et al. 2015). Additionally, VR can be used to deliver traditional therapeutic interventions, such as exposure therapy, in a virtual environment. Virtual reality exposure therapy may be as effective as exposure in imagination therapy in reducing depression and anxiety (Gamito et al. 2010). Overall, however, there is less evidence for VR use in domains of psychopathology other than dementia and cognitive impairment.

Electronic Health Records

Originally developed in the 1960s, EHR systems have only become standard practice in recent years (Atherton 2011). EHRs allow for more efficient storage and communication of health information, and, with effort, they can move us into a new age of connected and coordinated medical care. Additionally, novel data-processing algorithms can be applied to the clinical information in EHRs to gather population-level data and extract information from a larger number of patients than would have been possible with paper records.

Geriatric patients often present with highly complex clinical pictures and tend to be heavy users of general care and specialty services. Care coordination across providers within a patient's care team is especially important for patients with four or more chronic conditions, which is likely to be most of the geriatric patient population (Burton et al. 2004). For this reason, geriatric patients may benefit most from increased care coordination using EHR systems. Care coordination has been split into three concrete dimensions for empirical study: timely access to complete information, treatment goal agreement, and role/responsibility agreement. A study of primary care clinicians and EHR use showed that those with ≥6 months of EHR use reported more timely access to complete information and more treatment goal agreement with other clinicians compared with clinicians not using an EHR and with those who had <6 months of EHR use (Graetz et al. 2009). Although EHR systems aggregate and consolidate patients' medical information, their benefits cannot be realized immediately, as suggested by the previously mentioned data, nor without effort on behalf of the clinician.

The broad implementation of EHRs has not come without some resistance and barriers. First, the standardization of clinical information is necessary for communication between clinicians. One effort to address this barrier has been the development of the Continuity of Care Record (CCR), which provides a snapshot of the most relevant information about a patient. The CCR was developed as a national standard to facilitate information exchange during referrals so that the new provider understands the patient's status and reason for referral. However, a second and potentially more difficult barrier to address is the willingness and readiness of clinicians to use the EHR in their daily practice. The decision to adopt an EHR system comes with a significant up-front cost for implementing the technology and training staff, both clinicians and administrators, to use it most effectively. Additionally, clinicians' perceptions of the existing levels of care coordination may influence how valuable they perceive the EHR to be and therefore influence their willingness to learn how to use it (Burton et al. 2004).

An additional benefit of storing clinical information in an EHR is the ability to analyze and work with data in a way not feasible with paper records. Natural language processing, which involves the use of machine learning to extract information from written or spoken language, can be applied to EHRs. They contain both structured fields for storing information, such as ICD diagnostic codes, and free text fields for providers to input clinical notes. However, the geriatric population often experiences adverse health issues not captured by structured EHR fields because they do not fit into a specific diagnostic category. These issues can be referred to as "geriatric syndromes" and include common problems such as falls, malnutrition, dementia, urinary incontinence, or lack of social support. Natural language processing may be able to analyze clinical notes from free text fields and extract geriatric-specific health data, which can eventually contribute to risk stratification models for the geriatric population. Practice with identifying geriatric syndromes can also inform models of extra, nonclinical information from EHRs, such as social determinants of health (Chen et al. 2019).

The use of EHRs is increasingly being mandated and accompanied by payer incentives, yet a growing body of literature indicates that challenges such as poor cross-communication between EHR systems, heavier burdens of documentation, and functional inefficiency may be contributing to breakdowns in care and physician burnout.

Technology Policy in Geriatric Psychiatry

A major barrier to implementing new technologies in geriatric psychiatry is the willingness of insurance companies, Medicaid, and Medicare to reimburse for services, especially telepsychiatry. Currently, private insurance covers telemedicine in only 32 states. In 48 states, Medicaid programs will reimburse for only some telepsychiatry services, and Medicare only reimburses for telepsychiatry services if the community is considered rural (American Psychiatric Association 2020). Expanding reimbursement for telepsychiatry across all states and communities would greatly benefit older adults, even those who live in more urban areas and are mobility deficient. A 2019 bill introduced in the U.S. House of Representatives seeks to allow providers to be reimbursed by Medicare for mental health care services conducted using telemedicine. This bill, called the Mental Health Telemedicine Expansion Act, would require the patient and provider to have had an in-person assessment of need for the services before beginning telemedicine for the services to be covered. Although one visit does not appear to be a great barrier, it still presents a barrier to care (Wicklund 2019).

Policy support could overcome barriers to care, as exemplified early on during the COVID-19 pandemic when the relaxation of Health Insurance Portability and Accountability Act (HIPAA) restrictions on nonsecure videoconferencing platforms was issued. Further policy change with regard to supporting and training clinicians in using such platforms to enhance psychotherapy would be beneficial in further improving access to care (Torous and Wykes 2020). In addition, designing methods for patient support in using videoconferencing platforms would further enable this medium. Providing guidance for patients, especially within the geriatric population, could offer tools to overcome barriers to access as well. Patients with less technology fluency could gain technical abilities with using videoconferencing platforms through staff assistance. Developing standardized methods for patient guidance in platforms that eventually become conventionally used or authorizing use of widespread platforms with which patients may already have experience would streamline and accelerate the process of meeting the needs of the geriatric population.

Ethics and Privacy

The rise of the digital era at the turn of this century succeeded foremost in pushing the boundaries of communication. Digitization meant the sharing of information at a breakneck speed—megabytes of data could be sent and received in a matter of seconds—and the storage of vast amounts of data. There was even a certain automation to the design that added layers of efficiency to the digital space. Despite this revolutionary shift, certain sectors have been slower than others in joining the movement. The health care industry has largely continued to rely on an offline work flow in accordance with HIPAA laws, which were also ratified at the turn of the century. As the computer and technological interventions grow in popularity, however, it has become apparent that HIPAA needs to clearly outline the boundaries for this new technology in health care. In the following sections we broadly explore the principles that frame personal health information (PHI) in conducting research, with a special emphasis on vulnerable, older adult patients. We also outline the process for obtaining informed consent from older adults for the collection and protection of PHI and assessing the risks versus benefits of emergent technology in the digital age. Last, we elaborate on further considerations that various stakeholders must address to help this field realize its full potential.

Personal Health Information and Research

PHI is identifying information, but not all identifying information is PHI. According to the U.S. Department of Health and Human Services, data are only classified as PHI if they are tied to an individual's health information. For example, although individuals' name, age, address, and phone number may identify them, these would not be considered PHI unless that information is also tied to the individuals' medical history (U.S. Department of Health and Human Services 2015). Three ethical principles can guide the decision-making framework that dictates the ways in which PHI may be collected, used, shared, and stored for research: respect for persons, beneficence, and justice. These principles highlight four considerations in digital health: privacy, the assessment of risk and benefit, access and usability, and data management (Nebeker et al. 2019). In the following section, we focus on privacy and risk and benefit in the context of conducting research in the vulnerable older adult population.

Ethical Principles of Conducting Research

In 2002, the federal government ratified the HIPAA Privacy Rule with the aim of protecting patient confidentiality while optimizing data sharing between covered entities and business associates. Covered entities include individuals or institutions directly involved in the provision of health care—whether that be treatments, payments, or administrative operations. Business associates are third-party vendors authorized to receive and use PHI. Broadly, three domains fall under protected information according to these privacy laws (HIPAA Journal 2020):

1. A patient's present or past physical or mental status
2. The health treatments and services a patient is rendered
3. Any payment made for the provision of health treatments or services

If PHI is protected by HIPAA, how may health data be used for purposes beyond the treatment of an individual, such as in research, marketing, and public health communication? Two conditions permit health data to move from the private to the public sphere: informed consent and deidentification.

During the informed consent process, patients are asked to give permission for their health information to be used for a particular purpose, such as research. Patients must fully understand why their data are being collected, used, and shared. Once consent is given, all information conveyed to the public must be deidentified. Deidentification strips the health data of any identifying information to protect patient privacy. There are two methods in the HIPAA Privacy Rule for achieving deidentification: expert determination and safe harbor. In the former method, an expert who is a covered entity determines and documents whether the health information in question is identifiable. The latter method involves removing 18 different identifying tags from PHI, including name, address, email, medical record number, photographs, and license numbers. Once PHI has been deidentified, it is no longer considered PHI and has lost the protection of the Privacy Rule. Although clinicians may not consider deidentification protocols in the course of routine care, these must be considered carefully in scenarios in which clinicians may be recommending the use of an application. Clinicians must also be aware of privacy risks that may exist with applications that patients may be using on their own and inform patients accordingly.

Conducting Digital Health Research in the Older Adult Population

Regarding digital health research, the issue of obtaining informed consent is particularly complex when working with vulnerable populations such as older adults. Aging may wear down an elderly person's capacity to give informed, meaningful, and voluntary consent. Therefore, researchers must affirm a patient's capacity. In severe cases of impairment, a health care proxy or legally authorized guardian may be needed to give consent on behalf of the patient, and the patient may only be able to deny *assent*. The underlying rationale for these considerations is to prevent coercion, safeguard privacy, and retain the highest possible autonomy of older adults.

In addition to privacy, it is necessary to consider the risk versus benefit of doing research with older adults. Research is voluntary and not clinical treatment. Patients participating in research must understand that outcomes are not guaranteed and, in blinded studies, the intervention is not guaranteed. In the case of technological research tools that capture new types of data inaccessible to traditional tools, patients must be informed of what data are being captured and how the data are being used, shared, and stored. Technology developed for treatment interventions must display a level of evidence to support safety, feasibility, and efficacy before patients can give meaningful consent. In research using emergent health technologies and tools, potential benefits must outweigh risks.

Further Consideration for Stakeholders

Implicit in the evaluation of risks and benefits in research protocols is an understanding of what those risks are. Although new technologies promise the potential for individualized care, improved diagnostics, and novel treatments, the laws and regulations around these new technologies remain largely underdeveloped. This deficit impacts both patients and researchers. For patient participants, there is no ethical standard for how technologies may use their data; for researchers, this lack of an ethical standard may lead to research misconduct if protocols do not take adequate steps to protect subjects (Pagoto and Nebeker 2019). The question remains: Who creates the ethical infrastructure to guide research of technological tools? Stakeholders must grapple with this issue before new health technologies are deployed in hospitals and clinics.

A New Geriatric Psychiatry

As a field, geriatric psychiatry has always reckoned with the fact that much of what is considered the norm in psychiatry simply does not apply to older adults. The criteria laid out in DSM-5 (American Psychiatric Association 2013) for several disorders may not accurately reflect the clinical presentation commonly seen. For example, major depressive disorder may be underdiagnosed in late life because older adults tend to have predominantly subsyndromal depressive symptoms, but this is not adequately characterized in DSM-5. However, newer technologies are enabling the assessment of each criterion listed in DSM independently and longitudinally with a greater density of data than was previously possible (Bader et al. 2020). This will facilitate a much more precision-based approach and enable us to overcome deficiencies in standardized diagnostic criteria. Although we anticipate that it will be several years, if not decades, before such technologically facilitated diagnosis and prognostic monitoring becomes the standard of care, in many ways adoption of this technology has begun already. Clinicians frequently use commercial wearable fitness monitors to track patients' sleep and assess the sedative impact of medications.

We also anticipate that technologies will begin to provide solutions to more complex challenges in late life, such as isolation, loneliness, frailty, and the need for more continuous monitoring for the most impaired older adults with late-stage dementia. The care of older adults is one of the primary drivers of increasing health care costs, and we anticipate that a new geriatric psychiatry will incorporate more technologies that can address these complex challenges, improve outcomes, and reduce the cost of care. The COVID-19 pandemic has accelerated the adoption of these new tools on the heels of scaled adoption of telemedicine. In this section, we project out new models of care and management approaches currently in proof-of-concept stage that may be adopted more widely over the forthcoming years or decades.

Integration of Clinical Assessment and Digital Information

Currently, clinicians rely on an in-person examination of their patients along with collateral information typically gathered by talking to family members or other providers or obtained from medical records. However, with aspects of our lives and our interactions happening digitally in larger and larger amounts, a body of digital collateral information will increasingly become accessible to clinicians, and this will be a factor in how diagnoses are made and care prognosis is monitored.

Incorporating Technologies Into Psychotherapy

With a growing demand for supportive and evidence-based manualized psychotherapies and a growing realization that these therapies can effectively be delivered via telemedicine, we anticipate that the next wave in the evolution of psychotherapy will be the incorporation of digital tools such as applications and chatbots into therapy. Available evidence demonstrates that these tools are most effective when supported by an actual clinician and are not meant to be used as substitutes for an actual therapist. However, they afford significantly wider access to therapy, even across borders, and provide real-time care and support. Many unanswered questions remain around the use of these tools in therapy, but we expect that as these questions are answered, digitally augmented psychotherapy for older adults will become more common.

Digital Connectivity to Target Isolation and Loneliness

Already, the arrival of digitally driven services such as ridesharing and the home delivery of groceries and essential supplies has allowed older adults with ambulation challenges and the inability to drive to obtain essential goods and services without relying on external supports. We anticipate that this digitally driven service industry will continue to grow. In addition, video-based communication platforms and, potentially, augmented and VR platforms may facilitate the creation of new modes of connectivity and interaction in which better integration of virtual and real environments will reduce limitations of physical distance by enhancing virtual presence.

Robotics-Based Support and Care

With an increasing need for care and support, especially for older adults with dementia, models of care have evolved toward either assisted living or more expensive and greater in-home support, much of which can lead to increased costs of care. Although the application of robotics to the care of older adults is in its infancy, there is a growing body of evidence around the use of the robot seal PARO, and other robotics-based approaches can serve a broad range of functions, from being a platform for virtual presence to aiding motility and fall prevention. We anticipate that with the population of older adults poised to grow, robotics will gain a more prominent role in aging care.

Conclusion

Changes in geriatric psychiatry follow the pattern of broader social changes and are occurring simultaneously with an increase in the digitalization of everyday life. The COVID-19 pandemic has likely accelerated this process. Although complex challenges must be overcome before most technologies can be considered the standard of care, the availability of digital tools for diagnostics, monitoring, and treatment delivery is already leading to a significant paradigm shift. Challenges in technology adoption and issues of privacy notwithstanding, we believe that geriatrics serves as a floor for how widely these technologies can be deployed, and, for certain technology such as passive sensing, geriatrics may even serve as the ceiling. With greater availability and wider use of technology, we expect that medical education and residency training, as well as clinical practice, will adopt more digital approaches, and these in turn will allow for more personalized, more accessible, and more equitably distributed care for older adults not just in the United States but worldwide.

Key Points

- There is a clear upward trend in the use of technologies to support the current standard of geriatric mental health care.

- The use of technology, including social media, mobile technologies, and wearables for older adults, has significantly increased in the past decade and provides a foundation for diagnostic and therapeutic targets.

- Digital phenotyping, which has been defined as "moment-by-moment quantification of the individual-level human phenotype in situ using data from personal digital devices," complements traditional methods of diagnosis.

- Wearables and noncontact prototype devices allow the passive, continuous collection of ecologically valid data.

- The uses of mobile application technologies are broad, and they can be platforms through which diagnosis and interventions can be delivered.

- The roles of robotics and virtual reality in intervention are expanding but require closer evaluation.

- Given the unique benefits and challenges within the geriatric population, the role of telemedicine in the care of older adults can be expanded with further investigation into building effective infrastructure.

- Telemedicine reimbursement is a great barrier to care that could be overcome by policy support. The Mental Health Telemedicine Expansion Act is under consideration at the time of this writing.

- Ethical concerns, including privacy and policy implications, are important to review as related to the broad-scale mental health application of technology.

Suggested Readings

Bader CS, Skurla M, Vahia IV: Technology in the assessment, treatment, and management of depression. Harv Rev Psychiatry 28(1):60–66, 2020

Cain AE, Depp CA, Jeste DV: Ecological momentary assessment in aging research: a critical review. J Psychiatr Res 43(11):987–996, 2009 19272611

Collier S, Monette P, Hobbs K, et al: Mapping movement: applying motion measurement technologies to the psychiatric care of older adults. Curr Psychiatry Rep 20(8):64, 2018

Husebo BS, Heintz HL, Berge LI, et al: Sensing technology to monitor behavioral and psychological symptoms and to assess treatment response in people with dementia. a systematic review. Front Pharmacol 10:1699, 2020

Narasimha S, Madathil KC, Agnisarman S, et al: Designing telemedicine systems for geriatric patients: a review of the usability studies. Telemed J E Health 23(6):459–472, 2017

Onnela JP, Rauch SL: Harnessing smartphone-based digital phenotyping to enhance behavioral and mental health. Neuropsychopharmacology 41(7):1691–1696, 2016

Vahia IV, Ressler KJ: Beyond the buzz: the maturing of technology use in geriatric psychiatry. Am J Geriatr Psychiatry 25(8):815–818, 2017

Vahia IV, Jeste DV, Reynolds CF: Older adults and the mental health effects of COVID-19. JAMA 324(22):2253–2254, 2020

Vahia IV, Kabelac Z, Hsu C-Y, et al: Radio signal sensing and signal processing to monitor behavioral symptoms in dementia: a case study. Am J Geriatr Psychiatry 28(8):820–825, 2020

References

Adrien BA, Kim HJ, Cray HV, et al: Training older adults to use telemedicine for mental health may have limited impact. Am J Geriatr Psychiatry 2021 34176731 Epub ahead of print

Au-Yeung WM, Miller L, Beattie Z, et al: Monitoring behaviors of patients with late-stage dementia using passive environmental sensing approaches: a case series. Am J Geriatr Psychiatry 2021 34039534 Epub ahead of print

Alexander NB, Mollo JM, Giordani B, et al: Maintenance of balance, gait patterns, and obstacle clearance in Alzheimer's disease. Neurology 45(5):908–914, 1995 7746405

American Psychiatric Association: Diagnostic and Statistical Manual of Mental Disorders, 5th Edition. Arlington, VA, American Psychiatric Association, 2013

American Psychiatric Association: Position Statement on Telemedicine in Psychiatry. Washington, DC, American Psychiatric Association, July 2018. Available at: https://www.psychiatry.org/File%20Library/About-APA/Organization-Documents-Policies/Policies/Position-2018-Telemedicine-in-Psychiatry.pdf. Accessed August 5, 2020.

American Psychiatric Association: What Is Telepsychiatry? Washington, DC, American Psychiatric Association, 2020. Available at: https://www.psychiatry.org/patients-families/what-is-telepsychiatry. Accessed August 5, 2020.

Anderson M, Perrin A: Tech adoption climbs among older adults. Pew Research Center, May 17, 2017

Asselbergs J, Ruwaard J, Ejdys M, et al: Mobile phone-based unobtrusive ecological momentary assessment of day-to-day mood: an explorative study. J Med Internet Res 18(3):e72, 2016

Atherton J: Development of the electronic health record. Virtual Mentor 13(3):186–189, 2011

Bader CS, Skurla M, Vahia IV: Technology in the assessment, treatment, and management of depression. Harv Rev Psychiatry 28(1):60–66, 2020 31913982

Bateson AD, Baseler HA, Paulson KS, et al: Categorisation of mobile EEG: a researcher's perspective. BioMed Res Int 2017:5496196, 2017 29349078

Ben-Zeev D, Young MA: Accuracy of hospitalized depressed patients? and healthy controls? retrospective symptom reports: an experience sampling study. J Nerv Ment Dis 198(4):280–285, 2010 20386257

Ben-Zeev D, Scherer EA, Wang R, et al: Next-generation psychiatric assessment: Using smartphone sensors to monitor behavior and mental health. Psychiatr Rehabil J 38(3):218–226, 2015 25844912

Burton LC, Anderson GF, Kues IW: Using electronic health records to help coordinate care. Milbank Q 82(3):457–481, 2004 15330973

Cain AE, Depp CA, Jeste DV: Ecological momentary assessment in aging research: a critical review. J Psychiatr Res 43(11):987–996, 2009 19272611

Chase JG, Starfinger C, Lam Z, et al: Quantifying agitation in sedated ICU patients using heart rate and blood pressure. Physiol Meas 25(4):1037–1051, 2004 15382840

Chen KY, Bassett DR Jr: The technology of accelerometry-based activity monitors: current and future. Med Sci Sports Exerc 37(11 suppl):S490–S500, 2005 16294112

Chen T, Dredze M, Weiner JP, et al: Extraction of geriatric syndromes from electronic health record clinical notes: assessment of statistical natural language processing methods. JMIR Med Inform 7(1):e13039, 2019 30862607

Chi YM, Cauwenberghs G: Wireless non-contact EEG/ECG electrodes for body sensor networks, in 2010 International Conference on Body Sensor Networks. IEEE, 2010, pp 297–301

Folstein MF, Folstein SE, McHugh PR: "Mini-mental state": a practical method for grading the cognitive state of patients for the clinician. J Psychiatr Res 12(3):189–198, 1975 1202204

Fortuna KL, Lohman MC, Gill LE, et al: Adapting a psychosocial intervention for smartphone delivery to middle-aged and older adults with serious mental illness. Am J Geriatr Psychiatry 25(8):819–828, 2017 28169129

Gamito P, Oliveira J, Rosa P, et al: PTSD elderly war veterans: a clinical controlled pilot study. Cyberpsychol Behav Soc Netw 13(1):43–48, 2010

García-Betances RI, Arredondo Waldmeyer MT, Fico G, Cabrera-Umpiérrez MF: A succinct overview of virtual reality technology use in Alzheimer's disease. Front Aging Neurosci 7:80, 2015 26029101

Gould CE, Hantke NC: Promoting technology and virtual visits to improve older adult mental health in the face of COVID-19. Am J Geriatr Psychiatry 28(8):889–890, 2020 32425468

Graetz I, Reed M, Rundall T, et al: Care coordination and electronic health records: connecting clinicians. AMIA Annu Symp Proc 2009:208–212, 2009

Guimond S, Keshavan MS, Torous JB: Towards remote digital phenotyping of cognition in schizophrenia. Schizophr Res 208:36–38, 2019 31047724

Guntuku SC, Ramsay JR, Merchant RM, Ungar LH: Language of ADHD in adults on social media. J Atten Disord 23(12):1475–1485, 2019 29115168

Harerimana B, Forchuk C, O'Regan T: The use of technology for mental healthcare delivery among older adults with depressive symptoms: a systematic literature review. Int J Ment Health Nurs 28(3):657–670, 2019 30666762

Hawkes E, Heintz H, Vahia IV: Digitally enhanced art therapy and mindfulness in older adults. Am J Geriatr Psychiatry 28(4):495–496, 2020

Hinrichs H, Scholz M, Baum AK, et al: Comparison between a wireless dry electrode EEG system with a conventional wired wet electrode EEG system for clinical applications. Sci Rep 10(1):5218, 2020 32251333

HIPAA Journal: HIPAA Privacy Laws. HIPAA Journal. Available at: https://www.hipaajournal.com/hipaa-privacy-laws. Accessed August 5, 2020.

Hobbs KW, Monette PJ, Owoyemi P, et al: Incorporating information from electronic and social media into psychiatric and psychotherapeutic patient care: survey among clinicians. J Med Internet Res 21(7):e13218, 2019 31301127

Hsu Y-L, Chung P-C, Wang W-H, et al: Gait and balance analysis for patients with Alzheimer's disease using an inertial-sensor-based wearable instrument. IEEE J Biomed Health Inform 18(6):1822–1830, 2014 25375679

Huguet A, Rao S, McGrath PJ, et al: A systematic review of cognitive behavioral therapy and behavioral activation apps for depression. PLoS One 11(5):e0154248, 2016 27135410

Jongstra S, Wijsman LW, Cachucho R, et al: Cognitive testing in people at increased risk of dementia using a smartphone app: the iVitality Proof-of-Principle Study. JMIR Mhealth Uhealth 5(5):e68, 2017 28546139

Jung MM, van der Leij L, Kelders SM: An exploration of the benefits of an animallike robot companion with more advanced touch interaction capabilities for dementia care. Front ICT 4:16, 2017

Kam JWY, Griffin S, Shen A, et al: Systematic comparison between a wireless EEG system with dry electrodes and a wired EEG system with wet electrodes. Neuroimage 184:119–129, 2019 30218769

Kim H, Lee S, Lee S, et al: Depression prediction by using ecological momentary assessment, actiwatch data, and machine learning: observational study on older adults living alone. JMIR Mhealth Uhealth 7(10):e14149, 2019

Komatsu H, Sekine Y, Okamura N, et al: Effectiveness of information technology aided relapse prevention programme in schizophrenia excluding the effect of user adherence: a randomized controlled trial. Schizophr Res 150(1):240–244, 2013 23998952

Kortelainen JM, Mendez MO, Bianchi AM: Sleep staging based on signals based on signals acquired through bed sensor. IEEE Transactions on Information Technology in Biomedicine 14(3):776–785, 2010

Kroll L, Böhning N, Müßigbrodt H, et al: Non-contact monitoring of agitation and use of a sheltering device in patients with dementia in emergency departments: a feasibility study. BMC Psychiatry 20(1):165, 2020 32295567

Lauderdale DS, Philip Schumm L, Kurina LM, et al: Assessment of sleep in the National Social Life, Health, and Aging Project. J Gerontol B Psychol Sci Soc Sci 69(suppl 2):S125–S133, 2014

Lin CT, Liao LD, Liu YH, et al: Novel dry polymer foam electrodes for long-term EEG measurement. IEEE Trans Biomed Eng 58(5):1200–1207, 2011 21193371

Lui JHL, Marcus DK, Barry CT: Evidence-based apps? A review of mental health mobile applications in a psychotherapy context. Prof Psychol Res Pr 48(3):199–210, 2017

Makdissi M, Collie A, Maruff P, et al: Computerised cognitive assessment of concussed Australian Rules footballers. Br J Sports Med 35(5):354–360, 2001 11579074

Maruff P, Thomas E, Cysique L, et al: Validity of the CogState brief battery: relationship to standardized tests and sensitivity to cognitive impairment in mild traumatic brain injury, schizophrenia, and AIDS dementia complex. Arch Clin Neuropsychol 24(2):165–178, 2009

Matthews CE, Hagströmer M, Pober DM, Bowles HR: Best practices for using physical activity monitors in population-based research. Med Sci Sports Exerc 44(1 suppl 1):S68–S76, 2012

McClain C, Vogels E, Perrin A, et al: The internet and the pandemic (online). Washington, DC, Pew Research Center, September 1, 2021. Available at: https://www.pewresearch.org/internet/2021/09/01/the-internet-and-the-pandemic. Accessed November 8, 2021.

McDowell K, Lin C-T, Oie KS, et al: Real-world neuroimaging technologies. IEEE Access 1:131–149, 2013

Morley JE: Telemedicine: coming to nursing homes in the near future. J Am Med Dir Assoc 17(1):1–3, 2016 26620072

Moyle W, Jones C, Murfield J, et al: Effect of a robotic seal on the motor activity and sleep patterns of older people with dementia, as measured by wearable technology: a cluster-randomised controlled trial. Maturitas 110:10–17, 2018 29563027

Mulvenna M, Gibson A, McCauley C, et al: Behavioural usage analysis of a reminiscing app for people living with dementia and their carers. Presented at the European Conference on Cognitive Ergonomics, Umea, Sweden, 2017

Narasimha S, Madathil KC, Agnisarman S, et al: Designing telemedicine systems for geriatric patients: a review of the usability studies. Telemed J E Health 23(6):459–472, 2017

Nebeker C, Torous J, Bartlett Ellis RJ: Building the case for actionable ethics in digital health research supported by artificial intelligence. BMC Med 17(1):137, 2019 31311535

Ng CL, Reaz MBI, Chowdhury MEH: A low noise capacitive electromyography monitoring system for remote healthcare applications. IEEE Sens J 20(6):3333–3342, 2020

Onnela J-P, Rauch SL: Harnessing smartphone-based digital phenotyping to enhance behavioral and mental health. Neuropsychopharmacology 41(7):1691–1696, 2016 26818126

Ozturkcan S, Merdin-Uygur E: Humanoid service robots: the future of healthcare? Journal of Information Technology Teaching Cases 2021. Available at: https://journals.sage-pub.com/doi/pdf/10.1177/20438869211003905. Accessed November 8, 2021.

Pagoto S, Nebeker C: How scientists can take the lead in establishing ethical practices for social media research. J Am Med Inform Assoc 26(4):311–313, 2019 30698793

Palmius N, Tsanas A, Saunders KEA, et al: Detecting bipolar depression from geographic location data. IEEE Trans Biomed Eng 64(8):1761–1771, 2017 28113247

Perry A, Tarrier N, Morriss R, et al: Randomised controlled trial of efficacy of teaching patients with bipolar disorder to identify early symptoms of relapse and obtain treatment. BMJ 318(7177):149–153, 1999 9888904

Pettersson AF, Olsson E, Wahlund L-O: Motor function in subjects with mild cognitive impairment and early Alzheimer's disease. Dement Geriatr Cogn Disord 19(5–6):299–304, 2005 15785030

Ramos-Ríos R, Mateos R, Lojo D, et al: Telepsychogeriatrics: a new horizon in the care of mental health problems in the elderly. Int Psychogeriatr 24(11):1708–1724, 2012 22687259

Rosenbaum L: Swallowing a spy: the potential uses of digital adherence monitoring. N Engl J Med 378(2):101–103, 2018 29281504

Sekhon H, Cray HV, Vahia IV: Robots in geriatric mental health: pipe dream or viable solution? Am J Geriatr Psychiatry 2021 Epub ahead of print

Shiffman S, Stone AA, Hufford MR: Ecological momentary assessment. Annu Rev Clin Psychol 4(1):1–32, 2008 18509902

Silva GE, Goodwin JL, Sherrill DL, et al: Relationship between reported and measured sleep times: the sleep heart health study (SHHS). J Clin Sleep Med 3(6):622–630, 2007 17993045

Smith RJ, Crutchley P, Schwartz HA, et al: Variations in Facebook posting patterns across validated patient health conditions: a prospective cohort study. J Med Internet Res 19(1):e7, 2017 28062392

Sposaro F, Danielson J, Tyson G: iWander: an Android application for dementia patients, in 2010 Annual International Conference of the IEEE Engineering in Medicine and Biology Society. IEEE, 2010, pp 3875–3878

Sun Y, Yu XB: Capacitive biopotential measurement for electrophysiological signal acquisition: a review. IEEE Sens J 16(9):2832–2853, 2016

Tan H-X, Tan H-P, Liang H: Technology-enabled medication adherence for seniors living in the community: experiences, lessons, and the road ahead, in Human Aspects of IT for the Aged Population: Applications in Health, Assistance, and Entertainment, Vol 10927. Edited by Zhou J, Salvendy G. Berlin, Springer, 2018, pp 127–141

Teo AR, Markwardt S, Hinton L: Using Skype to beat the blues: longitudinal data from a national representative sample. Am J Geriatr Psychiatry 27(3):254–262, 2019 30442532

Torous J, Wykes T: Opportunities from the coronavirus disease 2019 pandemic for transforming psychiatric care with telehealth. JAMA Psychiatry 77(12):1205–1206, 2020 32391857

Torous J, Kiang MV, Lorme J, Onnela JP: New tools for new research in psychiatry: a scalable and customizable platform to empower data driven smartphone research. JMIR Mental Health 3(2):e16, 2016

Troiano RP, Berrigan D, Dodd KW, et al: Physical activity in the United States measured by accelerometer. Med Sci Sports Exerc 40(1):181–188, 2008 18091006

Troiano RP, McClain JJ, Brychta RJ, Chen KY: Evolution of accelerometer methods for physical activity research. Br J Sports Med 48(13):1019–1023, 2014 24782483

Trull TJ, Ebner-Priemer U: Ambulatory assessment. Annu Rev Clin Psychol 9(1):151–176, 2013 23157450

U.S. Department of Health and Human Services: Guidance Regarding Methods for Deidentification of Protected Health Information in Accordance with the Health Insurance Portability and Accountability Act (HIPAA) Privacy Rule. Washington, DC, U.S. Department of Health and Human Services, 2015. Available at: https://www.hhs.gov/hipaa/for-professionals/privacy/special-topics/de-identification/index.html. Accessed August 5, 2020.

Vahia IV, Sewell DD: Late-life depression: a role for accelerometer technology in diagnosis and management. Am J Psychiatry 173(8):763–768, 2016 27477136

Vahia IV, Kabelac Z, Hsu C-Y, et al: Radio signal sensing and signal processing to monitor behavioral symptoms in dementia: a case study. Am J Geriatr Psychiatry 28(8):820–825, 2020 32245677

Velligan DI, DiCocco M, Bow-Thomas CC, et al: A brief cognitive assessment for use with schizophrenia patients in community clinics. Schizophr Res 71(2–3):273–283, 2004 15474898

Watkin L, Blanchard MR, Tookman A, Sampson EL: Prospective cohort study of adverse events in older people admitted to the acute general hospital: risk factors and the impact of dementia. Int J Geriatr Psychiatry 27(1):76–82, 2012 21360591

Wicklund E: Congress to try again on Medicare coverage for telemental health. MHealth Intelligence, March 7, 2019. Available at: https://mhealthintelligence.com/news/congress-to-try-again-on-medicare-coverage-for-telemental-health. Accessed August 5, 2020.

CHAPTER 26

Ethics in
Geriatric Mental Health

Daniel S. Kim, M.D.
Laura B. Dunn, M.D.

Although ethics are critical to the practice of all aspects and specialties in medicine—and ethics knowledge and skills are foundational to the comprehensive practices, professionalism, and identities of mental health professionals—the importance of ethics to the wise practice of geriatric mental health can hardly be overstated. Psychiatric and neurocognitive disorders affect the core aspects of being human (e.g., emotions, behaviors, thoughts, memories, insight, judgment). Disturbances in one or more of these aspects of a person's being can result, in various ways, in tensions among ethical principles. Older adults' strengths, vulnerabilities, needs, sociocultural characteristics, and relationships all factor into the ethical aspects of their care. Although many of the ethical issues encountered in geriatric psychiatry overlap with those commonly addressed in psychiatry, numerous issues are either unique to or occur more commonly in older adults. The ethical dilemmas and questions that arise in caring for the geriatric population are among the most complex challenges providers will face in their careers.

The unprecedented increase in the number of people with various forms of cognitive impairment—from mild cognitive impairment (MCI) to major neurocognitive disorders, including Alzheimer's disease (AD) and other dementias—is bringing a host of ethical dilemmas to the forefront of geriatric mental health. These issues appear in both clinical and research contexts and range from the nuances of obtaining meaningful informed consent to navigating the choppy waters of confidentiality to balancing ethical duties around beneficence, autonomy, and justice. The medical and psychiatric complexities that arise in geriatric mental health also bring ethical issues related to the end of life. Communicating disease prognosis, discussing goals of care, and helping patients and families cope with the unique challenges at the end of life may encompass a number of delicate ethical challenges for geriatric mental health providers.

Finally, other considerations that affect older adults and their loved ones—including ageism and stigma around mental illness and dementia—can influence, sometimes subtly and sometimes overtly, the perceptions and attitudes of patients about their illness and those of their families, medical providers, and other care providers. All of these factors bring added dimensions to any discussion of ethical issues in the care of older adults. Therefore, the objectives of this chapter are to

1. Provide an overview of the fundamental ethics knowledge and skills relevant to working with older adults in geriatric mental health contexts.
2. Discuss issues unique to older adults that have ethical implications.
3. Review concepts of and literature on decision-making capacity in older adults.
4. Describe important ethical considerations in the clinical care of older adults.
5. Discuss ethical aspects of research in geriatric mental health.

Ethics Knowledge and Skills in Geriatric Mental Health

Although the acquisition of a basic level of understanding of ethics concepts is assumed to be a fundamental part of the training of all medical and mental health professionals, the forms and content of this training vary widely. Most providers could likely cite the major ethics principles that are at the core of their professional ethical obligations, but it is less clear whether many would be able to describe the philosophical bases for these principles. Why is autonomy so important? Where does the notion of beneficence come from?

Understanding different theories of moral behavior—the basis of modern medical ethics—helps professionals apply the them and their attendant principles to address the challenges that they face in actual practice. Although a complete review of these theories is beyond the scope of this chapter, additional details can be found in the major texts of biomedical ethics (e.g., Beauchamp and Childress 2019; Jonsen 2008; O'Neill 2005). Geriatric mental health practitioners of all disciplines should be comprehensively trained not only in the core knowledge and competencies of their specific field but also in a set of essential ethical skills. As described in detail by Roberts (2016), these skills require not only initial instruction but also continuous attention, practice, and refinement over the course of a provider's career. These ethics skills can take on urgency and importance in the care of older adults with psychiatric and neurocognitive disorders. We describe and provide examples of each of these ethics skills in action.

First, the basic ability to identify ethical issues when they arise is vital to caring for older adults. This can take the form of an intuition—a sense that something is not right or a nagging worry that there may be more to the story. Paying attention to this sense, understanding what issues are at stake, taking the time to carefully examine the myriad potential contributing factors in the specific instance, and ultimately deciding on a course of action will almost always be the wisest path in caring for patients and can potentially be lifesaving. For example, consider the common scenario of an older adult who lives alone and continues to drive but has recently been noted by relatives and friends to be developing symptoms of cognitive impairment, and perhaps has gotten lost while driving or had one or two "fender benders" (i.e., seemingly small road accidents) that may be early indicators of decline in any of several cognitive domains. The alert clinician will need not only to consider what must be done in terms of a diagnostic workup, collateral information gathering, and functional skills assessment but also to be knowledgeable about under what circumstances and how to report the patient to the appropriate authorities, how to obtain further evaluation of the patient's driving skills, and how to discuss these issues with the patient and other involved persons. This scenario raises multiple ethically laden issues of patient autonomy, considerations of the public good, confidentiality, and legal responsibilities.

The second skill—the ability to appreciate the influence of one's own personally held values and beliefs on one's clinical approach and decision-making—can be illustrated by the case of a psychiatrist who is caring for an older adult with end-stage dementia and whose experiences with difficult end-of-life decision-making in her own family are affecting her ability to discuss all aspects of her patient's current situation openly with the patient's family. The influence of past experience on current behavior is often so ingrained that it may be difficult, in the moment, to understand and manage. This ethics skill, then, is something that astute providers are continuously monitoring at some level—and, ideally, can discuss with trusted colleagues.

The third skill—namely, having a clear-eyed perspective on one's own limitations in terms of knowledge, skills, and expertise—is obviously critical in all helping professions. However, in the case of psychiatry generally (National Council Medical Director Institute 2017)—and perhaps even more so in the special case of geriatric psychiatry (Juul et al. 2017)—the ongoing shortage of trained specialists may make this ethics skill even more challenging. For instance, when a provider is the only geriatric mental health specialist in the region, that provider may experience numerous pressures to care for patients whose needs the provider may feel underequipped to address. Recognizing that this is, in fact, an ethical issue is an important part of any decision about providing such care and can help the provider realize that he or she may need to consult with an appropriate colleague with the relevant expertise, do additional reading, or obtain additional training. Although resolving this kind of ethical dilemma is never easy, the essential skill of knowing one's limitations will help providers strike the most appropriate balance between trying to help the patient (beneficence) and ensuring that this help is not inadvertently harmful (nonmaleficence).

Identifying clinical situations likely to engender ethical issues (i.e., "high-risk situations") is the fourth essential ethics skill. Although these situations sometimes are readily apparent (e.g., the need for involuntary hospitalization of an imminently suicidal patient), in many other cases it can be more difficult to recognize the lurking ethical issues. In geriatric psychiatry, for example, family disagreement about the living situation or appropriate care of a patient with advanced dementia should be a signal that ethical considerations may be, or soon will become, critical to understand and address.

The fifth ethical skill is being willing and able to seek consultation, review ethics codes or guidelines, or otherwise gather additional knowledge, insights, or advice when dealing with an ethically challenging situation. In geriatric mental health, seeking expertise from a colleague or an expert in a given area may be necessary—even crucial—in particularly challenging cases. Obtaining guidance from colleagues, whether in the same or a related discipline, can be extremely useful. Legal expertise or consultation may also be needed at times, such as when a family is seeking to obtain guardianship of a patient.

Finally, proactively interweaving appropriate ethical safeguards into clinical or research activities is another crucial ethics skill. For example, informing patients and families at the outset of treatment about mandates to report elder abuse or neglect would be considered an ethical safeguard, as would having routine methods of obtaining and documenting informed consent for treatment (e.g., providing written and verbal information about black box warning for antipsychotics in dementia). Another common ethical safeguard that may be relatively neglected is informing patients and families about the limits of confidentiality for information that is documented in the electronic health record, particularly in the context of collaborative care and working within large health care organizations (Shenoy and Appel 2017). As psychiatry and mental health care continue to evolve, older adults and their families will benefit from clinicians who thoughtfully and skillfully navigate the ethical waters of emerging technologies and approaches.

Unique Aspects of Aging: Ethical Implications

The year 2010 marked the beginning of the "silver tsunami": the first of a growing wave of Baby Boomers—those born after World War II—to turn 65 years of age and officially join the ranks of senior citizens. With this growing cohort of older adults come added clinical and ethical challenges, imposed not only by increasing numbers but also by the unique cultural and demographic features of this large, distinctive generation of older adults. Although like most older adults the "Baby Boomers" are increasingly burdened with chronic health issues and functional limitations as they age, they may also have advantages over preceding generations. They tend to be more health care and technology savvy and less deferential to authority figures (including those in health care) and thus have higher expectations of "successful aging" (Rowe and Kahn 1987) as the new norm. Thus, the paternalistic approach of previous generations of clinicians seems particularly discordant when applied to this increasingly empowered geriatric population, who in principle appear ideally suited to the collaborative decisional process that is the reigning paradigm in patient care (Kahana et al. 2014)—a process contingent on identifying a patient's goals of care and dependent on intact decisional capacity and autonomy.

Nevertheless, although this newest cohort of older adults may particularly value their autonomy, they are still vulnerable to age-related clinical changes. Cognitive decline remains primarily a function of age and all too often is accompanied by the functional impairment that is a cardinal feature of dementia. Functional impairment may also be due to a decline in physical health and the accompanying limitations on independence that may require additional caregiver support. Finally, the increased psychosocial stressors of retirement, loss of loved ones, and other life transitions, as well as intrinsic physiological changes associated with later life, can contribute to significant psychiatric morbidity that may also increasingly limit an individual's independence late in life.

Meanwhile, practical remedies for these age-related ills (e.g., caregiver support, giving up driving, other safety measures) may be a particularly bitter pill for some older adults to swallow because of the potential conflict between other people's (including mental health professionals') goals of beneficence—to improve patients' health, safety, and quality of life—and the patients' goals of maintaining as much autonomy as possible. A state of autonomy implies that the person has capacity for self-governance and the agency to choose freely among a range of choices related to various domains of living. Autonomy is potentially jeopardized when the range of options is constrained or the agency to freely choose from that available range is unduly influenced by external factors. If, for example, a decline in physical health limits a person's driving abilities, beneficence may dictate curtailed driving despite the infringement on that person's independence. To take another example, the cognitive deficits or executive dysfunction associated with dementia or other neuropsychiatric conditions may limit a person's ability to weigh the risks and benefits of various health care choices—impairing his or her decisional capacity—and consequently beneficence may dictate designation of a proxy decision-maker.

Decision-Making and Older Adults

Capacity vs. Competency

Although the terms *autonomy*, *competency*, and *capacity* are often used interchangeably to address similar issues, they in theory address distinct components of the same overarching process. *Autonomy*, as noted, is the ethical principle that all individuals maintain the ability of self-government and agency. *Capacity* is the clinical assessment of a person's ability to weigh the various risks and benefits of a specific decision and make a choice based on their personal goals and life priorities. *Competency* is the legal construct that presumes a person is mentally capable of participating in a legal process or decision; the threshold of competency is determined by a legislature or court. Although the determination of competency is generally heavily influenced by a clinical assessment of capacity, at the end of the day it is strictly a legal determination.

Capacity to Make Medical Decisions

The assessment of a patient's medical decisional capacity is part and parcel of routine clinical care and is generally done informally, and often quite unconsciously. At times, however, the need for a formal evaluation is pressing, usually when there is a stark difference in opinion between the clinician and the patient regarding appropriate treatment. Such a difference in opinion would ideally not provoke a game of "heads I win, tails you lose" but rather would engender a sense of humility regarding the wide swath of human experiences and a sober consideration of the various reasons for such a difference in opinions, reasons ranging from different value systems to philosophical opposition to certain treatments to lastly—and most concerningly—a person's mental inability to make cogent decisions. It is strictly this last concern that should provoke the formal evaluation of an individual's decisional capacity and potential removal as decision-maker.

    The formal assessment of decisional capacity entails appraisal of four requisite abilities (known as the "Appelbaum criteria"): understanding (comprehension of relevant clinical information), appreciation (ability to relate clinical information to one's own circumstances), reasoning (ability to weigh information and reason through the consequences of a decision), and choice (ability to clearly and consistently communicate a decision) (Appelbaum and Grisso 1988). Understandably, the stringent application of this ideal model of decision-making may vary along a "sliding scale" depending on how routine or dire a clinical situation is or how safe or risky of a health care decision is needed. Thus, individuals with similar cognitive impairment may be adjudged to have differing levels of capacity—the assumption of their intact capacity might remain unchallenged—depending on the severity of their clinical condition and the relative risks versus benefits of the available treatment. For example, a treatment or procedure that has higher associated risk and clearer benefit, such as electroconvulsive therapy, would require a more rigorous evaluation for decisional capacity than an intervention with lower risk, such as engaging in psychotherapy.

Although older adults are more likely to be diagnosed with a neurodegenerative process or to experience serious sequelae from a neuropsychiatric disorder, such diagnoses do not, in and of themselves, determine incapacity. Patients with a formal diagnosis of dementia or serious mental illness such as schizophrenia, bipolar disorder, or severe depression may still possess decisional capacity regarding treatments ranging from pharmacotherapy to electroconvulsive therapy and interventions ranging from designating a health care power of attorney to psychiatric hospitalization. Although disease severity, age, and cognitive deficits may substantially impact patients' ability to make fully formed decisions about their psychiatric treatment, empirical evidence suggests that many people with severe mental illness continue to possess an intact ability to make informed treatment decisions (Okai et al. 2007).

Older adults' decisional capacity may fluctuate over time, however, so it is also crucial to conduct an ongoing series of decisional capacity assessments. Unfortunately, there is a dearth of studies examining the course of medical decision-making in older adults, making it difficult to predict when the threshold of decisional incapacity might be crossed. Okonkwo et al. (2008) addressed this information gap with a longitudinal examination of medical consent capacity in adults with MCI ($n=116$) and in healthy control subjects ($n=88$). Using the Capacity to Consent to Treatment Instrument (CCTI), an instrument that utilizes vignettes to assess decisional capacity, the authors noted a span of declining medical decision-making capacity over time in patients with MCI on the understanding component of decision-making capacity. However, these patients did not exhibit decrements over time on other components assessed by the CCTI. Notably, this decline in understanding accelerated as patients converted from MCI to AD.

Based on these findings and clinical observations, there appears to be a critical window during which consent capacity remains intact. For clinicians caring for patients with MCI and for their families, timely discussions of advance care planning and appointing surrogate decision-makers (i.e., options to consider proactively before or as the patient loses capacity) could be helpful, as could educating families about specific laws (which may vary by jurisdiction) regarding designating a surrogate decision-maker.

Decision Making for Sexual Activity and Intimacy

Another common dilemma associated with late life, particularly in long-term care facilities, involves sexuality and intimacy. Although ageist stereotypes may perpetuate a myth of the sexless lives of older adults, intimacy and sexuality remain a vital component of life for most older adults. The aging Baby Boomers, inculcated with the adage "make love not war" and reinvigorated by phosphodiesterase inhibitors such as sildenafil, may find that the long-term care facility provides ample opportunity to rediscover some of the hidden joys of communal living. However, sexual activity is not without risks for older adults. For one, older adults remain as vulnerable to sexual abuse as they do to other forms of abuse, and identifying sexual abuse can be challenging, particularly in the cognitively impaired older adult who may be unable to report such a crime or whose injuries might be attributed to physical vulnerabilities common in this population (Burgess and Phillips 2006). Another unexpected risk to many is sexually transmitted diseases (STDs). Compared with younger adults, older adults may not be as systematically screened for STDs by clinicians, who may be hesitant to raise these questions or who may assume that patients in this age group are not at risk. In addition, some older adults may be more reticent to discuss their sexual activity with their physician. Older adults may also be at higher risk because, given the absence of pregnancy, they are less likely to use condoms or to practice other forms of safe sex. This prophylactic lapse may have contributed to the Centers for Disease Control and Prevention finding in 2013 that people older than 55 years accounted for ~26% of the estimated 1.2 million people with HIV in the United States (Centers for Disease Control and Prevention 2017).

The risks of sexual activity are particularly fraught in older persons with cognitive impairment, who potentially lack the capacity to make informed choices regarding sexual intimacy, particularly in the long-term care setting where institutional priorities—and state legal standards—add an additional layer of complexity. Again, the central tension lies between the ethical principle of autonomy—respecting one's right to privately pursue physical intimacy and sexual activity—and beneficence—the need to protect a vulnerable person from nonconsensual sexual activity and harm. Arguably, the institutional tendency would be to err on the side of harm mitigation over individual autonomy, not only because of the risk of harm to the person but also because of the risk of family strife and potential litigation, particularly when the older person's autonomy is already diminished (Wilkins 2015). Yet this makes the objective, unbiased consideration of the older person's wishes and capacity to consent to sexual activity even more important to assess.

The American Bar Association and American Psychological Association (2008) coauthored guidelines on assessing patients' capacity for sexual consent. They suggested a balanced, interdisciplinary team approach, using multiple sources of information, including clinical interview to gather clinical data, determine sexual goals and values, and gauge decisional capacity; neuropsychological evaluation to determine cognitive status, including executive functioning; patient records to corroborate or expand on clinical data garnered from the clinical interview; and collateral sources of information such as family, friends, and caregivers to corroborate or expand on the person's relationship history, including sexual values and norms as well as daily behaviors, interactions, and relationships in long-term care. This capacity assessment should focus not only on identifying the patient's cognitive status and any clinical diagnoses that might affect judgment (e.g., bipolar disorder, impulse-control disorders), but also on the patient's awareness of the specific sexual activity in which he or she is choosing to engage and the parties with whom the patient is engaging in sexual activity, potential risks (e.g., STDs) associated with the activity being assessed, and whether the choice is free from undue influence or coercion.

Other Forms of Capacity: Living Independently, Financial Capacity, Driving

Geriatric mental health providers must also be versed in their legal and ethical obligations related to evaluating other domains of capacity in older adults. These include, for example, the capacity to live independently, to make financial decisions, to make or change one's will (i.e., testamentary capacity), and to drive. Because of the myriad medical and cognitive conditions that may compromise varied forms of decision-making, wise providers will understand that their role is to be alert to potential decrements in functional and decision-making abilities that may impair an older adult's capacity to function safely or effectively in a specific domain. It may be necessary to make referrals to other providers to do more comprehensive assessments of the specific abilities. Numerous screening and assessment tools are available to help providers assess these different domains, although it should be noted that with any assessment tool, clinical context and collateral information will often be needed in addition to the instrument itself.

The right to choose where and how one lives is fundamental to individuals' sense of dignity and freedom. Many older adults are fearful of losing their independence or of being placed against their will in an institutional setting; indeed, being able to live independently is among many older adults' primary life goals (Naik et al. 2005). Most would prefer to age in place (i.e., to continue to live as independently as possible in the community). Nursing homes and other residential care facilities are perceived by many older adults as placing numerous constraints and controls on their freedoms. These perceptions, although not always accurate, nevertheless are important to understand when assessing older adults' living situations. Therefore, geriatric mental health providers must not only be aware of the numerous medical, functional, and psychosocial dimensions of older adults' ability to live independently but also appreciate the ethical and legal aspects and consequences of losing this ability.

When assessing a person's capacity to live independently, there is no "gold standard" approach for determining this domain, although a variety of frameworks and methods have been proposed. Living independently requires a number of functional abilities—for example, the ability to plan (executive functioning), to execute appropriate judgment, and to navigate physical requirements in order to live safely. Therefore, assessment of a person's capacity to live independently necessitates a multidomain evaluative process that considers the individual's abilities to manage (either independently or with some level of assistance) both activities of daily living and instrumental activities of daily living, to provide for and maintain a safe home environment, to manage medical care, and to manage financial transactions using appropriate judgment (Naik et al. 2008). One model for this type of assessment process, described by Skelton et al. (2010), is the capacity assessment and intervention model, which includes a comprehensive geriatric assessment, use of several standardized assessment tools to assist in the evaluation of cognition and functional abilities, and an interdisciplinary team discussion of the findings and recommendations. This model illustrates the importance of gathering data and expertise from different kinds of providers (e.g., geriatrician, psychiatrist, psychologist or neuropsychologist, social worker, case manager) in order to develop as informed, judicious, and comprehensive an intervention plan as possible.

Financial capacity is one of the most important predictors of the ability to function independently, and impairments in financial capacity put older adults at risk of exploitation and major financial losses (Marson 2013). Financial capacity has been defined as "a medical-legal construct that represents the ability to independently manage one's financial affairs in a manner consistent with one's personal self-interest and values" (Marson 2013, p. 392). Risk factors for impaired financial capacity include neurodegenerative disorders, including MCI. Changes in financial skills, for example, were found to predict conversion from amnestic MCI to AD over 1 year of follow-up (Triebel et al. 2009). Various disorders common in late life may have differential effects on different subdomains of financial capacity. For example, patients with frontotemporal dementia may experience early declines in judgment that may affect their ability to wisely manage their money. In contrast, patients with MCI or early AD may forget to pay bills on time. When family members express concerns about an older adult's ability to manage finances, clinicians should be aware that this may be both a warning sign of worsening cognition and a flashing light indicating the need for enhanced ethical awareness.

As described by Marson (2013), clinicians should attend to the following five potential warning signs of declining financial capacity, noting that these should represent a change from the patient's prior level of functioning with regard to finances: 1) memory-related financial impairment (e.g., forgetting to pay bills); 2) disorganization, leading to misplacing important financial documents or missing important deadlines; 3) confusion, leading to impaired understanding of basic financial concepts that were previously understood (e.g., related to a mortgage or will); 4) math skills, manifesting as difficulty with basic daily financial tasks (e.g., calculating a tip); and 5) judgment, often showing up as poor decisions about investments or falling for financial schemes (e.g., "phishing" emails).

The ability to drive safely is another cherished marker of independence for many older adults. As with other forms of capacity, medical conditions (e.g., visual impairment and limited mobility) and cognitive impairment are risk factors for diminished driving ability. In addition, many older adults take medications that may contribute to diminished driving skills (e.g., reaction time). However, given that many older adults continue to drive safely, older age is not a de facto barrier to the capacity to drive. When concerns about driving are expressed by, for example, a patient's family members, the clinician should consider referral for additional testing (including on-road driver assessment or simulated driving conditions). Clinicians should also be aware of the specific legal obligations in their jurisdiction for reporting suspected impaired driving abilities and should consider their ethical duty to protect the patient (and in the case of driving, the public as well).

Appointment of Surrogate Decision-Makers

In cases in which an older adult is deemed through a legal process to lack decisional capacity—and thereby is legally incompetent—to make a specific decision or range of decisions, a surrogate or proxy decision-maker may be appointed to aid in navigating the various risks and potential benefits associated with any decision. Although the decision to designate a proxy decision-maker might be made with the best of intentions, such a step could nonetheless open the door for neglect, exploitation, and abuse—both financial and physical—of older adults by those who have been placed in a position of authority over them. Indeed, most U.S. states designate health care professionals as mandated reporters of potential abuse of older adults because this patient population is rightly deemed especially vulnerable to abuse, particularly—and unfortunately— by caregivers and legally designated proxy decision-makers (Aviv 2017).

The risk of abuse or neglect by a decision-maker may, in theory, be obviated by the designation of family members or other loved ones as the proxy decision-makers. Ideally, such a family member or loved one would also be the person who can best understand the patient's clinical situation and most clearly appreciate the patient's goals and values. Absent a court-appointed decision-maker or health care power of attorney document, most states have designated next of kin as decision-makers using various hierarchies of proximity to the person in question: typically, the person's spouse/domestic partner, then an adult child, a parent or a sibling, then possibly other relatives or close friends. If multiple parties have equal precedence (e.g., multiple adult children or multiple siblings) and a consensus decision is not achievable, then consultation with an institution's ethics committee would certainly be helpful; however, ultimately, a judicial review to determine the appropriate decision-maker may be necessary.

Unfortunately, the process for judicial designation of a proxy decision-maker—often labeled a "conservator" or "guardian"—is generally an onerous and lengthy one. Furthermore, once a conservatorship or guardianship has been enacted, it is often difficult to reverse, even after decisional capacity has been regained or even if next of kin disagree with decisions made by the conservator. This step should therefore be one of last resort if no other viable alternative is available. The far better option is to have a previously designated health care power of attorney, a legally documented decision by the person in question designating a specific proxy decision-maker for health care decisions. This document and designation are often paired with a living will or advance directive—a document outlining a person's health care preferences for end-of-life care or life-sustaining interventions, such as CPR, intubation and ventilation, or enteral (tube feeds) and parenteral (intravenous) nutrition. This not only allows individuals to explicitly designate the person (or persons) they think most capable to make health care decisions that accurately reflect their goals and values but also affords an opportunity for the frank discussion about these goals and values that all too often is avoided until it is too late. Prompting for such a discussion would ideally occur during routine longitudinal care provided by a person's primary health care clinician—the clinician who has the most robust relationship and most accurate clinical knowledge of the patient—and yet there, too, this conversation is often sidestepped until a health crisis or serious illness develops (Bernacki et al. 2014). Furthermore, delaying the conversation until it is compelled by a fraught situation may impede the sober discussion necessary to identify the goals and values that would ideally dictate the next steps in care.

The barriers to such a timely, sober discussion include practical challenges, such as time constraints in the primary care setting or a provider's lack of experience or education in conducting such a discussion, and more intangible concerns, such as a provider's fear of causing undue distress when the clinical need is not pressing (Bernacki et al. 2014). Yet an end-of-life discussion is unlikely to take happen without explicit prompting by a health care provider. Such a discussion affords the patient and clinician more than just an opportunity to identify an appropriate proxy decision-maker— thereby avoiding the legal complications of a court-appointed conservator; it also has clear clinical benefits. In a multisite longitudinal study by Wright et al. (2008), not only did timely discussion of end-of-life issues result in a marked decrease in unwanted end-of-life interventions such as ventilations, resuscitations, and intensive care unit (ICU) admissions but it also led to earlier and consequently longer enrollment in hospice—which is strongly correlated with higher patient quality of life—and decreased rates of major depressive disorder in bereaved caregivers.

On the opposite side of the spectrum of clinical challenges is the so-called unbefriended patient: the unknown, unrepresented, and incapacitated person with significant medical needs. Current estimates of the number of unbefriended patients in the United States vary widely, with studies in the ICU setting identifying numbers ranging from 5.5% to 16% (White et al. 2006). As the silver tsunami continues to crest, however, this challenging segment of the older adult population is forecast to increase in magnitude concomitantly. These patients frequently present with complications from chronic, often inadequately treated medical illnesses as well as comorbid psychiatric or neurocognitive disorders that contribute to their decisional incapacity. This challenge is made more dire when providers are confronted by a striking disconnect between the standard best-interests model of care—which inherently prioritizes long-term longevity over short-term discomfort—and a patient's apparent disagreement with such care. These challenging cases unavoidably provoke frustration and even helplessness in clinicians, which in turn could lead to errors in decision-making in terms of both over- and under-treating the patient. These errors are more likely absent a standardized approach to such cases, yet standards can vary widely from state to state and even county to county.

The American Geriatrics Society updated its position statement about unbefriended patients in 2016. They rightly noted that the best treatment for these patients is prophylactic: proactively identifying those at risk of becoming unbefriended and engaging them in both advance care planning and identifying surrogate decision-makers. Absent such foresight, however, the other necessary challenge to address remains the significant variation in legal standards and approaches to this population. The creation of a national legal standard in addressing unbefriended patients would obviate the ad hoc approach that unavoidably leaves clinicians vulnerable to errors in clinical decision-making and invariably lengthens the time necessary to make a consensus clinical decision. A systematic discussion of such cases ideally would include representatives from as wide an array of views as possible, particularly from those who may share the cultural background and values of the person in question, to ensure the best application of the standard best interests model of substituted decision-making in providing care to these patients (Farrell et al. 2017).

Ethical Issues in Clinical Care

Psychopharmacological Treatment

The central ethical tension in any treatment intervention is that between the principles of beneficence (the relief of suffering, enhancement of quality of life, and harm reduction to self or others) and nonmaleficence (avoiding harm). This tension is particularly evident with the use of psychopharmacological agents (i.e., antipsychotics, antidepressants, mood stabilizers, or sedative-hypnotics) in the cognitively impaired older adult. This population is uniquely vulnerable to a wide array of physical changes related to aging, as well as other age-related factors (e.g., diminished psychosocial support, functional impairment), and thus is more susceptible to medication-related side effects and adverse events.

All psychopharmacological agents are associated with potential side effects, some of which are highly risky or even fatal. Even medications generally considered quite safe, such as selective serotonin reuptake inhibitors, are associated with hyponatremia, decreased platelet aggregation, QT interval prolongation, and potentially higher risk of falls in older adults (Chemali et al. 2009). Other psychopharmacological agents such as antipsychotics are associated with even graver concerns and are labeled as such with an FDA black box warning that notes the increased risk of stroke and mortality associated with the use of antipsychotics in persons with dementia (Schneider et al. 2005). The primary use of psychopharmacological medications in this population is to address behavioral and psychological symptoms of dementia, which include behaviors such as agitation, aggression, sleep fragmentation, wandering, and resistance to care. Although use of psychotropic medications for these behaviors may have significant benefit for patients and their caregivers, their use remains off-label and therefore a form of clinical innovation. In this context, singular efforts should be undertaken not only to ensure that the anticipated benefits of a psychotropic medication outweigh the potential risks but also to ensure an optimal informed consent process is conducted with the patient or the surrogate decision-maker.

Autonomy is an ever-more-fragile ethical principle in this patient population that requires increasing efforts from both patient and provider to preserve. One must not presume that patients with mild to moderate stage of dementia, or even those with delirium, completely lack treatment decision-making capacity. Even when a patient has designated a surrogate decision-maker, constructive efforts to work with the cognitive strengths of the patient to maintain—as much as possible—the patient's autonomy remain an ethical imperative. These efforts might include steps such as repeated information sessions, use of visual materials, and presentation of information about proposed treatments and alternatives, including no intervention. In many circumstances, even in the context of an advanced neurocognitive disease, patients may still consent to certain aspects of their care (e.g., timing or format of medication) even if they are not fully capable of giving informed consent for treatment decisions. Adhering to the principle of autonomy in such circumstances reaffirms the importance of patients consenting to what they can as an ideal of clinical care.

Although progressive neurocognitive disorders presently do not have any disease-altering treatments, timely diagnosis nonetheless has considerable value. AD, for example, with a median survival after diagnosis of 4.2 years for males and 5.7 years for females (Larson et al. 2004) and an increasingly narrow window of decisional capacity, underscores the importance of diagnostic truth-telling (veracity) early in the care of patients with dementia. A timely discussion early in this progressive, irreversible illness allows the frank review of the patient's values and goals of care that is at the crux of ethically appropriate clinical care; it is the crucial step in maximizing the patient's autonomy in an illness that will ultimately end in the patient's decisional incapacity.

Polypharmacy is another all-too-common reality of late-life health care. Reduction in polypharmacy—*deprescribing*—can minimize harms by eliminating unnecessary or inappropriate medications, limiting side effects, decreasing drug–drug interactions, and reducing the pill burden that often contributes to nonadherence to necessary medications in older patients. The first critical step is identifying medications that may be inappropriate in this vulnerable population; resources such as the American Geriatrics Society's Beers Criteria can be helpful in this task (American Geriatrics Society 2015 Beers Criteria Update Expert Panel 2015). Next is the identification of "legacy prescriptions," medications initially prescribed for time-limited indications (e.g., proton pump inhibitors, bisphosphonates, antidepressants) (Mangin et al. 2018) that have been continued well past the period of intended treatment or that may have decreasing efficacy in a progressive illness. For example, given concerns for weight loss with cholinesterase inhibitors in patients with dementia, it is difficult to argue for maintaining these patients on these medications, particularly given the medications' overall modest benefit (Sheffrin et al. 2015). Last is the careful and judicious tapering and potential discontinuation of medications that are inappropriate or may have outlived their usefulness, keeping in mind the potential for discontinuation symptoms or resurgence of previously quiescent symptoms. Ongoing, thorough discussion and collaborative decision-making with the patient, if possible, as well as the family and proxy decision-makers, are critical throughout this process (Farrell and Mangin 2019).

End-of-Life Care

End-of-life care frequently becomes a nidus for ethical dilemmas. Geriatric mental health providers, regardless of their practice setting, should be familiar with these dilemmas and the growing evidence base that can inform patient and family decision-making. This is particularly important because research has shown that discussion of care preferences with patients—and documentation of those preferences in advance directives—is associated with lower rates of burdensome, painful, unwanted, or intrusive interventions at the end of life. For instance, compared with patients without advance directives, patients with severe dementia who had advance directives were less subject to aggressive end-of-life care, as evidenced by lower rates of in-hospital death and ICU stays (Nicholas et al. 2014).

Another example of a common ethical dilemma at the end of life is the issue of feeding and maintenance of basic nutrition. Many patients with moderate to severe cognitive impairment have difficulty maintaining weight due to reduced nutritional intake for multiple reasons, such as decreased appetite, early satiety, abdominal discomfort, or dysphagia. Despite this concern, placement of a permanent feeding tube is not recommended for patients with advanced dementia, even those with decreased nutrition and weight loss or those with dysphagia that may contribute to aspiration (Ganzini 2006). Studies have consistently shown that tube feeding does not prevent aspiration and may in fact increase the risk; furthermore, it has not been associated with weight gain or enhanced quality of life (Volicer and Simard 2015). On the contrary, tube feeding may cause greater discomfort and distress, which may lead to the increased use of physical or chemical restraints to maintain the feeding tube and to prevent medical complications from self-removal. A reduction in alertness and activity, greater social isolation, and worsened quality of life follow.

Until relatively recently, little was known about the clinical course and nature of care received at the end of life in patients with dementia. In the CASCADE study, a large prospective study of Boston-area nursing home residents ($N=323$ in 22 nursing homes) with advanced dementia conducted over 18 months, Mitchell et al. (2006) evaluated residents' clinical symptoms, complications, survival, and treatments. In addition—and of great ethical relevance—they assessed the understanding of the residents' health care proxies with respect to prognosis and expected clinical complications, assessed by a trained nurse interviewer. Some findings from this study are worth highlighting, because these findings should help inform how mental health professionals discuss dementia care with patients and their loved ones.

Among the residents followed, 55% died during the 18-month period (Mitchell et al. 2009). The 6-month mortality rate, adjusted for age, sex, and duration of disease, in residents who developed pneumonia was 47%; for residents who experienced a febrile episode, the corresponding mortality rate was 45%. Substantial proportions of patients experienced distressing symptoms at some point during the 18-month study period, as rated by their care providers; these symptoms included dyspnea (experienced by 46% of residents for ≥5 days per month), pain (39%), stage II or higher pressure ulcers (39%), agitation (54%), and aspiration (41%). Moreover, burdensome interventions (i.e., hospitalization, emergency department visits, parenteral therapy, or tube feeding) were common in the last 3 months of life, with 41% of residents who died having undergone at least one of these. One of the most important findings of this study, from an ethical perspective, was that in residents whose health care proxies understood the prognosis and expected clinical complications of advanced dementia, there was a significantly lower likelihood of burdensome interventions during the last 3 months of life compared with those whose proxies lacked this understanding. The study highlighted the need for greater attention to palliative care for persons with advanced dementia at the end of life.

Other studies have evaluated methods of conveying information about dementia to older adults in order to determine whether this information affected their preferences for different types of medical care. For example, in a randomized controlled trial that enrolled 200 older adults (≥65 years, mean age 75 years), Volandes et al. (2009) compared the effects of a verbal narrative describing advanced dementia ($n=106$) with the effects of the narrative plus a 2-minute video decision support tool on treatment preferences ($n=94$). The verbal description discussed the main characteristics of advanced dementia; the video showed an 80-year-old woman with dementia in a nursing home whose behaviors reflected these characteristics (i.e., inability to communicate, walk, or feed herself). In each condition, participants received the information about dementia and were asked their preferences for life-prolonging care (i.e., CPR, mechanical ventilation), limited care (i.e., hospitalization and antibiotics but not CPR), or comfort care (i.e., treatment to relieve symptoms). Findings included significant differences in the proportions of participants choosing the different categories of care. Specifically, among participants in the video-plus-narrative condition, 86% chose comfort care, 9% chose limited care, and 4% chose life-prolonging care. By comparison, in the narrative-alone condition, 64% opted for comfort care, 19% limited care, and 14% life-prolonging care. Higher education, greater health literacy, and being of white ethnicity were associated with a greater likelihood of choosing comfort care. These findings suggest that even the manner of conveying information about dementia may affect decision-making regarding the kinds of care that older adults would want for themselves in the future.

Physician-Assisted Suicide and Euthanasia

Physician-assisted suicide (PAS) and euthanasia have emerged during the past 15–20 years as important and contentious issues in medicine generally. Although these issues initially emerged in relation to terminal illnesses such as advanced cancer or degenerative neurological illnesses such as amyotrophic lateral sclerosis, in recent years the scope of indications for which PAS and euthanasia have been legalized in some jurisdictions has expanded (Emanuel et al. 2016). The implications of these developments for patients with psychiatric disorders generally, as well as for those with (or at risk for) neurocognitive disorders specifically, are potentially immense (Nicolini et al. 2020). PAS (also referred to as assisted dying, medical aid in dying, and physician-assisted death, among other terms) denotes a physician (or, in some jurisdictions, other types of providers) giving patients the information or means to end their own lives. *Euthanasia*, a distinct term, refers to the process by which a physician (or another health care provider) actively terminates a patient's life.

Although euthanasia remains illegal throughout the United States, PAS has made significant inroads and is now legal in some form in nine states and the District of Columbia and has been proposed in legislation in a number of other states. The American Medical Association (AMA) Code of Medical Ethics thus far remains clearly opposed to PAS and euthanasia, stating that these practices go directly against a physician's ethical duty to "do no harm" (i.e., the ethical obligation of nonmaleficence). The AMA's position is unequivocal, stating that a physician "(a) Should not abandon a patient once it is determined that a cure is impossible; (b) Must respect patient autonomy; (c) Must provide good communication and emotional support; and (d) Must provide appropriate comfort care and adequate pain control" (American Medical Association 2020). In a position statement that clearly referred to the AMA's position, the American Psychiatric Association (2016) explicitly noted that "a psychiatrist should not prescribe or administer any intervention to a non-terminally ill person for the purpose of causing death." This statement does not take a clear position with regard to terminally ill patients, however. In 2017, the American Psychological Association specifically acknowledged the numerous complexities surrounding the issue of "assisted dying" and defaulted to a neutral position at the time—that is, neither endorsing nor opposing the practice.

Against this backdrop of inconsistent ethics codes and widely varying public opinion, issues surrounding PAS and euthanasia that are specifically related to geriatric mental health should be noted. One major point—and something that often surprises physicians and mental health providers alike—is that a psychiatric or psychological evaluation of the patient requesting PAS (i.e., to assess for depression or other contributing psychological factors that could potentially be addressed) is rarely required by these laws (McCormack and Fléchais 2012). Instead, the laws allow the attending or consulting physician to decide whether such an evaluation is indicated (Oregon Health Authority 2020). Some have argued that psychiatrists should not serve as "gatekeepers," regardless of what one believes about the ethics of PAS (Sullivan et al. 1998). Data from states and countries that have had legalized PAS (and, in some cases, euthanasia) for some time suggest that such evaluations are rarely sought (Kim et al. 2016).

In Canada, both PAS and euthanasia are now legal. Euthanasia is available for individuals for whom a "reasonably foreseeable natural death" is expected. However, the question of whether eligibility for euthanasia may soon be expanded to include individuals with psychiatric illnesses remains open and hotly debated (Herx et al. 2020). Several commentators have expressed concerns about such an expansion. They worry such a move has the potential to send a message to individuals with chronic or severe mental illness that their life is not valued. Additional concerns include the minimal safeguards that have been put in place around euthanasia and the very real potential for moral distress for providers—particularly those who do not subscribe to the underlying premise of PAS or euthanasia (Herx et al. 2020).

In Europe, several countries allow PAS and euthanasia for psychiatric and neurocognitive disorders, including dementia. The total number of patients with psychiatric or neurocognitive disorders who have undergone euthanasia or PAS in these countries has increased dramatically over the past decade (Mangino et al. 2020). Although this increase is concerning by itself, data analyzed by researchers about the actual practices engaged in by physicians, including psychiatrists, in these countries have raised several concerning flags (Kim et al. 2016). Mangino et al. (2020) carefully reviewed 75 available reports (of 834 total dementia euthanasia or assisted suicide notifications between 2011 and 2018) of euthanasia performed in The Netherlands among adults with dementia. Although some patients (16 of 75) had made advance requests for euthanasia, 59 were "concurrent requests" (i.e., requests made by a patient who was already experiencing dementia). Patients were able to obtain euthanasia even when there was disagreement among physicians about their eligibility for it (in 25% of the 75 cases reviewed). Moreover, in 15% (n=9) of the 59 concurrent request cases, the patients had enough impairment that they were deemed "incompetent" by at least one evaluating physician. In these cases, patients' previous statements were used as evidence that they were competent to request euthanasia. In some cases, moreover, patients' body language was used to justify deeming them capable of requesting euthanasia or assisted suicide.

Particularly revealing in this study was the authors' finding that the specificity of applicability (i.e., regarding the circumstances under which the patient would want euthanasia) of some patients' advance directives was inadequate. They also noted that "although conceptually and legally there is a sharp boundary between advance and concurrent requests for (euthanasia/assisted suicide), in practice the boundary is not so clear" (Mangino et al. 2020, p. 474). Given that some of the patients who were classified as concurrent requests had significant cognitive and functional impairment and yet were still eventually deemed capable for making the specific decision regarding euthanasia/assisted suicide, the authors concluded that the model for assessing decision-making capacity appears to be different from the functional Appelbaum criteria (described earlier). This is a dramatic change, and geriatric mental health practitioners must understand its potential impact on the care of older adults with serious psychiatric or neurocognitive disorders. In particular, we should ask: What are the consequences of *not* applying the widely accepted ethics principle of the sliding scale to life-ending decisions? Decisions to undergo some potentially life-saving procedures (e.g., electroconvulsive therapy) often require a much higher threshold of decision-making capacity. The debate and discussion around PAS and euthanasia are certain to continue for the foreseeable future, and geriatric mental health providers are encouraged to read broadly to understand the various arguments, particularly as they pertain to older adults with psychiatric and neurocognitive disorders.

Elder Mistreatment: Abuse, Neglect, Exploitation

Although definitions of elder mistreatment or abuse vary somewhat, the following consensus definition from an expert panel convened by the National Research Council of the National Academies of Sciences provides a useful guide (Bonnie and Wallace 2002). Under this definition, elder mistreatment is defined as "intentional actions that cause harm or create a serious risk of harm (whether or not harm is intended) to a vulnerable elder by a caregiver or other person who stands in a trust relationship to the elder." This includes "failure by a caregiver to satisfy the elder's basic needs or to protect the elder from harm" (Bonnie and Wallace 2002, p. 40).

Elder mistreatment is, unfortunately, prevalent—with rates of some form of mistreatment, neglect, abuse, or exploitation ranging from 10% to 20% lifetime prevalence, depending on the sampling and ascertainment methods used. The actual rates may be even higher, given reluctance among older adults to report their concerns and the inadequate training among providers in recognizing potential abuse. One review reported the prevalence of any form of physical, emotional, verbal, or sexual abuse or financial exploitation or neglect to be ~10% (Lachs and Pillemer 2015). In a large survey of community-dwelling older adults (≥60 years) among a randomly selected national sample (N=5,777), Acierno et al. (2010) reported the 1-year prevalence rates of various forms of mistreatment or neglect as follows: physical abuse, 1.6%; sexual abuse, 0.6%; emotional abuse, 4.6%; current financial abuse by a family member, 5.2%; and potential neglect, 5.1%. Interestingly, low social support and previous exposure to at least one traumatic event were consistently found to correlate with the various forms of abuse.

The perpetrators of elder abuse are most often the patient's spouse or adult children; friends or neighbors may also be perpetrators, particularly of financial exploitation (Peterson et al. 2014). In addition, perpetrators are more likely to be male; to be socially isolated; to have financial, employment, or substance use problems; and to have physical or mental health conditions. Other risk factors for abuse include dementia, poor physical health, female sex, lower income, and living with a large number of household members besides a spouse (Cooney et al. 2006, Lachs and Pillemer 2015). There is a need for greater research into the prevalence, risk factors, nature, prevention, and screening of elder abuse involving people with dementia, especially given the growing number of older adults who have or will develop dementia (Cooney et al. 2006, Wiglesworth et al. 2010).

Ethical Issues in Research

The need for improvement in the understanding, evaluation, and treatment of psychiatric and neurocognitive disorders affecting older individuals necessitates ongoing research into these disorders. One aspect of clinical research that invokes ethical dimensions is the enrollment of patients who may lack decision-making capacity or who may have other types of vulnerability in the research context. Research ethics includes a range of issues in addition to informed consent and decision-making capacity. While issues around investigator training and conflicts of interest, ethics review committees, and safety monitoring, to name a few, are relevant in the bigger picture, we focus here specifically on issues of consent and capacity.

Numerous regulations, declarations, and codes of ethics exist to guide the conduct of research with humans worldwide, although a complete discussion of these codes is beyond the scope of this chapter. From a broad perspective, it is perhaps most important to note the ethical principles that have been most widely accepted as essential to the design, conduct, review, and oversight of research. In the United States, the Belmont Report laid the foundations, through an articulation of fundamental principles and examples of their operationalization, for the current framework of regulations that have been designed with the goal of protecting human participants (National Commission for the Protection of Human Subjects of Biomedical and Behavioral Research 1979). The first of these fundamental principles is "respect for persons," which has two complementary requirements—namely, that patients "be treated as autonomous agents" and that "persons with diminished autonomy are entitled to protection." From the perspective of geriatric mental health research, the implications are both highly relevant and often challenging. Determining when a person has "diminished autonomy" is not always straightforward.

The second fundamental principle is beneficence, further elaborated in the Belmont Report as encompassing two general rules that investigators must follow—namely, "1) do not harm; and 2) maximize possible benefits and minimize possible harms." The third and final principle is that of justice—illustrated by the question "Who ought to receive the benefits of research and bear its burdens?" Justice is one of the more abstract—yet arguably one of the most important—ethical questions in research because it can be extraordinarily difficult for a given investigator to ensure "fair" distribution of burdens and benefits. Nevertheless, awareness of this principle and ongoing consideration of the distribution of the benefits and burdens of research are critical to the ultimate goal of research—to improve the lives of as many individuals as possible through advances in knowledge.

Respect for persons directly leads to the requirement for informed consent for research, because respecting autonomy necessitates that individuals be empowered to make voluntary, informed decisions about whether to participate in research. In situations of diminished autonomy, as is often the case in research involving older adults (e.g., in studies focused on cognitive disorders or in any study enrolling individuals from populations in which a subset are likely to have impaired cognition), the investigative team will need to consider how to protect individuals with diminished autonomy (e.g., through procedures to seek appropriate surrogate consent). In the context of research, the "three components" model of informed consent continues to be the most widely accepted framework for ensuring or evaluating the adequacy of informed consent. Specifically, these requisite components are 1) information disclosure or sharing (i.e., a complete description, in language decision-makers can understand, of the research project's purpose, procedures, risks, and potential benefits as well as alternatives to participation); 2) decision-making capacity; and 3) voluntariness of participation (i.e., a free choice, made without coercion) (Appelbaum and Grisso 2001).

Decision-making capacity research is widely defined or operationalized as consisting of four component abilities: 1) understanding (comprehending the provided information about the research project); 2) appreciation (applying that information to the person's own situation, including awareness that the person may not benefit directly from participation); 3) reasoning (weighing the information and considering the consequences of the decision to participate); and 4) expression of choice (communicating a choice, including the stability of that choice over time). In the case of research, this amounts to a stable decision regarding participation (Appelbaum and Grisso 2001).

In terms of geriatric mental health research, there are several key points to emphasize about assessment of capacity for research. First, this model should be thought of as a guide rather than a recipe. Although several tools are available to help researchers assess research-related decision-making capacity, there is still no clear gold standard instrument, and investigators may want to seek guidance from their institutional ethics review committee. Second, the level of capacity sought from participants should follow the sliding scale model (i.e., threshold for capacity should be higher for higher-risk or higher-stakes decisions). Finally, laws, regulations, and other guidance about when and how to assess capacity for research decision-making are relatively sparse, as is legal guidance about the role of surrogate decision-makers in research decision-making (DeMartino et al. 2017). Therefore, protection of older adults with diminished capacity for research decision-making, as required by the principle of respect for persons, can be complicated. When a potential participant retains at least some ability relevant to research decision-making capacity yet also clearly has certain limitations (e.g., patients with MCI), investigators may wish to implement additional safeguards as part of the consent process and study procedures. For example, one common method used by researchers is to either require or encourage the involvement of a study "partner" (sometimes, but not always, a relative of the patient), who is present for the consent process and attends study visits.

However, as neurodegenerative disorders progress over time, patients inevitably will lose the capacity to make research decisions. Determining at what point this loss of capacity has occurred is challenging, although there is some evidence that this occurs, in the case of AD, at some point during the transition from mild to moderate AD (Kim and Karlawish 2003). Therefore, when research involves individuals with levels of impairment that are almost certainly associated with impaired decision-making capacity, such as moderate to severe AD, enrollment of research participants requires further safeguards. Usually this involves obtaining informed consent from a surrogate decision-maker as well as "assent" (i.e., agreement to participate, even without a complete understanding of the decision) from the patient. Who can legally serve as surrogate decision-maker can be unclear, however, particularly given that many jurisdictions are silent on this issue, even when there are laws regarding who can make treatment decisions on behalf of a patient.

Typically, investigators have resolved this issue by obtaining assent from the impaired patient while concurrently obtaining consent from a surrogate decision-maker. How surrogates interpret and enact their role in these decision-making processes and the extent to which they involve the patient in the actual decision have been examined in several studies. For instance, in an interview-based study of cognitively impaired individuals and their surrogate decision-makers who were considering enrolling in one of six dementia-related research protocols, Black et al. (2013) found that patients and their surrogates frequently disagreed when asked how the decision to participate was made; however, it was also noted that the patients (generally with mild to moderate dementia) did participate to some extent in the decision-making process.

Conclusion

One of the most challenging yet fulfilling aspects of caring for older adults rests in the recognition, assessment, and intervention in ethically relevant situations. Older adults with psychiatric and neurodegenerative disorders may present with obvious or subtle impairments that place them at risk of poor decision-making and at further risk of specific harms. The attentive clinician seeks to proactively prevent these situations. In reality, patients often present when these situations have already begun to unfold or are already causing significant problems. Therefore, the importance of both knowledge and skills related to ethical issues in late life remains paramount in the excellent care of older adults.

Key Points

- Older adults' decisional capacity is NOT a unitary status and is domain- and decision-specific. Capacity for specific decisions may still be preserved despite increased disease burden, functional limitations, and cognitive decline. Capacity must be considered in the context of the specific clinical decision at hand, with its associated risks and benefits. More severe disease states and treatments associated with higher risks and greater benefits require a closer scrutiny of decisional capacity.

- Respect for an older person's autonomy is best preserved by timely discussions about the patient's goals of care, health care values, quality of life considerations, and end-of-life wishes.

- Even individuals who may lack decisional capacity for certain health care decisions may still be capable of appointing a surrogate decision-maker.

- Capacity for functional independence is fundamental to maintenance of autonomy; the loss of markers of independence (e.g., the ability to drive oneself) is often the primary fear of older age. Multidomain evaluations can identify potential hurdles to independence that may be mitigated by practical interventions to preserve the core of independence while also ensuring safety.

- Older adults may maintain decisional capacity regarding sexual activity and yet be uniquely vulnerable to both sexual abuse and sexually transmitted diseases. An assessment of capacity for sexual consent is best done by an interdisciplinary team using multiple sources of information, including clinical interview, collateral sources, and neuropsychological evaluation.

- End-of-life care frequently prompts the most tangled of ethical dilemmas, particularly in the cognitively impaired individual who has not previously discussed end-of-life wishes. Absent a previous discussion, the comfort and well-being of a patient with dementia are often best served by an open discussion with the patient and family of the risks and benefits of end-of-life interventions, using multiple streams of information, such as oral discussion plus video.

Suggested Readings

Balasubramaniam M, Gupta A, Tampi RR (eds): Psychiatric Ethics in Late-life Patients: Medicolegal and Forensic Aspects at the Interface of Mental Health. Berlin, Springer International Publishing, 2019
Bloch S, Green SA (eds): Psychiatric Ethics. London, Oxford University Press, 2021

Catic AG: Ethical Considerations and Challenges in Geriatrics. Berlin, Springer International Publishing, 2017

Roberts LW: A Clinical Guide to Psychiatric Ethics. Washington, DC, American Psychiatric Association Publishing, 2016

References

Acierno R, Hernandez MA, Amstadter AB, et al: Prevalence and correlates of emotional, physical, sexual, and financial abuse and potential neglect in the United States: the National Elder Mistreatment Study. Am J Public Health 100(2):292–297, 2010 20019303

American Bar Association, American Psychological Association: Assessment of Older Adults with Diminished Capacity: A Handbook for Psychologists. Washington, DC, American Psychological Association, 2008

American Geriatrics Society 2015 Beers Criteria Update Expert Panel: American Geriatrics Society 2015 updated Beers criteria for potentially inappropriate medication use in older adults. J Am Geriatr Soc 63:2227–2246, 2015 26446832

American Medical Association: Physician-Assisted Suicide. Chicago, IL, American Medical Association, 2020. Available at: https://www.ama-assn.org/delivering-care/ethics/physician-assisted-suicide. Accessed June 1, 2020

American Psychiatric Association: Position Statement on Medical Euthanasia. Arlington, VA, American Psychiatric Association, December 2016

American Psychological Association: Resolution on Assisted Dying and Justification. Washington, DC, American Psychological Association, August 2017. Available at: https://www.apa.org/about/policy/assisted-dying-resolution. Accessed July 7, 2021.

Appelbaum PS, Grisso T: Assessing patients' capacities to consent to treatment. N Engl J Med 319(25):1635–1638, 1988 3200278

Appelbaum PS, Grisso T: MacCAT-CR: MacArthur Competence Assessment Tool for Clinical Research. Sarasota, FL, Professional Resource Press, 2001

Aviv R: How the elderly lose their rights. The New Yorker, October 9, 2017. Available at: https://www.newyorker.com/magazine/2017/10/09/how-the-elderly-lose-their-rights. Accessed June 15, 2020.

Beauchamp TL, Childress JF: Principles of Biomedical Ethics, 8th Edition. New York, Oxford University Press, 2019

Bernacki RE, Block SD, American College of Physicians High Value Care Task Force: Communication about serious illness care goals: a review and synthesis of best practices. JAMA Intern Med 174(12):1994–2003, 2014 25330167

Black BS, Wechsler M, Fogarty L: Decision making for participation in dementia research. Am J Geriatr Psychiatry 21(4):355–363, 2013 23498382

Bonnie RJ, Wallace RB (eds); Panel to Review Risk and Prevalence of Elder Abuse and Neglect: Elder Abuse: Abuse, Neglect, and Exploitation in an Aging America. Washington, DC, National Academies Press, 2002

Burgess AW, Phillips SL: Sexual abuse, trauma and dementia in the elderly: a retrospective study of 284 cases. Vict Offenders 1:193–204, 2006

Centers for Disease Control and Prevention: HIV Surveillance Report, Vol 29. Atlanta, GA, Centers for Disease Control and Prevention, 2017. Available at: http://www.cdc.gov/hiv/library/reports/hiv-surveillance.html. Accessed June 30, 2020.

Chemali Z, Chahine LM, Fricchione G: The use of selective serotonin reuptake inhibitors in elderly patients. Harv Rev Psychiatry 17(4):242–253, 2009 19637073

Cooney C, Howard R, Lawlor B: Abuse of vulnerable people with dementia by their carers: can we identify those most at risk? Int J Geriatr Psychiatry 21(6):564–571, 2006 16783768

DeMartino ES, Dudzinski DM, Doyle CK, et al: Who decides when a patient can't? Statutes on alternate decision makers. N Engl J Med 376(15):1478–1482, 2017 28402767

Emanuel EJ, Onwuteaka-Philipsen BD, Urwin JW, Cohen J: Attitudes and practices of euthana-sia and physician-assisted suicide in the United States, Canada, and Europe. JAMA 316(1):79–90, 2016 27380345

Farrell B, Mangin D: Deprescribing is an essential part of good prescribing. Am Fam Physician 99(1):7–9, 2019 30600973

Farrell TW, Widera E, Rosenberg L, et al: AGS position statement: making medical treatment decisions for unbefriended older adults. J Am Geriatr Soc 65(1):14–15, 2017 27874181

Ganzini L: Artificial nutrition and hydration at the end of life: ethics and evidence. Palliat Sup-port Care 4(2):135–143, 2006 16903584

Herx L, Cottle M, Scott J: The "normalization" of euthanasia in Canada: the cautionary tale con-tinues. World Med J 66:28–39, 2020

Jonsen AR: A Short History of Medical Ethics. New York, Oxford University Press, 2008

Juul D, Colenda CC, Lyness JM, et al: Subspecialty training and certification in geriatric psychi-atry: a 25-year overview. Am J Geriatr Psychiatry 25(5):445–453, 2017 28214074

Kahana E, Kahana B, Lee JE: Proactive approaches to successful aging: one clear path through the forest. Gerontology 60(5):466–474, 2014 24924437

Kim SY, Karlawish JH: Ethics and politics of research involving subjects with impaired deci-sion-making abilities. Neurology 61(12):1645–1646, 2003 14694022

Kim SY, De Vries RG, Peteet JR: Euthanasia and assisted suicide of patients with psychiatric disorders in the Netherlands 2011 to 2014. JAMA Psychiatry 73(4):362–368, 2016 26864709

Lachs MS, Pillemer KA: Elder abuse. N Engl J Med 373(20):1947–1956, 2015 26559573

Larson EB, Shadlen MF, Wang L, et al: Survival after initial diagnosis of Alzheimer disease. Ann Intern Med 140(7):501–509, 2004 15068977

Mangin D, Lawson J, Cuppage J, et al: Legacy drug-prescribing patterns in primary care. Ann Fam Med 16(6):515–520, 2018 30420366

Mangino DR, Nicolini ME, De Vries RG, Kim SYH: Euthanasia and assisted suicide of persons with dementia in the Netherlands. Am J Geriatr Psychiatry 28(4):466–477, 2020 31537470

Marson DC: Clinical and ethical aspects of financial capacity in dementia: a commentary. Am J Geriatr Psychiatry 21(4):392–400, 2013 24078779

McCormack R, Fléchais R: The role of psychiatrists and mental disorder in assisted dying prac-tices around the world: a review of the legislation and official reports. Psychosomatics 53(4):319–326, 2012 22748750

Mitchell SL, Kiely DK, Jones RN, et al: Advanced dementia research in the nursing home: the CASCADE study. Alzheimer Dis Assoc Disord 20(3):166–175, 2006 16917187

Mitchell SL, Teno JM, Kiely DK, et al: The clinical course of advanced dementia. N Engl J Med 361(16):1529–1538, 2009 19828530

Naik AD, Schulman-Green D, McCorkle R, et al: Will older persons and their clinicians use a shared decision-making instrument? J Gen Intern Med 20(7):640–643, 2005 16050860

Naik AD, Lai JM, Kunik ME, Dyer CB: Assessing capacity in suspected cases of self-neglect. Geriatrics 63(2):24–31, 2008 18312020

National Commission for the Protection of Human Subjects of Biomedical and Behavioral Re-search: The Belmont Report: Ethical Principles and Guidelines for the Protection of Human Subjects of Research. Washington, DC, U.S. Department of Health, Education, and Welfare, April 18, 1979. Available at: https://www.hhs.gov/ohrp/regulations-and-policy/belmont-report/read-the-belmont-report/index.html. Accessed July 7, 2021.

National Council Medical Director Institute: The Psychiatric Shortage: Causes and Solutions. Washington, DC, National Council Medical Director Institute, March 29, 2017. Available at: https://www.thenationalcouncil.org/wp-content/uploads/2017/03/Psychiatric-Shortage_National-Council-.pdf. Accessed April 30, 2020

Nicholas LH, Bynum JP, Iwashyna TJ, et al: Advance directives and nursing home stays asso-ciated with less aggressive end-of-life care for patients with severe dementia. Health Aff 33(4):667–674, 2014 24711329

Nicolini ME, Kim SYH, Churchill ME, Gastmans C: Should euthanasia and assisted suicide for psychiatric disorders be permitted? A systematic review of reasons. Psychol Med 50(8):1241–1256, 2020 32482180

Okai D, Owen G, McGuire H, et al: Mental capacity in psychiatric patients: systematic review. Br J Psychiatry 191:291–297, 2007 17906238

Okonkwo OC, Griffith HR, Copeland JN, et al: Medical decision-making capacity in mild cognitive impairment: a 3-year longitudinal study. Neurology 71(19):1474–1480, 2008 18981368

O'Neill O: Autonomy and Trust in Bioethics. Cambridge, UK, Cambridge University Press, 2005

Oregon Health Authority: Frequently Asked Questions: Oregon's Death With Dignity Act (DWDA). Salem, OR, Oregon Health Authority, 2020. Available at: https://www.oregon.gov/oha/ph/providerpartnerresources/evaluationresearch/deathwithdignityact/pages/faqs.aspx. Accessed June 10, 2020

Peterson JC, Burnes DP, Caccamise PL, et al: Financial exploitation of older adults: a population-based prevalence study. J Gen Intern Med 29(12):1615–1623, 2014 25103121

Roberts LW: A Clinical Guide to Psychiatric Ethics. Washington, DC, American Psychiatric Association Publishing, 2016

Rowe JW, Kahn RL: Human aging: usual and successful. Science 237(4811):143–149, 1987 3299702

Schneider LS, Dagerman KS, Insel P: Risk of death with atypical antipsychotic drug treatment for dementia: meta-analysis of randomized placebo-controlled trials. JAMA 294(15):1934–1943, 2005 16234500

Sheffrin M, Miao Y, Boscardin WJ, Steinman MA: Weight loss associated with cholinesterase inhibitors in individuals with dementia in a national healthcare system. J Am Geriatr Soc 63(8):1512–1518, 2015 26234945

Shenoy A, Appel JM: Safeguarding confidentiality in electronic health records. Camb Q Healthc Ethics 26(2):337–341, 2017 28361730

Skelton F, Kunik ME, Regev T, Naik AD: Determining if an older adult can make and execute decisions to live safely at home: a capacity assessment and intervention model. Arch Gerontol Geriatr 50(3):300–305, 2010 19481271

Sullivan MD, Ganzini L, Youngner SJ: Should psychiatrists serve as gatekeepers for physician-assisted suicide? Hastings Cent Rep 28(4):24–31, 1998 9762536

Triebel KL, Martin R, Griffith HR, et al: Declining financial capacity in mild cognitive impairment: a 1-year longitudinal study. Neurology 73(12):928–934, 2009 19770468

Volandes AE, Paasche-Orlow MK, Barry MJ, et al: Video decision support tool for advance care planning in dementia: randomised controlled trial. BMJ 338:b2159, 2009 19477893

Volicer L, Simard J: Palliative care and quality of life for people with dementia: medical and psychosocial interventions. Int Psychogeriatr 27(10):1623–1634, 2015 25573531

White DB, Curtis JR, Lo B, Luce JM: Decisions to limit life-sustaining treatment for critically ill patients who lack both decision-making capacity and surrogate decision-makers. Crit Care Med 34(8):2053–2059, 2006 16763515

Wiglesworth A, Mosqueda L, Mulnard R, et al: Screening for abuse and neglect of people with dementia. J Am Geriatr Soc 58(3):493–500, 2010 20398118

Wilkins JM: More than capacity: alternatives for sexual decision making for individuals with dementia. Gerontologist 55(5):716–723, 2015 26315314

Wright AA, Zhang B, Ray A, et al: Associations between end-of-life discussions, patient mental health, medical care near death, and caregiver bereavement adjustment. JAMA 300(14):1665–1673, 2008 18840840

Index

*Page numbers printed in **boldface type** refer to boxes, figures, and tables.*